Occupational Lung Disorders

This book is dedicated to the
memory of my father and mother.

Occupational Lung Disorders

Second Edition

W Raymond Parkes,
MD, FRCP, MFOM, DIH
Pneumoconiosis Medical Panel,
Department of Health & Social Security,
London

Honorary Clinical Lecturer,
(Professorial Unit, Thoracic Medicine),
Cardiothoracic Institute, Brompton Hospital,
London

with a foreword by
Margaret Turner-Warwick,
DM, PhD, FRCP
Professor of Medicine (Thoracic Medicine),
Cardiothoracic Institute, London

Butterworths
London Boston Durban Singapore Sydney Toronto Wellington

First published 1974
Second Edition 1982
Reprinted 1983

British Library Cataloguing in Publication Data

Parkes, W. Raymond
Occupational lung disorders. – 2nd ed.
1. Lungs – Dust diseases
I. Title
616.2'44 RC773

ISBN 0-407-33731-8

Typeset by Scribe Design Limited, Gillingham, Kent
Printed and bound in Great Britain by
William Clowes (Beccles) Limited, Beccles and London

Contents

Quidem enim tanti operis vtilitatem temptaui tractare et ordine certo doctorum precedencium sententias sub compendio redigere desideraui, plus fuit ex desiderio simplicioribus mihi similibus proficiendi quam ex cupiditate alicuius inanis iactancie procurande. Que circa prouidus lector simplicitati compilatoris parcat corrigendo. Et discat potius deliberata ratione emendare.

(My object, in wishing to reduce the opinions of the most distinguished teachers into one abridgement, was more the desire of assisting simpletons such as myself, than any passion to indulge in empty-headed ostentation. Wherefore, let the prudent reader spare the simpleness of the compiler by correcting the book and let him learn to amend its faults with mature deliberation.)

From *Breviarium Bartholomei* by Johannes de Mirfeld of St. Bartholomew's Priory, Smithfield. Medical Austin friar, died 1407. (*His Life and Works.* By Percival Horton-Smith Hartley and Harold Richard Alridge (1936), Cambridge University Press.)

Foreword

Technological sophistication in industry continues with geometric expansion and it is not surprising that the first edition of *Occupational Lung Disorders* published in 1974 has already needed to be greatly extended and updated.

It is perhaps partly due to the educational success of the first edition that chest physicians now expect to obtain a detailed occupational history as a routine and recognize that labelling a patient's job is no longer enough. However, obtaining a meaningful work record requires knowledge of both the technological aspects of the occupational hazard and an understanding of the medical implications. The importance of this book is not, however, limited to the medical profession. It is equally needed by all of those responsible for control and prevention of occupational hazards, including epidemiologists, hygienists, management and government departments responsible for the working environment of our industrialized country. For all of these, a detailed, comprehensive and well referenced text is essential and this second edition provides just such information.

Three new chapters have been added, namely 'Occupational Asthma'—a field which is perhaps one of the most rapidly advancing in the whole of medicine; 'Non-neoplastic Disorders due to Metallic, Chemical and Physical Agents' and 'Lung Cancer and Occupation'. The importance of each of these is self-evident.

Raymond Parkes not only has a unique understanding of the occupational background and the medical problems involved, but also has a particular appreciation of the medico-legal aspects of the subject which makes the text of particular practical value for a very wide range of readers. He has also made it virtually a life-time's work, collecting accurate data, innumerable elegant illustrations and obscure but relevant, as well as carefully selected but better recognized, references.

The Publishers should be congratulated for recognizing the importance of the subject and supporting an elaborated text at a time when constraints of various forms are all about us. If the reward is better understanding of occupational lung disease and, in consequence, a better working environment for our people, investment and endeavour will have been well worth while.

Margaret Turner-Warwick
Professor of Medicine (Thoracic Medicine)

Preface

In the seven years since this book first appeared there have been notable developments in the study of occupational disorders of the lung. This fact and the omission of some important respiratory hazards from the first edition, together with the encouraging reception accorded to it suggested that another edition, attempting to incorporate relevant advances and redress previous defects, might now be acceptable. Thus, the book has been almost completely rewritten and expanded with the addition of much new material, both textual and illustrative, while some dead wood has been cast aside. Among the additions, which it is hoped will be of value, are occupational respiratory infectious diseases and zoonoses, fungous disorders, and the effects of high altitude, fire smoke and changes in ambient pressure. Rather more attention than previously has been paid to disorders occurring outside the UK, in North America and elsewhere: for example, pulmonary mycoses. There are two new chapters: one on 'Occupational Asthma'—a topic of increasing interest; and another which gives separate, but brief consideration, to 'Lung Cancer and Occupation'.

However, the original objective and character of the book are unchanged; that is, as a practical guide and a modest, if enlarged, reference book intended for fellow clinicians, industrial medical officers, radiologists, pathologists and for those preparing for examinations in Occupational Health. It also aims to correlate the identity and nature of specific hazards with the clinico-pathological features of their effects on the lungs, together with some discussion of experimental and theoretical aspects of pathogenesis. The sequence of sections on pathology, pathogenesis and clinical features has been varied in some chapters for clarity of discussion.

Integration of a variety of non-medical disciplines and a wide clinical experience of both industrial and general lung disease is required of the physician in this specialty for effective diagnosis and prophylaxis. But to achieve this is an increasingly formidable demand on one individual. Thus, as indicated in the original preface, collaboration with experts in important ancillary fields is invaluable, if not essential: for example, mineralogists, mining engineers, metallurgists, industrial chemists and hygienists, physicists and epidemiologists. Moreover, the clinician should never fail to take a detailed, chronological history of the patient's working life to establish the *nature* of his occupation; a time-consuming, but necessary, procedure which may also require precise identification of processes involved in specific industries. In the UK doctors of the Employment Medical Advisory Service, who are deployed throughout the country, are highly expert in this field and give invaluable advice. Only in this way, on the one hand, will failure to recognize an occupational origin of lung disease be avoided and, on the other, wrongful attribution of disease to occupation and consequent lack of relevant treatment, prevented.

Details of various technical procedures referred to in the text and some additional information are included in the Appendix. Threshold limit values for individual substances have, with a few exceptions, been deleted and only brief mention of hygienic measures made. The reason for this is that, in general, both are of limited interest to clinicians and they comprise a large and changing subject which is properly dealt with by specialized texts on occupational hygiene. As before the question of compensation is not discussed because of its complexity, different modes of definition and legal interpretation, and other non-medical considerations, all of which vary from country to country.

Needless to say, a book of this type could not be undertaken without the generous and patient advice and criticism of many medical colleagues and specialists in other fields both here and overseas. They are referred to in the Acknowledgements and my debt to all is immeasurable. My thanks are once again due to Professor Turner-Warwick for contributing the Foreword.

Finally, it must be made clear that none of the statements, interpretations or opinions, whether of others or myself, in any part of the book are necessarily held or espoused by the Department of Health and Social Security in the UK.

W. Raymond Parkes

Acknowledgements

Once again experts in many different disciplines have graciously given me their valuable and unstinting advice and criticism during the preparation of the typescript, some for the second time. I am deeply grateful to all and hope that the result approaches their expectations. Certainly whatever errors or defects there may be are mine and not theirs. My debt to all acknowledged in the first edition continues in this.

Mr G. Berry: Mr W. A. Bloor, British Ceramic Research Association: Dr P. M. Bretland: Dr W. Rhind Brown, Pneumoconiosis Medical Panel, Glasgow: Dr P. Sherwood Burge, who generously provided the greater part of *Tables 12.1* to *12.6*): Dr A. B. Christie: Professor A. L. Cochrane: Dr J. E. Cotes: Dr R. N. Crockett, Mineral Resources Division, Institute of Geological Sciences, London: Mr A. S. Davidson, FRCS: Dr C. N. Davies, University of Essex: Dr J. Dickenson, Kathmandu: Dr D. H. Elliott, OBE, Consultant, Underseas Activities, Shell, UK Ltd: Professor Charles Fletcher, CBE: Dr P. Haslam: Professor A. G. Heppleston: Mr D. E. Highley, BSc, Minerals Strategy and Museum Division, Institute of Geological Sciences, London: Dr K. F. W. Hinson: Professor D. S. Jackson, Manchester: Dr M. Jacobsen, Institute of Occupational Medicine, Edinburgh: Dr W. Jones Williams: Dr J. Lacey, Rothamsted Experimental Station, Harpenden: Mr R. L. Langford, Institute of Geological Sciences, London: Mr R. J. Merriman, BSc, Petrology Unit, Institute of Geological Sciences, London: Dr Klara Miller: Dr Donald N. Mitchell: Dr A. J. Newman Taylor: Professor J. Pepys: Dr G. Rooke, Pneumoconiosis Medical Panel, Manchester: Dr W. J. Smither: Professor Margaret Turner-Warwick: Professor J. Zussmann.

My thanks again are also due to the outstanding photographic expertise of Mr K. G. Moreman. And it is a pleasure to recognize the continued support and guidance of Butterworths' editorial staff.

I am particularly grateful to my wife not only for typing almost all of both editions but also for her sterling forbearance over a prolonged period of domestic disruption and accumulations of bundles of papers in remarkable places.

Abbreviations

ANA antinuclear antibody
DAT differential agglutination test
DIPF diffuse interstitial pulmonary fibrosis
FEV forced expiratory volume
FEV_1 forced expiratory volume in one second
FRC functional residual capacity
FVC forced ventilatory capacity
HDI hexamethylene diisocyanate
IgA(E,G,M) immunoglobulin A (E,G,M)
iu international unit
MAC maximum allowable concentration
MDI diphenylmethane diisocyanate
NDI naphthalene diisocyanate
PEFR peak expiratory flow rate
PVP polyvinyl-pyrollidone
RF rheumatoid factor
RV residual volume
SCAT sheep-cell agglutination test
TDI toluene diisocyanate
Tl lung gas transfer (ml min^{-1} $torr^{-1}$)
TLC total lung capacity
TLV threshold limit value
UDS unit density sphere
VC vital capacity
WL working level (radioactivity)
WLM working level month

Units and quantities

Å ångström(s) Å = 10^{-1} nm
atomic number number of negatively charged electrons in an uncharged atom or the number of protons in its nucleus
Bq becquerel name for reciprocal second for measurement of radionuclide activity (numbers of nuclear transformations per second)
Ci curie = $3.7 \times 10^{10}\ s^{-1}$
g gramme(s)
h hour
half-life (biological) time taken for the content in a biological system of a marked substance to fall to half its original value
half-life (radioactivity) time in which the amount of a radioactive nuclide decays to half its initial value
in inch(es)
J joule = $m^2.kg.s^{-2}$
kg kilogramme(s)
l litre(s)
m metre(s)
m milli- ($10^{-3}\times$)
m^2 square metre(s)
m^3 cubic metre(s)
MeV mega electron volt(s) 1eV $\approx 1.602\ 189 \times 10^{-19}$J
mmHg millimetres of mercury pressure (torr)
mppcf million particles per cubic foot
μm micrometre(s) (10^{-6} m)
n nano- ($10^{-9}\times$)
nm nanometre(s) (10^{-9} m)
Pa Pascal = $m^{-1}.kg.s^{-2}$
ppm parts per million
psi pounds per square inch
s second
S Svedberg unit = 10^{-13} s
ton long ton = 1.016 tonnes
tonne metric ton = 1000 kg (1 Mg) = long ton × 1.01605
torr 1 Torr ≈ 1 mmHg ≈ 133 Pa

1 Introductory Considerations

TERMINOLOGY

To begin with, it is necessary to have a clear idea of what we mean by 'pneumoconiosis' because a variety of general definitions and descriptions have been current—and still are—since Zenker coined the term in 1866. In some instances they have been conditioned by the compensation standards employed by various countries in which case they are rarely scientifically adequate. There are some authorities today who advocate outright rejection of the term but, as it has been in use for more than a century, this is hardly practical and the necessity of defining and classifying pneumoconiosis from the medical standpoint, cannot be avoided. As Card (1967) has written: 'That the concept of disease is a mental construct and belongs logically to the class of useful fictions should not blind us to its practical utility. If we accept this mode of analysis of our experience and we wish to diagnose, that is, assign a group of data to a particular disease, we must be able to define the disease.'

'Pneumoconiosis'—Proust's (1874) modification of Zenker's term 'pneumonokoniosis' (πνεύμων, lungs; κωηὶος, dust, όσις, state of)—simply means 'dusty lung'. Thus, semantically, any dust-ridden state of the lungs or disease process resulting from it may legitimately be called 'pneumoconiosis'. Now, while classification may be done in a variety of ways according to the purpose for which it is intended, the most appropriate method of defining and classifying 'pneumoconiosis' for medical purposes rests upon morbid anatomical changes, and thus embraces a variety of lung disorders.

Following this principle the Industrial Injuries Advisory Council (1973) recommended that the term 'pneumoconiosis' should be taken to mean permanent alteration of lung structure due to the inhalation of mineral dust and the tissue reactions of the lungs to its presence, but should not include bronchitis and emphysema. This recommendation can be usefully expanded as follows: *'pneumoconiosis' is defined as the non-neoplastic reaction of the lungs to inhaled mineral or organic dust and the resultant alteration in their structure excluding asthma, bronchitis and emphysema.* There are three key words in this definition: *dust, lungs* and *reaction.*

DUST

Dusts consist of solid particles of mineral or organic origin dispersed in air and, as such, are distinct from vapours, fumes and smoke (these terms are defined in Chapter 3), although all these categories are commonly embraced by the general term *aerosol.* Hence, by definition, pneumoconiosis does not include lung disorders such as oedema or pneumonia caused by inhaled aerosols other than dusts.

LUNG

Strictly anatomically, the term 'lung' does not include the pulmonary (visceral) or parietal pleural membranes which are of different embryological origin from that of the lung parenchyma and, although it is convenient and customary to include the pulmonary pleura in this term, the parietal pleura is clearly distinct. To regard the parietal pleura as 'lung' is contrary to established embryological and anatomical knowledge, and thus, terminologically inaccurate. Hence, disease which *arises in*, or *primarily* involves, the parietal pleura—whatever its cause—should not be classed or described as 'lung disease' or pneumoconiosis (cf. parietal pleural plaques and asbestos exposure, Chapter 9).

This obvious point has to be made for, whereas the separate identities of (for example) the parietal pericardium and the heart, and the dura mater and the brain remain descriptively unscathed, there is a tendency for current usage in the field of occupational lung disease to lose sight of the distinction between parietal pleura and lung. And this does not contribute to clarity of thought or communication.

REACTION

The lungs react to inhaled dust in a variety of ways which are discussed in Chapter 4 but, briefly, the reaction may be transient as, for example, in the case of the acute fibrosing 'alveolitis' or granuloma formation of farmers' lung, or give rise to permanent reticulin proliferation or collagenous fibrosis.

To avoid misunderstanding at the outset it is important to emphasize that to pathologists, by common consent, 'fibrosis' means excessive production of collagen fibres (or scarring) and not proliferation of reticulin fibres (*see* Chapter 4). Dusts which cause fibrosis are termed *fibrogenic.*

Both inorganic (mineral) and organic dusts may be classified according to the type of reactions they produce and individual diseases placed into these categories (*Table 1.1*).

The foregoing definition of pneumoconiosis thus includes harmless as well as potentially harmful changes in the lungs and in the following pages it refers both to innocuous dust accumulation and to dust-induced disease confined to the gas exchanging region of the lungs (that is, the acini) but which, in some instances (for example, extrinsic allergic 'alveolitis') may also involve non-respiratory bronchioles.

Beryllium disease is a special case for, in addition to being a pneumoconiosis, it is also a systemic disorder and may be caused by beryllium fume as well as dust.

Because functional changes in the larger airways of the lungs caused by the inhalation of cotton and certain other vegetable dusts (that is, the 'byssinosis' group of diseases) are not associated with any characteristic morbid anatomical features, they are not classified under 'pneumoconiosis' and are considered separately in Chapter 12.

Improper terminology, sometimes encountered, includes the use of 'silicosis' as a general term for all forms of pneumoconiosis, and 'pneumoconiosis' to refer exclusively to coal pneumoconiosis. 'Mixed dust fibrosis' (*see* Chapter 7), incidently, means pneumoconiosis caused by the combination of free silica with substantial quantities of other dusts such as coal, carbon or iron oxides, and *not* to different types of pneumoconiosis (for example, silicosis and beryllium disease) in one individual.

During the past 100 years the incidence of silicosis and the pneumoconiosis of coal miners steadily increased in most major industrial countries until the 1950s, since when it has undergone a downward trend, while asbestosis has become increasingly more frequent, and disorders of the extrinsic allergic 'alveolitis' type (hypersensitivity pneumonia)—for example, farmers' lung—have only recently been properly recognized. These trends are reflected in *Table 1.2* which shows newly diagnosed compensation cases in Britain. Figures such as these, of course, are crude in that they are selective. Similar trends have occurred in other major industrial countries. But in newly developing countries the hazards which cause some of these diseases have only recently arisen and, if not properly controlled, could lead to new endemic areas of pneumoconiosis.

In short, pneumoconiosis and other dust-induced diseases are an important medical problem from the standpoint of differential diagnosis, and as a cause of respiratory disability and, sometimes, premature death in certain occupations.

ANATOMY

Some familiarity with the basic features of lung anatomy and cytology is necessary for an understanding of the pathogenesis and behaviour of the different types of pneumoconiosis and other occupational lung diseases.

LUNG AIRWAYS

From the trachea downwards each branch of the airways divides progressively into two daughter branches the length

Table 1.1 A Classification of Pneumoconiosis with some Examples

Type of dust	*Lung reaction*		*Examples*
Mineral	No fibrosis—'inert' Local macrophage accumulation; little structural change; mild reticulin proliferation		Soot Iron (siderosis) Tin (stannosis) Barium (baritosis) Early stages of coal pneumoconiosis
	Sarcoid-type granulomas		Beryllium disease
	Foreign body granulomas		Talc
	Collagenous fibrosis	nodular or massive	Quartz and certain other forms of free silica (silicosis) 'Mixed dust' fibrosis Later stages of coal pneumoconiosis
		diffuse interstitial	Asbestos (asbestosis) 'Talc' pneumoconiosis Beryllium disease Hard metal disease
Non-mineral (organic) e.g. actinomycete spores, avian and animal proteins	No fibrosis Transient 'interstitial pneumonia' or sarcoid-type granuloma formation (acute extrinsic allergic 'alveolitis')		Farmers' lung Mushroom workers' lung Bagassosis Bird fanciers' lung
	Collagenous fibrosis (chronic extrinsic allergic 'alveolitis'—diffuse interstitial pulmonary fibrosis)		Farmers' lung Bagassosis Bird fanciers' lung

Table 1.2 Numbers of New Cases of Major Types of Pneumoconiosis and Byssinosis in Selected Attributable Industries Diagnosed in the UK by the Pneumoconiosis Medical Panels

Industry	*1951*	*1954*	*1960*	*1963*	*1966*	*1969*	*1972*	*1975*	*1976*	*1978*	*1979*
Coal mining	3035	4449	3279	2268	937	624	632	683	575	476	538
Asbestos (i.e. asbestosis)	15	31	29	67	114	134	125	143	172	123	125
Refractories	20	26	16	24	14	16	25	9	9	5	9
Pottery	135	345	50	76	27	31	23	24	17	10	12
Slate mining and splitting	34	21	43	38	51	38	28	30	62	44	53
All foundries	156	256	99	86	55	40	41	31	35	29	19
Cotton (byssinosis)	43	73	403	354	149	78	48	156	102	78	75
Flax (byssinosis)	—	—	—	—	9	—	—	—	—	—	—

These figures which are derived from HM Department of Health and Social Security Annual statistics are a crude index of trends in that they record disease diagnosed for the first time in workers and ex-workers in the specified industries. The number of workers 'at risk' in most industries (the denominator) is not known. But see *Figure 8.2* for coal pneumoconiosis

and diameter of which are not necessarily uniform. The average diameter of daughter branches is smaller than that of the parent branch but, over the complete number of some 23 generations, the total cross-section and volume of the airways system increase progressively while the individual airways become smaller.

Bronchi are characterized by the presence of variable amounts of cartilage in their walls; the continuations of these airways without cartilage to the alveolar areas of the lung constitute the *bronchioles*. The last three or four (rarely, up to eight) generations of bronchioles which carry a variable number of *alveoli* (alveolus, a little hollow) in their walls are named *respiratory bronchioles* because they are capable of gas exchange. The *terminal bronchiole* is the last airway without alveoli before the first respiratory bronchiole (*Figure 1.1*). This diagram is not drawn to scale, the airways of the respiratory unit being shown disproportionally large by comparison with the conducting airways, and the distance between generations four and 17 spans the greater length of the lung. The small airways are about 2 mm in diameter or less.

The lining of the airways as far as the terminal bronchiole consists of epithelial cells which are of pseudo-stratified, columnar and ciliated type. Situated irregularly between them are mucus-secreting *goblet cells* opening to the surface. Goblet cells are plentiful proximally but become progressively fewer in number distally until, in the bronchioles, they are extremely scanty—at least in health.

Mucous glands are found only in bronchi and lie between the epithelium and cartilage. Their total volume is substantially greater than that of the goblet cells and it is likely that they produce the greater part of mucus secretion in health and disease (Reid, 1960). Increased activity is expressed by enlargement. This enlargement is the structural basis of chronic bronchitis, and the comparison of gland thickness to bronchial wall thickness is a valuable practical index of its presence and degree of severity (Reid, 1960) (*see* p.17).

Secreted mucus spreads as an uneven layer on the cilia which possess an auto-rhythmic stroke directed proximally and advancing the layer in that direction; this process is often referred to as the 'ciliary escalator'. Although this is an efficient arrangement for removal of inhaled foreign particles it may be impaired or destroyed by some noxious agents, and excess mucus in chronic bronchitis may sometimes impose an undue burden upon the cilia.

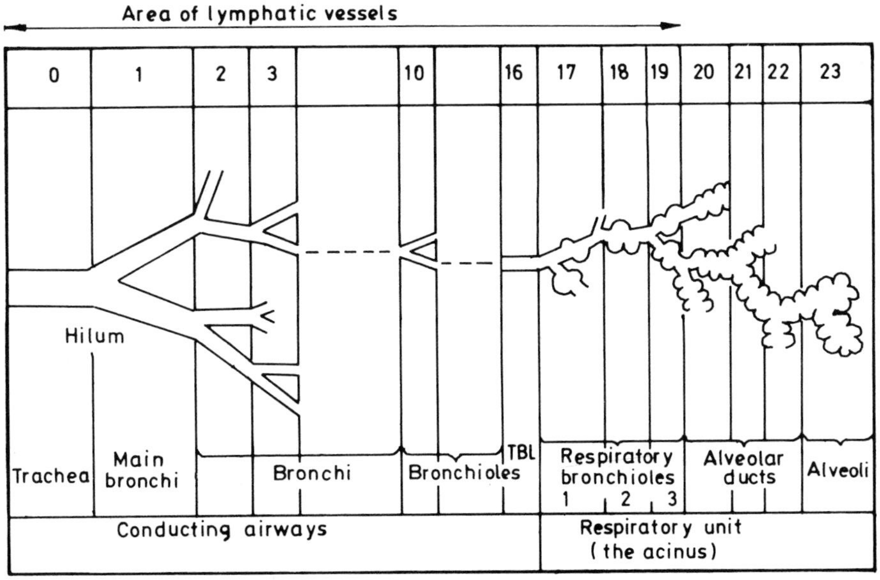

Figure 1.1 Conducting airways and respiratory unit (not to scale). The zones of the bronchi and bronchioles are truncated. The relative size of the respiratory unit is greatly enlarged; this is in fact about one-sixth of the distance from hilum to distal alveoli. Figures at the heads of the columns indicate the approximate number of generations from trachea to alveoli. (Modified, with permission, from Weibel, 1963)

The respiratory unit

The most distal respiratory bronchioles end in *alveolar ducts* which open into the *alveolar sacs* with clusters of alveoli (*Figure 1.1*). *Alveoli,* and their contained gas, are so closely in contact with the alveolar capillaries as to be integral with them.

The respiratory bronchioles, alveolar ducts and alveoli, therefore, comprise a respiratory unit—the *acinus* (a berry) (*Figure 1.1*). The size and shape of acini vary but they are from 0.5 to 1.0 cm in length.

Lobules consist of a variable number of respiratory units (from three to five) which may be partly bound by connective tissue. Their shape and size are very variable.

Alveoli are, on average, about 0.15 mm in diameter, approximately 300 million in number (possibly more) and their total surface area, which is proportional to lung volume, of the average order of 143 m² (±12) (Gehr, Bachofen and Weibel, 1978). Obviously, therefore, the lungs possess great resiratory reserve. About 40 per cent of alveoli appear to be located on the respiratory bronchioles and alveolar ducts (Pump, 1969).

Small tubular communications—the accessory bronchiolo–alveolar communications of Lambert (1955)—exist between some terminal and respiratory bronchioles and neighbouring alveoli. These accessory air inlets, as they appear to be, probably contribute to collateral ventilation, and dust particles or dust-containing macrophages may be found in them and in contiguous alveoli.

Alveolar walls are composed of a number of differing cell types which are variously responsible for gas exchange, disposal of inhaled foreign material, and immunological activity within the lung. Their appearance, distribution and relationships have been established by electron microscopy and six groups of cells can be distinguished morphologically in human lungs (Brooks, 1966). This is shown diagrammatically in *Figure 1.2* and microscopically in *Figure 1.3*.

(1) *Type I cells or squamous pneumocytes* These are flat and extremely thin epithelial cells which form a continuous layer (about 0.2 μm thick away from their

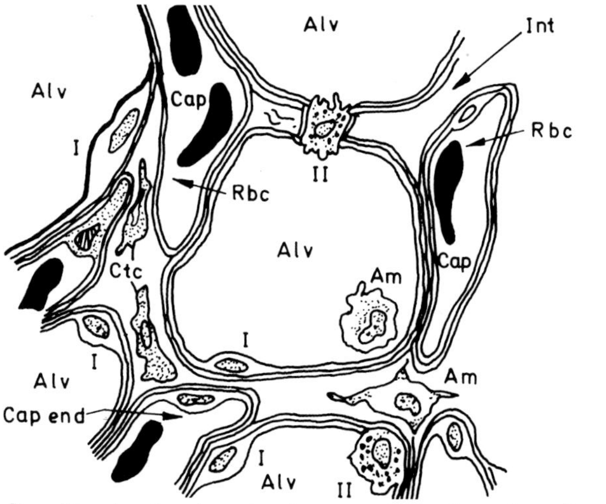

Key: Alv, alveolus; Am, alveolar macrophage; Cap end, capillary endothelial cell; Ctc, connective tissue cell; Int, interstitial 'space'; Rbc, red blood cell; I, Type I cells; II, Type II cells.

Figure 1.2 Diagram of the cells of the alveoli. (By courtesy of Dr R. E. Brooks and the Editor of American Review of Respiratory Diseases*)*

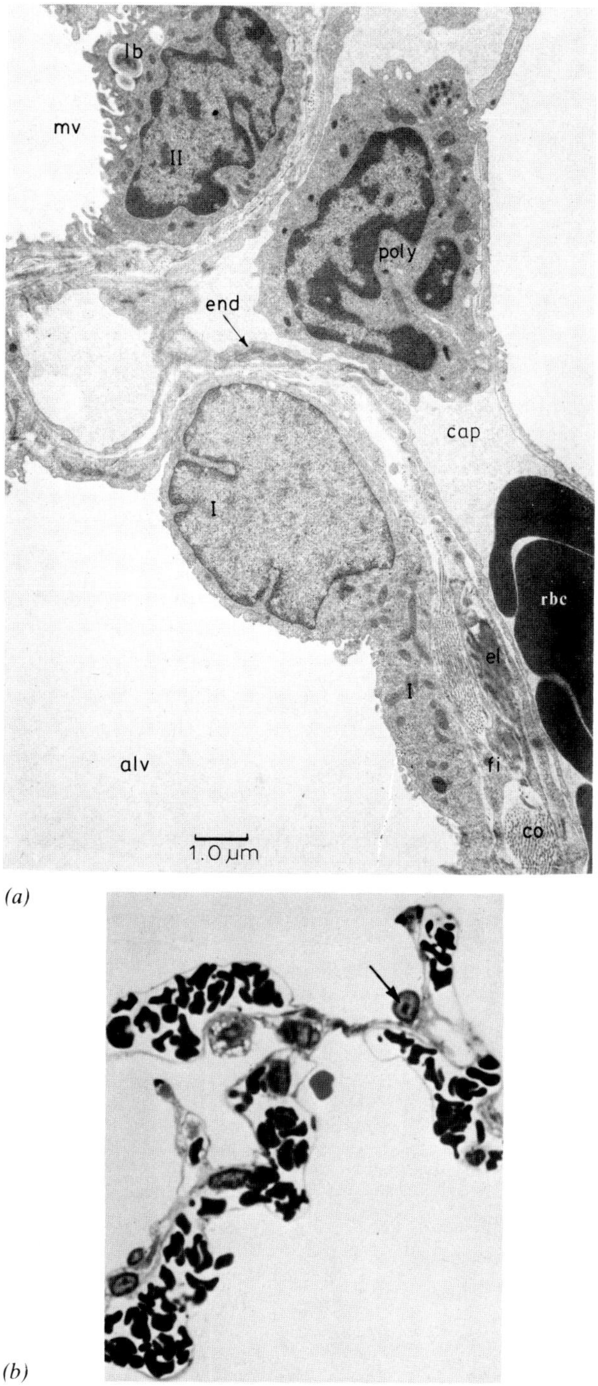

(a)

(b)

Figure 1.3 (a) Electron micrograph of part of rat alveolar wall showing a polymorph and red blood cells (rbc) in a capillary (cap) lined by endothelial cell (end). Most of the alveolus (alv) is lined by processes from the Type I pneumocyte (I). The top left of the picture shows a Type II pneumocyte (II) characterized by its lamellated bodies (lb) and microvilli (mv). The interstitium contains collagen (co) and elastin (el); a fibroblast (fi) can be seen. (Original magnification × 15 000, reproduced at × 7500; fixation, glutamic acid and osmium tetroxide; stain, uranyl acetate and lead hydroxide). (b) Part of a rat alveolar wall showing red blood cells in a capillary. A type II pneumocyte can be recognized by its vacuolated cytoplasm and a Type I pneumocyte is arrowed. (1 μm section; magnification × 675; stained toluidine blue.) Note: the morphology of rat and human lung is similar. (By courtesy of Professor Lynne Reid) nuclei and invisible by light microscopy) over the alveolus apart from sporadic interruption by Type II cells. Both types of cell rest on a tenuous, but continuous, basement membrane composed of reticulin fibres (*see* Chapter 4). Type I cells, which cover 95 per cent of the alveolar surface and through which gases are transferred across the alveolar–capillary interface, also possess phagocytic properties (*see Figure 1.4* and Chapter 3, p.50).

(2) *Type II cells or granular pneumocytes* These are round or cuboidal cells set here and there in the alveolar walls and they are characterized by concentric lamellar organelles known as lamellar bodies. They elaborate and secrete surfactant and are usually regarded as having no phagocytic activity (Heppleston and Young, 1973; Hook and Di Augustine, 1976) but there is reason to believe that this is not correct (Lauweryns and Baert, 1977) (*see* p.50).
Type I cells are very susceptible to injury whereas Type II cells are robustly resistant and have the capacity to proliferate and differentiate into Type I cells, thereby restoring alveolar walls to normality (Adamson and Bowden, 1974; Stephens *et al.*, 1974). However, if the activity of the injurious agent is continuous, Type II cells line the alveolar walls and do not undergo differentiation. Lauweryns and Baert (1977) suggest that phagocytosis by both cell types is provoked by different sets of circumstances.

(3) *Alveolar macrophages* These cells, which under normal circumstances have a ruffled surface and few filopodia, lie in contact with Type I cells or in small groups within the alveolus but are distinct from Type II cells (*Figures 1.4* and *1.5*). They are actively mobile and phagocytic and contain a variable number of phagosomes with ingested material (*see* Chapter 4). They originate outside the lungs from precursor cells (promonocytes) in the bone marrow and from peripheral blood monocytes (that is, promonocyte→monocyte→macrophage) thus forming a distinct cell line (van Furth, 1970) to which the term 'mononuclear phagocyte system' has been given. The macrophages, which have a spherical equivalent diameter ranging from 12 to 20 μm, enter the alveolar interstitium from the blood stream and undergo division and biochemical changes which distinguish them from other phagocytic mononuclear cells. They are able to migrate to terminal bronchioles and lymphatic vessels (Lauweryns and Baert, 1977) and appear to be maintained in continuous supply by migration and division of their fellows in the interstitium (Bowden, 1976). They also perform an immunological role by processing ingested particles which render them antigenic and capable of inducing immunological reactions via T and B lymphocytes (*see* Chapter 4, p.56), and by protecting lymphoid tissue from antigenic stimuli. However, as one of their transport routes is along lymphatic channels and through small, peribronchiolar nodules of lymphatic tissue it seems likely that they may participate in local immune reactions (Lauweryns and Baert, 1977).

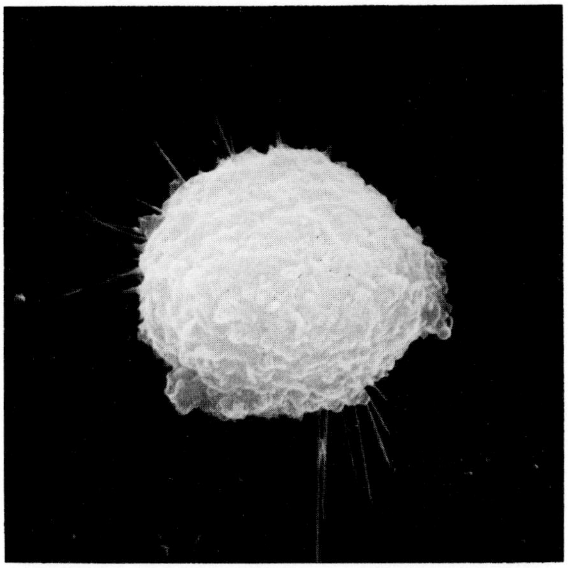

Figure 1.4 Scanning EM of a normal resident alveolar macrophage from the rat. Appearances similar to the human cell. Note normal surface membrane ruffles and very few filopodia (spine-like projections). (Original magnification × 6000). (Courtesy of Dr K. Miller and the Editor of J. Reticuloendothelial Soc.*) (*see Figure 4.1*)*

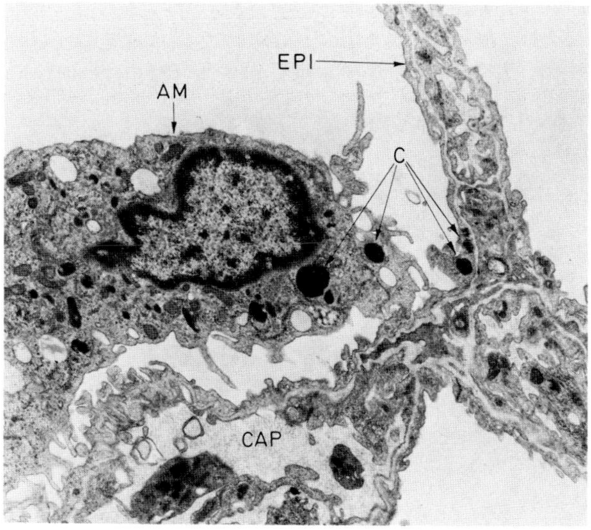

Figure 1.5 Alveolar macrophage containing inhaled carbon particles which are also present in the cytoplasm of a Type I cell en route to the interstitium. AM, alveolar macrophage; EPI, Type I pneumocyte; C, carbon particles; CAP, capillary. (EM original magnification × 14 000.) (Courtesy of Dr D. H. Bowden and the Editor of Environ. Hlth Perspectives*)*

(4) *Endothelial cells* In the capillaries these rest on a basement membrane of reticulin. The capillaries, of course, contain the cellular elements of the blood.

(5) *Connective tissue cells* Fibroblasts.

(6) *Leucocytes and lymphocytes in the interalveolar septa* Leucocytes are infrequent in the normal lung but different populations of lymphocytes are more numerous both within the septa and in bronchial lavage fluids and play an important immunological role (*see* Chapter 4, p. 76 and Addendum, p.88).

This arrangement—shown in the electron micrograph (*Figure 1.3*) of rat lung which is similar to human lung—provides intimate proximity of alveolar gas and capillary blood (gas/blood 'interface') and the opportunity for alveolar macrophages to ingest exogenous and endogenous material (*see* Chapters 3 and 4). Cells containing dust migrate from the alveoli to the ciliary 'escalator' and are subsequently expelled in the sputum or into the bronchiolar lymph vessels from which they pass to regional lymph nodes (*see* Chapter 3).

LUNG FRAMEWORK

The cellular elements of the lung are supported mainly by reticulin, elastic and collagen fibres. Reticulin fibres are the main support of alveolar walls which are reinforced by elastic fibres with collagen less well represented. As already stated, both basement membranes consist of reticulin fibres which are also found in the ground substance of the alveolar septa between the capillary and pulmonary epithelial cells.

The rest of the lung also has a framework of reticulin, collagen and elastic fibres.

SURFACE ACTIVE AGENT (SURFACTANT)

This is a substance which reduces surface tension and lines the walls of the alveoli and those of the respiratory and terminal bronchioles (Niden, 1973), and is secreted by Type II cells (Hook and Di Augustine, 1976; Mason, 1977) though the non-ciliated bronchiolar Clara cells may be an alternative or additional source (Smith, Heath and Moosavi, 1974). It is a lipoprotein containing saturated dipalmitoyl lecithin which, *in vitro,* is one of the most stable surface active agents known; it has the unusual property of its surface tension rising when it is stretched and falling nearly to zero when compressed. Almost certainly this prevents the lung collapsing when its transpleural pressure is reduced (as in expiration) and allows alveoli of different sizes to remain open at the same transpleural pressure (Pattle, 1968).

By enveloping deposited particles surfactant may facilitate their transport in the lungs but there is, as yet, no evidence that alteration in its properties is involved in the pathogenesis of any form of occupational lung disease (Niden, 1973) other than, possibly, alveolar silicolipoproteinosis due to inhalation of quartz particles (*see* Chapter 7, p.168). But its activity is impaired by cigarette smoke (*see* p.14).

BLOOD SUPPLY

Pulmonary arteries conveying venous blood and bronchial arteries conveying arterial blood into the lungs are closely associated with the bronchi and all are enveloped by a common connective tissue sheath the *broncho-arterial bundle.*

Pulmonary arteries accompany the bronchi—although they branch more frequently—and do not become capillaries until they reach the respiratory bronchioles, at which point they form an increasingly rich plexus in intimate proximity to the alveolar epithelium so that only the thickness of the pulmonary epithelial cells, the two basement membranes and a fine tissue space separate alveolar gas from capillary blood (*Figure 1.3*). This thickness away from cell nuclei may be as little as 0.2 μm. The capillary surface area is equal to that of the alveoli, that is, some 70 to 80 m^2 (Weibel, 1963).

LYMPHATICS

These are evident in the vicinity of respiratory bronchioles and there are lymph capillaries ('juxta-alveolar lymphatics') between the alveolar walls and interlobular, pleural, peribronchial and perivascular connective tissue, but not in the alveolar walls themselves; they are important channels for elimination of particles from the lungs (Lauweryns and baert, 1977). Anastomoses exist between lymph vessels in the walls of blood vessels and those in bronchial walls (Trapnell, 1963, 1964). Lymph moves in the interstitial tissue 'spaces' which are under sub-atmospheric pressure and so enters lymph vessels and bronchi.

Lymphatic tissue is distributed strategically and extensively throughout the respiratory tract: in the tonsils and pharyngeal region; in hilar and trancheobronchial lymph nodes; in the smaller nodes scattered along the bronchial tree, and the dense lymphoid aggregates which form cuffs around respiratory bronchioles and their arteries—the 'lympho-epithelial organs' of von Hayek (1960). All these depots are rich in phagocytes and immunologically active lymphocytes which are of capital importance in determining the responses the lungs may make to inhaled aerosols. Because of the arrangement of valves in the lymph vessels lymph flows centrally via the distally situated nodes to the hilar nodes.

PHYSIOLOGY

A detailed discussion of lung physiology and the principles, definitions and techniques of lung function testing is out of place here. (There are some excellent books available on the subject, for example, Bates, Macklem and Christie, 1971; West, 1977; Cotes, 1979.) But as the performance and appraisal of lung function tests is commonly an integral part of the diagnosis and follow-up of suspected and known cases of industrial disease, a brief summary of the patterns of abnormal function and reference to a few important practical points is, perhaps, indicated.

PATTERNS OF DISORDERED LUNG FUNCTION

Restrictive syndrome

This consists in the inability of the lungs to expand as fully as they should from any cause, such as: the effects of left ventricular failure, impairment of full movement of the chest wall (as for example, the sequelae of haemothorax), and by diffuse interstitial fibrosis ('fibrosing alveolitis') of the lungs from whatever origin, including asbestosis.

Vital capacity (VC) and *forced vital capacity* (FVC) are reduced but the proportion, or percentage, of FVC which can be expelled in one second (that is, *forced expiratory volume* in one second or FEV_1) remains normal or is increased provided that there is no co-existent airways obstruction. VC is, in fact, a most valuable simple discriminating test of the presence of parenchymal lung disease in asbestos workers (*see* Chapter 9).

Total lung capacity (TLC) is reduced because the distensibility of the lungs is diminished so that in the case of diffuse interstitial fibrosis, the elastic recoil is greater than normal and its reciprocal, *compliance,* reduced. Compliance can be measured during breath holding in which case it is referred to as *static compliance*, or during regular breathing when it is known as *dynamic compliance;* the observed value should be related to the size of the lung with which it varies directly.

Obstructive syndrome

Chronic non-specific lung disease—by which is meant asthma, emphysema and chronic obstructive bronchitis with or without emphysema—usually causes a greater or lesser degree of obstruction to air flow due to narrowing of larger or smaller airways. It may be reversible, as in the case of asthma, or irreversible, as in chronic obstructive bronchitis and some types of emphysema.

Obstruction to air flow occurs chiefly on expiration—but to some extent on inspiration—and in emphysema of panlobular type (*see* p. 15) it may exist only during expiration. Resistance to air flow in the airways is increased and the degree of obstruction is readily determined by measuring the FEV_1/FVC percentage which is reduced. This percentage varies widely in normal subjects according to age and height, the range being about 55 to 99 per cent in males and 64 to 98 per cent in females.

Normally FVC and VC have closely similar values but, in the presence of obstruction of air flow, FVC may be substantially smaller than VC because forced expiration increases airway narrowing more than unforced expiration.

Airflow obstruction raises the airways resistance; it also gives rise to uneven distribution of inspired air which results in an increase in the inequality of the ratio of ventilation to blood flow which normally exists in the lungs. In normal lungs ventilation and blood flow (perfusion) are not quite equally matched and either one is greater than the other in different parts of the lungs. These differences in *ventilation–perfusion ratio* are the chief reason why normal oxygen tension of arterial blood is not 100 mmHg, but varies from 95 to 97 mmHg. Hence, lung disease which impairs ventilation or causes a local or general reduction in perfusion will give rise to arterial oxygen desaturation.

When emphysema is the cause of airflow obstruction—'air trapping'—the normal elastic recoil tendency of the lungs is reduced and *residual volume* (RV) increased, thereby occupying a greater percentage of TLC than normal; and TLC is also increased. This increase in RV, however, is not specific for emphysema as it also occurs in other forms of chronic non-specific lung disease. Both RV and TLC are affected by age (*see* p. 10).

Resistance to air flow in the intrathoracic airways is composed of central and peripheral components: the former consisting of airways greater than 2 mm in diameter and the latter, those less than 2 mm in diameter which are chiefly respiratory bronchioles and offer a large cross-sectional area. Total pulmonary resistance is the sum of these two components. In normal subjects peripheral resistance accounts for only 10 to 15 per cent of total resistance and is negligible at lung volumes greater than 80 per cent of VC (Macklem and Mead, 1967). It is, therefore, possible for disease of peripheral airways to exist with little or no change in total resistance and with normal routine spirometric values, though the lungs are then less distensible (Mead, 1970). Disease involving the peripheral airways—whatever its nature—is almost invariably unevenly distributed so that only a proportion of the airways is affected. Such a scattered increase in airways resistance with decreased distensibility of the lungs will tend to cause some imbalance of the ventilation–perfusion ratio. Thus, sometimes routine spirometry and standard tests of airways resistance may not detect an increase in peripheral resistance. For this reason further indices have been developed.

(1) *Frequency dependent dynamic compliance* This is based on the principle that dynamic compliance will fall during faster breathing rates in the presence of increased resistance to air flow in the small airways. Though theoretically a sensitive test it is impractical for routine use, uncomfortable for the patient, difficult to measure, and the results appear to differ according to the manner in which they are expressed (Morgan, Lapp and Morgan, 1974).

(2) *Closing volumes* Ventilation of the lower parts of the lungs decreases with age due, apparently, to the small airways in these zones closing in advance of those in other zones (Milic-Emili *et al.*, 1966). Closure occurs earlier and more extensively in a number of disease conditions. The test is believed to measure the point in expiration at which the small airways close down. Although there are a variety of methods for its performance the basic principle is the same: that of continuously monitoring the concentration of a marker gas—such as helium or xenon introduced as a 'bolus' at the start of full inspiration—or of 'resident' lung nitrogen in the exhaled air. In both instances because the small airways in the lung bases close first, while the gas continues to flow from the upper parts of the lungs, a sudden increase in its concentration is recorded at this juncture. This is shown by an upswing of the end (phase 4) of the washout curve. The volume at which this occurs is the *closing volume* and it lies between the onset of phase 4 and RV; when related to TLC, it is called the *closing capacity* and is comprised of closing volume and RV. The single breath nitrogen washout technique is the most practical for routine use at present (Buist, 1973).
Unfortunately the original promise that this test would prove sensitive in detecting early airways disease and be of value in monitoring industrial health has not been fulfilled. Apart from the fact that closing volume is increased in cigarette smokers (Bates, 1972; Buist, Van Fleet and Ross, 1973), thoracic deformity (Bjure *et al.*, 1970), obesity (Craig *et al.*, 1971) and asymptomatic asthma (McCarthy and Milic-Emili, 1973) abnormal closing volume has not been found consistently in patients with mild airways obstruction (Abboud and Morton, 1975) and there are practical difficulties in deciding precisely at which point closure commences and in its measurement and interpretation (Cochrane *et al.*, 1974). Indeed, when applied to a randomly selected population, abnormality of closing volume is found in only a very small proportion of individuals in whom respiratory dysfunction would not *otherwise* have been suspected or already diagnosed (Knudson *et al.*, 1977).

(3) *Forced (maximal) expiratory flow rate* Measurement of the flow rate between 25 to 75 per cent of FVC (forced mid-expiratory flow $FEF_{50\%}$ is a fairly sensitive indication of early airways obstruction when compared with normal, and is even more so when it is measured between 75 and 85 per cent of FVC ($FEF_{75-85\%}$) (Morris, Koski and Breese, 1975). But here again there is a disadvantage in that the normal range is considerably wider than that of FEV_1 though this is reduced when consecutive readings over a period of time in one individual are compared with

his initial performance. Thus, whilst the maximum expiratory flow volume curve (MEFV) may be the most discriminative test of small airways obstruction when groups or populations of subjects are studied (Green, 1976) it has too large a variability for useful application to individuals (Cochrane, Prieto and Clark, 1977).

In summary: although it is often claimed that these tests may detect airways obstruction at an unprecedently early stage and that increased closing volume and reduced dynamic compliance are evidence of bronchiolitis, proof of this is lacking (Morgan, Lapp and Morgan, 1974); indeed, there is no certainty as to what closing volume signifies, measured as it is by indirect methods. This matter has been discussed at some length in order to make clear that the performance of these tests is, at present, largely heuristic and that their clinical value in the diagnosis and interpretation of occupational and other forms of lung disease has not yet been established. Prospective longitudinal epidemiological studies are required to establish if they possess any prognostic value (Milic-Emili, 1976). The FEV, therefore, remains the index of choice and, in fact, appears to reflect small airways disease fairly well (Thurlbeck, 1980); it should be measured in all circumstances when airways obstruction is suspected.

Nasal air flow

The nose accounts for approximately one-half of the total respiratory resistance to air flow (Proctor, 1977) and increased resistance to air flow in the nasal airways causes significant reduction in pulmonary function and increase in the work of breathing (Ogura *et al.*, 1966). Indeed, there is evidence that tracheobronchial resistance is increased by irritation of the nasal passage due, possibly, to activation of an unidentified neural reflex pathway (Kaufmann and Wright, 1969). Contrariwise, nasal airflow resistance is increased in patients with chronic lower airways obstruction (Cohen, 1969 and 1970; Nolte and Ulmer, 1966); and it is of interest that, under these conditions, bronchodilator drugs applied to the nasal passages alone lessen airflow resistance both in them and in the intrathoracic airways (Cohen, 1969).

Disease causing partial or complete obstruction of the nasal passages, therefore, can be expected to increase the funtional burden of diseased lungs and, hence, any respiratory disability. However, chest and industrial physicians seem rarely to consider the contribution made by nasal disease to total airways resistance (that is, the sum of nasal and intrathoracic airways resistance) nor to look for it as a routine. The point is important because relief of the nasal disorder may reduce total respiratory disability significantly (Ogura *et al.*, 1966), whereas failure to recognize it will result in disability being attributed solely to bronchopulmonary disease (*see also* Chapter 3, p.47).

Impairment of gas exchange

Exchange of gases across the alveolar–capillary interface is impaired when ventilation is reduced in relation to blood flow either locally or generally. This may occur in diseases causing the 'restrictive' or 'obstructive' patterns of functional disorder, or when blood flow is reduced relative to ventilation. The appearance of diffuse interstitial fibrosis (from whatever cause) under the light microscope may give the impression that resistance to diffusion of gases across the interface would unfailingly result, but this is often not so to any significant degree.

The diffusing capacity of the lungs (Dl) or, preferably, the *gas transfer factor* (Tl) (Cotes, 1979) is a function of alveolar gas, the alveolar–capillary interface or membrane component (Dm) and the volume of blood in the capillaries; that is, $\frac{1}{\mathrm{Tl}} = \frac{1}{\mathrm{Dm}} + \frac{1}{\theta \mathrm{Vc}}$ mm Hg/ml/min where θ is the rate of reaction of the test gas carbon monoxide with oxyhaemoglobin and Vc is the volume of blood in the alveolar capillaries. Providing that the conditions of measurement of Tl are properly controlled it is a reliable and reproducible test (Cotes and Hall, 1970), the recommended technique being the single breath carbon monoxide test. Because lung volumes are used in the calculation of Tl and larger volumes are associated with higher Tl values a correction can be made by dividing Tl by the alveolar volume at which the measurement is made. The resulting index (Tlco/Va) is the *differential coefficient of carbon monoxide,* Kco. Although impairment of gas diffusion due to increased interface resistance alone is unusual, in the early stages of diffuse interstitial fibrosis and granulomatous lung disease Tl and arterial oxygen saturation may be reduced during exercise, though normal at rest, and associated with hyperventilation without there being any abnormalities of other aspects of lung function. This may be encountered, for example, in the early stages of asbestosis, chronic beryllium disease and chronic extrinsic allergic 'alveolitis'.

It should be emphasized that in the diagnosis or assessment of progression of disease Tl values must *never* be considered in isolation but related to the lung volumes and the presence or absence of a restrictive defect or airflow obstruction. Reduction in Tl in association with abnormalities of other aspects of lung function occurs in diffuse interstitial fibrosis from whatever cause and in emphysema (both symptomatic and asymptomatic) in which some alveolar–capillary surface is lost and distribution of gas may be altered, but not in simple chronic bronchitis (bronchial catarrh) (Gelb *et al.,* 1973; Cotes, 1976). Apart from abnormalities in the ventilation–perfusion ratio Tl is also influenced by a variety of other conditions which may have to be taken into account when it is being assessed: for example, it is *reduced* by heavy meals, smoking, anaemia (Cotes *et al.,* 1972), acute alcohol ingestion and chronic alcoholism (Banner, 1980), chronic left ventricular failure, the prior inhalation of oxygen and by high ambient temperature; and *increased* by exercise, polycythaemia, hypoxia and increase in lung size which may be present in some cases of acromegaly (Evans, Hipkin and Murray, 1977). A normal Kco in the presence of reduced Tl indicates preservation of alveolar function and, therefore, excludes diffuse interstitial pulmonary fibrosis of any significance in the majority of cases.

The effects of impaired gas diffusing capacity are the same irrespective of the underlying cause and can be summarized as follows:

(1) Increased frequency of ventilation on effort; that is, the minute ventilation is increased relative to oxygen uptake.
(2) Diminished diffusion of gas across the alveolar–capillary interface either at rest or on exercise, or under both conditions.
(3) Hypoxaemia on exercise.

Hyperventilation

Disease of the lung parenchyma, panlobular emphysema (rarely chronic obstructive bronchitis) and skeletal diseases which restrict thoracic movement, if sufficiently severe, may cause hyperventilation on exercise or at rest. Hyperventilation may be present at rest as well as on effort due to acute exposure to high altitude, left ventricular insufficiency and the granulomatous (or 'proliferative') stage of extrinsic allergic 'alveolitis', beryllium disease and sarcoidosis. It is out of proportion to reduction in VC and may be of reflex origin mediated by the vagus nerve and due to involvement of lung receptors—possibly the 'deflation receptors' of Paintal (1970)—by the disease process. Some support for this is given by the fact that the breathlessness is reduced by vagus nerve block (Guz *et al.,* 1970) and steroid therapy (Cotes, Johnson and McDonald, 1970). It is important to recognize this possibility in order that dyspnoea from this cause is not dismissed as psychoneurotic. By contrast, this effect does not occur with established fibrosis, for example, asbestosis.

Hypoventilation

Reduction in the volume of ventilation/minute impairs alveolar ventilation which in turn leads to hypoxaemia due to ventilation–perfusion imbalance, and also to carbon dioxide accumulation (hypercapnia) in the arterial blood. It may be caused by depression of activity of the respiratory control centre in the reticular formation of the medulla oblongata due to local lesions or the action of inhibiting drugs, by pronounced weakness of the respiratory muscles (for example, old age and myopathies), and by excessive obesity and severe kyphoscoliosis or ankylosing spondylitis which also impair chest movement. The lungs themselves may be either free of disease or the seat of unrelated disease.

Mixed patterns

Disturbance of lung function usually consists of more than one of the foregoing categories.

PRACTICAL POINTS RELATING TO ROUTINE LUNG FUNCTION TESTS

The simpler tests of ventilatory function can be done in the consulting room, chest clinic, home, factory, or the hospital ward side-room; the more elaborate can only be done in the laboratory. The most valuable of all simple tests for routine use are FEV_1, FVC and VC. Of these FEV_1, which fulfils all the criteria for choice of lung function tests (Cotes, 1979), provides the best *single* test there is for assessment of respiratory disability, and the presence and severity of airways obstruction is given by its percentage of the FVC.

There are various instruments available for the performance of these tests but it is important that the one employed is robust, has a good capacity, as low a resistance to air flow as possible, and an accurate automatic timing device; and furthermore, that its maintenance and calibration should be simple and carried out regularly.

Because these tests are frequently done by non-physiologists (including physicians, nursing and non-medical personnel) it is important that every detail of their performance is properly carried out. The subject must remove heavy or tight clothing, lumbar belts and loose dentures; be comfortably seated before the apparatus; make the deepest possible inspiration and then close his mouth firmly round the mouthpiece, taking care not to obstruct it with his tongue. He must blow without hesitation as forcefully as possible down the tube; make two or three preliminary attempts before recording a number of blows, of which the mean of the best three is taken as the result; and rest for about 30 seconds between each blow. It is not necessary to blow much beyond one second until the last blow when FVC is tested and then forceful expiration must be pressed to the utmost. This is best done last as it is more exhausting and sometimes provokes a paroxysm of coughing. VC is performed in the same way but with a slow expiratory effort. Clipping of the nose, which is not otherwise necessary when performing these tests, is required in persons with cleft palate.

One observer, rather than a number, should do the tests and it is advisable that checks are made to establish that his results have consistent agreement with those of a known reliable observer or laboratory.

The other commonly used single breath test which reflects ventilatory capacity is the *peak expiratory flow rate* (PEFR). This varies with the interval of time during which it is recorded, but it is normally taken as the maximum expiratory flow that can be sustained for a period of 10 ms. Used alone it is less discriminative than other single breath tests. Portable instruments for its measurement (such as the Wright peak flow meter or peak flow gauge) tend to vary in their characteristics so that comparison of results from different instruments is not always satisfactory (Wright, 1974). Nonetheless, the test is useful for detecting possible changes in airways obstruction in a series of observations in an individual over a short period of time: for example, during a working day or shift, or when assessing the effect of a bronchodilator drug (*see* Chapter 12).

When spirometric tests are repeated in individuals over a period of time—as is the case in surveys of workers in the field—the individual may be used as his own control when subsequent test values are compared with his initial values, providing that changes due to age are taken into account. But it is important to remember that there are diurnal and seasonal variations in ventilatory function which is higher in the afternoon after a morning shift, and slightly lower during the evening and night shifts; and is significantly lower in the winter than in the summer months (Guberan *et al.,* 1969; McKerrow and Rossiter, 1968). Hence, repeated tests should be done at the same time in a working day or in a year. Providing that these normal variations and changes in smoking habits can be excluded, a fall in FVC or FEV_1 of 200 ml or more over a year suggests the possibility of lung disease, and a similar fall in the course of a working shift—especially if present in a number of workers—may reflect the presence of some harmful agent in the factory air.

Records of all tests should include the subject's age, height, sex, racial group and smoking habit. Prediction of reference values is related to the first four of these. The importance of smoking is referred to later.

Prediction formulas or nomograms should be derived from data from the same racial group as the subject tested and, as far as possible, from a kindred population. Considerable differences, for which correction should be made, exist in many aspects of lung function between white Europeans and coloured Africans (Rossiter and Weill, 1974a). When recording results, the source of the reference values should be stated; this applies equally to all lung function tests. Acceptable prediction indices and tables are available for the UK (Cotes, 1979), the USA (Kory *et al.*, 1961; Boren, Kory and Syner, 1966; but these do not distinguish racial groups) and India (Rao *et al.*, 1961; Cotes, 1979). Normal values for the gas transfer factor are reviewed by Cotes and Hall (1970). Care is required, however, in the use of such indices: for example, the reference populations may differ in certain respects from the individual or group being tested; and, the decline of ventilatory capacity, and other tests, with age is not necessarily as uniform as most regression equations suggest (Oldham, 1970).

Inter-laboratory variation of reference values, especially for gas transfer, are often very large and may invalidate comparison of physiological data at different times in the same subject.

Standardization

There is much variability in the results of lung function tests if scrupulous attention is not paid to apparatus, technique and diurnal and seasonal variations (Hruby and Butler, 1975). Not only must apparatus used outside the laboratory be generally acceptable but it must be frequently calibrated against a known standard. This means that the timing units of direct reading spirometers should be calibrated daily, as should the technical features of other apparatus.

The temperature of the room where tests are performed must be kept at a reasonably constant level in keeping with that of the country in which they are being performed, and at least one hour should have elapsed between the subject's last smoking or receiving bronchodilator drugs and performance of the test, and two hours between a main meal and the test.

INFLUENCE OF AGE ON LUNG FUNCTION

There is evidence that from the fifth decade onward, alveolar volume decreases and airway volume increases—both significantly. In other words there is 'a shift in pulmonary air-space volume from alveoli to ducts which is often called "ageing emphysema" if the shift is marked enough' (Weibel, 1968). This is likely to explain certain of the changes of values in lung function tests associated with age, although weakness of the respiratory muscles contributes.

The elastic recoil of the lungs gradually becomes reduced. In men the RV increases from an average of about 1.5 l at the age of 20 to about 2.2 l at the age of 60, but TLC does not increase significantly. In women, however, TLC is apt to decline. In both sexes RV as a percentage of TLC increases from about 25 per cent at 20 years of age to about 37 per cent at 60 years of age. The values of FEV_1 and VC fall with increasing age. In normal, non-smoking Caucasian males the decrease in FEV_1 is about 0.031/year and comparable changes occur in VC (Cotes, 1979). The rate of decline in FEV_1 in smokers is larger but reverts to the normal rate if they stop smoking though recovery of damage already done does not occur (Fletcher *et al.*, 1976).

The capacity for transfer of gases across the alveolar-capillary interface is reduced by about 33 per cent between the ages of 20 and 60 years due primarily to some loss of interface and to a decrease in alveolar capillary blood vessel volume which is also responsible for a less progressive reduction in Tl (Cotes, 1979).

Most parameters of lung function are closely related to age throughout life; a fact which must always be taken into account when the possible effects of lung disease upon function are assessed.

INFLUENCE OF SMOKING ON LUNG FUNCTION

Tobacco smoke has a significantly deleterious effect on lung function which is most pronounced with cigarette smoking.

First, there is increased airways resistance which is observed as an acute effect lasting for about an hour after smoking both in habitual smokers and non-smokers (McDermott and Collins, 1965; Stirling, 1967); and second, there is a chronic effect characterized by a high correlation of airways obstruction with cigarette smoking in both sexes and all age groups.

Therefore, FEV_1/FVC per cent and FVC are, on average, lower in smokers than non-smokers; it has been shown that the mean annual decline of FEV_1 in a UK population is between 0.05 and 0.10 l/year in smokers (Higgins and Oldham, 1962) compared with approximately 0.03 l in non-smokers and, as indicated earlier, closing volume is increased in smokers. In those of 50 years of age and over this appears to be due to loss of elastic recoil, but in younger smokers, to changes in the small airways (Bode *et al.*, 1975); and, in fact, respiratory bronchiolitis of irregular distribution has been demonstrated in young smokers (Niewoehner, Kleinerman and Rice, 1974). However, increased closing volume appears to be poorly related to respiratory symptoms, FEV_1 being more reliable in this respect (McDermott, Gilson and Ridley, 1975).

Airways obstruction in smokers, however, is not always accompanied by symptoms (Franklin and Lowell, 1961) even though chronic obstructive bronchitis is very much more prevalent among smokers than non-smokers.

Vital capacity, TLC and compliance (that is, 1/elastic recoil) are lower, and RV_1 RV/TLC percentage, gas mixing index and non-elastic resistance higher in smokers than in non-smokers (Zwi, Goldman and Levin, 1963; Krumholz, Chevalier and Ross, 1964). By comparison with non-smokers Tl and Kco are significantly reduced in smokers at rest and on effort, but whether this is due to anatomical changes (for example, emphysema) or to altered blood volume in the lung capillaries is uncertain (Frans *et al.*, 1975; Krumholz, Chevalier and Ross, 1964; van Ganse, Ferris and Cotes, 1972). All these changes of function are found in both sexes and are of significant order; they tend to be greater the larger the cigarette consumption and are well established after ten years of smoking. Furthermore, impairment of gas transfer occurs even in seemingly healthy smokers who have no evident impairment of ventilatory function or airways abnormality (Rankin, Gee and Chosy, 1965).

Stopping smoking, however, results in a lessening of airflow obstruction and both inspiratory and expiratory resistance, but not in improvement of VC (Wilhelmsen, 1967). Tl and Kco values return to levels found in non-smokers in most cases (Frans *et al.*, 1975).

Women smokers are affected in the same way as men but less severely. Pipe and cigar smoking cause a similar pattern of functional impairment to that of cigarettes though of significantly less severity, except when subjects inhale.

It is clear, then, that because of the profound effect smoking has upon the lungs, a detailed history of smoking habits must never be omitted. This should show whether a person is a *non-smoker* (that is, has never smoked), a *smoker,* or an *ex-smoker* and the duration of smoking in years and the number of cigarettes or grammes of tobacco smoked; if an ex-smoker, the year of stopping should be ascertained. Cigarette, pipe and cigar smoking should be shown separately. And, finally, smoking history and its effects must always be considered when interpreting the results of lung function tests.

APPLICATION OF LUNG FUNCTION TESTS IN OCCUPATIONAL LUNG DISEASE

Diagnosis

Lung function tests themselves are not diagnostic of any particular disease, but in many cases they form a necessary part of diagnostic criteria.

Whereas the standard tests of lung volumes, ventilation, gas distribution and transfer are not required in every case or at each examination, the basic ventilatory tests are indispensable in all.

Function tests may provide some guide to prognosis in cases (for example) of asbestosis, chronic beryllium disease and chronic obstructive bronchitis; they evaluate the response to treatment of reversible disorders, such as acute extrinsic allergic 'alveolitis' from any cause, and those which are present coincidently with a pneumoconiosis. When the effects of increasing age are allowed for, periodic tests are helpful in establishing whether or not disease has progressed and, if so, to what extent.

Prevention of disease

Determination of FEV_1 and FVC when a worker is about to enter any industry which may be hazardous to the lungs is essential in establishing a point of reference for later similar tests, and subsequently to detect the onset of incipient lung disease as early as possible. Data of this sort from a large number of individuals in an industry can be related to conditions of their work and exposure to dust or to physical or chemical agents. This not only provides essential prospective data about the health of a working population, but is a valuable contribution to the health of the individual worker.

More comprehensive tests may be indicated in workers in some industries (for example, those where there is exposure to asbestos or beryllium compounds) whose FVC or FEV_1 show an unexpected fall.

When a particular occupational environment is under investigation for a possible hazard the rate at which a test value changes with time may be of greater significance and help than an absolute value. It has been shown that in the case of a new or suspected potential hazard, the effect on FEV_1 may be established in a shorter time by its being measured prospectively (that is, a longitudinal study) once or twice a year over a period of not less than three nor more than five years than by observing its value on one occasion only—that is a cross-sectional study. But in a situation where workers are known to have been exposed to a potential hazard for several years a cross-sectional study is more appropriate. This general principle applies to other lung function tests (Berry, 1974). In some circumstances serial measurements over a working shift may also be informative (*see* Chapter 12).

The application of physiological tests to industrial lung disease is surveyed in detail by Cotes (1966, 1975a).

EMPHYSEMA

The term emphysema—ἐμφυσᾶν, to inflate or puff up—is descriptive of altered form without implying the cause or pathogenesis of this alteration. Like anaemia, emphysema of the lungs is a morphological complex comprising not one disease process but a number.

The terminology of emphysema was much confused until the definitions of the Ciba Foundation Guest Symposium (1959) in the UK and the American Thoracic Society (1962) were proposed, since when there has been fairly good, if not complete, agreement.

The definition of emphysema given by Reid (1967), which rests on structural and not functional abnormality, has the merit of simplicity and avoids implication of pathogenesis:

> Emphysema is a condition of the lung characterized by increase beyond the normal in the size of air spaces distal to the terminal bronchiolus, i.e. the acinus.

As a general rule air spaces are said to be emphysematous if they measure more than 1 mm in diameter.

Although air spaces of increased size are found in some cases of diffuse interstitial pulmonary fibrosis (fibrosing alveolitis) as 'honeycomb lung' and might, therefore, be classed as emphysema, the lesions are distinguished by commonly involving terminal and non-respiratory bronchioles as well as acini, and by gross and microscopical features which are referred to in Chapter 4.

Only those types of emphysema which are common in adult life are briefly described as they are most likely to be associated with a pneumoconiosis or other occupational lung disorders. The classification used throughout is that of the Ciba Foundation Guest Symposium and much of what follows rests on the work of Reid (1967).

The unit of description used by Reid (1967) is the acinus, but some other pathologists (for example, Wyatt, Fletcher and Sweet, 1961; Gough, 1968; Heard, 1969) prefer to employ the lobule for this purpose as it can usually be seen with the unaided eye in lung slices, partly delineated by fibrous septa. Hence the terms 'centriacinar' and 'panacinar' are taken as equivalent, respectively, to 'centrilobular' and panlobular. Although the acinus cannot be distinguished by the unaided eye its use is more consistent with the accepted definition of emphysema. However, as the terminology based on the lobule is so widely current it will be used throughout this book, but with this reservation continually in mind.

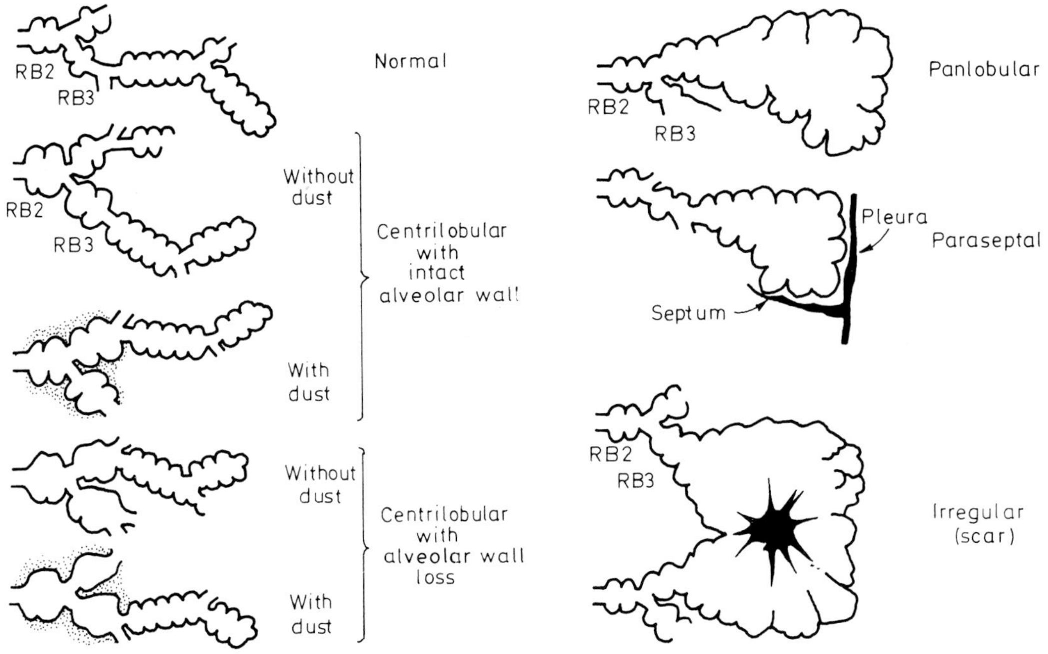

Figure 1.6 Diagram of the anatomical sites of different types of emphysema

The types of pathological changes which may be found are described, according to their dominant position in the lobule or acinus, as follows (*Figure 1.6*).

(1) Enlargement of alveoli in or near the centre of the lobule or acinus; *centrilobular (centriacinar) emphysema.*
(2) Enlargement of alveoli throughout the lobule or acinus: *panlobular (panacinar) emphysema.*
(3) Enlargement of alveoli at the periphery of the acinus only and contiguous with connective tissue septa or sheaths: *paraseptal (periacinar) emphysema.*
(4) Enlargement of alveoli which does not involve the acinus universally, is not characteristically located in one part of it, and is associated with scars; *scar, paracicatricial or irregular emphysema.*

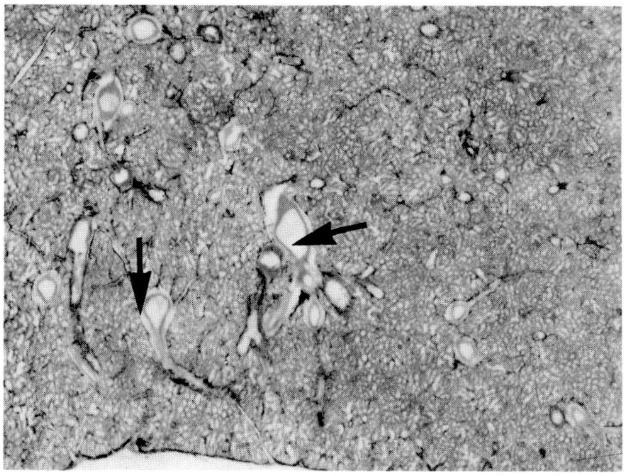

Figure 1.7 Normal lung. Alveolar spaces are less than 1 mm in diameter. Arrows indicate bronchi. (From paper-mounted section, natural size)

In a recent revision of this classification centrilobular emphysema is referred to as *proximal acinar emphysema* and paraseptal emphysema as *distal acinar emphysema* (Heppleston, 1972; Thurlbeck, 1976).

Each of these types may be localized or widespread, of slight or severe degree, and more than one type may be found in the same lung. The characteristic appearances of centrilobular and panlobular emphysema are shown in the accompanying illustrations compared with normal lung (*Figures 1.7* to *1.12*). *Figures 1.7* to *1.9* are natural-size photographs of lung sections and *Figures 1.10* to *1.12* are slightly magnified photomicrographs of the same types of emphysema.

Abnormal enlargement of alveoli may be caused by:

(1) Atrophy of their walls due to causes which are not understood.
(2) Destruction of their walls may sometimes result from inflammatory disease, although in most cases the cause is obscure. However, some cases of panlobular emphysema which has a predilection for the lower parts of the lungs, and is usually accompanied by chronic bronchitis and the onset of dyspnoea on exertion before the fifth decade are now known to be associated with an inherited deficiency of the enzyme α_1-antitrypsin carried by an autosomal recessive gene. The incidence of homozygous deficiency in these cases may be as much as 18 per cent (Leading article, 1971) or even higher (Hutchinson *et al.*, 1971). The pathogenesis of the emphysema remains to be explained but cigarette smoking appears to have an important contributory effect (Leading article, 1971). Immunological processes may be of importance in other types.

It is possible to separate types of emphysema into those with 'air trapping' (or airways obstruction) and those without. Air trapping is revealed by physiological tests during life and observations of the lungs at operation or post-mortem examination when they fail to deflate normally in whole or in part. It is a common and important cause of functional impairment.

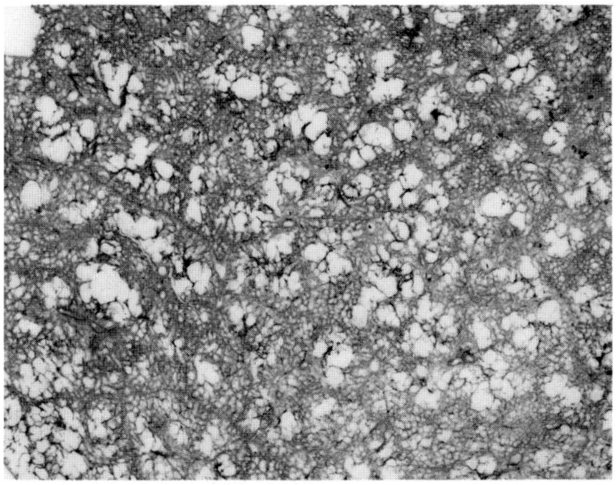

(a)

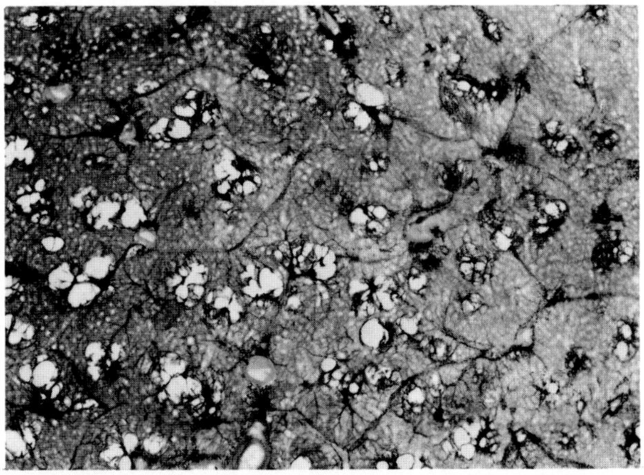

(b)

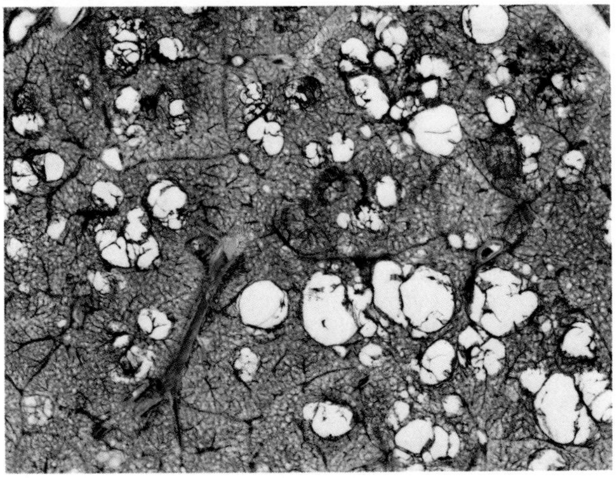

(c)

Figure 1.8 Examples of centrilobular emphysema. Note that the intervening lung is normal in all three. (From paper-mounted sections, natural size.) (a) Slight to moderate without dust pigmentation. (b) Slight to moderate with dust pigmentation. (c) Moderately severe with very slight pigmentation

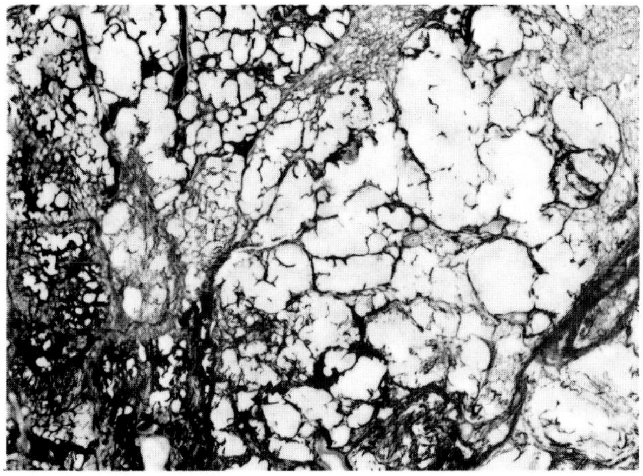

Figure 1.9 Moderate to severe panlobular emphysema. Little normal lung remains. (From paper-mounted section, natural size)

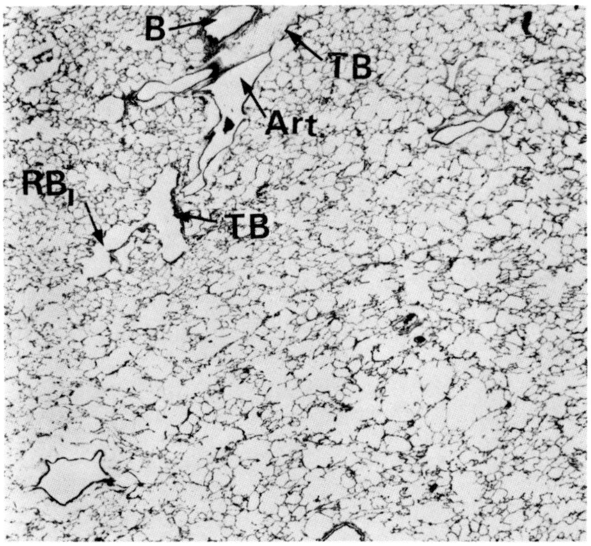

Figure 1.10 Microsection of normal lung: (art) pulmonary artery; (b) bonchiole; (tb) terminal bronchiole; (rb_1) first respiratory bronchiole. (Magnification × 10; by courtesy of Dr David Lamb)

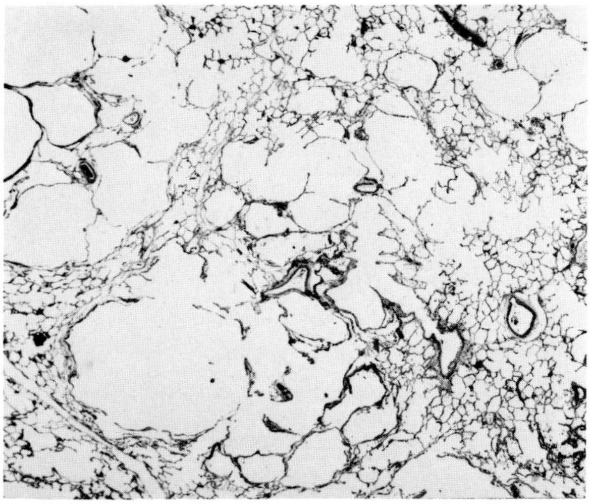

Figure 1.11 Microsection of centrilobular emphysema; normal lung between the lesions. (Magnification × 10; by courtesy of Dr David Lamb)

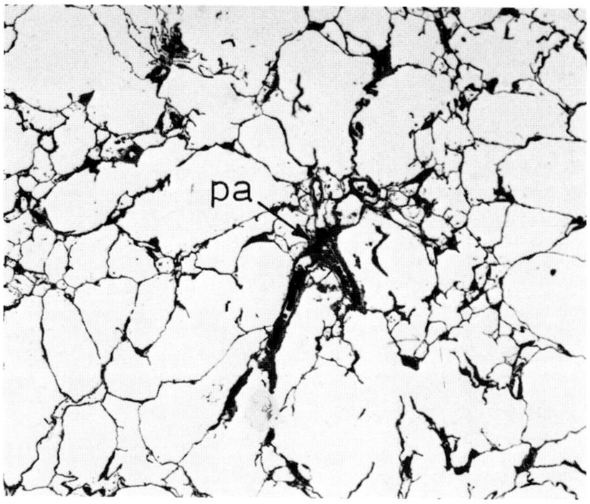

Figure 1.12 Microsection of panlobular emphysema; (pa) pulmonary artery. (Magnification × 10; by courtesy of Dr David Lamb)

Centrilobular (centriacinar) emphysema

This consists of a localized enlargement of the alveoli of respiratory bronchioles and, to some extent, of the walls of these bronchioles. The walls of the distended alveoli either remain intact, though distorted, or are lost to a variable degree. These two states can be referred to respectively as *'distensive' and 'destructive' centrilobular emphysema* (Heard, 1969), but it is to be understood that 'distensive' and 'destructive' are used here in a descriptive sense and do not imply pathogenesis. When the walls are intact ('distensive' centrilobular emphysema) the lesions appear to the naked eye as small isolated holes across which tenuous strands of the walls of enlarged alveoli are visible, but the basic alveolar structure persists. The holes vary from 1 mm to 4 mm diameter and the surrounding alveoli are normal

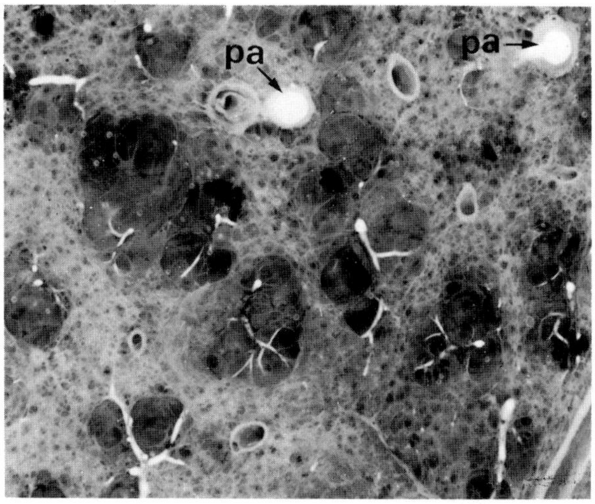

Figure 1.13 Centrilobular emphysema showing minute arteries coursing across the emphysema spaces which appear dark because of their depth; (pa) pulmonary arteries. (Barium-gelatin preparation; magnification × 3; by courtesy of Dr B. E. Heard and the Editor of Thorax*)*

(*Figure 1.8a, b*). When the walls are lost ('destructive' centrilobular emphysema) the holes are larger and may reach 1 cm or more in diameter (*Figure 1.8c* and *Figure 1.11*). Traversing strands are absent or very few, but small arteries may be seen coursing across them (*Figure 1.13*). Alveoli immediately surrounding these holes tend to be flattened and form a thin encircling wall; otherwise the neighbouring lung appears normal.

Both types of lesion may be present in the one lung and both may contain pigment or inhaled dust particles (for example, soot, coal, carbon, hematite and foundry dust according to the nature of past exposure) and, in these circumstances and especially when the dust is coal, the 'distensive' type with intact alveolar walls has been referred to as 'focal emphysema' (Heppleston, 1947). The lesions of centrilobular emphysema, therefore, may be of distensive type with or without dust, or of destructive type with or without dust. The quantity of pigment in the lungs of urban smokers appears to be significantly greater than in those of urban non-smokers (Pratt and Kilburn, 1971).

Centrilobular emphysema of both types is characteristically distributed in the upper two-thirds of the lungs, particularly in the posterior apical segments, but may be scattered throughout the lungs. It does not appear to be associated with air trapping (Reid, 1967).

Pathogenesis

(1) Both the 'distensive' and 'destructive' forms are found throughout the world. they have been observed in Jamaica, where there is virtually no air pollution, in at least 45 per cent of male autopsies (Hayes and Summerell, 1969) and in association with soot and pigment in the lungs of male Londoners (Heard and Izukawa, 1963). Centrilobular emphysema is found in the lungs of persons with no known history of chronic respiratory disease during life and who die of other causes (Snider, Brody and Doctor, 1962), as well as in those of persons known to have had chronic respiratory disease. It is more common in men than in women and is not found in children.

(2) There is a strong correlation between centrilobular emphysema and cigarette smoking (for example, Anderson *et al.*, 1966); indeed, by observing this type of emphysema in whole lung sections (*see* Appendix), and without other information, it has been found possible to distinguish those of smokers from those of non-smokers with statistically significant accuracy (Anderson and Foraker, 1967). The presence of respiratory bronchiolitis of irregular distribution in young smokers—which is referred to on pp. 10 and 18—may, perhaps, be a precursor of this type of emphysema.Cigarette smoke inhaled by experimental animals lowers the surface tension and increases the surface compressibility of surfactant (Webb *et al.*, 1967) which may diminish the stability of alveoli and thus render them likely to dilate (Miller and Bondurant, 1962).

(3) Chronic bronchitis, being a common disorder, is often present in lungs with 'distensive' or 'destructive' centrilobular emphysema—with or without dust. It has been suggested that bronchitis is the cause of 'destructive' centrilobular emphysema (Leopold and Gough, 1957), but this is open to doubt for the following reasons. This form of emphysema is often found in the lungs of persons

who did not have chronic respiratory disease. Chronic obstructive bronchitis, like centrilobular emphysema, is closely correlated with cigarette smoking, but either may exist independently of the other. And chronic bronchitis, determined by the Reid gland/wall ratio (p.17), is present uniformly throughout the lungs whereas centrilobular emphysema is distributed in sporadic fashion mostly in the upper halves of the lungs (Greenburg, Bousby and Jenkins, 1967). Furthermore, Reid and Millard (1964) were unable to find any significant correlation between severe chronic bronchitis and this type of emphysema. In short, chronic bronchitis does not appear to be the predominant cause.

However, bronchiolitis in the form of inflammatory changes and some loss of muscle and elastic fibres in the bronchioles leading into affected acini has been reported (Leopold and Gough, 1957; Heard, 1969), though complete obliteration rarely occurs. But it has not been shown that these changes are characteristically associated with 'destructive' centrilobular emphysema, and the apparent absence of a clear relationship between the presence of severity of bronchiolar stenosis and the degree of emphysema suggests that anatomical obstruction is not primarily responsible (Heppleston, 1972).

(4) 'Focal emphysema' is 'distensive' centrilobular emphysema with pigment and dust and, particularly in the case of coal dust, has been causally attributed to this (Heppleston, 1953, 1972). It is postulated that accumulation of dust in respiratory bronchioles weakens their walls and allows them to dilate. But the existence of 'focal emphysema' as a separate entity is controversial and the possibility that dusts may be preferentially deposited in already existing emphysema lesions rather than in normal lung is not excluded. This question is discussed in more detail in Chapter 8.

(5) 'Destructive' centrilobular emphysema has also been attributed to the inhalation of high concentrations of cadmium fume; and emphysema of unspecified type, to exposure to nitrogen dioxide. These questions are considered in Chapter 13.

In summary: on present evidence the most important factor in the pathogenesis of centrilobular emphysema appears to be cigarette smoking (Anderson, Dunnill and Ryder, 1972).

Clinical features

'Distensive' centrilobular emphysema is not responsible for any respiratory symptoms nor for any detectable impairment of lung function. This is not surprising when it is recalled that the lesions involve only a small fraction of the total alveolar surface, and do not cause air trapping.

'Destructive' centrilobular emphysema cannot be identified as such during life by physiological tests. But it has been suggested on theoretical grounds that abnormal enlargement of respiratory bronchioles may cause impairment of gas diffusion to the acini they supply (Staub, 1965; Horsfield, Cumming and Hicken, 1966), although the presence of this type of emphysema post mortem in individuals with no respiratory symptoms or physiological abnormality during life suggests that in many cases at least it does not cause significant functional deficiency. However, when the lesions are numerous and large, reduction of effective alveolar ventilation with increased ventilation–perfusion inequality may result. Dyspnoea and impaired lung function are most likely to be due to co-existent chronic obstructive bronchitis.

This type of emphysema even when extensive cannot be detected on standard chest radiographs although it may be demonstrated by bronchography.

Panlobular (panacinar) emphysema

This is the commonest type of emphysema associated with the retention or 'trapping' of air within the acinus. It occurs in any part of the lungs, the lower halves as much as the upper, but with a preferential tendency for the anterior and basal regions; it may be local or general, and vary from a slight to gross order of severity. The affected parts of the lungs do not deflate normally when the thorax is opened at necropsy, and the lung substance may be so attenuated that when cut it sags away from blood vessels and airways. To the naked eye the earliest stage reveals enlarged air spaces in part or all of the lobule anywhere in the lung; the most severe stage shows extensive loss of structure and dilatation of lung parenchyma (*Figure 1.9*). Microscopy (*Figure 1.12*) shows breakdown of alveolar walls which are consequently much reduced in number throughout the acinus and, in the more severe grades, respiratory bronchioles are also involved (*Figure 1.6*). Pigment or dust apparently deposited after formation of the emphysema may be present in surviving alveolar walls (*Figure 1.14*). Centrilobular and panlobular emphysema may both occur in the same lung.

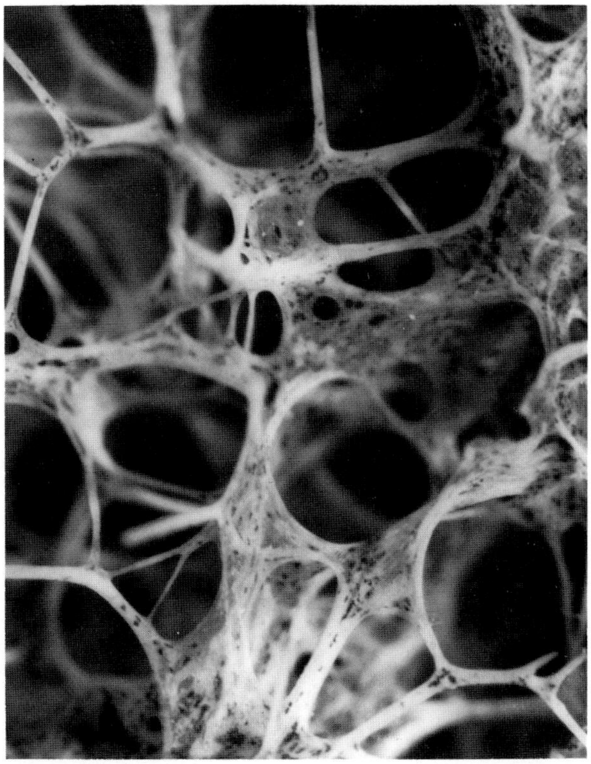

Figure 1.14 Severe panlobular emphysema with extensive alveolar wall loss and pigment in the surviving walls; city dweller's lung (Magnification × 22.4; courtesy of Dr B. E. Heard)

Pathogenesis

(1) Panlobular emphysema is not causally related to any form of pneumoconiosis.
(2) In adult life it is commonly found in association with chronic bronchitis and, therefore, with smoking, and is a disease of the second half of life. The frequency of this association is significantly higher than can be explained by chance. But panlobular emphysema may occur in the absence of chronic bronchitis in this age group and, rarely, in young men and women when it is known as *primary emphysema,* the cause of which is obscure (Reid, 1967). Contrawise, chronic obstructive bronchitis is often present in the absence of this type of emphysema.
(3) *Alpha-1-antitrypsin deficiency* The protein alpha-1-antitrypsin (α-1-AT) is one of the chief serum inhibitors of a wide range of proteolytic enzymes including leucocyte and bacterial proteases the primary function of which is to digest the debris of inflammatory exudates. Hence, it protects the lungs from attack by these enzymes. But if serum α-1-AT is severely deficient alveolar membranes are unprotected and are likely to be destroyed, resulting in emphysema (Lieberman, 1973). More than 20 different types of α-1-AT—known as Pi types—have been identified (Cox and Celhoffer, 1974) but only a small number of these alleles are linked with low serum levels; the ZZ (homozygote) genotype being most commonly associated with severe deficiency, and the MZ and MS (heterozygote) genotypes, with minor deficiency. It is homozygous individuals, therefore, who are apt to develop emphysema which is of panlobular type involving the lower lobes predominantly, and its incidence is especially high among smokers. An association between heterozygotes of MZ type and emphysema is controversial but it may predispose to airflow obstruction (Cox, Hoeppner and Levison, 1976; Hutchinson, 1976). The possibility that exposure of individuals with severe α-1-AT deficiency to irritant gases might increase their chance of developing emphysema requires investigation but, at present, is no more than speculative.

Clinical features

There is gradually increasing breathlessness on effort and, ultimately, at rest. There are no abnormal physical signs until the disease is fairly advanced. Before it reaches this stage it cannot be detected in chest radiographs, but it presents a characteristic appearance when widespread and severe (*see* Chapter 5). Its effect on lung function is referred to on p.7.

Paraseptal (periacinar) emphysema

This takes the form of rows of small bullae typically distributed along the margins of the lungs; the anterior margins of the upper and middle lobes and lingula, and the costophrenic margin of the lower. It is also contiguous with connective tissue septa, blood vessels and bronchi. The lesions are characterized by loss of the walls of alveoli at the periphery of the acinus and they contain little or no lung tissue; neighbouring alveoli and the rest of the lung are normal. Bullae may become very large (Edge, Simon and Reid, 1966; Reid, 1967).

Important features are:

(1) It does not cause airways obstruction and is, therefore, symptomless and rarely associated with impairment of respiratory function.
(2) It can often be clearly recognized on chest radiographs.
(3) It tends to cause spontaneous pneumothorax or enlarging bullae. Although large bullae may cause impairment of ventilation and blood flow of adjacent lung, resulting in dyspnoea, this does not necessarily occur (Davies, Simon and Reid, 1966); lung function may be nearly normal with disease advanced enough to be seen on the radiograph.
(4) It is not causally related to any type of pneumoconiosis, but may contain dust and pigment.

Irregular (or scar) emphysema

In the USA this is referred to as *paracicatricial emphysema* (cicatrix, a scar). It has two possible primary causes in adult life.

(1) Complete or partial destruction of alveoli by an inflammatory process with subsequent resolution and the formation either of a central, contracted, collagenous scar surrounded by enlarged and distorted alveoli, or of an area of interstitial scarring between alveoli. Some loss of capillary blood vessels is apt to occur in the lesions.
(2) Over-inflation of the alveoli on a large scale may be caused by retraction of a scar in neighbouring lung tissue (as is seen, for example, in healed tuberculosis). When severe, many alveoli are lost with consequent reduction in alveolar surface.

It is not to be confused with *compensatory emphysema* which is characterized by over-inflation of otherwise normal lung to occupy an adjacent area from which lung tissue has been lost due, for example, to segmental or lobar collapse or resection.

Irregular emphysema may be associated with the fibrotic nodules and confluent fibrotic lesions of some types of pneumoconiosis, especially coal pneumoconiosis (Chapter 8) when it is sometimes incorrectly referred to as 'focal emphysema'.

Irreversible airways obstruction may be present, but not always, and the disease is often detectable in chest radiographs.

Before leaving the question of emphysema in general, Heard's (1966) practical interpretation of the morbid anatomical appearances should be noted:

> We believe that emphysema should, like atherosclerosis, be accepted as a common and, in small amounts, unimportant necropsy finding. . . . There is a danger that too much importance be attached to small amounts of emphysema in problematical cases, forgetting the commonness of emphysema at necropsy anyway. There is a great reserve of activity in lungs, and a patient is not necessarily disabled by the surgical removal of the whole of one lung. On these grounds it would seem unwise to attribute pulmonary insufficiency to emphysema that involves less than half the area of a slice of prepared lung.

There are three factors which are quantitively related to death in chronic airways obstruction and to the weight or mass of the right ventricle: they are the total amount of emphysema, the amount of panlobular, but not of centrilobular, emphysema and the degree of reduction in the lumen of small airways (Scott, 1976).

Diffuse interstitial pulmonary fibrosis with 'honeycomb' cysts ('honeycomb lung')—the features of which are described in Chapter 4, p. 79—should not, as a rule, be confused with emphysema, though localized areas of emphysema which have previously been involved in an inflammatory process may occasionally present a superficial resemblance to 'honeycombing' on gross inspection.

It is important at this point to emphasize that, in order to make an accurate post-mortem assessment of the type, distribution and extent of emphysema, lungs should be perfused with fixative until their size is equivalent to their position in full inflation during life, after which they can be cut in sections for inspection (*see* Appendix).

CHRONIC BRONCHITIS

Chronic bronchitis, once regarded as pre-eminently the 'English Disease', is now known to be common in many parts of the world thanks to the standardization of terminology and examination technique exemplified by Fletcher *et al.* (1964). Because of the widespread belief that chronic bronchitis may be caused in some circumstances by occupational air pollution this will be discussed in some detail preceded by a brief review of current knowledge of chronic bronchitis in general.

Unfortunately, the subject is much confused by having a variety of different meanings attributed to the term *chronic bronchitis*. For example, chronic airflow obstruction in the absence of sputum production is often referred to as 'chronic bronchitis', and the World Health Organization (1975) has compounded confusion by proposing this vague definition: 'Chronic bronchitis is a non-neoplastic disorder of structure or function of the bronchi usually resulting from prolonged or recurrent exposure to infectious or non-infectious irritation'.

DEFINITION AND CLASSIFICATION

The definition of chronic bronchitis, unlike that of emphysema, rests on abnormality of function and not of anatomy: that is, chronic bronchitis is 'a condition of chronic or recurrent excess of mucus secretion in the bronchial tree' (Ciba Foundation Guest Symposium, 1959). This implies the persistent production of any sputum, expectorated or swallowed, which may or may not be accompanied by cough; and 'chronic' has been defined as 'occurring on most days for at least three months in the year for at least three successive years' (Medical Research Council, 1965). The American Thoracic Society (1962) adopted a similar definition.

In the UK the Medical Research Council (1965) classified chronic bronchitis as follows.

(1) *Chronic simple bronchitis:* chronic or recurrent increase in the volume of mucoid bronchial secretion sufficient to cause expectoration.
(2) *Chronic mucopurulent bronchitis:* chronic bronchitis in which the sputum is persistent or intermittently mucopurulent when this is not due to localized bronchopulmonary disease.
(3) *Chronic obstructive bronchitis:* chronic bronchitis in which there is persistent widespread narrowing of the intrapulmonary airways, at least on expiration, causing increased resistance to air flow.

A standard questionnaire for diagnosis and simple methods of assessing ventilatory function were proposed in 1960 and 1965 and have been widely used and elaborated since. Of course, other causes of chronic sputum production and cough must be excluded: that is, other chronic bronchopulmonary diseases (for example, bronchiectasis and tuberculosis) and disease of the nasal passages and paranasal sinuses which may cause expectoration of 'post-nasal drip' secretions. Evidence of such exclusion is not always provided, however, in reported epidemiological and clinical studies of chronic bronchitis. The prevalence of chronic sinusitis is greater in smokers than in non-smokers (Wilson, 1973) but there is no apparent relationship between chronic bronchitis and chronic sinusitis (Burton and Dixon, 1969).

The mucous hypersecretion of chronic simple bronchitis (the causes of which are discussed in the section on Pathogenesis, p. 18) is aptly referred to as 'bronchial catarrh' (Fletcher *et al.*, 1976). Identification of airflow obstruction has depended upon FEV_1 and FEV_1/FVC or, for epidemiological purposes, PEFR. Forced expiratory flow rates are not superior to FEV_1 and its ratio to FVC in detecting obstruction of central airways (Hankinson, Reger and Morgan, 1977). But early obstruction due to narrowing of small peripheral airways (that is, non-cartilagenous, non-alveolated airways less than 2 mm in diameter in the fully inflated lung) which may be present in subjects with chronic bronchitis (Matsuba and Thurlbeck, 1973) is not detected by these tests. However, although closing volume and $FEF_{75\%}$ are more sensitive tests of airflow obstruction in small airways this sensitivity is compromised by their lack of reproducibility which renders them less suitable for studies of large populations than FEV_1 and FVC (Cochrane, Prieto and Clark, 1977). In short, as indicated earlier (p.8), FEV_1 remains, overall, the best simple index of airflow obstruction for routine use.

Increased production of bronchial mucus is reflected at autopsy in enlargement of bronchial mucous glands which can be assessed by Reid's gland/bronchial wall ratio (Reid, 1967); the average value of the index in normal lungs is 0.26, and in those with chronic bronchitis 0.59 (Reid, 1960). However, the proportion of mucous glands in the bronchial walls is more accurately estimated by the point-counting technique adopted by Dunnill, Massarella and Anderson (1969); and a less tedious, though seemingly accurate, method based on radial intercepts has been described by Alli (1975). The chief factor in the enlargement of bronchial glands appears to be an increase in their cell numbers (that is, hyperplasia rather than hypertrophy) with enlargement of their acini caused by engorgement with mucus (Douglas, 1980).

Prevalence

Assessment of comparative prevalence in different countries and even in different parts of the same country is fraught with difficulty caused by the varying diagnostic criteria which have often been used during life and for death certification from which mortality rates are calculated. It is certain that 'chronic bronchitis' on some death certificates—especially in countries where the diagnosis is fashionable—may be inaccurate. Furthermore, mortality from chronic bronchitis, which is due primarily to irreversible airways obstruction, cannot be readily related to past prevalence studies during life in which attention has often been concentrated on the criterion of sputum production.

Variation in answers by subjects to questions, differences between observers, inaccuracy in the use of standard questionnaires and failure to exclude other respiratory disease may all cause erroneous or discordant results. It should also be borne in mind that workers in occupations traditionally supposed to be associated with chronic lung disease may, in good faith, give more false positive answers to the questionnaire than workers in occupations with no such recognized association.

Smoking is the most important factor affecting prevalence which has been shown to be greatly increased in smokers compared with non-smokers in both rural and urban areas of Britain and the USA, and in women as well as men. Although some 6 per cent of non-smoking men have chronic cough and phlegm there is a two-fold increase of chronic bronchitis in ex-smokers, a four-fold increase in light and moderate smokers (20 cigarettes or less/day) and, approximately, a six-fold increase in heavy smokers (more than 20 cigarettes/day) (Thurlbeck, 1976). Prevalence is higher in smokers who inhale than in those who do not (Rimington, 1974).

Environmental air pollution also appears to have some effect in that chronic cough and sputum with dyspnoea, and impaired ventilatory function has been found to be more frequent in cities than in rural areas irrespective of smoking habits (College of General Practitioners, 1961; Holland and Reid, 1965). However, a higher prevalence in Britain compared with Norway and Denmark where general air pollution was lower was attributed almost entirely to smoking (Mork, 1962; Olsen and Gilson, 1960).

The question of occupation is considered later.

PATHOGENESIS

By far the most important cause of chronic bronchitis is cigarette smoking which greatly increased in most western countries after 1920 (*Table 1.3*). The correlation of smoking and chronic bronchial catarrh with bronchial mucous gland enlargement and airflow obstruction is established but atmospheric pollution is less well correlated.

Fletcher *et al.* (1976) have provided evidence that mucus hypersecretion and airflow obstruction caused by smoking are independent effects. Some individuals have only bronchial catarrh (chronic simple bronchitis) which is not disabling; some have bronchial catarrh and airflow obstruction; and others, airflow obstruction with little or no bronchial catarrh. This absence of a clear relationship between respiratory symptoms (chronic cough and expectoration) and an irreversible decline in ventilatory function (apparently due mainly to changes in the smaller airways) in smokers has also been observed by Martin *et al.* (1973) and Oxhøj, Bake and Wilhelmsen (1976) and implies that the cause of mucus hypersecretion and cough differs from that of irreversible reduction in ventilatory function and may be due to differences in constitutional susceptibilities.

The small peripheral airways in patients with chronic bronchitis but no evidence of emphysema or respiratory disability during life have been found to be generally narrowed resulting in a significant loss of lumen, though the number of airways is not reduced. These changes, however, are not necessarily due to, or a complication of, chronic bronchitis and may be an effect of cigarette smoking (Thurlbeck, 1976). Indeed, respiratory bronchiolitis of irregular distribution has been found to be common in young smokers but not in non-smokers of comparable age; it may be reversible if smoking is stopped (Niewoehner, Kleinerman and Rice, 1974). In fact there are three distinct cigarette-related lesions: large airways disease, small airways disease and respiratory bronchiolitis (Thurlbeck, 1980).

Table 1.3 Cigarette Consumption per Adult per Annum in Selected Years in Six Countries (Data by courtesy of Tobacco Research Council)

Year	*UK*	*USA*	*S. Africa*	*Australia*	*Germany*	*France*
1920	1080	610	380	610	NA	NA
1930	1380	1370	520	610	680	NA
					(West Germany)	
1940	2020	1820	720	640	NA	610
1950	2180	3250	1170	1280	630	930
1960	2760	3780	1080	2440	1630	1320
1965	2680	3800	1080	2680	2100	1510
1968	2900	3700	1290	2780	2280	1680
1970	3050	3650	1360	2910	2510	1830
1971	2910	3560	1350	2900	2660	1880
1972	3090	3650	1350	2950	2650	1886
1973	3230	3850	1380	3080	2610	1920
1974	3210	3690	NA	NA	2610	1970
1975	3090	3710	NA	NA	2540	2060
1976	3040	3840	NA	NA	NA	2010
1978	2870	NA	NA	NA	NA	NA

NA: No information available
Adult: Population aged 15 years and over
Figures do not include hand-rolled cigarettes, cigars or cigarillos
(The Tobacco Research Council was dissolved mid-1978)

Fletcher and Peto (1977) have suggested, therefore, that bronchial catarrh and airflow obstruction, whether in the larger or smaller airways (the site of irreversible airflow obstruction), should be regarded as separate entities and that, instead of using 'chronic bronchitis' as an all-embracing term, a clear distinction should be made between *bronchial hypersecretion* and *airflow obstruction* (Fletcher and Peto, 1977).

Contrary to the widely held opinion that simple bronchitis predisposes to chronic mucopurulent bronchitis (which has never been demonstrated with any certainty) Fletcher *et al.* (1976) found that although mucus hypersecretion predisposes to episodes of chest infection these give rise only to a temporary increase in expectoration and are not a cause of persistent mucus hypersecretion nor of airflow obstruction; indeed, early intensive treatment of bacterial infection in chronic bronchitis has been shown not to affect the rate of decline of ventilatory function (Medical Research Council Working Party, 1966). The frequent association of bronchial catarrh and of airflow obstruction is explained by the fact that both are caused by a common factor—smoking; but there is no evidence that either predisposes to the other. These authors also showed that some smokers are more susceptible than others to developing severe airflow obstruction and, though the reason for this is uncertain, it may be related to unidentified social and genetic factors (Cohen *et al.*, 1977; Larson *et al.*, 1970). Interestingly, recent observations suggest that patients who die of chronic obstructive bronchitis (that is, with 'severe irreversible airways obstruction') are deficient in plasma and other cells containing IgA in the respiratory tract whereas those with 'incidental chronic bronchitis' are normal in this respect (Soutar, 1977).

It is known that the prevalence of chronic obstructive bronchitis increases as social class declines in both men and their wives (Medical Research Council Special Committee, 1966), and this may be related partly to a residual influence of social class in childhood among those who remain more or less in the same class throughout life (Kiernan *et al.*, 1976); and also to parental smoking habits and respiratory illness during infancy and childhood (Holland *et al.*, 1977).

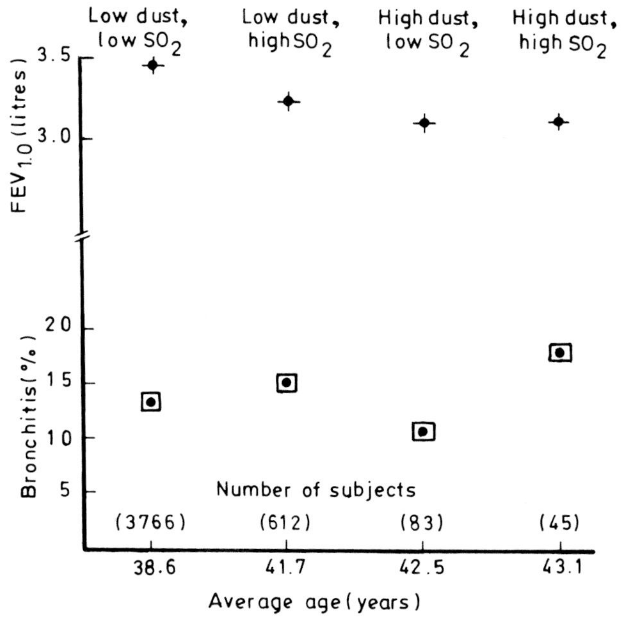

Figure 1.15 Relationship of ventilatory capacity and simple bronchitis to air pollution in a South Wales steel works survey. (By courtesy of Dr J. C. Gilson and the Hon. Editors of Proceedings of the Royal Society of Medicine*)*

Chief among the polluting substances in the atmosphere are smoke and sulphur dioxide, but noxious organic substances are sometimes produced by unusual photochemical meteorological conditions. However, rather than being a primary cause of chronic bronchitis, it appears probable that these environmental factors affect the severity of *existing* bronchitis and may precipitate exacerbations (Thurlbeck, 1976).

So far, then, it can be said that chronic simple and chronic obstructive bronchitis are caused mainly by smoking and that, to a lesser extent, chronic obstructive bronchitis is linked with social and, possibly genetic factors. But, in the context of this book, there remains the important question as to whether occupational exposure is also capable of causing disabling chronic bronchitis. In considering this the foregoing points and the distinction between bronchial catarrh and airflow obstruction, and of impaired respiratory function and respiratory disability (*see* p. 24) must ever be borne in mind. In addition, it must be stressed that airflow obstruction in the absence of chronic bronchial catarrh is not, by definition, chronic bronchitis.

CHRONIC BRONCHITIS AND OCCUPATION

Dusts and irritant fumes undoubtedly cause bronchial catarrh and the inhalation of inert dusts (for example, carbon) by mouth causes *transient* bronchoconstriction (Anderson *et al.*, 1979). However, the important question is: do dusts and irritant fumes, as is often supposed, also cause disabling and irreversible airflow obstruction?

Although there is an increased prevalence of persistent sputum production in foundry floor men compared with non-foundry men there is no evident association between work in foundry or smelter atmosphere (containing dust and sulphur dioxide fume) and airflow obstruction when age and smoking are accounted for (Brinkman, Block and Cress, 1972; Lloyd Davies, 1971; Lowe, Campbell and Khosla, 1970; Lebowitz, Burton and Kaltenborn, 1979; Mur *et al.*, 1979) except (in one of these surveys) among workers with bronchial catarrh who had one or more attacks of chest illness per year and in whom the effects of smoking and working in a foundry environment appeared to be additive (Lloyd Davies, 1971) (*Figure 1.15*). The production of sputum in the first hour of exposure at work is greater among foundry men than non-foundry men but is especially influenced by smoking habits (Lloyd Davies, 1971).

Chronic simple bronchitis (bronchial catarrh) was observed chiefly in smokers among South African gold miners exposed to rock dust, but the dust exposure apparently had no effect on ventilatory function (FEV_1) (Sluis-Cremer, Walters and Sichel, 1967a and b). A study of miners in 50 metal ore mines in the USA which was concerned primarily with analysis of FEV_1 showed that years under ground had little effect upon it compared to the natural fall with age and that attributed to smoking, although some effect was evident in subjects with established silicosis (US Public Health Service, 1963). However, bronchial catarrh is not an invariable feature of mining, for no association between mucus hypersecretion and dust exposure was found by Paul (1961) in Rhodesian copper miners.

Among workers exposed to siliceous and other dusts in the English pottery industry the prevalence of persistent cough and sputum was no higher than might have been expected in other working populations though the proportion of individuals with bronchial catarrh and reduced ventilatory function (FEV_1 and FEV_1/FVC) was greater amongst smokers and ex-smokers. 'Simple pneumoconiosis' (categories 2 and 3) was the only condition specifically related to dust exposure (Fox *et al.*, 1975).

The most extensive study of this problem, however, has been carried out in coal miners and it is more appropriate to consider it here than in Chapter 8.

The immediate results of inhaling coal dust are cough, increased secretion of mucus and airways resistance which are both acute and transient (McDermott, 1962); and a small but significant decrease in FEV_1, FVC and $FEF_{75\%}$ has been recorded at the end of a working shift underground in smoking coal miners, but only in $FEF_{75\%}$—which is less discriminative—in non-smoking miners (Lapp *et al.*, 1972). Chronic simple bronchitis (cough and sputum) is common in coal miners (Higgins, 1972; Kibelstis *et al.*, 1973; Minette, 1971; Rae, Walker and Attfield, 1971; Ulmer and Reichel, 1972) and appears to be related to duration of dust exposure (Kibelstis *et al.*, 1973; Minette, 1971; Rae, Walker and Attfield 1971) and the presence of pneumoconiosis (Rae, Walker and Attfield, 1971), though in some studies its prevalence is independent of radiographic category (Minette, 1971). Always, however, the effect of smoking is dominant.

The situation regarding airflow obstruction is somewhat inconsistent. In a series of surveys in England, Wales and the USA in the 1950s and 1960s miners and ex-miners were found to have a higher prevalence of cough, sputum and breathlessness and a lower average FEV than non-miners though the magnitude of the difference varied in different places (Higgins, 1972). A survey of a large number of American coal miners showed that reduction in ventilatory capacity was related primarily to cigarette smoking and that the effect of dust exposure was minimal as mean FEV values for non-smoking miners at the coal face and on the surface were respectively, 98 and 102 per cent of predicted values; in fact, the effect of cigarette smoking was five to six times greater than exposure to dust (Kibelstis *et al.*, 1973). Again, coal miners with chronic simple bronchitis and 'simple' coal pneumoconiosis in West Germany, were not found to have more airways obstruction than miners without either (Ulmer and Reichel, 1972). Although Lowe and Khosla (1972) observed more cough and sputum and poorer ventilatory capacity in ex-coal miners than in other men working in a South Wales steelworks, once again smoking was a more important factor than coal mining; and it was unlikely that the ex-miners were representative of the mining population from which they came. In contrast to the findings of Kibelstis *et al.* (1973) Hankinson *et al.* (1977) observed a slight reduction in maximal expiration flow rates in American miners with simple bronchitis (phlegm production only) which was related to years spent underground but not to category of pneumoconiosis or smoking; however, the magnitude of the change appears too small to be of clinical significance. Rogan *et al.* (1973) reported that increasing severity of 'bronchitis symptoms' (that is, cough and phlegm, chest illness and breathlessness on exertion) in British coal miners with category 0 to 3 radiographs was associated with a greater loss of FEV than could be accounted for by their estimated dust exposure, smoking and age, and that this loss was not related to category; they suggested that these findings may imply that once early bronchitis symptoms are present ventilatory capacity may deteriorate independently of factors which initiate the disease process. The lapse rate of the men, and other selection effects, in this study, however, make interpretation of the results most difficult. But, in any case, this suggestion is at odds with the observation of Fletcher *et al.* (1976), already referred to: namely, that mucus hypersecretion does not predispose to airflow obstruction; though it is not inconsistent with their conclusion that the association of the two disorders may be due to linked susceptibilities.

It is evident, therefore, that there is some discrepancy in different studies as to whether chronic simple bronchitis is related to, or independent of, radiographic category or is associated with airflow obstruction. In this respect Cochrane's recent (1976) comments are important. He criticized data derived from a large number of subjects in different geographic areas for lacking necessary 'within area comparisons' (or controls) and inclusion of ex-miners, and stressed the distorting effects that this may have because of the variety of influences which may affect both miners and non-miners living in different localities.

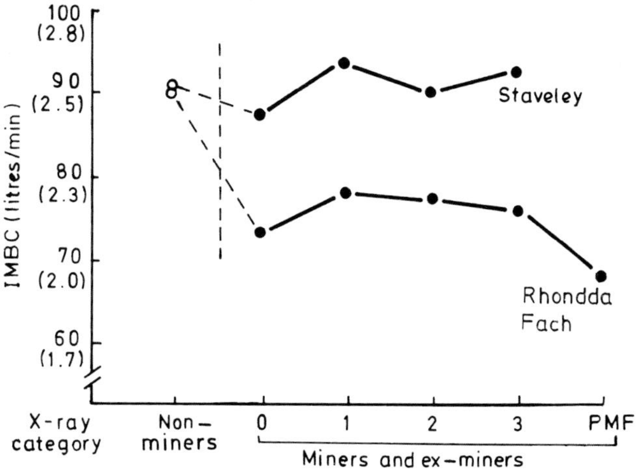

Figure 1.16 Mean indirect maximum breathing capacity (IMBC) (l/min) related to radiographic category of coal pneumoconiosis. (Random samples of males aged 55 to 64 in Staveley (Derbyshire) and the Rhondda Fach (S. Wales). (Figures in parenthesis are FEV_1 equivalents). (Courtesy of Professor A. L. Cochrane and Editor of the Proceedings of the Royal Society of Medicine*)*

This is exemplified in *Figure 1.16* which shows that ventilatory values can be significantly different in two different populations of miners yet unaffected by increasing radiographic category in both. It is difficult, therefore, on present evidence to see how the results of the studies of Hankinson, Reger and Morgan (1977) and Rogan *et al.* (1973), neither of which employed control groups of non-miners of comparable socio-economic status are compatible with the lack of significant relationship between radiographic category of 'simple' pneumoconiosis and FEV levels observed by others and the well-established correlation between radiographic category of 'simple' pneumoconiosis and the coal dust content of the lungs. It is also of interest that when Hankinson, Reger and Morgan, (1977) abstracted 100 non-smoking, non-bronchitic miners from those in the study just referred to and matched them with a control population of non-miners of comparable number and socio-economic status no significant differences were found in maximal expiratory flow rates.

In a recent review of the subject Morgan (1978) showed an association between slight impairment of ventilatory capacity and expectoration. But the effect is trivial and no causal relationship between severity of expectoration and degree of impairment of ventilatory capacity is demonstrated.

Chronic bronchitis (mucus hypersecretion), with or without airflow obstruction, and coal pneumoconiosis may occur independently. Dust particles larger than 5 μm aerodynamic diameter, which are deposited chiefly in the larger or dead space airways, are undoubtedly capable of causing mucus hypersecretion. But, of miners with similar dust exposures, why should some have bronchitis without pneumoconiosis and others pneumoconiosis with or without bronchitis? Assuming this question to be valid and not based on epidemiological artefacts no simple answer is to hand. The differences may be related to one or more of the following variables: patterns of respiration and whether individuals are predominantly nose or mouth breathers, smoking habits, individual susceptibility to cigarette smoke or to inhaled dust, and efficiency of ciliary clearance.

In short, there appears to be no consistent and clear association between the presence of chronic cough and phlegm and significant airflow obstruction or respiratory disability in coal miners; and, in fact, Gilson (1970) found no relationship between these features and radiographic category and dust content of the lungs (*see Figure 8.20*) nor with the number of years spent underground (*Figure 1.17*).

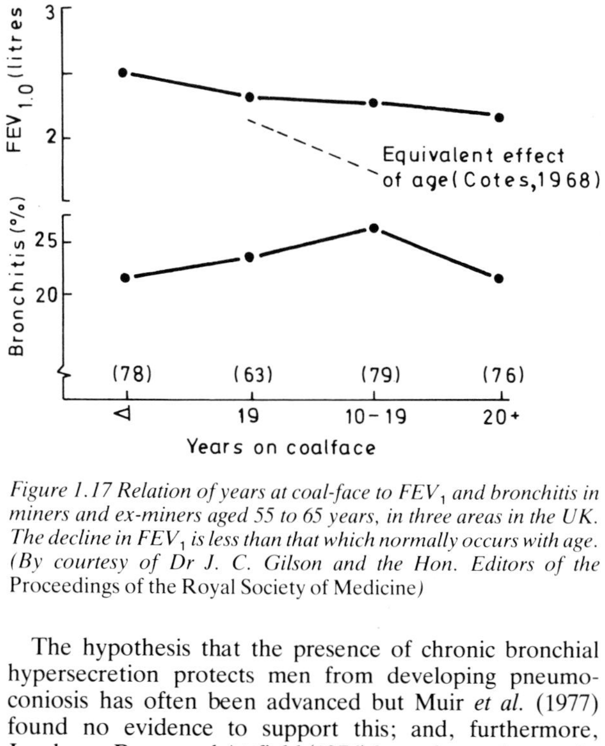

Figure 1.17 Relation of years at coal-face to FEV_1 and bronchitis in miners and ex-miners aged 55 to 65 years, in three areas in the UK. The decline in FEV_1 is less than that which normally occurs with age. (By courtesy of Dr J. C. Gilson and the Hon. Editors of the Proceedings of the Royal Society of Medicine*)*

The hypothesis that the presence of chronic bronchial hypersecretion protects men from developing pneumoconiosis has often been advanced but Muir *et al.* (1977) found no evidence to support this; and, furthermore, Jacobsen, Burns and Attfield (1976) have shown that smoking does not modify the effect that exposure to airborne dust has on the development of pneumoconiosis assessed radiographically.

When social status is considered a similar higher prevalence of chronic cough and sputum and reduced ventilatory function to that among coal miners and foundry workers compared with agricultural workers was found in the wives of the men in these groups (Higgins *et al.*, 1959). On the other hand, in another study in West Virginia coal miners in which the groups were watched for educational level there were no differences in prevalence of chronic simple bronchitis and lowered ventilatory function between miners and non-miners (Enterline and Lainhart, 1967). Higgins and Cochrane (1961) concluded that dust exposure seems unlikely to account for the excess of respiratory symptoms in miners compared with the rest of the community and that the finding in miners' wives points to an effect of social rather than occupational factors in miners. And, although, it has been argued (Lowe, 1968) that higher death rates from 'bronchitis' compared with non-miners and their wives must be due to occupation, re-analysis of the same data by Gilson (1970) failed to identify any other influential factor than that of social class.

The term '*industrial bronchitis*' has recently been introduced to refer to bronchial catarrh, with or without ventilatory impairment, in dusty occupations. This is particularly unfortunate in that it not only implies a separate species of 'bronchitis' but it is sometimes used, indefensibly, to connote airflow obstruction in the absence of phlegm production. If a special term is desired *occupational bronchial catarrh* might be preferable but this could only refer to a disorder capable of diagnosis in individuals who have never smoked and in whom no other cause of bronchial catarrh can be identified.

To summarize

Although there is no doubt that *chronic 'simple bronchitis'* (that is, persistent phlegm production without airflow obstruction which does not cause respiratory disability and which usually disappears when occupational exposure ceases) is caused by the inhalation of dusts and certain irritant fumes and gases, there is, at present, no convincing evidence to show that *chronic obstructive bronchitis* (that is, persistent bronchial catarrh *and* airflow obstruction—so common in the general population) nor associated respiratory disability are directly and consistently attributable to such exposure. The principal causes of 'obstructive bronchitis' appear to be smoking and social factors, and, although general environmental pollution may provoke exacerbation of existing bronchitis, it has not been clearly shown to be an initiating cause. A synergistic relationship between smoking and inhaled dust has been postulated but not proven, though in Britain it appears that smokers are more likely to suffer from the effects of air pollution than non-smokers (Royal College of Physicians Report, 1970); and a possibility of synergy between smoking and exposure to foundry manganese dust has been reported (Šarić and Lučić-Palaić, 1976). There is some evidence in experimental animals that such an effect might occur (Boren, 1964) but further investigation of the problem is needed.

It must be emphasized that in any consideration of chronic bronchitis in relation to occupation it is essential to distinguish clearly:

(1) between chronic cough with phlegm and permanent airflow obstruction; and
(2) between reduction in ventilatory function and dyspnoea (respiratory disability).

These important distinctions have not always been made in many published reports, and the habit of referring to airflow obstruction without chronic bronchial catarrh as 'chronic bronchitis' cannot be justified. It is evident, too, even from this brief review, that the greatest care is required in the methodology of surveys and in the standardization of all criteria used in the investigation of this problem.

The question of a possible relationship between chronic airflow obstruction and exposure to the oxides of nitrogen (so-called 'nitrous fumes') is discussed briefly in Chapter 13.

SOME PRACTICAL POINTS IN MEDICAL EXAMINATION

HISTORY TAKING

Occupational history

An inscription on a bell in an old Suffolk church which reads *Ars Incognita Imperitus Contemnitur* (an unknown art is considered unimportant by those who do not practise it) is relevant to the taking of an occupational history. For, although this is an essential part of the medical examination, it is commonly inadequately done or, worse, omitted altogether.

It cannot be too strongly emphasized that a carefully detailed history of the patient's present and previous occupations is the means by which, on the one hand, attention may be directed to the occupational nature of his lung disease or, on the other, to the fact that the disease in question cannot be occupational because it can be shown that he never worked in a relevant occupation or its immediate environment.

The work history must be taken in strictly chronological order starting with details of the first job on leaving school and progressing step by step to the present job or retirement. As far as possible no gaps or uncertainties should exist when it is complete, and the nature of the materials to which a worker has been exposed must be established. When a man has done a number of jobs which sound innocuous it is easy to accept this at face value with the result that a hazardous process remains unidentified; equally, not all processes which are imagined to be dangerous are so. It is also necessary to form some idea of the intensity of a man's exposure to a hazard (that is, whether dust or fume concentrations were in general high or low) as well as the duration of this exposure.

The description of a job or the name given to it by the worker may conceal its true nature and, therefore, an unexpected hazard. For example, a *bricklayer* may have worked with refractory bricks (not house bricks) containing high concentrations of free silica and, furthermore, may have used asbestos fibre or rope for grouting; a *stoker* may not only have stoked a factory, power station or hospital boiler but may also have been exposed to free silica dust produced when cleaning ('scaling') its tubes, or to an intermittent asbestos risk during the stripping, mixing and reapplication of lagging materials around the boiler and neighbouring pipes by laggers working in his immediate vicinity; a *labourer* in a factory producing poultry meal may have worked for years at a flint crushing mill and so have been exposed to the risk of silicosis; a man may describe himself as a *scrap-metal worker* but only on further enquiry does it become clear that his work involved the melting down of beryllium alloys; a *welder* may be exposed to cadmium fumes from cadmium-plated metals; and a *clerk* or a *housewife* may have been an asbestos worker many years previously.

Exposure of a worker to a hazardous aerosol from a nearby process and the disease which may result from it is often referred to as being *para-occupational.*

The popular description of a job may give no clue to its identity or to the nature of the work involved. It should be a rule, therefore, to establish precisely what the job entails and the materials used if these are not self-evident. The possibility of multiple risks operating in the one work process, or of a man having worked in different hazardous industries must be kept in mind. Such carefully detailed history is especially important in identifying the cause of occupational asthma (*see* Chapter 12).

The worker should also be asked whether, in what way and over what period of time, protective measures were used: in particular, local exhaust and general ventilation and the wearing of respirators and protective clothing. This enables the physician to obtain some impression of the concentrations of dust to which the man may have been exposed.

Enquiry as to whether any fellow workers have lung disease may provide help both in diagnosis and in identifying a previously unrecognized hazard.

Environmental history

Due to contamination outside the factory by harmful industrial materials, lung disease has sometimes been caused in persons who have never worked in the industry concerned. Non-occupational exposure has resulted from the discharge of dusts (such as beryllium and asbestos) by exhaust ventilation systems and smoke stacks into the atmosphere around a factory, and by the dumping in the open air of dangerous materials. Sources such as these are now generally controlled (*see* Chapter 3), but may still occur from time to time. Under these circumstances both sexes of all ages may have been potentially at risk in the past. Hence, some present-day adults may have been subjected to such exposures in childhood or adolescence. Disease contracted in this way is referred to as *neighbourhood disease.*

Domestic history

Potentially hazardous dusts shaken from a worker's overalls at home during cleaning or preparation for laundering, may be (or may have been in the past) a possible source of disease risk to his family. Asbestos and beryllium compounds have chiefly been indicted.

Details of hobbies should also be sought. Eliciting a history of bird fancying (chiefly budgerigars and pigeons) is especially important in those cases in which there has been repeated exposure for, under these conditions, chronic extrinsic allergic 'alveolitis' of insidious onset may occur and its relationship with the cause is apt to be unsuspected.

Soldering, work with certain woods or epoxy resin hardeners and keeping of small pet animals may be responsible for asthma which may require differentiation from occupational asthma (*see* Chapter 12).

Smoking habits

Accurate information about past and present smoking habits must always be obtained and recorded. People fall into one of three groups: smokers, ex-smokers and non-smokers. Cigarette, cigar and pipe smoking must be distinguished and its duration and the question of inhaling established.

It is usual to record cigarette consumption as the number smoked/day, but for comparison with other types of smoking it is helpful to note that one manufactured cigarette is approximately equivalent to 1 g of tobacco and that 1 oz (28 g) of tobacco/week, therefore, equals 4 g daily, whether smoked in a pipe or hand-rolled cigarettes (Higgins, 1959). Another method of recording (especially in the USA) is the '*pack year*' which is defined as one packet of 20 cigarettes/day for one year.

Nasal symptoms

The subject should be asked directly if he complains of 'nasal catarrh' during the greater part or all of the year and, if so, for how many years; and whether he is aware of discharge collecting in the back of his throat (post-nasal 'drip') especially when lying down. It is surprising how rarely individuals having a chest examination volunteer symptoms of even advanced upper respiratory disease.

PHYSICAL SIGNS

Nasal airways obstruction

The simple manoeuvre of getting the subject to inhale briskly with closed mouth first through one nostril and then the other while the opposite nostril is compressed shut with the finger is sufficient to establish the presence of significant obstruction (in the absence of acute infection) and whether this is bilateral or unilateral, partial or complete. In many individuals with post-nasal 'drip' the palatopharyngeal 'gag' reflex, which protects the lower respiratory tract, is unusually sluggish as stroking the uvular region with a spatula demonstrates. In any examination for possible chronic lung disease these simple routine observations should not be omitted.

A simple, sensitive method of measuring the volume of air inspired through the mouth and nose using a standard Vitalograph and the expression of the ratio of these values as a reproducible 'nasal patency index' has been described by Davies (1978).

The lungs

There are no physical signs which are pathognomonic of any one form of occupational lung disease. Certain fibrogenic types of pneumoconiosis (silicosis and coal pneumoconiosis, for example) may reach an advanced stage and yet present no abnormal physical signs.

Adventitious sounds

Throughout this book the long-established term 'crepitations' (Latin, *crepitare*: to crackle) rather than 'rales' or 'crackles' is used for the crackling sounds which may be heard in the lungs. 'Fine' crepitations have a high pitch and frequency (approximately 700 Hz); medium crepitations, somewhat lower pitch and frequency (approximately 400 Hz), and coarse crepitations, still lower pitch and frequency (approximately 250 Hz) (Murphy, 1975). Fine, and to a lesser extent medium, crepitations are associated with, and are a valuable sign of, diffuse interstitial pulmonary fibrosis (*see* Chapter 4, p. 75) including asbestosis and they occur during and usually in the latter part of inspiration, being best heard during maximal inspiration following maximal expiration (*Figure 1.18*). Forgacs (1967) has suggested that an inspiratory crepitation is generated by the explosive opening of a closed airway at the moment when a critical transmural pressure develops due to inspiratory inflation of the lung causing an increasing radial traction force on the airway. This has received some experimental support in patients with established asbestosis and other forms of intrapulmonary fibrosis (Nath and Capel, 1974).

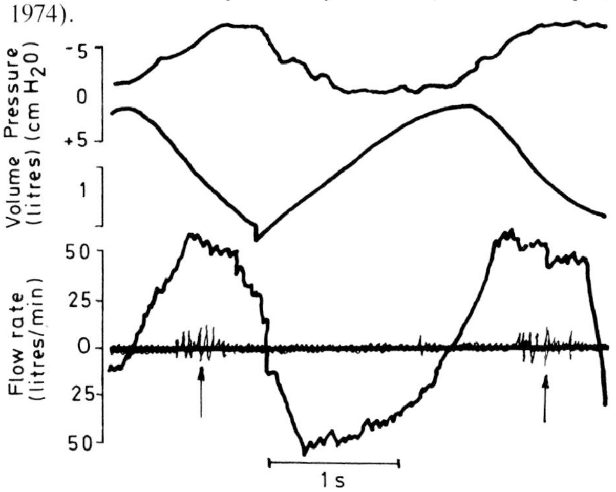

Figure 1.18 Simultaneous recording of inspiratory crepitations, airflow rate and transpulmonary pressure in a patient with diffuse intrapulmonary fibrosis and scleroderma. A pair of repetitive crepitations in two breaths are displayed. The pattern was repeated in nine successive breaths. The base line of the sound channel is the zero mark for the flow rate signal, hence this signal indicates the start and end of inspiration as it passes through the base line. (Courtesy of Drs Nath and Capel and the Editors of Thorax*)*

It is of particular practical importance that the crepitations of diffuse interstitial pulmonary fibrosis (including asbestosis), severe chronic bronchitis with airflow obstruction, and bronchiectasis can be differentiated clinically. In diffuse fibrosis fine to medium crepitations occur in mid or early inspiration, continue to its end, are crisp and persistent and are not heard in expiration; in severe chronic obstructive bronchitis they are of medium quality and confined to early inspiration; whereas in bronchiectasis they are medium to coarse, occur in the early and mid phases of inspiration but fade at its end, are profuse and are usually present during expiration. Furthermore, the crepitations of chronic obstructive bronchitis and bronchiectasis are altered after coughing and are often heard with the stethoscope at the mouth whereas those of diffuse fibrosis are not (Trail, 1948; Nath and Capel, 1980).

These sounds must be sought meticulously and systematically with the stethoscope over the lungs anteriorly, laterally and posteriorly while the subject inhales and exhales as deeply as possible, otherwise this important sign may be missed. Even so, their detection depends upon the efficiency of the clinician's ear, the quality of his stethoscope and the ability of the patient to breathe deeply. In some cases of advanced fibrosis maximal inspiratory volume may be too small for the changes which cause the sounds to develop, in which case they will be absent or few. There is some evidence that time-expanded phonogram wave forms may be able to identify fine basal crepitations in individuals with early asbestosis (and other types of interstitial pulmonary fibrosis) before they can be detected stethoscopically and in advance of any other evidence of the disease (Murphy, 1975). It remains to be seen, however, whether such a method will be of practical use for diagnosis in the field or clinic. This important sign is discussed further in Chapter 9 (p. 256).

RESPIRATORY DISABILITY

It should be recalled that *dyspnoea*, or breathlessness, is the subjective sensation of discomfort caused by the necessity for increased respiratory effort to a point beyond which it obtrudes unpleasantly into consciousness, and that it has causes other than diseases of the lungs and pleura. For example: anaemia and obesity; congenital and acquired heart disease; metabolic disturbances such as hyperthyroidism and the acidosis of diabetes mellitus and uraemia; and severe kyphoscoliosis. Sometimes one or other of these disorders may be overlooked as the cause of dyspnoea in a patient who also happens to have an occupational lung disease. In which case dyspnoea may be wrongly attributed to this and not to the true cause which remains untreated. Indeed, the dramatic nature of abnormal radiographic appearances in some pneumoconiosis cases may be an effective distraction in this respect.

It is also necessary to emphasize that *impairment of any of the functional components of respiration* is not necessarily associated with *respiratory disability*—that is, dyspnoea of greater or lesser degree—and that the two require to be clearly distinguished. Disability can be properly defined as

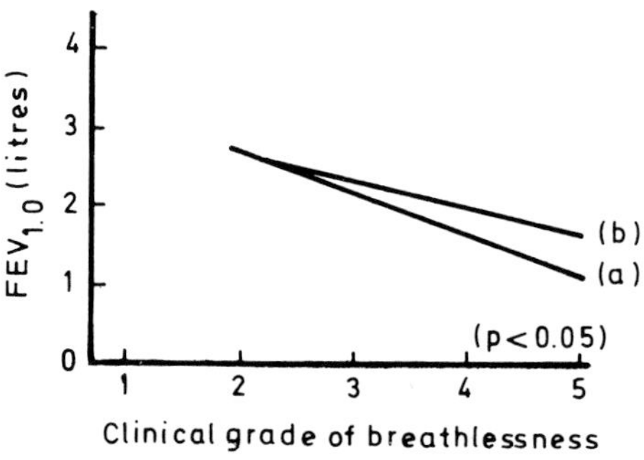

Figure 1.19 Relationship of forced expiratory volume (FEV_1) to grade of breathlessness (G) for coal workers seen (a) for research purposes, and (b) applying for compensation. Line (a) is described by: $FEV_1 = 3.67 - 0.51$ G, SD 0.69. Both groups were matched for age, height, weight and radiographic category of pneumoconiosis. (Courtesy of Dr J.E. Cotes and the Editor of Bull. Physiopath. Resp.*)*

an individual's want of, or incapacity for, competent bodily power. A recent suggestion that symptomless impairment of FEV should be described as 'disability' is, therefore, unfortunate for, although a slight fall in FEV_1 may be associated in some individuals with a small reduction of capacity for maximal, or extreme, effort this is not normally regarded as disability in the accepted sense. Clinical grades of breathlessness (such as those of Fletcher, 1952) are of practical value in assessing disability for they have little observer variation and correlate fairly well with ventilatory capacity; though they may lack reliability in the case of individuals examined for compensation purposes who may exaggerate their breathlessness, as exemplified in *Figure 1.19* (Cotes, 1975b).

Breathlessness on exertion in patients with lung disease is due mainly to reduction in ventilatory capacity, and there appears to be a better correlation between breathlessness and the dyspnoeic index than any other simple combination of tests. The *dyspnoeic index* is the ratio of ventilation during standard exercise to the maximal breathing capacity (that is, the maximal volume of air a subject can breathe/minute), and these indices are themselves correlated with FEV_1, Tl and the fall in oxygen tension during exercise. Therefore, FEV_1, Tl and genuine submaximal exercise are the most relevant tests in this context (Cotes, 1975b).

PRICK SKIN TESTS AND BRONCHIAL PROVOCATION TESTS

These are often necessary in the investigation of occupational asthma when the identity of the allergen is uncertain or unknown, and may be required to establish that a known industrial allergen is indeed the cause of a worker's asthma. The prick test can also be used to identify potentially sensitive persons before they enter an industry (*see* Chapter 4, p. 58, and Chapter 12).

BIOPSY

Examinations of a scalene node may help to resolve a difficult diagnosis especially in the presence of generalized systemic disease. Sarcoid-like granulomas of beryllium disease and silicotic nodules may sometimes be identified.

Sampling of lung or pleura by any technique must always be fully justified on the grounds of being essential either to diagnosis (and this usually means exclusion of non-occupational disease) or to the control of treatment and never solely for research or other interests. All available methods have a roughly similar incidence of complications to which the patient should not be unnecessarily exposed. In general, thoracotomy is preferable to drill and needle methods (although more unpleasant for the patient) because the most appropriate site for sampling can be selected by inspection and palpation of lung or pleura, and a larger and more representative sample of tissue obtained.

As a rule, it can be said that if the occupational and medical history, physical examination and appropriate investigations are carefully carried out and their results accurately and logically analysed, sampling of the intrathoracic tissues in suspected cases of any type of pneumoconiosis should rarely be necessary. It is axiomatic that inspection of earlier chest radiographs is an integral part of investigation, and this alone may often prevent embarrassing mistakes.

ROUTINE MEDICAL EXAMINATIONS

Before entering work in an industry with a known dust, fume, gas or atmospheric pressure hazard the prospective employee should have a clinical examination, chest radiograph and assessment of FEV_1 and FVC. A basic reference point for future examination is thus established. In general, this examination should exclude persons with chronic chest disease and, where relevant, those with an allergic (or atopic) diathesis. Chronic nasal obstruction should be looked for and if present and severe, corrective surgery advised; acceptance of individuals with chronic nasal obstruction into work having a potential aerosol hazard is probably undesirable. Ideally, allergic individuals should not be taken into an industry with a known risk of occupational asthma (*see* Chapter 12), and all aspirants to such an industry should be screened for allergy.

Established workers exposed to a potential risk of developing lung disease should be examined regularly; an interval of two years is probably most satisfactory for the majority of industries, but, in the case of possible exposure to asbestos or beryllium, a shorter interval is desirable. In some industries, such as those with a 'silica' risk, a chest radiograph is all that is required; but in others, in particular those involving asbestos, clinical, radiographic and physiological examination is mandatory.

Details of examinations must be fully recorded and the records kept readily available. To have maximal prospective value, each worker's record must include a description of his job and the nature of materials used (that is, their analysis and origin) and, whenever possible, the concentration of the relevant dust or fume in his environment. Changes in his work must also be noted. This demands close cooperation between medical, engineering and production departments and safety personnel. It is clear that such cooperation not only ensures the best information upon the incidence and behaviour of disease in the factory population, but also confers the greatest long-term advantage on the worker.

The necessity for these examinations should always be explained to the workers concerned. If this is done few will fail to understand that they are done for their benefit and will cooperate accordingly.

EPIDEMIOLOGY

Epidemiological methods play a key role in occupational medicine; in identifying hazards and disease; in defining the incidence or prevalence of disease in specified occupations; in detecting change (or absence of change) in lung function in workers in a given industry; in correlating the prevalence of disease with levels of exposure to a particular hazard; in establishing hygiene standards and the control of known hazards by studying the value of preventive measures; and in identifying increased mortality in an industrial process from a specific disease. Morbidity and mortality statistics are obtained by two basic techniques; by referring to past industrial health and other records (*retrospective investigation*) or by studying groups of workers or ex-workers progressively over a period of time (*prospective investigation*). The latter may be conducted over a short period or repeated at regular intervals over a long period. In both methods it is necessary that control populations are validly matched in all relevant respects: for example, age, sex, race, smoking habits, social status andd locality of residence.

It is not appropriate to discuss methods and techniques—many excellent texts are available, for example, Schilling (1981) and Weill (1975)—but the reader should be familiar with some important sources of error which may be found in epidemiological investigations. The validity and quality of the information obtained will only be as good as the accuracy of the methodology.

When ventilatory function is studied in workers in a particular industry it should be compared with a properly matched control population of the same social class in the same geographical area at similar times of day and year and not with predicted normal values derived from other populations; that is, 'within-area comparisons' should be made (*see* p. 20). Similarly, investigation of the incidence of a malignancy in an industry must compare this with the incidence in a control population of similar social class living in the same area and not solely with its national incidence, otherwise an unsuspected, local oncogenic factor may be overlooked and an excess of cancer wrongly attributed to the industrial process.

Mortality rates for a specified disease in a particular industry rely on death certificates, or similar documents, which may not record that disease if death was due to some unrelated cause. Hence, it is a common practice in mortality studies to 'correct' certificates where possible by finding evidence of the disease in hospital, general practioner or post-mortem records. Clearly, it is inadmissible to compare results obtained in this way with overall national mortality rate for the disease which are derived from *uncorrected* certificates for, in this way, an apparently higher rate in the industrial population will be attributed to the industrial exposure. The magnitude of error which may occur is exemplified by a recent study of death certification in the UK which showed that when the cause of death given on 191 death certificates was compared with hospital notes, consultants' opinions and post-mortem findings there was a major discrepancy in 20.4 per cent of the certificates and a minor, but epidemiologically important, discrepancy in 28.7 per cent. A similar situation was found in a study in New York State in 1955 (Medical Services Study Group of the Royal College of Physicians of London, 1978).

In any calculations designed to predict the risk of developing a particular disease over a long period of time adjustment must be made for other 'competing' diseases which may cause death prematurely—that is, before the disease under study has an opportunity to develop.

Prospective studies of the response of exposed workers to a specific hazard involve the measurement of exposure and of reponse in the workers. Measurement of exposure rests upon accurate determination of concentrations of 'respirable' aerosol in the air of the working area, the content of the aerosol and the duration of exposure (*see* Chapter 3). The techniques used and their methods of standardization must, of necessity, be valid. Response, in the case of dusts, is usually measured by lung function tests suitable to field conditions (for example, FEV_1) and, commonly, by chest radiography. Possible pitfalls in lung function surveys have been referred to earlier but it should be noted here that when reduction in lung function is related to dust exposure respiratory symptoms or disability are not necessarily implied or present. The techniques of X-ray surveys and their application to dust dose-related prevalence or incidence of radiographic abnormality are complex and outside the intention of this book, but two important points must be made. *First,* the validity of the results obtained rests upon the technical quality of the films, the experience and ability of the observers, and the level of consistency of repeated observations by individual and multiple observers. The degree of disagreement which may occur in individuals is referred to as *intra-observer error* and in a team, as *inter-observer error.* Good agreement in a team, however, does not necessarily imply a high level of expertise and the production of valid results. *Second,* a slight, but real change in radiographic appearance which might be unimportant in an individual may be epidemiologically significant in a group if its occurrence is shown to increase smoothly and consistently with increasing exposure. The standard UICC system used for the categorization of radiographs in epidemiological studies is described in Chapter 5.

REFERENCES

Abboud, R. and Morton, W. J. (1975). Comparison of maximal midexpiratory flow, flow volume curves and nitrogen closing volumes in patients with mild airway obstruction *Am. Rev. resp. Dis.* **111,** 405—417

Adamson, Y. R. and Bowden, D. H. (1974). The type 2 cell as progenitor of alveolar epithelial regeneration. *Lab. Invest.* **30,** 35—42

Alli, A. F. (1975). The radial intercepts method for measuring bronchial mucous gland volume. *Thorax* **30,** 687—692

American Thoracic Society (1962). Statement on definitions and classification of chronic bronchitis, asthma and pulmonary emphysema. *Am. Rev. resp. Dis.* **85,** 762—768

Anderson, A. E. Jr. and Foraker, A. G. (1967). Predictability of smoking habits, sex and age in urbanists from their macroscopic lung morphology. *Am. Rev. resp. Dis.* **96,** 1255—1258

Anderson, A. E. Jr., Hernandez, J. A., Holmes, W. L. and Foraker, A. G. (1966). Pulmonary emphysema. Prevalence, severity and anatomical patterns in macrosections with respect to smoking habits. *Archs envir. Hlth* **12,** 569—577

Anderson, I., Lundqvist, G. R., Proctor, D. F. and Swift, D. L. (1979). Human response to controlled levels of inert dust. *Am. Rev. resp. Dis.* **119,** 619—627

Anderson, J. A., Dunnill, M. S. and Ryder, R. C. (1972). Dependence on the incidence of emphysema on smoking history, age and sex. *Thorax* **27,** 547–551

Banner, A. S. (1980). Alcohol and the lung. *Chest* **77,** 460–461

Bates, D. V. (1972). Air pollutants and the human lung. *Am. Rev. resp. Dis.* **105,** 1—13

Bates, D. V., Macklem, P. T. and Christie, R. V. (1971). *Respiratory function in disease,* 2nd edition. Philadelphia; Saunders

Berry, G. (1974). Longitudinal observations. Their usefulness and limitations with special reference to forced expiratory volume. *Bull. physiopath. esp.* **10,** 643—656

Bjure, J., Grimby, G., Kasalicky, J., Lindh, M. and Nachemson, A. (1970). Respiratory impairment and airway closure in patients with untreated idiopathic scoliosis. *Thorax* **25,** 451—456

Bode, F. R., Dosman, J., Martin, R. R. and Macklem, P. T. (1975). Reversibility of pulmonary function abnormalities in smokers. A prospective study of early diagnostic tests of small airways. *Am. J. Med.* **59,** 43—52

Boren, H. G. (1964). Carbon as a carrier mechanism for irritant gases. *Archs envir. Hlth* **8,** 119–124

Boren, H. G., Kory, R. C. and Syner, J. C. (1966). The Veterans Administration—Army cooperation study of pulmonary function II. The lung volume and its subdivisions in normal men. *Am. J. Med.* **41,** 96—114

Bowden, D. H. (1976). The pulmonary macrophage. *Envir. Hlth Perspect.* **16,** 55—60

Brinkman, G. L., Block, D. L. and Cress, C. (1972). Effects of bronchitis and occupation on pulmonary ventilation over eleven year period. *J. occup. Med.* **14,** 615—620

Brooks, R. E. (1966). Concerning the nomenclature of the cellular elements in respiratory tissue. *Am. Rev. resp. Dis.* **94,** 112—113

Buist, A. S. (1973). Early detection of airways obstruction by the closing volume technique. *Chest* **64,** 495—499

Buist, A. S., Van Fleet, D. L. and Ross, B. B. (1973). A comparison of conventional spirometric tests and the test of closing volume in an emphysema screening center. *Am. Rev. resp. Dis.* **107,** 735—743

Burton, P. A. and Dixon, M. F. (1969). A companion of changes in the mucous glands and goblet cells of nasal, sinus and bronchial mucosa. *Thorax* **24,** 180—185

Card, W. (1967). Towards a calculus of medicine. In *Medical Annual,* pp. 9—21. Bristol; Wright

Ciba Foundation Guest Symposium (1959). Terminology, definitions and classification of chronic pulmonary emphysema and related conditions. *Thorax* **14,** 286—299

Cochrane, A. L. (1976). An epidemiologist's view of the relationship between simple pneumoconiosis and morbidity and mortality. *Proc. R. Soc. Med.* **69,** 12—14

Cochrane, A. L. and Higgins, I. T. T. (1961). Pulmonary ventilatory functions of coal miners in various areas in relation to the X-ray category of pneumoconiosis. *Br. J. prev. soc. Med.* **15,** 1—11

Cochrane, G. M., Prieto, F. and Clark, T. J. H. (1977). Intra-subject variability of maximal expiratory flow volume curve. *Thorax* **32,** 171—176

Cochrane, G. M., Prieto, F., Hickey, B., Benetar, S. R. and Clark, J. H. (1974). Early diagnosis of airways obstruction. *Thorax* **29,** 389—393

Cohen, B. M. (1969). Nasal airways resistance and the effects of bronchodilator drugs in expiratory airflow disorders. *Respiration* **26,** 35—46

Cohen, B. M. (1970). The nasal respiratory handicap of expiratory airflow disease: the response to bronchodilator aerosols. *Respiration* **27,** 406—416

Cohen, B. H., Diamond, E. L., Graves, C. G., Kreiss, P., Levy, D. A., Menkes, H. A., Permutt, S., Quaskey, S. and Tockman, M. S. (1977). A common familial component in lung cancer and chronic obstructive pulmonary disease. *Lancet* **2,** 523—526

Cole, C. (1967). Bronchitis in foundry men—an analytical description of some clinical experience. *Ann. occup. Hyg.* **3,** 277—282

College of General Practitioners (1961). Chronic bronchitis in Great Britain: a national survey. *Br. med. J.* **2,** 973—979

Cotes, J. E. (1966). Tests of lung function in current use; proposals for their standardisation. In *Respiratory Function Tests in Pneumoconiosis,* pp. 93—140. Occupational Safety and Health Series, No 6. Geneva; ILO

Cotes, J. E. (1975a). Respiratory and cardiac function tests in relation to occupational lung disease. *Bull. physiopath. resp.* **11,** 561—568

Cotes, J. E. (1975b). II. Assessment of disablement due to impaired respiratory function. *Bull. physiopath. resp.* **11,** 210P–217P

Cotes, J. E. (1976). Lung ventilation and gas exchange in asymptomatic emphysema. *Prog. resp. Res.* **10,** 117—132

Cotes, J. E. (1979). *Lung Function.* 4th Ed. Oxford; Blackwell

Cotes, J. E., Dabbs, J. M., Elwood, P. C., Hall, A. M., McDonald, A. and Saunders, M. J. (1972). Iron deficiency anaemia: its effect on transfer factor for the lung (diffusing capacity) and ventilation and cardiac frequency during sub-maximal exercise. *Clin. Sci.* **42,** 325–335

Cotes, J. E. and Hall, A. M. (1970). The transfer factor for the lung; normal values in adults. *Panminerva med.* 327—343

Cotes, J. E., Johnson, G. R. and McDonald, A. (1970). Breathing frequency and tidal volume; relationship to breathlessness. In *Breathing: Hering-Breuer Centenary Symposium,* Edited by R. Porter, pp. 297–314. London; Churchill

Cox, D. W. and Celhoffer, L. (1974). Inherited variants of α_1-antitrypsin: a new allele, PiN. *Can. J. Genet. Cytol,* **16,** 297–303

Cox, D. W., Hoeppner, V. H. and Levison, H. (1976). Protease inhibitors in patients with chronic obstructive pulmonary

disease: the alpha-1-antitrypsin heterozygote controversy. *Am. Rev. resp. Dis.* **113,** 601–617
Craig, D. B., Wahba, W. M., Don, H. F., Coutuse, J. G. and Becklake, M. R. (1971). Closing volume and its relationship to gas exchange in seated and supine positions. *J. appl. physiol.* **31,** 717—721
Davies, G. M., Simon, G. and Reid, L. (1966). Pre- and post-operative assessment of emphysema. *Br. J. Dis. Chest.* **60,** 120—128
Davies, H. J. (1978). Measurements of nasal patency using a Vitalograph. *Clin. Allergy* **8,** 517–523
Dick, R., Heard, B. E., Hinson, K. F. W., Kerr, I. H. and Pearson, M. C. (1974). Aspiration needle biopsy of thoracic lesions: an assessment of 227 biopsies. *Br. J. Dis. Chest* **68,** 86—94
Douglas, A. N. (1980). Quantitative study of bronchial mucous gland enlargement. *Thorax* **35,** 198–201
Dunnill, M. S., Massarella, G. R. and Anderson, J. A. (1969). A comparison of the quantitative anatomy of the bronchi in normal subjects, in status asthmaticus, in chronic bronchitis and in emphysema. *Thorax* **24,** 176—179
Edge, J., Simon, G. and Reid, L. (1966). Periacinar (paraseptal) emphysema: its clinical, radiological and physiological features. *Br. J. Dis. Chest* **60,** 10–18
Enterline, P. E. (1967). The effects of occupation on chronic respiratory disease. *Archs envir. Hlth* **14,** 189—198
Enterline, P. E. and Lainhart, W. S. (1967). The relationship between coal mining and chronic nonspecific respiratory disease. *Am. J. publ. Hlth* **57,** 484–495
Evans, C. C., Hipkin, L. J. and Murray, G. M. (1977). Pulmonary function in acromegaly. *Thorax* **32,** 322—327
Evans, M. J., Cabral, L. J., Stephens, R. J. and Freeman, G. (1973). Renewal of alveolar epithelium in the rat following exposure to nitrogen dioxide. *Am. J. Path.* **70,** 175–190
Fletcher, C. M. (1952). The clinical diagnosis of pulmonary emphysema—an experimental study. *Proc. R. Soc. Med.* **45,** 577–578
Fletcher, C. M., Jones, N. L., Burrows, B. and Niden, A. H. (1964). American emphysema and British bronchitis. *Am. Rev. resp. Dis.* **90,** 1–13
Fletcher, C. M. and Peto, R. (1977). The natural history of chronic airflow obstruction. *Br. med. J.* **1**, 1645–1648
Fletcher, C. M., Peto, R., Tinker, C. and Speizer, F. E. (1976). *The natural history of chronic bronchitis and emphysema.* Oxford; Oxford University Press
Forgacs, P. (1967). Crackles and wheezes. *Lancet* **2,** 203–205
Fox, A. J., Greenberg, M., Ritchie, G. L. and Barraclough, R. N. J. (1975). *A survey of respiratory disease in the pottery industry.* London; HMSO
Franklin, W. and Lowell, F. C. (1961). Unrecognised airway obstruction associated with smoking: a probable forerunner of obstructive pulmonary emphysema. *Ann. intern. Med.* **54,** 379–386
Frans, A., Stañescu, D. C., Veriter, C., Clerbaux, T. and Brasseur, L. (1975). Smoking and pulmonary diffusing capacity. *Scand. J. resp. Dis.* **56,** 165—183
Gehr, P., Bachofen, M. and Weibel, E. R. (1978). The normal human lung: ultrastructure and morphometric estimation of diffusion capacity. *Resp. Physiol.* **32,** 121–140
Gelb, A. F., Gold, W. M., Wright, R. R., Bruch, H. R. and Nadel, J. A. (1973). Physiologic diagnosis of subclinical emphysema. *Am. Rev. resp. Dis.* **107,** 50–63
Gilson, J. C. (1970). Occupational bronchitis. *Proc. R. Soc. Med.* **63,** 857–864
Goldman, A. L. (1976). Cigar inhaling. *Am. Rev. resp. Dis.* **113,** 87–89
Gough, J. (1968). The pathogenesis of emphysema. In *The Lung.* Edited by A. A. Liebow and D. E. Smith, p. 109–133. Baltimore; Williams nd Wilkins
Green, M. (1976). Small-airway tests and prevalence of emphysema. *Proc. R. Soc. Med.* **69,** 133
Greenburg, S. D., Bousby, S. F. and Jenkins, D. E. (1967). Chronic bronchitis and emphysema: correlation of pathologic findings. *Am. Rev. resp. Dis.* **96,** 918–928
Guberan, E., Williams, M. K., Walford, J. and Smith, M. M. (1969). Circadian variation of FEV in shift workers. *Br. J. ind. Med.* **26,** 121–125
Guz, A., Noble, N. I. M., Eisele, J. H. and Trenchard, D. (1970). Experimental results of vagal block in cardio-pulmonary disease. In *Breathing; Hering-Breuer Centenary Symposium,* edited by R. Porter, pp. 315–336. London; Churchill
Hankinson, J. L., Reger, R. B., Fairman, R. P., Lapp, N. L. and Morgan, W. K. C. (1977). Factors influencing expiratory flow rates in coal miners. In *Inhaled Particles and Vapours IV,* edited by W. H. Walton, pp. 737–752. Oxford; Pergamon Press
Hankinson, J. L., Reger, R. B. and Morgan, W. K. C. (1977). Maximal expiratory flows in coal miners. *Am. Rev. resp. Dis.* **116,** 175–186
Hayes, J. A. and Summerell, J. M. (1969). Emphysema in a non-industrialised tropical island. *Thorax* **24,** 623–625
Heard, B. E. (1966). Disease of the Lungs. In *Recent Advances in Pathology,* 8th edition, edited by C. V. Harrison p. 363. London; Churchill
Heard, B. E. (1969). *Pathology of Chronic Bronchitis and Emphysema.* London; Churchill
Heard, B. E. and Izukawa, T. (1963). Dust pigmentation of the lungs and emphysema in Londoners. *Fortschr. der Staublungen forschung,* edited by H. Reploh and W. Klosterkötter, pp. 249–255. Dislaken
Heppleston, A. G. (1947). The essential lesion of pneumoniosis in Welsh coal miners. *J. Path. Bact.* **59,** 453–460
Heppleston, A. G. (1953). The pathological anatomy of simple pneumoniosis in coal workers. *J. Path. Bact.* **66,** 235–246
Heppleston, A. G. (1972). The pathological recognition and pathogenesis of emphysema and fibrocystic disease of the lung with special reference to coal workers. *Ann. N.Y. Acad. Sci.* **200,** 347–369
Heppleston, A. G. and Young, A. E. (1973). Uptake of inert particulate matter by alveolar cells: an ultrastructural study. *J. Path.* **111,** 159–164
Higgins, I. T. T. (1959). Tobacco smoking, respiratory symptoms and ventilatory capacity. *Br. med. J.* **1,** 325–329
Higgins, I. T. T. (1972). Chronic respiratory disease in mining communities. *Ann. N.Y. Acad. Sci.* **200,** 197–210
Higgins, I. T. T. and Cochrane, A. L. (1961). Chronic respiratory disease in a random sample of men and women in the Rhondda Fach in 1958. *Br. J. ind. Med.* **18,** 93–102
Higgins, I. T. T., Cochrane, A. L., Gilson, J. C. and Wood, C. H. (1959). Population studies of chronic respiratory disease. A comparison of miners, foundry workers and others in Stavely, Derbyshire. *Br. J. ind. Med.* **16,** 155–268
Higgins, I. T. T., Higgins, M. W., Lockshin, M. D., and Canale, N. (1968). Chronic respiratory disease in mining communities in Marion County, West Virginia. *Br. J. ind. Med.* **25,** 165–175
Higgins, I. T. T. and Oldham, P. D. (1962). Ventilatory capacity in miners: a five-year follow up study. *Br. J. ind. Med.* **19,** 65–76
Holland, W. W., Colley, J. R. T., Leeder, S. R., Crokhill, R. and Halil, T. (1977). Comment absorber en épidémiologie l'étude de la bronchite chronique et de ses signes precurseurs chez l'enfant. *Rev. fr. Mal. resp.* **5,** 87–94
Holland, W. W. and Reid, D. S. (1965). The urban factor in chronic bronchitis. *Lancet* **1,** 445–448
Hook, G. E. R. and Di Augustine, R. P. (1976). Secretory cells of the peripheral pulmonary epithelium as targets for toxic agents. *Envir. Hlth Perspect.* **16,** 147–156
Horsfield, K., Cumming, G. and Hicken, P. (1966). A morphologic study of airway disease using bronchial casts. *Am. Rev. resp. Dis.* **93,** 900–906
Hruby, J. and Butler, J. (1975). Variability of routine pulmonary function tests. *Thorax* **30,** 548–553
Hutchinson, D. C. S. (1976). Homozygous and heterozygous alpha-1-antitrypsin deficiency: prevalence in pulmonary emphysema. *Proc. R. Soc. Med.* **69,** 130–131
Hutchinson, D. C. S., Cook, P. J. L., Barter, C. E., Harris, H. and

Hugh-Jones, P. (1971). Pulmonary emphysema and α_1-antitrypsin deficiency. *Br. med. J.* 1, 689–694
Industrial Injuries Advisory Council (1973). *Pneumoconiosis and Byssinosis.* London; HMSO
Jacobsen, M., Burns, J. and Attfield, M. D. (1976). Smoking and coal workers' simple pneumoconiosis. In *Inhaled Particles IV,* edited by W. H. Walton, pp. 759–771. Oxford; Pergamon Press
Kaufmann, J. and Wright, G. M. (1969). The effect of nasal and nasopharyngeal irritation on airway resistance in man. *Am. Rev. resp. Dis.* **100,** 626–630
Kibelstis, J. A., Morgan, E. J., Reger, R., Lapp, N. L., Seaton, A. and Morgan, W. K. C. (1973). Prevalence of bronchitis and airway obstruction in American bituminous coal miners. *Am. Rev. resp. Dis.* **168,** 886–893
Kiernan, K. E., Colley, J. R. T., Douglas, J. W. B. and Reid, D. D. (1976). Chronic cough in young adults in relation to smoking habits, childhood environment and chest illness. *Respiration* **33,** 236–244
Knudson, R. J., Lebowitz, M. D., Burton, A. P. and Knudson, D. E. (1977). The closing volume test: evaluation of nitrogen and bolus methods in a random population. *Am. Rev. resp. Dis.* **115,** 423–434
Kory, R. C., Callahan, R., Boren, H. G. and Syner, J. C. (1961). The Veterans Administration–Army Cooperative Study of Pulmonary Function. 1. Clinical spirometry in normal men. *Am. J. Med.* **30,** 243–258
Krumholz, R. A., Chevalier, R. B. and Ross, J. C. (1964). Cardiopulmonary function in young smokers. *Ann. intern. Med.* **60,** 603–610
Lambert, M. W. (1955). Accessory bronchiolo-alveolar communications. *J. Path. Bact.* **70,** 311–314
Lapp, N. L., Hankinson, J. L., Burgess, D. B. and O'Brien, R. (1972). Changes in ventilatory function in coal miners after a work shift. *Archs envir. Hlth* **24,** 204–208
Larson, R. K., Barman, M. L., Kueppers, F. and Fudenberg, H. H. (1970). Genetic and environmental determinants of chronic obstructive pulmonary disease. *Ann. intern. Med.* **72,** 627–632
Lauweryns, J. M. and Baert, J. H. (1977). Alveolar clearance and the role of the pulmonary lymphatics. *Am. Rev. resp. Dis.* **115,** 625–683
Lawther, P. J. (1967). Air pollution and chronic bronchitis. *Medna thorac.* **24,** 44–52
Leading article (1971). Enzyme deficiency and emphysema. *Br. med. J.* **3,** 655–656
Leading article (1976). Natural history of chronic bronchitis. *Br. med. J.* **1,** 1297–1298
Lebowitz, M. D., Burton, A. and Kaltenborn, W. (1979). Pulmonary function in smelter workers. *J. occup. Med.* **21,** 255–259
Leopold, J. C. and Gough, J. (1957). The centrilobular form of hypertrophic emphysema and its relation to chronic bronchitis. *Thorax,* **12,** 219–235
Lieberman, J. (1973). Alpha-1-antitrypsin. *J. occup. Med.* **15,** 194–197
Lloyd Davies, T. A. (1971). *Respiratory disease in Foundrymen. Report of a Survey, Dept. of Employment.* London; HMSO
Lowe, C. R. (1968). Chronic bronchitis and occupation. *Proc. R. Soc. Med.* **61,** 98–102
Lowe, C. R., Campbell, H. and Khosla, T. (1970). Bronchitis in two integrated steel works. III. Respiratory symptoms and ventilatory capacity related to atmospheric pollution. *Br. J. ind. Med.* **27,** 121–129
Lowe, C. R. and Khosla, T. (1972). Chronic bronchitis in ex-coal miners working in the steel industry. *Br. J. ind. Med.* **29,** 45–49
McCarthy, D. S. and Milic-Emili, J. (1973). Closing volume in asymptomatic asthma. *Am. Rev. resp. Dis.* **107,** 559–570
McDermott, M. (1962). Acute respiratory effects of the inhalation of coal dust particles. *J. Physiol. Lond.* **162,** 53P
McDermott, M. and Collins, M. M. (1965). Acute effects of smoking on lung airways resistance in normal and bronchitic subjects. *Thorax* **20,** 562–569
McDermott, M. Gilson, J. C. and Ridley, N. (1975). Closing volume and the single breath nitrogen index in a Danish population—a ten year follow up. *Bull. physiopath. resp.* **11,** 41P–45P
McKerrow, C. B. and Rossiter, C. E. (1968). An annual cycle in ventilatory capacity of men with pneumoconiosis and of normal subjects. *Thorax* **23,** 340–349
Macklem, P. T. and Mead, J. (1967). Resistance of central and peripheral airways measured by a retrograde catheter. *J. appl. Physiol.* **22,** 395–401
Martin, R. R., Lemelin, C., Zutter, M. and Anthonisen, M. R. (1973). Measurement of 'closing volume' application and limitation. *Bull. physiopath. resp.* **9,** 979–995
Mason, R. J. (1977). Phospholipid synthesis in primary cultures of type II alveolar cells. *Am. Rev. resp. Dis.* **115,** (Supplement), 352
Matsuba, K. and Thurlbeck, W. M. (1973). Disease of small airways in bronchitis. *Am. Rev. resp. Dis.* **107,** 552–558
Mead, J. (1970). The lung's 'quiet zone'. *New Engl. J. Med.* **282,** 1318–1319
Medical Research Council Committe on Aetiology of Chronic Bronchitis (1960). Standardised questionnaires on respiratory symptoms. *Br. med. J.* **2,** 1665
Medical Research Council on the Aetiology of Chronic Bronchitis (1960). Questionnaire on respiratory symptoms and instructions for use. Dawlish; Holman
Medical Research Council Committee on the Aetiology of Chronic Bronchitis (1965). Definition and classification of chronic bronchitis for clinical and epidemiological purposes. *Lancet,* **1,** 775–779
Medical Research Council Special Committee (1966). Chronic bronchitis and occupation. *Br. med. J.* **1,** 101–102
Medical Research Council Working Party on Trials of Chemotherapy in Early Chronic Bronchitis. (1966). *Br. med. J.* **1,** 1317–1322
Medical Services Study Group of the Royal College of Physicians of London (1978). Death certification and epidemiological research. *Br. med. J.* **2,** 1063–1065
Middle article. (1966). Chronic bronchitis and occupation. *Br. med. J.* **1,** 101–102
Milic-Emili, J. (1976). Prevalence of emphysema: physiological features. *Proc. R. Soc. Med.* **69,** 132
Milic-Emili, J., Henderson, J. A. M., Dolovich, M. B., Trop, D. and Kaneko, K. (1966). Regional distribution of inspired gas in the lung. *J. appl. Physiol.* **21,** 749–759
Miller, D. and Bondurant, S. (1962). Effects of cigarette smoke on the surface characteristics of lung extracts. *Am. Rev. resp. Dis.* **85,** 692–696
Minette, A. (1971). Role de l'empoussierage professionel dans la production des bronchites chroniques des mineurs de charbon. In *Inhaled Particles III,* edited by W. H. Walton, pp. 873–881. Old Woking, Surrey; Unwin Bros. Ltd
Morgan, W. K. C. (1978). Industrial bronchitis. *Br. J. ind. Med.* **35,** 285–291
Morgan, W. K. C., Lapp, N. L. and Morgan, E. J. (1974). The early detection of occupational lung disease. *Br. J. Dis. Chest* **68,** 75–85
Mork, T. (1962). A comparative study of respiratory disease in England and Wales and Norway. *Acta med. scand.* **172,** Suppl. 384
Morris, J. F., Koski, A. and Breese, J. D. (1975). Normal values and evaluation of forced end-expiratory flow. *Am. Rev. resp. Dis.* **111,** 755–762
Muir, D. C. F. (1975). Pulmonary function in miners working in British collieries: epidemiological investigations by the National Coal Board. *Bull. physiopath. resp.* **11,** 403–414
Muir, D. C. F., Burns, J., Jacobson, M. and Walton, W. H. (1977). Pneumoconiosis and chronic bronchitis. *Br. med. J.* **2,** 424–427
Mur, J-M., Mereau, P., Cavelier, C., Pham, Q. T. and Castet, P. (1979). Ateliers de fonderie et fonction respiratoire. *Arch. Mal. Prof.* 587–595

Murphy, R. L. H. (1975). Human factors in chest auscultation. In *Human Factors in Health Care,* edited by R. M. Pickett and T. J. Triggs, pp. 73–88. Massachusetts and London; Lexington Books
Myrvik, Q. N. (1973). The role of the alveolar macrophage. *J. occup. Med.* **15,** 190–193
Nath, A. R. and Capel, L. H. (1974). Inspiratory crackles and mechanical events of breathing. *Thorax* **29,** 695–698
Nath, A. R. and Capel, L. H. (1980). Lung crackles in bronchiectasis. *Thorax* **35,** 694–699
Niden, A. H. (1973). Pulmonary surfactant. *J. occup. Med.* **15,** 181–185
Niewoehner, D. E. Kleinerman, J. and Rice, D. B. (1974). Pathologic changes in the peripheral airways of young cigarette smokers. *New Engl. J. Med.* **291,** 755–758
Nolte, D. and Ulmer, W. T. (1966). Messung der Nasen-Resistance mittels Granzkörperplethysmographie. *Med. thorac.* **23,** 349–357
Ogura, J. H. Togawa, K., Dammkoehler, R., Nelson, J. R. and Kawasaki, M. (1966). Nasal obstruction and the mechanics of breathing. *Archs Otolar.* **83,** 135–150
Oldham, P. D. (1970). The usefulness of normal values. In *Parvminerva Medicine,* edited by P. Archangeli, pp. 49–56
Olsen, H. C. and Gilson, J. C. (1960). Respiratory symptoms, bronchitis and ventilatory capacity in men: an Anglo-Danish comparison with special reference to difference in smoking habits. *Br. med. J.* **1,** 450–456
Oxhøj, H., Bake, B. and Wilhelmsen, L. (1976). Spirometry and flow-volume curves in 10-year follow up in men born in 1913. *Scand. J. resp. Dis.* **57,** 310–311
Paintal, A. S. (1970). The mechanism of excitation of Type J receptors and the J reflex. In *Breathing: Herring-Breuer Centenary Symposium,* edited by R. Porter, pp. 59–76. London; Churchill
Pattle, R. E. (1968). The surface active lining of the lung. *J. R. Coll. Physns* **2,** 137–140
Paul, R. (1961). Chronic bronchitis in African miners and non-miners in Northern Rhodesia. *Br. J. Dis. Chest* **55,** 30–34
Pratt, P. C. and Kilburn, K. H. (1971). Extent of pulmonary pigmentation as an indicator of particulate environmental air pollution. In *Inhaled Particles, 3,* pp. 661–669, edited by W. H. Walton. Woking; Unwin
Proctor, D. F. (1977). The upper airways. 1 Nasal physiology and defense of the lungs. *Am. Rev. resp. Dis.* **115,** 97–129
Proust, A. (1874). *Bull. Acad. Méd.,* Ser. 2, **3,** 624
Pump, K. K. (1969). Morphology of the acinus of the human lung. *Dis. Chest* **56,** 126–134
Rae, S., Walker, D. D. and Attfield, M.D. (1971). Chronic bronchitis and dust exposure in British coal miners. In *Inhaled Particles III,* edited by W. H. Walton, pp. 883–894. Old Woking, Surrey, Unwin Bros. Ltd
Rankin, J., Gee, J. B. L. and Chosy, L. W. (1965). The influence of age and smoking on pulmonary diffusing capacity in healthy subjects. *Medna thorac.* **22,** 366–374
Rao, M. N., Sen Gupta, A., Saha, P. N. and Sita, Davi, A. (1961). *Physiological norms in Indians.* New Delhi; India Colonial Medical Research Spec. Rep. Ser. 38
Reid, D. D. (1969). The beginnings of bronchitis. *Proc. R. Soc. Med.* **62,** 311–316
Reid, D. D., Anderson, D. O., Ferris, B. G. and Fletcher, C. M. (1964). An Anglo-American comparison of the prevalence of bronchitis. *Br. med. J.* **2,** 1487–1491
Reid, L. (1960). Measurement of bronchial mucous gland layer; a diagnostic yardstick in chronic bronchitis. *Thorax* **15,** 132–141
Reid, L. (1967). *The Pathology of Emphysema.* London; Lloyd Luke
Reid, L. and Millard, F. J. C. (1964). Correlation between radiological diagnosis and structural lung changes in emphysema. *Clin. Radiol.* **15,** 307–311
Rimington, J. (1974). Cigarette smokers' chronic bronchitis: inhalers and non-inhalers compared. *Br. J. Dis. Chest* **68,** 161–165
Rogan, J. M., Attfield, M. D., Jacobson, M., Rae, S., Walker, D. D. and Walton, W. H. (1973). Role of dust in the working environment in development of chronic bronchitis in British coal miners. *Br. J. ind. Med.* **30,** 217–226
Rossiter, C. E. and Weill, H. (1974a). Ethnic differences in lung function: evidence of proportional differences. *Int. J. Epidemiol.* **3,** 55–61
Rossiter, C. E. and Weill, H. (1974b). Synergism between dust exposure and smoking: an artefact in the statistical analysis of lung function. *Bull. physiopath. resp.* **10,** 717–725
Royal College of Physicians Report (1970). *Air Pollution and Health.* London; Royal College of Physicians
Šarić, M. and Lučić-Palaić, S. (1976). Possible synergism of exposure to air-borne manganese and smoking habit in occurrence of respiratory symptoms. In *Inhaled Particles and Vapours IV,* edited by W. H. Walton, pp. 773–778. Old Woking, Surrey; Unwin Bros. Ltd.
Schilling, R. S. F. (1981). (Ed.) *Occupational Health Practice.* 2nd edn. London; Butterworths
Scott, K. W. M. (1976). A pathological study of the lungs and heart in fatal and non-fatal chronic airways obstruction. *Thorax* **31,** 70–79
Sharp, J. T., Paul, O., McKean, H. and Best, W. R. (1973). A longitudinal study of bronchitic symptoms and spirometry in a middle-aged male industrial population. *Am. Rev. resp. Dis.* **108,** 1066–1077
Sluis-Cremer, S. K., Walters, K. G. and Sichel, H. B. (1967a). Chronic bronchitis in miners and non-miners; an epidemiological survey of a community in the gold mining area in the Transvaal. *Br. J. ind. Med.* **24,** 1–12
Sluis-Cremer, S. K., Walters, K. G. and Sichel, H. B. (1967b). Ventilatory function in relation to mining experience and smoking in a random sample of miners and non-miners in a Witwatersrand town. *Br. J. ind. Med.* **24,** 13–25
Smith, P., Heath, D. and Moosavi, H. (1974). The Clara cell. *Thorax* **29,** 147–163
Snider, G. L., Brody, J. S. and Doctor, L. (1962). Subclinical pulmonary emphysema. *Am. Rev. resp. Dis.* **85,** 666–683
Soutar, C. A. (1977). Distribution of plasma cells and other cells containing immunoglobulin in the respiratory tract in chronic bronchitis. *Thorax* **32,** 387–396
Staub, N. C. (1965). Time dependent factors in pulmonary gas exchange. *Medna thorac.* **22,** 132–145
Stephens, R. J., Sloan, M. A., Evans, M. J. and Freeman, G. (1974). Early response of lungs to low level of ozone. *Am. J. Pathol.* **74,** 31–58
Stirling, G. M. (1967). Mechanisms of bronchoconstriction caused by cigarette smoking. *Br. med. J.* **2,** 275–277
Thurlbeck, W. M. (1976). *Chronic Airflow Obstruction in Lung Disease. Volume 5 Major Problems in Pathology,* edited by James L. Bennington. Philadelphia; W. B. Saunders
Thurlbeck, W. M. (1980). Smoking, airflow limitation and the pulmonary circulation. *Am. Rev. resp. Dis.* **122,** 183–186
Tobacco Research Council (1978). Personal communication
Tobacco Research Council (1972). *Tobacco Consumption in Various Countries.* Research Paper No. 6. 3rd edition, edited by G. F. Todd
Trail, R. (1948). *Chest Examination,* p. 57. Edinburgh; J. and A. Churchill
Trapnell, D. H. (1963). The peripheral lymphatics of the lung. *Br. J. Radiol.* **36,** 660–672
Trapnell, D. H. (1964). Radiological appearances of lymphangitis carcinomatosa of the lung. *Thorax* **19,** 251–260
Ulmer, W. T. and Reichel, G. (1972). Epidemiological problems of coal worker's bronchitis in comparison with the general population. *Ann. N.Y. Acad. Sci.* **200,** 211–219
United States Public Health Service Publications (1963). No. 1076. *Silicosis in the Metal Mining Industry: a Revaluation 1958–1961.* Washington; US Government Printing Office
Van Furth, R. (1970). Origin and kinetics of monocytes and macrophages. *Semin. Hematol.* **7,** 125–141

Van Ganse, W. F. Ferris, B. G., Jr. and Cotes, J. E. (1972). Cigarette smoking and pulmonary diffusing capacity (transfer factor). *Am. Rev. resp. Dis.* **105,** 30–41

von Hayek, H. (1960). *The Human Lung.* Trans. by V. E. Krahl. New York; Hafner

Webb, W. R., Cook, W. A., Lannis, J. W. and Shaw, R. R. (1967). Cigarette smoke and surfactant. *Am. Rev. resp. dis.* **95,** 244–247

Weibel, E. R. (1963). *Morphometry of the Lung.* New York; Academic Press

Wiebel, E. R. (1968). Airways and respiratory surface. In *The Lung,* edited by A. A. Liebow and D. E. Smith. Baltimore; Williams and Wilkins

Weill, H. (1975). Epidemiologic methods in the investigation of occupational lung disease. *Am. Rev. resp. Dis.* **112,** 1–6

West, J. B. (1977). *Regional Differences in the Lung.* New York, San Francisco, London; Academic Press

Wiles, F. J. and Faure, M. H. (1977). Chronic obstructive lung disease in gold miners. In *Inhaled Particles IV,* edited by W. H. Walton, pp. 727–734. Oxford; Pergamon Press

Wilhelmsen, L. (1967). Effects of broncho-pulmonary symptoms, ventilation and lung mechanics of abstinence from tobacco smoking. *Scand. J. Resp. Dis.* **48,** 407–414

Wilson, R. W. (1973). Increased prevalence of sinusitis among smokers compared with non-smokers. *J. occup. Med.* **15,** 236–244

World Health Organisation (1975). Memoranda. Epidemiology of chronic non-specific respiratory diseases. *Bull. Wld Hlth Org.* **52,** 251–259

Wright, B. M. (1974). Peak flow meter and peak flow gauge. *Lancet* **2,** 1151

Wyatt, J. P., Fischer, V. W. and Sweet, H. (1961). Centrilobular emphysema. *Lab. Invest.* **10,** 159–177

Zenker, F. A. (1866). *Staubinhalations Krankheiten der Lungen*

Zielhuis, R. L. (1970). Tentative emergency exposure limits for sulphur dioxide, sulphuric acid, chlorine and phosgene. *Ann. occup. Hyg.* **13,** 171–176

Zwi, S., Goldman, H. I. and Levin, A. (1964). Cigarette smoking and pulmonary function in healthy young adults. *Am. Rev. resp. Dis.* **89,** 73–81

2 Elements of Geology and Geochemistry

The medical worker in the field of industrial lung disease often encounters mineral and rock names with which he may not be familiar, or he may be unaware of the composition of some well-known substance. A basic knowledge of geology should enable him to decide what the nature and composition of a particular natural mineral or rock is likely to be. This not only saves time and points further enquiry in the right direction but also helps to establish rational thinking about pathogenesis and to avoid mistaken diagnosis.

According to the theory of the formation of the Earth put forward by Urey (1952) oxygen actively combined with silicon, aluminium, magnesium, iron, calcium and potassium atoms (themselves forged by thermonuclear processes) within nebulous gas to form complex silicates, and with hydrogen to form water. Hydrogen combined with nitrogen and carbon to form fundamental units of organic structure.

The Earth consists of a superficial *crust* a few miles thick which rests on a denser mass, the *mantle,* nearly 2000 miles thick, and a central *core* which is probably solid but behaves in some respects as if in a molten state. Molten rock material, or *magma* (which contains gases and steam), also exists as pockets within the crust and mantle or is extruded on to its surface as volcanic lava.

Chemically, the 'average' composition of the crust consists of about 27.7 per cent silicon, 46.6 per cent oxygen, 8 per cent aluminium and 16.2 per cent in aggregate of calcium, iron, magnesium, potassium and sodium. This gives a total of 98.5 per cent, the remainder consisting of all the other elements.

In our present context it is the crust and its rocks which are of importance. The crust is considered to have an upper and lower zone; the upper zone, which is confined to continents, is composed largely of *si*lica and *al*umina (SIAL); and the lower zone, which is present beneath both continents and oceans, is predominantly *si*lica and *ma*gnesia (SIMA)

Rock means 'any mass or aggregate of one or more kinds of mineral or of organic matter, whether hard and consolidated or soft and incoherent, which owes its origin to the operation of natural causes. Thus granite, basalt, limestone, clay, sand, silt and peat are all equally termed rocks' (Geikie, 1908).

The ingredients available for rock formation are known as *minerals.* A mineral is probably best defined as an inorganic homogeneous substance which occurs naturally and has distinct crystal structure, chemical composition and physical properties. Minerals may crystallize in different *habits* or forms under different physical conditions: for example, prismatic, acicular, asbestiform and platy for single crystals; columnar, radiating, granular, massive and foliated for crystalline aggregates (Zoltai and Wylie, 1979).

Silicon and oxygen are the two most important elements in the crust and form a fundamental SiO_4 tetrahedral unit consisting of a central silicon ion with oxygen ions attached three-dimensionally at the four 'corners' of a tetrahedron. All forms of 'silica'—that is, silicon dioxide $(SiO_2)_x$—are composed of these tetrahedra joined by common oxygen atoms so that each crystal consists of a giant molecule with an average stoicheiometric formula of SiO_2. Being uncombined they are referred to as 'free silica'. The tetrahedra are linked in various ways by —Si—O—Si— chains, and the manner in which metallic cations are included in this linkage decides their form and characteristics.

The distinction between 'free' and 'combined' silica is important. *Combined silica* is SiO_2 in combination with various cations as silicates. *Free silica* is the most widespread substance in nature with a fibrogenic potential for the lungs, but examples of combined silica which are fibrogenic (mainly and most importantly the asbestos group of minerals) are of more restricted distribution. It should be noted that many reported chemical analyses of rocks make no distinction between 'combined' and 'free' silica and only the total SiO_2 content may be shown. Under these circumstances the quantity of 'free' silica remains unknown.

Free silica (silicon dioxide) occurs in three forms: *polymorphic crystalline, cryptocrystalline* (that is, minute crystals) and *amorphous* (that is, non-crystalline).

The principal crystalline phases of silica are:

(1) *quartz* which is stable up to 867 °C but is capable of metastable existence at higher temperatures;
(2) *tridymite* which is stable from 867 to 1470 °C and capable of metastable existence both above 1470 °C and below 867 °C;
(3) *cristobalite* which is stable from 1470 °C up to its melting point of 1723 °C but is capable of metastable existence at any temperature below 1470 °C. *Opaline–silica* is a variety of cristobalite (Sosman, 1965).

Pure quartz when heated to temperatures between 867 °C and 1470 °C is nearly always converted to cristobalite and not to tridymite unless a catalyst is present.

Two naturally occurring, crystalline forms of silicon dioxide are of interest in the pathogenesis of silicosis: *coesite* and *stishovite* which respectively have tetrahedral and octahedral configurations (*see* Chapter 4, p. 66). Both were apparently formed by high, shock-wave pressures and high temperatures due to the impact of meteorites on hard sandstone terrain (Chao, Fahey and Littler, 1962).

The cryptocrystalline forms of free silica—which consist of minute grains of quartz cemented together with amorphous silica—include *flint, chert* and *chalcedony* (a variable mineral which is differently named according to its colour as, for example, *agate, cornelian* and *onyx*) in which the crystal size is about 400 Å (Å = Ångstrom unit; 10 Å = 1 nm) (Drenk, 1959). These are sometimes incorrectly referred to as 'amorphous silica'. As in the case of quartz the rate of conversion of this form of silica into cristobalite is greatly influenced by temperature, but at given higher temperatures (1200 to 1400 °C) the rate of change is, in general, much greater than that of pure quartz.

The most important form of amorphous silica from the point of view of lung disease is *diatomite* (or *kieselguhr*) which consists of myriads of skeletons of diatoms (*see* Chapter 9). Finely divided amorphous silica changes to cristobalite at all temperatures between 1000 and 1723 °C but in the pure, dry state conversion to tridymite does not apparently occur though, in the presence of a flux or of water, tridymite may be produced between 867 and 1470 °C without the intermediate formation of cristobalite. Another amorphous form, *vitreous silica,* is produced when any of the crystalline phases of silica is melted to form liquid silica and then quickly cooled. If, however, vitreous silica is heated above 1000 °C devitrification with the formation of cristobalite occurs.

These phase changes in silica are relevant to the severity of resulting lung disease as the fibrogenic potential of crystalline silica appears to increase in ascending order from quartz to cristobalite to tridymite (*see* Chapters 4 and 7). Examples of possible industrial sources of cristobalite and tridymite are fired silica (refractory) bricks and other highly siliceous ceramic products, fired insulation bricks, used refractory bricks and foundry sands, and straight and flux calcined diatomite (*see* Chapter 7).

TYPES OF ROCK

Silicon does not exist free in nature. Free silica, therefore, is the principal rock-forming constituent and the proportions in which it is present determines the nature of many rocks.

There are three principal types of rocks.

IGNEOUS ROCKS

These are the primary rocks of the crust which were formed from magma either by rapid extrusion of magma on to the Earth's surface or by intrusion of magma within the crust (igneous = fiery); in the first case cooling occurred quickly and in the second, slowly. The rate of cooling determined the size of the rock crystals: the quicker the cooling, the smaller the crystals; and the slower the process, the larger the crystals. Granite is an important example.

SEDIMENTARY ROCKS

Sedimentary rocks are formed in two ways:

(1) By the gradual breakdown of igneous or older sedimentary and metamorphic rocks (*see* next section) by the action of wind, sun, water, frost and ice in weathering and corrosion processes to form deposits of debris such as sand and mud.
(2) By the deposition in former seas or swamps of the shells of marine organisms, rotting vegetation and chemical substances.

Slow or cataclysmic earth movements altered the levels of both types of accumulation and new sediments were deposited on top of them squeezing out their water and compressing them into rocks such as sandstone, limestone and coal.

METAMORPHIC ROCKS

Metamorphism implies change of form, structure and constitution in already existing igneous and sedimentary rocks. This change is brought about in four ways:

(1) By a local and substantial rise in temperature caused by the intrusion of magma which bakes the neighbouring rocks (*thermal metamorphism*).
(2) By movement of the crust which applies shearing or thrusting forces to the rocks and so distorts them that the formation of new minerals results (*dynamic metamorphism*).
(3) By percolation of hot water through rocks, and steam and gases through the magma which causes important chemical changes (*hydrothermal metamorphism*).
(4) By a combination of thermal and dynamic metamorphism (*regional metamorphism*).

Composition

For the most part all such rocks are composed of *silicate minerals:* that is, silicon dioxide in various combinations with the oxides of other elements such as aluminium, calcium, iron, magnesium and potassium.

The proportion of silica which was available in the original magma determined the form which igneous rocks were to take and it varied from approximately 30 to 75 per cent.

Where the percentage of silicon dioxide was very low, iron and magnesium, which have a strong affinity for it, combined with all that was available, especially if they were predominant among the cations. This gave rise to the 'ferro-magnesian' group of minerals (such as the *olivine group*). When a large quantity of uncombined iron remained, this was deposited as iron ore; when the percentage of silica was of intermediate order, iron and magnesium again combined with it, but, if their concentration was low, aluminium, potassium, sodium and calcium combined with the available remaining silica to produce the *feldspar group* of minerals. Where the percentage of silicon was high, all available cations were absorbed and an excess of silica left which crystallized as quartz.

Acid and basic rocks

Silica-rich magmas are termed 'acid' and those having little silica but large quantities of bases, such as aluminium, iron and magnesium, are termed 'basic'. Four magma types are distinguished according to their total or '*combined*' silica content.

Ultrabasic	from 30 to 44 per cent silica	(basalts)
Basic	from 45 to 54 per cent silica	(andesites)
Intermediate	from 55 to 64 per cent silica	
Acid	from 65 to 75 per cent silica	(rhyolites)

The more acid the rock, therefore, the more free silica it contains. The proportions of free silica in any rock can only be expressed in general terms. It is practically impossible to give numerical values which are valid for a given rock type found in any one area or globally. Rocks which contain no quartz do not contain free (uncombined) silica.

Among the igneous rocks the quartz content of the acid group (chiefly the granite family) may be as much as 30 per cent; in some rocks of the intermediate group, the content is negligible, while in others it may be up to 5 per cent. *Quartz is absent from rocks of the basic and ultrabasic groups.*

CLASSIFICATION OF IGNEOUS ROCKS

The common igneous rocks can be classified in eight groups.

Olivine group

These have the lowest proportion of silica and are, therefore, generally confined to ultrabasic and basic rocks. They are iron and magnesium silicates and contain no aluminium.

Pyroxene group

The most important member is *augite* which possesses more silica than the previous group and is a calcium magnesium iron aluminium silicate. It has a single chain structure.

Amphibole group

The silica content is not substantially different from the pyroxene group. *Hornblende* is the commonest member and is a complex calcium magnesium iron and sodium silicate and, like *tremolite* (calcium magnesium silicate), it has a double chain structure which lends itself to the formation of long fibres. *Actinolite* differs from tremolite in containing a considerable quantity of iron but it, too, may be of fibrous habit. *Amosite* and *crocidolite* asbestos also belong to this group (*see* pp. 38 and 39).

Micas and clay group

This group is generally associated with acid rocks such as granite. The structure of micas is of the sheet lattice type which gives them their well-known characteristic of cleavage into layers. Important members of the group are *biotite*, a complex silicate of magnesium, aluminium, potassium and iron found in many igneous and metamorphic rocks; and *muscovite* (potassium aluminium silicate), the common white mica. *Sericite*, once thought to be important in the pathogenesis of coal pneumoconiosis, is a secondary muscovite which may be produced by the alteration of orthoclase feldspar. And *vermiculite*, which possesses important industrial properties, is a natural alteration product of biotite and phlogopite micas.

The clay group of minerals contributes to the majority of the sedimentary rocks and is produced by the breakdown of feldspar and ferro-magnesium minerals. They are hydrous aluminium silicates of sheet lattice type.

Feldspar group

Members of this group are the most common of all the rock-forming minerals and the most important constituents of igneous rocks. Chemically they are silicates of aluminium with either potassium, sodium or calcium, or a combination of these three. They fall into two main series:

(1) *Orthoclase feldspars* which are potassium rich and usually occur in 'acid' rocks with a high percentage of quartz.
(2) *Plagioclase feldspars* which contain variable proportions of sodium and calcium. Sodium plagioclases occur in more 'acid' rocks and are, therefore, frequently associated with orthoclase, whereas calcium plagioclases are found in the 'basic' rocks.

This is the most appropriate place to note that because the feldspar minerals, which are extensively used in the ceramic industry, are commonly associated with significant amounts of quartz they may cause silicosis but, in the absence of quartz, they do not give rise to collagenous fibrosis in the lungs of experimental animals (Goldstein and Rendall, 1970; Mohanty *et al.*, 1953).

Feldspathoid group

Members of this group are composed of the same elements as the feldspars but in different proportions and they play a similar, though subordinate, part in rock formation. Their proportion of free silica is very low and that of alkalis, such as sodium and potassium, high.

Quartz group

As already stated, when silica is present in abundance and all other substances have entered into combination with it a variable amount remains and crystallizes as quartz. This almost pure free silica is found in such important igneous rocks as *quartz-porphyry*, *rhyolite* and *granite*. The sedimentary and metamorphic rocks which were subsequently formed from them also have a high silica content.

Volcanic glasses

These are volcanic lavas of which the following are important examples. *Pumice* and *pumicite* (volcanic ash): these are light coloured, silicic glasses formed by volcanic explosions which have accumulated as pyroclastic rocks in massive heaps or sheets around extinct volcanic vents; the only difference between them is their particle size, pumice being more and pumicite less than 2 to 3 mm in diameter. Pumice is usually a pure frothy glass but occasionally it contains small crystals of quartz and feldspar. *Perlite:* this is a volcanic silicate glass of rhyolytic composition which consists of minute spheroids a few millimetres in diameter. Because of its content of combined water it possesses the property of rapid expansion ('popping') when heated to between 760 and 1200 °C. Small amounts of quartz may be found in some ores (*see* Chapter 9, p. 317).

Crystalline structure

The order of crystallization of these rocks depended primarily on the composition of the magma: for example, in a magma rich in silicon dioxide, quartz tended to crystallize first—hence, quartz-prophyries. Similarly, in basic rocks, feldspar often crystallized before pyroxene. Within the ferro-magnesian and feldspar groups, therefore, fairly well-defined sequences are observed. For example:

Ferromagnesian minerals		*Feldspars*
Olivine	Plagioclose	Calcium feldspar
↓		↓
Pyroxene		Sodium calcium feldspar
↓		↓
Amphibole		Sodium potassium feldspar
↓		
Biotite		

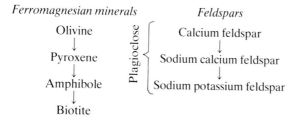

It is worth noting, as a general principle, that some minerals cannot occur together in rocks. In particular, quartz is not present in rocks of the olivine group (other than those which are almost pure iron-olivine) or in the feldspathoid group. Rocks which contain quartz are often classified as 'oversaturated'; those with little or no quartz but which contain olivine and feldspathoids, as 'undersaturated'.

NON-SILICATE ROCKS

Non-silicate minerals are also rock-forming and are important constituents of certain sedimentary and metamorphic rock types. They fall into the following groups.

Carbonates

These are the predominant non-silicates and they consist of *calcite* ($CaCO_3$—the chief constituent of limestone) *dolomite* ($MgCO_3.\ CaCO_3$—which constitutes dolomite limestone) and *siderite* ($FeCO_3$). *Marbles* are metamorphosed calcite or dolomite. Siderite occurs in some coal measures (*see* p. 38).

Haloids and sulphates

Rock salt (NaCl), *anhydrite* ($CaSO_4$), and *gypsum* ($CaSO_4.2H_2O$) which were deposited by evaporation of lakes and land-locked seas, and *fluorspar* (CaF_2) contain no free silica unless by contamination.

Oxides and sulphides

These are mainly iron minerals and their most important representatives are *magnetite* (Fe_3O_4) and *iron pyrites* (FeS_2).

The principal rocks can now be briefly described.

IGNEOUS ROCKS

The rate at which the original magma cooled determined the degree and form of its crystallization and, therefore, the 'texture' or fundamental structure of the igneous rock. Magma which solidified within the crust is called 'intrusive'.

Three primary categories of igneous rocks are recognized:

(1) *Extrusive or volcanic* which are glassy or fine grained ('grain' refers to crystal size) because they cooled very rapidly.
(2) *Minor intrusive or hypabyssal* which, being fairly near the surface of the crust, cooled rather more slowly and are medium grained.
(3) *Major intrusive or plutonic* (after Pluto, the god of the Underworld) are deep below the surface, cooled very slowly and are medium to coarse grained.

Intrusive rocks reach the surface of the crust through the action of earth movements and the erosion and disruption of overlying rocks.

SEDIMENTARY ROCKS

Sedimentary rocks fall broadly into three categories.

(1) *Fragmental rocks*

As the chief ingredients of these were produced mechanically by attrition and erosion they are classed according to the nature and size of the fragments.

(a) *Rudaceous (that is, rubbly) rocks* These are composed of granules, pebbles or boulders which, when rounded by wear produce *conglomerates;* but if angular, are called *breccias*. The fragments are cemented together by a mineral such as secondary silica, leached out from elsewhere, or by mud.

(b) *Arenaceous (arena = sand) rocks* The raw materials of these are sands and silts cemented by siliceous and clay substances. The chief members of this group are the *sandstones* and they are composed predominantly of quartz grains.

(c) *Argillaceous (argilla = clay) rocks* These consist essentially of naturally plastic clay minerals which invariably contain significant quantities of free silica derived from older quartz-bearing rocks—so-called detrital quartz—as well as other detrital minerals (*see Table 2.2*). They are laid down as clays and when consolidated become rocks. They form an important group and, according to the degree or stage of their consolidation, fall into three principal types. (i) *Clays*, the most important of which industrially are china clay, ball clay, fuller's earth, bentonites and fireclays. Some quartz is present: the quantity in fuller's earth is very small, variable in ball clays and fireclays, and moderate in bentonite. Commercial kaolins contain very little though there may be appreciable amounts in the raw material from which they are produced. (ii) *Mudstone or claystone* which is an indurated, massive, unlaminated, argillaceous sediment. (iii) *Shales*, which have the property of splitting readily into layers or laminae, consist of arenaceous shales (containing much sand), carbonaceous (black) shales associated with coal measures, and oil shales (saturated with bituminous matter). All contain varying, often large, quantities of detrital quartz. In some coal measure shales it may exceed 8 per cent and in mudstones and shales used for the manufacture of bricks and pipes and similar materials may be up to 60 per cent.

It is important to point out that the term *fuller's earth*, which refers to the property of absorbing grease and oil, is a source of serious semantic confusion because it is used for a number of different clays possessing this property, from various parts of the world. The most effective 'fulling' clays, however, are rich in the mineral montmorillonite, which contains loosely bonded exchangeable cations, and it is the nature of these cations—either calcium or sodium—which defines the two principal varieties of montmorillonite: calcium montmorillonite is known as fuller's earth and sodium montmorillonite, as *bentonite*. Bentonite, which is much less common than fuller's earth, is a highly plastic clay derived, as an alteration product, from volcanic ash and its main source is the USA. When in contact with water calcium montmorillonite has low swelling, and sodium montmorillonite high swelling properties. Unfortunately, the former—known as fuller's earth in the UK—is referred to as 'non-swelling' bentonite in the USA; and the latter is known as bentonite in the UK and as 'swelling' bentonite in the USA. To add to the confusion 'fuller's earth' is used in the USA to refer to *palygorskite (attapulgite) clays* (amphibole relatives) which are not related to the montmorillonites although they possess some similar properties and were, in fact, originally introduced to substitute fuller's earth from England (Highley, 1972). These terminological differences undoubtedly explain the disparity in reports as to whether or not fuller's earth causes lung disease, for other minerals associated with the different clays vary both qualitatively and quantitatively— quartz in particular. The problem is discussed in Chapter 9.

(2) *Rocks of organic origin*

(a) *Limestones* These are chiefly of organic origin and consist mostly of calcium carbonate. Small amounts of magnesium carbonate are often present but when this reaches significant proportions the rock is referred to as dolomite limestone or *dolomite*. Many different types of organism have contributed to their formation including among others corals, crustacea, foraminifera, molluscs and algae. The calcium carbonate of some limestones, however, is entirely of chemical origin. In general they do not contain any free silica but small amounts are sometimes present as an impurity. However, flint occurs as nodules in some chalk deposits, and chert in some limestone deposits.

Rottenstone and wollastonite are found in association with limestone and are used in industrial processes.

Rottenstone is a siliceous-argillaceous limestone from which calcium carbonate has been removed in solution. It contains up to 15 per cent quartz and 85 per cent alumina, and has been used in industry as a refractory material and as a filler.

Wollastonite is a naturally occurring calcium metasilicate ($CaSiO_3$) formed mainly by contact metamorphism of quartz-bearing limestone and by silica-bearing emanations from igneous intrusions (often granite) reacting with pure or impure limestone. It is used in some countries as a substitute for flint, quartz, sand, feldspar and china clay (*see* p. 317) in ceramic-bonded abrasives, and in other industries (Andrews, 1970).

(b) *Carbonaceous rocks* Lignite and coals were formed from the accumulation of rottting vegetation (trees, ferns, giant club mosses) in swampy conditions and subsequent inundation by sediment and solute-bearing river, lake or sea waters which overlaid it with deposits destined later to become sandstone, shale or limestone. The subsequent raising of the area or drop in sea level caused by earth movements allowed forest vegetation to take root once again, so that the cycle was repeated, not once but many times in succession.

Most plant tissues possessed a high proportion of carbohydrates and many hydrocarbons in the form of resins, waxes, oils and fats together with mineral salts originally absorbed from the soil. Their residue, therefore, contains at least 50 per cent carbon, not more than 44 per cent oxygen and 6 per cent hydrogen.

Where dead vegetation accumulated in stagnant water in conditions of poor oxygen supply, decomposition was slow and plant structure remains clearly distinguishable. In this way *peat* was formed. When organisms such as unicellular algae, spores and pollen grains petrified in deeper waters and mingled with inorganic muds a jelly-like carbonaceous slime, *sapropel*, resulted.

Peat and sapropel are the basis of all coals which may be classified according to *type* and *rank*, although no classification devised so far has proved to be uniformly satisfactory for coals of both the northern and southern hemispheres. The types of vegetation and other organic materials, the condition prevailing at the time of their deposition and regional tectonic disturbances are responsible for this variability.

As earlier layers of peat and sediment subsided and were successively overlain by new layers, so they became subjected to increasing pressure and temperature as well as to chemical changes. These processes gave rise to the different coal types first by gradual change of peat to *brown coal* and *lignite* which, by comparison with peat, have a slight increase in carbon and loss of oxygen; then to *bituminous coal* well known as house and gas coals which are much richer in carbon content but poorer in oxygen and volatiles (*sub-bituminous coals* are intermediate between these two); and, finally, to *anthracite coals* which contain some 95 per cent carbon and less than 5 per cent oxygen and volatile materials (*Table 2.1*).

The progression of the lignite–anthracite series of coals from low carbon and high oxygen content and volatile residue at the one end of the scale to high carbon and low oxygen and volatile contents at the other defines the *'rank'* of coal; the former being classed as low rank and the latter, high. This variation is due to the degree of alteration (diagenesis and metamorphorphism) produced in the original peat-coal deposits following their burial under younger rocks over long periods of time. As a generalization high rank coal is the oldest and low rank coal the most recent in geological age. The fixed carbon content of coal, by contrast, with its content of volatile matter, increases with depth in vertical succession at any point in a coal field (Hilt's law) due to temperature increasing with depth and to variation in the non-carbon content which is very low in coals of intermediate and high rank. The rank of coal may have some bearing on the pathogenesis of coal pneumoconiosis (*see* Chapter 8).

non-protein amino acids and other compounds; and, although diamino and non-amino acids are present in lignite and sub-bituminous coal, only negligible quantities of non-amino acids are present in bituminous and anthracite coals. Similarly, carbohydrates—cellulose, sugars and lignins—are decomposed and depolymerized by the coalification and ageing processes. By contrast, lipids—that is, aliphatic hydrocarbons, alcohols and esters, aromatic hydrocarbons and terpinoids—are geologically more stable and, because of this, some were the source of essentially pure deposits such as petroleum as long ago as the Palaeozoic Age (Mueller, 1972); but they are not immunogenically active.

Therefore, it can be concluded that organic material possessing immunogenic potential is very unlikely to have survived and to exist in bituminous and anthracite coals.

The wide variability in the physical and chemical properties of coal has to be taken into account in the interpretation of *in vitro* experiments on its biological action.

Table 2.1

Coal type	*Rank*	*Composition (%) (dry mineral matter-free basis)* *Carbon*	*Hydrogen*	*Oxygen*
Peat		50–65	5–7	30–40
Lignite	(Low)	65–75	5–6	20–30
Sub-bituminous	↓	75–80	5–6	13–20
Bituminous	(Intermediate)	80–90	4.9–5.7	5–15
Semi-bituminous	↓	90–92	4.5–4.9	4–5
Anthracite	(High)	92–95	2–4	2–4

Coal types differ in their content of bark, wood and plant fragments, spore cases (exines), leaf cuticles, resin and algal bodies: algal bodies are found mainly in low rank coals and spore cases (megaspores and microspores) tend to be more numerous in intermediate and high rank coals. The original constituents of all these organisms were, of course, proteins, polysaccharides and lipids, and because these entities in bacteria and fungal spores and hyphae are a known cause of extrinsic allergic 'alveolitis' (*see* Chapters 4 and 11) it is sometimes suggested that coal dusts may be capable of causing this disorder. The question, then, is: do potentially immunogenic organic elements survive the coalification process?

It is generally accepted that organic matter in sediments is extensively altered with the passage of time. Large populations of micro-organisms, fungi and streptomycetes are present in the surface layer of peat but at depths ranging from 180 to 325 cm below the surface few or no viable organisms are found because of lack of oxygen and other factors (Given, 1972). This suggests that there are likely to be no viable organisms at greater depths. In coal proper most vegetable remains are crushed, compacted, carbonized and mineralized but, because of their resistance to alteration, spore cases may survive intact and are either empty or filled with mineral matter. The mineralization or 'petrification' process may also occur in plant cells forming fossils. In the process of fossilization the original protein hydrolyses to its constituent amino acids which, in turn, break down into

By virtue of their origin coal seams are closely associated with strata of such sedimentary rocks as sandstone, mudstone, shale, siltstone, fireclay and, occasionally limestone. Such variation in rock types is responsible for the range of dust compositions found in different coal mines and in different parts of the same mine. But the amount of free silica in coal itself is usually very low and it may be absent. In passing it should be noted that siliceous sandstones, known as *ganisters*, which are the seat-earths of some coal seams and have a very high quartz content, have been specially mined in the UK for refractory materials particularly in Yorkshire and Durham, but this has now ceased. However, compact quartzites in the Millstone Grit (that is, coarse sandstone with beds of shale) of South Wales and Durham are still worked on a small scale for refractory bricks.

(c) *Siliceous earths* These consist of the fossilized remains of myriads of diatoms deposited in fresh-water or marine conditions of unusual purity. Organisms such as diatoms, radiolaria, and siliceous sponges secreted the silica of their skeletons which has, seemingly, unique and distinctive physical properties and, as already stated, is amorphous.

The degree of consolidation of these deposits which are known as *diatomite, diatomaceous earth* or *kieselguhr* is variable. The term *'tripolite'*, which has also been applied to diatomite, is no longer in general use and must be distinguished from *tripoli* which is a chalecodonic quartz and contains no diatoms.

The amorphous silica content of the siliceous earths is very high ranging from about 58 to 90 per cent. Examples from North America are especially high.

(3) *Non-framental rocks of chemical origin*

These include 'evaporites' which are, for the most part, precipitates of desiccated seas and lakes; they include

Table 2.2 Classification of some Common Sedimentary Rocks

	Group character	*Type*	*Main features of composition*
Mechanical origin	Rudaceous	Conglomerate	Quartz content similar to parent rock; iron oxides (e.g. limonite, hematite); sometimes calcite or dolomite
		Breccia	Mixed rock fragments; calcite and limonite with fine silt or mud in matrix
	Arenaceous	Sandstone	Quartz, muscovite, and feldspar rock particles cemented by siliceous, ferruginous, calcareous, argillaceous and carbonaceous matter
		Gritstone	Similar to sandstone. Particle slightly different in shape
		Arkose	Sandstone or gritstone with about 25 per cent feldspars of various sorts. Siliceous and ferruginous content
		Quartzite	Sandstone or gritstone with detrital quartz cemented by secondary silica
		Ganister	Highly siliceous. Quartz, cherts, orthoclase, feldspar, clay minerals such as kaolinite ($Al_2Si_2O_5(OH)_4$). Hematite and limonite are accessory minerals
		Siltstone	Fine-grained, compact detritus from rivers, lakes and glacial action. Quartz, muscovite, feldspars and iron ores with siliceous, ferruginous and calcareous cementing material
	Argillaceous	Clay	Fine-grained, earthy material, plastic when wet; hard when dry. Consists of orthoclase and plagioclase feldspars, muscovite and occasionally a little quartz (*see* note)
		Fuller's earth	Mainly montmorillonite [$(Mg.Ca)O.Al_2O_3.5SiO_2(5–8)H_2O$] but also small amounts of feldspar, mica, glauconite and apatite may be present. Quartz rare except in intercalated sand layers
		Volcanic clay	Bentonite: sodium montmorillonite with quartz, cristobalite, feldspar, mica, apatite and ferro-magnesian minerals
		Residual clay	Formed *in situ* from rock decomposition. Very finely divided: for example, bauxite (hydrous aluminium oxides) and china clay (kaolin) (*see* note)
		Mudstone	Consolidated, non-fissile clay with similar constituents. Usually from beneath coal seams ('seat-earths')
		Fireclay	Contains quartz, feldspars, mica, secondary silica and iron compounds. Quart content high
		Shale	Indurated, laminated, fine-grained clay mineral matter; contains quartz, mica, iron ores, secondary silica, calcite and iron oxides. Quartz content moderate
	Calcareous-argillaceous	Marl	Unconsolidated, non-laminated calcareous clay. Composition as clays but more calcareous materials as matrix. Quartz content small and variable
		Calcareous shale	Consolidated, laminated clay with such calcareous material, i.e. consolidated marl with similar composition
Organic origin	Calcareous	Limestone	$CaCO_3$ mainly of organic origin (e.g. corals, crustacea, molluscs, algae, foraminifera), occasionally iron ores. Very small quantities of free silica may be present
		Dolomite	Limestone with large quantity of $Ca.Mg(CO_3)_2$, much of organic origin; also variable hematite
		Oolitic and pisolitic limestone	Limestone, more chemical than sedimentary in origin, with large characteristic grains of $CaCO_3$ found in successive layers round nucleus of shell fragments or quartz grains. ('Grains' resemble fishroe or peas.) Small and variable amounts of free silica
		Chalk	Almost pure $CaCO_3$. No free silica, but nodules of flint in some chalk deposits
	Siliceous	Chert and flint	Crystalline and cryptocrystalline silica (microcrystalline quartz) often aggregated into 'nodules' in chalk. Very high free silica content with traces of limonite
		Siliceous earth	Group of siliceous deposits of organic origin. Total silica content (amorphous only) of diatomite ranges from 58 to 90 per cent. Some iron salts and calcareous matter. No crystalline or cryptocrystalline free silica
	Carbonaceous	Carbonaceous rocks	Peat, lignite, coal, anthracite and cannel. Variable but usually small amounts of iron ore (pyrite, siderite, limonite) and clays (e.g. kaolinite). No free silica but may be present in adjacent strata

Table 2.2 (cont.)

Group character		*Type*	*Main features of composition*
Chemical origin	Calcareous	Calcium carbonate (calcite)	$CaCO_3$ but some impurity such as limonite. Traces of free silica are rare and accessory
		Dolomite (partly)	Occurring as mineral, not limestone replacement. $Ca.Mg(CO_3)_2$ with some iron impurities
	Ferrugineous	Bedded iron ores	From aqueous solutions in mudstones, limestones, primary hematite, magnesite. Variable quartz content
		Bog iron ores	Negligible quartz
	Saline	Chlorides	Mainly rock salt (NaCl) with many other impurities but negligible quartz
		Sulphates	Gypsum, anhydrite, barytes ($BaSO_4$), celestine ($SrSO_4$). Rarely free of rock impurity from slight mineral contamination due to variable amounts of sands, marls, clays, shales, and limestones: therefore, small quantities of free silica may be present

NOTE: The majority of true clays contain very little free silica and what there is depends upon the nature of the parent rock. Clays with particle size greater than 2 μm (μm = 1/1000 mm) may contain a small quantity (occasionally up to 10 per cent) but those of smaller particle size contain as insignificant quantity.
'Free silica' refers to crystalline or cryptocrystalline forms unless otherwise stated.
Table freely adapted, by permission of the publishers, from Milner, H. B. (1962). *Sedimentary Petrography*, Vol. 2. London: Allen and Unwin

calcite, rock salt, apatite, anhydrite, gypsum, and a form of calcium carbonate known as *aragonite*.

Iron from aqueous solutions or iron-storing bacteria is found in two main forms:

(a) Bedded iron ore (bedded ironstones) in which iron was deposited in mudstones and limestones in the form of *glauconite* (hydrated silicate of iron and potassium), *hematite* (Fe_2O_3) and *limonite* ($2Fe_2O_3.3H_2O$). Hematite is, in addition, probably formed by processes other than sedimentation, namely hydrothermal, in areas such as Cumberland. These ores are sometimes intimately associated with beds of chert, so that a high concentration of free silica may be encountered when they are mined.

(b) *Bog iron ores* which consist mostly of limonite deposited in swampy ground and underlaid by clay; free silica is absent. Siderite forms the clay-ironstone of many coal measures, in Britain, notably those of South Wales and Durham.

The more important sedimentary rocks relevant to this study are shown with their main compositional characteristics in *Table 2.2*.

METAMORPHIC ROCKS

Examples of metamorphic rocks which are encountered in industry are:

(1) *The asbestos group* 'Asbestos' includes minerals of different origins. Firstly, crystals of ultrabasic rocks such as *peridotite* (an intrusive igneous rock composed mainly of olivine) and of *serpentine* (hydrous magnesium silicate often containing iron) which is itself a derivative of such ferro-magnesian minerals as olivine, pyroxenes and amphiboles, were altered by enormous forces of hydrothermal and dynamic metamorphism to fibrous magnesium silicate or *chrysotile*, the commonest form of asbestos.

Secondly, minerals of the amphibole and pyroxene groups were transformed by the same forces into *crocidolite*, the fibrous form of riebeckite (hydrous iron sodium silicate) and *amosite*, the fibrous form of grunerite (hydrous iron magnesium silicate)—their host rock usually being a sedimentary ironstone; also *tremolite* (hydrous calcium magnesium silicate), *actinolite* (hydrous calcium magnesium iron silicate) and *anthophyllite* (magnesium iron silicate). The host rock of these three is sedimentary as well as igneous by virtue of hydrothermal metamorphism of impure dolomite (magnesium-rich) limestones (Hodgson, 1977).

Asbestos minerals are frequently of fibrous habit.

Correct understanding of the terms 'fibre', 'fibrous' and 'asbestos' is most important as their use in medical and hygienist literature is often much at variance with mineralogical definitions.

A *'fibre'* is a single, acicular crystal or elongated polycrystalline aggregate resembling organic fibres: that is, having circular cross-section, flexibility, axial lineation and a high *aspect* (length–breadth) *ratio*. It is not always possible to distinguish microscopically between acicular, crystals, needle-like cleavage fragments and asbestiform fibres. The term *'fibrous'* refers to a mineral compound of parallel, radiating or interlaced aggregates of fibres from which the fibres can usually, but not always, be separated. 'Asbestiform' is reserved for a special type of fibrous habit.

'Asbestos' was the term originally used for the fibrous form of actinolite, the massive microcrystalline variety of which is a type of jade (nephrite), because it was thought, incorrectly, to be a distinct mineral. Although the term might justifiably be applied to non-silicate minerals which crystallize in fibrous habit, 'asbestos' is now understood as a collective mineralogical term which refers to the unusual crystallization of certain silicate minerals in a special type of fibrous habit—*asbestiform*—in which the fibres have extreme length–breadth ratios, are flexible, have a higher tensile strength than crystals in other habits of the same mineral and are aggregated in parallel or radiating bundles from which the fibres can easily be separated (Zoltai, 1978; Zoltai and Wylie, 1979). (*See also* Chapter 9, p. 233).

Talc (*see* next section) and serpentine share a common origin from metamorphosed ultrabasic rocks but, in the majority of talc deposits, talc has replaced serpentine; hence, chrysotile is rarely found as an accessory mineral.

(2) *Talc (french chalk)* This is a hydrated magnesium silicate which was formed by the same metamorphic processes applied to dolomite limestones and ultrabasic igneous rocks in magnesium carbonate. It may take the form of flat, flaky plates, granules or short fibres (which may be due to pseudo-morphing). The process was closely akin to that of the production of asbestos minerals and, in fact, the amphiboles actinolite, anthophyllite and tremolite may be present as accessory minerals with talc which is then often referred to as *asbestine;* and, in addition, chlorites, calcite, dolomite, magnesite, magnetite, pyrite, pyrophyllite (*see* next section) and quartz may be present. The amount of quartz varies from negligible to about 20 per cent in some deposits (Weiss and Boettner, 1967).

Analysis of bulk talc samples imported into Great Britain has shown that quartz is a fairly common contaminant in minor amounts (1 to 2 per cent by weight) though it exceeded 5 per cent in one sample; and although tremolite was uncommon it was present as a major phase (more than 30 per cent by weight) in one sample. No other varieties of asbestos minerals were detected (Pooley and Rowlands, 1977).

It must be emphasized, however, that tremolite occurs in blocky acicular, fibrous (non-asbestos) and asbestos forms and that only the last of these varieties can be classed as asbestos; and, furthermore, that there are no commercial sources of tremolite asbestos since it is found rarely in Nature and then only in small quantities. Thus, any description of tremolite must clearly define its variety (Campbell *et al.,* 1979). This is discussed further in Chapter 9.

Hence, some examples of 'talc' may contain substantial quantities of quartz and others may consist to a large extent of tremolite or talcose anthophyllite. This wide variation in the identity and quantity of accessory minerals which depends upon the source of the talc deposits is undoubtedly an important determinant of the pathogenesis and variable characteristics of 'talc' pneumoconiosis (*see* Chapter 9).

Neither the flaky nor the 'fibrous' habit of talc is lost by grinding.

For industrial use talcs which are virtually free of all impurities are known as 'high grade' and those in which impurities may be as much as 50 per cent, as 'low grade'. The term *steatite (soapstone)* has long been applied to an impure, massive form of talc which can be quarried in large blocks, but is now often used to designate especially pure forms of talc for industry.

Pyrophyllite (hydrous aluminium silicate) is closely similar in origin, structure and properties and is commercially included with, and defined as, talc. However, aluminium replaces magnesium in its composition and, unlike talc, it does not fuse when fired.

(3) *Kaolin (china clay)* This is finely divided aluminium silicate derived from the feldspars of igneous rocks by weathering and sedimentation (as in Georgia and South Carolina, USA) or by hydrothermal attack (as in Cornwall and Devon). Therefore, most of the commercial china clay of the USA is not metamorphic in origin.

In the most advanced stage of the hydrothermal process only quartz may remain unaltered in powdery feldspar so that it is found in variable, but significant quantities. This is the form of china clay most suitable to the ceramic industry.

(4) *Quartzites* These are the result of thermal or dynamic metamorphism cementing sandstones. They, therefore, consist of a mosaic of quartz crystals and their free silica content is consequently very high.

(5) *Slates* Slates, shales and mudstones (which contain quartz grains and clay minerals) were compressed by lateral forces so that reorientation of their crystalline structure allows easy and fine cleavage. The quartz content of all slates is usually high, being about 30 to 45 per cent by weight. The production of commercial slate powders results in a slight loss so that, for example, powdered Cornish slate contains about 25 per cent and powdered North Wales slate, 30 per cent quartz.

(6) *Schists* These resulted from the effects of regional metamorphism upon argillaceous and certain metamorphic rocks and include mica-schists and talc.

(7) *Marbles* These were produced by thermal and dynamic metamorphism of limestone. If the limestone was pure (dolomite, for example) a pure marble with negligible free silica content resulted, but if it was impure, marbles with variable silicate composition were produced; for example, *forsterite* (magnesium silicate of the olivine group). Marbles, therefore, are not a source of free silica.

(8) *Mineral ores* Mineral ores originated in a number of ways; early crystallization from magma and then separation for example, *chromite* ($FeCr_2O_4$); percolation and subsequent solidification of magmatic gas or liquid in pockets within native rock which was frequently of igneous type (for example, *beryl, copper, gold, lead, silver, tin, zinc*); and by subterranean waters dissolving scattered minerals and depositing these elsewhere in increased concentration.

It is evident, therefore, that mineral ores are apt to be found deposited in 'pockets' and 'veins' among rocks of widely differing type and composition.

(9) *Graphite* a soft black form of carbon, is found disseminated mostly in mica-schists, micaceous quartzites, and occasionally in various igneous rocks. For this reason, although some graphite is pure carbon and, therefore, lacks combined and free silica, it may contain various impurities derived from the associated rock minerals, especially in the mined material. These include feldspars, pyrites, iron oxides, muscovite and quartz; their amount varies according to the origin of the graphite deposit. The amount of quartz is usually low, but may be about 2 per cent and an example as high as 11 per cent has been reported (Parmeggiani, 1950).

EARTH MOVEMENTS

The various rock types have not remained in the order in which they were formed. The effects of weathering and enormous pressures due to earth movements caused by earthquakes and volcanic activity folded, dislocated and fractured the crust. The effects of movements are exemplified by simple folds, overfolds, faults and thrusts of sedimentary rocks, the original strata of which were thereby extensively displaced and intermingled.

This means that in tunnelling and mining or quarrying for a mineral in a particular stratum, a variety of different and unrelated materials may be encountered, from which it is evident that the composition of dusts produced by these processes will vary from locality to locality.

PRODUCTS OF ACTIVE VOLCANIC ERUPTIONS

Violent eruptions produce pyroclastic fragments consisting of the following:

(1) *Ash:* that is, pulverized lava composed of crystals, glass or rock fragments, or a mixture of all three less than 4 mm in diameter. The finest particles are dusts.
(2) *Lapilli* or small stones.
(3) *Blocks and 'bombs',* which are larger rocks up to boulder size.

These fragments are formed from erupting fluid magma and from the fracture and ejection of old rocks and lava in the walls of the volcano's conduit by the force of the eruption. It is the composition of volcanic ash and dust which is of interest here.

As noted earlier (p. 33), magmas consist of various gradations of molten *basalts, andesites* and *rhyolites*. The temperature at the vent of the conduit is likely to range from 750 to 1200 °C so that, although free silica may be present as crystals of quartz, tridymite and cristobalite in the resulting ash, it is very largely converted into glass by rapid cooling on ejection.

The average size of air-fall ash deposit fragments at any point decreases exponentially with the distance from the vent, the largest and heaviest thus being nearest. The distances at which ash-falls occur depend upon the severity of the eruption. When very violent the ash cloud is projected miles into the air and fall-out occurs over enormously large areas (often hundreds of miles) and is most concentrated down-wind. The finest and furthest travelled ash derived from siliceous magmas (rhyolites and andesites) commonly consists largely of glass shards; some rock minerals such as feldspar may be present but free silica (mainly cristobalite) forms a very small part. Particles less than 1 μm in size are rare. If the existing rocks lining the conduit are siliceous some free silica fragments may be present transiently in the local atmosphere. Long, flexible fibrous particles or threads are a feature of the air-fall dust and ash of some eruptions often at very great distances. These are formed of basalitic glass and are known as Pele's hair—after the legendary goddess of Hawaiian volcanoes.

The amount of free silica (chiefly cristobalite) in ash in the vicinity of the Mount St Helens eruption (Washington State, USA) in March, 1980 is reported to range from 2 to 7 per cent and no fibrous particles have been observed (Merchant, 1980). An X-ray diffraction trace of air-fall ash from this eruption is shown in *Figure 2.1*.

Thus, it can be reasonably concluded that exposure to air-fall ash—which, of course, is likely to be short—does not present a pneumoconiosis hazard, though at best it is a significant nuisance and at worst, in high concentrations near the source of an eruption, may cause acute respiratory distress or asphyxia in unprotected individuals especially if ash clouds are projected at high speed near ground level. However, when the eruption has ceased personnel in certain occupations (such as bulldozer and truck drivers, forestry and agricultural workers, geologists and volcanologists) may have a more prolonged exposure to dust from deposited ash although rainfall may soon change the ash into a cement-like texture.

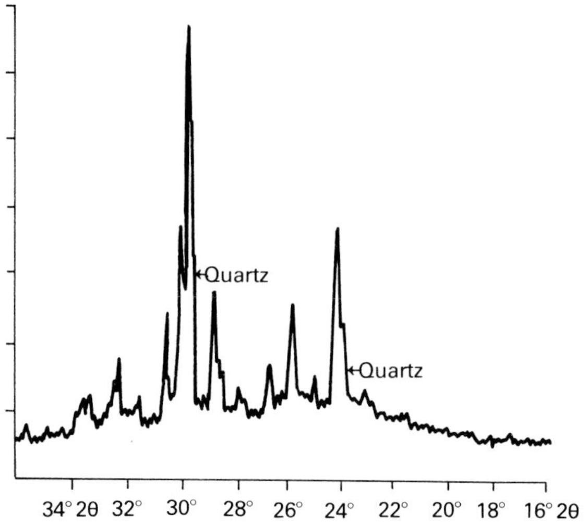

Figure 2.1 An X-ray diffraction trace of volcanic ash erupted on 18th May 1980 from Mount St Helens, Washington State, USA, collected at Great Falls, Montana. The main crystalline phase present is a feldspar which is responsible for most of the diffraction peaks. Quartz forms approximately 2 per cent of the total volume of ash and produced the two peaks indicated on the trace. Much of the ash is composed of non-crystalline glass shards which do not produce diffraction peaks. (Published by permission of the Director, Institute of Geological Sciences, London)

Another danger of volcanic activity which is not confined to the immediate vicinity of an eruption is the presence of toxic gases (*see* Chapter 13). These include sulphur dioxide, sulphur trioxide, hydrogen sulphide, chlorine and hydrogen chloride in varying proportions, and also carbon dioxide. They are present in ash clouds, and unexpected jets of gas may be expelled from innocent-looking cooling lava flows distant from the centre of the eruption. The predominant gas in the early stages of an eruption is sulphur dioxide but hydrogen sulphide is more common later. Not all eruptions are short and violent; some grumble on for years with episodic emissions of these and other gases. Steam vents (*fumaroles*) which may be found in the vicinity of both active and dormant volcanoes often produce high concentrations of carbon dioxide and sulphur dioxide.

Sulphur dioxide, hydrogen sulphide and carbon dioxide are the most hazardous of volcanic gases because, being heavier than air, they hug the ground and accumulate in hollows and can thus cause acute respiratory disease or asphyxia in man and animals. Carbon dioxide is especially dangerous as it is odourless and non-irritant and its presence is likely to be unsuspected.

ROCK NAMES

The local names attached to similar rocks in different regions of the British Isles vary greatly and are sometimes the cause of confusion; a valuable key to their meanings—and, therefore to the identity of the rocks—is provided by Arkel and Tomkeieff (1953).

SOME COMMON USES OF ROCKS AND MINERALS

The following, presented in brief note form, is not intended to be comprehensive but to give some indication of the range of use of these materials.

ABRASIVES

Diamond, corundum (natural crystallized Al_2O_3), emery (corundum with iron oxides); garnet (that is, *almadine*—iron aluminium silicate) which may contain a minute amount of free silica and is usually heated at temperatures up to 1000 °C before use; and *grossularite*—calcium aluminium silicate—in which there is no quartz; quartz, quartzite, sandstone and tripoli; fine grade pumice, pumicite, diatomite, iron oxides (as jeweller's rouge, 'crocus' and black rouge for polishing precious metals and gem stones); talc and zircon ($Zr\ SiO_4$) which is used for 'sandblasting' and burnishing. Feldspar has recently been used in abrasive soaps.

Although abrasive grains are used directly for some purposes (such as 'sandblasting') it is necessary, before they can be efficiently employed, to combine them with some bonding material and then to press them into required shapes such as grinding wheels or discs (*bonded abrasives*); or to apply the grains to a backing material of paper or cloth (*coated abrasives*). The commonest bonded abrasives consist of grains mixed with clay, flint or feldspar shaped and then fired at about 1270 °C for a few days (*vitrified bonds*). It is possible, therefore, that quartz, tridymite or cristobalite may be present in some bonds though they are unlikely to be released in significant amount during use. Rubber, resinoid and shellac bonding is also employed.

A brief list of the applications of the more important abrasives some of which, however, are synthetic, may be useful at this point.

Fused alumina (aluminium oxide): the most commonly used in a wide variety of bonded, coated and grain forms (*see* Chapter 14).

Fused alumina-zirconia: employed for heavy duty grinding wheels (*see* Chapter 6).

Silicon carbide: extensively used in bonded and coated abrasives (*see* Chapter 6).

Boron carbide: manufactured from boric acid and coke in an electric arc furnace and used chiefly in moulded form, but also for lapping and polishing. Not known to be hazardous to the lungs.

Cubic boron nitride: a product of high temperature and pressure technology, second only to diamond in hardness, is used for specialized grinding wheels in which it is superior to alumina and diamond. No hazard to the lungs known.

Diamond: the hardest substance known, is employed mainly for shaping and maintaining other cutting and grinding materials of lesser hardness, in resin-bonded wheels for grinding tungsten carbide ('hard metal') tools, and impregnated in wire saws for cutting ceramics and plastics. It is without danger to the lungs.

Emery: used for buffing and other applications (*see* Chapter 6).

Corundum: use now largely limited to grinding glass lenses (*see* Chapter 13).

Garnet: high-grade coated almadine is employed for wood work and grinding glass.

Quartz: still in use for the manufacture of sand paper and, in the USA but not in the UK, for sandblasting. Silica flour is used in abrasives in the USA.

BUILDING MATERIALS

Gravels and crushed flint or chert for concrete; sand for cement mortar and plaster; marl for cement; limestones for lime, Portland cement and plaster. There are many different types of cements but, for the most part, they consist of limestones and clay or slate. Sandstone, shale and mudstone are employed as a source of silica in some cements. Gypsum is added to retard the setting time. Crushed pumice, perlite and exfoliated vermiculite are used in light-weight concrete, and both pumice and pumicite are combined in pozzolan–portland cements in the USA.

Aggregates (that is, crushed rocks of various types or blast furnace slag) are mixed with sand and cement to make concrete.

Gypsum is widely used for plaster (plaster of Paris) and to manufacture plaster board. Perlite, ground pumice, pumicite and exfoliated vermiculite are employed in acoustic and other types of plaster and as loose-fill insulation.

Of separate but great importance is asbestos (of one type or another) which, when added as a lightweight aggregate, produces a cement from which corrugated roofing, pipes, wall sheets and sections of pipe-covering materials are moulded or pressed; it is also used in millboards and putties, as fillers in floor tiles and sprayed in suspension on to walls and ceilings.

BUILDING AND MONUMENTAL STONES (DIMENSION STONE)

Granite (and other igneous rocks), sandstones, limestone, dolomite and marble.

ROOFING MATERIALS

Materials crushed into granular form and applied as fillers in asphaltic or bituminous mixtures include: limestone, calcined flint, chert, mica, slate dust, quartzite, gravels, asbestos, low grade talc and diatomite. These are used in the manufacture of damp course materials as well as roofing felts, and finely ground slate (slate flour) may also be added to the rubber mix to provide 'body'.

Talc powder is also employed in the manufacture of roofing felt to prevent adhesion when rolled.

Slate cut into blocks by circular saws and split to desired thickness by chisel and mallet.

ROAD CONSTRUCTION MATERIALS

Some igneous rocks, limestone dolomite, most members of

the rudaceous and arenaceous sedimentary rock groups, chert, flint, ganister and quartzite crushed to size are used to fill or aggregate asphalt and concrete for highways, pavements, airfield runways and the like. Asbestos has also been used as a filler for asphalt.

CERAMICS

There are three ceramic groups: (1) refractory and technical; (2) earthenware, chinaware and stoneware; (3) structural clay products.

Refractory and technical

(1) *A refractory ceramic* is a substance possessing the ability to resist high temperatures and changes of temperature without loss of physical or chemical identity.

Bricks and cements for the lining of furnaces and kilns may have to withstand temperatures of 1500 °C or more and mortars and crucibles may be required to resist temperatures of in excess of 3000 °C.

Materials used are: fireclays; ganisters; quartz and chert; graphite; magnesite; olivine rock as forsterite; chromite; alumina (bauxite); sillimanite minerals (anhydrous aluminium silicate) and zircon.

(2) *Technical ceramics* are employed in the electronic and other specialized industries, for example, metallurgy, atomic reactors and other forms of nuclear engineering, electrical and radio engineering, cutting tools, aircraft, missiles and spaceships.

The materials used are selected for their special dielectric, thermal conductivity and low neutron absorption properties according to their required purpose; refractory properties are secondary. Examples are: alumina which has great toughness, and excellent thermal conductivity and qualities of electrical insulation; carborundum (a synthetic compound, silicon carbide); beryllium oxide, widely used in nuclear engineering, thorium oxide and zirconium dioxide; uranium and plutonium oxides for ceramic fuels. A mixture of talc (or pyrophyllite), china clay or ball clay and a flux, usually barium carbonate, fired at about 1400°C, is used extensively for low-loss electroceramics such as valve holders, insulators and condenser plates in the radio and television industry. Beryllium oxide (beryllia) possesses all the necessary properties in high degree and is increasingly important in modern technology (*see* Chapter 10).

Earthenware, chinaware and stoneware

Both non-plastic and plastic materials are required. Non-plastic materials include quartz, flint and feldspar; plastic materials include china clay, ball clay, fire clay and red clay.

Enamel glazes are prepared from sands and sandstones of very high quartz content.

Wollastonite is used extensively in the USA, Finland and Denmark as a substitute for these ingredients in the ceramic mix and in glazes.

Structural clay products

Those include building and engineering bricks of all sorts, floor and roof tiles, drain pipes and chimney pots. Clays and shales are the chief ingredients but silica sand, and wollastonite are used in various combinations in the manufacture of wall tiles. The use of wollastonite without flint, or with a small quantity only, has reduced the risk of silicosis (Andrews, 1970). Talc or pyrophyllite is the main ingredient in some body formulas, but not in the UK.

FILLERS

Fillers are substances which are used to fill the voids within a material and to modify its chemical or physical properties (for example, its viscosity) and also to lower the cost. According to their function, therefore, they are also referred to as *extenders* when they aid even spreading of paint pigments without impoverishing their colour. In general, they require to be finely divided so that a substantial proportion of their particles are less than 10 μm in size.

Some important materials in which they are used are as follows.

Asphalt and concrete: limestones, clays, silica, mica, slate dusts, asbestos (in some countries), diatomite and talc.

Gramophone records (before 1948 in the UK): rottenstone, finely ground slate and barytes.

Paints: barium sulphate (barytes), titanium dioxide, exfoliated vermiculite, calcined diatomite, gypsum, china clay, mica, pyrophyllite and crystalline silica usually in the form of fine sand or powdered slate. Talc in the form of *asbestine* (*see* p. 39) is used in paint primers and fillers, and as an extender to improve suspending and spreading powers. It should be noted, however, that, in the UK, some grades of talc used for these purposes and which do not apparently contain fibrous minerals are being referred to as *asbestine*. Asbestos is employed in bitumen paints and mastics.

Paper: china clay, natural and calcined diatomite, gypsum and talc may be added at the stage of the beater process, and barytes is used in heavy printing papers and playing cards, and titanium dioxide as a pigment. Diatomite also functions as an extender of white pigment.

Pesticides: a 'carrier' is needed to sustain the physical properties and efficiency of the active chemical agent; clays, fuller's earth, diatomite, pyrophyllite and talc are among those used.

Plastics: asbestos, mica or talc are added to some thermosetting and amino-resins; asbestos only to laminated and some polyvinyl chloride plastics. Barytes, titanium dioxide and exfoliated vermiculite are also used. Diatomite, crystalline silica and alumina are constituents of silicone resins.

Rubber (natural and synthetic): fillers have two functions here. Apart from increasing bulk for the sake of cheapness, they also improve one or more of the physical properties of the rubber. Carbon black is most commonly used but others of importance are china clay (the particles of which are usually less than 2 μm diameter), other clay powders, slate powder, barytes, graphite, gypsum, diatomite, ground mica, talc (both as a filler and extender in heat-resistant mixes) and asbestos.

Textiles: fillers are often added to the starch, glue or synthetic sizes and include clays, gypsum and talc.

MOULDING AND FOUNDRY FACING MATERIALS

Quartzose sands of high quartz content are bonded with clays such as halloysite ($Al_2O_3.2SiO_2.2H_2O$), illite (a mica-like clay), kaolinite and montmorillonite. Zircon sand bonded with oil is now used because of its high resistance to thermal shock and to reduce the 'silica' risk, and there is an increasing use of olivine sand. Natural graphite is employed extensively for facings.

GLASS

Quartz sands of exceptionally high purity and uniform grain size are employed with lime in glass manufacture. For special glasses there is a wide range of other materials such as lithium, boron and strontium; and barium carbonate is used extensively in the UK in the glass of television screens as a barrier to X-radiation.

PIGMENTS

The iron oxides are among the most important in relation to quantities used. They are of natural and synthetic origin. The natural oxides are: *yellow iron oxide pigments* such as ochres, siennas and limonite; *red iron oxide pigments* such as hematite and calcined siderite; *brown iron oxide pigments* such as umbers and calcined siderite; and *black iron oxide pigments* such as magnetite. They occur in areas of fracture and fault in rocks like quartzite and limestone, in shales and in certain clays. Hence, variable amounts of quartz are likely to be associated with the raw material so that a silica risk may exist in some mining and beneficiation processes. But quartz is likely to be present in only very small amounts, if at all, in the final pigments because its presence in appreciable quantities makes grinding difficult and the end-result unsuitable for most manufacturing purposes. Some dustiness may occur in the grinding and calcining processes. Calcination is necessary to eliminate organic matter in minerals from some sources.

Natural iron oxide pigments are used in paints and coatings, stains, rubber, plastics, concrete products, polishing rouges (*see* Abrasives), paper, ceramics and fertilizers.

Synthetic iron oxide pigments, which are gaining rapidly in importance, are free of quartz and organic matter. All the colours corresponding to the natural oxides can be synthesized and are variously used in paints, especially for the motor car industry, and enamels; in magnetic recording tapes and electronic materials; in plastics, rubber, floor tiling and linoleum; and as a colouring agent for dog foods.

The particle size distribution of the natural ground iron oxide pigments ranges from about 0.4 to 40 μm and is mostly about 10 μm; whereas that for the synthetic oxides is about 0.2 to 4 μm and is chiefly concentrated in the 0.4 to 4 μm range (Hancock, 1975).

Other synthetic pigments include carbon black, which is used in printing inks and gramophone records, and those containing antimony and cadmium. Heavy metal impurities, however, are considerably less (about a tenth) in synthetic than in natural oxides (Hancock, 1975).

Titanium dioxide and barium salts also have a wide range of uses as pigments (*see* Chapter 6).

COSMETICS AND PHARMACY

These industries are major users of high quality talc from France, Italy and China which is employed after purification by elutriation or acid treatment in 'talcum', baby and face powders, and as a dusting powder for various pharmaceutical purposes and for polishing tablets. Despite purification small quantities of 'free silica' may occasionally be found in some samples in the USA (Cralley *et al.*, 1968). The question of possible contamination with asbestos minerals is discussed in Chapter 9.

DUSTING AGENTS

Medium to low grade talc is used to prevent adhesion of surfaces in the manufacture of rubber materials, roofing felts, linoleum, corks and 'chewing gum'. It is employed in the leather industry not only as an anti-adhesive but also to absorb oil. The previously widespread use of talc in the rubber industry in the UK has declined in recent years and only small quantities are now used. Other applications of talc are in the production of polished rice, corn and barley, and in promoting free flow of dry fire-extinguishing powders (*see* Chapter 9).

Finely ground scrap or flake mica is employed as an anti-adhesive.

HEAT INSULATION MATERIALS

Mixes of various compositions for application to boilers, pipes and joints, bulkheads and other parts of ships include asbestos of various types, diatomite, kaolinite, magnesite, and mineral wools (*see* Chapter 9).

Other uses of asbestos materials

As the asbestos minerals are known to be of great medical importance, reference to some uses other than those already mentioned should be made:

(1) Spinning and weaving fibres for textiles such as fireproof suits and ropes. Chrysotile and, to a lesser extent, crocidolite are used.
(2) In gaskets, brake linings, clutch facings, insulating blocks, welding rod coatings and cooking mats. Again, mainly chrysotile and occasionally crocidolite are employed.
(3) Filters for beer, fruit juices, plasma, wine, pharmaceutical and other liquids. Chrysotile is most commonly used and diatomite is sometimes added. Anthophyllite and tremolite are also, but less often, employed.
(4) Mixes of chrysotile, amosite or anthophyllite in an adhesive medium are sprayed under pressure on to walls and ceilings in buildings for fire protection and modification of acoustics. The method is also used in ships. Asbestos is a frequent ingredient of coloured dressings for the outside of houses and other buildings.
(5) Chrysotile, crocidolite and amosite are (or have been) compounded with resins to impregnate paper or millboard for use in aeroplane wings, motor-car bodies, small boats and missile nose cones; and with waterproofing resins and other materials to make caulking compounds.

Crocidolite seems to have been used in cigarette filters in the USA but not in the UK (Tobacco Research Council, 1968).

REFERENCES

Andrews, R. W. (1970). *Wollastonite.* Institute Geol. Sci. London; HMSO

Arkel, W. J. and Tomkeieff, S. I. (1953). *English Rock Terms.* London; Oxford University Press

Campbell, W. J., Steel, E. B., Virta, R. L. and Eisner, M. H. (1979). Characterization and cleavage fragments and asbestiform amphibole particulates. In *Dusts and Disease (Occupational and Environmental Exposures to Selected Fibrous and Particulate Dusts)*, edited by Richard Lemen and John M. Dement, pp. 275–285. Pathotox Publishers Inc.

Chao, F. C. T., Fahey, J. J. and Littler, J. (1962). Stishovite, SiO_2, a very high pressure new mineral from Meteor Crater, Arizona. *J. geophys. Res.* **67,** 419–421

Cralley, L. J., Key, M. M., Gorth, D. H., Lainhart, W. S. and Ligo, R. M. (1968). Fibrous and mineral content of cosmetic talcum products. *Am. ind. Hyg. Ass. J.* **29,** 350–354

Drenk, K. (1959). *X-ray Particle Size Determination and its Aplication to Flint.* Pennsylvania State University; X-ray and Crystal Structure Laboratory

Geikie, J. (1908). *Structural and Field Geology,* 2nd edition, p. 32. London; Oliver and Boyd

Given, P. H. (1972). Biological aspects of the geochemistry of coal. In *Advances in Organic Geochemistry 1971,* edited by H. R. von Gaertner and H. Wehner, pp. 69–92. Braunschweig; Pergamon Press

Goldstein, B. and Rendall, R. E. G. (1970). The relative toxicities of the main classes of minerals. In *Pneumoconiosis. Proceedings of International Conference. Johannesburg. 1969,* edited by H. A. Shapiro, pp. 429–434. Cape Town, South Africa; Oxford University Press

Hancock, K. R. (1975). Mineral Pigments. In *Industrial Minerals and Rocks,* 4th edition, edited by S. J. Lefond *et al.*, pp. 335–357. New York; American Institute of Mining, Metallurgical and Petroleum Engineers, Inc.

Highley, D. E. (1972). Fuller's earth. *Mineral Dossier No. 3.* Mineral Resources Consultative Committee. London; HMSO

Highley, D. E. (1974). Talc. *Mineral Dossier No. 10. Mineral Resources Consultative Committee. London; HMSO*

Hodgson, A. A. (1977). Nature and paragenesis of asbestos minerals. *Phil. Trans. R. Soc., Lond.* **286,** 611–624

Merchant, J. A. (1980). Personal communication

Milner, H. B., Ward, A. M. and Higham, F. (1962). *Sedimentary Petrography. Vol. II.* London; George Allen and Unwin Ltd

Mohanty, G. P., Roberts, D. C., King, E. J. and Harrison, C. V. (1953). The effect of felspar, slate and quartz on the lungs of rats. *J. Path. Bact.* **65,** 501–512

Mueller, G. (1972). Organic geochemistry. In *The Encyclopaedia of Geochemistry and Environmental Sciences,* edited by R. W. Fairbridge, pp. 812–818. New York; Van Nostrand Reinhold Co

Parmeggiani, L. (1950). Graphite pneumoconiosis. *Br. J. ind. Med.* **7,** 42–45

Pooley, F. D. and Rowlands, N. (1977). Chemical and physical properties of British talc powders. In *Inhaled Particles IV,* edited by W. H. Walton and B. McGovern, pp. 639–646. Oxford, New York; Pergamon Press

Sosman, R. B. (1965). *The Phases of Silica,* 2nd edition. New Brunswick, New Jersey; Rutgers University Press

Tobacco Research Council (1968). Personal communication

Urey, H. C. (1952). *The Planets; Their Origin and Development.* New Haven, Conn.; Yale University Press

Weiss, B. and Boettner, E. A. (1967). Commercial talc and talcosis. *Archs envir. Hlth* **14,** 304–308

Zoltai, T. (1978) History of asbestos-related mineralogical terminology. *Proceedings of Workshop on Asbestos: Definitions and Measurement Methods,* edited by C. C. Gravitt, P. D. Lafleur and K. F. Heinrich. Nat. Bureau Standards Spec. Publ. 506. Washington; US Government Printing Office. Library of Congress Category Card No: 78-600109

Zoltai, T. and Wylie, A. G. (1979). Definitions of asbestos-related mineralogical terminology. *Ann. N.Y. Acad. Sci.* **330,** 707–709

3 Inhaled Particles and their Fate in the Lungs

A detailed discussion of this highly technical subject is beyond the scope and purpose of this book. Nevertheless some basic knowledge of the behaviour of inhaled particles is necessary to appreciate the sizes at which they are likely to reach the depths of the lungs (and hence require detection and control in the work environment), and the forces which govern their deposition and retention in the lungs, and subsequent elimination.

Substances of diverse nature and physical form, once airborne, may reach the upper and lower airways of the lungs in inspired air. Their ability to do this depends on their physical properties. The more a material (such as rock) is broken down, finely divided and dispersed the more likely are its particles to be airborne and, therefore, capable of inhalation. But there are types of particulate clouds, other than those produced by attrition of rock, which have a wide range of particle size; everyday language speaks of 'dusts', 'fumes', 'smokes' and 'mists', and it is important that these should be distinguished.

Dust, in daily speech, means tiny particles which have settled on a surface, can be readily disturbed and are visible in a shaft of sunlight. It is more properly defined as consisting of solid particles dispersed in air (or other gaseous media) due to mechanical disintegration of rocks, minerals and other materials by such impulsive forces as drilling, blasting, crushing, grinding, milling, sawing and polishing; or to the agitation or breaking down of organic materials such as cotton fibres, pollens and fungal spores.

The approximate size ranges of some different types of particles are shown for comparison in *Table 3.1*.

Rock dusts vary greatly in size depending upon the sort of material worked, the process involved, the magnitude of the sample of dust taken and the time for which a dust cloud has been airborne. The majority of asbestos particles are fibrous and are produced by handling, disintegrating, carding (that is, combing out or disentangling) and weaving of amosite, chrysotile and crocidolite, their length usually ranging from 5 μm to 100 μm; but, in addition, a substantial proportion are non-fibrous, small and compact. (*See* p. 46 for the distinction between 'fibrous' and 'compact' particles.)

Fumes consist of metal oxides formed by heating metals to their melting points. Particle size ranges from 0.1 μm to 1 μm diameter at source, but aggregation of these particles readily occurs and, although these aggregations are often of large diameter, they have very low densities. This term is often used to refer to clouds of acid droplets but strictly speaking these should be classed as *vapours*.

Mists are liquid droplets formed by the condensation of vapours or the 'atomization' of liquids around appropriate nuclei. Many particles are less than 0.1 μm diameter and therapeutic mists are usually less than 10 μm, but some droplets may be up to 500 μm diameter.

The term *aerosol* is now commonly used to embrace airborne particles in all of these categories and so includes both dispersed particles and droplets.

Potentially dangerous particles, therefore, vary in size from those just small enough to enter the upper respiratory tract down to gas molecules.

Table 3.1 Comparison of Particle Sizes

Material	*Dimension range*
Sand grains	200–2000 μm diam
Cement dusts	4– 100 μm diam
Pollens	10– 100 μm diam
Fungal spores	2– 100 μm length 0.5– 7 μm diam
Actinomycete spores	0.6–2.5 μm length
*Rock dusts	1– 10 μm diam
Tobacco smoke	0.2– 2 μm diam
Viruses	28 nm– 0.2 μm diam

*Particles of flint, sandstone, shale, coal and other rock dusts produced by such processes as drilling, blasting shovelling, chiselling and milling

PROPERTIES OF DUSTS

The majority of dust particles are not spherical but of irregular shape and, according to their composition, exist either individually or as aggregations. Particles which approximate to a sphere (for example: bituminous coal, some clays, and some spores) are referred to as *compact;* and those whose length exceeds their diameter, as *fibrous* (for example: chrysotile and crocidolite asbestos). The United States Occupational Safety and Health Administration (1974) has stipulated, in this context, that a *fibre* has a length to diameter ratio of 5:1 or more but a ratio of 3:1 or more is commonly used by industrial hygiene laboratories and by pathologists. However, mineralogists regard a particle as a fibre when its length to diameter ratio (aspect ratio) is 10:1 or more. This important point is discussed in more detail in Chapters 2 and 9.

All particles have a small but independent motion of their own and their primary characteristic, when airborne, is a tendency to settle under the influence of gravity. The gravitational force exerted on a particle is equal to its mass multiplied by acceleration due to gravity. Against this, for a particle in motion, is opposed the force due to the viscosity of air which exactly balances the mass of a particle when it has accelerated to its terminal rate of fall—an effect which is greater for large than for small particles. Other things being equal the terminal velocity of a particle due to gravity is roughly proportional to its density and the square of its diameter for diameters between 0.5 and 50 μm. Hence, a spherical particle of unit density and 50 μm diameter falls through air at a speed of 73 mm/s whereas one of 5 μm diameter falls through air at a speed of about 0.78 mm/s. The terminal settling velocity—*free-falling speed*—is an important determinant of the aerodynamic behaviour of particles in the airways of the lungs and is related to their size, shape, surface characteristics and density. It is not their *apparent* size which decides the manner in which particles behave, but their aerodynamic properties. The particle sizes of importance in pneumoconioses are those which behave as if they were *unit density spheres* (UDS) of 0.5 to 10 μm diameter. An aggregation of dust particles with a total diameter of (say) 20 μm may be porous and, hence, of low density so that the settling velocity may be equivalent to that of a UDS of only 5 μm diameter; this enables it to penetrate deeply into the lung. The aerodynamic diameter of such a particle is, therefore, 5 μm compared with its microscopic diameter of 20 μm.

The term *aerodynamic diameter,* now in general use, therefore, denotes the diameter of the UDS which falls under gravity at the same speed as the particle or aggregate considered. If the particle is nearly spherical and of density ρ, then its aerodynamic diameter is its actual diameter multiplied by $\sqrt{\rho}$. In the case of the 20 μm aggregate just referred to ρ is equal to 0.5g/cm³, assuming that it is a compact aggregate, because the loose packing of its constituent particles renders it porous. If the particle or aggregate is not compact in shape, then a shape factor has to multiply $\sqrt{\rho}$ in order to obtain the aerodynamic diameter. The use of this term is limited to particles with UDS diameters from 0.5 to 50 μm which approximately obey Stokes' law of air resistance (*see* Appendix, p. 508). Even within this range the behaviour of a particle in the airways of the lungs is not wholly governed by its aerodynamic diameter; particles of extreme shape (fibres, plates, chain aggregates) and particles of extremely low density, ρ, are more likely to entangle themselves with the bronchial epithelium than the respective aerodynamic diameters would indicate. This is a geometrical effect known as *interception* (*see* p. 47).

Particles smaller than 1 μm diameter are referred to as *submicron particles* and are apt to remain airborne for long periods of time; hence they may present a special hazard if their concentration is sufficiently high.

BEHAVIOUR OF INHALED PARTICLES

Aerosols inhaled into the respiratory tract closely follow the movement of the air in which they are suspended, and the depth to which they penetrate into the lung depends not only upon their physical characteristics (size, density, shape and aerodynamic properties) but also upon the volume of each respiration. Once a particle comes in contact with the wall of an airway or an alveolus it cannot again become airborne, and it is then said to be *deposited.* Because the majority of inhaled particles less than 1 μm diameter are expelled in exhaled air (*Figure 3.1*) their concentration in the inhaled air must be high to enable some of them to be deposited in the lungs. The total number of particles exhaled differs from the total number inhaled during steady breathing by the number deposited in the dead space airways during inhalation and exhalation, and the number retained in the alveolar regions. This applies to repeated breaths only and not to a single breath.

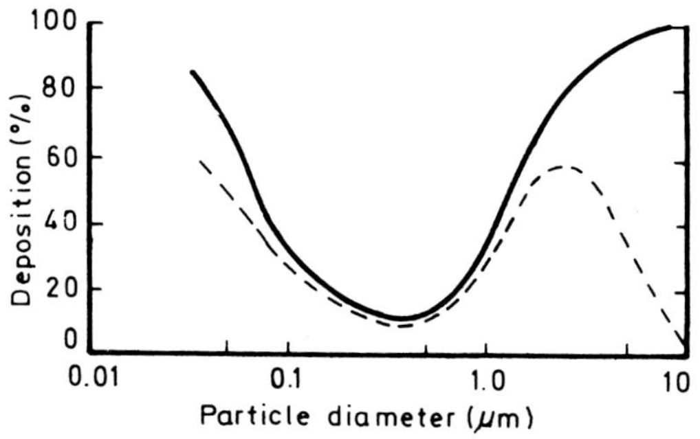

Figure 3.1 Deposition curves of compact particles during mouth breathing. The dotted curve represents particle deposition in the alveolar region of the respiratory tract (alveolar deposition); maximum deposition is seen to lie in the 2 μm to 5 μm range. The continuous curve represents deposition throughout the respiratory tract from nose to alveoli (total deposition). Below 0.1 μm diameter there is again some tendency for alveolar deposition to increase. (From Clinical Aspects of Inhaled Particles, *by courtesy of Dr D. C. F. Muir and the publishers, Heinemann)*

The composition of particles, whether in the solid or liquid state, does not influence their deposition.

There are four ways in which solid particles are deposited—sedimentation, inertial impaction, interception and diffusion.

Sedimentation

Sedimentation is settlement influenced by gravity. It is determined by the density and diameter of particles (density

× diameter²). Under some circumstances the form of airflow in a tube may influence sedimentation but, for practical purposes, it has no effect upon particle sedimentation in the lungs which occurs predominantly at low velocities. Particles deposited in this way have aerodynamic sizes of about 2 μm or less. Deposition in the larger airways is chiefly due to sedimentation.

The free-falling speed of fibrous particles is determined by the square of their diameter and is little influenced by their shape or length. Gravitational settlement of fibres occurs only in large airways and it limits the diameter of fibres which can penetrate to small airways to less than 3 μm (Timbrell, 1970). In small airways, therefore, deposition of fibres is not determined by their falling speed, but by their length and shape (*see* Interception).

Inertial impaction

When an airstream carrying fairly large particles has its direction changed by the curving or branching of airways (as in nasal cavities and large airways of the lungs) the particles tend to follow their original path in the airstream and, in consequence, impinge upon the walls. Impaction of particles in this way is related to their density × diameter², the diameter and change of direction of the tube, and the rate of air flow in the tube.

This is the primary mechanism of deposition in the nose and is important in large airways for compact particles larger than 10 μm. Particles smaller than this are able to penetrate to the small airways and alveoli.

Interception

This concerns particles of irregular shape (for example, mica plates) or of fibrous habit (such as asbestos) in which the length and shape of the particles—their aerodynamic diameter—is more important than their falling speed.

The lower the length/diameter ratio of a fibrous particle the closer its behaviour resembles that of a compact particle, but the longer a fibre the less likely it is to behave in this way. Hence, long fibres of small diameter (less than 3 μm), unlike compact particles, avoid sedimentation and impaction in larger airways and are intercepted by collision with the walls of terminal and respiratory bronchioles particularly at their bifurcations. This explains the fact that asbestos fibres as long as 200 μm may be found in this region.

Chrysotile fibres are frequently curled, a property which increases their likelihood of collision with the walls of narrow airways, mainly at their bifurcations. Amphibole fibres, on the other hand, are always straight and rigid, and this favours their orientation parallel to the axis of the airways by the aerodynamic forces so that they penetrate deeper into the lung. Crocidolite (blue asbestos) fibres reach the periphery of the lung having suffered little sedimentation *en route* (Timbrell, Pooley and Wagner, 1970). Mathematical predictions of the influence of fibre shape on deposition in the airways indicate that it is about twice as great for straight fibres in ordered orientation as for irregular (curled) fibres in random orientation (Harris and Timbrell, 1977).

The variable depth of penetration by different types of asbestos fibre may be significant in determining which types are likely to cause disease. This is discussed further in Chapter 9.

Diffusion

This effect, which is exhibited by very small particles (less than 0.1 μm diameter) and which is independent of their density, influences their deposition significantly in the region beyond the terminal bronchioles and also upon the wall of the trachea; indeed, it may be responsible for their complete deposition (*Figure 3.1*). It does not affect the behaviour of larger particles.

Because the diffusion forces of oxygen and carbon dioxide operate in opposite directions and are almost equal they are unlikely to have any effect on the movement and deposition of particles in the region beyond the terminal bronchiole.

INFLUENCE ON DEPOSITION OF AERODYNAMIC SIZE AND PATTERNS OF RESPIRATION

The aerodynamic size of particles is a decisive factor in determining how far they can penetrate into the respiratory tract and the probability of their deposition.

NASAL AIRWAYS

These are of great importance in removing particles, vapours and gases from inhaled air before they can gain access to the lower respiratory airways. Very few compact particles larger than 20 μm and only about half of those 5 μm in diameter pass the nasal filter during breathing at rest, due mainly to impaction, and many particles of smaller size are also removed (Proctor *et al.*, 1969). Deposition of many particles 5 μm or less in diameter is increased in transit due to their humidification which causes them to grow in size; but if nasal breathing is impossible (as is the case in obstructive disease of these airways, in the inhalation of tobacco smoke which bypasses them, and in permanent tracheostomy) the number of these particles reaching the pulmonary airways and alveoli is much greater than would otherwise be the case. Habitual mouth breathing, therefore, allows an increased number of particles to reach the lower airways and alveoli (Albert and Lippmann, 1972) and, indeed, a relationship between the incidence of pneumoconiosis in miners and nasal filtering efficiency was suggested by Lehman in 1935.

Peak air flows through the nose are approximately 1.0 l/s. Therefore, factors which lower this rate, such as nasal disease or other causes of increased nasal resistance to air flow, and work loads which demand high ventilation rates result in a change from nasal to mouth breathing (Proctor *et al.*, 1973). Resistance to air flow is increased by low ambient air temperatures (Salman *et al.*, 1971). Nasal mucociliary activity which clears deposited materials backwards to the pharynx where they are swallowed, so enhancing the defence mechanism, is unaccountably defective in about one-third of normal subjects. Whether or not this defect contributes to the future development of lung disease remains to be established (Proctor *et al.*, 1973). Certainly nasal resistance varies widely among apparently normal subjects (Proctor, 1977).

PULMONARY AIRWAYS AND ALVEOLI

It is of particular practical importance both in regard to the causation and prevention of bronchopulmonary disease to know whether inhaled mineral or organic particles are likely to be deposited on the mucociliary surface of the dead space airways or on alveolar walls. Although precise knowledge of the size range of compact particles which reach the alveoli has not yet been achieved, it is clear that the volume and frequency of respiration play a significant role.

Earlier experimental work on human adults breathing compact particles through the mouth suggested that alveolar deposition is maximal at an aerodynamic diameter greater than 2μm (Altshuler, Palmes and Nelson, 1967), but less than 4 μm (Lippmann and Albert, 1969). These results and the observations of the Task Group on Lung Dynamics (1966) are the basis of most published deposition curves typical example of which is shown in *Figure 3.1*. However, recent studies have demonstrated that for particles between 0.2 and 0.5 μm total depositions are two or more fold less than the Task Force predictions, and that for particles between 0.5 μm and 2.5 μm there is less rapid increase in deposition than predicted (Davies, 1974). *Figure 3.2* shows these differences for this size range compared with *Figure 3.1*. During steady (quiet) breathing only 10 to 15 per cent of

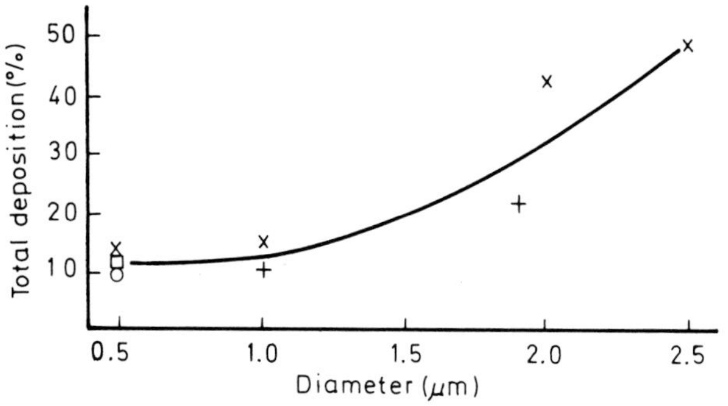

Figure 3.2 Deposition of aerosols of spherical particles in the lungs. Recent experimental data. ○ *Muir and Davies, 1967.* □ *Davies, Heyder and Subba Ramu, 1972.* + *Heyder, Gebhart, Heigwer, Roth and Stahlhofen, 1973.* × *Davies, Lever and Rothenburg, 1977. (By courtesy of Dr C.N. Davies and Editor of* Chemistry and Industry*)*

0.5 μm compact particles are retained in the lungs but all of these are deposited in the alveoli, the rest being exhaled in spite of having travelled down and up a distance of about 40 cm from mouth to airways whose diameters may be as small as 0.5 μm. Deposition of 1 μm particles under similar breathing conditions is practically the same (Davies, 1974).

The tidal volume of each respiration and the frequency of the respiratory cycle profoundly influence the behaviour of particles in the airways. The greater the tidal volume the deeper the mass flow of transporting air penetrates into the lungs, whereas with increasing frequency of respiration the deposition of compact particles decreases (Muir and Davies, 1967). Both tidal volume and respiration frequency are increased by effort, and it is the *minute volume* (that is, the product of tidal volume and number of breaths per minute) which is the most important factor determining the *total volume* of particles deposited. In short, the increase in minute volume which accompanies heavy physical effort results in a greater deposition of particles than occurs when the subject is at rest or performing light work.

Hence, different breathing patterns, which are determined by work load, impose significant individual variations in deposition which are not evident in *Figure 3.1*, so that in effect this is a rigid 'model' of only limited practical value; furthermore, because the mechanical factors of sedimentation and impaction vary with differences in breathing pattern it is impossible to be dogmatic as to which mechanism of deposition predominates. However, Davies (1979) is preparing a set of tables based upon a recently elaborated formula (Davies, Lever and Rothenberg, 1977) which are capable of predicting nasal, total lung and alveolar deposition of compact particles in the 0.5 μm to 10 μm range for any breathing pattern. These tables will be of great practical value in the work of industrial hygienists and physicians. An example of the quantitative range of deposition during different breathing patterns for particles of various sizes predicted by the tables is shown in *Table 3.2*.

Increasing gravitational force (G) causes an almost linear increase in total deposition of 2.0 μm particles from about 20 per cent at 0 G to about 45 per cent at 2 G (Hoffman and Billingham, 1975). As a similar trend undoubtedly exists for particles of other sizes this observation is relevant to a variety of aerospace conditions.

The size range of particles likely to be deposited in the alveolar regions and the size-selecting characteristics of the respiratory tract are particularly relevant to the design specification of dust sampling instruments and in deciding the maximal allowable concentrations of specified dusts in a work environment (*see* Threshold Limit Values).

Dust particles recovered after death from the lungs of coal miners have a wide range of sizes but the majority are about 1 μm (Cartwright, 1967; Leiteritz, Einbrodt and Klosterkötter, 1967). This is due largely to the breakdown of aggregations of particles which individually are approximately 1 μm diameter.

The distribution in the lungs of inhaled air carrying dust particles is of particular interest in relation to the zonal preference of certain types of pneumoconiosis. Although it is virtually simultaneous in all zones during normal breathing, the lower zones are ventilated more than the upper when breathing from FRC but, at lung volumes approaching RV, ventilation of the upper zone is greater than the lower (Milic-Emili, Henderson and Kaneko, 1968). It is not known to what extent these events at the extremes of tidal volumes determine the zonal distribution of deposited particles.

Other mechanisms which have been suggested as influencing particle deposition are turbulence in the upper airways and surges of air flow in the lower airways synchronous with the heart beat (West, 1961). There is little evidence to support or refute these contentions.

Deposition of particles of a given size shows great variation between subjects examined under almost identical conditions due to factors other than differences in ventilatory patterns and nasal filtration efficiency. Firstly, the normal human respiratory tract is not structurally uniform and there is considerable variability between individuals in the total number of alveoli and the dimensions of airways (Angus and Thurlbeck, 1972; Lapp *et al.*, 1975; Thurlbeck and Haines, 1975). Secondly, deposition tends to occur more proximally than distally in cigarette smokers due, probably, to the bronchoconstrictive effect of tobacco

Table 3.2 Effect of Breathing Patterns on Deposition

	V_t cm^3	F min^{-1}	*Aer. diam. (μm)**	*Site of deposition, % inhaled particles* Nose	Lungs	Dead space	Alv.
SEDENTARY BREATHING PATTERN							
In nose, out mouth	500	15	0.5	2	10.5	0	10.5
Min. vol. 7.5 l			1.0	6	11.8	0.1	11.7
			2.0	26	28.3	12.2	16.1
			5.0	57	30.1	21.7	8.4
ACTIVE BREATHING PATTERN							
In and out mouth	2000	25	0.5	0	11.5	0	11.5
Min. vol. 50 l			1.0	0	13.3	1.0	12.3
			2.0	0	55.5	28.8	26.7
			5.0	0	100.0	72.1	27.9

V_t = Tidal volume; F = Breathing frequency; Min. vol. = minute volume; Aer. diam. = aerodynamic diameter; Lungs include larynx
*Values for particles larger than 2.5 μm tentative at present (1980)
By courtesy of Dr C. N. Davies

smoke (Lippmann, Albert and Peterson, 1971; Sanchis *et al.*, 1971); and indeed, uniform 5 μm particles have been shown to penetrate less deeply into bronchitic lungs than into normal lungs (Thomson and Pavia, 1974). Penetration of particles in patients with airways obstruction is directly related to the volume of particles inspired per breath and to FEV_1; and inversely related to inspiratory flow rate (Pavia *et al.*, 1977).

Particles of cigarette smoke which range from 0.18 to 1.5 μm in diameter would, due to their size, suffer negligible deposition on the walls of the airways. However, they are hygroscopic and by absorbing water from the air in the lungs (which has an almost 100 per cent humidity), if held in the airways for a few seconds during inhalation, they increase significantly in size and are deposited on their walls: for example, a particle of 0.4 μm diameter will grow to 1.1 μm (Davies, 1974). This process is undoubtedly important in the genesis of bronchial carcinoma, and may well be significant for some other aerosols.

CLEARANCE OF PARTICLES FROM THE LUNGS

Both inert and cytotoxic insoluble particles which are deposited in the conducting airways above the terminal bronchioles are eliminated either in a free (that is, extracellular) state or within alveolar macrophages via the mucociliary 'escalator' and by reflex cough, and are expectorated in sputum or swallowed. In this way the majority of particles are cleared in the first hour after deposition. However, in the gas-exchanging region distal to the terminal bronchioles the behaviour of inert and cytotoxic particles appears to be different.

Inert particles deposited in alveoli tend to remain in the alveolar area and to be eliminated mainly by the bronchial route. They are engulfed by macrophages which migrate from the alveoli over the non-ciliated zone of the respiratory bronchioles to the mucociliary 'escalator' in the terminal bronchioles. It is not understood how they are able to bridge this gap but it has been suggested that a proximal movement of surfactant may be responsible, and that respiratory movements facilitate migration (Kilburn 1968); certainly dust tends to accumulate in less mobile parts of the lungs, such as the bronchiolovascular regions. Particles lodged in the interstitium may be carried by macrophages in tissue fluids to the lymphatics whence they travel to intrapulmonary and hilar lymph nodes, but others are retained, or 'stored', in the interstitial site for years. Therefore, by contrast with insoluble particles deposited in ciliated airways the time taken for the clearance of similar particles from the peripheral non-ciliated regions is prolonged.

Cytotoxic dusts, for example free silica dusts, behave differently. Their lethal effect upon macrophages (*see* Chapter 4) appears to be decisive so that particles deposited distal to the terminal bronchioles have a greatly limited chance of being transported by these cells to the mucociliary 'escalator' and eliminated. Most of them, therefore, penetrate into the interstitium whence some are removed by the lymphatic system (possibly mainly in an extracellular state) to the regional lymph nodes but many are carried only a limited distance from their point of entry where they provoke local fibrogenesis. Those particles which reach the 'escalator' are probably transported and removed in the extracellular state.

It appears that if a small quantity of quartz (3 to 4 per cent) is intermingled with inert dusts their penetration into the interstitium is facilitated and their bronchial elimination reduced (Klosterkötter and Bünemann, 1961).

Smaller insoluble particles tend to travel to hilar lymph nodes more quickly than larger ones (Nagelschmidt *et al.*, 1957), but quartz particles reach the lymphatics more rapidly than non-toxic particles, such as titanium oxide, of similar size (Klosterkötter and Bünemann, 1961). Furthermore, some small particles may pass into the blood stream; this explains the occasional presence of silicotic lesions in the liver and spleen and other organs.

The efficiency with which insoluble dusts are removed from the lungs varies, therefore, according to whether they are inert or cytotoxic as well as upon the load or concentrations of particles imposed upon the elimination routes. Soluble particles dissolve readily and pass into the capillary blood, or, possibly, are bound to lung tissue proteins. Hence, both insoluble and soluble particles, if possessed of antigenic potential, may cause immunological reactions in airways, alveolar walls and local lymphatic tissue, or systemically (*see* Chapter 4).

Clearance of fibres appears to be related to their lengths rather than to their diameters (*see* Chapter 9).

The process by which inert and cytotoxic particles pass from the alveolar lumen through the alveolar wall into the adjacent interstitium is not clear. Direct breaching of the walls has been suggested, especially in alveoli in the bronchiolovascular regions (Gross and Westwick, 1954; Spencer, 1968), and probably occurs in the case of inert particles smaller than 50 nm diameter but not of larger particles (such as may reach human alveoli) which are either taken up by phagocytic Type I cells (see *Figure 1.5*, p. 5) or are incorporated into the interstitium when these cells are damaged and before they are able to regenerate (Bowden, 1976; Hapke and Pedersen, 1968; Heppleston and Young, 1973; Sanders *et al.*, 1971). The question as to whether dust laden alveolar macrophages *re-enter* alveolar walls appears to be unresolved (Bowden, 1971), although there is suggestive affirmative evidence (Stirling and Patrick, 1980); but, macrophages already in the walls ingest particles which have gained access to the interstitium and leave via the lymphatics (Lauweryns and Baert, 1977).

A comprehensive synoptic review of alveolar clearance has been made by Lauweryns and Baert (1977).

Elimination of particles from the lungs occurs in rapid and slow phases. The rapid phase is usually complete in about 24 hours and is accounted for by the clearance of particles which have been recently deposited in the ciliated airways either by their transportation by the mucociliary stream or by their solution and subsequent passage into the blood stream. The slow phase takes months—up to 300 days in the case of 5 μm particles (Booker *et al.*, 1967). Inert particles which are not removed within months appear as if stored in the lungs although, in fact, they are slowly eliminated over a period of many years; indeed, the appearance of coal or hematite dusts, for example, in the sputum of men who have been away from dust exposure for years is well known both to them and their physicians. The period during which particles are resident in the lungs is especially important if they are radioactive (*see* Chapter 14).

The effect of cigarette smoking on the efficiency of mucociliary clearance, as observed by various workers, is complex and, to some extent, contradictory but, briefly, seems to be as follows. Early clearance of radioactive labelled particles from the lungs of smokers tends to be reduced by comparison with non-smokers (Sanchis *et al.*, 1971; Pavia, Thomson and Pocock, 1971) but at 24 hours the clearance rates are similar (Albert *et al.*, 1975). However, smoking a few cigarettes has been shown to produce transient decrease in the *total* time required for bronchial clearance in both smokers and non-smokers, due to acceleration of deep bronchial clearance in the absence of convincing evidence of a reduced rate of elimination from the upper bronchial tree (Albert *et al.*, 1975). Nonetheless, there is little doubt that cigarette smoke is ciliatoxic (Kennedy and Elliot, 1970) and that it reduces the rate of ciliary beat and increases production of bronchial mucus.

THRESHOLD LIMIT VALUES

In industry (especially where there are processes using potentially dangerous materials) it is important to know if an inhalable aerosol is generated and exists in the ambient air, and if so in what concentration. If such an aerosol cannot be completely eradicated at source it is necessary to devise a method capable of defining a concentration level in the atmosphere which should not be exceeded if health is not to be endangered.

Clinical and epidemiological experience and animal experiments have shown that some aerosols have greater disease-producing potential than others; and some individuals are more susceptible to them (and, therefore, have a greater liability to disease) than others. That is, a more dangerous aerosol may provoke disease at very low concentrations in a short period of time whereas another, less dangerous, may require fairly high concentrations over a long period. It is possible from such studies to find an approximate empirical level of concentration of a potentially hazardous airborne aerosol which will not cause lung disease in workers exposed to it over a period of a working life. This empirical level is the *Threshold Limit Value (TLV)* of the aerosol. Concentration is expressed either as particles/cm^3 or as millions of particles per cubic foot (mppcf). In some countries, however, standards are based on levels which are not to be exceeded—so-called *Maximum Allowable Concentrations (MAC)*. Permissible levels of both TLVs and MACs are based upon the type of dose response for each substance in man and animals which is used as an index (Hatch, 1972).

In the UK and the USA TLVs for the majority of airborne contaminants are related to the time that a worker is exposed to a particular risk and they refer to *time-weighted* concentrations during a seven or eight hour 'working day' and a five day (40 hour) 'working week'. In some countries—for example, the USSR—continuous exposure is measured. Although time-weighted average concentration is the most practical method of controlling most hazardous materials, substances which have a rapid action (for example, toluene diisocyanate and nitrogen dioxide, *see* Chapters 12 and 13) are best controlled by a *Ceiling Limit* (MAC) which should not be exceeded at any time.

Threshold limit values of all hazardous substances are reviewed and published annually by the Committee on Threshold Standards of the American Conference of Governmental Industrial Hygienists (ACGIH) and by the Department of Employment and Productivity in the UK as 'Technical Data Notes', but other countries also issue their own standards referring either to general lists of substances or to individual materials. The International Labour Office publishes TLVs employed in most countries of the world. Recommendations are also made by the American National Institute of Occupational Safety and Health and the British Occupational Hygiene Society.

It should be understood that a TLV does not indicate a definitive dust concentration to which it is *safe* to be exposed, and above which it is not. Obviously, freedom from the effects of a dangerous dust is certain only when it is absent from the environment. But the TLV assumes that, if individual hazardous materials can be prevented from exceeding a certain empirically determined level at any time, then below this level it is unlikely to cause disease during the period of a working life; in the majority of cases this has been well borne out by experience. As far as possible concentrations of dusts or fumes should at all times be kept below their TLVs.

The question arises as to whether it is preferable to measure average or 'peak' aerosol concentrations in the worker's environment. Whereas average concentrations can be readily related to the period of a working life there is much evidence to suggest that 'peak' measurements of some substances (especialy certain harmful dusts) are more significantly correlated with risk to health. For example, it has been urged (Roach, 1966) that sampling time should be related to the biological half-life in the body of the sampled particles so that in the case of soluble or radioactive particles, absolute—not average—'peak' values should be determined. Nevertheless, because cumulative deposition appears to be roughly the same with both high and low concentrations of environmental dust when the values of 'dust concentration × time of exposure' are similar (Klosterkötter, 1968), determination of average exposure should give a satisfactory indication of cumulative deposition (and hence the risk of certain types of pneumoconiosis) which may be expected to occur in the lungs.

The naturally-occurring gases radon and thoron constitute an important potential hazard to the lungs; radon and radon 'daughters' are found in uranium mines, some other types of mine and, occasionally, in tunnelling works (*see* Chapter 14). Decay of the unstable atoms of these gases releases α particles and the remaining decay product, which has the property of a solid, may adhere to aerosol (dust) particles. Radioactive aerosols are the most hazardous of all and they have the lowest concentration which can be tolerated indefinitely.

Alpha particles have low energy and when deposited in the airways or alveoli are absorbed within a few micrometres distance from their source; that is, in neighbouring cells. Gamma particles possess much greater energy and so pass through the tissues to leave the body, and hence are less damaging to cells. The TLV for α-emitters, therefore, is lower than that for γ-emitters.

Of non-radioactive aerosols beryllium is the most toxic and other substances fall into a scale of decreasing toxicity.

Emergency exposure limits have been proposed for the calculation of risks to rescue workers and the neighbouring population which might result from slight exposure to large scale air pollution: for example, accidents in transport and dangerous chemicals (Zielhuis, 1970).

Inert substances

Particles of inert substances are sometimes referred to as 'Nuisance Particulates' mainly because they may have an irritant effect in the upper respiratory tract. They do not cause fibrotic pneumoconiosis, although this may occur if fibrogenic or radioactive contaminants are associated with them. Some inorganic examples are chalk, Portland cement, corundum, emery, gypsum, iron oxides, limestone and silicon carbide.

The TLVs of most of the aerosols, gases and fumes discussed in this book are not, however, given because in many cases they are under frequent review and they are of limited interest to most physicians.

SAMPLING

The frequency of sampling required differs according to whether the potential hazard is subject to a 'ceiling' or 'time-weighted' limit: a single short period of sampling is sufficient in the former case, but a number of samples taken throughout the period of the work shift are necessary in the latter.

The underlying principles of instruments for sampling atmospheric dusts varies according to the nature and TLV of the dust to be analysed; whether particle counting (which is usually size-selective) or compositional analysis is required; the siting of instruments in the work environment, and the duration of sampling planned. Hence, there are many different types of instrument, both portable and static. Samples may be obtained from the workers' immediate environment ('breathing zone'), from the locality of the work process ('source zone'), or from the general factory atmosphere ('background zone'); and they can be either of very brief duration and taken at random ('grab samples') or of prolonged duration.

Identification of radioactive gases and aerosols and the assessment of the degree of their radioactivity requires instruments of special design to separate dust particles, radioactive particles and gas.

The prospective as well as the immediate value of analyses of sampling data is apparent in the protection afforded the worker, in the identification of faulty methods of dust suppression and in computation of the worker's possible total exposure to a specific dust hazard over his working life.

The complexities of sampling instruments and sampling strategy and of the details of the many techniques for protecting the worker and for the disposal of dusts and fumes are beyond the scope and competence of this book. A comprehensive account of sampling instruments is given by the American Conference of Government Industrial Hygienists (1977). (*See also* Schilling, 1981.)

PROTECTION

The basic principles of protection can be briefly summarized.

(1) Substitution of the hazardous material by another without hazard, or a modification of the process designed to render the material innocuous. If neither of these is possible one or more of the following is employed.
(2) Complete enclosure of the process from the work atmosphere.
(3) Partial enclosure of the process with exhaust ventilation applied locally and to the 'background' air of the factory.
(4) High-velocity exhaust ventilation applied to the source of fume and dust.
(5) Suppression of dust by wet processes.
(6) Protective clothing and respirators. Respirators are, however, a last line of defence and, for the most part, unsatisfactory in that their use depends upon workers' cooperation. The protection given by some designs is inadequate.
(7) Good factory 'housekeeping' to prevent, by appropriate cleaning and disposal methods, accumulation of dust about workrooms and its dispersal in the atmosphere.
(8) Efficient storage and transport methods of dangerous materials (for example, asbestos and chlorine) so that accidental spilling and leakage does not occur.
(9) Controlled disposal of potentially dangerous waste substances.

REFERENCES

Albert, R. E. and Lippmann, M. (1972). Factors influencing dust retention in the pulmonary parenchyma. *Ann. N.Y. Acad. Sci.* **200**, 37–45

Albert, R. E., Lippmann, M. and Briscoe, W. (1969). The characteristics of bronchial clearance in humans and the effects of cigarette smoking. *Archs envir. Hlth* **18**, 738–755

Albert, R. E., Peterson, H. T., Bohning, D. E. and Lippmann, M. (1975). Short-term effects of cigarette smoking on bronchial clearance in humans. *Archs envir. Hlth* **30**, 361–367

Altshuler, B., Palmes, E. D. and Nelson, D. (1967). Regional aerosol deposition in the human respiratory tract. In *Inhaled Particles and Vapours*, Vol. 2, edited by C. N. Davies, pp. 323–355. Oxford; Pergamon

American Conference of Government Industrial Hygienists (1977). *Air Sampling Instruments Manual*, 5th edition, Cincinnati; ACGIH

Angus, G. E. and Thurlbeck, W. M. (1972). Number of alveoli in the human lung. *J. appl. Phys.* **32**, 483–485

Booker, D. V., Chamberlain, A. C., Rundo, J., Muir, D. C. F. and Thomson, M. L. (1967). Elimination of 5 μ particles from the human lung. *Nature, Lond.* **215**, 30–33

Bowden, D. H. (1971). The alveolar macrophage. In *Current Topics in Pathology*, edited by H. W. Altmann *et al.*, pp. 1–36. Berlin, Heidelberg, New York; Springer-Verlag

Bowden, D. H. (1976). The pulmonary macrophage. *Envir. Hlth Perspect.* **16**, 55–60

Cartwright, J. (1967). Airborne dust in coal miners: the particle-size—selection characteristics of the lung and the desirable characteristics of dust sampling instruments. In *Inhaled Particles and Vapours*, Vol. 2, edited by C. N. Davies, pp. 393–406. Oxford; Pergamon

Davies, C. N. (1974). Deposition of inhaled particles in man. *Chem. Ind. (June)* 441–444

Davies, C. N. (1979). Personal communication

Davies, C. N., Heyder, J. and Subba Ramu, M. C. (1972). Breathing of half-micron aerosols 1. experimental. *J. appl. Physiol.* **32**, 591–600

Davies, C. N., Lever, M. J. and Rothenberg, S. J. (1977). Experimental studies of the deposition of particles in the human lungs. In *Inhaled Particles IV*, edited by W. H. Walton, pp. 151–160. Oxford; Pergamon Press

Gross, P. and Westwick, M. (1954). The permeability of lung parenchyma to particulate matter. *Am. J. Path.* **30**, 195–213

Hapke, E. J. and Pederson, H. J. (1968). Cytoplasmic activity in Type 1 pulmonary epithelial cells induced by macroaggregated albumin. *Science* **161**, 380–382

Harris, R. L., Jr. and Timbrell, V. (1977). the influence of fibre shape in lung deposition—mathematical estimates. In *Inhaled Particles IV*, edited by W. H. Walton, pp. 75–88. Oxford, New York, Toronto, Sydney; Pergamon Press

Hatch, T. F. (1972). Permissable levels of exposure to hazardous agents in industry. *J. occup. Med.* **14**, 134–137

Heppleston, A. G. and Young, A. E. (1973). Uptake of inert particulate matter by alveolar cells: an ultrastructural study. *J. Path.* **111**, 159–164

Heyder, J., Gebhart, J., Heigwer, G., Roth, C. and Stahlhofen, W. (1973). Experimental studies of the total deposition of aerosol particles in the human respiratory tract. *J. aerosol. Sci.* **4**, 191–208

Hoffman, R. A. and Billingham, J. (1975). Effect of altered G levels on deposition of particulates in the human respiratory tract. *J. appl. Physiol.* **38**, 955–960

Kennedy, J. R. and Elliott, A. M. (1970). Cigarette smoke: the effect of residue on mitochondrial structures. *Science* **168**, 1097–1098

Kilburn, K. H. (1968). A hypothesis for pulmonary clearance and its implications. *Am. Rev. resp. Dis.* **98**, 449–463

Klosterkötter, W. (1968). Pneumoconiosis of coalworkers: results, problems and practical consequences of recent research. In *Pneumoconiosis*. Report on a Symposium at Katowice, pp. 99–109. Copenhagen; World Health Organization

Klosterkötter, W. and Bünemann, G. (1961). Animal experiments on the elimination of inhaled dust. In *Inhaled Particles and Vapours*, Vol. 1, edited by C. N. Davies, pp. 327–341. Oxford; Pergamon

Lapp, N. L., Hankinson, J. L., Amandus, H. and Palmes, E. D. (1975). Variability in the size of airspaces in normal human lungs as estimated by aerosols. *Thorax* **30**, 293–299

Lauweryns, J. M. and Baert, J. H. (1977). Alveolar clearance and the role of the pulmonary lymphatics. *Am. Rev. resp. Dis.* **115**, 625–683

Lawrie, W. B. (1967). Some aspects of dust, dust sampling, the interpretation of results, and an approach to the methods of suppressing dust clouds. In *Course on Dust Prevention in Industry*, pp. 4–45. Occ. Safety and Hlth Ser. No. 8. Geneva; ILO

Lehman, G. (1935). The dust filtering efficiency of the human nose and its significance in the causation of silicosis. *J. ind. Hyg.* **17**, 37–40

Leiteritz, H., Embrodt, H. J. and Klosterkötter, W. (1967). Grain sizes and mineral content of lung dust of coal miners compared with mine dusts. In *Inhaled Particles and Vapours*, Vol. 2, edited by C. N. Davies, pp. 381–390. Oxford; Pergamon

Lippmann, M. and Albert, R. E. (1969). The effect of particle size on the regional deposition of inhaled aerosols in the human respiratory tract. *Am. ind. Hyg. Ass. J.* **30**, 257–275

Lippmann, M., Albert, R. E. and Peterson, H. T. (1971). The regional deposition of inhaled aerosols in man. In *Inhaled Particles III*, edited by W. H. Walton, pp. 105–120. Woking; Unwin

Milic-Emili, J., Henderson, J. A. M. and Kaneko, H. (1968). Regional distribution of pulmonary ventilation. In *Form and Function in the Human Lung*, edited by G. Cumming and L. B. Hunt, pp. 66–75. London; Livingstone

Muir, D. C. F. and Davies, C. N. (1967). The deposition of 0.5 μ diameter aerosols in the lungs of Man. *Ann. occup. Hyg.* **3**, 161–173

Nagelschmidt, G., Nelson, E. S., King, E. J., Attygalle, D. and Yoganathan, M. (1967). The recovery of quartz and other minerals from the lungs of rats; a study in experimental silicosis. *Archs ind. Hlth* **16**, 188–202

Pavia, D., Thomson, M. L., Clarke, S. W. and Shannon, H. S. (1977). Effect of lung function and mode of inhalation on penetration of aerosol into the human lung. *Thorax* **32**, 194–197

Pavia, D., Thomson, M. L. and Pocock, S. J. (1971). Evidence of temporary slowing of mucociliary clearance in the lung caused by tobacco smoking. *Nature* **231**, 325–326

Proctor, D. F. (1977). The upper airways. I Nasal physiology and defence of the lungs. *Am. Rev. resp. Dis.* **115**, 97–129

Proctor, D. F., Anderson, I., Lundqvist, G. and Swift, D. L. (1973). Nasal mucociliary function and indoor climate. *J. occup. Med.* **15**, 169–174

Proctor, D. F., Swift, D. L. Quinlan, M., Salmon, S., Takagi, Y. and Evering, S. (1969). The nose and man's atmospheric environment. *Archs envir. Hlth* **18**, 671–680

Roach, S. A. (1966). A more rational basis for air sampling programmes. *Am. ind. Hyg. Ass. J.* **27**, 1–12

Salman, S., Proctor, D. F., Swift, D. L. and Evering, S. A. (1971). Nasal resistance: Description of a method and effect of temperature and humidity changes. *Ann. otolar.* **80**, 736–743

Sanchis, J., Dolovich, M., Chalmers, R. and Newhouse, M. T. (1971). Regional distribution and lung clearance mechanisms in smokers and non-smokers. In *Inhaled Particles III*, edited by W. H. Walton, pp. 183–188. Woking; Unwin

Sanders, C. L., Jackson, T. A., Adee, R. R., Powers, G. J. and Wehner, A. P. (1971). Distribution of inhaled metal oxide particles in pulmonary alveoli. *Archs intern. Med.* **127**, 1085–1089

Schilling, R. S. F. (1981). *Occupational Health Practice*, 2nd edn. London; Butterworths

Spencer, H. (1968). Chronic interstitial pneumonia. In *The Lung*, edited by A. A. Liebow and D. E. Smith, pp. 134–150. Baltimore; Williams and Wilkins

Stirling, C. and Patrick, G. (1980). The localisation of particles retained in the trachea of the rat. *J. Pathol.* **131**, 309–320

Task Group on Lung Dynamics. (1966). Deposition and retention models for internal dosimetry of the human respiratory tract. *Hlth Phys.* **12**, 173–207

Thomson, M. L. and Pavia, D. (1974). Particle penetration and clearance in the human lung. *Archs envir. Hlth* **29**, 214–219

Thomson, M. L. and Short, M. D. (1969). Mucociliary function in health, chronic obstructive airway disease, and asbestosis. *J. appl. Physiol.* **26**, 535–539

Thurlbeck, W. M. and Haines, J. R. (1975). Bronchial dimensions and stature. *Am. Rev. resp. Dis.* **112**, 142–145

Timbrell, V. (1970). The inhalation of fibres. In *Pneumoconiosis. Proceedings of the International Conference, Johannesburg, 1969*, edited by H. A. Shapiro, pp. 3–9. London and Capetown; Oxford University Press

Timbrell, V., Pooley, F. D. and Wagner, J. C. (1970). Characteristics of respirable asbestos fibres. In *Pneumoconiosis. Proceedings of the International Conference, Johannesburg, 1969*, edited by H. A. Shapiro, pp. 120–125. London and Capetown; Oxford University Press

United States Occupational Safety and Health Administration (1974). Field Memorandum. No. 74–92. Washington, D.C.; Dept. of Labor

Walton, W. H. and Hamilton, R. J. (1972). The measurement of airborne dust. In *Medicine in the Mining Industries*, edited by J. M. Rogan, pp. 145–165. London; Heinemann

West, J. B. (1961). Observations on gas flow in the human bronchial tree. In *Inhaled Particles and Vapours*. Vol. 1, edited by C. N. Davies, pp. 3–7. Oxford; Pergamon

Zielhuis, R. L. (1970). Tentative emergency exposure limits for sulphur dioxide, sulphuric acid, chlorine and phosgene. *Ann. occup. Hyg.* **13**, 171–176

4 Fundamentals of Pathogenesis and Pathology

INTRODUCTION

There are a limited number of ways in which the lungs may react to foreign agents depending to a large extent upon their nature and properties. Toxic gases and fumes may cause acute haemorrhagic tracheobronchitis and bronchiolitis, pulmonary oedema, haemorrhagic pneumonitis and destruction of alveolar epithelium. Dusts provoke reactions which range from a trivial local aggregation of cells at one end of the scale to striking and often progressive collagenous fibrosis or widespread, but resolvable, cell accumulations or granulomas at the other (*see Table 1.1*, p. 2). Some substances in all these categories may be capable of inducing asthma. The character and severity of reactions are determined by at least three basic factors.

(1) The nature and properties of the dust.
(2) The amount of dust retained in the lungs and the duration of exposure to it; that is, a dose × time relationship.
(3) Individual idiosyncrasy and immunological reactivity of the subject.

Each of these poses complex problems. Whereas the identity and physicochemical characteristics of inhaled dusts are usually known, the reasons for the differing patterns of events which follow their retention are not completely understood. In a general way it can be said that the extent of disease likely to be produced by a dust of fibrogenic potential is proportional to the amount of dust and the period of time over which it is inhaled; a large dose over a short period and a small dose continued over a long period are both liable to cause disease.

The possible end-results of reactions caused by different dusts have been broadly distinguished in Chapter 1. Inorganic (mineral) dusts either have or do not have an intrinsic fibrogenic potential and organic dusts may be fibrogenic in the lungs of hypersensitive subjects (*see* Chapter 11). Obviously, a simple, all-embracing concept of the pathogenesis of the different types of pneumoconiosis and other occupational diseases cannot be expected because, on the one hand, the composition of inhaled and potentially noxious substances, and, on the other, the reaction of the body to them, differ both qualitatively and quantitatively.

In the encounter between the lungs and extraneous agents, cell components of the gas exchanging regions of the lungs (including alveolar macrophages and Type I and II cells) are crucial, not only because some have the capacity to remove dust particles, but because of their active role in pathogenesis. Immunological reactions are important in disease caused by inhaled fungal spores and a wide variety of other foreign proteins, and may also be identified in association with some cases of inorganic pneumoconiosis—an association which, however, is not yet fully understood. For these reasons and also because of the rapidity of developments in this field a brief outline of basic cytological and immunological principles is justified.

Non-fibrotic pneumoconiosis is described as 'inert', or 'benign', because it does not damage the structure of the lungs nor cause progressive disease as may pneumoconiosis due to a fibrogenic dust.

RELEVANT CYTOLOGICAL FEATURES

The different types of pulmonary cells have been enumerated in Chapter 1.

Macrophages

The intracellular lysosomal system of these cells plays a fundamental role in pathogenesis (*Figure 4.1a*).

Lysosomes (lytic bodies) belong to the group of minute units known collectively as 'organelles' which, among their other activities, produce catalytic enzymes, ribonucleic acid and the structural protein precursors of tropocollagen (*see* p. 63). They are also referred to as *storage granules* or *primary lysosomes*, and are tiny vesicles bounded by membranes of lipoprotein.

Macrophages ingest foreign materials (such as dust particles) by invagination of their boundary membrane (phagocytosis) and the vesicle formed is known as a *phagosome (Figure 4.1b)*. Primary lysosomes then migrate on to its wall and discharge their enzymes within; it is now referred to as a *secondary lysosome* or *digestive vacuole*. These events resemble those of a rudimentary intestinal tract in that the contents are ingested, digested and the residue subsequently extruded from the cell. But in other instances digestion of particles is incomplete and they remain within the cell as *residual bodies*. Normally the membrane of secondary lysosomes remains intact until the contents are extruded from the cell and escape of enzymes into the cytoplasm, which would result in autodigestion and consequent cell death, does not occur.

Ingested foreign particles may be innocuous to the membranes of secondary lysosomes in which case they either pass harmlessly through the cell or remain within it as 'residual bodies' until the natural death of the cell releases

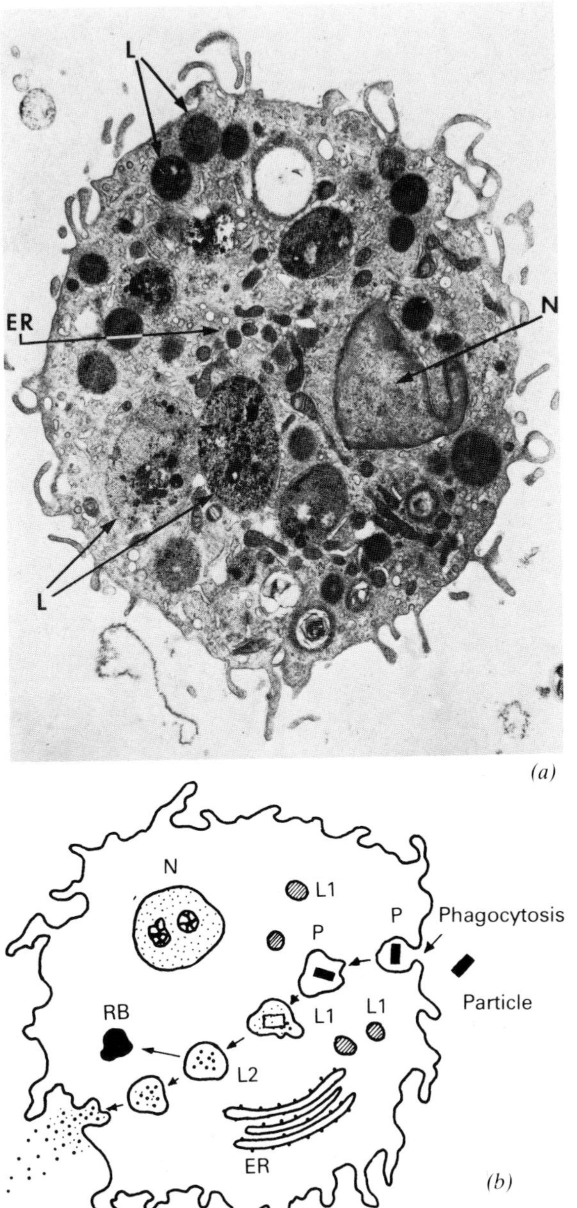

Figure 4.1 (a) Internal structure of a human alveolar macrophage from lung lavage fluid. The arrows indicate numerous lysosomes in the cytoplasm (L), endoplasmic reticulin (ER) and the nucleus (N). Magnification × 6800. (By courtesy of Miss Ann Dewar.) (See also *Figure 1.4*). *(b) Simplified diagram of an alveolar macrophage ingesting a particle.* (See also Figures 1.4 *and* 4.4.) *A primary lysosome (L1) is attached to phagosome (P) and is discharging its enzymes into it. The secondary lysosome (L2) either forms a residual body (RB) or discharges its contents outside the cell. (ER, endoplasmic reticulum with ribosomes; N, nucleus)*

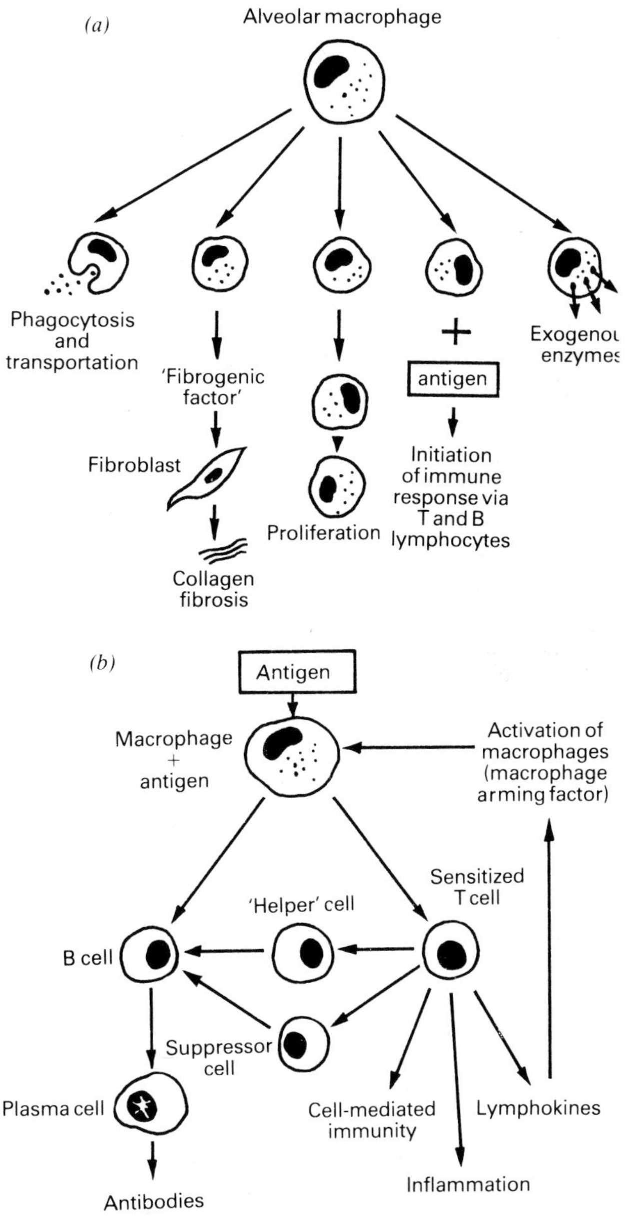

Figure 4.2 (a) Scheme of the activities of alveolar macrophages. (b) Scheme of interrelationships between macrophages, and T and B lymphocytes in cell-mediated and humoral immune responses

these bodies and they are engulfed once again by other cells or survive as fragmentary extracellular 'residual bodies'. But if they have noxious properties (such as quartz possesses in high degree) the membrane structure is damaged and the secondary lysosome ruptures, releasing its enzymes into the cytoplasm. Death and disruption of the cell then follow and the released particles are taken up again by other cells and the cycle repeated.

Alveolar macrophages play a central role in pulmonary affairs (*see* Chapter 1). Apart from their scavenging and carrying extraneous particulates out of the lungs or (possibly) into their alveolar walls, possessing membrane receptors for complement (Reynolds *et al.*, 1975), processing particulate antigens which stimulate T lymphocyte activity and, in turn, being activated by these cells (*see* next section) they probably release fibrogenic factors following ingestion of certain minerals (for example, free silica). Their phagocytic properties are depressed by a variety of extrinsic and intrinsic agents, in particular by tobacco smoke (Green *et al.*, 1977). By contrast their content of the proteolytic enzymes protease and elastase-like esterase is greatly increased in cigarette smokers compared with non-smokers (Harris *et al.*, 1975). Hence it is possible that uncontrolled release of these enzymes in the case of α_1-antitrypsin deficiency causes alveolar wall breakdown and emphysema and explains the rapid rate of development of emphysema in some smokers (*Figure 4.2a*) (*see* Chapter 1).

Lymphocytes

There are two main groups of these cells: thymus dependent lymphocytes (T cells) and peripheral lymphoid tissue dependent lymphocytes (B cells). They are responsible for all aspects of specific immunity (*see* next section): the T cells for cell-mediated immunity and the B cells for humoral immunity, their reaction with antigens operating via different mechanisms. Interaction of antigen with antigen-specific T cells results in a number of effects. These cells acquire cytotoxicity for other cells carrying the antigen and release soluble mediating substances known as *lymphokines*. Lymphokines possess a variety of important properties: inhibition of the migration of macrophages (*Migration Inhibition Factor—MIF*) which confines them to the site of reaction and activates their lysosomal systems. Lymphocyte transformation and increased mitosis in other 'non-sensitized' lymphocytes, increase of capillary permeability and the tissue response of delayed (Type IV) hypersensitivity may occur. In addition, T cells are responsible for the release of a 'specific macrophage arming factor' which empowers macrophages to immobilize cells carrying the specific antigen (*Figure 4.2b*).

There are also small populations of cells which do not possess the properties of T or B lymphocytes and are known as 'null' cells.

Although T and B cells have different immunological functions either group may augment or suppress the activity of the other. For example: T cells act as 'helper cells' and influence the differentiation of B cells into antibody-producing plasma cells, but they also act as 'suppressor' cells which inhibit antibody production. Thus, antibodies produced by B cells against an antigen may enhance or impair T cell activity to the same antigen. Reduction in the T cell population which occurs with age may, on the one hand, permit uncontrolled production of circulating antibody by B cells against the tissues of a variety of organs or, on the other hand, depress the stimulus to antibody production by B cells against new antigens (Stobo and Tomasi, 1975). Imbalance of the functional interrelationships between the two cell populations, therefore, may well have an important influence on the development and the mode of evolution of lung disease due to exogenous agents with increasing age.

Plasma cells

These cells and their precursors, plasmablasts, are produced by the transformation of B cells (*Figure 4.2b*). Plasma cells contain an abundance of *ribosomes* (organelles) related to endoplasmic reticulum, which synthesize circulating antibodies as well as other proteins and are, therefore, the chief source of these antibodies (Nossal, 1964). Large collections of these cells in a lesion imply significant local antibody activity.

Plasma and other cells containing IgA are present in much larger numbers than those containing IgG or IgE (*see* p. 57) in the lobar bronchi of smokers compared with non-smokers, but not in the peripheral parts of the lungs (Soutar, 1976).

Lymphocytes, macrophages and plasma cells are, therefore, involved in the various complex immunological reactions of health and disease. These reactions and their relevance to occupational disorders of the lungs are summarized briefly in the next section.

Eosinophils

These are associated with immediate, Type I, IgE (reagin) mediated allergic reactions though their role is uncertain. There is some evidence that they suppress or terminate these reactions by releasing a histamine inhibiting substance. They have phagocytic properties, possess surface receptors for IgG and complement components C3b and C4, and are altered chemotactically by the C5a component and by mast cell- and basophil cell-derived chemotactic factors. Tissue eosinophilia, therefore, may be related to mast cell activity and to complement-dependent reactions involving either the classic or alternative pathways (Turner-Warwick, 1978) (*see* next section).

Fibroblasts

Organelles in these cells elaborate *tropocollagen* the elementary unit from which all collagen structures are synthesized (*see* section on Reticulin and Collagen).

IMMUNOLOGICAL CONSIDERATIONS

It is now evident that immunological reactions underlie certain types of occupational lung disease either directly and causally as, for example, in the extrinsic allergic group of disorders (*see* Chapters 11 and 12), or indirectly as in some cases of diffuse interstitial fibrosis and the 'rheumatoid' variants of pneumoconiosis (*see* later in this chapter). The reader will find the compact review of the immunology of respiratory disease by Turner-Warwick (1978) of great help in this field.

TERMS AND CONCEPTS

On entering the body, micro-organisms and some alien substances act as *antigens* (or *allergens*) and stimulate the production of specific immunoglobulins—*antibodies*—which react with them in several different ways and play a prime role in the protection of the host from foreign invasion. The antigen–antibody reaction is commonly termed the *immune reaction* (*immunis* = free, exempt) because it frees the body of noxious agents. But although many antibodies are protective in that they aid the neutralization or destruction of foreign antigens, others react with antigens in such a way as to give rise to hypersensitivity diseases such as hay fever, eczema and asthma; and yet others play no active role in the destruction of antigen nor in pathogenesis, and are merely 'markers' of the underlying events. For this reason the term *allergy* ἄλλοσ = other; ἔργον = work), coined originally by von Pirquet to indicate an increased tissue response dependent upon an interaction between antigens and antibodies and including reactions which are harmful as well as protective to the host, appears preferable to 'immune reaction'.

Antibodies are γ-globulins which have been classified by electrophoretic, ultracentrifuge and immunological methods. They are referred to as *immunoglobulins* (Ig) and are categorized as follows:

(1) *IgG* is the major immunoglobulin in man accounting for 800 to 1600 mg/ml of the total serum immunoglobulins. It has four subclasses, three of which fix complement. *Complement,* incidentally, consists of an enzyme system of serum proteins which are essential for certain antigen-antibody reactions. It has nine components designated as C1 to C9 (*see* p. 58).
(2) *IgA* contributes 150 to 420 mg/ml to total serum immunoglobulins. It is the major Ig component of secretions in the respiratory tract, though IgG is also found in smaller amounts, and is increased in smokers due, probably, to augmentation of the B lymphocyte population (Sharp, Warr and Martin, 1973).
(3) *IgM* accounts for 50 to 200 mg/ml of total serum immunoglobulins and fixes complement.
(4) *IgE* constitutes only 17 to 450 ng/ml of the total immunoglobulins. It is intimately associated with anaphylactic or reaginic antibody activity (*see* next section).
(5) *IgD,* which has some of the properties of IgG but is incompletely defined, accounts for 0 to 0.4 mg/ml.

(These values are those of normal European adults.)

An antigen provokes appropriate cells to manufacture and release antibody. But antigen is not always of extrinsic origin and, under certain circumstances, the body's own cellular components may provoke the production of antibodies. Antigens, whether extrinsic or 'intrinsic', do not necessarily *react* with antibody and they may do no more than stimulate its production. Under normal circumstances antibodies are not directed against the body's own cells and proteins which are 'recognized' as 'self'; that is, their antigenic potential is tolerated or ignored. But under abnormal conditions antibodies may be directed against 'self' cells or proteins resulting in an *auto-allergic* reaction; the reacting antibodies are then referred to as *auto-antibodies*. There are various hypotheses to explain the underlying mechanism of auto-immune reactions; one of these is that the body's tolerance of its own antigens fails. This presumed failure of *antigen* (or *immune*) tolerance may be causally related to at least some of the manifestations of so-called auto-immune diseases, and it appears likely that it may be involved in the pathogenesis of some forms of pneumoconiosis.

There are two fundamental modes of allergic (or immune) reaction:

(1) *Antibody-mediated immunity* In response to antigen antibody globulins are produced by plasma cells and circulate freely in body fluids and, on reacting with antigen, may produce tissue damage in a variety of ways. IgA-containing plasma cells are found in large numbers in the lymphoid tissue of the upper respiratory tract (Tomasi *et al.*, 1965).
(2) *Specific cell-mediated immunity* This is determined primarily by T lymphocyte activity, the resulting response being referred to as *'delayed hypersensitivity'*, and is exemplified by the tuberculin reaction against proteins of the tubercle bacillus.

ALLERGIC (IMMUNE REACTIONS) WITH TISSUE DAMAGING POTENTIAL

Four fundamental types of tissue damaging reaction are recognized (Gell, Coombs and Lachmann, 1975). However, it is important to bear in mind that, although each reaction type has its characteristic features, different types may either occur together or independently. The classification, therefore, is based on initiating events only (Coombs, 1974).

Immediate, anaphylactic and reagin-dependent reaction (Type I)

IgE antibody (often known as *reaginic antibody*) attaches itself to mast and basophil cells for a period of days or weeks and on contact with antigen causes rapid release of pharmacologically active mediators (*anaphylatoxins*) such as histamine, slow reacting substance A and various plasma kinins which, in turn, are responsible for the clinical manifestations of urticaria, hay fever and 'extrinsic' asthma. These are 'immediate' reactions.

It is customary to use the terms *atopy* or *atopic status* to denote a constitutional or hereditary tendency to the development of immediate hypersensitivity states—for example, asthma. However, because 'extrinsic' asthma may be caused by a different reaction (Type III) and Type I reactions may, in some instances, be mediated by IgG short-term sensitizing antibody (STS) and not by IgE (Parish, 1970), it has been suggested that 'atopy' should be confined to the immunological reactivity of the allergic subject in whom reaginic antibody is readily produced in response to common allergens in the environment (Pepys, 1975). But this reactivity, it must be remembered, does not necessarily correlate with clinical symptoms.

Prick skin tests using extracts of allergens are an important means of identifying the responsible allergen or allergens, and positive responses correlate well with the presence of specific IgE in the serum (Stenius *et al.*, 1971). These and other clinical tests which are employed to indicate the types of immune responses present in the patient are discussed later.

Cytolytic or cytotoxic reaction (Type II)

This indicates immunological reactions where antibody reacts with antigen which is either a natural constituent of tissue not recognized by the body as 'self' (that is, a *complete antigen*) or is formed by *haptens* which are protein-free chemicals of low molecular weight which are capable of binding on to cell or other body protein to form an antigen complex. Haptens, therefore, may also be referred to as *incomplete antigens*. IgG and IgM antibodies have both been implicated and, in many cases, complement is also involved in the destruction of target cells or tissues.

Examples of Type II responses are blood transfusion reactions, drug induced purpura and haemolytic anaemia; and immunoglobulins and complement have been demonstrated in the basement membrane of alveoli and the glomeruli of the kidneys in cases of Goodpasture's syndrome (that is, glomerulonephritis with lung haemorrhage and haemoptysis), and basement membrane antibodies present in the serum have been shown to react with lung and kidney. Some evidence has been offered that circulating lung-reactive antibodies—apparently of IgA class—are present in a variety of lung diseases and may have pathogenic significance (Burrell, Wallace and Andrews, 1964; Burrell *et al.*, 1966; Burrell *et al.*, 1974), but this has not been generally confirmed. The problem is referred to again under *Lung Reactive Antibodies* (p. 61).

Immune complex (Arthus Type) reaction (Type III)

Circulating precipitating antibodies (*precipitins*), which are commonly present in man indicating immunological evidence of exposure to particular allergens, react with antigen. The nature of this reaction is determined by the relative amounts of antigen and antibody involved, the concentrations of antigen being critical. The antibodies are of IgG and IgM classes. When antigen is present in tissue spaces microprecipitins are frequently formed in and around small blood vessels. In other circumstances an excess of *circulating* antigen is exposed to antibody so that soluble antigen–antibody complexes are precipitated in the walls of blood vessels. Hence, both types of reaction are associated with vasculitis.

Complement is crucial to the development of the Arthus reaction. It comprises an enzymatic system of serum proteins which plays either an essential or an intermediate part in a variety of biological reactions. It has nine components—denoted as C1 to C9—which react in different sequences according to the type of activity promoted. Activation of C3 appears to be the most significant part of the complement sequence and it is initiated by two different routes both of which give rise to C3 converting enzymes (C3 convertases) (Lachmann, 1975). The first of these routes, the *classic pathway of complement activation*, is promoted by antigen–antibody complexes which involve components C1, C4 and C2 and lead to the cleavage of C3 and the production of C3b fragment, which is initially chemotactic for polymorphonuclear leucocytes and has the capacity to cause macrophages to liberate tissue damaging enzymes. The second or *alternative pathway of complement activation* also results in the generation of C3b but involves components of the properdin enzyme system without antigen–antibody intervention and is capable of being activated by many substances such as mouldy hay dust, thermophilic actinomycetes, zymosan (a constituent of yeast cell walls), Gram negative bacteria and some inorganic substances. Hence, the Type III reaction can be initiated by either mode of activation but in the case of the classic pathway antibodies are involved whereas in that of the alternative pathway they are not. This is of particular importance in extrinsic allergic 'alveolitis' (*see* Chapter 11) and may be in other disorders of extrinsic origin.

The Arthus reaction occurs between four and 12 hours after introduction of antigen and lasts for about 24 to 36 hours; it is often referred to as a 'late' reaction. It apparently takes place in bronchial and peribronchial tissues, in alveolar walls and, probably, in the upper respiratory tract and plays an important part in the pathogenesis of the extrinsic allergic 'alveolitis' type of lung diseases following inhalation and, possibly, ingestion of foreign protein antigens (*see* Chapter 11), and in 'late' extrinsic asthma (*see* Chapter 12). In such cases the Arthus reaction can be produced in the patient's skin by intradermal injection of the antigen.

Type I, Type II and Type III reactions are all examples of antibody-mediated tissue responses.

Cell mediated reaction: delayed hypersensitivity (Type IV)

This reaction is mediated by specifically sensitized T lymphocytes and is entirely independent of circulating antibodies. Antigen-specific receptors on those cells react with antigen which is either freely dispersed or bound to other exogenous cells (for example, homografts) or to the subject's own cells. The reaction releases factors—referred to already on p. 56—which cause the pathological features of the lesions of delayed hypersensitivity. These lesions develop in 24 to 48 hours (earlier in highly sensitive individuals) and last for a few days.

Well known responsible antigens are tuberculin, histoplasmin, brucellin and a variety of viral antigens such as measles. Cell mediated immunity occurs in some cases of beryllium disease (*see* Chapter 10), in extrinsic allergic 'alveolitis' (*see* Chapter 11) and, probably, in the genesis of zirconium granulomas (*see* Chapter 6).

From the clinical point of view it is important to appreciate that an antigen may provoke more than one type of tissue-damaging immunological response.

Clinical identification of the allergic reaction types

It is convenient at this point to make brief mention of the techniques employed though their application is discussed further in the relevant places (Chapters 11 and 12).

(1) Prick skin tests

This is used to detect Type I reactions. Extracts of allergens are pricked superficially into the skin in such a manner as not to draw blood and, in relevantly sensitized individuals, result in an immediate weal and flare. The use of three or four common allergens is sufficient to identify most atopic subjects who, in the UK, number about 30 per cent of the population (Pepys, 1977). But the test cannot be used as the sole means of *certain* identification of clinical allergies. When it is negative a positive response can sometimes be obtained by injecting antigen intracutaneously—enough to raise a bleb. The reaction is inhibited by antihistamines but not by corticosteroids.

The intracutaneous route is also used to identify Type IV reactions which occur about 48 hours after injections.

(2) Intradermal tests

Type III reactions are detected by injection of antigen. An immediate reaction occurs followed by diffuse, painless, non-irritant swelling in six to eight hours. Biopsy of the lesion reveals perivascular cuffing by mononuclear or polymorphonuclear cells, and the presence of IgG and complement is identified by immunofluorescent techniques. It is suppressed by corticosteroids.

(3) Bronchial provocation tests (Pepys and Hutchcroft, 1974)

After a controlled dose of relevant allergen is inhaled an immediate but brief bronchoconstrictive response occurs in Type I reactions which can be measured by a disproportionate fall in FEV_1 compared with FVC values. It is reversed by isoprenaline and prevented by sodium cromoglycate or isoprenaline given before the test, but not by corticosteroids. A variety of chemical fumes, vapours and dusts can provoke immediate asthmatic reactions when inhaled and are similarly blocked by sodium cromoglycate but not by corticosteroids. However, this test cannot distinguish between an agent acting as a bronchial irritant or as an allergen (*see* Chapter 12).

Two forms of 'late' response can occur usually between four to eight hours after inhalation. The first is an asthmatic reaction with an associated fall in FEV_1 ('non-immediate asthma'). The second occurs in the peripheral gas-exchanging region of the lungs and is accompanied by a restrictive ventilatory defect and, in some cases, a fall in gas transfer; and by malaise, fever, leucocytosis and inspiratory crepitations. Small discrete opacities due to bronchiolo-alveolitis may appear in the chest radiograph if the challenge dose is high—an undesirable effect which should never be deliberately provoked (*see also* Chapter 11, p. 366).

Bronchial challenge tests are invaluable in the diagnosis of uncertain cases of extrinsic allergic bronchiolo-alveolitis and in identifying previously unrecognized causes of this disease or of occupational asthma (*see* Chapters 11 and 12). But it must be stressed that they should be done only under strict control in hospital conditions commencing with minute doses of the provocative agent and with the ready availability of appropriate drugs for reversal of a serious reaction.

(4) Lymphocyte function tests

These *in vitro* tests on blood lymphocytes are of proven value in the detection of delayed, Type IV, hypersensitivity (David, Lawrence and Thomas, 1964; David and Schlossman, 1968). They include:

(a) *Lymphocyte transformation test* In this test lymphocytes cultured in the presence of a mitogen, such as phytohaemagglutinin or of an antigen to which they are specifically primed, undergo blastogenic transformation.
(b) *Macrophage migration inhibition factor test (MIF)* This detects a factor which impairs the migration of macrophages and is produced when T lymphocytes are incubated with a priming antigen.

Auto-allergy (auto-immunity)

Because of the possibility that auto-allergy may play a part in the pathogenesis of some forms of pneumoconiosis this concept is briefly considered.

Antigen tolerance is established in a short period before and just after birth. This is exemplified experimentally by the effect of injecting bovine serum albumin as antigen into newborn rabbits which do not thereafter produce antibody to the same antigen injected in later life. In order to be tolerated, therefore, antigen must be in contact with the antibody-producing system at this crucial period, otherwise antibodies will be produced against it.

Alteration or denaturation of host antigen by chemical, physical or biological means, or the presence of foreign antigens which bear close structural resemblance to the host antigen, but are not identical with it, may weaken or destroy antigen tolerance. Similarly, complex antigens produced by the combination of host haptens with exogenous materials may have the same effect.

Tissue-damaging antibodies resulting from these changes are of two types (Hijmans *et al.*, 1961):

(1) those reacting with a specific tissue component of a particular organ or system of organs—*organ-specific antibodies.*
(2) those reacting with cellular components which are common to many organs—*non-organ-specific antibodies.*

Organ-specific antibodies are implicated in such disease as Hashimoto's thyroiditis (reacting with thyroglobulin) and pernicious anaemia (reacting with antigens of gastric parietal cells) but, although lung reactive antibodies have been demonstrated in various lung disorders (*see* p. 61), there is as yet no evidence that any involve organ-specific antigens.

Non-organ-specific antibodies are circulating antibodies which may be associated with a number of connective tissue disorders involving the lungs (for example, pleuro-pulmonary systemic lupus erythematosus, rheumatoid disease, systemic sclerosis and cryptogenic diffuse interstitial fibrosis) and with some types of fibrogenic pneumoconiosis—for example, silicosis and asbestosis. They are separable into two major groups: *antinuclear antibodies* and *rheumatoid factors.*

ANTINUCLEAR ANTIBODIES (ANA)

In systemic lupus erythematosus many different organs of the body are involved and antibodies are directed at a variety of cytoplasmic and nuclear antigens. The antigens in this and other diseases in which circulating ANAs are found are located in the nuclei of different cell types and the antibodies may be immunoglobulins of IgG, IgA or IgM class, and IgD and IgE have also been reported. The main methods of their detection are: immunofluorescent techniques for broad routine screening of ANA activity; and immunoprecipitation or radioimmunoassay tests for deoxyribonucleic acid (DNA)-binding antibodies. Unlike systemic lupus erythematosus in which ANAs detected by immunofluorescence are invariably present and in high titre, their prevalence and titres in the other diseases with which they are associated are lower and they have no diagnostic significance (*see Table 4.1*). It must be noted, however, that ANAs are found in low titres (1:10 and over) in about 5 per cent of normal men and women in the UK, and in titres of 1:16 or more in 2 per cent of men over 40 years of age (Beck, 1963); in elderly females the prevalence is higher and may reach about 20 per cent in those over 80.

The characteristics of ANAs in these various lung disorders differ considerably (*see Table 4.2*) suggesting that the stimulus to their formation and persistance is different and that their role in stimulating or increasing tissue damage is also likely to vary. And consonant with this is the fact that there are substantial differences in the early clinical and microscopical features of these diseases even though the end-stage appearances of diffuse interstitial fibrosis are often similar. Additional reasons for believing that ANAs are of specific origin are that they develop early in the course of disease and persist, and are not increased in such fibrotic disorders as sarcoidosis or chronic extrinsic allergic 'alveolitis' (*see Table 4.3*). The higher prevalence and different characteristics of ANAs in severe silicosis compared with asbestosis correlate with the fact that the *in vitro* cytotoxicity of quartz greatly exceeds that of asbestos (*see* later in this chapter). The presence of ANAs in the pneumoconioses is, however, unrelated to co-existent chronic bronchitis unless this is recurrent, severe and purulent (Hodson and Turner-Warwick, 1976).

There is experimental support for the concept that these antibodies are capable of intensifying some pre-existing pathological processes because the production of certain types of ANA has been shown to worsen inflammatory lesions in rats (Hughes and Rowell, 1970). There is reason to believe that this may occur in human disease, as immunofluorescence localized to nuclei of alveolar lining cells or intra-alveolar macrophages or both has been observed in patients with cryptogenic fibrosing 'alveolitis' (*see* p. 75 *et seq.*) all of whom had circulating ANAs (Turner-Warwick, Haslam and Weeks, 1971; Turner-Warwick, 1975). And the same class of ANA immunoglobulin has been found in the alveolar walls as in the serum of patients with cryptogenic diffuse pulmonary fibrosis (Nagaya, Elmore and Ford, 1973).

Table 4.1 Prevalence of ANA and RF in some 'Connective Tissue' Disorders of the Lung

Disorder	*Total no.*	*ANA*	*RF*	
		Prevalence %	*Total no.*	*Prevalence %*
Pleuropulmonary SLE	30	30(100%)	18	7(39%)
'Rheumatoid lung'	36	16(44%)	34	23(68%)
Systemic sclerosis with lung involvement	14	10(71%)	14	0(0%)
CFA	97	33(34%)	97	14(14%)
CFA (Kang *et al.*, 1973)	9	5(56%)	9	1(11%)

CFA = Cryptogenic fibrosing 'alveolitis'
(Data from Kang *et al.*, 1973 and Turner-Warwick, 1978)

RHEUMATOID FACTORS (RFs)

These are a group of circulating anti-IgG antibodies each of which possesses slightly different specificities for parts of the antigenic complex in the crystallizable fragments (Fc) of IgG molecules. Classic RFs, which are present in the

Table 4.2 Variable Characteristics of ANA in Different Lung Diseases

	SLE	*CFA*	*Asbestosis*	*Silicosis*
Age related	no	no	yes	no
Mean titres	1/80–1/160	1/20–1/40	1/20	1/20–1/40
Ig Type	mixed G/M/(A)	lone and mixed	especially M	especially G
Immunofluorescent pattern	diffuse	diffuse	diffuse	diffuse
Farr binding Ds DNA	23%	6%	0%	9%
Precipitins ss DNA	57%	36%	22%	41%
Complement fixing	39%	34%	0%	14%
Nucleoprotein antibody	61%	12%	7%	5%

CFA = Cryptogenic fibrosing 'alveolitis'
Ds DNA = Double stranded
ss DNA = Single stranded
Farr binding = Radioimmunoassay technique for measuring antibodies in absolute amounts
(Haslam, 1976)

Table 4.3 Prevalence of ANA and RF in some Fibrotic Pneumoconioses and Extrinsic Allergic Alveolitis

	Total no.	*ANA*	*Total no.*	*RF*
Silicosis (sandblasting)	39	17(44%)	40	3(8%)
Asbestosis	75	19(25%)	75	17(23%)
Asbestosis (Kang *et al.*, 1973)	32	11(34.4%)	32	8(25%)
Asbestos exposure (normal radiographs)	75	2(3%)	75	2(3%)
Coal pneumoconiosis (all categories)	109	19(17%)	71	5(7%)
Coal pneumoconiosis (Kang *et al.*, 1973)	31	8(25.8%)	31	2(6.5%)
Coal pneumoconiosis (Lippmann *et al.*, 1973)	156	53(34%)	53	9 (6%)
Extrinsic allergic 'alveolitis'	54	2(4%)	57	3(5%)

(Data from Kang *et al.*, 1973; Lippmann *et al.*, 1973; Turner-Warwick, 1978)

majority of patients with rheumatoid arthritis, are antibodies of the IgM class and are detected by their ability to agglutinate sheep or human red cells coated with a sub-agglutinating quantity of anti-erythrocyte IgG antibody raised in the rabbit. This is the principle of the sheep cell agglutination test (SCAT) or Rose–Waaler test, the human erythrocyte agglutination test (HEAT) and the differential agglutination test (DAT). Polystyrene or bentonite particles coated with human IgG form the basis of the latex fixation test (LFT) and the bentonite fixation test (BFT) which also detect RFs of IgM class and, although more sensitive, simpler and more convenient to use than the other tests, they are less specific. The titre levels at which these tests are customarily considered to be positive are 1:32 for the SCAT, 1:16 for the DAT and 1:20 for the LFT. However, as minor variations in technique influence the results, these should be regularly compared with standard sera of known potency (Anderson *et al.*, 1970).

Rheumatoid factors in SCAT titres of 1:32 or more are present in 1.6 to 5.4 per cent of men and women in normal random European populations (Ball and Lawrence, 1961) and, though their prevalence does not appear to increase with advancing age, titres in healthy individuals born before 1892 are, in general, higher than in those born after 1942 (Lawrence 1967). And there appears to be a genetic tendency—probably due to multiple additive genes—for multivalent RFs to occur in certain families, the members of which, with this trait, are more likely, than those without, to develop rheumatoid arthritis (Lawrence, 1973). This may have some bearing on the occurrence of 'rheumatoid' pneumoconiosis.

Apart from the strong association of RFs with rheumatoid arthritis these antibodies are found in a significant proportion of cases of other disorders such as systemic lupus erythematosus, systemic sclerosis, Sjögrens disease, lymphoproliferative disorders, diffuse interstitial pulmonary fibrosis, silicosis, coal pneumoconiosis and asbestosis but their activity is more restricted (*see Tables 4.1* and *4.3*). Why autologous IgG in individuals with these disorders is particularly immunogenic is not known but subtle structural differences between normal native and 'rheumatoid' native IgG molecules are probably sufficient to provoke antibody formation (Johnson and Faulk, 1976). The mechanisms by which such changes may be produced in some pneumoconioses is also not understood, nor is it apparent why they are not found in the chronic, fibrotic stage of extrinsic allergic 'alveolitis', when they can occur transiently in its acute stage and also sarcoidosis and tuberculosis. Evidently RFs arise as a result of a variety of different stimuli of uncertain nature. When administered to rabbits they have been shown to accentuate vascular injury in pre-existing granulomas (de Horatius and Williams, 1972) and it is possible that this occurs in human 'rheumatoid lung' (de Horatius, Abbruzzo and Williams, 1972); but, in general, there is no clear evidence that they participate in the genesis of lung disease in man.

It is interesting to compare the prevalence of RF in cryptogenic diffuse interstitial pulmonary fibrosis (fibrosing 'alveolitis') and asbestosis (*Tables 4.1* and *4.3*) with earlier observations that one in five patients (20 per cent) with diffuse interstitial pulmonary fibrosis have rheumatoid arthritis (Doctor and Snider, 1962) and, conversely, that among patients with rheumatoid arthritis 33 per cent have evidence of diffuse interstitial fibrosis whereas among those with osteoarthritis there is none (Popper, Boddonoff and Hughes, 1972).

Anti-IgG auto-antibodies of IgG class have also been identified in IgM RF positive and negative rheumatoid subjects and in a variety of other disorders but at present their clinical significance is not clear.

Although ANAs and RF are antibodies directed against different antigens they may be found together in one clinical disorder.

Pleural effusion and pulmonary nodules with or without necrosis and cavity formation (so-called 'necrobiotic' nodules) may occur in association with rheumatoid arthritis in individuals who have had no exposure to industrial dusts. The effusion is often characterized by an abnormally low glucose content which otherwise is only encountered in tuberculous effusions (Calnan *et al.*, 1951; Scadding, 1969). And nodules are histologically identical with rheumatoid subcutaneous nodules and have also been found in other viscera including the dura mater, tongue and pharynx (Maher, 1954; McInnes and Littman, 1977). It is important, therefore, that similar effusions and necrobiotic nodules may also occur independently or together in individuals with some types of pneumoconiosis (especially coal pneumoconiosis) associated with circulating RFs, often in the absence of arthropathy.

LUNG REACTIVE ANTIBODIES

The important question as to whether organ-specific antibodies arise in the pneumoconioses is, as yet, unresolved.

Both reticulin and collagen possess distinctive antigenic activity. Extracts of the reticulin component of human liver and renal cortex are antigenic in rabbits and give a characteristic immunofluorescent staining pattern with human antireticulin antibody (Pras *et al.*, 1974). Circulating antibodies to natural and denatured collagen occur in man although their true prevalence in health and disease remains to be clarified. Auto-antibodies against denatured collagen are present in some rheumatic and chronic disorders associated with collagen breakdown (for example, rheumatoid arthritis, systemic lupus erythematosus, Sjögren's disease, scleroderma and emphysema); and they have been found in rheumatoid synovial tissues and fluids (Holborow *et al.*, 1977).

It is interesting, therefore, that Burrell (1972) reported identifying antilung connective tissue antibodies in the IgA fractions of serum in a majority of coal miners with massive fibrosis and in the pneumoconiotic lesions themselves (*see* Chapter 8), the reactive antigen apparently being insoluble collagen in alveolar basement membrane (Hagedorn and Burrell, 1968). And other observations suggest that lung connective tissue antibodies could be involved in the pathogenesis of silicosis (Lewis and Burrell, 1976) (*see* Chapter 7). Furthermore, collagen has been shown experimentally to incite cell-mediated immunity (Senyk and Michaeli, 1973), and there is also experimental evidence to suggest that delayed hypersensitivity to lung connective tissue antigens develops in response to pulmonary damage caused by tuberculosis, coal pneumoconiosis and beryllium disease in animals (Cate and Burrell, 1974).

In cryptogenic diffuse interstitial pulmonary fibrosis the amount of Type I collagen relative to Type II is increased although it is not clear whether this is due to a preferential increase in synthesis of Type I or degradation of Type III, or to both (Seyer, Hutchinson and Kang, 1976): and, in addition, peripheral blood T lymphocytes from patients with this disease are sensitized by Type I collagen to produce MIF and to induce specific cytolysis of collagen-coated sheep red blood cells—phenomena not observed in non-fibrotic lung disease nor in normal individuals (Kravis *et al.*, 1976). However, there is nothing to suggest that lung collagen is antigenically distinct from collagen in other organs. This is discussed further at the end of this Chapter (p. 64).

In short, the fact that both circulating antibodies and cell-mediated reactivity to collagen have been shown to occur has important implications in the consideration of fibrotic occupational lung disease and, although these immune responses may be secondary to injury caused by the inhaled aerosols, they could well be decisive in determining the subsequent course of the disease process.

To summarize

Circulating precipitating antibodies associated with an Arthus (Type III) reaction due to activation of complement by the classic pathway are a feature of many, but not all, cases of extrinsic allergic 'alveolitis' (*see* Chapter 11).

The fact that both ANAs and RFs are often found in some individuals with certain types of non-occupational and occupational fibrosis of the lungs but not in others suggests that these non-organ-specific antibodies do not arise simply as a consequence of a common insult to the lungs. They may occur for a number of different, and as yet unidentified, reasons under different circumstances. This prompts speculation as to whether certain inhaled mineral dusts when retained in the lungs might, by virtue of their cytotoxic or other effects and resultant fibrogenesis, cause the formation of these antibodies which, under appropriate conditions, could accelerate or modify the disease process. An adjuvant or intensifying effect might then be the most likely mechanism. That immunological activity may occur, is supported by the fact that an important histological feature of some cases of coal and other types of pneumoconiosis, which undergo rapid progression or have atypical radiographic appearances during life, is the presence of abundant plasma cells and lymphocytes in the lesions. It is interesting to speculate whether imbalance between T and B cell populations—outlined on p. 56—might influence pathogenesis, especially as there is evidence that macrophages may carry membrane-bound antigens which facilitate macrophage–lymphocyte interaction capable of stimulating lymphocytes to differentiate into antibody-secreting cells, and so prime the host for a secondary response (Askonas and Jarošková, 1970).

Proof that organ-specific antibodies participate in the genesis of occupational and other lung disease in man has not yet been provided but cell-mediated immunity is now known to occur in beryllium disease and extrinsic allergic 'alveolitis' (*see* Chapters 10 and 11 respectively).

THE MAJOR HISTOCOMPATIBILITY SYSTEM

The discovery of the major histocompatibility (H-2) system in the mouse (Lilly, 1970) prompted the identification of a similar 'tissue type' antigen system in man. The antigens of this system are present on the cell membranes of lymphocytes and a wide variety of other cells, and are now referred to generically as the *human—leucocyte—antigen*, or *HLA, system*.

HLA antigens of any individual are apparently determined by two closely linked autosomal genes and, as each of these genes is highly polymorphic, a large number of allelic forms have been identified. Four major gene loci are now recognized and, according to World Health Organization nomenclature, are given the prefix HLA and classified as A, B, C and D; at each locus the number of alleles is 19, 20, 5 and 6 respectively (Bodmer, 1975a). This nomenclature has replaced systems recommended at earlier international 'workshops' and the speed with which the changes have occurred has caused some confusion.

The antigenic groups of the system can be segregated into at least three categories. *First,* antigens determined by the HLA A, B and C loci which act as primary targets for cytotoxic T lymphocytes and are detected serologically. *Second,* a serologically detectable group closely associated with HLA A and B loci which are present primarily on B lymphocytes—but not on T lymphocytes—and are referred to as Ir-type (that is, *immune-response* associated) antigens. And *third,* antigens associated with HLA D which are identifiable by special mixed lymphocyte culture tests, the responding cells being primarily T lymphocytes (Bach, Bach and Sondel, 1976).

The different combination of HLA antigens found are governed by a complicated genetic inheritance specified by the two autosomal genes and, within a given family, the number of genetic recombinations is limited, but in the population at large the chance of recombination may be greatly increased. This phenomenon, known as *linkage disequilibrium*, consists in the tendency for genes that are linked to occur together in a population with a greater frequency than might be expected. The incidence of individual HLA antigens, therefore, differs in different racial groups.

Apart from the importance of HLA antigens in tissue transplantation it is now evident that certain of them are associated with specific human diseases if the gene determining the disease is closely linked to the HLA gene on the same chromosome. Most of the associations which have been detected so far have been with the alleles of the B series; for example, ankylosing spondylosis and Reiter's syndrome with B27, psoriasis with B13 and W17, and gluten sensitive enteropathy (coeliac disease) with B8. However, because of the statistical complexity of the gene relationship it is improbable that 100 per cent concordance between HLA genes and disease will be encountered except in disease inherited according to simple Mendelian principles. The closest association observed to date is between ankylosing spondylosis and HLA B27 which is present in 96 per cent of cases compared with 5 to 10 per cent of control subjects (Oliver, 1977), but even a weak association of HLA antigen and a particular disease may point to the presence of a gene concerned in the pathogenesis of the disease which is situated close to the HLA locus on the chromosome. How this association is related to pathogenesis is not yet known.

Four possible mechanisms have been suggested and are summarized by Bodmer (1975b) as follows:

(1) Molecular mimicry resulting in tolerance due to cross reaction with foreign, pathogen associated antigens.
(2) Interaction with receptors for viruses or other pathogens.
(3) Pick-up of antigen by a pathogen from cell membranes.
(4) Association with immune response genes.

The last possibility appears to be most generally favoured. That an immune response gene which confers suceptibility may be associated with autoimmune disease is well exemplified by autoimmune thyroiditis in the mouse in which antibody to thyroglobulin is controlled by an H–2 linked gene and the level of antibody is related to the severity of the disease (Vladutiu and Rose, 1971). However, such a clear relationship has not yet been observed in human disease but would be expected to be difficult to identify, and may have to await improved techniques for the analysis of mixed lymphocyte culture reactions (Vladutiu and Rose, 1974). Nevertheless, there is suggestive evidence that the HLA system may influence the development of certain occupational lung diseases in some individuals or groups of individuals. The matter is referred to again in the chapters dealing with coal pneumoconiosis, asbestosis, extrinsic allergic 'alveolitis', and in the section on diffuse interstitial fibrosis on p. 76.

Although 'the game of chasing statistically significant associations which may have little biological and clinical relevance' must be avoided (Ceppellini, 1973), it is likely that understanding of associations between the HLA system and occupational disease will prove to be of practical value. For these reasons: specific antigens may identify individuals who, on the one hand, are unduly susceptible or, on the other hand, are relatively resistant to developing the disease in question; and, in individuals in whom the disease is established, may earmark those in whom it is either likely to progress or remain quiescent. Hence, the rationale of both prevention and prognosis could well be significantly advanced.

RETICULIN AND COLLAGEN

The distinction between these connective tissue components is important in the study of occupational and non-occupational disease of the lungs, and the difference between them must be recognized in the interpretation of both normal and abnormal micro-anatomy.

Most connective tissues consist of fibres, cells and a matrix or ground substance, and there are three types of fibres: reticulin, collagen and elastin of which the first two only will be discussed here. Fibroblasts are intimately associated with reticulin and collagen and are scattered between their fibres and matrix.

Fundamental differences between reticulin and collagen are revealed by light microscopy.

Reticulin is the term given to extracellular fibres which are fine, branched and coloured faintly red (or not at all) by van Giesen's connective tissue stain, magenta by periodic acid Schiff (a strong reaction) and black by silver impregnation; and they are isotropic under polarized light.

Collagen, which appears to the naked eye as white fibrous tissue, consists of bundles of non-branched fibres of uniform diameter coloured bright red with van Giesen's stain, slightly pink with periodic acid Schiff (a negative reaction), and yellow or brown with silver impregnation. Mature and hyalinized collagen is refringent under polarized light.

Under the electron microscope, however, both types of fibre have a similar cross-striated structure and the matrix between them is apparently indistinguishable (Chvapil, 1967), although there are important immunological differences.

There is a continuous network of connective tissue fibres composed mainly of collagen extending from the pulmonary pleura to the peribronchial and peritracheal regions. Reticulin fibres form part of the basement membranes of the alveoli and capillaries, and they are present in small quantities in alveolar walls.

The molecular precursors of both types of fibre are synthesized by fibroblasts and converted into *tropocollagen* which has the capacity to polymerize and aggregate spontaneously into fibrils. It contains the amino acids hydroxyproline and hydrolysine which determine the final structure of the fibres. Extracellular collagen is composed of polypeptide chains (α_1 and α_2 chains) wound round each other in helical form. At least five genetically distinct collagen types have been identified in various tissues and, although α_1 chains in collagen types II, III and IV are identical they each have, due to genetic polymorphism, a different primary structure. Thus:

Type I is composed of two α1 (I) chains and one 2 chain expressed symbolically as $[\alpha 1(I)]_2\alpha_2$, and is present in nearly all connective tissues and most parenchymal organs.
Type II $[\alpha 1(II)]_3$ containing three α1 chains is found only in cartilage and, therefore, in the trachea and bronchi.
Type III $[\alpha 1(III)]_3$ appears to be reticulin (Crystal *et al.*, 1976).

Type IV $[\alpha 1(IV)]_3$ forms the non-fibrous collagen of basement membranes.
Type V $[(\alpha A)\ (\alpha B)_2]$ which is also present in basement membranes and the interstitium of parenchymal organs and is associated with smooth muscle cells (Madri and Furthmayr, 1980).

Types I and III, approximately in the ratio 2:1, are the two major forms of collagen in the lung parenchyma (Seyer, Hutchinson and Kang, 1976) with smaller amounts of Types IV and V (Kravis *et al.*, 1976; Madri and Furthmayr, 1980).

Both reticulin and collagen possess distinctive antigenic activity. Extracts of the reticulin component of human liver and renal cortex are antigenic in rabbits and give a characteristic immunofluorescent staining pattern with human antireticulin antibody (Pras *et al.*, 1974). Circulating antibodies to natural and denatured collagen occur in man although their true prevalence in health and disease remains to be clarified. Auto-antibodies against denatured collagen are present in some rheumatic and chronic disorders associated with collagen breakdown (for example, rheumatoid arthritis, systemic lupus erythematosus, Sjögren's disease, scleroderma and emphysema) and they have been identified in rheumatoid synovial tissues and fluids (Holborow *et al.*, 1977). Moreover, collagen has been shown, experimentally, to incite cell-mediated immunity (Senyk and Michaeli, 1973).

In cryptogenic and other forms of diffuse interstitial pulmonary fibrosis the ratio of Type I to Type III collagen is increased although it is not clear whether this is due to a preferential increase in synthesis of Type I or to degradation of Type III, or to both (Seyer, Hutchinson and Kang, 1976; Madri and Furthmayr, 1980). This disorder is discussed further at the end of this chapter.

In short, the fact that circulating antibodies and, possibly, cell-mediated reactivity to collagen occur has important implications in the consideration of fibrotic occupational lung disease and, although these immune responses may be secondary to injury caused by inhaled aerosols, they could well be decisive in determining the subsequent course of the disease process.

The confusion to which the term *reticulation* may give rise if used to describe proliferation of reticulin fibres is discussed in Chapter 5. And it should be noted, too, that *fibrosis* in the sense used by the pathologist is, by general consent, an histological term which denotes an excess of collagen fibres and not proliferation of reticulin fibres. *Reticulum,* by the way, refers to a fine network formed by *cells* and has no relevance to the present context.

In order to indicate the microscopic degree of fibrosis present in human lungs, a modification of the system suggested by Belt and King (1945) for grading in experimental animals can be used.

Grade 1 Cellular lesions; loose reticulin; no collagen.
Grade 2 Cellular lesions; compact reticulin with or without a few collagen fibres.
Grade 3 Lesions somewhat cellular, but mostly collagenous.
Grade 4 Acellular collagen.

Using this scale, Grade 2 when collagen is present, indicates very slight or negligible fibrosis; Grade 3, moderate fibrosis, and Grade 4, severe fibrosis. This grading, of course, expresses the *degree* of fibrosis in the area sampled and not the *extent* of its distribution in the lungs.

BASIC REACTIONS OF THE LUNGS TO INHALED PARTICLES

As described in Chapter 3 the acini are the most significant sites of deposition of mineral and organic aerosols although deposition of fungal spores and other organic particles on the walls of non-respiratory bronchioles is important in the pathogenesis of extrinsic allergic 'alveolitis', and on larger airways in that of extrinsic asthma.

MINERAL DUSTS

Within the alveolar walls, macrophages rapidly converge upon extracellular particles and engulf them. If the number of particles is large the elimination mechanisms described in Chapter 3 may fail, and dust particles and dust-containing macrophages collect in the interstitium—especially in perivascular and peribronchiolar regions. If these aggregations remain *in situ,* Type I pneumocytes grow over them so that they become enclosed and completely interstitial in position but, in the case of inert dusts and coal and quartz dusts, they are strictly localized in these regions. According to the amount of dust and cell accumulation the alveolar walls either protrude to a greater or lesser degree into the alveolar spaces or obliterate them altogether. Meanwhile, a delicate supporting framework of fine reticulin fibres develops between the cells, but in the case of dusts with fibrogenic potential, proliferation of collagen fibres subsequently occurs.

Inert dusts, such as carbon, iron, tin and titanium remain within macrophages in these lesions until they die at the end of their normal life span when the particles are released and reingested by other macrophages; secondary lysosomes are unharmed in the process (*see Figure 1.5*). But the lesions are not static and some dust-laden macrophages continually migrate to lymphatics or to bronchioles whence they are eliminated. Migration is increased by infection or oedema of the lung.

Some fibrogenic dusts, most notably crystalline silica, cause rapid destruction of macrophages followed by formation of proliferative collagenous fibrosis in *localized* lesions. By contrast asbestos dusts, which are less cytotoxic, cause a *diffuse* collagenous fibrosis in the walls of terminal and respiratory bronchioles spreading distally into alveolar walls; that is, a diffuse interstitial fibrosis or fibrosing bronchiolo-alveolitis (*see* Theories of pathogenesis).

To summarize, there are four different basic types of lesion caused by the alveolar deposition of mineral dusts.

(1) Plastering of the walls of the alveoli of respiratory bronchioles to a greater or lesser degree by dust particles.
(2) A small, *localized* interstitial—that is, mainly peribronchiolar—lesion consisting of accumulations of dust, macrophages and a mild proliferation of reticulin without collagenous fibrosis. This is caused by inert dusts, for example, iron (siderosis); many of the discrete lesions of coal pneumoconiosis are of this sort.
(3) A localized, *nodular,* peribronchiolar interstitial lesion of collagenous fibrosis caused by particles of quartz, flint and certain other fibrogenic dusts.
(4) A *diffuse* interstitial fibrosis of bronchiolar and alveolar walls, the most important example of which is asbestosis.

The chief characteristics of (2), (3) and (4) are described in more detail in Chapters 6, 7 and 9 respectively.

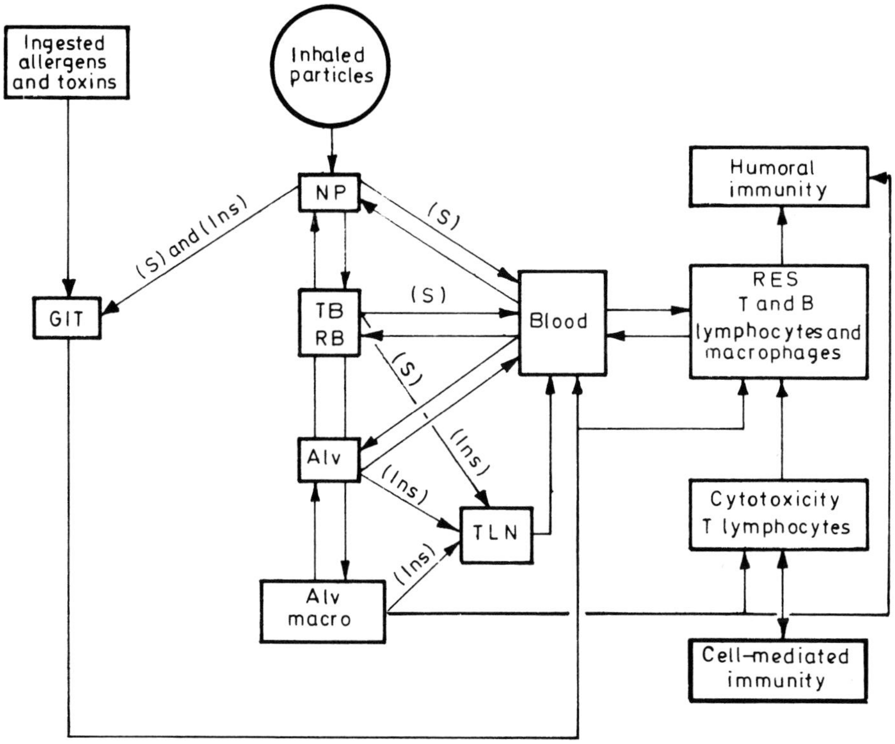

Figure 4.3 Diagram showing the possible fates and influence of inhaled aerosols and ingested materials. Alv. alveolus; Alv. macro. alveolar macrophages; GIT gastrointestinal tract; Ins insoluble particles; NP nasopharynx; RB red blood cell; RES reticulo-endothelial system; S soluble particles; TB terminal bronchioles; TLN thoracic lymph nodes. (Adapted from Kilburn, 1968; by courtesy of the Editor of American Review of Respiratory Diseases*)*

In addition, certain metallic aerosols—such as chromium salts, cobalt, nickel and complex salts of platinum—deposited on the walls of bronchi and smaller airways may cause asthma (*see* Chapter 12).

The possible fates of inhaled and ingested aerosols and the train of events they may initiate are summarized in *Figure 4.3*.

ORGANIC DUSTS

Protein particles, such as the spores of the thermophilic actinomycete *Micropolyspora faeni* from mouldy hay and straw or dust from the droppings and feathers of certain birds, may act as antigens and provoke Type I, III or IV allergic reactions. These and other protein aerosols can cause immediate asthma mediated by a Type I reaction in sensitized (atopic) individuals but, in others, asthma of delayed onset due, probably, to a Type III reaction; or, in the case of cotton or flax dusts, an asthma-like reaction (byssinosis) in which no allergic reactions or distinctive histopathology have yet been identified (*see* Chapter 12). They may also result in the development of pneumonitis or sarcoid-type granulomas which, in some cases, is followed by diffuse interstitial fibrosis (extrinsic allergic 'alveolitis') provoked by activation of complement by the classic pathway in sensitized individuals or by activation of the alternative pathway in non-sensitized individuals (*see* Chapter 11); circulating precipitating antibodies are present in the former but absent in the latter. Sarcoid-type granulomas are also a feature of beryllium disease caused by inorganic (metallic) compounds. However, an important distinction exists in that the granulomas in extrinsic allergic 'alveolitis' occur only in acute disease and are evanescent, whereas they are often present in the chronic stages of beryllium disease and sarcoidosis.

The granulomas in both instances appear to be the expression of a Type IV reaction: T lymphocytes are sensitized by proteins or by beryllium compounds and incite accumulation of macrophages and their transformation into epithelioid and giant cells. These points are discussed in detail in Chapters 10 and 11.

SOME THEORIES OF THE PATHOGENESIS OF MINERAL PNEUMOCONIOSIS AND EXPERIMENTAL OBSERVATIONS

Precisely why particles of one material provoke collagenous fibrosis or other disease processes—such as sarcoid-type granulomas—whereas those of another do not is poorly understood, but one thing is clear: the form that the lesions of each type of pneumoconiosis takes is primarily determined by particular attributes of the inhaled particles and by cellular and humoral responses to them; and, possibly, concomitant infection in the lung may sometimes play a part. Recent advances in cytology, enzyme chemistry, histochemistry and immunology have identified some important features of the sequence of pathogenic events following exposure to certain mineral dusts both in man and under experimental conditions.

Many theories to explain the fibrogenesis of different types of pneumoconiosis have been elaborated but only those relevant to current knowledge are discussed.

SILICOSIS

Theory of piezoelectric effect

This suggested that minute electrical currents caused by mechanical stresses on quartz crystals may damage tissue cells (Evans and Zeit, 1949), but precisely how was not made clear. Against this it was shown that substances other than quartz which possess piezoelectric activity were non-fibrogenic, whereas tridymite, which lacks this activity, is strongly fibrogenic. However, recent work has resuscitated and modified the theory. It is postulated that emission of electrons from the edges of the tetrahedral crystals of silicon dioxide (Chvapil, 1974) or electric charge-transfer between the crystals and cell membranes (Robock, 1968) initiate the cell damage which provokes fibrogenesis.

The solubility theory

This theory—originally elaborated by Kettle (1926) and widely favoured until recently—postulated that crystalline silica passes slowly into solution in tissue fluids producing silicic acid which causes fibrosis. However, there are many reasons why this theory is untenable. There is a significant difference in the fibrogenic potential of different types of free silica, the severity and speed of fibrosis being greatest due to tridymite then, in descending order, to cristobalite, quartz and least of all, to vitreous silica although the solubility of all is similar (King *et al.*, 1953; Stöber, 1968). Quartz etched with hydrofluoric acid is much less soluble than unetched quartz yet is more fibrogenic (Engelbrecht *et al.*, 1958). Furthermore, of the submicron polymorphic forms of silicon dioxide which have similar solubilities to quartz coesite causes little fibrosis and stishovite behaves as an inert dust (Brieger and Gross, 1967; Strecker, 1965) (*see also* Chapter 2, p. 32). Finally, silicic acid, when allowed to permeate from diffusion chambers into the peritoneal cavities of animals while quartz particles are excluded, does not cause fibrosis (Curran and Rowsell, 1958; Allison, Clark and Davis, 1977).

Holt (1957) modified this theory—the so-called Extended Solubility Theory—by postulating that silicic acid is absorbed on to the protein of collagen precursors causing them to polymerize into collagen. But there has been no satisfactory evidence to support this either.

It appears, then, that the ability of free silica to cause fibrosis depends fundamentally on two conditions: (1) particular types of crystal or particle structure and their surface properties; and (2) intimate contact with cells.

The process of fibrogenesis and the control of collagen synthesis are of general medical importance and, for some years past, the effect of free silica on cells *in vitro* and in animals has been used as a model to investigate this wider problem as well as specifically the genesis of silica-induced disease. In addition, there is now much evidence which points to involvement of immunological processes at some stage in the silicotic process. Hence, there are two, possibly interrelated, concepts of pathogenesis—cellular and immunological—which may also be applicable to other types of pulmonary disease believed to be caused by inhaled aerosols.

Theory based on cytotoxicity and collaboration of macrophages and fibroblasts

Both non-cytotoxic particles—such as titanium dioxide (rutile), diamond and amorphous carbon—and cytotoxic particles of quartz when added to macrophages in a culture medium containing serum are quickly ingested by the cells and enveloped in their phagosomes (*Figures 4.4* and *4.5a*). The resulting digestive vacuoles (secondary lysosomes) which contain non-cytotoxic particles remain intact and the cells undamaged, whereas those which contain quartz soon rupture or become permeable and release their contents into the cytoplasm (*Figure 4.5b*). Thereupon, the macrophages become round and immobile, and disintigrate discharging all their contents—particles, enzymes and other constituents (*Figure 4.6*)—which are then re-ingested by other viable macrophages and the process repeated (Allison, Harington and Birbeck, 1966; Nadler and Goldfischer, 1970). A similar train of events has been demonstrated in experimental animals by a double-dusting inhalation technique using both inert and toxic quartz dusts (Heppleston, 1963) though the effects on macrophages are less dramatic since the concentration of mineral particles is generally less than in '*in vitro*' experiments (Bruch and Otto, 1967). It seems likely that similar events also occur in man.

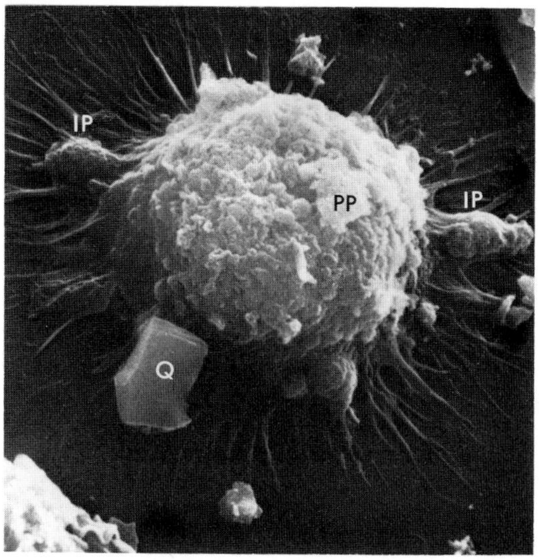

Figure 4.4 Scanning electron micrograph of macrophage showing phagocytosis of quartz after addition of particles. Note prominent filopodia associated in places with ingested particles (IP). PP, partly ingested particles; Q, extra-cellular quartz particle. (Original magnification × 5400. Courtesy of Dr K. Miller and Editor of Environ. Res.*). Compare with* Figure 1.4

Macrophages, therefore, are affected in dissimilar ways by different materials. Inert particles, after phagocytosis, do not appear to interfere with the normal life-span of the cells; whereas particles of crystalline silica continue to destroy macrophages until the particles are incarcerated by proliferating collagenous tissue which presumably prevents a state of perpetual cell destruction. For this reason macrophages probably play a minor role in eliminating quartz and other forms of fibrogenic crystalline silica particles from the lungs.

When macrophages are present by themselves in a millipore diffusion chamber (from which cells or particles larger than 1 μm diameter cannot escape) placed in the peritoneal cavity of an animal no fibrosis of the peritoneum occurs, but when both macrophages and quartz particles (> 1 μm diameter) are present together in the chamber significant synthesis of collagen in the visceral and parietal peritoneum results. The degree of fibrogenesis is more pronounced with

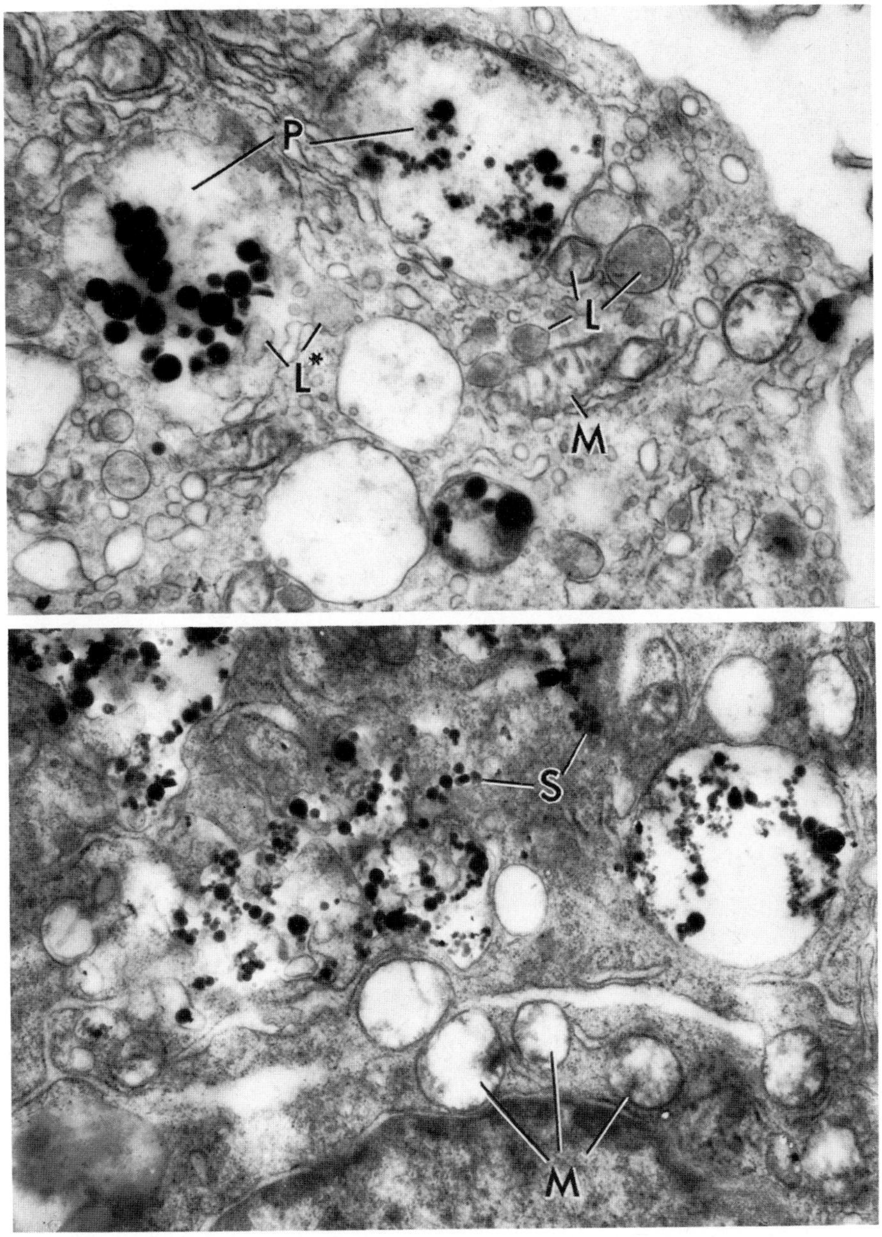

Figure 4.5 (a) Electron micrograph of a macrophage showing quartz particles in phagosomes (P). There are numerous lysosomes (L) some of which are apparently attached to a phagosome (L). The structure of the cytoplasm and mitochondria (M) is well preserved. (b) Phagosomes in the centre of the field have disrupted, releasing the quartz particles (S) into the cytoplasm, the detail of which is becoming obscured. The phagosome on the right of the field is still intact. Mitochondria (M) above the nucleus are swollen and degenerating. (Original magnification × 24 000, reproduced at × 19 200; by courtesy of Dr A. C. Allison)*

lower concentrations of quartz which are not rapidly cytotoxic than with higher concentrations which kill most of the cells. These observations imply that macrophages which have ingested an insufficient amount of quartz to kill them secrete a factor which stimulates fibroblasts to synthesize collagen (Allison, Clark and Davies, 1977).

Quartz particles affect macrophages in two distinctly different ways. When the particles are added to the cells in a serum-free medium the majority are damaged within an hour due to interaction with the plasma membrane, and lysosomal and cytoplasmic enzymes (such as lactate dehydrogenase) are released. When, however, the encounter occurs in a medium containing serum the cytotoxic process is delayed because serum proteins coat the particles so that they do not harm the plasma membrane and only when this coating is digested away in secondary lysosomes is the surface of the particles exposed to interact with the lysosomal membrane (Allison, Clark and Davies, 1977). In explanation of this interaction it has been suggested that the numerous strong hydroxyl (silanol) groups of silicic acid on the surfaces of quartz crystals act as hydrogen donors in hydrogen bonding reactions with the membranes of the secondary lysosomes causing irreversible injury (Allison, 1971); and the importance of the absorption properties of silanol groups in the fibrogenic activity of quartz dusts—which apparently differs in quartz from different geological sites—has, in fact, been demonstrated by physical methods such as chemoluminescence intensity and infrared spectroscopy (Kriegseis *et al.*, 1977). This harmful effect and that of cell membrane damage is blocked by coating the particles with aluminium or polyvinyl pyridine-N-oxide (PVPNO) (Nash, Allison and Harington, 1966), or by treating macrophages with PVPNO before or shortly after exposure (Allison, Harington and Birbeck, 1966). The polymer

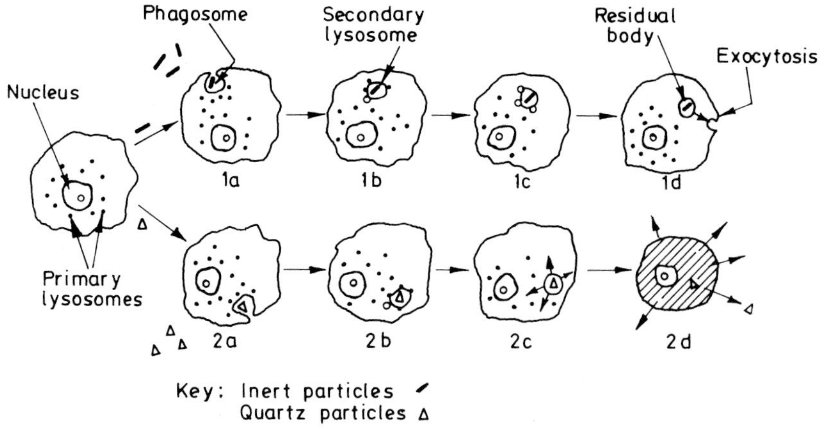

Figure 4.6 Diagram of intracellular events after ingestion of inert and noxious particles. (1a) Macrophages ingesting inert particles by endocytosis to form a phagosome; (1b, 1c) primary lysosomes have migrated on to the wall of the phagosome (now known as a secondary lysosome) and are discharging their enzymes into it; (1d) residual body is formed if the particles are wholly or partly undigested. Some bodies attach to the cell wall and discharge their contents by exocytosis. (2a, b) macrophage ingesting quartz particles and formation of secondary lysosome; (2c) membrane of secondary lysosome damaged and rendered permeable, resulting in leakage of enzymes into the cytoplasm which is thus broken down and the cell rounds up and dies (2d), releasing the particles and the enzymes

enters the secondary lysosomes with the particles and reacts with them when their protein coating has been digested away. The protective effect of PVPNO—which also inhibits fibrogenesis in animals which have inhaled quartz dust (Klosterkötter, 1968)—may be due to their forming strong hydrogen bonds preferentially with the silanol groups before these can damage the cell membranes (Allison, 1968) or to their interfering with normal collagen synthesis (Kilroe-Smith, 1974). On the other hand, it has been suggested that the cause of lysosomal disruption is lipid peroxidation at membrane level, possibly initiated by one or other of the mechanisms proposed by the modified piezo-electricity theory; however, there is evidence that the action of quartz is not due to its peroxidative properties (Chvapil, 1974; Kilroe-Smith, 1974). It is clear, therefore, that the exact reason for membrane damage is still to be discovered.

Among the constituents released from dying macrophages is a factor (or factors) which stimulates an increased production of hydroxyproline (HOP), but not deoxyribonucleic acid (DNA), by cultured fibroblasts suggesting that this factor augments the function, but not proliferation, of these cells. This response is inhibited by PVPNO and does not occur when quartz particles are applied directly to fibroblasts nor when fibroblasts are cultured with extracts of normal macrophages (Allison, 1973). It appears, then, that the effect of free silica within macrophages is to produce or activate a relatively soluble substance—possibly in lysosomes—which is capable of stimulating collagen formation and may act in low concentration (Burrell and Anderson, 1973; Heppleston and Styles, 1967). Aalto, Polita and Kulonen (1976) confirmed these observations and also showed that subcellular particles of disintegrated *untreated* macrophages when exposed to crystalline silica produce a collagen stimulating factor; and Nourse *et al.* (1975) using a different technique observed that collagen synthesis occurred only in actively dividing fibroblasts. However, Harington, Allison and Badami (1975) did not substantiate these findings due, possibly, to the methods they employed. There is also *in vitro* evidence that antibody reacting with macrophages causes them to release a factor which stimulates collagen synthesis (*see* p. 71).

Although Harington (1963) suggested that the fibrogenic factor might be a lipid or lipoprotein, Kilroe-Smith *et al.* (1973) have shown that it is almost certainly of non-lipid nature. The pulmonary reaction induced in rats by the inhalation of fairly heavy concentrations of quartz or cristobalite consists, however, not of the formation of silicotic nodules, but of exudation into the alveolar space of a material which appears identical histologically, histochemically and ultrastructurally with that found in human alveolar lipoproteinosis (*Figure 4.7a* and *b*) (Heppleston, Wright and Stewart, 1970; Corrin and King, 1970; Heppleston and Young, 1972). Though macrophages are a prominent feature in the early stages of the reaction, most of the alveolar material is acellular and has a high phospholipid content. Electron microscopy shows that it contains numerous extracellular osmiophilic bodies similar to those normally found as inclusions in Type II epithelial cells—which, are greatly increased in number—and osmiophilic lamellae consisting of phospholipid in a liquid-crystalline phase arranged in parallel, concentric, quadratic and hexagonal patterns in which quartz particles are enmeshed (*Figure 4.8*) (Heppleston and Young, 1972). Chemically the lungs of these animals show a great overall increase in lipid content compared with controls.

The inferences drawn from these observations are that only lipid-free material from the dusted macrophages provokes fibrosis whereas the production of excess lipids by Type II cells—possibly due to the stimulus of some other factor also released from the damaged macrophages—inhibits the formation of silicotic fibrotic nodules apparently because there is insufficient contact between the quartz particles and macrophages to produce significant concentrations of the fibrogenic factor. It appears, in fact, that the rate at which quartz particles accumulate in the alveoli is of crucial importance as exposure of animals to low quartz

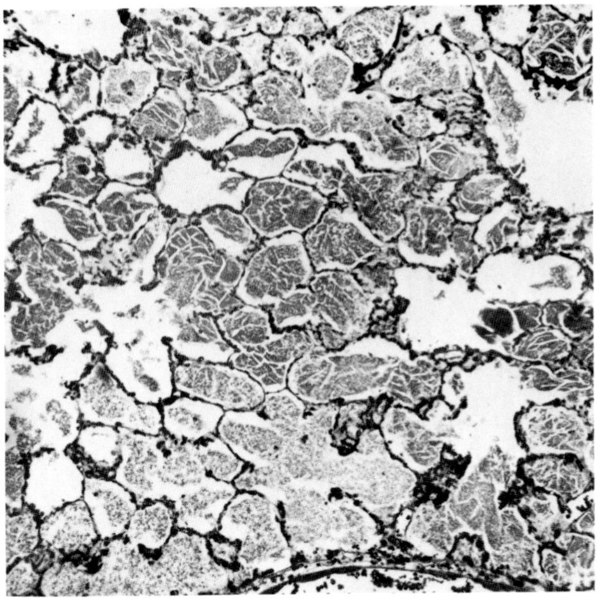

(a)

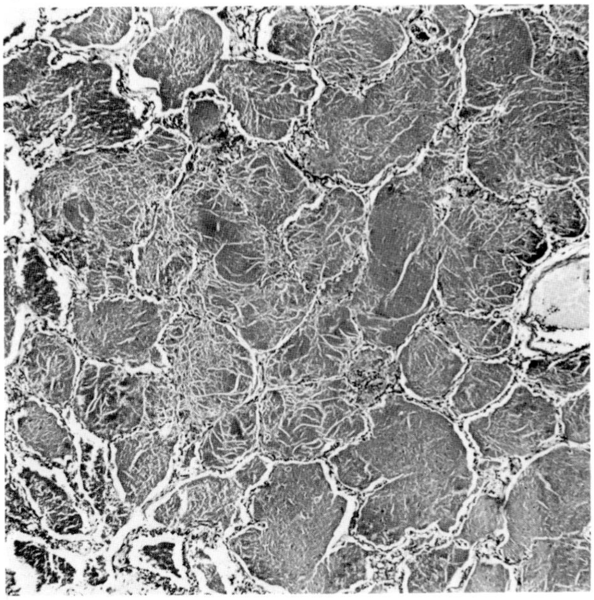

(b)

Figure 4.7a and b Alveolar silico-lipoproteinosis. *Dense granular material fills most of the alveoli. Alveolar walls remain intact and show little increase in cellularity. (a), rat lung (original magnification × 100); (b), human lung (original magnification × 40). The similarity of the two is evident. (Courtesy of Professor A.G. Heppleston)*

concentrations for a few hours a day over a long period causes the development of silicotic nodules, whereas exposure to high concentrations for most of the day for a short period results in lipoproteinosis (Heppleston, 1973). This is consonant with the types of occupational exposure associated with the variants seen in human disease (*see* Chapter 7). An increase in Type II cells occurs early in the genesis of lipoproteinosis while intact macrophages are still present in the alveoli, and they appear almost certainly to be the chief source of the lipid accumulation of which a significant part is dipalmitoyl lecithin, the major component of lung surfactant (Heppleston, Fletcher and Wyatt, 1974); but the silica–macrophage reaction itself also contributes some lipids (Munder *et al.*, 1966). The pronounced accumulation of this material in the alveoli may be due to its formation outstripping the capacity of macrophages to remove it (Heppleston, Fletcher and Wyatt, 1974).

Lipid production in the lungs probably exerts a stimulating effect, both locally and systemically, on recruitment of macrophages to replace those lost in the encounter with free silica (Heppleston, 1973; Civil and Heppleston, 1979).

Although these experimental observations have greatly

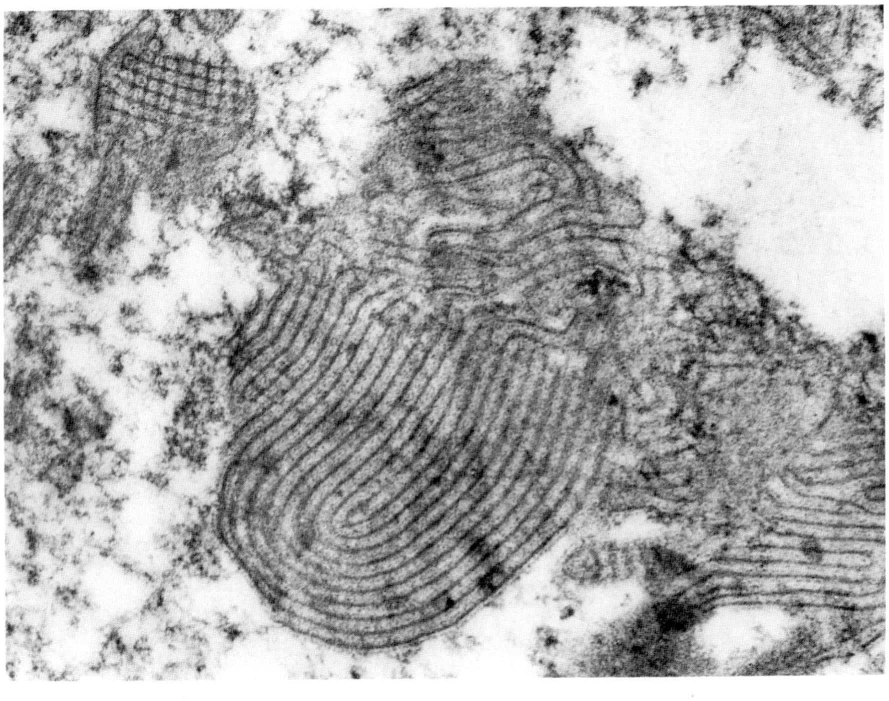

Figure 4.8 Alveolar material from a long-surviving quartz-dusted rat showing a quadratic lattice and parallel lamellae. The formation has a periodicity of about 45 nm and represents a longitudinal section of the lattice. (EM, magnification × 60 000). (Courtesy of Professor A. G. Heppleston and Editor of J. Path.*)*

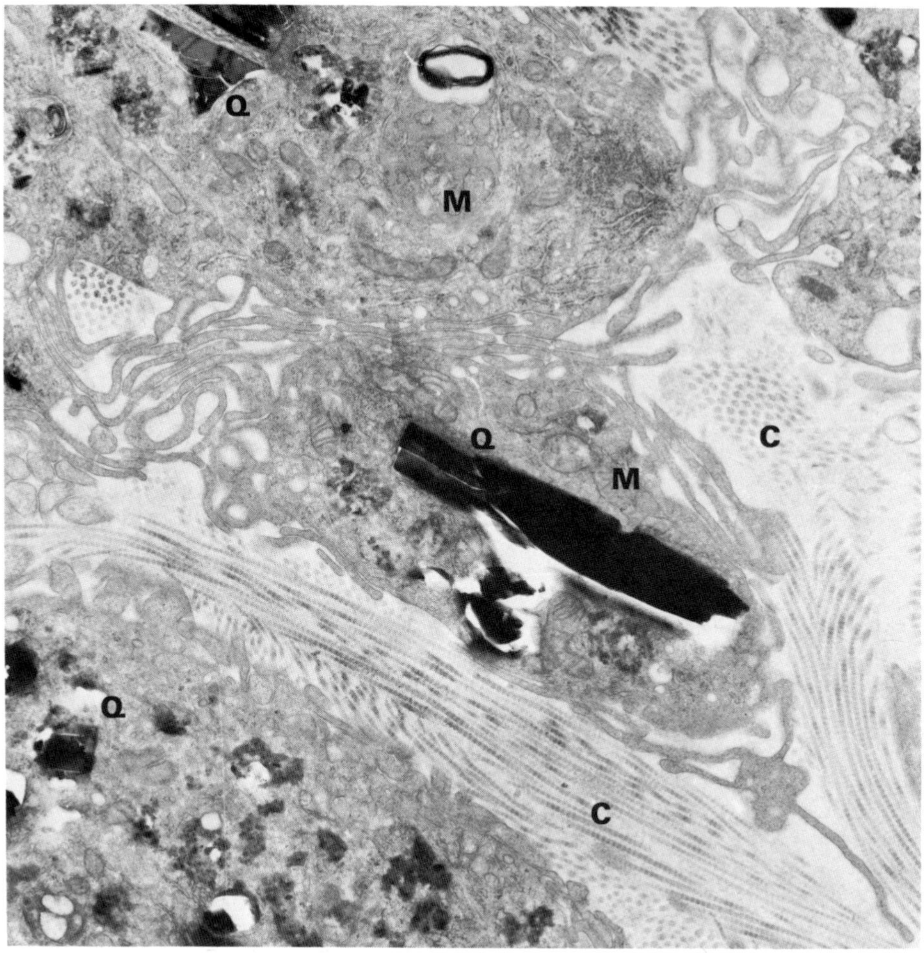

Figure 4.9 Electron micrograph of cellular constituents of a silicotic nodule. Bundles of young collagen fibres (C) are seen in close proximity to macrophages (M) containing quartz particles (Q). (Original magnification × 14000). (Courtesy of Dr D. H. Bowden and the Editor of Environ. Hlth Perspect.*)*

advanced knowledge of the biological activity of free silica they do not yet furnish a wholly comprehensive explanation of the pathogenesis and evolution of silicosis in man. But the effects of quartz appear to be biphasic and to alter the proportions of both stimulating and inhibiting factors liberated from macrophages (Heppleston, 1978; Aho *et al.*, 1979); so that the secretions of living macrophages as well as products of dying or disrupted cells are probably important in determining the development of fibrosis. In any event electron microscopy of the cellular constituents of silicotic nodules has demonstrated macrophages containing quartz particles in close proximity to young collagen fibres (*Figure 4.9*). Furthermore, prolonged biological activity of siliceous dusts in the lungs is implied by the finding that, in comparison with control subjects, significantly increased numbers of Type II pneumocytes are present in broncho-alveolar lavage fluid of silicotic patients years after their last exposure to dust (Schuyler *et al.*, 1980).

Theory based on immunological reactions

There are three possible ways in which free silica particles might cause immunological reactions.

(1) By acting as an antigen

Unlike organic dusts (Chapter 11) which may provoke an Arthus (Type III) reaction mineral dusts—including free silica—do not act in this way. Theoretically, they may function as a hapten to produce a Type II allergic response, but no satisfactory evidence to support this has been produced. Although some workers, notably Kashimura (1959), have apparently demonstrated antibodies against quartz in experimental animals, this observation has not been confirmed (Voison *et al.*, 1964), and the results of the earlier experiments may have been due to bacterial contamination of quartz particles.

(2) By producing an auto-antigen

They may modify the structure of some body protein and thereby produce antigen. Proteins absorbed on to the surface of quartz are denatured (Scheel *et al.*, 1954) and, by virtue of this, may conceivably acquire antigenic potential. Gamma globulins are most likely to be involved and when denatured in various ways they have been shown to produce antibodies in experimental animals (Milgrom and

Witebsky, 1960; McClusky, Miller and Benacerraf, 1962). However, Jones and Heppleston (1961) failed to demonstrate antibodies to whole serum or γ-globulin by immunofluorescence in experimental silicotic nodules, and there is no convincing evidence of such auto-antigenic activity in man.

Recent work has offered evidence that lung connective tissue antibodies stimulate quartz-exposed macrophages to release a factor which stimulates synthesis of collagen—a substance possessing antigenic potential (*see Lung Reactive Antibodies*, p. 61 and *Reticulin and Collagen*, p. 63—by fibroblasts resulting in the production of more antigen (Lewis and Burrell, 1976). This is of particular interest in view of that fact that the existence of human auto-antibodies against denatured collagen now seems to be well authenticated in some disorders associated with collagen breakdown, and it has been suggested that anticollagen antibody might stimulate fibroblasts to synthesize and secrete more collagen (Holborow *et al.,* 1977). If the presence of these events is substantiated they would imply 'collaboration' between the immediate cytotoxic effect of free silica and a secondary and later contributory antigen–antibody reaction.

(3) By acting as an adjuvant

They may, like Freund's adjuvant, facilitate an allergic reaction which would not otherwise occur (Pernis and Paronetto, 1962). In experimental animals the induction of hypersensitivity causes larger and more clearly demarcated silicotic lesions (due to powdered quartz) than in control animals (Powell and Gough, 1959).

Although experimental work (Thiart and Engelbrecht, 1967) has indicated that the ground substance of silicotic nodules in rats consists, not of γ-globulins but of β-globulins derived from macrophages killed by quartz, human silicotic nodules (*see* Chapter 7) apparently contain IgG and IgM which are found in the hyaline and among collagen fibres and may be bound to them (Pernis, 1968). Plasma cells around the periphery of actively developing lesions are believed to be the source of the immune globulins. These features vary widely in lesions from different subjects and in different lesions in the same subject: and in some they cannot be identified at all. They appear to be most prominent in actively evolving lesions and absent from old inactive lesions. The nodules contain a variable amount of hyaline in which there is no more than about 40 per cent collagen (Vigliani and Pernis, 1963).

It is possible, therefore, that immunoglobulins may play a role in the evolution of the later stages of silicosis, especially in the formation of conglomerate masses (*see* Chapter 7). In this respect it is of interest that amyloid lesions, in which auto-immune phenomena are thought to play a part, also contain variable amounts of IgG (Schultz *et al.*, 1966) and complement, and there are similarities in the hyaline of both types of lesion (Pernis, 1968). However, it may be that the presence of globulins is due simply to permeation of serum proteins which remain sequestered in the lesions (Heppleston, 1969). In view of the lack of agreement in reported observations a possible adjuvant effect of quartz or other types of free silica cannot be said to have been proved.

Inhalation of crystalline silica by mice is reported to result in decreased T-lymphocyte activity in mediastinal lymph nodes but in increased activity in the spleen; and in reduction of B lymphocyte activity in both of these sites (Miller and Zarkower, 1974a). However, administration by the intravenous route does not apparently demonstrate unequivocal evidence of a direct effect on these cells although macrophage function is, in general, depressed (Levy and Wheelock, 1975). Alveolar macrophages of rats which have inhaled quartz show an increase of surface receptor sites for IgG and the C3 component of complement (Miller and Kagan, 1977). Hence, the possibility that inhalation of free silica might alter the development and expression of acquired immunity is obviously important and continues to be investigated.

To summarize

The silicotic process appears to be *initiated* by the cytotoxic effect of free silica on alveolar macrophages and the release of fibrogenic factor(s) from these cells. Antigen–antibody reactions have not, until recently, been regarded as playing a pathogenic role in man but there is increasing reason to believe that such reactions may develop at a later stage in the evolution of the disease in some cases. These reactions may be the result of an adjuvant effect or, as seems more likely, of the development of anticollagen antibodies against denatured collagen stimulating increased collagen production.

COAL PNEUMOCONIOSIS AND 'MIXED DUST FIBROSIS'

Fibrogenesis in coal pneumoconiosis, unlike silicosis, appears to be determined in some way chiefly by the amount of total dust in the lungs. Whether or not the small and variable quantities of quartz which may be associated with coal dust contribute to this is controversial and the problem is discussed further in Chapter 8. Coal particles are not cytotoxic to alveolar or peritoneal macrophages (Collet *et al.,* 1967; Harington, 1972). From animal experiments, also, it appears that as the concentration of quartz in coal dust is increased the degree of resultant fibrosis is more pronounced though the histological appearances of the lesions do not resemble silicotic nodules. Aluminium silicates associated with the coal apparently reduce the fibrogenic potential of quartz (Martin *et al.,* 1972). However, it is far from certain that this simple pathogenic model applies to man in whom advanced disease may exist in lungs which contain a large quantity of coal dust but only small amounts of quartz or none at all (*see* Chapter 8).

On the basis of mineralogical examination of human lungs, Nagelschmidt (1960) suggested that smaller amounts of relatively insoluble dusts, such as coal and hematite, are required for a given severity of fibrosis the more quartz they contain; and, conversely, larger amounts of dust, the less quartz they contain. This is illustrated in *Figure 4.10*.

An additional feature which may have pathogenic importance in both silicosis and coal pneumoconiosis is that *organic* iron (as ferritin) is taken up by macrophages in the same way as quartz and shortens their life-span. Indeed, accumulation of organic iron occurs in both silicotic lesions and those of coal pneumoconiosis (Otto and Maron, 1959). The source of this non-haem iron is probably mainly

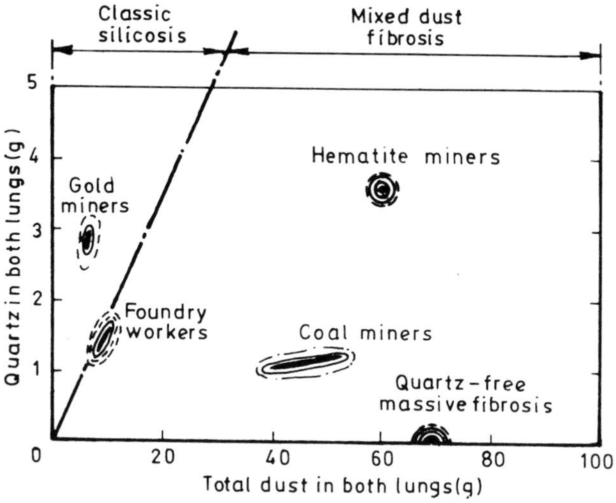

Figure 4.10 Average values of total dust and quartz in lungs with advanced forms of different dust diseases. (From Nagelschmidt (1960). Br. J. ind. Med. **17**, *247 by courtesy of HMSO)*

endogenous; experimentally, iron accumulates in macrophages which have ingested a mixture of carbon and 2 per cent quartz (Collet *et al.*, 1967) or mucoid substances, and it is thought likely to originate from plasma transferrin (McCarthy, Reid and Gibbons, 1964). Iron in this form is not identified by routine iron stains (*see* Chapter 6, p. 115). Whether or not it influences collagen synthesis in these and in any of the pneumoconioses, it has a significant effect upon determining their appearances on the chest radiograph (*see* Chapter 5). Inorganic iron, by contrast, when mixed with quartz *inhibits* its fibrogenic potential (*see* Chapter 7, p. 159).

It has been suggested that coal dust may act as an adsorbing surface for serum proteins thereby denaturing them to a form capable of reactions with antibodies—for example, rheumatoid factor—but this has not been confirmed experimentally. Nonetheless, coal dust does adsorb serum proteins to a significant degree which is unrelated to its rank so that large quantities of protein accumulate in lungs with a high dust content—a point which may favour the 'total dust hypothesis' of the pathogenesis of coal pneumoconiosis (Wagner, 1972). Evidence that auto-antibody activity, in which the chief antigenic components are reticulin and collagen, participates in the pathogenesis of the disease appears to rest mainly on the presence of crystalline silica and not upon coal or carbon dust alone (Burrell, 1972).

Inhalation of carbon dust by mice is reported to cause depression of T lymphocyte activity in their mediastinal lymph nodes but enhancement in their spleens (Miller and Zarkower, 1974b); whereas, in man, coal pneumoconiosis appears to be associated with impaired responsiveness of T cells in the peripheral blood (Dauber, Finn and Daniele, 1976).

Viral interferon and coal dust

The synthesis of interferon by human and simian cells exposed to coal dust of any rank is apparently partly or completely inhibited, but this effect is largely prevented if either the dust or the cells are pre-treated with PVPNO (Hahon, 1974). Whether or not these observations have any relevance to coal pneumoconiosis in man remains to be demonstrated.

Pathogenesis is discussed further in Chapter 8.

Influence of coexisting tuberculosis

For many years it has been believed that tuberculosis enhances the progress of lesions of silicosis and coal pneumoconiosis and, in the case of free silica, this has been demonstrated in experimental animals (Chapter 7, p. 145). It is possible that, if such an effect exists in man, it may be caused by an adjuvant influence of live or dead tubercle bacilli upon the production of non-specific antibody which becomes localized, not only where the bacilli are situated, but also in the pneumoconiotic lesion. On the other hand, the growth of tubercle bacilli is increased in the presence of crystalline silica through the intermediary of macrophages (Allison and Hart, 1968) (*see* Chapter 8) and cell-mediated (Type IV) allergic responses are apparently potentiated in animals exposed to tridymite (Pernis and Paronetto, 1962).

A direct influence of the tuberculous inflammatory process in causing the development of the confluent masses ('progressive massive fibrosis') of coal and carbon pneumoconiosis in man has been suggested for years but not convincingly demonstrated, although it is possible that it may initiate these lesions in a proportion of cases and subsequently die out. The problem is discussed in more detail in Chapter 8.

Various 'opportunist' mycobacteria, distinct from *M. tuberculosis,* are found in some cases of fibrotic pneumoconiosis which seems to favour their growth. *M. avium* is probably the most important of these as it is poorly sensitive to antibiotic agents and carries a poor prognosis (Marks, 1970). *M. kansasii,* a photochromogen, is also pathogenic for man, and work with guinea pigs has shown that its pathogenicity is enhanced by quartz and coal dusts (Policard *et al.*, 1967). No evidence has been forthcoming to show that these organisms play any part in the formation or enhancement of pneumoconiotic lesions.

Only in the case of *M. kansasii* infection is there evidence of a definite rather than a fortuitous association with dust. Exposure to a particular dust at, or shortly before, the time of diagnosis of the infection appears to be more important to its development than the presence of an established pneumoconiosis. This may indicate either that the organism is inhaled with the dust or that the dust diminishes the lungs' defences against the organism (British Thoracic and Tuberculosis Association, 1975). However, not all cases with this infection have been exposed to a dust hazard (Marks, 1975).

The technique for classifying tubercle bacilli and other mycobacteria cultured from clinical specimens has been auhoritatively reviewed by Marks (1976). Thirteen different opportunist organisms are now identifiable.

ASBESTOSIS

The pathogenesis of asbestosis appears to be different from that of both silicosis and coal pneumoconiosis. The various types of asbestos are distinguished in Chapters 2 and 9. Irrespective of asbestos type short fibres (less than about 10 μm) are readily and completely ingested by macrophages and, like quartz particles, are enclosed in secondary

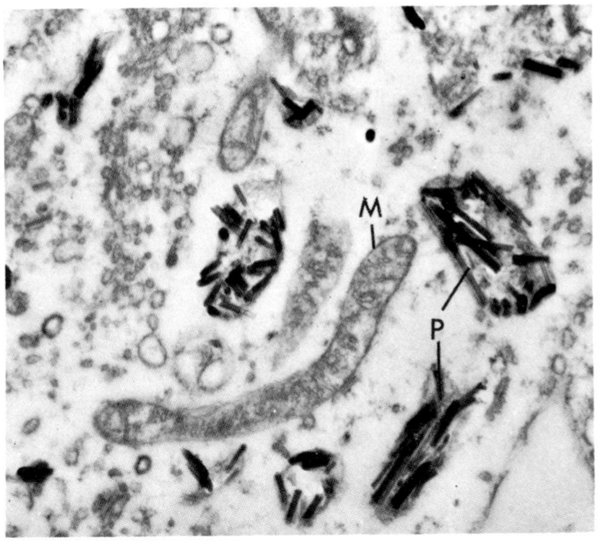

Figure 4.11 Electron micrograph of a segment of a macrophage that has ingested asbestos particles. These are grouped in phagosomes (P) which remain intact; mitochondria (M) are still well preserved. (By courtesy of Dr A. C. Allison)

lysosomes (*Figure 4.11*) whereas long fibres (more than 30 μm) are never completely engulfed and a number of cells may be attached to one fibre. Stereoscan electron microscopy shows apparent continuity of their cytoplasm; sometimes they fuse to form foreign body giant cells. Fibres of intermediate length (5–20 μm) may or may not be completely ingested by the cells (Allison 1973) (*Figure 4.12*).

As in the case of quartz two types of cytotoxic activity occur: an early effect (for example, haemolysis) which follows shortly after fibres come in contact with the plasma membrane of cells in saline media but is greatly inhibited by the presence of serum proteins; a late effect due to the interaction of ingested fibres with the membranes of secondary lysosomes. Chrysotile and anthophyllite fibres have, in general, been found to be more active in both types of reaction than crocidolite and amosite (Allison, 1973)—although this has not been confirmed by all observers (Parazzi *et al.*, 1968; Pernis and Castano, 1971)—but, compared with crystalline silica, the cytotoxicity of all types of asbestos is mild (Allison, 1971). This contrast between the effects of silica and asbestos is reflected in the different behaviour of alveolar macrophages from normal rats when exposed *in vitro* to quartz particles and crocidolite fibres. Phagocytosis of quartz is extremely rapid and the cells develop long, tenuous filopodia whereas phagocytosis of crocidolite is much slower and filopodia are less prominent (Miller, Handfield and Kagan, 1978) (*Figure 4.4*).

The mechanism by which fibroblasts are stimulated to synthesize collagen is far from clear but again macrophages probably play a key, intermediary role. For example, in the presence of asbestos fibres they selectively release large amounts of lysosomal enzymes (Davies *et al.*, 1974), and a direct effect on fibroblast cell membranes may occur (Hext *et al.*, 1977; Richards *et al.*, 1977). However, there is strong evidence that the fibrogenic potential of asbestos fibres is chiefly determined by their length: that is, fibres longer than 10–20 μm may be fibrogenic whereas those which are shorter are not (Timbrell and Skidmore, 1968; Beck *et al.*, 1971; Webster, 1970; Allison, 1973; Rendall, 1972; Bruch, 1974; Gross, 1974; Robock and Klosterkötter, 1977; Wright

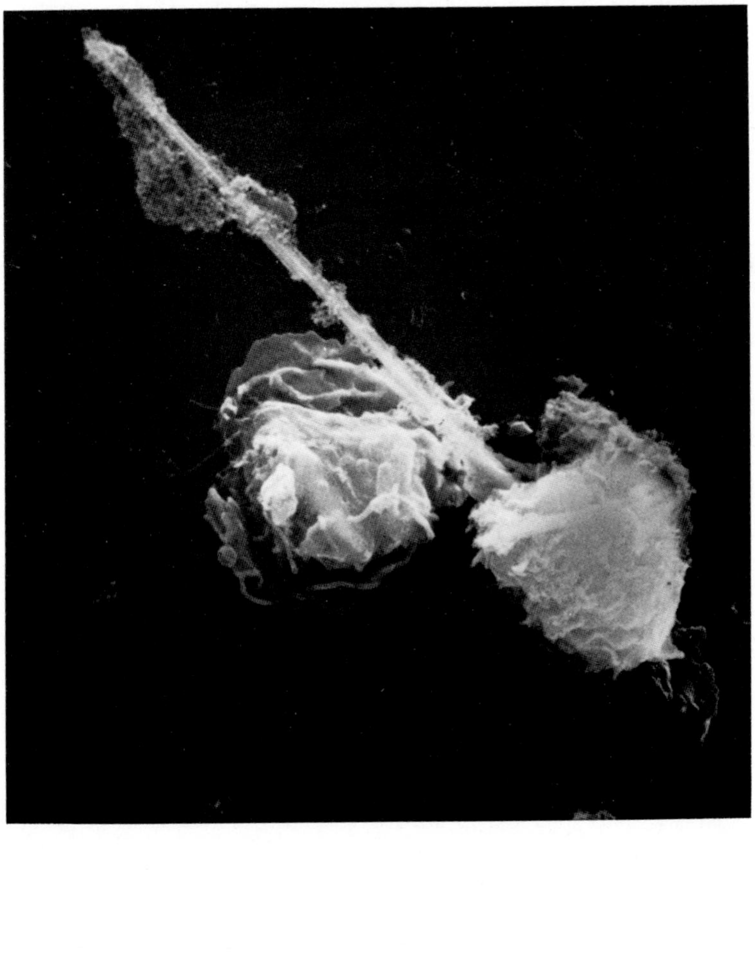

Figure 4.12 Scanning electron micrograph showing attempted phagocytosis of a crocidolite fibre by several alveolar macrophages. The cell at the upper end of the fibre is dead. (Original magnification × 1440). (Courtesy of Dr K. Miller and the Editor of Environ. Hlth*)*

and Kuschner, 1977) (*see also* Chapter 9, p. 254). Furthermore, long curly fibres are more likely than short, straight fibres to be intercepted at respiratory bronchiolar level where the fibrosis commences (*see* Chapter 3, p. 47). Incompletely ingested fibres increase the permeability of the macrophage cell membrane (Beck, Holt and Manojlovic, 1972) allowing both prolonged interaction with plasma membranes and leakage of enzymes and other cell products, and these may initiate the train of fibrogenic events. They also impair the ability of the cells to transport them from the lungs, whereas short fibres (less than 15 μm) —unlike quartz particles—are readily carried away by intact macrophages to the airways and hilar lymph nodes. Thus, it appears that when fibres are short enough to be completely engulfed by macrophages they have little or no fibrogenic or oncogenic potential (Gross, 1974; Harington, Allison and Badami, 1975). Although Wagner *et al.* (1974) reported the development of asbestosis, of lung cancers related to the severity of asbestosis and of occasional pleural mesotheliomas in rats exposed to the four major asbestos types with *mean* fibre lengths ranging from 5.3 μm to 9.0 μm, fibres up to and in excess of 150 μm were also present in the dust clouds (Skidmore, 1977). A similar inhalation experiment with three different types of asbestos—chrysotile, crocidolite and amosite—gives additional support to the concept of long fibres being more fibrogenic than short in that chrysotile dust clouds contain many more fibres greater than 20 μm in length than the amphibole clouds and cause more fibrosis (Davis *et al.*, 1978). The major body of evidence, therefore, indicates that the length of asbestos fibres is the decisive factor in the production of asbestosis and malignant mesothelioma in animals and man; though small fibre-diameter (less than 1 μm) appears to be important in the genesis of mesothelioma (*see* Chapter 9).

The injury caused to cell membranes by chrysotile and anthophyllite is believed to be due to their high magnesium content (Allison, 1973), but this does not explain the fibrogenic effect of crocidolite which is magnesium-free. Alternatively, there is evidence that the surface charge of fibres is the principal responsible factor and that this is more pronounced for chrysotile than for the amphiboles (Light and Wei, 1977). This effect may also result in lipid peroxidation which appears to be one of the reactions by which membrane damage is caused by asbestos (Gabor and Anca, 1975).

A significant feature revealed by electron microscopy is the development of an electron-dense matrix around asbestos particles in secondary lysosomes; this may protect the lysosomal membranes from damage and account for the difference between their comparatively mild cytotoxicity, on the one hand, and strong haemolytic effect, on the other (Allison, 1971). Iron-containing pigment collects in the vacuoles and is important *in vivo* in the formation of 'asbestos bodies' (*see* p. 239).

There is also reason to believe that immunological events may be related in some way to pathogenesis. The presence of circulating RF and ANA in a substantial number of individuals with asbestosis has been referred to already on pp. 60 and 61. The normal receptor sites for IgG and the C3 component of complement on the surface of macrophages (Reynolds *et al.*, 1975) are apparently increased in cells which have ingested crocidolite fibres shorter than 5 μm, although these surface changes are in no way specific. Furthermore, changes in serum immunoglobulins and circulating T lymphocytes have been reported in individuals with asbestosis (intrapulmonary fibrosis). These points are discussed in Chapter 9.

The interesting observation that chrysotile, amosite, crocidolite and anthophyllite fibres inhibit the production of viral interferon by human and simian cells—an effect which, as in the case of coal (*see* p. 72), can be reduced or abolished by pre-treatment of the fibres or the cells with PVPNO (Hahon, Booth and Eckert, 1977)—has not, as yet, been shown to have any relevence to human asbestos-related disease.

In short, the pathogenesis of asbestosis and other forms of asbestos-related disease appears to be determined by a complex interplay between asbestos fibres, cells and, possibly, immunological events which is gradually being elucidated.

BERYLLIUM DISEASE

Beryllium is a powerful adjuvant to antibody production in experimental animals and there is little doubt that immunological reactivity plays an important role in human beryllium disease. This is discussed in Chapter 10.

CONCLUSIONS

The occurrence, evolution and characteristics of lung diseases caused by the inhalation of extraneous particles depend not only upon the nature of the particles and the dose and duration of their inhalation, but also upon their effects on macrophages and, indirectly, on fibroblasts; and, in some instances, upon alteration of T and B lymphocyte function and the development of antigen–antibody response—that is, a 'host response'. The end-result of the inhalation of fibrogenic dusts in the various types of pneumoconiosis is likely to depend as much upon complex cellular or humoral reactions to them as upon some direct fibrogenic potential of the dust. The patterns of these reactions appear to vary qualitatively and quantitatively in different subjects. The relevance of immunological reactions in the development and evolution of various occupational disorders of the lung can be summarized in this way.

(1) Non-organ-specific auto-antibody activity occurs at some stage, and to a varying degree, in the course of the pathogenesis of silicosis, coal pneumoconiosis and asbestosis, but its significance is not yet properly understood. In addition, T lymphocyte function may also be depressed in these diseases.
(2) An Arthus (Type III) reaction resulting from activation of complement by the classic or the alternative pathways plays a major role in the pathogenesis of acute extrinsic allergic 'alveolitis' provoked by certain organic dusts (for example, farmers' lung and bird fanciers' lung). But the total tissue response appears to be more complex and to involve—in some cases at least—a Type I reaction which acts as a trigger mechanism for the development of the Type II reaction which, in turn, may be followed by a Type IV, cell-mediated response (*see* Chapter 11).
(3) Cell-mediated immunity is apparently involved in the development of beryllium disease in which there is also an increase in serum immunoglobulins (*see* Chapter 10).

(4) The possibility that antibodies to natural or denatured collagen or collagen–anticollagen immune complexes might play an important part in the genesis of certain fibrotic pneumoconioses seems real and calls for investigation (*see* p. 64).
(5) Extrinsic asthma has a variety of occupational causes and may be of immediate onset resulting from reaginic (IgE) or non-reaginic (STS–IgG) Type I reactions or of 'late' (non-immediate) onset due to a Type III reaction. A long delay in onset after exposure to the allergen may indicate involvement of a Type IV reaction but this remains to be established (*see* Chapter 12).
(6) It seems likely that HLA type may exert some influence on individual susceptibility or resistance to the development or progression of a pneumoconiosis and other form of occupational lung disorder such as extrinsic allergic 'alveolitis'.

Use of cell culture for testing cytotoxicity of various mineral dusts is invaluable as a convenient and reproducible technique. However, because uniform standardization of methodological detail has been lacking and the results of experiments in the hands of some workers has, therefore, been in doubt there is need to correct this situation on an international basis (Harington, 1972). This has been achieved to some extent in the case of standard reference samples of the asbestos minerals for experimental use (Timbrell, Gilson and Webster, 1968).

DIFFUSE INTERSTITIAL PULMONARY FIBROSIS (DIPF) AND FIBROSING ALVEOLITIS

These terms describe certain non-specific features of lung disease but other terms are also used, so that confusion of meaning is apt to occur. The disease consists of bilateral, diffuse fibrosis which chiefly affects the gas-exchanging regions of the lungs from the terminal bronchioles onwards (that is, the acini), and may or may not be associated with cyst formation of varying severity. It represents the end-stage of antecedent acute or subacute disease provoked by a great variety of causes which fall into three main categories: non-occupational, occupational and unknown (cryptogenic).

As fibrosis of non-occupational origin and unknown cause appears to be increasing in prevalence (Rosenow, 1972; Spencer, 1975) there may be considerable difficulty in identifying specific pathogenesis both clinically and pathologically and, therefore, in diagnosis. This difficulty is enhanced in individuals who have been exposed to an occupational respiratory hazard—for example, the asbestos minerals. Hence, when the clinician sees a patient with diffuse pulmonary fibrosis and a history of work in a known occupational risk he may be tempted, without detailed investigation, to attribute the disease (incorrectly) to that risk; or, on the other hand, if he overlooks a relevant occupational hazard he may wrongly relegate the disease to some other cause. It seems desirable, therefore, to attempt some clarification of this important difficulty. Individual occupational disorders are described in later chapters.

Because antecedent disease does not necessarily progress to fibrosis and may resolve completely Scadding (1964) proposed the general term 'diffuse fibrosing alveolitis' to embrace all stages of the continuum and Scadding and Hinson (1967) distinguished two fundamental types of lesion:

(1) At one extreme (*acute*) alveolar walls are little, if at all, thickened by fibrosis but numerous mononuclear cells, either Type II pneumocytes or alveolar macrophages, occupy the air spaces. They called this '*desquamative*' fibrosing alveolitis. It is usually distributed more or less uniformly in the lungs, but may be patchy.
(2) At the other extreme (*chronic*) alveolar walls are much thickened by fibrosis and intra-alveolar cells are few. This they termed '*mural*' fibrosing alveolitis and it is distributed irregularly in the lungs being sometimes fairly localized.

There are many intermediate stages or patterns between these two extremes but the predominantly acellular fibrotic, mural type corresponds to an end-stage commonly referred to as *diffuse interstitial pulmonary fibrosis* (DIPF)—the term used throughout this book.

However, Liebow, Steer and Billingsley (1965) and Liebow (1975) described the antecedent pathological changes in other terms:

(1) Usual or 'classic' interstitial pneumonia (UIP).
(2) UIP with bronchiolitis obliterans.
(3) Desquamative interstitial pneumonia (DIP).

The early stage of UIP consists of congestion and oedema of the alveolar walls and damage to or destruction of Type I pneumocytes and alveolar, capillary endothelial cells with leakage of plasma constituents into the alveolar spaces and production of hyaline membranes and fibrin. The later stages are identical with mural fibrosing alveolitis of Scadding and Hinson. In some cases bronchiolitis obliterans is superimposed on the disease process at one stage or another. DIP consists primarily of large cellular accumulations in alveolar spaces with less striking changes—usually infiltration by lymphocytes and plasma cells—in the walls.

But, in addition, chronic oedema of alveolar walls due to chronic left ventricular failure and chronic renal disease (Spencer, 1975), and widespread sarcoid-type granuloma formation such as occurs in beryllium disease and extrinsic allergic alveolitis (*see* Chapters 10 and 11 respectively) may result in mural fibrosing alveolitis or DIPF. There is, therefore, a wide range of acute and subacute pathological features which antecede the common, irreversible end-stage DIPF, although in many cases the earlier stages may resolve completely either spontaneously or with treatment.

In spite of this multiplicity of terms for the earlier stages in the continuum DIPF appears the most satisfactory for the final stage. 'Alveolitis' is a useful shorthand term for the intermediate stages provided it is understood that the disease process it describes is not limited to the alveoli but commonly involves the walls of respiratory bronchioles and sometimes terminal bronchioles; that Arthus (Type III) reactions of extrinsic allergic disease frequently occur in adjacent small blood vessels, and that sarcoid-type granulomas are found in both bronchiolar and alveolar walls in acute and chronic beryllium disease and extrinsic allergic disease. The general term 'extrinsic allergic alveolitis' introduced by Pepys (1969) to describe the acute and chronic phases of allergic disease caused by inhaled organic antigens is firmly established but the irreversible end-stage is, of course, DIPF.

The historical development of these terms can be summarized schematically as follows:

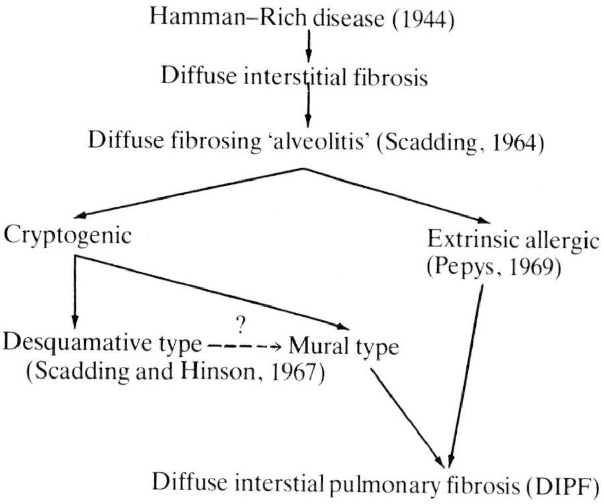

And their equivalence with the other terms in general use appears to be as follows:

Desquamative fibrosing 'alveolitis'	= DIP
Hamman–Rich disease	= UIP
Mural fibrosing 'alveolitis'	= UIP (with or without bronchiolitis obliterans)
Late mural fibrosing 'alveolitis'	= DIPF
Diffuse pulmonary alveolar fibrosis (Scadding, 1974)	= DIPF

PATHOGENESIS

As indicated in Chapter 3 potential pathogenic agents, both inorganic and organic, may reach the alveolar walls in inhaled air or via the capillary blood stream when absorbed from the intestines or introduced intravenously. The lungs can concentrate many drugs and some are known to cause UIP, desquamative fibrosing 'alveolitis' and DIPF; and acute and chronic allergic processes may occur in relation to treatment. It is probable that a proportion of cases of cryptogenic DIPF represents the end-result of unrecognized drug reactions and of antecedent UIP or desquamative fibrosing 'alveolitis' due to other causes (Davies, 1969; Rosenow, 1972; Gillett and Ford, 1978). The possibility that avian and other antigens absorbed from normal gut or the gut of gluten sensitive enteropathy may cause or precipitate exacerbation of existing extrinsic allergic 'alveolitis' is discussed in Chapter 11. It has been stressed that the antecedents of end-stage DIPF may be any form of UIP or mural fibrosing 'alveolitis', or of a variety of other diseases, especially those characterized by miliary or disseminated granulomas (Liebow, 1975); and an additional cause in recent years may be incomplete resolution of pneumonic exudates due to inhibition of inflammatory cell activity by antibiotic drugs (Auerbach, Mims and Goodpasture, 1952). And corticosteroids may also have played a part. Furthermore, DIPF is well known to be associated with a number of 'connective tissue disorders' (*Table 4.4*). But in many cases there is no identifiable cause (cryptogenic DIPF) though, occasionally, some are familial (familial pulmonary fibrosis); which raises the question of genetic predisposition, even of a 'fibrotic gene' (Bitterman and Crystal, 1980; Hughes, 1964).

The percentage of lymphocytes in broncho-alveolar lavage fluid is reported to be increased in patients with sarcoidosis and extrinsic allergic 'alveolitis' but not in those with cryptogenic pulmonary fibrosis alone or with pulmonary fibrosis associated with collagen vascular disease or eosinophilic granuloma. However, in cryptogenic

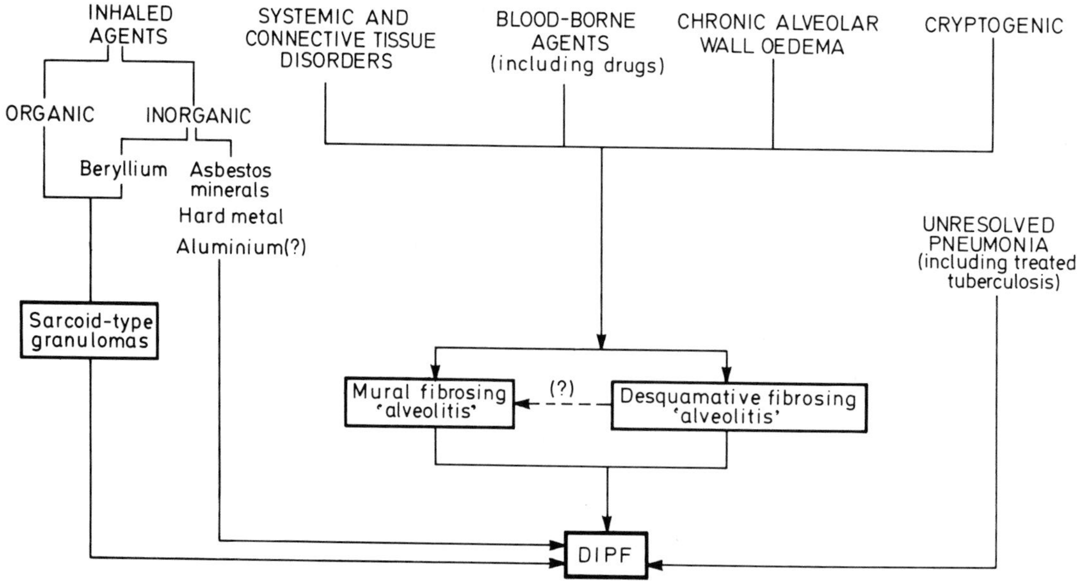

Figure 4.13 Schema of possible pathways of pathogenesis of DIPF

Table 4.4 Some Causes of Diffuse Interstitial Pulmonary Fibrosis (DIPF)

(1) LONE DIPF	
(a) *Inhaled materials*	
Inorganic	Asbestos minerals (Chapter 9) Beryllium metal and compounds (Chapter 10) 'Hard metal disease' (Chapter 13) 'Aluminium lung' (Chapter 13) Mercury vapour (Chapter 13)
Organic	Fungal spores (Chapter 11) Avian serum proteins (Chapter 11) Other foreign proteins (Chapter 11) Toluene diisocyanate (Chapter 11) Hairsprays (?) (Chapter 11)
(b) *Ingested or parenterally administered materials*	
Drugs	Bischloroethylnitrosourea (Durant *et al.*, 1979; Malato and Tuveri, 1980) Bleomycin Busulphan Chlorambucil Cyclophosphamide 5-Fluorouracil and mitomycin C (Stockley and Brookes, 1978) Gold salts (Geddes and Brostoff, 1976; Terho, Torkko and Valta, 1979) Hexamethonium* Mecamylamine* Melphelan (Codling and Chakera, 1972) Methotrexate (Bedrossian, Miller and Luna, 1979) Methysergide Nitrofurantoin (Sovijärvi *et al.*, 1977) Pentolinium* Practolol (Erwteman, Braat and van Aken, 1977) Vincristine
Other	Avian proteins ? (Ingested) Kerosene Paraquat (Chapter 11)
(c) *Incomplete resolution of pneumonias*	
(d) *Ionizing radiation*	
(e) *Chronic oedema of alveolar walls*	Chronic left ventricular failure Chronic renal failure
(2) ASSOCIATED SYSTEMIC DISEASE	Sarcoidosis Rheumatoid disease Systemic sclerosis Systemic lupus erythematosus Dermatomyositis Sjögren's disease Idiopathic pulmonary haemosiderosis Polyarteritis nodosa Histocytosis X Multiple neurofibromatosis Tuberose sclerosis Hyperglobulinaemic renal tubular acidosis
(3) FAMILIAL PULMONARY FIBROSIS	

*No longer employed in treatment of systemic hypertension

pulmonary fibrosis there is a relatively high percentage of neutrophil granulocytes compared with the other disease categories and, as these cells produce collagenase, they could be responsible for degrading Type III collagen (Weinberger *et al.*, 1978; Gell, 1980). Although considerable overlap of cell levels in these various disease types exists further investigation may show distinctive cellular differences in patients with lone cryptogenic pulmonary fibrosis, pulmonary fibrosis with collagen vascular disease, and asbestosis. Indeed, a hint of a possible difference in asbestosis has been observed by Haslam *et al.* (1980). There are also large numbers of broncho-alveolar lymphocytes and differences in the ratio of T and B cells compared with their ratio in the peripheral blood in cryptogenic pulmonary fibrosis and extrinsic allergic 'alveolitis', suggesting that the lungs may function as relatively independent immune organs (Reynolds *et al.*, 1977). In all such investigations it is, of course, necessary to take the effects of smoking on cell populations into account (*see* Addendum, p. 88).

The possibility that auto-allergic, delayed, hypersensitivity to collagen—perhaps denatured in some way—may be involved is supported by the report that antibodies to Type I collagen have been found in patients with cryptogenic pulmonary fibrosis (Kravis *et al.*, 1976).

The observation that the desquamative stage of cryptogenic fibrosing 'alveolitis' (DIP) is significantly associated with IgG deposition in alveolar walls and capillary walls and with raised serum levels of immune complexes whereas the acellular, diffuse fibrotic stage is not would, if confirmed, support an immunological pathogenesis in some cases of desquamative fibrosing 'alveolitis' (Dreisen *et al.*, 1978).

Examples of the diverse causes of DIPF are summarized in *Table 4.4* and their possible modes of action indicated in *Figure 4.13*. With regard to extrinsic allergic 'alveolitis' it is worth noting that in Britain approximately 12 per cent of the population are computed to be in contact with budgerigars (parakeets) and that between 65 and 900/100 000 are likely to have the disease (Hendrick, Faux and Marshall, 1978) (*see* Chapter 11).

PATHOLOGICAL FEATURES

Macroscopic appearances

In many cases (*excluding* those of asbestosis) when disease is advanced the surface of the pulmonary pleura is studded with multiple small, soft, hob-nail protuberances or 'air blebs' caused by underlying cysts and may resemble the surface of cirrhotic liver. Unlike most cases of asbestosis diffuse thickening of the pleura is, in general, slight or absent.

When cut the lungs show an irregular pattern of light or dark grey or brown coloured fibrosis which may be predominant in their lower or upper halves or, in some cases, involves all zones. Occasionally the fibrosis is black due to accumulated carbon. It is usually patchy and tends to be concentrated in the peripheral subpleural zones or towards the centres of the lobes, but both distributions may co-exist. In general, there is a sharp demarcation between the fibrotic areas and adjacent normal lung. Honeycomb cysts varying from 2 to 15 mm or more in diameter may also be present in the areas of fibrosis except where this is most dense; they are bilateral but not necessarily equally so, may be localized or widespread and larger cysts are more apt to occur away from the immediate periphery of the lobes (Heppleston, 1956) (*Figures 4.14* and *4.15*). The hallmark of the DIPF of *asbestosis* is that it is sited peripherally in the lower lobes, the middle lobe and lingula. Only occasionally (and then in advanced disease) does it involve more central zones or extend to the basal regions of the upper lobes. Its demarcation from normal lung is usually ill-defined. Cysts are

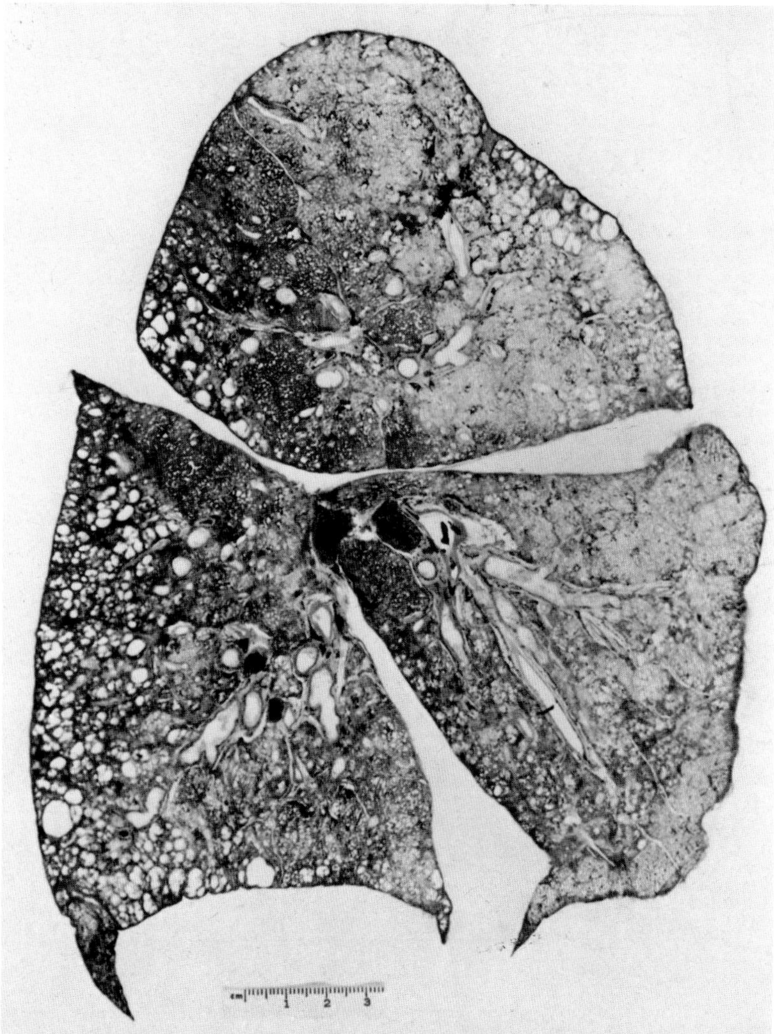

Figure 4.14 Whole section of right lung showing extensive, non-pigmented DIPF with multiple cysts up to 8 mm diameter in original section. Note the extent of involvement of the lower and upper lobes. The DIPF is sharply defined from adjacent normal lung. Diagnosis: cryptogenic fibrosing 'alveolitis'. No occupational risk. (Compare with Figure 9.12*)*

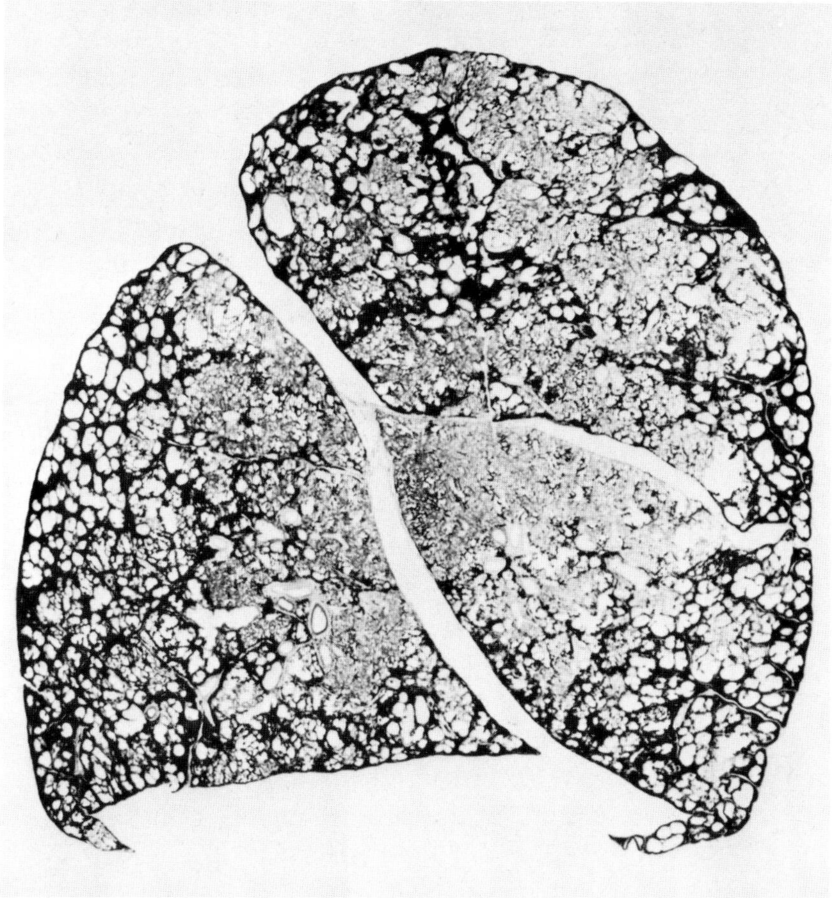

Figure 4.15 Widespread, black pigmented DIPF with cysts up to 1.0 cm diameter in original section. Sharp demarcation from adjacent lung. Coal miner for 20 years. No coal pneumoconiosis. (Compare with Figure 9.12.*)* See Figure 8.42 *for radiographic appearances*

uncommon but, when present, rarely exceed about 3 mm in diameter (*see* Chapter 9 and *Figure 9.12*).

Microscopic appearances

Alveolar walls are much thickened by collagen fibrosis, and in some areas the alveolar spaces are obliterated. A relative increase in Type I and a decrease in Type III collagen (reticulin) in cryptogenic DIPF has already been referred to on p. 64. Large numbers of lymphocytes and plasma cells may be present in the alveolar walls, and there are many macrophages in air spaces adjacent to the fibrosis. Where the fibrosis is uniformly black the individual has usually had significant exposure to carbon in some form (for example, soot, coal, graphite) and macrophages in the vicinity are often laden with black pigment which is probably carbon but may also be related (at least in part) to pigment from cigarette smoke. The blackening suggests that the fibrosis occurred in an already dusty or pigmented lung, but there is no known pathogenic significance attached to this.

Unlike emphysema honeycomb cysts have no crossing strands and are lined by flattened, cuboidal, ciliated or non-ciliated columnar epithelium. The cysts consist of localized bronchiolectasis caused by dilatation of both terminal and respiratory bronchioles. Valvar obstruction at the point where bronchioles enter the cysts may contribute to their pathogenesis (Heppleston, 1956); they may also be formed by greatly enlarged alveolar ducts.

Proliferation of *smooth muscle* in large or small bundles is often present in varying degree in the fibrotic areas as a lattice work among the cysts or in parallel groups beneath the pulmonary pleura and also in the walls of vessels, especially those of lymphatics (Davies *et al.*, 1966; Heppleston, 1956; Herbert *et al.*, 1962; Liebow, Loring and Felton, 1953; Ovenfors *et al.*, 1980) (*Figure 4.16*). This appears to be due to active hyperplasia or production of muscle cells as the muscle bundles are often distant from their normal locations, and electron microscopy suggests that immature, multipotential mesenchymal cells in alveolar walls may differentiate into smooth muscle cells (Fraire *et al.*, 1973), and that normal myofibroblasts (non-muscle cells) can assume the characteristics of smooth muscle cells (Evans, Kelley and Adler, 1980). *Elastic tissue*, either as single strands or dense tangled masses, is often prominent due, partly, to compaction of normal elastic tissue resulting from collapse and obliteration of alveolar spaces and respiratory bronchioles but in the denser areas it is frequently excessive probably as a result of active hyperplasia—'elastosis' (Heppleston, 1956) (*Figure 4.17*). Furthermore, *lymph follicle hyperplasia*—sometimes with germinal centres—may be present as a survival from antecedent desquamative fibrosing 'alveolitis' in which it is a common feature (Scadding and Hinson, 1967) (*Figure 4.18*). However, all these hyperplasic changes are not necessarily seen in any one case. In DIPF associated with generalized neurofibromatosis there is hyperplasia of neurilemmal cells in the intrapulmonary nerves especially in

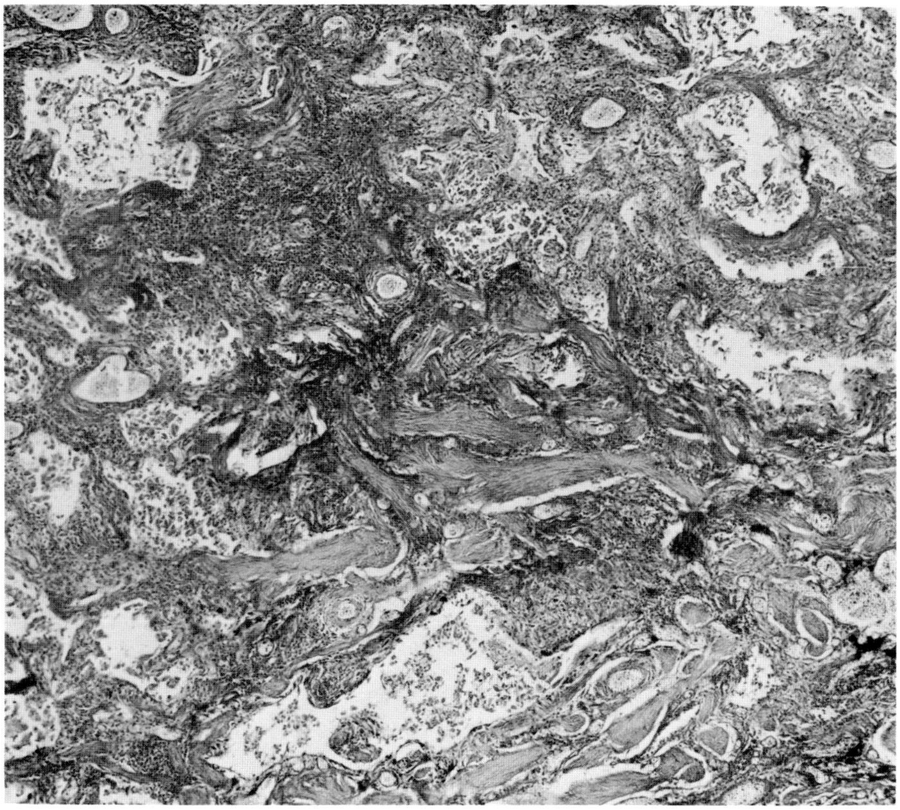

Figure 4.16 DIPF with well marked muscular hyperplasia. Muscle bundles are especially prominent in the middle and lower right quadrant of this field. Elsewhere alveolar walls are fibrotic. Note cellularity and cyst formation. No granulomas. A small number of asbestos bodies present in other sections but not in this. (Original magnification × 60. Picro-Mallory stain.)

Naked eye: there was moderately extensive DIPF with cysts from 2–10 mm diameter, more in the upper lobes than the lower. (See Figure 9.24 *for the radiographic appearances and further details)*

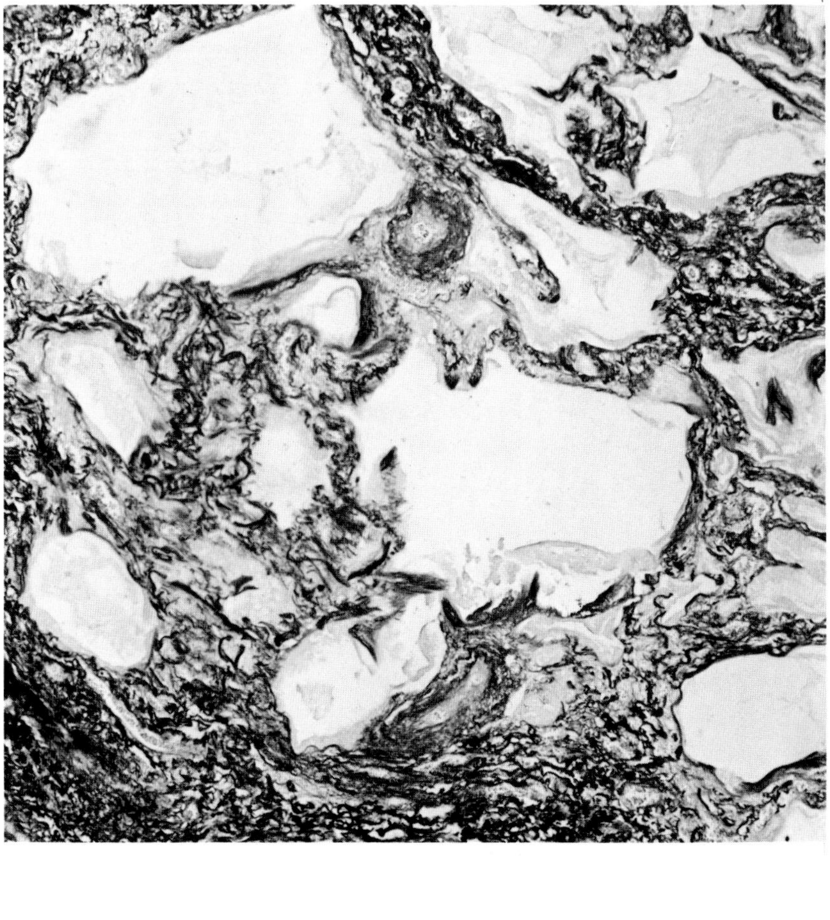

Figure 4.17 DIPF with substantial increase of elastic fibres (dense wavy lines) especially in areas of collagenous fibrosis (less dense) and multiple cysts. Occasional asbestos bodies seen in 30 μm sections but not in this. No granulomas. (Original magnification × 60. Elastic van Giesen stain).

Naked eye: scattered irregular fibrosis with many cysts up to 6 mm diameter distributed more in the upper lobes than the lower.

Female aged 70 at time of death. Worked in an asbestos processing factory for 12 months 35 years earlier in 1944

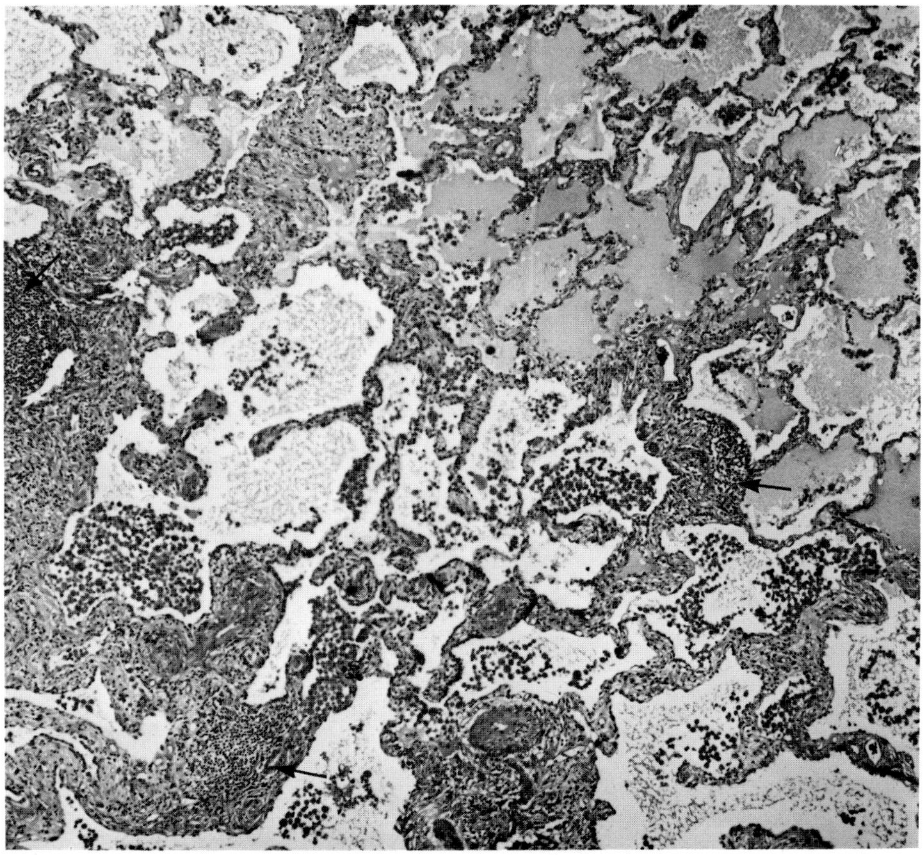

Figure 4.18 DIPF (mural type fibrosing 'alveolitis') with lymph follicle hyperplasia (arrowed). Moderate patchy fibrosis of alveolar walls and occasional 'honeycomb' cysts. (Original magnification × 60. H and E stain.)

Naked eye: there was irregular fibrosis in all lobes with cysts from 2 to 10 mm diameter more in the upper than the lower. No granulomas. No asbestos bodies identified. (See Figure 9.23a *and* b *for radiographic appearances and details)*

periarterial branches, and glomus-like structures in small branches of the pulmonary veins, in addition to smooth muscle hyperplasia (Spencer, 1977).

By contrast, in asbestosis smooth muscle proliferation of and lymph follicle hyperplasia are absent and although there may be some compaction of the elastic fibres of fibrotic alveolar walls, hyperplasia does not seem to occur. Also, there is no accumulation of lymphocytes and plasma cells in alveolar walls, and remnant areas of UIP or DIP which may be found in lungs with DIPF due to other causes are not seen. In addition, of course, asbestos or ferruginous bodies are *readily* identifiable in, and adjacent to, the fibrosis and elsewhere in the lungs (*see* Chapter 9).

Active sarcoid-type granulomas or follicular scars of healed lesions may persist in the lungs and hilar lymph nodes in sarcoidosis and chronic beryllium disease, but are not seen in chronic extrinsic allergic 'alveolitis' (*see* Chapters 10 and 11).

In recent years an increasing number of lungs, referred to us as cases of asbestosis, have shown many of the macro- and microscopical features just described instead of, or in addition to, the appearances which, over many years, have been regarded as indicative of asbestosis even though some asbestos (or 'ferruginous') bodies and a history of occupational exposure to asbestos have usually been present. There are three possible explanations for this:

(1) The disease is not asbestosis in spite of the evidence of asbestos exposure. In many cases this is supported by the uncharacteristic distribution of fibrosis, the presence of multiple large honeycomb cysts, of hyperplasia of smooth muscle, lymph follicles and elastic, and, occasionally, by remnants of active fibrosing 'alveolitis'. And, of course, there is no reason why an asbestos worker should not develop an unrelated lung disease. When the asbestos fibre content of these lungs has been quantified it is often not much in excess of values found in random samples of the urban population (*see* Chapter 9).

(2) Both asbestosis and some other form of DIPF are present concurrently. This is a rare occurrence but occasional cases are seen. The fibre content of the lungs is then likely to be high.

(3) The disease seen represents a hitherto unrecognized variant of asbestosis. This is improbable. In the past pathologists experienced in the study of asbestosis have not described these changes as a feature of the disease (*see*, for example: Gloyne, 1932–33; Caplan *et al.*, 1965; Hourihane and McCaughey, 1966; Spencer, 1977); and Heppleston (1956) in his authoritative study of 'honeycomb lung' did not mention asbestosis. In short, there is no convincing evidence to support this explanation.

It is noteworthy that in many of these cases past asbestos exposure appears to have been fairly low.

The profusion of asbestos bodies in microsections is a reasonably good index of the total number of uncoated asbestos fibres in the lungs even though most of these are invisible by light microscopy (Ashcroft and Heppleston, 1973 (*see* Chapter 9, p. 239). But they are also present in small numbers—about 20 or less per 1.5 cm² field in 30 μm sections (Doniach, Swettenham and Hathorn, 1975; McPherson and Davidson, 1969; Um, 1971)—in from 20 to 90 per cent of non-fibrotic lungs of city dwellers (*see* Chapter 9, p. 240). Therefore, it is to be expected that asbestos bodies may also be found in the lungs of a proportion of cases with unrelated disease including DIPF which is not asbestosis. In this respect it is of interest that Ashcroft and Heppleston (1973) showed that whereas mild to moderate asbestosis is directly related to the amount of asbestos dust retained in the lungs—and, hence, to the profusion of asbestos bodies—the changes which they considered to be those of severe asbestosis exhibit no such relationship. Their 'severe asbestosis' consisted of areas of solid fibrosis and of multiple large honeycomb cysts (similar to *Figures 4.14* and *4.15*) which they suggested might be the sequelae of non-specific inflammatory disease resulting from inadequate antibiotic treatment. While this is probably true of some cases, in others an equally plausible explanation is that the disease—especially when its distribution and form are atypical—is, in fact, DIPF of different origin in which the presence of asbestos bodies (and fibres) is fortuitous. Similarly, the finding of scanty 'ferruginous bodies' thought to contain asbestos fibres in a reported case of desquamative fibrosing 'alveolitis' (Corrin and Price, 1972) does not prove asbestos to have been the cause of the disease.

The following point is worth considering in this respect. It is customary to regard groups of asbestos bodies or their fragments in areas of fibrosis as proof that the fibrosis is caused by asbestos. However, as animal experiments have shown, development of fibrosis in the lungs may locally impede the natural clearance of both compact and fibrous particles ultimately enclosing them in some areas so that their removal may become impossible. And there is evidence that this occurs in man (*see* Chapter 9, p. 254). One can envisage, therefore, that DIPF associated with asbestos (or 'ferruginous') bodies may not necessarily be asbestosis but could be due to some other cause.

However, it has been suggested that minute asbestos fibres or fibrils beyond the resolution of light microscopy may be responsible for some cases of 'idiopathic interstitial fibrosis' (Gaensler and Addington, 1969; Miller *et al.*, 1975). Miller and his colleagues based this view on a case of an individual with no known exposure to potentially pathogenic dusts who had diffuse honeycomb fibrosis in which asbestos bodies and fibres were not demonstrated by the light microscope although minute chrysotile fibres averaging 27.5 nm in diameter and less than 100 nm (0.1 μm) in length were observed by electron microscopy. But, as already stated (p. 73 *et seq.*), current evidence indicates that asbestos fibres small enough to be completely engulfed by macrophages are not fibrogenic. In any case, the development of asbestosis is determined by the product of intensity and duration of dust exposure (*see* Chapter 9, p. 253).

The significance of the lung content of asbestos bodies and fibres in asbestosis and in individuals with no occupational exposure is discussed in Chapter 9.

It has been claimed that a variety of other inorganic dusts and cotton fibres found in the lungs may induce DIPF (Rüttner, Spycher and Engeler, 1968; Rüttner, Spycher and Sticher, 1973), but satisfactory proof of a causal relationship was not substantiated; indeed, the 'cotton fibres case' appears rather to be one of unrelated extrinsic allergic alveolitis.

In short, it seems clear that the detection of various minerals—even those with known pathogenic potential—in diseased lungs does not *necessarily* prove a causal relationship. Indeed, much of the extrinsic foreign material detected in the lungs by highly sensitive techniques is likely to be without pathogenic significance. Research into this important problem continues but ensuing results demand critical appraisal.

To summarize

The pathological differentiation between DIPF of occupational and non-occupational origin rests upon the macro- and microscopical features of the disease and on thorough investigation of past occupational exposure and exclusion of the various other possible causes of DIPF (*Table 4.4*). Microsections should be taken from different parts of both lungs (including adjacent normal-appearing lung which may contain remnants of antecedent fibrosing 'alveolitis') and from the hilar lymph nodes. Mineralogical studies may be helpful but should not be allowed to eclipse clinico-pathological judgement. (*See* Appendix.)

Perhaps, in the near future, the cytology and Ig content of bronchoalveolar washings may prove to be of value in differential diagnosis.

Some of the pathological features which help to distinguish different causes of DIPF are summarized in *Table 4.5*. Two important points to be borne in mind are that DIPF and pleural disease associated with rheumatoid arthritis rarely occur together in the same patient (Turner-Warwick and Evans, 1977); and that titres of circulating RF are usually substantially higher in cases of DIPF with rheumatoid arthritis than in lone cryptogenic fibrosing 'alveolitis' and asbestosis. The radiographic appearances which may assist differential diagnosis are discussed in Chapter 9.

POST-MORTEM EXAMINATION OF LUNGS

Sound practical knowledge of the pathology of occupational diseases of the lung is only achieved by correlating, whenever possible, observations made during life with the morbid anatomical features of the lungs after death. As Morgagni wrote two centuries ago: 'those who have dissected many bodies, have at least learned to doubt when the others, who are ignorant of anatomy and do not take the trouble to attend to it, are in no doubt at all'. No opportunity, therefore, should be lost to study lungs removed after death and relate the findings to the industrial history, symptomatology and clinical, physiological, radiological and other data obtained during life. Modern techniques for preparing lungs for making paper-mounted whole sections for permanent record contribute greatly to this end. These and some other technical considerations,

Table 4.5 Pathological Features of Different types of DIPF Summarized

	*Cryptogenic and non-allergic**	*Chronic extrinsic allergic 'alveolitis'** (Hypersensitivity pneumonia)	*Asbestosis*
GROSS FEATURES			
Diffuse thickening of pulmonary pleura	Uncommon (unless infected)	Fairly common	Very common
Multiple pleural cysts (air blebs)	Common	Fairly common	Absent
Distribution in lung: predominantly 'lower zones' (i.e. lower lobes, middle lobe and lingula)	Uncommon except in cryptogenic disease	Uncommon Usually 'upper and mid zones' (upper lobes). Generalized in severe disease	Invariable Lower part of upper lobes affected in advanced disease
Lobar distribution: peripheral (sub-pleural) vs central	Peripheral usual but may be slight. Central zones of upper and lower lobes commonly involved. Peripheral zone spared in some cases	Peripheral and central zone involement usual	Peripheral invariable More central involvement unusual
Demarcation from normal lung	Well-defined; sharp, especially CFA	Well-defined	Ill-defined
Honeycomb cysts	Common (2 to 15 mm diameter or more)	Common (2 to 15 mm diameter or more)	Uncommon (seldom more than 3 mm diameter)
MICROSCOPIC FEATURES			
Asbestos bodies in lung	Absent or small numbers	Absent or small numbers	Numerous (i.e. readily found)
Smooth muscle proliferation	Fairly common; may be pronounced	Fairly common	Absent
Follicular lymphoid hyperplasia	Common	Fairly common	Absent
Elastin apparent increase due to compaction or real increase due to hyperplasia	Often prominent especially when fibrosis severe	Fairly common especially when fibrosis severe	Exceptional
Features of desquamative fibrosing 'alveolitis' (DIP) in adjacent lung	Occasional	Rare	Absent
Sarcoid-type granulomas lungs lymph nodes	Absent except in sarcoidosis and chronic beryllium disease	Absent. Seen only in acute and sub-acute disease	Absent

*Note: These disorders may occur in asbestos workers

including polarized light microscopy and a simple method of lung preservation for electron microscopy are referred to in the Appendix.

REFERENCES

Aalto, M., Potila, M. and Kulonen, E. (1976). The effects of silica-treated macrophages on the synthesis of collagen and other proteins *in vitro*. *Expl Cell Res.* **97,** 193–202

Aho, S., Peltonen, J., Jalkanen, M. and Kulonen, E. (1979). Effect of silica on a culture of rat peritoneal macrophages. *Ann. occup. Hyg.* **22,** 285–296

Allison, A. C. (1968). Lysosomes and the responses of cells to toxic materials. In *Scientific Basis of Medicine Annual Reviews,* pp. 18–30. (Br. Postgrad. Med. Fed.) London; Athlone Press

Allison, A. C. (1971). Effects of silica and asbestos on cells in culture. In *Inhaled Particles 3,* edited by W. H. Walton, pp. 437–441. Woking; Unwin

Allison, A. C. (1973). Experimental methods—cell and tissue culture: effects of asbestos particles on macrophages, mesothelial cells and fibroblasts. In *Biological Effects of Asbestos,* edited by P. Bogovski, J. C. Gilson, V. Timbrell and J. C. Wagner, pp. 89–93. Lyon; International Agency for Research on Cancer

Allison, A. C., Clark, I. A. and Davies, P. (1977). Cellular interactions in fibrogenesis. *Ann. rheum. Dis.* **36** (Suppl) 8–13

Allison, A. C. and Hart, P. D. (1968). Potentiation by silica of the growth of *Mycobacterium tuberculosis* in macrophage cultures. *Br. J. exp. Path.* **49,** 465–476

Allison, A. C., Harington, J. S. and Birbeck (1966). An examination of the cytotoxic effects of silica on macrophages. *J. exp. Med.* **124,** 141–154

Anderson, S. G., Bentzon, M. W., Houba, V. and Krag, P. (1970). International Reference preparation of rheumatoid arthritis serum. *Bull. Wld Hlth Org.* **42,** 311–318

Ashcroft, T. and Heppleston, A. G. (1973). The optical and electronic microscopic determination of pulmonary asbestos fibre concentration and its relation to the human pathological reaction. *J. clin. Path.* **26,** 224–234

Askonas, B. A. and Jarošková, L. (1970). Antigen in Macrophages and Antibody Induction. In *Mononuclear Phagocytes,* edited by R. van Furth, pp. 595–610. London and Edinburgh; Blackwell Scientific Publications

Auerbach, S. H., Mims, O. M. and Goodpasture, E. W. (1952). Pulmonary fibrosis secondary to pneumonia. *Am. J. Path.* **28,** 69–87

Bach, F. H., Bach, M. L. and Sondel, P. M. (1976). Differential function of major histocompatability complex antigens in T-lymphocyte activation. *Nature* **259,** 273–281

Ball, J. and Lawrence, J. S. (1961). Epidemiology of the sheep cell agglutination test. *Ann. rheum. Dis.* **20,** 235–245

Beck, E. G., Bruch, J., Friedricks, K. H., Hilscher, W. and Pott, F. (1971). Fibrous silicates in animal experiments and cell culture—morphological cell and tissue reactions according to different physical chemical influences. In *Inhaled Particles 3*, eduted by W. H. Walton, pp. 477–487. Woking; Unwin

Beck, E. G., Holt, P. F. and Manojilović, N. (1972). Comparison of effects on macrophage cultures of glass fibre, glass powder and chrysotile asbestos. *Br. J. ind. Med.* **29,** 280–286

Beck, J. S. (1963). Auto-antibodies to cell nuclei. *Scott. med. J.* **8,** 373–388

Bedrossian, C. W. M., Miller, W. C. and Luna, M. A. (1979). Methotrexate-induced diffuse interstitial pulmonary fibrosis. *Southern Med. J.* **72,** 313–318

Belt, T. and King, E. J. (1945). *Chronic Pulmonary Disease in South Wales Coal Miners.* III. Experimental Studies. MRC. SRS. No. 250. London; HMSO

Bitterman, P. B. and Crystal, R. G. (1980). Is there a fibrotic gene? *Chest* **78,** 549–550

Bodmer, W. F. (1975a). Histocompatibility testing international. *Nature* **256,** 696–698

Bodmer, W. F. (1975b). The HL-A system and its association with immune response and disease. *Ann. Rheum. Dis.* **34,** Suppl. 1. 13–16

Brieger, H. and Gross, P. (1967). On the theory of silicosis III. *Archs envir. Hlth* **15,** 751–757

British Thoracic and Tuberculosis Association (1975). Opportunist mycobacterial pulmonary infection and occupational dust exposure: an investigation in England and Wales. A Report of the Research Committee. *Tubercle* **56,** 295–310

Bruch, J. (1974). Response of cell cultures to asbestos fibres. *Environ. Hlth. Perspect.* **9,** 253–254

Bruch, J. and Otto, H. (1967). Elektronenmikroskopische Beobach-tungen and Alveolarmacrophagen in der Rattenlunge nach Quarz-staubinhalation. *Ergebnusse und Untersuchungen auf dem Gebeit der Staub-und Silikosebekaempf in Steinkohlenbergbau* **6,** 141–148. Defmold, W. Germany; Bosman

Burrell, R. (1972). Immunological aspects of coal worker's pneumoconiosis. *Ann. N.Y. Acad. Sci.* **200,** 94–105

Burrell, R. and Anderson, M. (1973). The induction of fibrogenesis by silica-treated alveolar macrophages. *Envir. Res.* **6,** 389–394

Burrell, R., Esber, H. J., Hagadorn, J. E. and Andrews, C. E. (1966). Specificity of lung reactive antibodies in human serum. *Am. Rev. resp. Dis.* **94,** 743–750

Burrell, R., Flaherty, D. K., De Nee, P. B., Abrahams, J. L. and Gelderman, A. H. (1974). The effect of lung antibody on normal lung structure and function. *Am. Rev. resp. Dis.* **109,** 106–113

Burrell, R., Wallace, J. P. and Andrews, C. E. (1964). Lung antibodies in patients with pulmonary disease. *Am. Rev. resp. Dis.* **89,** 697–706

Calnan, W. L., Winfield, B. J. O., Crowley, M. F. and Bloom, A. (1951). Diagnostic value of the glucose content of serous pleural effusions. *Br. med. J.* **1,** 1239–1240

Caplan, A., Gilson, J. C., Hinson, K. F. W., McVittie, J. C. and Wagner, J. C. (1965). II. Pulmonary study of observer variation in the classification of radiographs of asbestos-exposed workers and the relation of pathology and x-ray appearances. *Ann. N.Y. Acad. Sci* **132,** 379–386

Cate, C. C. and Burrell, R. (1974). Lung antigen induced cell-mediated immune injury in chronic respiratory disease. *Am. Rev. resp. Dis.* **109,** 114–123

Cavagna, G. and Nichelatti, T. (1963). The protective influence of polyvinyl-pyridine-N-oxide in experimental silicosis. *Medna Lav.* **54,** 621–627

Ceppellini, R. (1973). Discussions. In *General Control of Immune Responsiveness,* edited by H. O. McDevitt and M. Landy, pp. 333–338. New York; Academic Press

Chvapil, M. (1967). *Physiology of Connective Tissue,* p. 230. London; Butterworths

Chvapil, M. (1974). Pharmacology of fibrosis and tissue injury. *Envir. Hlth Perspect.* **9,** 283–294

Civil, G. W. and Heppleston, A. G. (1979). Replenishment of alveolar macrophages in silicosis: implication of recruitment by lipid feed-back. *Br. J. exp. Path.* **60,** 537–547

Codling, B. W. and Chakera, T. M. H. (1972). Pulmonary fibrosis following therapy with melphalan for multiple myeloma. *J. clin. Path.* **25,** 668–673

Collet, A., Martin, J. C., Normand-Renet, C. and Policard, A. (1967). Recherches infra-structurales sur l'évolution des macrophages alvéolaires t leurs réactions aux poussières minérales. In *Inhaled Particles and Vapours,* II, edited by C. N. Davies, pp. 155–162. Oxford; Pergamon

Coombs, R. R. A. (1974). Immunopathological Mechanisms. (Symposium in Number 14). *Proc. R. Soc. Med.* **67,** 525–530

Corrin, B. and King, E. (1970). Pathogenesis of experimental pulmonary alveolar proteinosis. *Thorax* **25,** 230–236

Corrin, B. and Price, A. B. (1972). Electron microscopic studies in desquamative interstitial pneumonia associated with asbestos. *Thorax* **27,** 324–331

Crystal, R. G., Fulmer, J. D., Roberts, W. C. Moss, M. L., Line, B. R. and Reynolds, H. Y. (1976). Idiopathic pulmonary fibrosis. Clinical, histologic, radiographic, physiologic, scintographic, cytologic and biochemical aspects. *Ann. intern. Med.* **85,** 769–788

Curran, R. C. and Rowsell, E. V. (1958). The application of the diffusion-chamber techniques to the study of silicosis. *J. Path. Bact.* **76,** 561–568

Dauber, J. H., Finn, D. R. and Daniele, R. P. (1976). Immunologic abnormalities in anthrosilicosis. *Am. Rev. resp. Dis.* **113,** 94

David, J. R., Lawrence, H. S. and Thomas, L. (1964). Delayed hypersensitivity *in vitro* III. The specificity of hapten protein conjugates in the inhibition of cell migration. *J. Immunol.* **93,** 279–282

David, J. R. and Schlossman, S. F. (1968). Immunochemical studies on the specificity of cellular hypersensitivity. *J. exp. Med.* **128,** 1451–1459

Davies, D., McFarlane, A., Darke, C. S. and Dodge, O. G. (1966). Muscular hyperplasia ('cirrhosis') of the lung and bronchial dilations as features of chronic diffuse fibrosing alveolitis. *Thorax* **21,** 272–289

Davies, P., Allison, A. C., Ackerman, J., Butterfield, A. and Williams, S. (1974). Asbestos induces selective release of lysosomal enzymes from mononuclear phagocytes. *Nature* **251,** 423–425

Davies, P. D. B. (1969). Drug-induced lung disease. *Br. J. Dis. Chest* **63,** 57–70

Davis, J. M. G., Beckett, S. T., Bolton, R. E., Collings, P. and Middleton, A. P. (1978). Mass and number of fibres in the pathogenesis of asbestos-related lung disease in rats. *Br. J. Cancer* **37,** 673–688

de Horatius, R. J., Abruzzo, J. L. and Williams, R. C. Jr. (1972). Immunofluorescent and immunologic studies of rheumatoid lung. *Archs intern. Med.* **129,** 441–446

de Horatius, R. J. and Williams, R. B. (1972). Rheumatoid factor accentuation of pulmonary lesions associated with experimental diffuse proliferative lung disease. *Arth. Rheum.* **15,** 293–301

Doctor, L. and Snider, G. L. (1962). Diffuse interstitial pulmonary fibrosis associated with arthritis. *Am. Rev. resp. Dis.* **85,** 413–422

Doniach, I., Swettenham, K. V. and Hathorn, M. K. S. (1975). Prevalence of asbestos bodies in a necropsy series in East London: association with disease, occupation and domiciliary address. *Br. J. ind. Med.* **32,** 16–30

Dreisen, R. B., Schwarz, M. I., Theofilopoulus, A. N. and Stanford, R. E. (1978). Circulating immune complexes in the idiopathic interstitial pneumonias. *New Engl. J. Med.* **298,** 353–357

Durant, J. R., Norgard, M. J., Murad, T. M., Bartolucci, A. A. and Langford, K. H. (1979). Pulmonary toxicity associated with bischloroethylnitrosourea (BCNU). *Ann. intem. Med.* **90,** 191–194

Englebrecht, F. R., Yoganathan, M., King, E. J. and Nagelschmidt, G. (1958). Fibrosis and collagen in rat's lungs produced by etched and unetched free silica dusts. *Archs ind. Hlth* **17,** 287–294

Erwteman, T. M., Braat, M. C. P. and van Aken, W. G. (1977). Interstitial pulmonary fibrosis: a new side effect of practolol. *Br. med. J.* **2,** 297–298

Evans, J. N., Kelley, J. and Adler, K. B. (1980). Contractile properties of parenchymal tissue in pulmonary fibrosis. International Colloquium on Pulmonary Fibrosis, February, 1980. University of London

Evans, S. M. and Zeit, W. (1949). Tissue response to physical forces II. The reponse of connective tissue to piezoelectrically active crystals. *J. Lab. clin. Med.* **34,** 592–609

Fraire, A. E., Greenberg, S. D., O'Neal, R. M., Weg, J. G. and Jenkins, D. E. (1973). Diffuse interstitial fibrosis of the lung. *Am. J. clin. Path.* **59,** 636–647

Gabor, S. and Anca, Z. (1975). Effect of asbestos on lipid peroxidation in the red cells. *Br. J. ind. Med.* **32,** 39–41

Gaensler, E. A. and Addington, W. W. (1969). Asbestos and ferruginous bodies. *New Engl. J. Med.* **280,** 488–492

Gallop, P. M., Blumerfeld, O. O. and Seifter, S. (1972). Structure and metabolism of connective tissue proteins. *Ann. Rev. Biochem.* **41,** 617–672

Geddes, D. M. and Brostoff, J. (1976). Pulmonary fibrosis associated with hypersensitivity to gold salts. *Br. med. J.* **1,** 1444

Gee, J. B. L. (1980). Cellular mechanisms in occupational disease. *Chest* **78,** 384–387 (Supplement)

Gell, P. G. H., Coombs, R. R. A. and Lachmann, P. J. (1975). *Clinical Aspects of Immunology,* 3rd edition. Oxford; Blackwell

Gillett, D. G. and Ford, G. T. (1978). Drug-induced lung disease. In *The Lung, Structure, Function and Disease,* edited by William M. Thurlbeck and Murray, R. Abell, pp. 21–42. Baltimore; The Williams and Wilkins Company

Gloyne, S. R. (1932–33). The morbid anatomy and histology of asbestos. *Tubercle (Edin).* **14,** 445–451; 493–497; 550–558

Green, G. M., Jakab, G. J., Low, R. B. and Davis, G. S. (1977). Defense mechanisms of the respiratory membrane. *Am. Rev. resp. Dis.* **115,** 479–514

Gross, P. (1974). Is short fibered asbestos dust a biological hazard? *Archs envir. Hlth.* **29,** 115–117

Hagadorn, J. E. and Burrell, R. (1968). Lung reactive antibodies in IgA fractions of sera from patients with pneumoconiosis. *Clin. exp. Immunol.* **3,** 263–267

Hahon, N. (1974). Depression of viral interferon induction in cell monolayers by coal dust. *Br. J. ind. Med.* **31,** 201–208

Hahon, N., Booth, J. A. and Eckert, H. L. (1977). Antagonistic activity of poly (4-vinylpyridine-N-oxide) to the inhibition of viral interferon induction by asbestos fibres. *Br. J. ind. Med.* **34,** 119–125

Hammon, L. and Rich, A. R. (1944). Acute diffuse interstitial fibrosis of the lungs. *Bull. Johns Hopkins Hosp.* **74,** 117–212

Hankinson, J. L., Reger, R. B., Fairman, R. P., Lapp, N. L. and Morgan, W. K. C. (1976). Factors influencing expiratory flow rates in coal miners. In *Inhaled Particles IV,* Ed. W. H. Walton, pp. 737–752. Oxford; Pergamon Press

Harington, J. S. (1963). Some biological actions of silica: their part in the pathogenesis of silicosis. *S. Afr. med. J.* **37,** 451–456

Harington, J. S. (1972). Investigative techniques in the laboratory study of coal worker's pneumoconiosis: recent advances at the cellular level. *Ann. N.Y. Acad. Sci.* **200,** 817–834

Harington, J. S., Allison, A. C. and Badami, D. V. (1975). Mineral fibres: chemical, physicochemical and biological properties. *Advances in Pharmacology and Chemotherapy* **12,** 291–402

Harris, J. O., Olsen, G. N., Castle, J. R. and Maloney, A. (1975). Comparison of proteolytic enzyme activity in pulmonary alveolar macrophages and blood leukocytes in smokers and non-smokers. *Am. Rev. resp. Dis.* **11,** 579–586

Haslam, P. L. (1976). Antibody and lymphocyte responses to cell nuclei in human lung disease. Thesis for Ph. D., University of London

Haslam, P. L., Turton, C. W. G., Heard, B., Lukoszek, A., Collins, J. V., Salsbury, A. J. and Turner-Warwick, M. (1980). Bronchoalveolar lavage in pulmonary fibrosis: comparison of cells obtained with lung biopsy and clinical features. *Thorax* **35,** 9–18

Heppleston, A. G. (1956). The pathology of honeycomb lung. *Thorax* **11,** 77–93

Heppleston, A. G. (1963). Deposition and disposal of inhaled dust. The influence of pre-existing pneumoconiosis. *Archs envir. Hlth* **7,** 548–555

Heppleston, A. G. (1969). Pigmentation and disorders of the lung. In *Pigments in Pathology,* edited by M. Wolman, pp. 33–73. New York and London; Academic Press

Heppleston, A. G. (1971). Observations on the mechanism of silicotic fibrogenesis. In *Inhaled Particles and Vapours, III,* edited by W. H. Walton, pp. 357–369. Woking: Unwin

Heppleston, A. G. (1973). The biological response to silica. In *Biology of the Fibroblast,* edited by E. Kulonen and J. Pikkarainen, pp. 529–537. London and New York; Academic Press

Heppleston, A. G. (1978). Cellular reactions with silica. In *Biochemistry of Silicon and Related Problems.* Nobel Symposium 40. Edited by G. Benz and I. Lindquist, pp. 357–359. New York; Plenum Publishing Corporation

Heppleston, A. G., Fletcher, K. and Wyatt, I. (1974). Changes in the composition of lung lipids and the 'turnover' of dipalmitoyl lecithin in experimental alveolar lipo-proteinosis induced by inhaled quartz. *Br. J. exp. Path.* **55,** 384–395

Heppleston, A. G. and Styles, J. A. (1967). Activity of a macrophage factor in collagen formation by silica. *Nature (London)* **214,** 521–522

Heppleston, A. G., Wright, N. A. and Stewart, J. A. (1970). Experimental alveolar lipo-proteinosis following the inhalation of silica. *J. Path.* **101,** 293–307

Heppleston, A. G. and Young, A. E. (1972). Alveolar lipo-proteinosis: an ultrastructural comparison of the experimental and human forms. *J. Path.* **107,** 107–117

Herbert, F. A., Nahurias, B. B., Gaensler, E. A. and MacMahon, H. E. (1962). Pathophysiology of interstitial pulmonary fibrosis. *Archs intern. Med.* **110,** 628–648

Hext, P. M., Hunt, J., Dodgson, K. S. and Richards, R. J. (1977). The effects of long-term exposure on lung fibroblast strains to chrysotile asbestos. *Br. J. exp. Path.* **58,** 160–167

Hijmans, W., Doniach, D., Roitt, M. and Holborow, E. J. (1961). Serological overlap between lupus erythematosus, rheumatoid arthritis and thyroid auto-immune disease. *Br. med. J.* **2,** 909–914

Hinson, K. F. W. (1970). Diffuse pulmonary fibrosis. *Hum. Path.* **1,** 275–288

Hodson, M. E. and Turner-Warwick, M. (1976). Autoantibodies in patients with chronic bronchitis. *Br. J. Dis. Chest* **70,** 83–88

Holborow, E. J., Faulk, W. P., Beard, H. K. and Conochie, L. B. (1977). Antibodies against reticulin and collagen. *Ann. rheum. Dis.* **36** (Suppl), 51–56

Holt, P. F. (1957). *Pneumoconiosis. Industrial Diseases of the Lung caused by Dust,* pp. 138–141. London; Edward Arnold

Hourihane, D. O'B. and McCaughey, W. T. E. (1966). Pathological aspects of asbestosis. *Postgrad. med. J.* **42,** 613–622

Hughes, E. W. (1964). Familial interstitial pulmonary fibrosis. *Thorax* **19,** 515–525

Hughes, P. and Rowell, N. R. (1970). Aggravation of turpentine-induced pleurisy in rats by 'homogenous' and 'speckled' anti-nuclear antibodies. *J. Path.* **101,** 141–155

Johnson, P. M. and Faulk, W. P. (1976). Rheumatoid factor: its nature, specificity and production in rheumatoid arthritis. *Clin. Immunol. Immunopath.* **36,** 414–430

Jones, J. H. and Heppleston, A. G. (1961). Immunological observations in experimental silicosis. *Nature* **191,** 1212–1213

Kang, K. Y., Yagura, T., Sera, Y., Yokoyama, K. and Yamamura, Y. (1973). Antinuclear factor in pneumoconisis and idiopathic pulmonary fibrosis. *Med. J. Osaka Univ.* **23,** 249–256

Kashimura, M. (1959). A study of the antibody produced after intravenous administration of particulate silicic acid in suspension. *Bull. Hyg. Lond.* **34,** 636–637

Kettle, E. H. (1926). Experimental silicosis. *J. ind. Hyg. Toxicol.* **8,** 491–495

Kilroe-Smith, T. A. (1974). Peroxidative action of quartz in relation to membrane lysis. *Envir. Res.* **7,** 110–116

Kilroe-Smith, T. A., Webster, I., van Drimmeten, M. and

Marasas, L. (1973). An isoluble fibrogenic factor in macrophages from guinea pigs exposed to silica. *Environ. Res.* **6,** 298–305

King, E. J., Mohanty, G. P., Harrison, C. V. and Nagelschmidt, G. (1953). The action of different forms of pure silica on the lungs of rats. *Br. J. ind. Med.* **10,** 9–17

Klosterkötter, W. (1968). Pneumoconiosis of coal workers: results, problems and practical consequences of recent research. In *Pneumoconiosis.* (Report of Symposium at Katowice, June 1967, pp. 99–109.) Copenhagen; WHO

Kravis, T. C., Ahmed, A., Brown, T. E., Fulmer, J. D. and Crystal, R. G. (1976). Pathogenic mechanisms in pulmonary fibrosis. Collagen-induced migration inhibition factor production and cytotoxicity mediated by lymphocytes. *J. clin. Invest.* **58,** 1223–1232

Kriegseis, W., Biederbick, R., Boese, J., Robock, K. and Scharmann, A. (1977). Investigations for the determination of the cytotoxicity of quartz dust by physical methods. In *Inhaled Particles and Vapours IV,* edited by W. H. Walton, pp. 345–357. Oxford; Pergamon Press

Lachman, P. J. (1975). The immunochemistry of complement. In *The Immune System,* edited by M. J. Hobart and I. McConnell, pp. 56–75. Oxford; Blackwell

Lange, A., Smolik, R., Zatoński, W. and Szymańska, J. (1974). Autoantibodies and serum immunoglobulin levels in asbestos workers. *Int. Arch. Arbeirmed.* **32,** 313–325

Lawrence, J. S. (1965). Surveys of rheumatic complaints in the population. In *Progress in Clinical Rheumatology,* edited by A. St J. Dixon. London; Churchill

Lawrence, J. S. (1967). Genetics of rheumatoid factor and rheumatoid arthritis. *Clin. exp. Immunol.* **2,** 769–783

Lawrence, J. S. (1973). Rheumatoid factor in families. *Sem. Arthr. Rheum.* **3,** 177–188

Levy, M. H. and Wheelock, E. F. (1975). Effects of intravenous silica on immune and non-immune functions of the murine host. *J. Immunol.* **115,** 41–48

Lewis, D. M. and Burrell, R. (1976). Induction of fibrogenesis by lung antibody-treated macrophages. *Br. J. ind. Med.* **33,** 25–28

Liebow, A. A. (1975). Definition and Classification of Interstitial Pneumonias in Human Pathology. *Prog. resp. Dis.* **8,** 1–33. Basel; Karger

Liebow, A. A., Loring, W. E. and Felton, W. L. (1953). The musculature of the lungs in chronic pulmonary disease. *Am. J. Path.* **29,** 885–911

Liebow, A. A., Steer, A. and Billingsley, J. G. (1965). Desquamative interstitial pneumonia. *Am. J. Med.* **39,** 369–404

Light, W. G. and Wei, E. T. (1977). Surface change and hemolytic activity of asbestos. *Envir. Res.* **13,** 135–145

Lilly, F. (1970). The Role of Genetics in Gross Virus Leukemogenesis. *Bibliotheca Haemotalogica* **36,** 213

Lippmann, M., Eckert, H. L., Hahon, N. and Morgan, W. K. C. (1973). Circulating antinuclear and rheumatoid factors in coal miners. *Ann intern. Med.* **79,** 807–811

McCarthy, C., Reid, L. and Gibbons, R. A. (1964). Intra-alveolar mucus—removal by macrophages: with iron accumulation. *J. Path. Bact.* **87,** 39–47

McClusky, R. T., Miller, F. and Benacerraf, B. (1962). Sensitisation to denatured autologous gammaglobulin. *J. exp. Med.* **115,** 153–273

McInnes, G. T. and Littman, C. D. (1977). Rheumatoid nodule of pharynx. *Br. med. J.* **1,** 685

McPherson, P. and Davidson, J. K. (1969). Correlation between lung asbestos count at necropsy and radiological appearances. *Br. med. J.* **1,** 355–357

Madri, J. A. and Furthmayr, H. (1980). Collagen polymorphism in the lung. *Human Pathology* **11,** 353–366

Maher, J. A. (1954). Dural nodules in rheumatoid arthritis. *Archs Path.* **58,** 354–359

Marks, J. (1970). New mycobacteria. *Hlth Trends* **2,** 68–69

Marks, J. (1975). Occupation and Kansasii infection in Cardiff residents. *Tubercle* **56,** 311–313

Marks, J. (1976). A system for the examination of tubercle bacilli and other mycobacteria. *Tubercle* **57,** 207–225

Martin, J. C., Daniel-Moussard, H., Le Bouffant, L. and Policard, A. (1972). The role of quartz in the development of coal worker's pneumoconiosis. *Ann. N.Y. Acad. Sci.* **200,** 127–141

Melato, M. and Tuveri, G. (1980). Pulmonary fibrosis following low-dose 1,3-bis (2-chloroethyl)-1-nitrosourea (BCNU) therapy. *Cancer* **45,** 1311–1314

Milgrom, F. and Witebsky, E. (1960). Studies on the rheumatoid and related serum factors. *J. Am. med. Ass.* **174,** 56–63

Miller, A., Langer, A. M., Teirstein, A. S. and Selikoff, I. J. (1975). 'Non-specific' interstitial pulmonary fibrosis. *New Engl. J. Med.* **292,** 91–93

Miller, K. and Kagan, E. (1977). The *in vivo* effects of quartz on alveolar macrophage membrane topography and on the characteristics of the intrapulmonary cell population. *J. reticuloendothel. Soc.* **21,** 307–316

Miller, K., Handfield, R. I. M. and Kagan, E. (1978). The effect of different mineral dusts on the mechanism of phagocytosis: a scanning electron microscope study. *Envir. Res.* **15,** 139–154

Miller, S. D. and Zarkower, A. (1974a). Alterations of murine immunological responses after silica dust inhalation. *J. Immun.* **113,** 1533–1543

Miller, S. D. and Zarkower, A. (1974b). Effects of carbon dust inhalation on the cell-mediated immune response in mice. *Infect. Immunity* **9,** 534–539

Morgagni, G. B. (1769). *De Sedibus et Causis Morborum,* Vol. 1. Book 2, p. 396. Letter 16. Trans. by B. Alexander

Munder, P. G., Mododell, M., Ferber, E. and Fischer, H. (1966). Phospholipoide in quarzgeschadigten Makrophagen. *Biochem. Z.* **344,** 310–313

Nadler, S. and Goldfischer, S. (1970). The intracellular release of lysosomal contents in macrophages that have ingested silica. *J. Histochem. Cytochem.* **18,** 368–371

Nagaya, H., Elmore, M. and Ford, C. D. (1973). Idiopathic interstitial fibrosis. *Am. Rev. resp. Dis.* **107,** 826–830

Nagelschmidt, G. (1960). The relationship between lung dust and lung pathology in pneumoconiosis. *Br. J. ind. Med.* **17,** 247–259

Nash, T., Allison, A. C. and Harington, J. S. (1966). Physiochemical properties of silica in relation to its toxicity. *Nature, Lond.* **210,** 259–261

Nossal, G. J. V. (1964). How cells make antibodies. *Scient. Am.* **211,** 106–115

Nourse, L. D., Nourse, P. N., Botes, H. and Schwartz, H. M. (1975). The effects of macrophages isolated from the lungs of guinea pigs dusted with silica on collagen biosynthesis by guinea pig fibroblasts in cell culture. *Envir. Res.* **9,** 115–127

Oliver, R. T. D. (1977). Histocompatability antigens and human disease. *Br. J. hosp. Med.* **18,** 449–459

Otto, H. and Maron, R. (1959). Zur Histologie der Eisenablagerungen bei Porzellinersilikoson. *Arch. Gewerbepath. Gewerbehyg.* **17,** 117–126

Ovenfors, C-O., Dahlgren, S. E., Ripe, E. and Ost, A. (1980). Muscular hyperplasia of the lung: a clinical, radiographic and histopathological study. *Am. J. Roentgenol.* **135,** 703–712

Parazzi, E., Pernis, B., Secchi, G. C. and Vigliani, E. C. (1968). Studies on *in vivo* cytotoxicity of asbestos dusts. *Medna Lav.* **59,** 561–576

Parish, W. E. (1970). Short-term anaphylactic IgG antibodies in human sera. *Lancet* **11,** 591–592

Pepys, J. (1969). *Hypersensitivity Diseases of the Lungs due to Fungi and Organic Dusts.* Basel and New York; Karger

Pepys, J. (1975). Atopy. In *Clinical Aspects of Immunology,* edited by G. H. Gell, R. R. A. Coombs and P. J. Lachmann, p. 877. Oxford; Blackwell

Pepys, J. (1977). Clinical and therapeutic significance of patterns of allergic reactions of the lungs to extrinsic agents. *Am. Rev. resp. Dis.* **116,** 573–588

Pepys, J. and Hutchroft, B. J. (1974). Bronchial provocation tests in etiological diagnosis and analysis of asthma. *Am. Rev. resp. Dis.* **112,** 829–859

Pernis, B. (1968). Silicosis. In *Textbook of Immunopathology*, Vol. I, edited by P. A. Miescher and H. J. Muller-Eberhard, pp. 293–301. New York and London; Grune and Stratton

Pernis, B. and Castano, P. (1971). Effetto dell' asbesto sulle cellule in vitro. *Medna Lav.* **62,** 120–129

Pernis, B. and Paronetto, F. (1962). Adjuvant effect of silica (tridymite) on antibody production. *Proc. Soc. exp. Biol. Med.* **110,** 390–392

Policard, A., Gernez-Rieux, C., Taquet, A., Martin, J. C., Devalder, J. and Le Bouffant, J. (1967). Influence of pulmonary dust load on the development of experimental infection by *Mycobacterium kansasii. Nature, Lond.* **216,** 177–178

Popper, M. S., Bogdonoff, M. L. and Hughes, R. L. (1972). Interstitial rheumatoid lung disease. *Chest* **62,** 243–249

Powell, D. E. B. and Gough, J. (1959). The effect on experimental silicosis of hypersensitivity induced by horse serum. *Br. J. exp. Path.* **40,** 40–43

Pras, M., Johnson, G. D., Holborow, E. J. and Glynn, L. E. (1974). Antigenic properties of a non-collagen reticulin component of normal connective tissue. *Immunology* **27,** 469–478

Price, T. M. L. and Skelton, M. O. (1965). Rheumatoid arthritis with lung lesions. *Thorax* **11,** 234–240

Rendall, R. E. G. (1972). Quoted by Timbrell, V. (1973). Physical factors as etiological mechanisms. In *Biological Effects of Asbestos,* edited by P. Bogovski, J. C. Gilson, V. Timbrell and J. C. Wagner, pp. 295–303. Lyon; International Agency for Research of Cancer

Reynolds, H. Y., Atkinson, J. P., Newball, H. H. and Frank, M. M. (1975). Receptors for immunoglobulin and complement on human alveolar macrophages. *J. Immunol.* **114,** 1813–1819

Reynolds, H. Y., Fulmer, J. D., Kazmierowski, J. A., Roberts, W. C., Frank, M. M. and Crystal, R. G. (1977). Analysis of cellular and protein content of broncho-alveolar lavage fluid from patients with idiopathic pulmonary fibrosis and chronic hypersensitivity pneumonitis. *J. clin. Invest.* **59,** 165–175

Richards, R. J., Hext, P. M., Desai, R., Tetley, T., Hunt, J., Presley, R. and Dodgson, K. S. (1977). Chrysotile asbestos: biological reaction potential. In *Inhaled Particles and Vapours IV,* edited by W. H. Walton and B. McGovern; pp. 477–490. Oxford; Pergamon Press

Robock, K. (1968). A new concept of the pathogenesis of silicosis: Luminescence measurements and biochemical cell experiments with SiO_2 dusts. *Staub Reinhalt. Luft.* **28,** 15–26

Robock, K. and Klosterkötter, W. (1977). The biological effect of asbestos and asbestos cement products. In *Inhaled Particles and Vapours IV,* edited by W. H. Walton and B. McGovern, pp. 447–452. Oxford; Pergamon Press

Rosenow, E. C. III. (1972). The spectrum of drug-induced pulmonary disease. *Ann. intern. Med.* **77,** 977–991

Roszman, T. L. and Rogers, A. S. (1973). The Immunosuppressive potential of products derived from cigarette smoke. *Am. Rev. resp. Dis.* **108,** 1158–1163

Rüttner, J. R., Spycher, M. A. and Engeler, M-L. (1968). Pulmonary fibrosis induced by cotton fibre inhalation. *Path. Microbiol.* **32,** 1–14

Rüttner, J. R., Spycher, M. A. and Stichner, H. (1972). Diffuse 'asbestos-like' interstitial fibrosis of the Lung. *Path. Microbiol.* **38,** 250–257

Rüttner, J. R., Spycher, M. A. and Sticher, H. (1973). The detection of aetiological agents in interstitial pulmonary fibrosis. *Human Path.* **4,** 497–512

Sakabe, H. and Koshi, K. (1967). Preventative effect of polybetaine on the cell toxicity of quartz particles. *Ind. Hlth* **5,** 181–182

Savel, H. (1970). Clinical hypersensitivity to cigarette smoke. *Archs envir. Hlth (Chicago)* **21,** 146–148

Scadding, J. G. (1964). Fibrosing alveolitis. *Br. med. J.* **2,** 686–941

Scadding, J. G. (1969). The lungs in rheumatoid arthritis. *Proc. R. Soc. Med.* **62,** 227–238

Scadding, J. G. (1974). Diffuse pulmonary alveolar fibrosis. *Thorax* **74**, 271–281

Scadding, J. G. and Hinson, K. F. W. (1967). Diffuse fibrosing alveolitis (diffuse interstitial fibrosis of the lungs). Correlation of histology at biopsy with prognosis. *Thorax* **22,** 291–304

Scheel, L. D., Smith, B., Van Riper, J. and Fleischer, E. (1954). Toxicity of silica. *Archs ind. Hyg.* **9,** 29–36

Schultz, R. T., Calkins, E., Milgrom, F. and Witebsky, E. (1966). Association of gamma globulin with amyloid. *Am. J. Path.* **48,** 1–17

Schuyler, M. R., Gaumer, H. R., Stankus, R. P., Kaimal, J., Hoffman, E. and Salvaggio, J. E. (1980). Bronchoalveolar lavage in silicosis. Evidence of Type II cell hyperplasia. *Lung* **157,** 95–102

Senyk, G. and Michaeli, D. (1973). Induction of cell-mediated immunity and tolerance to homologous collagen in guinea pigs: demonstrations of antigen-reactive cells for self-antigen. *J. Immunol.* **111,** 1381–1388

Seyer, J. M., Hutchinson, E. T. and Kang, A. H. (1976). Collagen polymorphism in idiopathic chronic pulmonary fibrosis. *J. clin. Invest.* **57,** 1495–1507

Sharp, P. M., Warr, G. A. and Martin, R. R. (1973). Effects of smoking on bronchial immunoglobulins. *Clin. Res.* **21,** 672

Skidmore, J. W. (1977). Personal communication

Soutar, C. A. (1976). Distribution of plasma cells and other cells containing immunoglobulin in the respiratory tract of normal man and class of immunoglobulin contained therein. *Thorax* **31,** 158–166

Sovijärvi, A. R. A., Lemola, M., Stenius, B. and Idänpään-Heikkilä, J. (1977). Nitrofurantoin-induced acute, subacute and chronic pulmonary reactions. *Scand. J. resp. Dis.* **58,** 41–50

Spencer, H. (1975). Pathogenesis of interstitial fibrosis of the lung. In *Alveolar Interstitium of the Lung, Prog. Resp. Res.* **8,** 34–44

Spencer, H. (1977). *Pathology of the Lung,* 3rd edition. Oxford; Pergamon Press

Stalder, K. and Stöber, W. (1965). Haemolytic activity of suspensions of different modifications and inert dusts. *Nature, Lond.* **207,** 874–875

Stenius, B., Wide, L., Seymour, W. M., Holford-Strevens, V. and Pepys, J. (1971). Clinical significance of specific IgE to common allergens. I *Clin. Allergy* **1,** 37–55

Stöber, W. (1968). On the theory of silicosis. IV. *Archs envir. Hlth* **16,** 706–707

Stobo, J. D. and Tomasi, T. B. (1975). Aging and the regulation of immune reactivity. *J. chron. Dis.* **28,** 437–440

Stockley, R. A. and Brookes, V. S. (1978). Interstitial lung disease in a patient treated with 5-fluorouracil and mitomycin C. *Br. med. J.* **2,** 602

Strecker, F. J. (1965). Histoplysiologische Untersuchungen zur 'silicotischen Gewebsreaktion' im *Intraperitonealtest und zur Gewebswirkung von Coesit und Stischowit. Beitr. Silikoseforsch. S. Bd Grundfragen Silikoseforsch.* **6,** 55–83

Terho, E. O., Torkko, M. and Valta, R. (1979). Pulmonary disease associated with gold therapy. *Scand. J. resp. Dis.* **60,** 345–349

Thiart, B. F. and Engelbrecht, F. M. (1967). Globulins in silicotic lungs. *S. Afr. med.* **41,** 731–733

Timbrell, V., Gilson, J. C. and Webster, I. (1968). UICC standard reference samples of asbestos. *Int. J. Cancer* **3,** 406–408

Timbrell, V. and Skidmore, J. W. (1968). Significance of fibre length in experimental asbestosis. In *International Konferenz uber die biologischen Wirkungen des Asbestos,* edited by Holstein and Anspach, pp. 52–56. Dresden

Tomasi, T. B. Jr., Tan, E. M., Solomon, A. and Prendergast, R. A. (1965). Characteristics of an immune system common to external secretions. *J. exp. Med.* **121,** 101–124

Torrigiani, G., Roitt, I. M., Lloyd, K. N. and Corbett, M. (1970). Elevated IgG antiglobulins in patients with seronegative rheumatoid arthritis. *Lancet* **1,** 14–16

Turner-Warwick, M. (1975). Immunology of interstitial lung disease. In *Alveolar Interstitium of the Lung, Prog. Resp. Res.* **8,** 59–65

Turner-Warwick, M. (1978). *Immunology of the Lung.* London; Edward Arnold

Turner-Warwick, M. and Evans, R. C. (1977). Pulmonary manifestations of rheumatoid disease. *Clinics rheum. Dis.* **3,** 549–564

Turner-Warwick, M. and Haslam, P. (1971). Antibodies in some chronic fibrosing lung diseases. 1. Non-organ-specific autoantibodies, *Clin. Allergy,* **1,** 83–95

Turner-Warwick, M., Haslam, P. and Weeks, J. (1971). Antibodies in some chronic fibrosing lung diseases. *Clin. Allergy* **1,** 209–219

Um, C. H. (1971). Study of the secular trends in asbestos bodies in London. 1936–1966. *Br. med. J.* **2,** 248–251

Vigliani, E. C. and Pernis, B. (1963). Advances in tuberculosis research. In *Fortschritte der Tuberkulose-forschung,* Vol. 12, edited by H. Birkhauser, H. Bloch, and G. Canetti, pp. 230–279. Basel and New York; Karger

Vladutiu, A. O. and Rose, N. R. (1971). Autoimmune murine thyroiditis relation to histocompatability (H-2) type. *Science* **174,** 1137–1139

Vladutiu, A. O. and Rose, N. R. (1974). HL-A antigens: association with disease. *Immunogenetics* **1,** 305–328

Voisin, G. A., Collet, A., Martin, J. C., Daniel-Moussard, H. and Toulet, F. (1964). Propertés immunologiques de la silice et des composés du beryllium: les formes soluble comparées aux formes insoluble. *Revue fr. Étud. clin. biol.* **9,** 819–828

Wagner, J. C. (1972). Etiological factors in complicated coal workers' pneumoconiosis. *Ann. N.Y. Acad. Sci.* **200,** 401–404

Wagner, J. C., Berry, G., Skidmore, J. W. and Timbrell, V. (1974). The effects of inhalation of asbestos in rats. *Br. J. Cancer* **29,** 252–269

Webster, I. (1970). The pathogenesis of asbestosis. In *Pneumoconiosis. Proceedings of the International Conference. Johannesburg. 1969,* edited by H. A. Shapiro, pp. 117–119. Cape Town: Oxford University Press

Weinberger, S. E., Kelman, J. A., Elson, N. A., Young, R. C., Jr., Reynolds, H. Y., Fulmer, J. D. and Crystal, R. G. (1978). Bronchoalveolar lavage in interstitial lung disease. *Ann. intern. Med.* **89,** 459–466

Williams, R. C. and Kunkel, H. G. (1962). Rheumatoid factor, complement, and conglutin aberrations in patients with subacute bacterial endocarditis. *J. clin. Invest.* **41,** 666–675

Wright, G. and Kuschner, M. (1977). The influence of varying lengths of glass and asbestos fibres on tissue response in guinea pigs. In *Inhaled Particles and Vapours IV,* edited by W. H. Walton and B. McGovern, pp. 455–472

Addendum to page 77

Recent work has confirmed that neutrophils and eosinophils are the predominant cell types in bronchial lavage fluid from patients with cryptogenic DIPF, and that there may be a slight increase in lymphocytes which, however, is substantially less than in the granulomatous disorders. Neutrophils and eosinophils may also be increased in asbestosis, though to a much smaller degree; but lymphocytes are not increased (Turner-Warwick *et al.*, 1981). A significant excess of histamine, which correlates with increased neutrophil and eosinophil counts, is also present in lavage fluid, and mast cells (its most likely source) are readily identifiable by biopsy of thickened alveolar walls. Histamine, by causing capillary damage, may be an important reason for the influx of inflammatory cells into alveolar walls and air spaces (Haslam *et al.*, 1981). Whether or not similar changes occur in other fibrosing disorders, and, if so, to what degree, remains to be established.

Haslam, P. L., Cromwell, O., Dewar, A. and Turner-Warwick, M. (1981). Evidence of increased histamine levels in lung lavage fluids from patients with cryptogenic fibrosing alveolitis. *Clin. exp. Immunol.* **44**, 587–593

Turner-Warwick, M., Haslam, P. L., Lukoszek, A., Townsend, P., Allan, F., Du Bois, R. M., Turton, C. W. G. and Collins, J. V. (1981). Cells, enzymes and interstitial lung disease. *J. Roy. Coll. Phys. Lond.* **15**, 5–16

5 The Chest Radiograph

Although the diagnosis of a pneumoconiosis necessarily involves an analysis of occupational history, physical examination and lung function tests, the chest radiograph is without doubt the most informative single investigation available.

The general principles of chest radiography and radiology are admirably discussed, respectively, in *Clark's Positioning in Radiography* (1979) and by Simon (1973) among others. But when the pneumoconioses are under consideration it is particularly important that certain principles which determine the appearance of the chest radiograph should be understood if errors of interpretation are to be avoided.

Chest radiography is employed both for clinical and epidemiological purposes: the first to establish diagnosis, prognosis and guidance of treatment; the second to estimate prevalence and behaviour of disease in different communities. Our concern here is mainly with the first. Whichever the purpose, however, the highest possible standard of radiographic technique must always be sought.

RELEVANT X-RAY PHYSICS

X-rays used for diagnostic purposes are electromagnetic radiations normally within the 0.1 Å to 1 Å wavelength range (0.01 nm to 0.1 nm) which travel in straight lines but, on encountering matter, may be absorbed or scattered in various amounts and directions by its atoms.

The *atomic number* (that is, the number of electrons around the nucleus in an uncharged atom) of an element decides its character. It is the average atomic number of a body tissue—*not* its atomic weight—which is responsible for the extent to which incident X-rays of given energy will be absorbed or scattered by different tissues and, hence, for the appearance of the radiographic image.

ABSORPTION AND SCATTER

The amount of absorption and scatter is also determined by the number of atoms per unit volume and consequently by the density or specific gravity of the material. Therefore, both X-ray absorption and scatter are significantly less in air than in fluids such as blood or pleural effusion.

Some X-rays pass through matter without interacting with its atoms but those which do interact are subject to a range of increasing effects. These are as follows: slight change in their direction with some loss of energy; interaction with electrons in their orbital shells; and complete absorption by atoms resulting in the emission of electrons and secondary radiation.

Detailed consideration of these processes is inappropriate here but the enunciation of two fundamental principles is important:

(1) Some radiation is totally or partly absorbed in the material while the remainder either has its direction changed or is degraded to lower energy radiation which is scattered in all directions.
(2) The amount of scatter is dependent upon the number of electrons/g of irradiated material and, allowing for density, this is much the same for most elements in biological materials with the exception of hydrogen which has about twice the number (Osborn, 1969).

PRODUCTION OF THE X-RAY IMAGE

The effect of X-rays upon the conventional X-ray film is to produce blackening when it is developed. Conversely, unexposed film is transparent and appears white when viewed against white light. Materials or tissues which absorb X-rays completely and prevent them reaching the film emulsion cast 'shadows' which appear white and these are conventionally regarded as of high density. Consequently the various tissues of the body, which have different absorptive capacities for X-rays, produce a range of effects from black (for example, air) when absorption is least, through tones of grey (for example, fat and muscle), to white (for example, bone) when absorption is greatest.

Hence, it is convenient to conceive of four basic degrees of radiographic densities: 'air', 'fat', 'water' (equivalent to blood and soft tissues), and 'bone'. With the exception of air the radio-opacity of different tissues is dependent more upon their effective atomic number than upon their specific gravity (Spiers, 1946) or chemical composition. The *effective atomic number* is an expression of the resultant total absorption of X-rays by atoms of the different elements in a material and it is dependent upon the percentage by weight, the atomic number and atomic weight of each element. In the low-voltage region where photo-electric absorption is important, the contribution made by any one element to the effective atomic number of the material as a whole depends on its atomic number raised to about the third power (Johns and Cunningham, 1969). The effective atomic number for fat is given as 5.9, for muscle and water as 7.4, for air as 7.6, and for bone as about 14; the atomic numbers of phosphorus and calcium are 15 and 20, respectively. Air, in spite of the value of its effective atomic number and for reasons given in the next section, is virtually radiolucent; fat (which contains less hydrogen than water) produces a grey effect; all body fluids, muscle and solid viscera have a similar radiographic density which is equivalent to that of water('water equivalent') and this produces a lighter grey effect than fat; and bone gives the densest, that is, the whitest, 'shadows' of all tissues. A radiograph of a normal shoulder (*Figure 5.1*) demonstrates these degrees of radio-opacity. The contrast between the various radiodensities makes the total image.

Within the diagnostic range of X-ray energy, the absorption of rays is apparently proportional to the second or third power of the effective atomic number (Osborn, 1969) which explains not only why bone stands out so clearly, but also why extraneous materials with higher atomic numbers than the tissues cast denser 'shadows'. It is on this account that some of these materials, notably iodine and barium, are

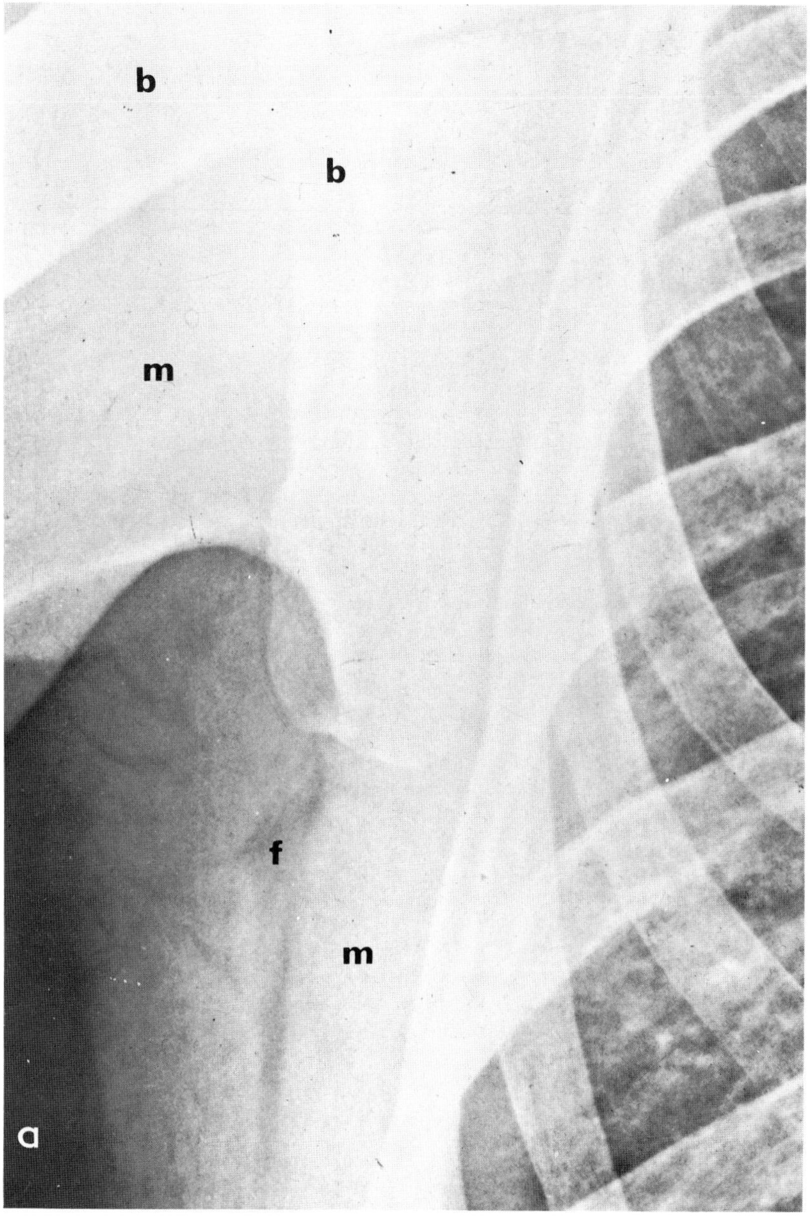

Figure 5.1 Radiograph of a normal shoulder showing the contrast between radio-opacity caused by bone (b), muscle (m), fat (f) and lung compared with air (a)

Table 5.1 Atomic Numbers of some Relevant Elements

Chief atomic constituents of body tissues and fluids		*Elements of exogenous origin*			
Hydrogen	1	Beryllium	4	Tin	50
Carbon	6	Carbon	6	Antimony	51
Nitrogen	7	Aluminium	13	Iodine	53
Oxygen	8	Silicon	14	Barium	56
Sodium	11	Titanium	22	Cerium	58
Phorphorus	15	Vanadium	23	Rare earth elements	58 to 71
Calcium	20	Chromium	24	Tungsten	74
		Manganese	25	Lead	82
		Iron	26	Thorium	90
		Zirconium	40		
		Silver	47		

introduced into the body as contrast media, but the importance of this principle in the present context is that heavy metals such as iron, tin, antimony and barium when retained in the lungs cast particularly dense shadows which contrast sharply with the surrounding lung (*see Figure 6.4*). *Table 5.1* sets out the atomic numbers of the major elements of the body and of some relevant extraneous elements.

In short, the image of the lung fields on the film is caused by the differential absorption of the X-ray beam by various lung constituents of both endogenous and exogenous origin. Hence, it is the *sum* of superimposed radiodensities of structures and lesions throughout the thickness of the chest.

THE EFFECT OF THE AIR CONTENT OF THE LUNGS

As the values of the effective atomic numbers given in the last section suggest, air, if compressed to unit density, would in fact absorb more X-rays than unit density muscle or unit density fat. But air in the lungs is not in this state and its volume in normal lungs causes their density to be nearer that of air than that of the surrounding soft tissues—or 'water equivalent'—by a factor of about 800 (Osborn, 1969). This is due to the fact that air contains practically no hydrogen unless, as is virtually the case in the lungs, it is saturated with water vapour when it contains only about 0.8 per cent hydrogen by weight in contrast to some 10 per cent in soft tissues (Osborn, 1969). Hence, because the ratio of air density to tissue density is normally 1:800 the absorption of X-rays by air and the lungs as a whole is very substantially less than by other tissues. Furthermore, the lungs cause negligible scatter of radiation because the number of electrons/cm^3 in their air is very small by comparison with the number of electrons/cm^3 of the surrounding tissues. Indeed, it is calculated that the scattering effect (*Scatter Attenuation Coefficient*) of air is almost 1000 times less than that of soft tissues whether these be fat, muscle, blood vessels or fibrous tissue (Osborn, 1969).

Therefore, lung tissue has negligible radiodensity in contrast to that of its pulmonary blood vessels and their blood, mediastinal and other soft tissues, and bone; an increase of soft tissue density within the lungs or the presence of radiodense dusts therefore produces additional contrasting opacities on the film. This has a direct and important bearing on an alleged obscuring effect which emphysema is wrongly, but often, supposed to have on the X-ray images of pneumoconiotic lesions (*see* this Chapter, p. 109).

SHARPNESS OF THE RADIOGRAPHIC IMAGE ON THE FILM

Sharpness in radiographs is limited by three factors:

(1) The penumbra around the image which is related to the size of the X-ray source and the distance of the subject from the film (*Figure 5.2*). This is reduced by increasing the distance between the X-ray source and the film, and by decreasing the size of the 'focal spot' in the X-ray tube.
(2) Movement of the subject. For example, slight body movement, failure to hold the breath, and normal movement of the heart and great vessels.
(3) Limitations imposed by film grain size and intensifying screens.

X-ray scatter within the lungs does not diminish sharpness of the image but excessive superficial fat and well-developed muscles may be responsible for sufficient absorption and scatter to cause reduction of contrast due to more or less uniform greyness of the total image. A much greater effect, of course, is produced by fluid—such as pleural effusion.

Appreciation of these points is of particular importance for the production of radiographs with the sharp definition required for investigation of all forms of pneumoconiosis, especially as these are sometimes represented by small or tenuous opacities.

THE STANDARD CHEST RADIOGRAPH

Conventionally, the routine chest film is a postero-anterior (PA) view and is usually 17 × 14 inches (42.5 × 35.0 cm). During X-ray exposure the subject's breath must be held in the deepest possible inspiration; the mid-expiratory position suggested by the International Labour Office (1959) is not desirable as it is not capable of accurate control and prevents full expansion and, hence, optimal visualization of the lung fields—a matter of importance in the examination of asbestosis subjects. The technique for taking good quality films is summarized in *International Classification of Radiographs of Pneumoconioses* (ILO, 1970). Too white (under-exposed) or too dark (over-exposed) films are to be avoided, and the quality of serial films should, as far as possible, be kept comparable. The kilovoltage range in common use is 60 to 80 kV and with standard speed films it produces high quality pictures

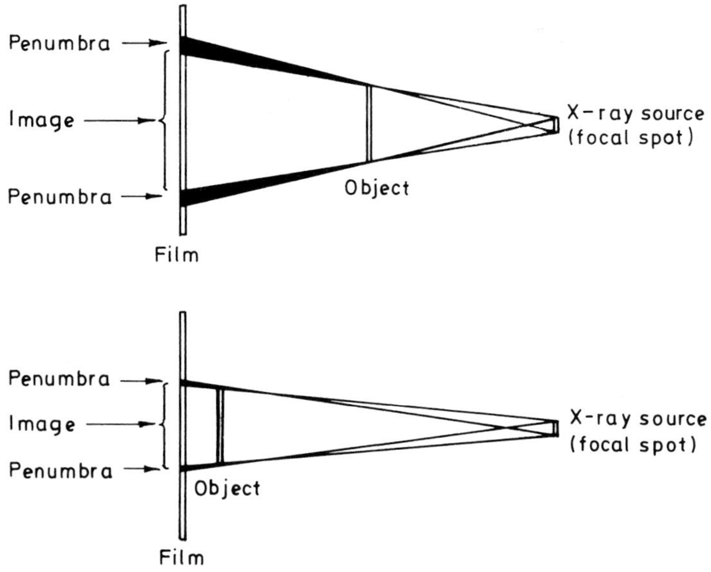

Figure 5.2 Diagram showing the effect of the position of an object on the size of the penumbra around its image on the film. The closer the object to the focal spot from which the X-rays emanate the larger the image produced. But, since the focal spot has a finite size, the penumbra is also larger, and this has the effect of blurring the edges of the image. This blurring effect can be decreased by reducing the object-film distance in relation to the focus-film distance or by reducing the size of the 'focal spot'. It is for this reason that chest films are customarily taken at 6 feet using a fine focal spot—preferably under 1 mm diameter

providing exposure time is less than about 0.08 s. It is claimed that the quality and detail of the standard postero-anterior view is increased by using 110 to 140 kV range and a very fine, stationary lead grid (Jackson, Bohlig and Kiviluoto, 1970), but this technique is not in general use.

Films must be of adequate size to include the whole of the thorax from the lung apices to just below the costophrenic angles and this applies equally to routine pneumoconiosis surveys as to investigation of the individual so that 14 × 14 inches (35 × 35 cm) films are unsatisfactory. In subjects with unduly large chests the lung bases may be incompletely visualized, in which case a wide basal view should be taken to include both costophrenic angles especially when asbestosis is suspected. Alternatively film size should be changed to 16 × 16 inches (40 × 40 cm) as suggested by Bohlig and Gilson (1973).

The subjects should be unclothed above the waist, and corsets and lumbar belts removed because, in addition to obscuring the lower lung fields, these limit maximal inspiratory descent of the diaphragm. Failure to remove clothing may lead to confusing artefacts which are often subtle so that vigilance is required if they are not to be interpreted as evidence of pathology—especially if the obvious clue of pins and buttons is absent and it is taken for granted that the subject was stripped to the waist when the film was taken. This problem is more likely to be encountered in periodic radiographic examinations of workers in industry than in clinical practice.

Consistency of technique is essential at all times in order to detect early radiographic changes and maintain a good comparative standard. This is particularly important in monitoring working industrial populations over a period of years.

PROCEDURE FOR INSPECTION OF THE CHEST RADIOGRAPH

Unless a systematic and consistent discipline for examining the film is followed, abnormalities may be overlooked or misinterpreted. It is also important to acquire the imaginative power of 'looking into' the two-dimensional film as if it were three-dimensional. If the quality and technique of the film is acceptable it can then be inspected by orderly stages.

Stage 1. Peripheral region

The soft tissues of the root of the neck, axillae, chest wall and diaphragm on both sides are studied and compared. The intense radio-opacity of the diaphragm must be carefully 'looked into' to detect abnormal opacities (such as localized pleural thickening) which are only slightly different in contrast.

Next, the skeleton is inspected; clavicles, ribs (posterior, lateral and anterior aspects), scapulae, spine and sternum. In this way the occasional clues which bone lesions may give to lung disease are not missed.

The costal margins of the lung fields should be followed from the lung apices to the costophrenic angles and then along the diaphragm to the cardiophrenic angles. In this respect one should be familiar with the lower 'companion shadows' of the lateral chest wall which may be seen for a few rib spaces above the costophrenic angles in a proportion of normal PA films. These are triangular opacities whose lateral aspects are continuous with the rib shadows and their medial aspects usually well defined and vertical, while their lower parts lack definition. They are bilateral although not necessarily symmetrically equal and are caused by the interdigitations of the serratus anterior and external abdominal oblique muscles (*Figure 5.3*). *Slight* rotation of the chest during exposure of the film makes these shadows more prominent on one side than the other, when they may be misinterpreted as pleural lesions if their true nature is not recognized. However, they disappear completely on oblique views.

Another important normal anatomical feature is extrapleural costal fat. This is distributed bilaterally beneath the parietal pleura immediately adjacent to the ribs. It varies in amount but in some subjects it is prominent and hangs in flap-like folds from the ribs. It tends to be most abundant posteriorly over the fourth to ninth ribs and although, as a

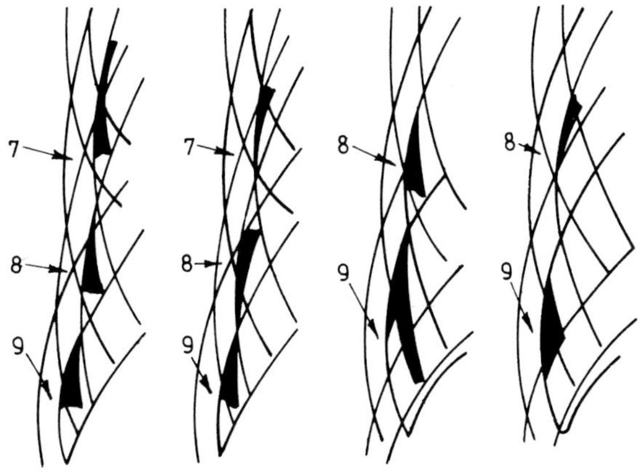

(a)

Figure 5.3 (a) Diagrams of different forms of normal muscle shadows—'companion shadows'—on the lateral chest wall. (Courtesy of Drs Fletcher and Edge and the Honorary Editor of Clinical Radiology*). (b) Radiograph of type C. (Courtesy of Dr L. Preger and Editor, Grune and Stratton*). These shadows are apt to be mistaken for pleural abnormalities, a point which may be important in an asbestos worker*

**Asbestos-Related Disease, Figure 2.22*

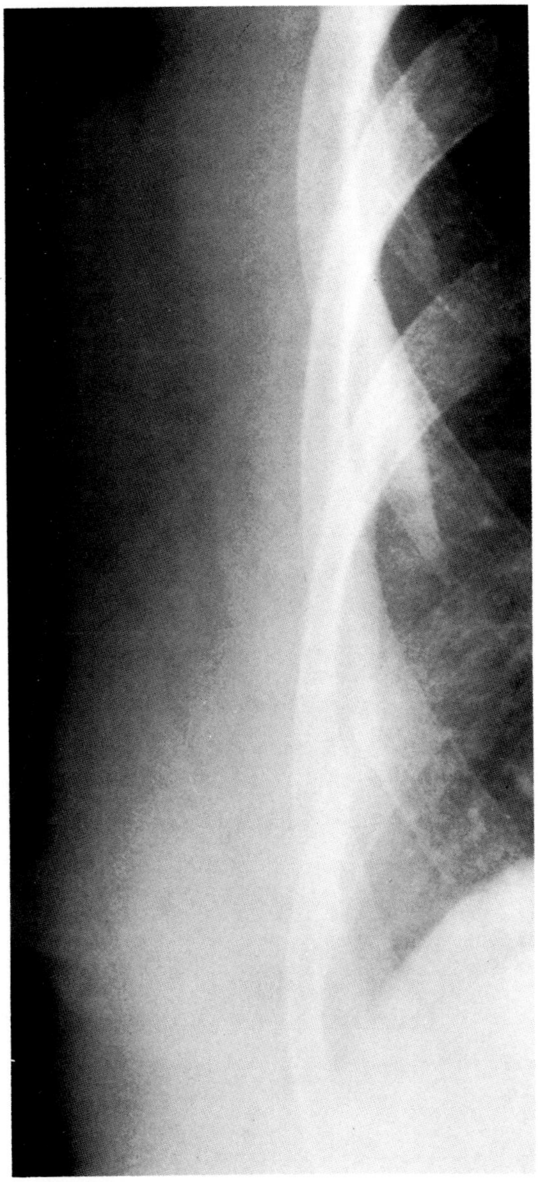

(b)

rule, not closely correlated with total body fat it may be excessive in some subjects in whom there has been a large gain in weight, including those with hypercorticosteroidism. The deposits cause an undulating opacification along the costal margins of the lung fields and may be wrongly interpreted as pleural thickening or hyaline plaque formation if the observer is unaware of this normal variant (Vix, 1974) (*see Figure 5.4a* and *b*). They are most clearly demonstrated by anterior oblique views (*see* p. 96).

Stage 2. Central region

The position, size and shape of the trachea, great vessels and heart are noted. The heart shadow, especially on the left, must be 'looked through' for any abnormal opacity which may be superimposed upon it.

Stage 3. Hilar region

The position, size and shape of the hilar shadows—which are caused by the basal pulmonary artery and proximal parts of the pulmonary veins—are examined and the size and distribution of the pulmonary arteries passing to the lung fields noted.

Stage 4. Lung fields

These should be examined in two stages. First, the pulmonary arteries ('lung markings') should be followed until they are no longer visible which is usually in the outer third of the lung fields, and their branching and size (whether unduly thick or narrow) noted. These appearances are produced by vessels which run roughly parallel to the plane of the film, but those running in the anterior-posterior plane, and at right angles to that of the film, appear as oval or round opacities. If this is not understood they are sometimes wrongly interpreted as round lesions of silicosis (or some other discrete pneumoconiosis) when there is a relevant occupational history.

Second, the vessels must, as far as possible, be ignored and the lung fields 'looked into' for opacities indicating lesions in the parenchyma, and their size, shape and distribution assessed. Corresponding regions in both fields must be compared throughout.

Each lung field is arbitrarily, but conveniently, subdivided into three zones by two horizontal lines, drawn respectively through the anterior ends of the second and fourth ribs. These demarcate upper, middle and lower zones to which the distribution of abnormal shadows can be referred.

(a)

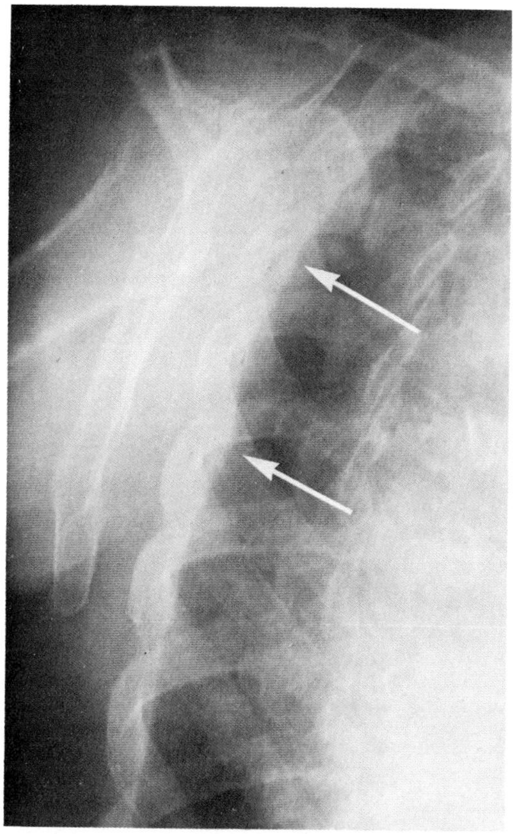

(b)

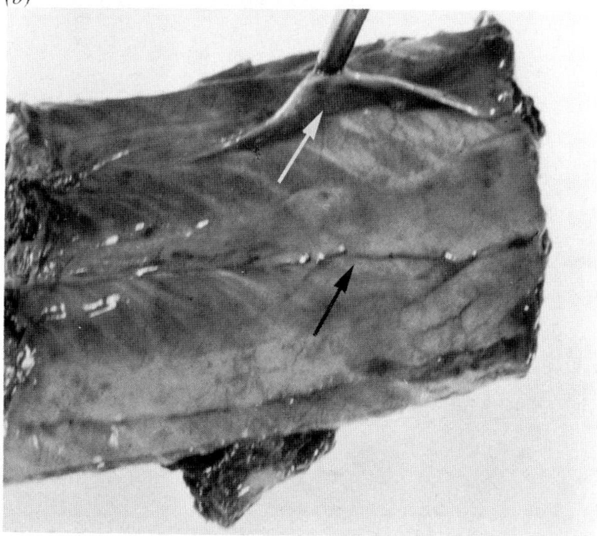

Figure 5.4 (a) Appearances caused by prominent extrapleural costal fat which may be mistaken for pleural disease. (b) Post-mortem appearances of flaps of costal fat (arrowed). (Courtesy of Dr Vernon Vix and Editor of Radiology*)*

SOME COMMON CAUSES OF ERROR IN INTERPRETATION

ROTATION OF THE SUBJECT

A consequence of incorrect positioning, this causes unequal radiotranslucency of the two lungs fields. For example, if the subject's chest is rotated to the right (that is, the right shoulder is closer to the film than the left) the right hilar region is more prominent than the left which is partly obscured by the heart shadow, and the left lung field is more radiotranslucent than the right. It is important, therefore, to be on the lookout for this fault during routine inspection by identifying asymmetry in the skeletal outlines.

FILM TAKEN IN EXPIRATION

The lower zones of a film taken at the end of expiration have a different appearance from those of a film taken in full inspiration due to condensation of tissue radiodensities, the reduced volume of air and elevation of the diaphragm (*Figure 5.5a* and *b*). If the technical error of such a film, or one taken in incomplete inspiration, is not identified, misinterpretation is likely to occur. An early stage of diffuse interstitial fibrosis may be diagnosed or, if this is already present (in the form of asbestosis, for example), it may be regarded as being more advanced than it really is and the elevated diaphragm construed as evidence of contraction of the lungs.

SOFT TISSUE SHADOWS

Prominence of both pectoral muscle shadows, or of one more than the other on the dominant side of a muscular man, can be recognized for what they are if the inspection procedure is carefully followed, otherwise pleural or intrapulmonary disease may be wrongly suspected. The effect of the interdigitations of serratus anteria and the external oblique muscle of the abdomen has been referred to already.

Large breasts tend to obscure the lower fields and when good visualization of these zones is important this can usually be achieved by lightly binding the breasts and taking another PA film using a Potter–Bucky diaphragm.

BRONCHOGRAPHIC CONTRAST MEDIA

The scattered, rather dense, opacities of variable size which sometimes persist for a period of time after bronchography are sometimes a source of confusion if their cause is not recognized. However, bronchography is less often used today than it was a few years ago and many clinics use water-soluble media which disperse quickly. Bronchography has no particular value in the diagnosis of any form of pneumoconiosis.

OTHER RADIOLOGICAL TECHNIQUES

LATERAL VIEW

A lateral view should always be taken when the individual is seen for the first time, not only to define the spatial relationship of abnormal shadows seen in the PA view, but also to show the configuration of the chest, the shape and level of the diaphragm and the dimensions of the retrosternal translucence.

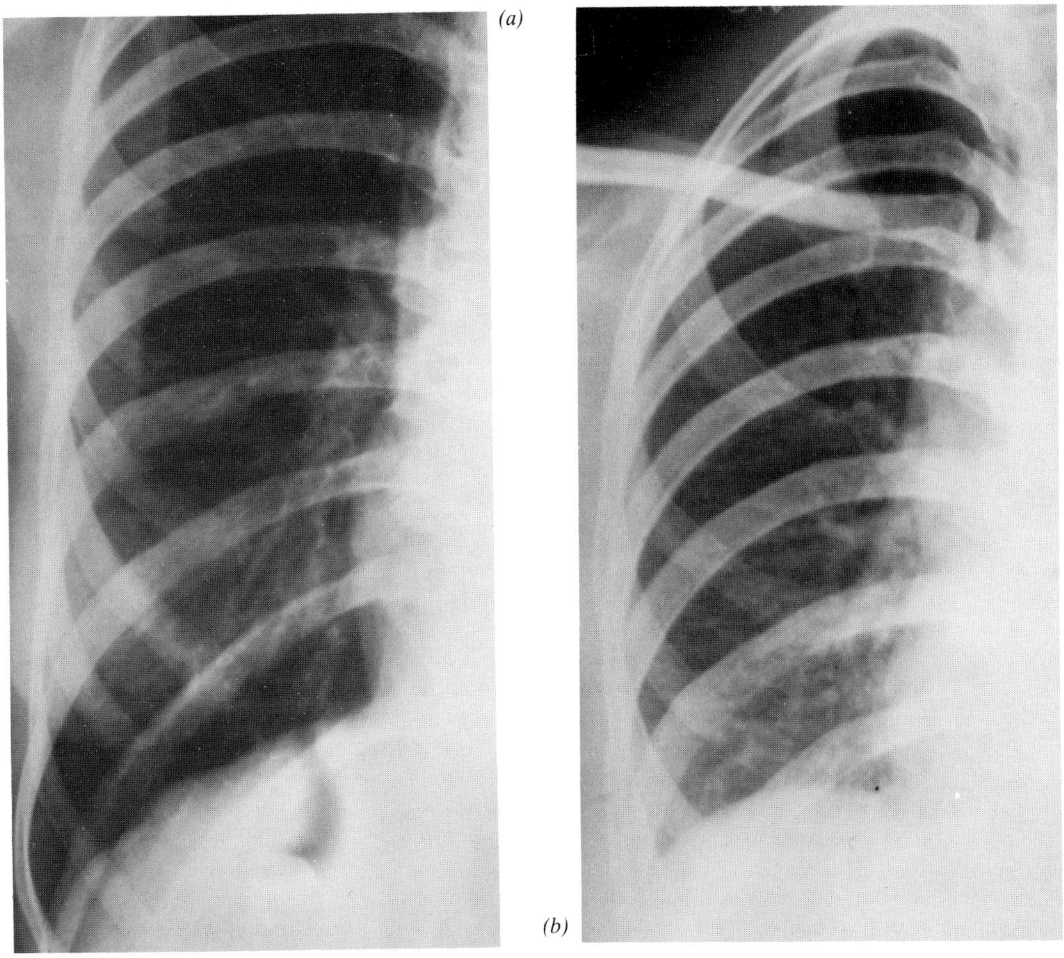

Figure 5.5 Difference in the appearances of the lower zones of normal lung fields in (a) inspiration compared with (b) expiration. The latter may be interpreted as mild diffuse interstitial fibrosis (for example, in asbestos workers)

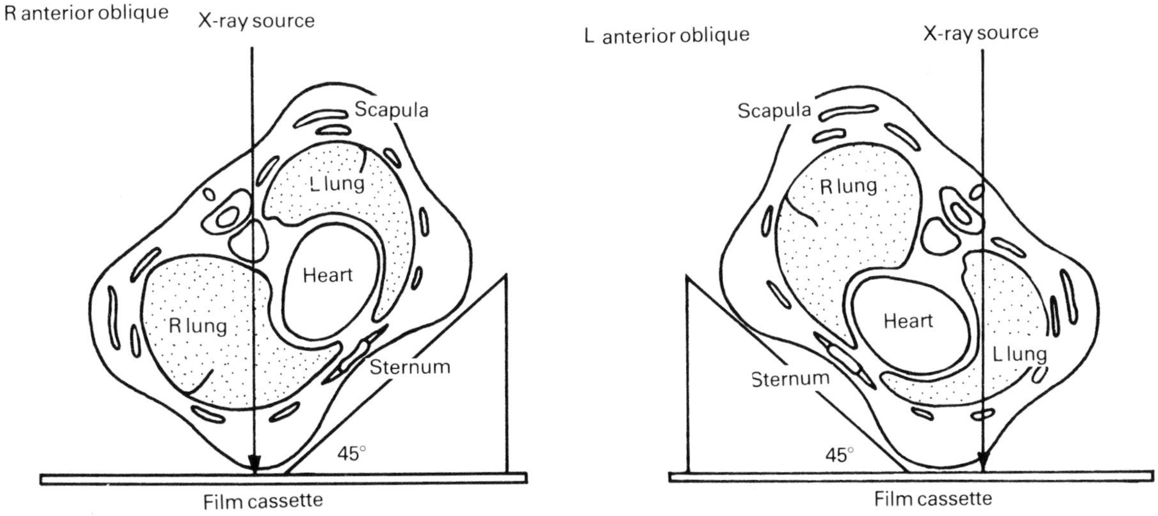

Figure 5.6 Positioning of the thorax for right and left anterior oblique views at 45 degrees showing why these provide invaluable complementary evidence to standard PA and lateral views of disease of the chest wall, pleura and lung. (Adapted with permission from Clark's Positioning in Radiography*)*

ANTEROPOSTERIOR VIEW (AP VIEW)

An AP view is invaluable for the clarification of uncertain or small and indistinct opacities seen in PA film because lesions which cause these may be situated rather more posteriorly than anteriorly in the lungs and are therefore more clearly defined.

RIGHT AND LEFT ANTERIOR (FIRST AND SECOND) OBLIQUE VIEWS (RAO AND LAO)

These are particularly helpful in demonstrating peripheral disease such as diffuse pleural thickening or tumour deposition and hyaline pleural plaques which may be poorly defined or even invisible in a PA view, and also in confirming or refuting the presence of diffuse intrapulmonary fibrosis especially in the lower lung fields (*see* Chapter 9). As a rule more informative oblique views are produced if the subject's chest is positioned at 45 degrees to the cassette rather than at the conventional 60 degree angle (McKenzie and Harries, 1970). In some cases the RAO is better taken with the subject at 35 or 40 degrees to the cassette to achieve optimal visibility by reducing the obscuring effect of the heart (*Figure 5.6*). For routine purposes, however, the LAO is usually the more helpful of the two views but both should be taken when a patient suspected of having asbestos-related pleural or intrapulmonary fibrosis is first examined (*see* Chapter 9).

MACRORADIOGRAPHY (MAGNIFICATION TECHNIQUE)

This employs a finer focus X-ray source—0.1 mm to 0.3 mm—than is used for the standard PA view, and the subject is placed midway between the source and the cassette (Bracken, 1964). It produces larger, but less distinct images than the standard film. It is sometimes used in the hope of detecting small discrete lesions of a pneumoconiosis before they give evidence of their presence in standard films. This is not borne out by general experience, and surveys have shown that macroradiographs of normal persons who have never been exposed to dust hazards may be interpreted as showing discrete pneumoconiotic lesions while those of persons who have been so exposed, may be regarded as normal. In practice, macroradiography offers no advantage over good quality PA and AP films examined first by naked eye and subsequently with a hand lens of × 2 or × 3 magnification. And this conclusion is corroborated by the good correlation which exists between appearances of standard PA view and post-mortem examination of the lungs (*see* this Chapter, p. 108).

APICAL VIEW

The apical view, also known as an apicogram or lordotic view, is often of value in clarifying poorly defined and partly obscured shadows in the regions of the upper lobe apices, and may be helpful in distinguishing pneumoconiotic masses from other lesions in this region.

TOMOGRAPHY

Recourse to this technique is rarely required in the diagnosis of any type of pneumoconiosis. It is sometimes helpful in differentiating a confluent pneumoconiotic mass from other lesions which may resemble it, and of identifying such a mass when partly obscured by heart or mediastinal shadows; lateral tomography may then be of value.

MASS MINIATURE RADIOGRAPHY (MMR)

It is unnecessary to emphasize in general what a valuable technique this is, but the use of 35 mm or 70 mm films is not satisfactory for the detection of the early stages of a discrete pneumoconiosis (for example, silicosis or coal pneumoconiosis) or of a diffuse interstitial fibrosis (such as asbestosis) as they are not easily discerned on such films. Full size, standard PA films are always to be recommended.

A disadvantage of all MMR techniques is that the dose of radiation to the subject is greater by a factor of three or four than with the standard PA view.

USE OF THE CHEST RADIOGRAPH IN INDUSTRY

As an essential part of pre-employment examination the chest radiograph serves the dual purpose of identifying existing chest disease and establishing an initial point of reference by which later radiographs may be compared.

(1) It enables the majority of industrial lung diseases to be identified at an early stage.
(2) It is an invaluable epidemiological tool for defining the incidence ('attack rate') and progression of a particular lung disease in a given industrial population. This technique has been applied extensively to the identification of new cases of coal pneumoconiosis and the detection of progression of existing cases in individual collieries in Britain (Liddell and May, 1966). It is similarly used in industries in which there is a risk of other forms of pneumoconiosis, although in some (especially those involving asbestos exposure), physiological tests are needed to augment the radiographic examination (*see also* p. 108).

INTERPRETATION OF THE PA RADIOGRAPH IN INDUSTRIAL LUNG DISEASE

The brightness of viewing boxes should not be less than that given by two 15-watt white fluorescent tubes. A film which is overexposed ('too-black') can usually be interpreted satisfactorily if viewed against a very bright white light rather than on a standard viewing box, but a much underexposed ('too-white') film is worthless.

As in the diagnosis of any lung disease, it is necessary first to establish *where* the lesions are (that is, their anatomical site) and then to deduce *what* they are (that is, their pathology). The anatomical placing of lesions demands a careful routine of inspection of the PA and lateral films as has already been described.

It must be emphasized that, in general, there is no radiographic appearance unique to any one type of pneumoconiosis. Radiographic diagnosis must be deductive in the light of all other relevant data, and the habit of 'spot' diagnosis in this branch of chest medicine is particularly apt to cause unfortunate mistakes.

Fundamentally, appearances in the lung fields caused by pneumoconioses are of two main types: discrete, roughly round opacities of small or large size (often referred to as 'nodular')—such as occur in siderosis, silicosis and coal pneumoconiosis; and fine to coarse linear, curvilinear, and irregular opacities which are sometimes accompanied by small ring shadows with central translucencies—such as occur in asbestosis, the fibrotic stage of extrinsic allergic 'alveolitis', chronic beryllium disease and cryptogenic diffuse interstitial fibrosis. When discrete, round opacities are very small and numerous they may present an ill-defined 'ground glass' appearance but, when viewed through a × 2 or × 3 hand lens are seen never to lose their identity completely. Indefinite, fine, net-like, irregular opacities are sometimes associated with retention of dusts of low atomic number—carbon, for example—and are caused mainly by superimposition of different radiodensities and not by the pathological process alone. The term '*reticulation*' is often applied to this appearance but if it is used it should be made clear that radiographic appearances are referred to and not the proliferation of reticulin fibres for which the same term is sometimes used by pathologists. This derives from the confusing statement of Belt and Ferris (1942): 'Dust reticulation may be defined as a dust-ridden state of the lungs corresponding to X-ray reticulation'. Such confusion of identity must be avoided for there is no correlation between the net-like irregular opacities and reticulin proliferation in the lungs. It is preferable not to use the term in either sense. '*Mottling*' is frequently employed as a vague term to describe appearances in the lung fields but it is uninformative unless used in the sense defined by the Ministry of Health (1952): that is, multiple discrete or semi-confluent shadows generally less than 5 mm in diameter, 'miliary mottling' consists of numerous discrete, well-defined shadows not exceeding 2 mm in diameter' which roughly correspond to the ILO categories for small round opacities (*see* next section).

Discrete or linear opacities are transient or permanent according to the nature of the underlying disease process and are due, therefore, to a large number of causes. A list of these—it makes no claim to be comprehensive—is given in *Table 5.2*.

It is clear, therefore, that failure to elicit a satisfactory occupational history and relate it to the radiographic and other features may result in non-occupational disease being wrongly interpreted as a pneumoconiosis so that appropriate treatment is delayed or not given, or in a pneumoconiosis being mistaken for non-occupational disease with the consequence of irrelevant treatment.

When an individual is first seen, whether in clinic, hospital or work-place, earlier radiographs must be obtained for comparison. This procedure is essential for confirming or refuting the diagnosis, in determining whether or not disease has progressed, and in identifying possible intercurrent disease such as carcinoma of lung.

Table 5.2 Some Causes of Discrete and Irregular Lung Opacities

Discrete	*Irregular or linear with or without 'honeycomb'*
INFECTIONS	
Chicken pox (healed calcified lesions) in adults	
Tuberculosis; miliary, acino-nodular (*)	
Blastomycosis(*)	
Coccidioidomycosis (*)	
Histoplasmosis (*)	
Torulosis (*)	
Schistosomiasis	
INHALATION	
Dusts	
Iron	
Silver	
Barium	
Tin	
Antimony	
Titanium	
Zirconium	
Cerium oxide	
Coal and carbon	
Free silica	Free silica (occasional)
China clay	
Asbestos	Asbestos
'Talc'	'Talc'
Beryllium (*)	Beryllium
	'Hard metal' (cobalt)
Actinomycetes, fungi and other organic materials (extrinsic allergic 'alveolitis') (*)	Actinomycetes, fungi and other organic materials (diffuse interstitial fibrosis)
Fumes and gases	
Oxides of nitrogen (*)	
Ozone (*)	
Phosgene (*)	
(*see Table 13.3*)	

Table 5.2 (continued)

Discrete	*Irregular or linear with or without 'honeycomb'*
ASPIRATION	
Dysphagia pneumonitis (*)	
Lipoid granuloma (*)	Lipoid granuloma
Diagnostic contrast media (bronchography) (*)	
ASSOCIATED WITH CARDIOVASCULAR DISEASE	
Alveolar oedema (*)	Diffuse interstitial oedema*
Mitral stenosis	
Haemosiderosis	
Miliary ossification	
Right-sided infective endocarditis (*)	
OF UNCERTAIN CAUSE	
Sarcoidosis (*)	Sarcoidosis
Associated with erythema nodosa	Cryptogenic diffuse interstitial fibrosis ('fibrosing alveolitis')
Idiopathic haemosiderosis	
Alveolar proteinosis (*)	
Microlithiasis	
ASSOCIATED WITH GENERAL CONSTITUTIONAL DISEASES	
	'Honeycomb lung' and diffuse interstitial fibrosis, (fibrosing 'alveolitis')
	Developmental
	Xanthomatosis
	Tuberose sclerosis
'Rheumatoid' pneumoconiosis	'Rheumatoid lung'
	Sjögren's syndrome
	Scleroderma (progressive systemic sclerosis)
	Generalized lupus erythematosus
	Cystic disease of the pancreas
RETICULOSIS AND BLOOD DISEASE	
Leukaemia	
Hodgkin's disease	
Lymphosarcoma	Lymphosarcoma
NEOPLASTIC	
Primary and secondary carcinoma	Lymphangitis carcinomatosa
Bronchiolar carcinoma	
ALLERGIC	
Extrinsic allergic 'alveolitis' (*)	Extrinsic allergic 'alveolitis'
Eosinophilic infiltration (*)	
Infiltration during asthma (*)	
Polyarteritis nodosa (*)	
ASSOCIATED WITH HEALED INFLAMMATORY DISEASE	
	Fibrosis
	Bronchiectasis

*Opacities which may be transient
(Modified from J. G. Scadding (1952) with the permission of Emeritus Professor Scadding and the Editor of *Tubercle*)

CLASSIFICATION OF PNEUMOCONIOSIS RADIOGRAPHS

It is important that the technique of interpreting as well as taking films should, as far as is practicable, be standardized—especially in the case of epidemiological surveys—in order to reduce to a minimum discrepancies between different observers. Hence various systems of classification have been proposed to standardize description of opacities but that proposed by the International Labour Office in 1959 and its subsequent modifications in 1970 and 1971 with sets of standard reference films has been generally adopted (Jacobsen and Gilson, 1972; Liddell, 1972). Shortly before this book went to press (and too late for comprehensive inclusion in the text) a further modification with a new set of standard films has been introduced. The Classification is designed to provide 'a means for recording systematically the radiographic abnormalities in the chest provoked by the inhalation of dusts' seen in standard (PA) radiographs (International Labour Office, 1980). In the main it seeks to do two things: to categorize *the size or form* of opacities and to indicate their *profusion or extent* in the lung fields. The 1971 version is displayed in *Table 5.3*.

The symbols p, q, r, s, t and u are used for small opacities, q being equivalent to m ('micronodular') and r to n ('nodular') in pre-1971 Classifications. In the 1980 version s, t and u irregular opacities are defined as having the same widths respectively as the diameters of p, q, and r round opacities. Furthermore, two letters are now used to indicate

Table 5.3 ILO U/C International Classification of Radiographs of Pneumoconioses 1971

I. Outline of classification

Feature	*Short classification*	*Extended classification*
No pneumoconiosis	0	Rounded, Irregular 0/–, 0/0, 0/1
PNEUMOCONIOSIS		
SMALL OPACITIES		
Rounded		
Profusion*	1, 2, 3	1/0, 1/1, 1/2; 2/1, 2/2, 2/3; 3/2, 3/3, 3/4
Type	p, q(m), r(n)	p, q(m), r(n)
Extent	—	zones: right, left; upper, middle, lower
Irregular		
Profusion*	1, 2, 3	1/0, 1/1, 1/2; 2/1, 2/2, 2/3; 3/2, 3/3, 3/4
Type	s, t, u	s, t, u
Extent	—	zones: right, left; upper, middle, lower
LARGE OPACITIES		
Size	A, B, C	A, B, C
Type	—	wd (well defined), id (ill defined)
PLEURAL THICKENING		
Costophrenic angle	—	Right, left
Walls and diaphragm		
Site		Right, left
Width	pl	a, b, c
Extent		1, 2
DIAPHRAGM OUTLINE	—	Ill defined: right, left
CARDIAC OUTLINE	—	Ill defined: 1, 2, 3
PLEURAL CALCIFICATION		
Site	plc	Walls, diaphragm, other; right, left
Extent		Length: 1, 2, 3

II. Details of classification

		Codes	*Definitions*
Small opacities	*Rounded* Profusion*		The category of profusion is based on assessment of the concentration (profusion) of opacities in the affected zones The standard films define the mid-categories (1/1, 2/2, 3/3)
		0/– 0/0 0/1	Category 0—small rounded opacities absent or less profuse than in Category 1
		1/0 1/1 1/2	Category 1—small rounded opacities definitely present but few in number
		2/1 2/2 2/3	Category 2—small rounded opacities numerous. The normal lung markings are usually still visible
		3/2 3/3 3/4	Category 3—small rounded opacities very numerous. The normal lung markings are partly or totally obscured
	Type	p, q(m), r(n)	The nodules are classified according to the approximate diameter of the predominant opacities p —rounded opacities up to about 1.5 mm diameteer q(m)—rounded opacities exceeding about 1.5 mm and up to about 3 mm diameter r(n) —rounded opacities exceeding about 3 mm and up to about 10 mm diameter
	Extent	RU RM RL LU LM LL	The zones in which the opacities are seen are recorded. Each lung is divided into three zones—upper, middle and lower
	Irregular Profusion*		The category of profusion is based on the assessment of the concentration (profusion) of opacities in the affected zones The standard films define the mid-categories
		0/– 0/0 0/1	Category 0—small irregular opacities absent or less profuse than in Category 1
		1/0 1/1 1/2	Category 1—small irregular opacities definitely present but few in number. The normal lung markings are usually visible
		2/1 2/2 2/3	Category 2—small irregular opacities numerous. The normal lung markings are usually partly obscured

Table 5.3 (continued)

		Codes	*Definitions*
		3/2 3/3 3/4	Category 3—small irregular opacities very numerous. The normal lung markings are usually totally obscured
	Type	s t u	As the opacities are irregular, the dimensions used for rounded opacities cannot be used, but they can be roughly divided into three types† s—fine irregular or linear opacities t—medium irregular opacities u—coarse (blotchy) irregular opacities
	Extent	RU RM RL LU LM LL	The zones in which the opacities are seen are recorded. Each lung is divided into three zones—upper, middle and lower—as for rounded opacities
	Combined Profusion*		When both rounded and irregular small opacities are present, record the profusion of each separately and then record the combined profusion as though all the opacities were of one type. This is an optional feature of the classification
Large opacities	Size	A B C	Category A—an opacity with greatest diameter between 1 cm and 5 cm, or several such opacities the sum of whose greatest diameters does not exceed 5 cm Category B—one or more opacities larger or more numerous than those in category A, whose combined area does not exceed the equivalent of one-third of the area of the right lung field Category C—one or more opacities whose combined area exceeds one-third of the area of the right lung
	Type	wd id	As well as the letter 'A', 'B' or 'C', the abbreviation 'wd' or 'id' should be used to indicate whether the opacities are well defined or ill defined
Other features	*Pleural thickening* Costophrenic angle	Right left	Obliteration of the costophrenic angle is recorded separately from thickening over other sites A lower limit standard film is provided
	Walls and diaphragm Site	Right left	
	Width	a b c	Grade a—up to about 5 mm thick at the widest part of any shadow Grade b—over about 5 mm and up to about 10 mm thick at the widest part of any shadow Grade c—over about 10 mm thick at the widest part of any shadow
	Extent	0 1 2	Grade 0—not present or less than Grade 1 Grade 1—definite pleural thickening in one or more places such that the total length does not exceed one-half of the projection of one lateral chest wall. The standard film defines the lower limit of Grade 1 Grade 2—definite pleural thickening in one or more places such that the total length exceeds one-half of the projection of one lateral chest wall†
	Diaphragm Ill defined	Right left	The lower limit is one-third of the affected hemidiaphragm. A lower limit standard film is provided
	Cardiac outline Ill defined (shagginess)	0 1 2 3	Grade 0—not present or up to one-third of the length of the left cardiac border or equivalent Grade 1—above one-third and up to two-thirds of the length of the left cardiac border or equivalent Grade 2—above two-thirds and up to the whole length of the left cardiac border or equivalent Grade 3—more than the whole length of the left cardiac border or equivalent
	Pleural calcification Site	Right left	
	Diaphragm Walls Other		Grade 0—no pleural calcification seen Grade 1—one or more areas of pleural calcification, the sum of whose greatest diameters does not exceed about 2 cm Grade 2—one or more areas of pleural calcification, the sum of whose greatest diameters exceeds about 2 cm, but not about 10 cm
	Extent	0 1 2 3	Grade 3—one or more areas of pleural calcification, the sum of whose greatest diameters exceeds about 10 cm

Symbols

ax —coalescence of small rounded pneumoconiotic opacities

bu —bullae

ca —cancer of lung or pleura

cn —calcification in small pneumoconiotic opacities

co —abnormality of cardiac size or shape
cp —cor pulmonale
cv —cavity
di —marked distortion of the intrathoracic organs
ef —effusion
em —marked emphysema
es —eggshell calcification of hilar or mediastinal lymph nodes
hi —enlargement of hilar or mediastinal lymph nodes
ho —honeycomb lung
k —septal (Kerley) lines kl(1980)
od —other significant disease. This includes disease not related to dust exposure, e.g. surgical or traumatic damage to chest walls, bronchiectasis, etc.
pq —pleural plaque (uncalcified)
px —pneumothorax
rl —rheumatoid pneumoconiosis rp(1980) (Caplan's syndrome)
tba —tuberculosis, probably active
tbu —tuberculosis, activity uncertain

*****Use of 12-point scale for small opacities.** The instructions are to classify the film in the usual way into one of the four categories, 0 to 3, and if, during the process, a neighbouring category is considered as a serious alternative, record this after the formal category. Thus category 2/1 is a film which is category 2, but category 1 was seriously considered as an alternative. The film which is without doubt a category 2, i.e. a mid-category closely similar in profusion to the standard film, would be classified as 2/2. In films within category 0, a subdivision is also possible. thus category 0/1 is a film which is category 0, but category 1 was seriously considered. Category 0/0 is a normal film without small opacities. Occasionally films look exceptionally 'normal', i.e. there is exceptional clarity of the normal architecture. Provision for these is made by the category 0/–. (Reproduced by permission of ILO)
†See text for changes in the 1980 revised version

whether small opacities are deemed to be of similar or of different size and shape; for example, q/q if all are round and between 1.5 and 3 mm diameter; and q/t if the q category is predominant but is accompanied by 'significant numbers' of irregular opacities. The profusion of small opacities according to the 1971 Classification is expressed by reference to the zones of the lung fields: Category 1 consists of relatively few small round opacities occupying no more than two zones of both lung fields; Category 2, more numerous opacities; and Category 3, very numerous opacities, which may partly or wholly obscure 'normal lung markings'. See *Figures 5.8* to *5.13*—which are *not* ILO standard films—for examples of the major categories. Surprisingly, in the 1980 version the standard films are intended to take precedence over the written definitions for the assessment of profusion. There are now three categories to denote the *extent* of pleural thickening. Otherwise the 1971 version is substantially unchanged.

The specifications of large opacities, Categories A, B and C which correspond to larger masses are the same in the 1971 and in the 1980 systems as in the old, and the method of distinguishing between Categories B and C is shown in *Figure 5.7;* category A is readily defined with a ruler.

When small 'round' opacities coexist with large opacities the category of the small opacities should be given first (for example, 2q) and that of the large opacity (or opacities) next (for example, B) so that the category denomination is then written 2qB. Categories A, B and C may be observed in the absence of accompanying small, round ('background') opacities, but this is not common.

There are numerous additional symbols which are shown in *Table 5.3*. This method of classification, it should be noted, does not specify any particular disease process nor imply degree of impairment of lung function or of respiratory disability.

It should be noted that the allotment of category indicates no more than a particular profusion of a certain type of opacity in the lung fields. It does not specify a diagnosis nor imply respiratory disability or impairment of lung function.

To be fully acquainted with the new Classification the reader should consult the text of the 1980 'Guidelines'.

PROGRESSION FROM LOWER TO HIGHER CATEGORIES OF PROFUSION

Because this sort of classification of radiographs is arbitrary, it gives only a semi-quantitative scale of increasing radiographic abnormality. It is conceivable that in reality there is

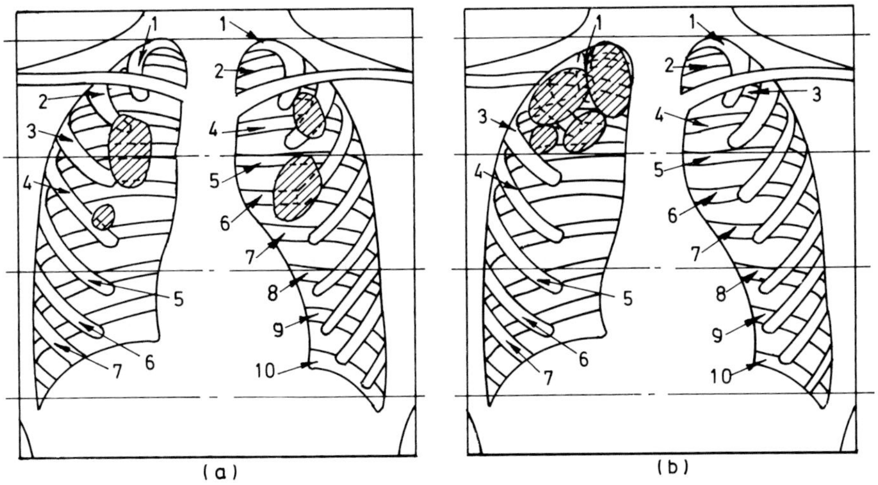

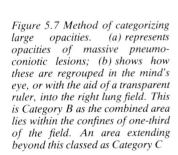

Figure 5.7 Method of categorizing large opacities. (a) represents opacities of massive pneumoconiotic lesions; (b) shows how these are regrouped in the mind's eye, or with the aid of a transparent ruler, into the right lung field. This is Category B as the combined area lies within the confines of one-third of the field. An area extending beyond this classed as Category C

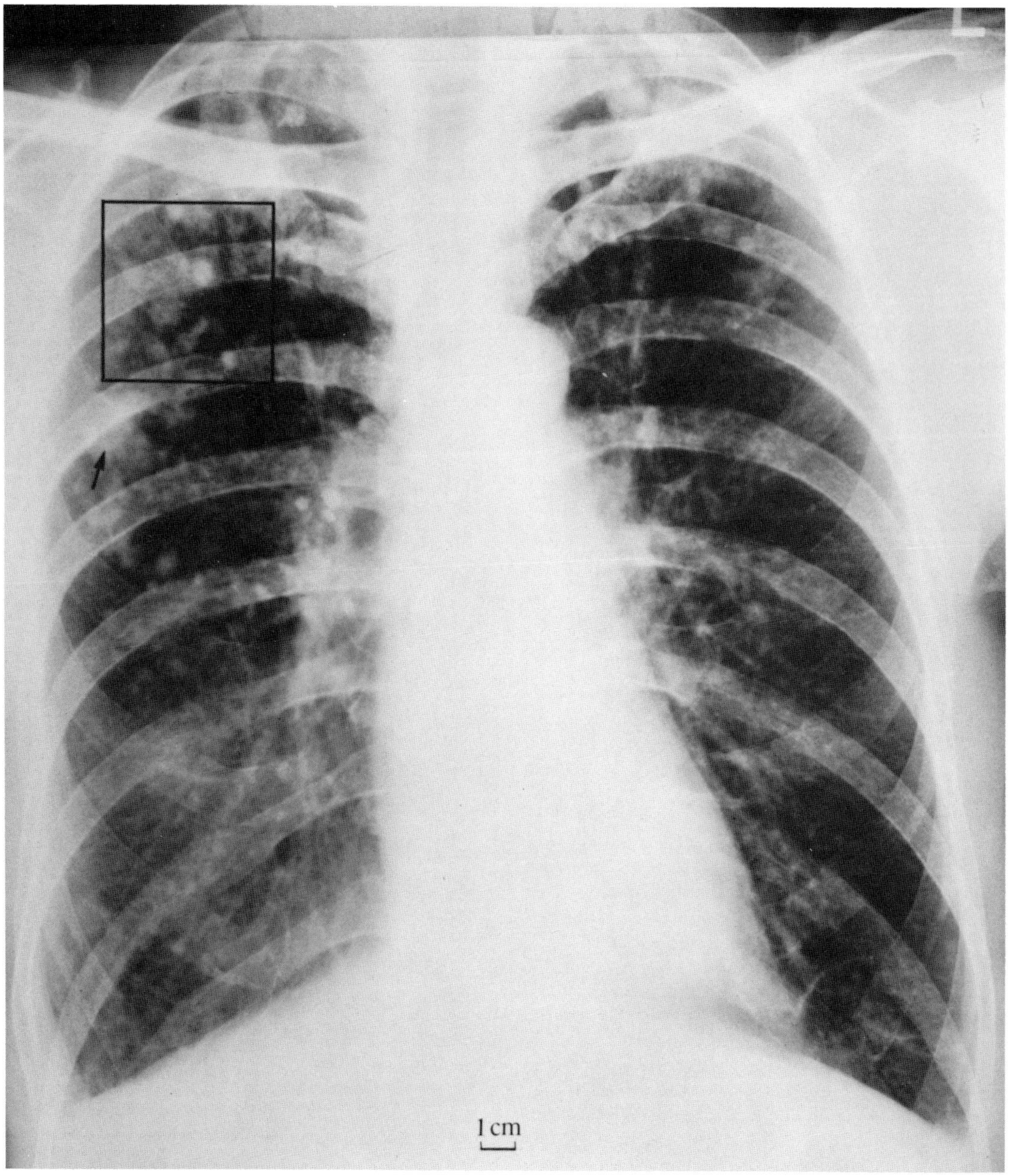

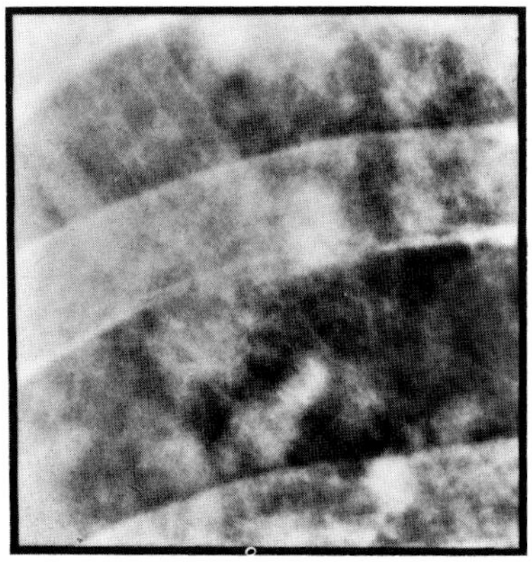

Figure 5.8 Category 1r(n)A. Opacities greater than 3 mm but less than 10 mm in diameter. The A opacity (arrowed) measures 2.0 × 1.5 cm. (Selected area, natural size)

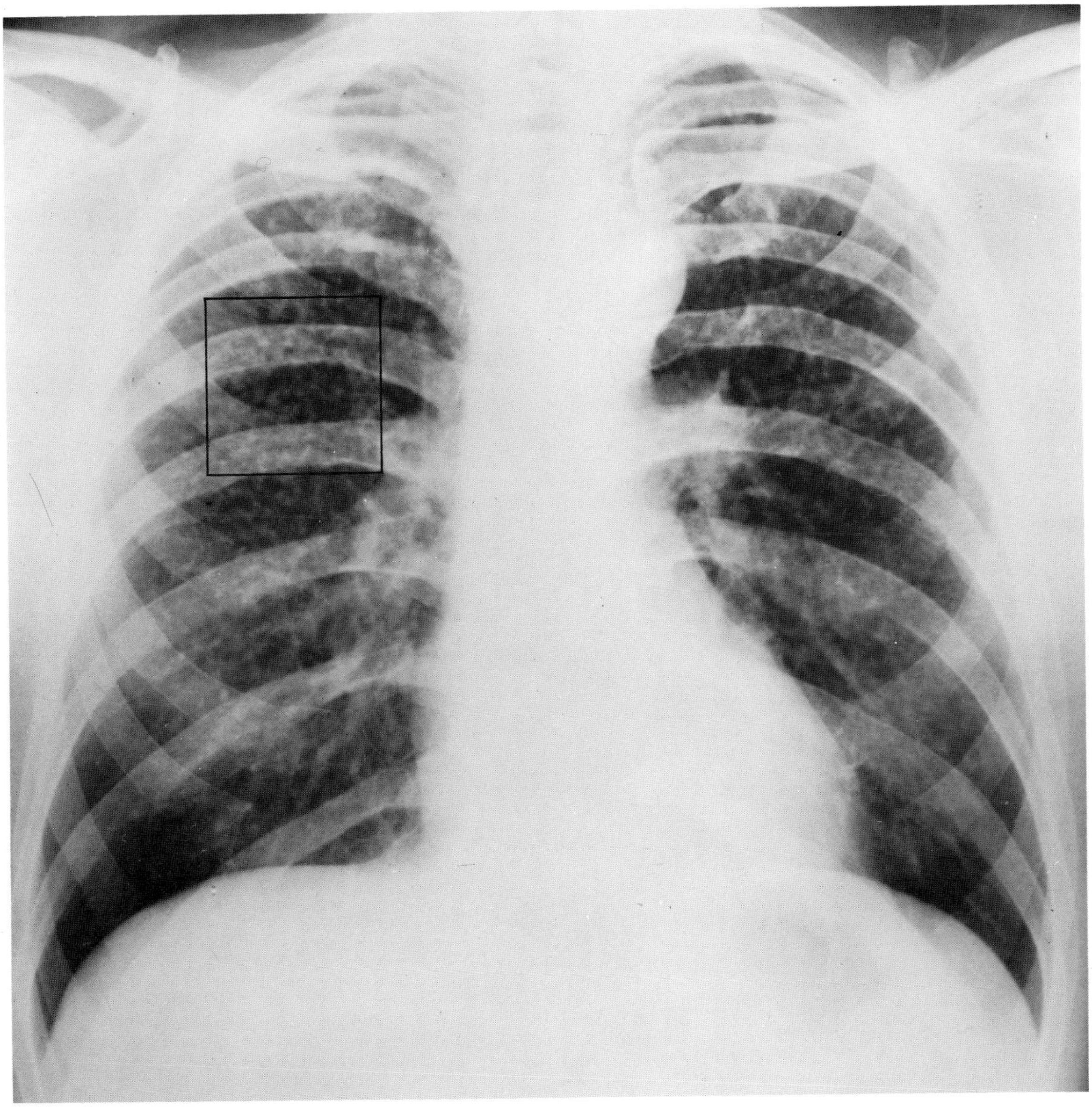

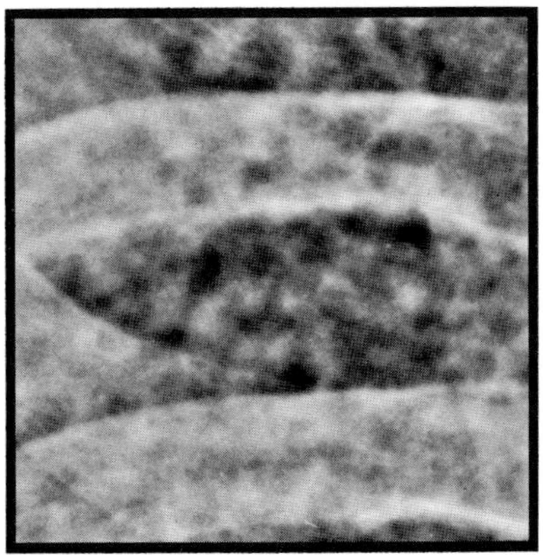

Figure 5.9 Category 2q(m). Opacities greater than 1.5 mm but less than 3 mm in diameter. (Selected area, natural size)

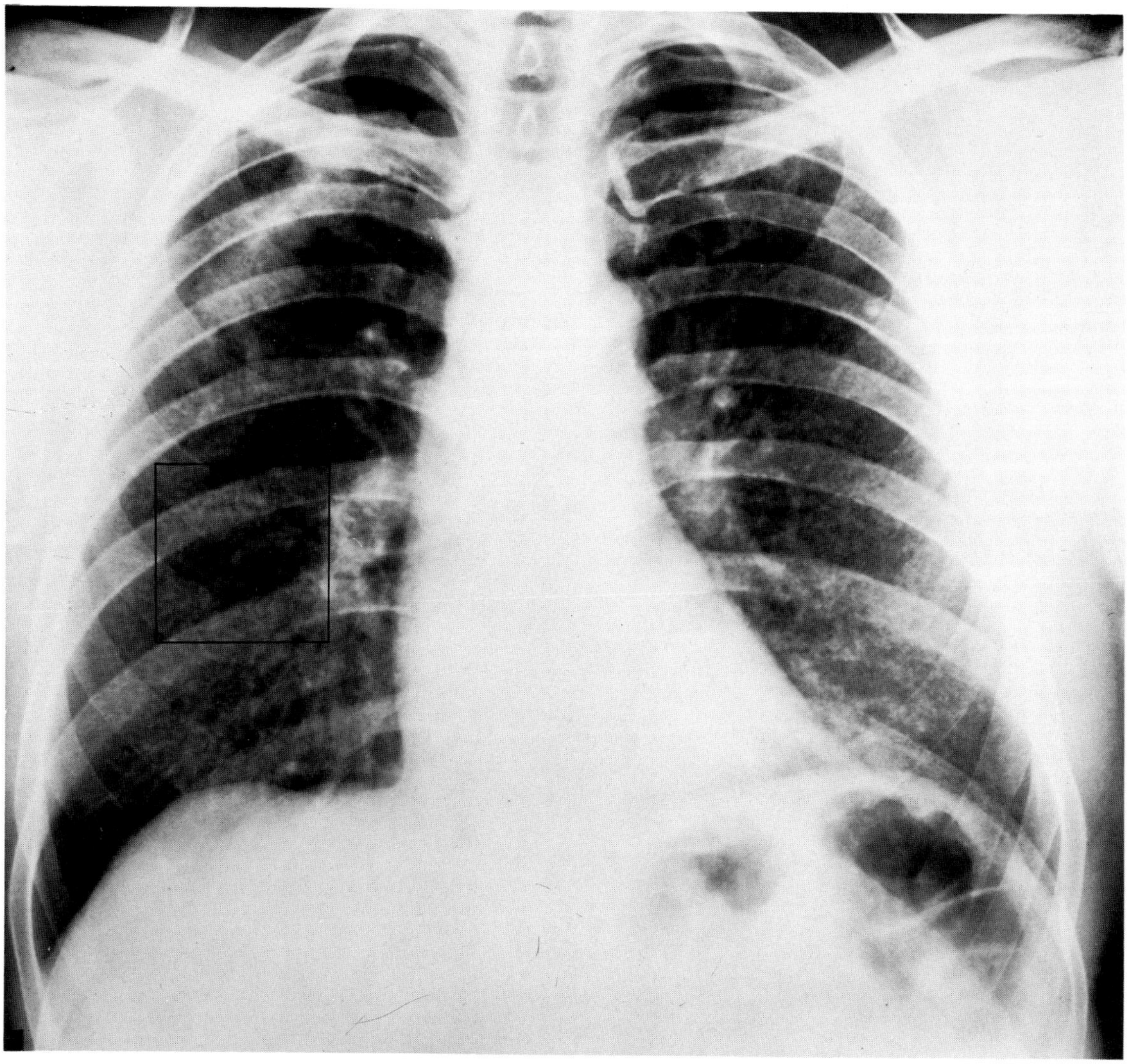

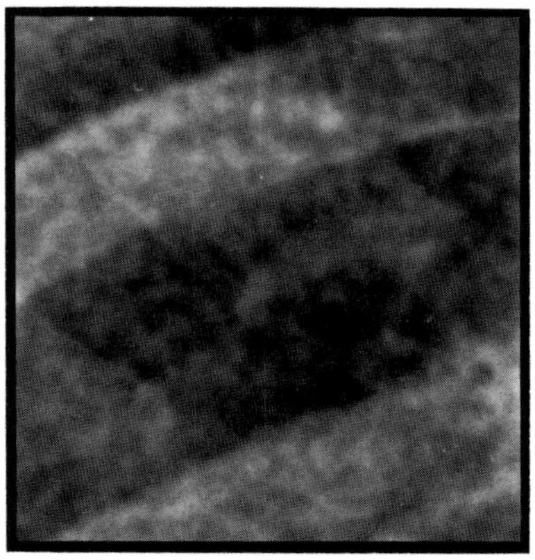

Figure 5.10 Category 3pB. Widespread small opacities not exceeding 1.5 mm in diameter. 'B' opacity in right upper zone is slightly more than 5 cm in its long axis; note the central density indicative of calcification. (See *Chapter 8*)

a continuum from normality along an abnormality scale; although, of course, a disease process may accelerate rapidly at one time, lag at another or remain permanently at a standstill at any one point. Because the four point profusion scale (category 0 to 3) was found to be insufficiently sensitive for assessment of progression for epidemiological purposes Liddell (1963) suggested that it be subdivided and converted into a 12 point scale which is, to some extent, a statistical abstraction. This modification was adopted by the British National Coal Board and subsequently introduced into the ILO/UC (1971) classification (*see Figure 5.14* and, for method of use, footnote to *Table 5.3*).

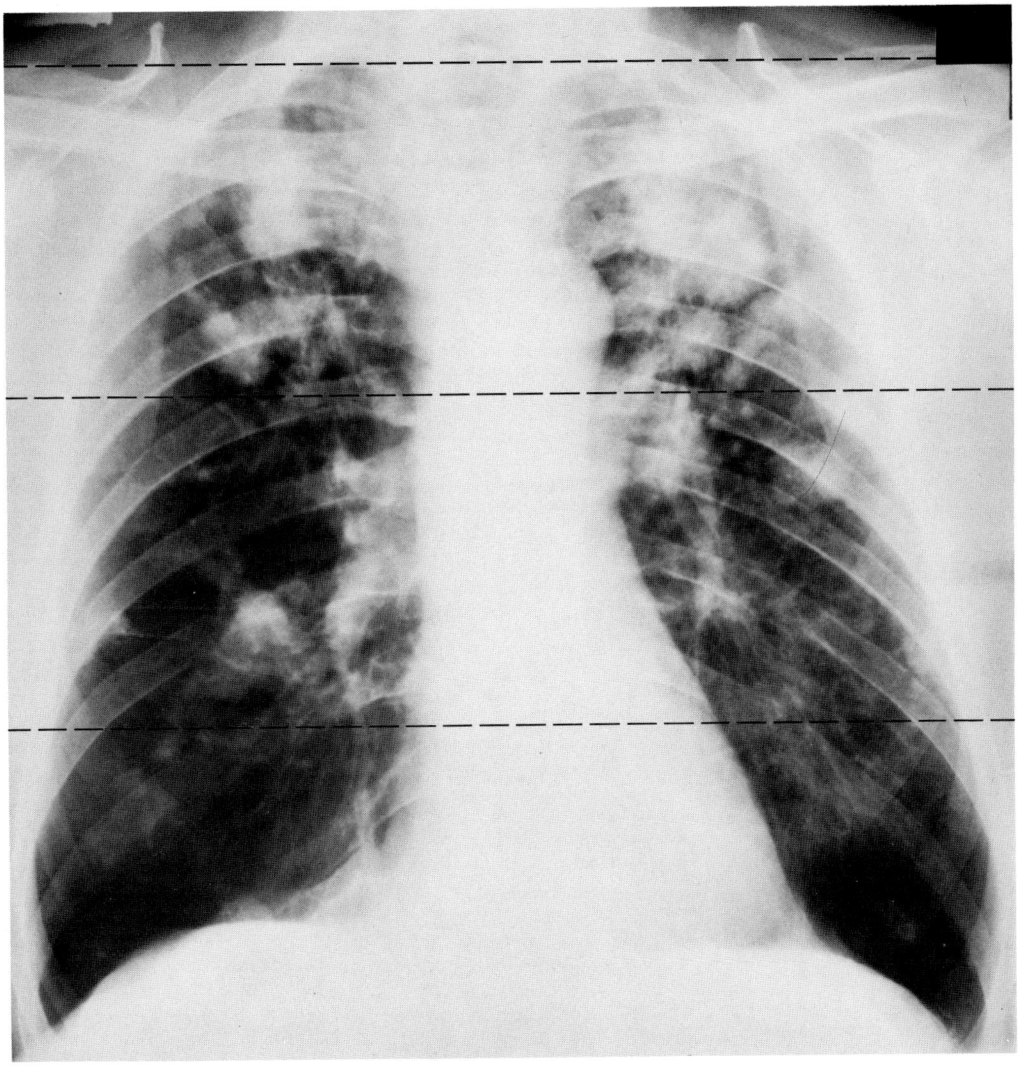

Figure 5.11 Category B with very few small, discrete opacities. All the large opacities can just be aggregated into the right upper zone and, thus, do not exceed one-third of the right lung field, as in Figure 5.6. *This is a case of Caplan's syndrome (*see *Chapter 8)*

The 1971 (and 1980) ILO Classification, therefore, is presented in 'short' and 'extended' forms: the short form closely resembles the old 1958 system, but the extended form incorporates the NCB elaboration of profusion for both 'round' and 'irregular' opacities. The short form is adequate in clinical practice and the extended form is appropriate for epidemiological and research studies.

RELEVANT ASPECTS OF PRODUCTION AND INTERPRETATION OF THE CHEST RADIOGRAPH

EFFECTS OF TECHNICAL QUALITY OF RADIOGRAPHS ON CATEGORY

There is a tendency when examining films which are too 'black' or too 'white' to relegate small discrete opacities to too low a category (Wise and Oldham, 1963; Pearson *et al.*, 1965), though too high a category is apt to be assessed in under-exposed films (Reger *et al.*, 1972); and the proportion of unsatisfactory films is greater as chest thickness (Liddell, 1961) or the ratio of body weight to sitting (stem) height increases (Pearson *et al.*, 1965). Three points follow from this.

(1) Film quality has an important effect on the category attributed to it (Reger *et al.*, 1972). There is need, therefore, for rigorous international standardization of radiographic technique and, although much effort is being directed to this end, the technical difficulties involved are considerable.
(2) The use of a standard set of films exemplifying each category is theoretically desirable but, in practice, it is difficult to provide satisfactory examples.
(3) If normal (Category 0) radiographs are excluded, observer error tends to be greater the lower the category. Category 1 is most likely to be obscured or lost by poor radiological technique. But, under clinical conditions,

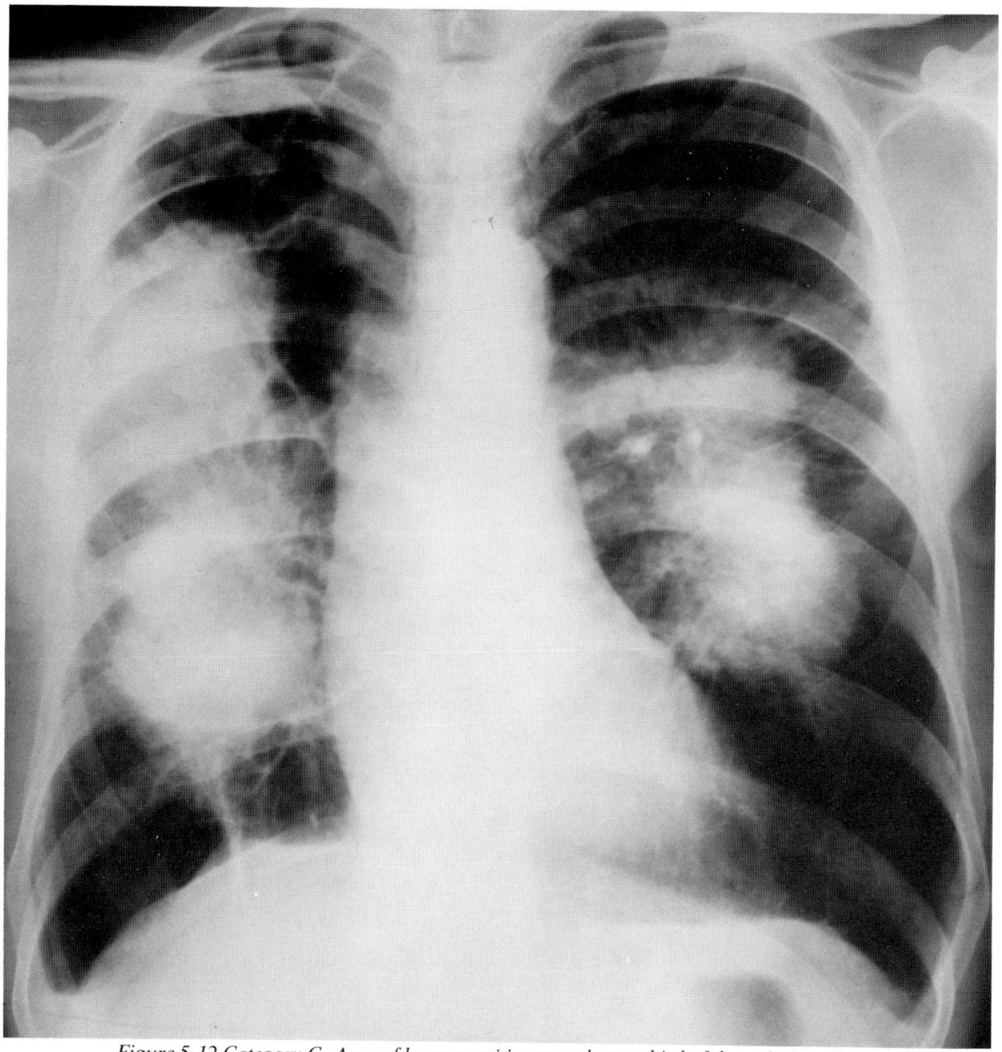

Figure 5.12 Category C. Area of large opacities exceeds one-third of the right lung field

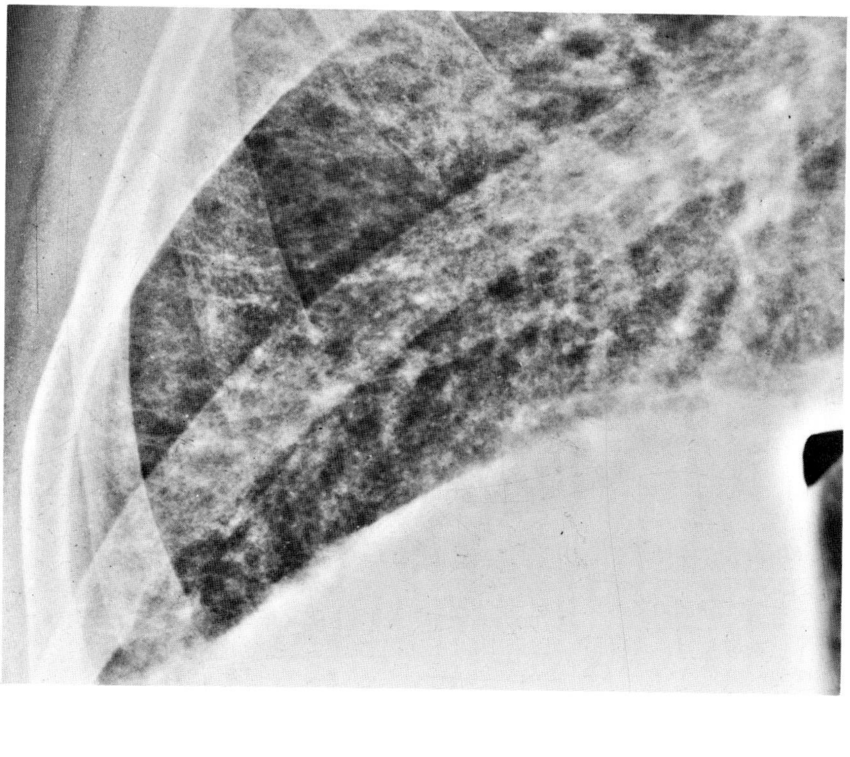

5.13(a)

Figure 5.13 Examples of irregular and linear opacities. (a) Category 's': fine type in right costophrenic angle. (b) Category 't': medium type (between fine and coarse) with some septal lines (Kerley Type B) in the left lower zone. (c) Category 'u': coarse type with appearances of 'honeycomb' cyst formation in the right mid zone. (Elaboration of the earlier ILO Classification of profusion of small opacities)

5.13(b)

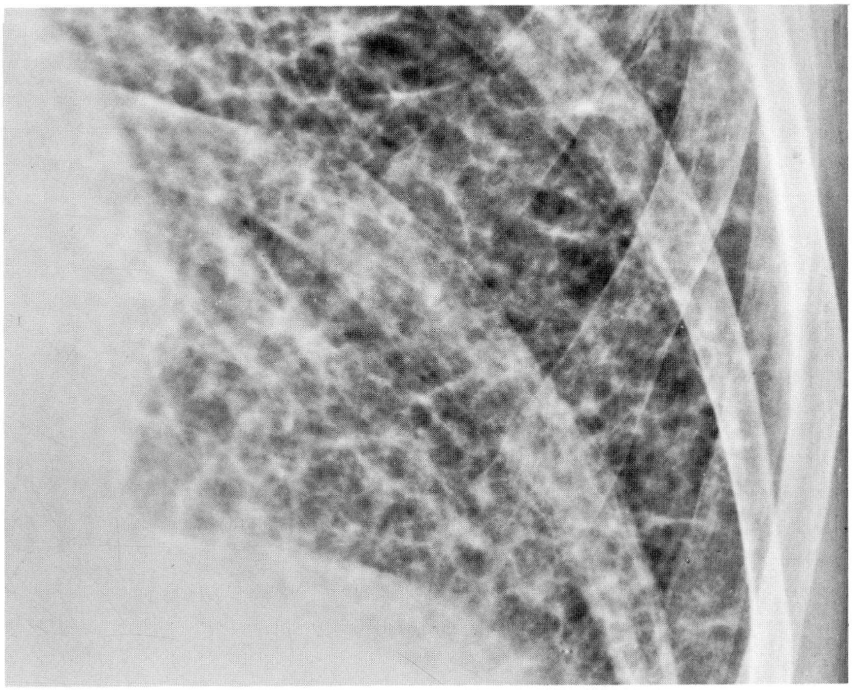

5.13(c)

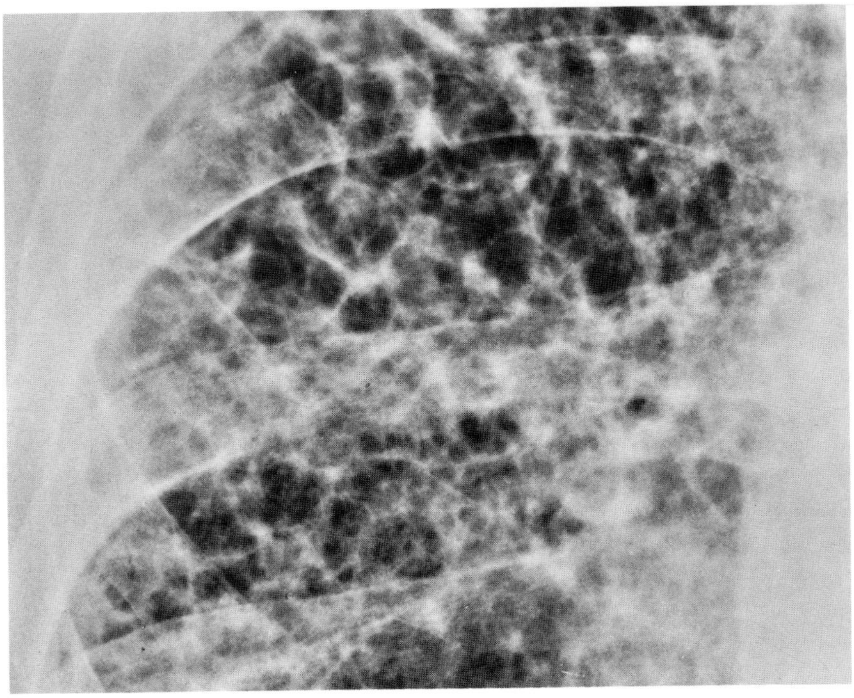

the general level of agreement becomes progressively better as the category increases.

Small round opacities, unless caused by substances of high atomic number, do not represent individual lesions, but the summation of normal and abnormal structures in the lungs. Their appearance is altered, therefore, by variation in the degree of inflation of the lungs, by slight rotation of the chest, and by excess of soft tissue shadow. If the soft tissue background is much increased it becomes difficult to interpret the significance of such opacities. Furthermore, nodular pulmonary lesions may appear to be 'cystic' on the film, and linear structures, 'nodular' (Carstairs, 1961).

THE USE OF CHEST RADIOGRAPHS IN EPIDEMIOLOGY

Even with films of consistently good quality there is considerable variation in the category assigned to individual films by different observers and by the repeated readings of

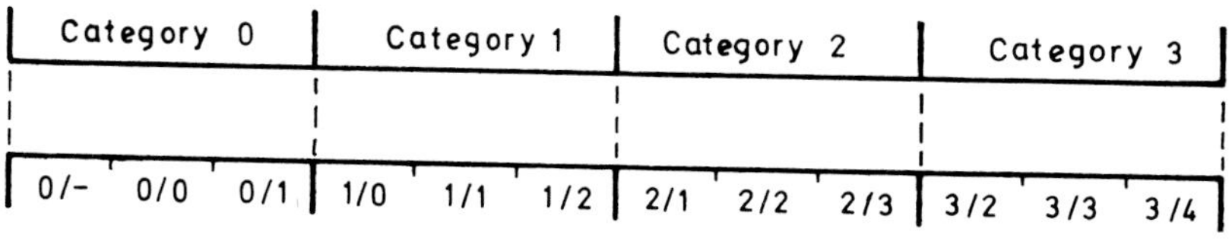

Figure 5.14 Elaboration of the earlier ILO classification profusion of small opacities. (By courtesy of Professor F. D. K. Liddell (Quebec) and Dr John Rogan, National Coal Board (Medical Research Memorandum, 4. 1966))

one observer, the discrepancies being greatest among multiple observers. For example, disagreement between groups reading films of coal pneumoconiosis has been shown to be due to poor film quality, lack of experience of the classification system and lack of familiarity with the radiographic appearances of the disease (Felson *et al.*, 1973); and sometimes, it must also be admitted, to lack of familiarity with normal variation of lung field patterns and the appearances of unrelated disease. The performances of individual readers of a group involved in an epidemiological study should, therefore, be tested and compared at the outset and, for this, multiple 'blind' readings are desirable. This is supported by evidence that perception of contrast in X-ray films by individual observers is an inherent ability which is not much affected by practice (Adrian-Harris, 1979).

There are two methods for reading serial films of individual subjects in whom progression of disease may have occurred: in the first, the films of each are inspected 'side-by-side' in chronological order; and, in the second, the films are separated and shuffled in with those of all subjects in the group being studied, thus producing a random collection of films. The relative accuracy of both techniques has been extensively investigated and evidence produced to indicate that the 'side-by-side' method causes bias in coal pneumoconiosis, tuberculosis and sarcoidosis (Amandus *et al.*, 1973; Reger, Petersen and Morgan, 1974). It is often urged, therefore, that the randomized method results in less bias in interpretation of progression or regression. However, Liddell (1974) has shown that there is substantially less error when three films are viewed by the 'side-to-side' method and are read together in sequence rather than in film groups of first and third, first and second or second and third.

Another source of difference in the interpretation of radiographs lies in the fact that certain category definitions in the ILO 1959 Classification have been altered in the ILO/UC 1971 Classification. In the former, 'suspect opacities' or 'increased lung markings' were allocated a separate category, Z; in the latter, this has been deleted and such appearances tend to be classed as 'rounded' or 'irregular' Category 1 opacities (Morgan and Reger, 1972). Again, profusion of small opacities in the 1959 system was assessed according to the extent of their distribution in the lung fields as follows:

Category 1 A small number of opacities in an area equivalent to at least two anterior rib spaces and at the most not greater than one-third of the two lung fields.

Category 2 Opacities more numerous and diffuse than in Category 1 and distributed over most of the lung fields.

Category 3 Very numerous profuse opacities covering the whole or nearly the whole of the lung fields.

The method of assessment in the ILO/UC 1971 system is less precise, as can be seen in *Table 5.3 Section II*. This may result, for example, in a film which would have been interpreted as Category 2 by the old system being interpreted as Category 3 by the new. Moreover, it remains to be seen what the comparative effect of using reference to standard films (as recommended by the 1980 Classification) as the preferred guideline for categorization will be. However, categorization of large opacities is unaffected.

Evidently, therefore, it is of the utmost importance that these sources of variability are taken into account in assessing radiographic prevalence or progression of a pneumoconiosis if these are not to be substantially over- or underestimated. Hence, comparison of prevalence between studies done at different times or with different observers and in different countries is not possible unless the standards of radiographic technique and method of film interpretation are known to be valid and similar. The most extensive investigations of this problem have been done in coal pneumoconiosis (*see* Chapter 8).

CORRELATION OF RADIOGRAPHIC APPEARANCES WITH PNEUMOCONIOTIC LESIONS

Correlation between the number and distribution of discrete opacities on chest radiographs and the number and distribution of small pneumoconiotic lesions observed post mortem is fairly good, in spite of the fact that the appearance of the radiograph is determined not only by the number and composition of the lesions but also by the superimposition of their own radiodensities and those of lung and chest wall structures.

Various factors operate to absorb X-rays in different types of lesion. The profusion and distribution of silicotic nodules (*see* Chapter 7) observed post mortem show close agreement with radiographic appearances and category; these appearances are due to the combined effect of the concentration of iron within the nodules (Otto and Maron, 1959) (referred to in Chapter 4), to collagen fibrosis, possibly to the content of free silica, and, in some cases, to deposition of calcium salts. In the case of coal pneumoconiosis, the higher the ILO category of small 'round' opacities the greater the number of foci of retained dust and the higher the proportion of fibrotic (collagen) nodules found in the lungs (Caplan, 1962). Rossiter (1972) has shown that the radiographic appearances in coal workers are most highly correlated with the mineral content of the lungs, although iron also makes a significant contribution. Due to their different X-ray mass absorption coefficients 1.6 g of iron and 5 g of other minerals in the lungs have an equal effect in increasing the category by one unit as 16 g of coal (Gilson, 1968). The category of discrete ('simple') coal pneumoconiosis correlates better with the non-haem endogenous iron content (which may accumulate during phagocytosis of dust particles) (*see* Chapter 8) than with the total iron content of the lungs (Bergman, 1970). It is probable, therefore, that the effect of iron upon category reflects variation in the amounts of coal and mineral present (Rossiter, 1972). Coal itself contributes very little to the appearances (*see* p. 128, Chapter 8).

As might be expected, correlation of radiographic abnormality with large conglomerate or pneumoconiotic masses of whatever cause is usually good.

Correlation of radiographic appearances and diffuse pulmonary fibrosis is not, on the whole, as good as that for discrete, round pneumoconiosis lesions, but it improves as the severity of the fibrosis increase from partial loss of alveolar wall architecture to its complete replacement by fibrous tissue sometimes with the development of multiple cystic spaces ('honeycombing') (Livingstone *et al.*, 1964) (*see Figure 5.13b*). It is difficult to detect the earlier stages on routine radiographs. These considerations apply not only to diffuse fibrosis of unknown cause or associated with connective tissue disorders but also to asbestosis, chronic beryllium disease and extrinsic allergic bronchioloalveolitis (*see* Chapters 4, 9, 10 and 11).

Experimental work designed to simulate linear opacities by radiographing increasing numbers of layers of plastic lattices placed at right angles to the X-ray beam has shown that, as the number of layers is increased, an appearance of discrete ('nodular' or 'mottled') opacities and ill-defined areas of relative translucency is produced—not more emphatic linear opacities (Carstairs, 1961) (*Figure 5.15*). This observation probably explains some of the discrete opacities and relative translucencies which may be seen in many cases of DIPF, and possibly also the small 'p' type opacities sometimes observed on the films of coal workers (*Figure 5.10*) who are subsequently found to have uniformly distributed emphysema in dust pigmented lungs without fibrosis (*see Figure 8.20*). These appearances may be due in some cases to the effective contrast between the increased volume of air in the numerous dilated air spaces on the one hand, and the surrounding lung tissue which possesses greater radiodensity than normal owing to the combined effect of mineral dusts, endogenous iron and coal, on the other (*see also* p. 197). In the case of inert dusts of high atomic number the opacities are denser and more clearly demarcated (*see* Chapter 6).

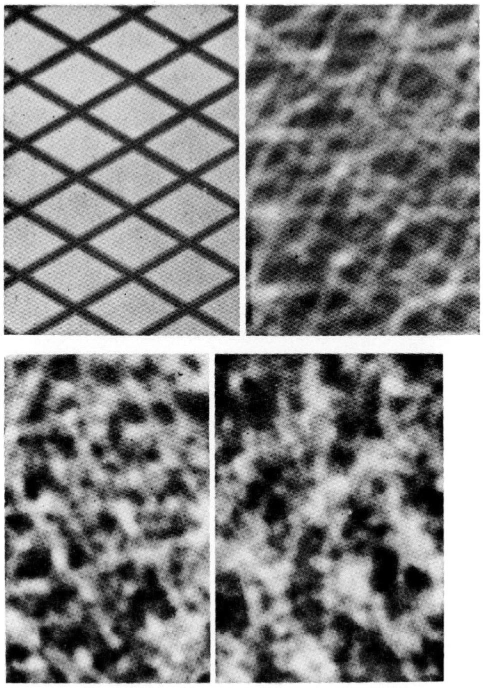

Figure 5.15 The effect produced by superimposing an increasing number of plastic lattices lying at right angles to the x-ray beam. The simple pattern produced by one layer becomes progressively 'nodular' in appearance with ill-defined areas of relative translucency. (By courtesy of Dr L. S. Carstairs and the Hon. Editors of Proceedings of the Royal Society of Medicine*)*

It is important to remember that, in general, respiratory symptoms and patterns of impaired lung function correlate very poorly with the radiographic appearances of pneumoconiosis.

ALLEGED OBSCURING EFFECT OF EMPHYSEMA

There is a fairly common belief, which has been current for more than 40 years (Rappaport, 1936, 1967; Ogilvie, 1970) that emphysema may obscure opacities which, in its absence, would have been caused by discrete (round) pneumoconiotic lesions with the result that an expected Category 2 or 3 would be converted to 0 or 1; or, contrariwise, that Category 0 could be produced in the presence of significant pneumoconiosis. This effect, it has been claimed, is produced by attenuation of X-rays due to their scatter by excess air in the lungs (Rappaport, 1936). From the physical principles already described on p. 91 it is evident that this cannot be true and that both absorption and scatter of X-rays by air are very substantially less than by the tissues or by minerals, so that an increased volume of air in the lungs will tend to *increase* the 'visibility' of the pneumoconiotic lesions. Confirmation of this is furnished by two observations: (1) when moderate or severe emphysema is present, Categories 0 to 1 are not correlated, post mortem, with an unexpectedly large number of pneumoconiotic lesions (Caplan, 1962); (2) the presence of 'focal' emphysema (which cannot be identified as such radiographically) is associated with over-assessment and not under-assessment of category (Rossiter *et al.*, 1967) due, probably, to the contrast effect referred to in the last section. And, of course, air is an effective 'contrast medium' in diagnostic radiology.

Displacement of lung in which there are pneumoconiotic lesions by distension of large emphysematous bullae is a different matter and is obvious radiographically.

KERLEY'S 'A' AND 'B' LINES

These lines were first described by Kerley, tentatively in 1933, dogmatically in 1950.

'A' lines

'A' lines are fine, not more than 1 mm thick, do not branch, are usually between 2 and 4 cm long and do not pass into the periphery of the lung to reach the pleural margin.

'B' lines

'B' lines are similarly fine, short (usually less than 2 cm), are almost perpendicular to the pleural margin with which their outer end is always in contact, and can occur anywhere in the lung fields but are usually in the lower zones (*Figures 5.13b* and *6.3*).

Both lines appear to be caused by increased radiodensity of connective tissue septa in the lungs: peripheral interlobular septa in the case of B lines and similar type septa in the depth of the lungs in the case of A lines (Trapnell, 1973). The increased radiodensity may be due to deposition of mineral dusts so that the lines are frequently present in the 'benign' pneumoconioses caused by inert dusts, especially those of high atomic number (*see* Chapter 6), and they are found more frequently in higher than in lower categories of coal pneumoconiosis (ILO Categories 3, A, B and C), B lines being more common than A (Trapnell, 1964); and both tend to be seen rather more often in the right lung than in the left (Rivers *et al.,* 1960). In my experience, however, they are present in less than half the cases of coal pneumoconiosis in these categories—a finding confirmed by Trapnell (1964) (*see Figure 8.24*).

The most common cause of these lines, however, is increased pulmonary venous pressure due to mitral stenosis and chronic left ventricular failure and, possibly, to allergic oedema (Prosser and Thurley, 1976); but they also result from infiltration of the septa by fibrosis, new growth, sarcoidosis and haemosiderin (haemosiderosis). It is important, therefore, to be aware of the fact that they may be associated with a number of different types of pneumoconiosis.

RADIOGRAPHIC APPEARANCES OF EMPHYSEMA

Due to its air trapping effect panlobular emphysema when widespread and severe is readily identified by the criteria of a low, flat diaphragm, increase in size and downwards extension of the retrosternal translucent area seen in the lateral film, a narrow, vertical heart shadow, prominent hilar vessels and unduly small arterial shadows in the mid and peripheral lung fields in the PA view (Simon, 1964). Although severe panlobular emphysema is virtually excluded by a normal radiograph, lesser degrees may fail to produce these characteristic signs or give rise to only some of them (Reid and Millard, 1964; Thurlbeck *et al.,* 1970).

On the other hand, centrilobular emphysema—whether or not associated with dust retention or pneumoconiosis—cannot be detected on standard radiographs even when it is widespread (Snider, Brody and Doctor, 1962), although it is claimed that severe grades accompanied by panlobular emphysema may sometimes be recognized (Laws and Heard, 1962).

Once established, bullae associated with local panlobular or paraseptal emphysema are usually readily recognized.

Chronic obstructive bronchitis or severe widespread panlobular emphysema may sometimes cause secondary polycythaemia in which case the pulmonary artery opacities in the middle of the lungs as well as at the hila become unduly large and prominent. Because of the 'end-on' appearance of such arteries on a PA radiograph a discrete pneumoconiosis (such as silicosis or coal pneumoconiosis) is sometimes incorrectly diagnosed; this may also occur with pulmonary artery plethora from other causes (for example, atrial septal defect).

CALCIFICATION OF THE PLEURA

Nowadays, pleural fibrosis and calcification (pleural 'plaques') are looked for in the radiographs of people who have been, or are thought to have been, exposed to an asbestos hazard (Chapter 9). When it is fairly widespread, pleural calcification is readily identified by virtue of a bizarre and irregular configuration (the so-called holly-leaf pattern) which does not correspond with any lobar or segmental distribution and which has an intensity of opacity contrasting strongly with the surrounding lung. But sometimes it is represented only by tiny opaque flecks, or short thin lines of opacity along the diaphragmatic and cardiac outlines or along the costal margin, or by small irregular areas in the lung fields. These are readily overlooked if a systematic search is not made. As described on p. 96, 45-degree anterior oblique views are helpful in defining these lesions.

Anterior oblique views 'incidentally' may also be of assistance in the investigation of malignant pleural mesothelioma (*see* Chapter 9).

It should not be forgotten, however, that calcification of the pleura, whether widespread or localized, may be due to past empyema, tuberculous pleurisy, haemothorax (as may follow chest injury), or may occur spontaneously in normal aged persons. Even when an individual has been exposed to asbestos, one or other of these may, in fact, be the true cause of the calcification. Calcification due to the first three of these causes is usually wholly or predominantly unilateral.

Calcification of costal cartilages will not be mistaken for pleural calcification if the routine for inspection is followed but the possibility of making this error must always be kept in mind; even the elect are sometimes deceived by it especially where the abnormal opacities are superimposed on the diaphragmatic shadow.

A DIRECT QUANTITATIVE RADIOLOGICAL TECHNIQUE

Direct detection of the nature and amount of an exogenous dust retained in the lungs of the living person is possible using the principle that every element has a definite 'absorption edge' which abruptly changes the transmission of X-rays through it. When radiation, with energies ranging above and below the energy of the 'absorption edge' of a given element, is passed through the lungs, alteration in its penetration due to the differential absorption effect of the element should be demonstrated (McCallum and Day, 1965). Theoretically, this offers a new dimension in radiographic identification of certain types of pneumoconiosis, but, in practice, it is in an experimental stage. It is limited to elements with atomic numbers greater than about 40 and, so far, has been applied only to antimony and tin (McCallum *et al.*, 1971).

OTHER INVESTIGATIVE TECHNIQUES

PERFUSION SCINTIGRAPHY

Colour scintigraphy using ^{131}I-labelled human albumin particles injected intravenously has demonstrated that irregular distribution of blood flow may exist in the vicinity of massive lesions of silicosis and coal pneumoconiosis (Schröder *et al.*, 1969), but this is not likely to be of practical use for purposes of routine investigation.

Similarly, gallium-67 scintigraphy has been used to complement chest radiography because this radioactive material is concentrated in regions of metabolic and mitotic activity. It may be able to indicate the presence of active disease in some types of pneumoconiosis but is of no help in differential diagnosis (Siemsen *et al.*, 1976).

XERORADIOGRAPHY

This electrostatic method of X-ray imaging has a wider latitude than conventional radiography so that simultaneous records of lung structure or lesions having a substantially different radiation absorption coefficient can be made, especially with high kilovoltage exposure (200 kV). Normal and abnormal linear opacities (such as those of DIPF) and pleural plaques (*see* Chapter 9) are better shown than on conventional radiographs, but demonstration of discrete, rounded opacities (as in silicosis) are poorly shown (Thomas and Sluis-Cremer, 1977).

However, for most purposes, the results obtained do not appear to be greatly superior to the combination of good quality PA and AO films. And the added disadvantage of increased radiation, the small size of radiographs and the limited availability of generators to produce the required unusually high kVs excludes this technique from practical use.

COMPUTER TECHNIQUES

Texture analysis

The 'reading' of films with discrete round opacities by computer is claimed to compare favourably with that of human observers and might be applicable to 'measuring pneumoconiosis in epidemiological work', and could be carried out very rapidly (Jagoe and Paton, 1975; Ledley, Huang and Rotolo, 1975). But further appraisal of the technique is essential (especially in respect of the accuracy with which the quality of films to be read is standardized and of other important variables) before it could be used with confidence.

Computerized tomography (whole-body scanning)

This technique is capable of revealing peripheral lesions in lung and pleura (for example, hyaline pleural plaques situated low down in the paravertebral gutter) and intrapulmonary fibrosis which may not be visible on standard chest radiographs (Katz and Kreel, 1979), although these are usually detectable on 45 degree AO films. However, though it produces interesting pictures, the interpretation of which in relation to underlying pathology is not always certain, it is neither a practical nor a necessary investigation of occupational lung disease for routine use; in any case, it is not accessible to most clinicians.

MAGNETOPNEUMOGRAPHY

X-radiation is not involved in this newly developed technique which appears to be capable of detecting the deposition of exogenous, iron-containing (ferrimagnetic) minerals in the lungs before it can be identified radiographically. (*See* Appendix.)

REFERENCES

Adrian-Harris, D. (1979). Aspects of visual perception in radiography. *Radiography* **45,** 237–243

Amandus, H. E., Reger, R. B., Pendergrass, E. P., Dennis, J. M. and Morgan, W. K. C. (1973). The pneumoconioses: methods of measuring progression. *Chest* **63,** 736–743

Belt, T. H. and Ferris, A. A. (1942). Histology of coal miner's pneumoconiosis. In *Chronic Pulmonary Disease in South Wales Coal Miners,* pp. 203–222. (Medical Research Council.) London; HMSO

Bergman, I. (1970). The relation of endogenous non-haem iron in formalin-fixed lungs to radiological grade of pneumoconiosis. *Ann. occup. Hyg.* **13,** 163–169

Bohlig, H. and Gilson, J. C. (1973). Radiology. In *Biological Effects of Asbestos,* edited by P. Bogovski *et al.,* pp. 25–30. Lyon; Int. Agency for Res. on Cancer

Bracken, T. J. (1964). The technique of macroradiography in the diagnosis of industrial disease of the chest. *Radiography* **30,** 291–298

Caplan, A. (1962). Correlation of radiological category with lung pathology in coal worker's pneumoconiosis. *Br. J. ind. Med.* **19,** 171–179

Carstairs, L. S. (1961). The interpretation of shadows in a restricted area of lung field in the chest radiograph. *Proc. R. Soc. Med.* **54,** 978–980

Clark's Positioning in Radiography (1979). 10th edition, Vol. 1. (Ilford Publication.) London; Heinemann Medical Books

Felson, B., Morgan, W. K. C., Bristol, L. J., Pendergrass, E. P., Dessen, E. L., Linton, O. W. and Reger, R. B. (1973). Observations on the results of multiple readings of chest films in coal miners' pneumoconioses. *Radiology* **109,** 19–23

Gilson, J. C. (1968). *Classification of Chest Radiographs and its Application to the Epidemiology of Pneumoconiosis.* (Report on a Symposium at Katowice, 1967.) Copenhagen; WHO

International Labour Office (1959). Meetings of Experts on the International Classification of Radiographs of the Pneumoconioses. *Occup. Saf. Hlth* **9,** No. 2

International Labour Office (1970). *International Classification of Radiographs of Pneumoconioses. (Revised 1968).* Occup. Saf. Hlth Series No. 22. Geneva; ILO

International Labour Office (1980). *Guidelines for the Use of ILO International Classification of Radiographs of Pneumoconioses.* Occup. Saf. Hlth Series No. 22 (Rev. 80). Geneva; ILO

Jacobson, G., Bohlig, H. and Kiviluoto, R. (1970). Essentials of chest radiography. *Radiology* **95,** 445–450

Jacobson, G. and Gilson, J. C. (1972). Present status of the UICC/Cincinnati Classification of Radiographic Appearances: report of a meeting held at the Pneumoconiosis Research Unit, Cardiff, Wales, 13–15 April, 1971. *Ann. N. Y. Acad. Sci.* **200,** 552–569

Jagoe, J. R. and Paton, K. A. (1975). Reading chest radiographs for pneumoconiosis by computer. *Br. J. ind. Med.* **32,** 267–272

Johns, H. E. and Cunningham, J. R. (1969). *The Physics of Radiology,* 3rd edition, pp. 210–211. Springfield; Thomas

Katz, D. and Kreel, L. (1979). Computed tomography in pulmonary asbestosis. *Clin. Radiol.* **30,** 207–213

Kerley, P. (1933). Radiology in heart disease. *Br. med. J.* **2,** 594–597

Kerley, P. (1950). In *A Textbook of X-ray Diagnosis,* Vol. 2, edited by S. C. Shanks and P. Kerley, pp. 404–405. London; Lewis

Laws, J. W. and Heard, B. E. (1962). Emphysema and the chest film: a retrospective radiological and pathological study. *Br. J. Radiol.* **35,** 750–761

Ledley, R. S., Huang, H. K. and Rotolo, L. S. (1975). A texture analysis method in classification of coal workers' pneumoconiosis. *Comp. biol. Med.* **5,** 53–67

Liddell, F. D. K. (1961). The effect of film quality on reading radiographs of simple pneumoconiosis in a trial of X-ray sets. *Br. J. ind. Med.* **18,** 165–174

Liddell, F. D. K. (1963). An experiment in film reading. *Br. J. ind. Med.* **20,** 300–312

Liddell, F. D. K. (1972). Validation of classifications of pneumoconiosis. *Ann. N. Y. Acad. Sci.* **200,** 527–551

Liddell, F. D. K. (1974). Assessment of radiological progression of simple pneumoconioses in individual miners. *Br. J. ind. Med.* **31,** 185–195

Liddell, F. D. K. and May, J. D. (1966). *Assessing the Radiological Progression of Simple Pneumoconiosis.* Medical Research Memorandum 4. National Coal Board Medical Service

Livingstone, J. L., Lewis, J. G., Reid, L. and Jefferson, E. E. (1964). Diffuse interstitial pulmonary fibrosis. *Q. Jl Med.* **23,** 71–103

McCallum, R. I. and Day, M. J. (1965). *In vivo* method of detecting antimony deposits in the lung by differential absorption of X-radiation. *Lancet* **2,** 882–883

McCallum, R. I. and Day, M. J., Underhill, J. and Aird, E. G. A. (1971). Measurement of antimony oxide dust in human lungs *in vivo* by X-ray spectrophotometry. In *Inhaled Particles 3,* edited by W. H. Walton, pp. 611–618. Woking; Unwin

MacKenzie, F. A. F. and Harries, P. G. (1970). Changing attitude to the diagnosis of asbestos disease. *Jl R. nav. med. Serv.* **56,** 116–123

Ministry of Health (1952). *Standardization of Terminology of Pulmonary Disease and Standardization of Technique of Chest Radiography.* London; HMSO

Morgan, W. K. C. and Reger, R. B. (1972). A comparison of two classifications of coal workers' pneumoconioses. *J. Am. med. Ass.* **220,** 1746

National Coal Board (1977). *Medical Service Annual Report 1975–76*

Ogilvie, C. M. (1970). Emphysema and coal worker's pneumoconiosis. *Br. med. J.* **3,** 769

Osborn, S. B. (1969). Personal communication

Otto, H. and Maron, R. (1959). Zur Histologie der Eisenablagerungen bei Porzeillinersilikosen. *Arch. Gewerbepath. Gewerbehyg.* **17,** 117–126

Pearson, N. G., Ashford, J. R., Morgan, D. C., Pasqual, R. S. H. and Rae, S. (1965). Effect of quality of chest radiographs on the categorization of coal worker's pneumoconiosis. *Br. J. ind. Med.* **22,** 81–92

Prosser, I. M. and Thurley, P. (1976). Septal lines in a case of asthma with eosinophilia. *Br. J. Radiol.* **49,** 176–177

Rappaport, I. (1936). The phenomena of shadow attenuation and summation in roentgenography of the lungs. *Am. J. Roentg.* **35,** 772–776

Rappaport, I. (1967). Overinflation of the lungs of coal miners. *Br. med. J.* **3,** 493–494

Reger, R. B., Petersen, M. R. and Morgan, W. K. C. (1974). Variation in the interpretation of radiographic change in pulmonary disease. *Lancet* **1,** 111–113

Reger, R. B., Smith, C. A., Kibelstis, J. A. and Morgan, W. K. C. (1972). The effect of film quality and other factors on roentgenographic categorization of coal workers' pneumoconioses. *Am. J. Roentgenol.* **115,** 462–472

Reid, L. and Millard, F. J. C. (1964). Correlation between radiological diagnosis and structural lung changes in emphysema. *Clin. Radiol.* **15,** 307–311

Rivers, D., Wise, M. E., King, E. J. and Nagelschmidt, G. (1960). Dust content, radiology, and pathology in simple pneumoconiosis of coal workers. *Br. J. Med.* **17,** 87–108

Rossiter, C. E. (1972). Relation between content and composition of coal worker's lungs and radiological appearances. *Br. J. ind. Med.* **29,** 31–44

Rossiter, C. E., Rivers, D., Bergman, I., Casswell, C. and Nagelschmidt, G. (1967). Dust content, radiology and pathology in simple pneumoconiosis of coal workers (Further Report). In *Inhaled Particles and Vapours, 2,* edited by C. N. Davies, pp. 419–434. London; Pergamon

Scadding, J. G. (1952). Chronic lung disease with diffuse nodular or reticular radiographic shadows. *Tubercle, Lond.* **33,** 352–355

Schröder, H., Magdeburg, W., Tewes, E. and Rockelsberg, I. (1969). Perfusion scintigraphy of the lungs in patients with silicosis and silicotuberculosis. *Germ. med. Mon.* **14,** 551–552

Siemsen, J. K., Grebe, S. F., Sargent, E. N. and Wentz, D., (1976). Gallium-67 scintigraphy of pulmonary diseases as a complement to radiography. *Radiology* **118,** 371–375

Simon, G. (1964). Radiology and emphysema. *Clin. Radiol.* **15,** 293–306

Simon, G. (1973). *Principles of Chest X-ray Diagnosis,* 3rd edition. London; Butterworths

Snider, G. L., Brody, J. S. and Doctor, L. (1962). Subclinical pulmonary emphysema. Incidence and anatomic patterns. *Am. Rev. resp. Dis.* **85,** 666–683

Spiers, F. W. (1946). Effective atomic number and energy absorption in tissues. *Br. J. Radiol.* **19,** 52–63

Thomas, R. G. and Sluis-Cremer, G. K. (1977). 200 kV xeroradiography in occupational exposure to silica and asbestos. *Br. J. ind. Med.* **34,** 281–290

Thurlbeck, W. M., Henderson, J. A., Fraser, R. G. and Bates, D. V. (1970). Chronic obstructive lung disease. A comparison between clinical roentgenologic, functional and morphologic criteria in chronic bronchitis, emphysema, asthma and bronchiectasis. *Medicine, Baltimore* **49,** 81–145

Trapnell, D. H. (1963). The peripheral lymphatics of the lung. *Br. J. Radiol.* **36,** 660–672

Trapnell, D. H. (1964). Septal lines in pneumoconiosis. *Br. J. Radiol.* **37,** 805–810

Trapnell, D. H. (1973). The differential diagnosis of linear shadows in chest radiographs. *Rad. clin. N. Am.* **11,** 77–92

Vix, V. A. (1974). Extrapleural costal fat. *Radiology* **112,** 563–565

Wise, M. E. and Oldham, P. O. (1963). Effect of radiograhic technique on readings of categories of simple pneumoconiosis. *Br. J. ind. Med.* **10,** 145–153

6 Inert Dusts

DEFINITION

Inert dusts are inorganic (mineral) dusts which, if insoluble, cause neither substantial proliferation of reticulin fibres nor give rise to collagenous fibrosis when retained in the lungs; and, if soluble, are not toxic locally or systemically. They are classed as 'inert dusts' or '*nuisance particulates*' by the ACGIH provided that they are free of toxic impurities and that their quartz content is less than 1 per cent.

IMPORTANCE OF INERT DUSTS AND FUMES

Their radiodensity ranges from high to low (*see Table 5.1*, p. 91). They may be inhaled in almost pure form or in association with fibrogenic dusts (usually free silica in the form of quartz) either as an intimate mixture produced simultaneously by one industrial process, or separately and at different times by different occupations. Dusts and fumes of low radiodensity give no evidence of their presence on a chest radiograph whereas those of high radiodensity cast small, round, well-defined and contrasted opacities throughout the lung fields and often cause pronounced opacity of hilar lymph nodes (due to their concentration in these sites) which may be misinterpreted as calcification.

It is, therefore, possible to consider inert dusts according to whether they are of high or low radiodensity and whether or not their presence is associated with that of a fibrotic pneumoconiosis (such as silicosis or asbestosis), in which case the lesions due to the inert dusts are morphologically distinct from the others. But inert dusts (most notably iron oxides) may modify the fibrogenic effect of quartz, and other forms of free silica, and cause 'mixed dust fibrosis' (*see* Chapter 7) which lacks the characteristic morphology of the silicotic nodule. As noted in Chapter 3, the presence of quartz in the lungs increases the retention and interstitial and lymphatic penetration of inert dusts, but reduces their elimination by the airways. If low radiodensity dusts are contaminated by quartz as an accessory mineral of parent rock both types of dust may be inhaled when such rocks are mined, quarried, crushed or used in industrial processes. It is necessary to be aware of this in order that an inert dust is not, on the one hand, wrongly considered to be fibrogenic or that, on the other, the presence of a free silica risk does not go unsuspected.

DUSTS OF HIGH RADIODENSITY BENIGN PNEUMOCONIOSIS

Pneumoconiosis caused by inert dusts has been referred to as 'benign' which is, perhaps, unfortunate as it implies that other forms of pneumoconiosis are necessarily 'malignant'. In order to produce radio-opacities, substances with lower atomic numbers will require to be present in the lungs in greater amount than those with higher atomic numbers. Hence, it is probable that greater concentration or duration of exposure of the former will be necessary for this to occur.

Siderosis is discussed first because it is the most common of these pneumoconioses; the others are less common if not rare.

IRON (ATOMIC NUMBER, 26): SIDEROSIS (σίδηρος, IRON)

Sources of exposure

Dust or fume of metallic iron and iron oxide may be encountered in the following processes, although their concentrations in many industries are limited by dust control measures.

(1) *Iron and steel rolling mills* in which metal strips are subjected to much agitation with the consequent production of rust and iron scale dust.
(2) *Steel grinding* produces metallic dust.

(3) *Electric arc and oxyacetylene welding* The high temperature of these types of welding when applied to iron gives rise to iron oxide fume and other fumes and gases. The concentration of fumes in the breathing zone is often high if welders work in confined and ill-ventilated places such as tanks, boilers, and the holds of ships. Siderosis of arc welders was first described by Doig and McLaughlin (1936).

Welding methods and their possible hazards are discussed in more detail in Chapter 13.

(4) *Polishing of silver and steel with iron oxide powder* The powder is usually an especially pure form of ferric oxide in a finely divided state and is often referred to as 'rouge' or 'crocus'. Polishing is done by means of power-operated buffing wheels of wool or cotton. Silver polishing is also likely to produce minute particles of metallic silver.

Ferric oxide is further used to polish glass, stone and cutlery.

(5) *Fettling (that is, scouring), chipping and dressing castings in iron foundries* Until recently this process was a common source of quartz as well as iron dust from attrition of burnt-on moulding sands adhering to the castings (*see* Chapter 7) and, therefore, liable to cause 'mixed dust fibrosis' or typical silicosis. Nevertheless, siderosis may occur alone when it may be wrongly diagnosed as silicosis.

A survey in a Sheffield steel foundry between 1955 and 1960 revealed that the average prevalence of siderosis among welders and burners in the fettling and grinding shops was 17.6 per cent (Gregory, 1970).

(6) *Boiler scaling* involves the cleaning of fireboxes, flues and water-tubes in enclosed spaces in the boilers of ships, factories, power stations and the like. A high concentration of dust is produced which contains iron and carbon, and, in coal-fired—but not oil-fired—boilers, silicates and small quantities of quartz derived from the coal. Although siderosis alone may be produced, mixed dust fibrosis may also occur.

(7) *Mining and crushing iron ores* The important ores are magnetite, hematite and limonite.

Magnetite occurs in several geological environments and ores of the mineral are frequently associated with quartz-bearing rock and contain quartz gangue (as in Northern Sweden, where the richest deposits are found). It is also found in beach sands. Therefore, quartz may sometimes be a substantial contaminant of the ore resulting in mixed dust fibrosis or silicosis in addition to siderosis in miners and crusher operators; but, again, siderosis may be observed alone.

Hematite, known also as 'specularite' and 'kidney ore', is mined chiefly in Cumberland and, until recently, in the Furness district of Lancashire where it occurs in limestone beds; but some deposits are associated with red ferruginous sandstone and are, therefore, liable to contamination by quartz. One of the largest sources in the world, near Lake Superior in Canada, is also partly contaminated by free silica because it contains interbedded layers of chert, but quartz is virtually absent from deposits at Bilbao and on the Quebec–Labrador border.

Limonite, including 'bog iron ore', is, for practical purposes, free from contaminating free silica.

It will be seen, therefore, that the likelihood of siderosis occurring alone, or accompanied by pure silicosis or 'mixed dust fibrosis' will depend to a large extent upon the geographical origin of the ore or the site from which it comes in any one deposit. Dust is produced during mining, loading, crushing and milling of the ores.

Hematite and limonite are used as pigments in paint manufacture and, together with magnetite, are added in finely divided form to certain fertilizers. It is possible, therefore, for workers in those industries to be exposed to iron oxide dusts.

(8) *Mining, milling and mixing emery and its use as an abrasive* Emery is an intimate mixture of hematite, magnetite and *corundum* (aluminium oxide, Al_2O_3) which, next to diamond, is the hardest natural mineral known. At one time emery came mainly from the Grecian Island of Naxos but today Turkey is the largest producer, and smaller quantities come from the USA. It is found most commonly in pockets or lenses in crystalline limestone, gneisses and schists, or as a deposit derived from these rocks by weathering. It contains insignificant quantities of quartz, and its abrasive quality is due mainly to the aluminium oxide present.

Because emery is apt to contain variable amounts of impurities (such as plagioclase feldspar) and a constant composition cannot, therefore, be relied upon, it has been very largely replaced by artificial abrasives—principally Carborundum and synthetic corundum (*see* pp. 130, 455). On account of its particular hardness, purity and resistance to heat, Naxos emery was used for grindstones, but Turkish emery, which is softer, is still employed in the making of coated abrasives such as emery cloths and papers for hand use, and buffing wheels and mops; and also in abrasive pastes and as a non-slip, wear-resisting component of concrete floors and road surfaces, and for polishing rice. High concentrations of emery dust have been, and occasionally still are, produced during the manufacture of most of these materials and the use of the different abrasive preparations for various polishing procedures (Bech, Kipling and Zundel, 1965; Foá, 1967).

Pneumoconiosis in emery workers, therefore, will almost certainly be siderosis unless there has also been exposure to some other dust hazard (for example, the coal-mining, pottery or asbestos industries).

(9) *Mining, pulverizing and mixing natural mineral pigments* Hematite and limonite have already been referred to as a source of pigments but others are the ferruginous earths—ochre, sienna and umber clays—which consist of iron and aluminium oxides with a variable amount of siliceous impurity. These clays are mined in the USA, the Persian Gulf, Turkey, Cyprus, France, Italy and Andalusia but pulverizing and mixing are usually done by the firm which imports them. Synthetic iron pigments prepared from iron oxides, however, are now much more important than the natural products (*see* p. 43).

Siderosis may occur alone in workers who pulverize and mix natural pigments which, at this stage, have been purified by screening, washing, and drying; and also in those engaged in some stages of the manufacture of synthetic pigments and in their use. But disease identical to the 'mixed dust fibrosis' of hematite miners (*see* p. 159) may be found among miners and in operatives involved in crushing and coarse-screening the ore when the quartz content of the clays or other parent rocks is substantial as is the case in Italy where it varies from 2 to 35 per cent (Champeix and Moreau, 1958), and in the Apt area of

France where it is as high as 50 per cent (Roche, Picard and Vernhes, 1958).

Pathology

The features of siderosis only are considered here. But it must be stressed that some workers exposed to metallic iron dust or iron oxide fume (such as welders, iron foundry men, boiler scalers and miners and millers of iron ores) may also have had significant exposure to other dusts such as quartz or asbestos so that siderosis may be complicated by the presence of 'mixed dust fibrosis' (*see* Chapter 7) or asbestosis.

Iron oxide dust inhaled by experimental animals is non-fibrogenic (Harding, Grant and Davies, 1947; Vorwald *et al.*, 1950), and natural emery introduced into the lungs or peritoneum of rats causes neither reticulin proliferation nor collagenous fibrosis (Mellissonos, Collet and Daniel-Moussard, 1966). It also exerts an inhibitory effect upon quartz fibrogenesis, which is referred to in Chapter 7, p. 159.

Macroscopic appearances

The pulmonary pleura is marbled a rust-brown colour but, in the case of hematite, the colour may be a deep brick-red. This is due to the deposition of iron oxide in the pleural lymphatics similar to the black pigmentation seen in the pleura of coal miners.

The cut surface of the lungs reveals grey to rust-brown coloured macules (*macula,* a stain or mark) from 1 to 4 mm in diameter which are impalpable and do not stand up from the surface in contrast to silicotic nodules. They are evenly distributed but may be difficult to distinguish as individual lesions if the lungs are generally dust stained. The appearance of the lungs and lesions where hematite is involved is particularly striking due to the brick-red coloration. Some hematite lungs may also exhibit discrete nodular fibrosis or massive fibrosis when quartz is associated with the iron oxide, but this is described in Chapter 7. Typical silicotic lesions are readily distinguishable by the naked eye.

Microscopic appearances

The fundamental lesion consists of a perivascular and peribronchiolar aggregation of dark pigmented iron oxide particles which are present both in macrophages and extracellularly in alveolar spaces and walls where they are mostly perivascular. Slight reticulin proliferation may be present but there is no collagenous fibrosis; and intra- and extracellular collections are also seen sub-pleurally and infiltrating interlobular septa (*Figure 6.1*). These particles, unlike the protein-bound endogenous iron haemosiderin are not stained, and, therefore, not identified, by Perl's Prussian Blue reaction. However, because haemosiderin, together with ferritin, is commonly associated with iron oxide deposition in the lungs a positive reaction may occur. But ferritin—which may be ingested by macrophages containing iron oxide in similar fashion to those containing carbon and quartz (*see* Chapter 4, p. 71)—must be separated from the protein apoferritin by a reducing agent, such as hydrosulphite, before it will take the stain. But it is possible, apparently, to distinguish between inorganic iron and ferritin and haemosiderin in human lungs by Mössbauer spectroscopy (Guest, 1976).

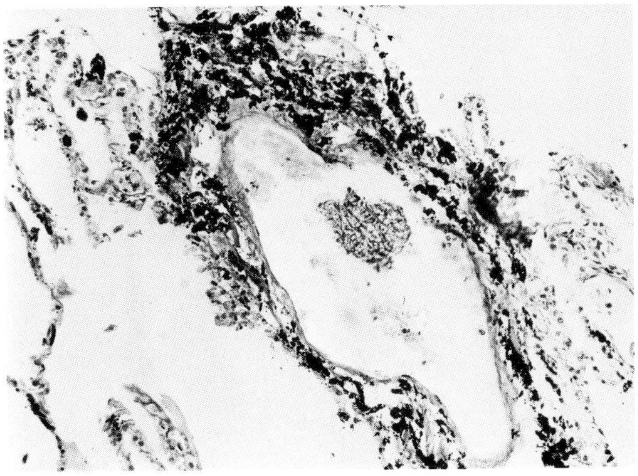

Figure 6.1 Siderosis. There is a perivascular 'cuff' of iron particles and dust-laden macrophages but no fibrosis. The alveolar walls and spaces are normal. (Original magnification × 225 reproduced at half-scale; H and E stain)

If fibrotic lesions are seen they are usually due to tuberculosis or to the additional presence of crystalline silica (Mosinger *et al.*, 1968).

Metallic silver, as well as iron, is present in the lungs of silver polishers. It is taken up as a vital stain by the elastic tissue, which appears grey-black in colour, in the walls and airways of arteries, and it is not fibrogenic. This is known as *argyro-siderosis* (Barrie and Harding, 1947). The silver (atomic number 47) contributes significantly to the effective atomic number of the mixture and, therefore, to the density and summation of opacities on the radiograph.

It has been suggested that the retention of iron dust may cause emphysema but there is no evidence to support this in man. In rabbits no major changes in the lysosomal enzymes of lung macrophages have been found following the inhalation of an iron oxide aerosol; that is, endogenous lytic enzymes capable of attacking alveolar walls were absent (Grant, Sorokin and Brain, 1976). The question of a possible relationship between iron oxides and bronchial carcinoma is referred to later.

Symptoms and physical signs

Apart from the production of reddish coloured sputum which sometimes follows exposure to these dusts, there are no symptoms or abnormal physical signs caused by siderosis, and if any are present they are due to some other cause.

Lung function

There is no impairment of any parameter of lung function (Fogh, Frost and Georg, 1969; Morgan and Kerr, 1963; Kleinfeld *et al.*, 1969; Teculescu and Albu, 1973) and, although a greater prevalence of airways obstruction has been reported among electric arc welders compared with non-welders (Hunnicutt, Cracovaner and Myles, 1964), this was related mainly to cigarette smoking. Impaired lung function in a subject with lone siderosis is due either to the effects of cigarette smoking or to non-industrial lung disease, or a combination of both.

Radiographic appearances

The absorptive capacity of iron for X-rays is considerably higher than that of non-iron lung constituents and of silicate minerals or coal deposits in the lungs; in fact, whereas the mass absorption coefficient for silicate minerals is three to five times greater than carbon, that of iron is 40 times greater (Safety in Mines Research, 1963).

The standard chest radiograph shows a variable, usually large, number of small opacities varying from 0.5 mm to about 2 mm in diameter; of striking density and associated with fewer fine, rather less dense, linear opacities (*Figure 6.2*). Large, confluent opacities do not occur. In some cases Kerley's B lines caused by the accumulation of iron in interlobular septa are prominent. The hilar lymph nodes may appear unusually radio-opaque due to their concentrated iron content, but they are not enlarged.

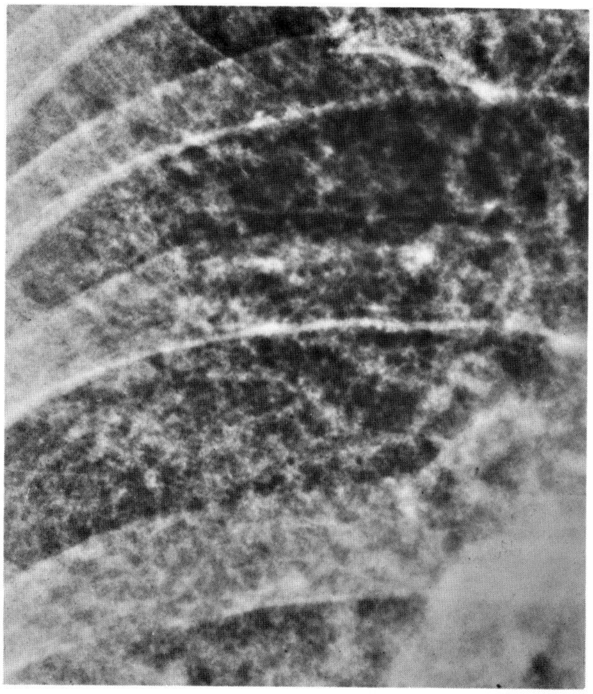

Figure 6.2 Siderosis in an emery worker. Numerous small fairly dense opacities evenly scattered throughout the lung fields. Category 3p. (Natural size)

Prolonged exposure to iron dust or fume is usually required to give these radiographic appearances, but in the event of exposure to high dust concentration they have been observed after as short a period as three years (Kleinfeld *et al.*, 1969).

Deposition of iron-containing (ferrimagnetic) dust or fume in the lungs can apparently be identified by magnetopneumography before it is detectable radiographically (*see* Appendix).

Diagnosis

This rests upon a history of work in processes known to give rise to iron dust or fume coupled with the radiographic appearances. Siderosis can be easily overlooked if the details of the work are not known as, for example, when it occurs in woodworkers who have used emery abrasives. Biopsy of lung tissue is rarely justifiable.

It is to be borne in mind that welders may have been exposed intermittently to free silica dust if, for example, they worked in the neighbourhood of fettling or sand-blasting operations in foundries (*see* Chapter 7), or to asbestos dust when working in the vicinity of insulation workers lagging boilers, pipes or other apparatus. Hence, nodular silicosis mixed dust fibrosis or asbestosis may be present together with siderosis in welders.

Differential diagnosis

Other inert dusts of high radiodensity (antimony, tin and barium, for example) may produce almost identical appearances. As a rule the size, density and uniform distribution throughout the lung fields of the opacities of siderosis distinguish them from those of nodular silicosis and coal pneumoconiosis which are larger, less dense, usually less well defined and commonly predominant in the upper and middle zones of the lung fields. Occasionally, tiny 'pin-head' opacities are observed in the radiographs of coal miners (*see* Chapter 8) but their density is generally less than those of siderosis.

Miliary tuberculosis is readily distinguishable because of the lack of industrial exposure, the illness of the patient and the fact that the opacities tend to be less dense, less well defined and often most profuse in the mid-zones of the lung fields.

Some cases of idiopathic sarcoidosis present a similar appearance but the lack of an industrial history, evidence of enlarged hilar lymph nodes and other clinical and investigatory features of this disorder readily establish the diagnosis. When, however, there is a history of relevant industrial exposure the differentiation may occasionally be sufficiently difficult to indicate lung biopsy, but this should rarely be necessary if the discipline of differential diagnosis is properly followed.

Cryptogenic pulmonary haemosiderosis, which is commoner in men than women and in which opacities similar to those of siderosis follow repeated capillary haemorrhages (Wynn-Williams and Young, 1956; Karlish, 1962), is distinguished by recurrent haemoptysis, hypochromic anaemia and, in some cases, finger clubbing and enlargement of liver and spleen. Haemosiderosis due to mitral stenosis is readily identified in most cases if the presence of the valve disease is recognized and, though differentiation is impossible in the occasional case of a worker with mitral stenosis who has been exposed to iron oxide dusts or fumes, this is of no practical importance.

Prognosis

After the worker leaves exposure, the iron dust is slowly eliminated from the lungs over a period of years. This is reflected in the partial or complete disappearance of radiographic opacities (Doig and McLaughlin, 1948); but the greater the quantity of dust the longer the period for its elimination.

The benign nature of siderosis has been clearly demonstrated in arc welders (Doig and McLaughlin, 1936; Morgan and Kerr, 1963).

Prevention

This depends upon effective suppression of dust or fume, and exhaust ventilation methods. In many of the processes already listed concentrations have been either eliminated or greatly reduced in recent years. Nevertheless, persons who have inhaled large quantities of iron dusts in the past will continue to have abnormal chest radiographs for many years or permanently.

Bronchial carcinoma and iron-dust inhalation

It has been suggested that inhaled iron dust may act as a carcinogen mainly on the grounds that a higher incidence of bronchial carcinoma has been calculated to be present in hematite-miners than in the general population (Faulds and Stewart, 1956), but the methods of reaching this conclusion were criticized by Doll (1959). However, other substances (such as tars) with known carcinogenic potential were present in some of the work processes and the smoking habits of the workers were not analysed. Nevertheless, recent work has confirmed that West Cumberland iron-ore miners have a lung cancer mortality about 70 per cent higher than 'normal' (Boyd *et al.*, 1970) and there is evidence of a similar lung cancer risk among iron-ore miners in Lorraine, France (Roussel *et al.*, 1964). This might seem to increase the suspicion that iron oxides are lung carcinogens. However, it has been shown that radon concentrations are unusually high in the Cumberland hematite mines (Duggan *et al.*, 1970) and may be the carcinogenic agency, although the identity of this is still regarded as obscure by Boyd *et al.* (1970) (*see* Chapter 14).

In short, there is no convincing evidence to incriminate exogenous iron as a pulmonary carcinogen.

TIN (ATOMIC NUMBER, 50): STANNOSIS (STANNUM, TIN)

Because the atomic number of tin is almost double that of iron its radiodensity is substantially greater.

Stannosis was first recognized in Germany during the Second World War. Shortly afterwards it was reported in Czechoslovakia (Barták and Tomečka, 1949), in the USA (Pendergrass and Pryde, 1948; Cutter *et al.*, 1949; Dundon and Hughes, 1950) and, in particular detail, in the UK (Robertson and Whittaker, 1955; Robertson *et al.*, 1961). It is much less common than siderosis because the possibilities of industrial exposure are limited. By 1959 over 150 cases were recorded in the world literature (Barnes and Stoner, 1959).

Origins of tin ore

The chief tin ore is *cassiterite*, tin oxide, from which tin must be recovered by smelting. The main tin fields of the world are in Malaysia, the UK, Thailand, Indonesia, Bolivia, Nigeria and Australia. The metalliferous region of South West England is the only indigenous source in the UK and production here has increased greatly in recent years after a long period of decline. In spite of this the UK is one of the world's largest importers and consumers of tin in various forms after the USA which possesses no workable tin deposits.

The ore is found only in association with granitic rocks which contain substantial quantities of quartz.

Sources of exposure and uses

Because the amount of tin in the crude ore is extremely small, mining procedures (drilling and loading of ore), crushing and screening are unlikely to cause stannosis, but the highly siliceous dust produced is a source of silicosis. Concentrates of cassiterite received by the smelters are largely freed of associated rock and the content of quartz, therefore, almost eliminated.

Processes likely to produce tin dust or fume are as follows: the emptying of bags of crude ore into skips; milling and grinding of ore (Oyanguren *et al.*, 1957); shovelling up of spilt ore; tipping of crushed ore into the calcination furnace; charging smelting furnaces with calcined ore (molten tin issuing from these furnaces gives off tin oxide fume) (Spencer and Wycoff, 1954); raking out of refinery furnaces which contain a high percentage of tin oxide and melting down tin scrap to recover tin oxide (Dundon and Hughes, 1950). Solid impurities are removed by heating the impure tin just above melting point. It is then drained off or separated by filtration; little tin oxide fume is likely to be evolved.

Tin dust produced by grinding, briquet making, smelting and casting contains 58 to 65 per cent tin and only 0.2 to 1 per cent quartz (Oyanguren *et al.*, 1957). High concentration of tin dust and fume are also produced by hearth tinning where the articles to be plated are dipped by hand into molten tin (Cole *et al.*, 1964). Tin plating is now done mainly by electrodeposition methods.

The greatest production of primary refined tin in 1972 was by West Malaysia and then in order, the UK, Thailand, Indonesia, Nigeria, Bolivia, Australia, Spain and the USA (Slater, 1974).

The uses of tin are extensive, the two most important being in tinplating and solders, but also in bronzes, bearing metals, various alloys (such as tin-lead, known as 'Babbitt', and aluminium tin), inorganic tin compounds (employed, for example, in ceramic glazes, vitreous enamels and tooth pastes) and organotins (that is, tin-based organic compounds) which are used in the manufacture of certain polyvinyl chloride articles in fungicides, pesticides, antifouling paints and paper manufacture (Slater, 1974). Wafers of metallic tin are reacted with chlorine to produce stannic chloride (used in electroplating salts) which is further processed into various organotins such as tributyl and dioctyl tin. Opportunity for exposure to metallic tin dust or oxide fume in this process is, however, negligible. Occasional exposure to the irritant vapours of stannic chloride and hydrochloric acid may occur during plant maintenance but simple precautions render this of minor order (Fysh, 1977). In the float glass process (*see* p. 137) plate glass is floated in molten tin in an enclosed bath, but there is no exposure to tin fume or dust at any stage (Cameron, 1970).

Pathology

Pneumoconiosis in tin-miners occurs in the form of nodular silicosis; stannosis is not seen.

Macroscopic appearances

In stannosis, naked-eye inspection of the cut surface of the lungs reveals numerous tiny (1 to 3 mm), grey-black dust macules, soft to the touch and not raised above the cut surface of the lung.

Microscopic appearances

Macrophages containing tin oxide dust particles are present in alveolar walls and spaces, perivascular lymphatics, and interlobular septa. The macules, like those of siderosis, consist of dense perivascular and peribronchiolar aggregations of dust-laden macrophages (*see Figure 6.1*). By light microscopy the intracellular particles are indistinguishable from carbon but they remain after micro-incineration (Robertson *et al.*, 1961) whereas carbon disappears; X-ray diffraction gives definitive identification. The tetragonal crystals of tin oxide exhibit strong birefringence but, as seen by the 'medical' microscope, this has no diagnostic significance (*see* Appendix) and it is important that it should not be taken to imply the presence of crystals of quartz which, in any case, is poorly birefringent. There is no excess of reticulin or collagen fibres even after 50 years' exposure to tin oxide (Robertson *et al.*, 1961).

The quartz content of the lungs is negligible and has been estimated as substantially less than 0.2 g/lung (Robertson *et al.*, 1961) and in the same cases the amount of tin was estimated as ranging from 0.5 to 3.3 g/lung—the former value related to a man with an 11-year exposure and the latter, one with 50 years. Dust particles, single or aggregated, recovered from the lungs are from 0.1 to 0.5 μm in diameter and closely resemble furnace fume particles in size and appearance (Robertson *et al.*, 1961).

The hilar lymph nodes appear black but are not fibrotic.

Although small quantities of tin oxide have been found in the spleen and liver of a man who had stannosis (Barták and Tomečka, 1949) there is no evidence that it has any systemic toxic effect.

Tin oxide does not cause fibrosis in the lungs (Robertson, 1960; Fischer and Zinnerman, 1969), liver or spleen (Fischer and Zinnerman, 1969) of experimental animals.

Symptoms and physical signs

There are no symptoms or abnormal physical signs due to the inhalation and retention of tin oxide dust.

Lung function

Lung function is unaffected (Robertson, 1960) and if there is any associated abnormality it is due to some other cause.

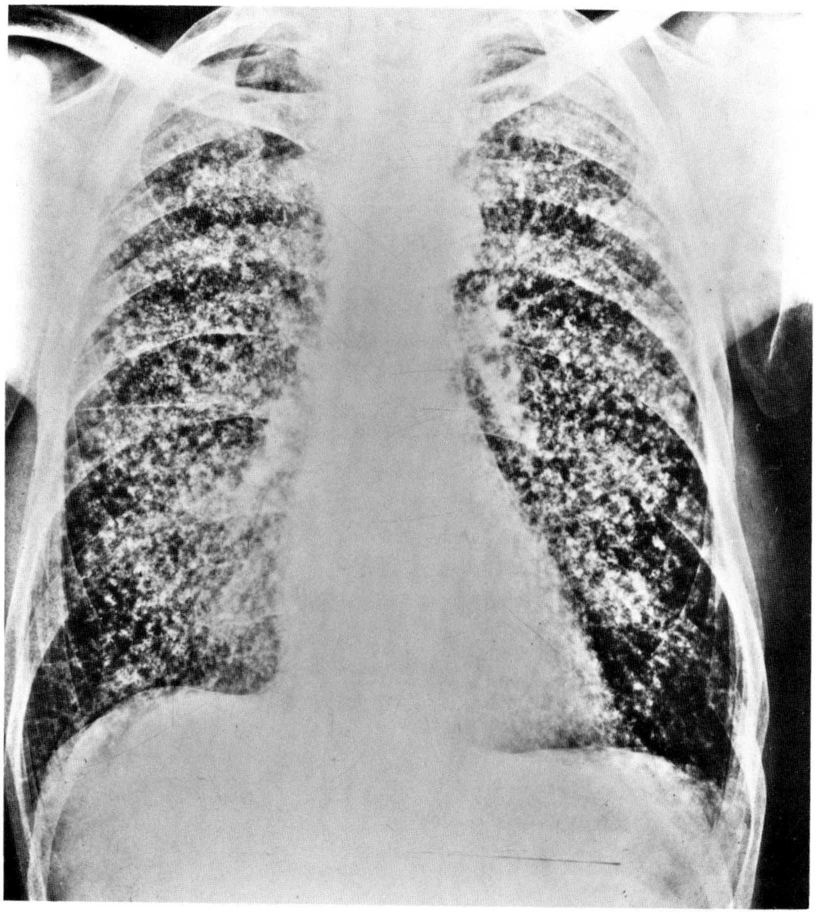

Figure 6.3 Stannosis in a furnace charger in a tin smelting works for 42 years. Note the density of the pulmonary and hilar node opacities. The Kerley-type B lines in the right costophrenic angle and sharp definition of the lesser fissure are also due to tin deposition

Radiographic appearances

When exposure to tin oxide dust has been heavy or prolonged numerous small, very dense opacities are scattered evenly throughout the lung fields; they may be somewhat larger (2 to 4 mm diameter) and more 'fluffy' or irregular in outline than those of siderosis—possibly due to the combined effect of superimposition and their greater radiodensity (*Figure 6.3*). Kerley's B lines are often clearly defined, and thin dense linear opacities may be seen in the upper lung zones. With lesser degrees of exposure, opacities are fewer, less dense and somewhat larger (Robertson, 1960).

Large confluent opacities do not occur and the hilar shadows, although unduly radio-opaque, are of normal size.

Diagnosis

The occupational history, lack of symptoms and physical signs and the striking density of the opacities on the radiograph are diagnostic. In the absence of a history and when opacities are fairly few they might be mistaken for silicosis, possibly for baritosis or for other causes of discrete bilateral lung lesions already referred to in *Table 5.2*, p. 97.

Prognosis

Stannosis has no known effect upon health or life span. It is possible, if sufficient time were to elapse after last exposure to the dust, that the opacities would gradually disappear but this has not been reported.

Prevention

This depends upon efficient dust suppression, exhaust ventilation and good factory 'housekeeping'.

BARIUM (ATOMIC NUMBER, 56): BARITOSIS

The most important compound is *barytes* ($BaSO_4$) known as *barite* in the USA. *Witherite* ($BaCO_3$) is less important.

Although baritosis ('barium lung') was first described by Fiori (1926) in Italy the subject of his report also appears to have had silicosis. One of the first accounts of pure baritosis was given by Arrigoni (1933), and reports from other countries followed over the years. A survey of a barium plant (related to duration of exposure) revealed the presence of baritosis in 48 per cent of 118 workers (Lévi-Vallensi *et al.*, 1966).

Barytes is widely distributed throughout the world together with other minerals and is often associated with igneous, sedimentary and metamorphic rocks. Therefore, such minerals as fluorite, calcite, limestone, witherite, quartz and chert may be intermixed according to the type of deposit in which the barytes is found. In the UK deposits are almost wholly of hydrothermal origin and may thus contain varying amounts of quartz derived from the hydrothermal fluids and not from the surrounding rocks in which they lie. It is evident then that barytes from some areas will contain variable and often significant quantities of free silica.

In 1969 the world's greatest producer of barytes was the USA (mainly from Nevada, Missouri, Arkansas and Georgia), followed in magnitude by Federal Germany, the USSR, Greece, Mexico, the Irish Republic and Canada. It is of particular interest that production by the Irish Republic (County Sligo) has increased almost 40-fold since 1961. The total output by the UK (chiefly as barytes recovered as a by-product of fluorspar production in Derbyshire) is now very small (Collins, 1972).

Until recently, the UK was the sole world supplier of *witherite* which was mined in Northumberland and Durham, but production ceased in 1969.

Sources of exposure and uses

During mining of the crude ore high concentrations of dust may be produced and, as indicated, in some areas this may contain either quartz in hydrothermal deposits or chert from neighbouring rocks. When mining is done by the opencast method the concentration of airborne dust is greatly reduced.

Barytes is supplied to various industries in crude form, as flotation concentrates from which contaminants have been removed, or in ground and purified form. With the exception of the crude form it is washed, leached out and then crushed or ground in the wet state. The chance of dust inhalation in these circumstances, therefore, is low, but during the drying and bagging of ground barytes, high concentrations of dust may be produced.

Ground barytes is used today chiefly as a weighting agent in muds circulated in the rotary drilling of oil and gas wells, and also as a filler, extender and weighting agent in heavy printing papers, paints, textiles, playing cards, clutch facings, brake linings, soap, linoleum, rubber and plastics. It was used in gramophone records until about 1948 when microgroove records were introduced. A large quantity of the world's barytes is employed in glass manufacture as a flux and to add brilliance, and, because it absorbs γ-radiation efficiently, in aggregates for special concrete ('atomic concrete') and bricks used for radioactivity shields. A hard variety of barytes is used in 'sand blasting' (Collins, 1972).

Barytes is almost the only source of barium used in the manufacture of numerous barium chemicals which, in the UK, is largely concentrated at Widnes in Lancashire. Both chemically precipitated barium sulphate, *blanc fixe,* (employed as an extender in high opacity white pigments, in 'fining' molten glass and coating photographic papers) and barium sulphate *BP* have a fine particle size and so may readily become airborne. Barium carbonate is employed in the UK in the production of glass for television sets (as a barrier to X-rays) and glass of high refractive index, in certain ceramic processes, in some welding rod coatings, and with titanium dioxide to yield barium titanate, the valuable piezo-electric properties of which are exploited in electronic ceramics, digital computers and sonar apparatus. Other barium salts also find a variety of uses: for example, in pyrotechnics, explosives and beet sugar refining.

Lithopone was widely used as a pigment and filler until recent years. It is made by roasting crude, 'silica free' barytes with carbon in a rotary kiln, leaching out the product and adding zinc sulphide and sulphate; the precipitate is washed, filtered dried and again calcined. At some stages of this process a mixture of barytes and carbon dusts may be present; coal was often used in the past as a source of carbon, and grinding this was a dusty process. Thus, there was the possibility of coal or carbon pneumoconiosis co-existing with baritosis. The production of lithopone in Lancashire ceased in 1969. It was used extensively in paints for many years but latterly has largely been replaced by titanium dioxide (*see* p. 127) which has superior properties; however, it is still the main pigment in oil bound distempers and some emulsion paints.

The likelihood of exposure to barium dust has evidently varied greatly according to the processes involved but, since barium compounds have such a wide application, mild degrees of baritosis may be more common than is realized. In general, quartz is absent from barytes used in industry but, if present, the amount is minute.

Pathology

Although this section is concerned with baritosis, it should be noted that if exposure has occurred to both barytes and 'free silica' dusts (as may be the case in some barytes mines) then both baritosis and silicosis may be present. But there is no evidence that the pathogenesis of the silicotic lesions is modified by barytes.

Macroscopic appearances

Many discrete grey macules are present in the pulmonary pleura and the cut surface of the lungs shows numerous discrete, impalpable macules which resemble those of stannosis. There are no nodules, no confluent massing and no evidence of fibrosis. Hilar lymph nodes are not enlarged.

Microscopic appearances

The appearances of the lesions are similar to those of stannosis and siderosis. The initial reaction is an insignificant mobilization of polymorphonuclear leucocytes but a brisk macrophage response together with a little intra-alveolar exudate. There is little increase of reticulin and no fibrosis. The lack of fibrotic reaction is confirmed in experimental animals (Huston, Wallach and Cunningham, 1952). Following accidental inhalation of barium meal, barium-containing macrophages fill the alveoli and small airways and some are present in alveolar walls.

It is claimed that barium can be identified by a special staining technique (Waterhouse, 1951) in which lung tissue is fixed with carefully neutralized 10 per cent formalin in 70 per cent alcohol and immersed in a 1 or 2 per cent solution of sodium rhodizonate in distilled water when an intense red colour is produced by barium compounds. As calcium reacts with this reagent under alkaline, but not neutral, conditions the test may not always be successful. If positive identification is important, X-ray diffraction or spectrographic methods are advisable. Barytes particles are moderately birefringent.

Symptoms and signs

Baritosis is symptomless and causes no abnormal physical signs. There are no systemic toxic effects due to absorption of barytes and most barium compounds from the lungs as they are poorly soluble and chemically inert.

Lung function

Impairment of lung function has not been recorded nor is it to be expected.

Radiographic appearances

The usual appearances consist of particularly dense, discrete small opacities sometimes of star-like configuration and usually about 2 to 4 mm diameter which are distributed fairly evenly throughout the lung fields, and may develop after only a few months' exposure to the dust (Pancheri, 1950). When the amount of retained barium dust is large (as may be the case after long periods of exposure) the opacities may be bigger and, indeed, large, irregular and densely opaque areas which may give an impression of confluent lesions may be seen. This is due to the superimposition effect of very many highly radiodense deposits. But lack of correlation between duration of exposure and intensity of radiographic abnormality is occasionally encountered and is not readily explicable (Doig, 1976). Kerley's B lines are often prominent and the hilar lymph nodes may be remarkably opaque, though not enlarged (*Figures 6.4a* and *6.5*). However, in the earlier stages of baritosis the opacities may be indistinguishable from those of nodular silicosis or coal pneumoconiosis (Doig, 1976).

As in the case of siderosis gradual clearing of the opacities occurs after industrial exposure has ceased, due to physiological elimination of the dust (Doig, 1976; Lévi-Valensi *et al.*, 1966; Wende, 1956) (*Figure 6.4*).

Diagnosis

A detailed work history presents the necessary clue and the density of the opacities should suggest the possibility of baritosis. But if exposure to the dust has been slight, or if opacities are few, confusion with other causes of discrete opacities may well occur.

It is important to remember that pneumoconiosis in barytes-miners is likely to be predominantly silicosis. For example, in the case of one such miner many characteristic silicotic nodules were found and analysis of the lung ash revealed about 15 per cent SiO_2 by weight but only 4 per cent $BaSO_4$.

Baritosis is rare and many men in whom it is first identified are now elderly and have left the responsible industry years previously. But sporadic new cases can be expected from some among the plethora of processes in which barium compounds are used. This means that consideration of baritosis may occasionally be important in differential diagnosis.

Prognosis

The presence of barytes or witherite in the lungs is not known to have any adverse effect upon health or life expectancy. Gradual clearance of opacities can be expected over the years after the worker has left exposure.

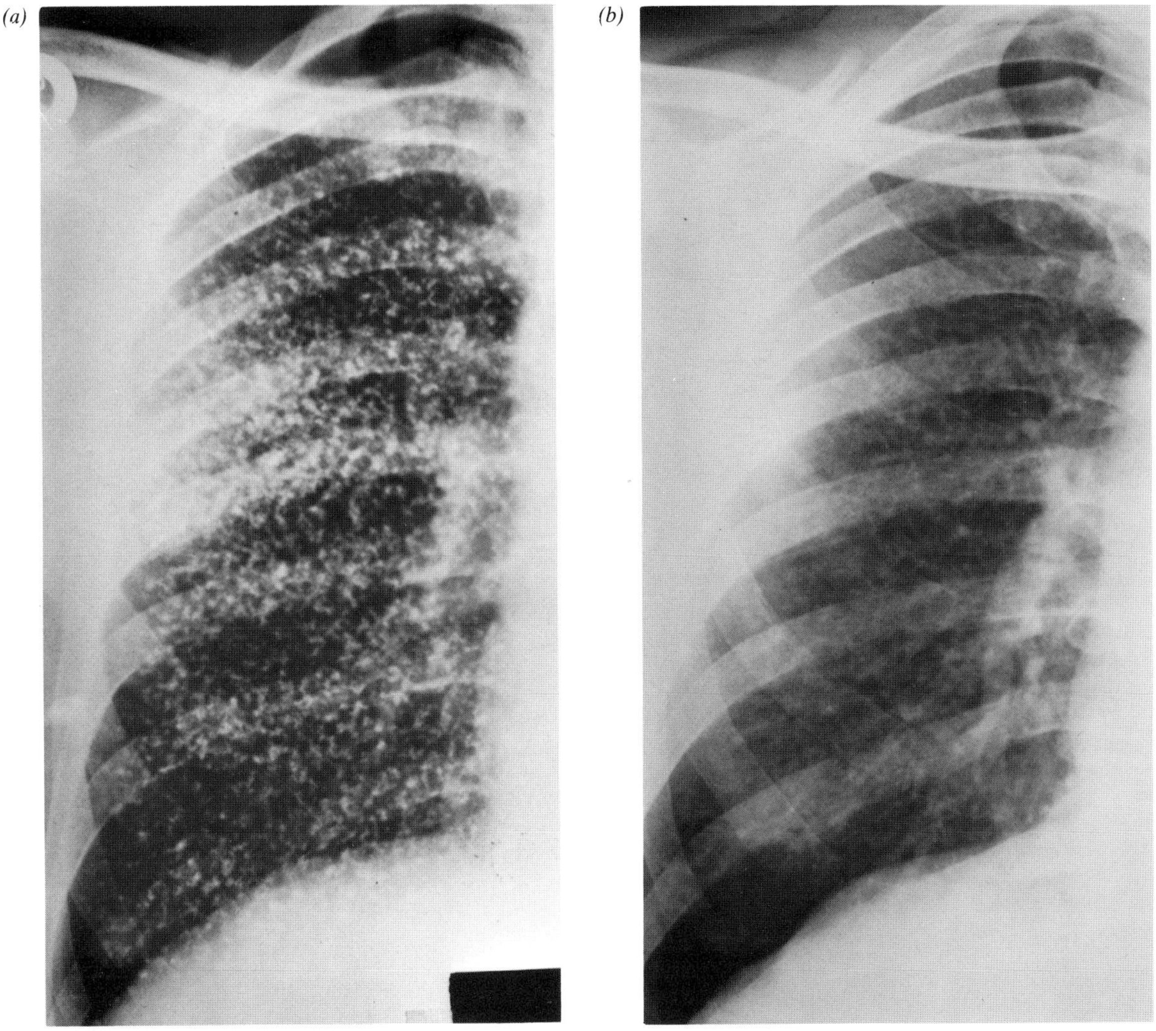

Figure 6.4 Very dense, discrete opacities in a miller and grinder of barytes for 15 years. These have steadily regressed in number and density over 18 years from 1961 due to cessation of exposure and normal pulmonary clearance. (a) 1961. (b) 1979. Ventilatory function tests normal throughout. (Films (a) and (b) by courtesy of Dr A.T. Doig and the Editors of Thorax.*) In most cases of baritosis the opacities are less striking than this*

ANTIMONY (ATOMIC NUMBER, 51)

Antimony occurs in metamorphic deposits in quartz veins of deep-seated origin which lie in or near intrusive rocks such as the granites and as deposits in limestone and shales. It is mined in South Africa, China, Bolivia, Algeria, Mexico and parts of Europe.

It is imported into other countries as *stibnite* (Sb_2S_3) ore or powder. Antimony metal, trioxide, pentoxide, trisulphate and pentasulphide are produced from the ore.

Sources of exposure and uses

Exposure to antimony dust may occur during mining, crushing the ore, and cleaning of extraction chambers which collect the oxide dust from roasting chambers (Renes, 1953). Exposure to fumes may occur among antimony alloy workers and Linotype setters, but is most important among men who smelt and refine the ore.

In the UK antimony is smelted near Newcastle-upon-Tyne in the largest smelting plant in Europe. The chief centres in the USA are in Pennsylvania and Texas (Cooper *et al.*, 1968). The metal and white antimony trioxide are produced.

Antimony dust apparently remains suspended in the air longer than might be expected of a heavy metal (Fairhall and Hyslop, 1947) which suggests that the particle size is small; and the fine white fume of antimony oxide which is produced during smelting consists of particles which, on average, are less than 1 μm diameter (McCallum *et al.*, 1971). Work in the baghouse or at the furnaces is associated with most dust or fume exposure. Pneumoconiosis due to the inhalation of quartz-free powdered antimony trioxide with a particle size of less than 5 μm is recorded (Klučík, Juck and Gruberová, 1962).

The metal is used chiefly as a component of lead alloys for battery plates, electrodes, pewter and printing type. Antimony oxides are employed as pigments for paints, glass

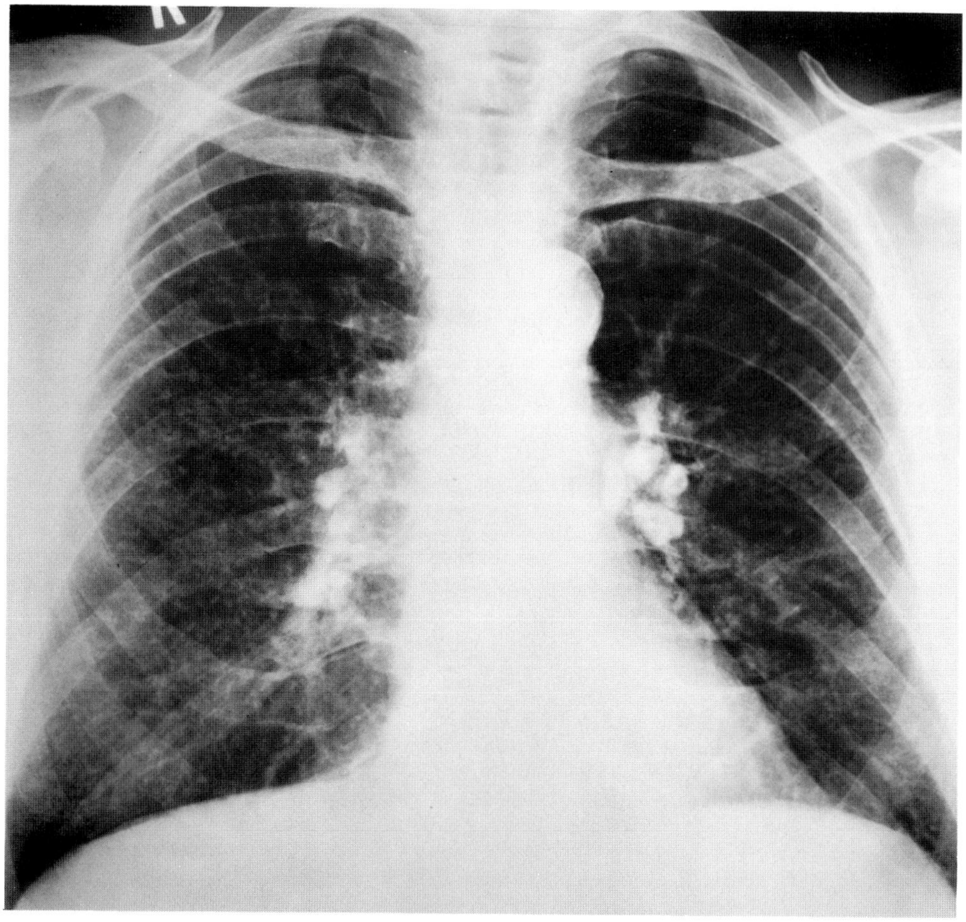

Figure 6.5 Dense opacity of hilar lymph nodes in a man who handled barium carbonate powder for 20 years. The pulmonary opacities, however, are not prominent

and fusable enamels; in the colouring and vulcanizing of rubber, in plastics and the red tips of matches.

Antimony trichloride and pentachloride are referred to briefly in Chapter 13 because, being highly toxic substances, they are not relevant to this chapter.

Pathology

Histological examination of the lungs of antimony workers has shown an accumulation of dust particles and dust-laden macrophages in alveolar walls and perivascular regions, but no fibrosis or inflammatory reaction (McCallum, 1967); the dust of antimony ore or the trioxide does not cause fibrosis in the lungs of experimental animals (Cooper *et al.*, 1968).

Small amounts of antimony have been detected in the urine of a worker some four years after he left the industry, suggesting that antimony is not fixed in the lungs and may be absorbed into the circulation in small quantities and excreted (McCallum, 1963).

Symptoms and physical signs

There are no symptoms or abnormal physical signs associated with the pneumoconiosis but those of acute chemical pneumonia or pulmonary oedema have occurred rarely in antimony smelters (Renes, 1953).

Some workers may develop rhinitis, perforation of the nasal septum or skin irritation with a popular and pustular rash in the vicinity of sebaceous and sweat glands of the forearms and thighs, especially in the flexures.

Lung function

There is no abnormality of lung function (McCallum, 1963).

Radiographic appearances

These consist of numerous small, dense opacities similar to those of siderosis which vary from ILO Categories 1p to 3p. Larger, confluent shadows are not seen but the hilar regions may be denser than normal (Cooper *et al.*, 1968; Klučík, Juck and Gruberóva, 1962; McCallum, 1963) (*Figure 6.6*).

A radiographic survey of 262 men in an antimony works between 1965 and 1966 revealed the presence of 44 cases (16.8 per cent) of antimony pneumoconiosis (McCallum *et al.*, 1971).

Using the differential X-ray absorption technique referred to in Chapter 5 in some of these workers McCallum *et al.* (1971) observed antimony values ranging from nil to just over 11 mg/cm^2 and these tended to rise the longer the period of employment in the industry and the higher the ILO Category recorded.

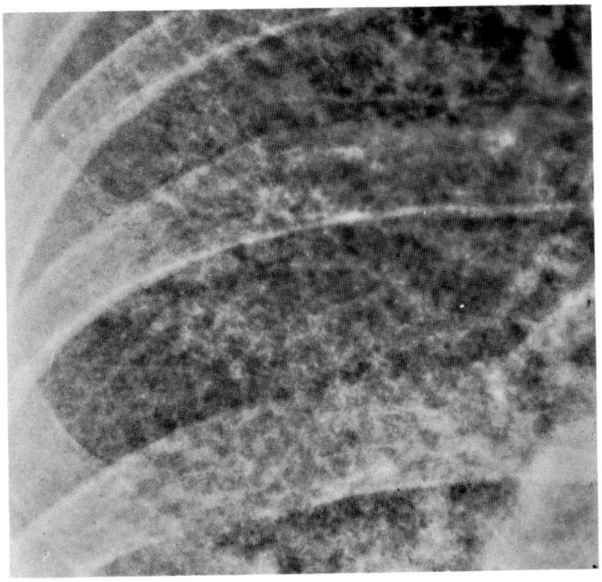

Figure 6.6 Category p opacities in an antimony process worker and weighman for 26 years. Approximately 425 µg/l of antimony was present in his urine. (Courtesy of Dr R. I. McCallum)

Abnormal chest radiographs have beeen reported in men mining and smelting antimony ore in Yugoslavia (Karajovic, 1957) but those of the miners appear to have been due to silicosis. The appearances of pulmonary oedema may be seen after heavy exposure to smelting fumes (Renes, 1953).

Diagnosis

Benign antimony pneumoconiosis is rare but if the clinician is not aware that antimony in the lungs causes radiographic abnormality, or if a history of industrial exposure to antimony is not obtained in the first place, errors in diagnosis (mainly in the direction of non-industrial disease) will probably occur.

The differential diagnosis is generally similar to that of siderosis (p. 116).

Prognosis

There is no known detrimental effect upon health or life expectancy.

Unlike siderosis and baritosis no evident diminution of radiographic appearances has yet been recorded.

ZIRCONIUM (ATOMIC NUMBER, 40) AND HAFNIUM (ATOMIC NUMBER, 72)

Zirconium (Zr) occurs most commonly as *zircon* ($ZrO_2.SiO_2$) and *baddeleyite* (ZrO_2). Both zirconium and hafnium (Hf) are closely geochemically associated in zircon, which is the principal ore mineral, in the ratio of 50 to 1. The two are not separated for use other than in nuclear applications (Ampian, 1975). Hafnium oxide is known as *hafnia*. In addition to hafnium, minor amounts of thorium, uranium and rare earth elements are commonly present in the mineral (Klemic, 1975).

Zircon, which is widely distributed in igneous and sedimentary rocks, is recovered commercially from beach sands and river gravels and is concentrated by magnetic and electrostatic separation techniques to remove accessory minerals such as ilmenite, rutile, magnetite and monazite; and quartz is removed by gravitation.

Zircon is very heavy, has a low solubility and remarkable refractory properties.

Sources of exposure and uses

Zircon dust or fume may be produced when zircon concentrate is dried and calcined to remove organic material; subsequent treatment with magnetic and roll separators to remove quartz and other impurities may also give rise to dust. Dust of zirconium compounds may be produced during many of the processes in which it is used. Quartz dust may be a hazard during the milling of the raw material and in the separation processes, but is otherwise absent.

Probably the largest use of zirconium is in alloy manufacture: with silicon and manganese in steel, and in nickel-cobalt and niobium-tantulum alloys which resist neutron bombardment. This is because zirconium imparts special alloying properties, structural stability at high temperatures, corrosion resistance and specific neutron absorption characteristics.

Zircon is of particular importance in the manufacture of technical refractory ceramics in the form of crucibles, tubes and boats and for high-temperature work in chemistry and metallurgy. It is increasingly, though not universally, used in foundry work in the form of oil-bonded 'sand', and for mould paints and parting powder in place of quartz sands and 'silica flour' (*see* Chapter 7). Not only does it eliminate the 'silica' risk—and so may be used for sandblasting—but it possesses the additional advantage of high resistance to thermal shock. In the interest of economy, recovery of zircon sand for re-use in foundries is likely to increase in the future. Zircon and various zirconium compounds are employed as opacifiers in ceramic enamels and in glasses and glazes because of their resistance to acid and to thermal shock; and to impart high dielectric strength to electrical porcelain such as sparking plugs. Zircon is also employed as a polishing agent for glass and television tubes and, in the form of 'pebbles', as a grinding medium in rotary mills. Aluminium oxide and zircon fused in an electric arc furnace produce 'alumina-zirconia' abrasives which are employed in heavy duty grinding wheels.

Zirconium dioxide—or *zirconia*—which is produced by reacting zirconium with dolomite at high temperature plays an important role in turbojet and rocket manufacture because it melts at about 2700 °C and, in stabilized form, can withstand temperatures in excess of 1900 °C. Some hafnia is invariably present in zirconia but is not a disadvantage to its use as a refractory.

Baddeleyite, which consists chiefly of zirconium dioxide with minor mineral impurities including hafnium up to 1.7 per cent, has similar properties to those of zirconia.

Zirconium is used in the production of photographic flash bulbs, in the surface reflecting material of 'space' satellites and in the chemical and nuclear reactor industries.

Hafnium is used mainly for control rods in naval and, to a lesser extent, in commercial nuclear reactors, and a small amount is employed in optical glass, flash bulbs and as an additive in refractory alloys.

Pathology

The possible biological effect of zircon was investigated in animals by Harding (1948) and Harding and Davies (1952). It was found to be remarkably inert in the lungs. Normal phagocytosis of dust particles and a slight accumulation of small cells occurred but there was no fibrosis or increase of reticulin. Numerous small dense opacities were present throughout the lung fields of radiographs of the animals' lungs due to the atomic number of the retained dust (Harding and Davies, 1952). These observations were confirmed by Reed (1956).

But zirconium-containing compounds can cause non-caseating granulomas in human skin when repeatedly applied in deodorants (Rubin *et al.*, 1956) or when injected experimentally into the skin of man and guinea pigs especially as sodium zirconium lactate (Shelley and Hurley, 1958; Epstein, Skahen and Krasnobrod, 1962; Turk and Parker, 1977). Although these granulomas have been referred to as 'allergic-type', delayed hypersensitivity has not been successfully demonstrated in animals (Epstein, 1967). This contrasts with the observation that beryllium salts (which cause sarcoid-type granulomas) induce delayed hypersensitivity in both man and animals (*see* Chapter 10). Experimental studies in the rabbit have demonstrated a striking difference between the effects of zirconium compounds and beryllium sulphate. Zirconium aluminium glycate and sodium zirconium lactate when introduced intradermally give rise to small 'foreign body type' (low turnover) granulomas without *in vivo* and *in vitro* evidence of delayed hypersensitivity, lymphocyte stimulation or production of macrophage inhibition factor (MIF). Whereas beryllium sulphate, as well as inducing local non-caseating granulomas, causes delayed skin reactivity and MIF after repeated injections. Furthermore, the zirconium compounds are much less toxic to alveolar macrophages than beryllium sulphate. Whatever the explanations of the differences between the effects of zirconium and beryllium compounds may be, these observations suggest that the zirconium compounds do not induce delayed hypersensitivity in man. It is possible, as mentioned in Chapter 10, that the insolubility of the zirconium salts limits their dispersal to and contact with immunologically competent cells (Kang *et al.*, 1977). There is no cross-sensitivity between beryllium and zirconium (Shelley and Hurley, 1971).

Electron microscopy of epithelioid and multinucleate giant cells in granulomas induced by repeated intradermal injection of sodium zirconium lactate shows that they have the same appearances as these cells in granulomas caused by this compound in human skin, but that their ultrastructure differs in a number of respects from similar cells observed in human sarcoidosis (Turk, Badenoch-Jones and Parker, 1978).

There is no radiographic nor, as far as I can discover, histopathological evidence to date indicating that zirconium or its compounds have caused granulomatous or fibrotic lung disease in man (Reed, 1956). But peribronchial granulomas have been induced in rabbits by the inhalation of zirconium lactate (Prior, Cronk and Ziegler, 1960) although, in another inhalation experiment with the same compound in three animal species, no granulomas and only minimal fibrosis were observed (Brown, Mastromatteo and Horwood, 1963).

No investigations into the effects of hafnium or hafnia appear to have been done.

Symptoms and physical signs

There is nothing at present to suggest that the inhalation of dust of zirconium or of zirconium compounds causes any clinical effects in man.

Lung function

Estimations of ventilatory function (FEV_1 and FVC) and gas transfer (Tl) in 11 zircon exposed workers with category 1 to 3 radiographic opacities were normal, though low normal Tl was observed in two. Repetition of the Tl test two to three years later in five of these men, four of whom were non-smokers, showed a decrease greater than that expected due to age, but there was no clear indication that this change was due to zircon in the lungs. There was no measurable defect in ventilatory capacity. Among 49 other workers with no evidence of pneumoconiosis who were employed in the

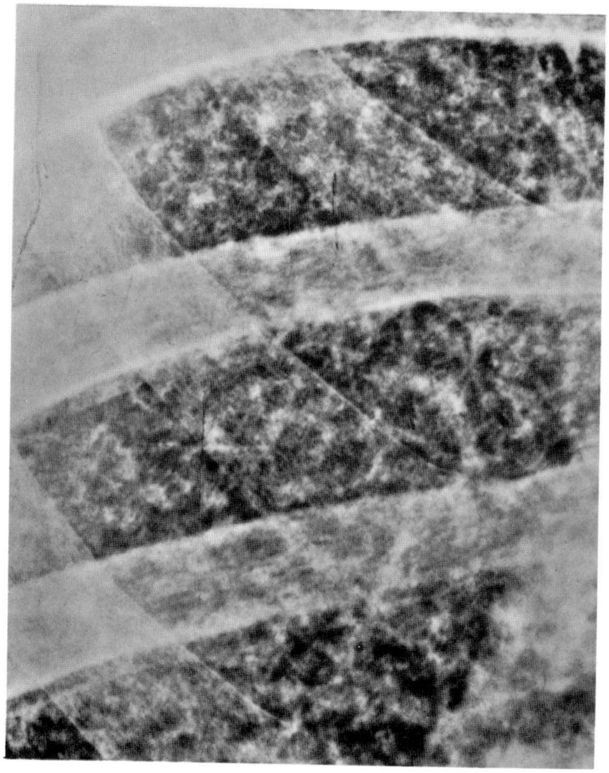

Figure 6.7 Category 'q' opacities in a worker exposed predominantly to zirconium silicate and oxide in a zircon processing plant for about ten years. (Courtesy of Dr R. I. McCallum)

same process ventilatory function tests were normal, both in smokers and non-smokers (McCallum and Leathart, 1975).

Radiographic appearances

A survey of workers in a factory processing zircon revealed a number with discrete pneumoconiotic opacities though many of the men had also been exposed to antimony, barium and titanium dust. But 12 men who had been exposed mainly to zirconium silicate and oxide dusts for periods of six to 26 years had small dense opacities ranging from category 1 to 3p. Progression from category 0 to early changes or from one category to a higher category was seen in four men over a period of years although, in general, category did not correlate well with duration of exposure (McCallum and Leathart, 1975) (*Figure 6.7*). By contrast no radiographic changes 'reasonably attributable to radio-opaque dusts' were found by Reed (1956) in 22 men who worked in a zirconium plant for one to five years; this could well have been due to the short period of exposure. McCallum (1977)—like Harding and Davies (1952) previously—has produced discrete opacities in the lung fields and dense hilar node shadows in cats (which remained fit and well) following prolonged exposure to pure zirconium silicate dust.

It is likely that the effective atomic number of zirconium compounds—and, hence, their absorptive capacity for X-rays—will exceed that of zirconium according to the amount of hafnium associated with them, though this will usually be small.

Diagnosis

The possibility of a symptomless and benign pneumoconiosis being caused by zirconium dusts should be borne in mind in view of the widespread use of these compounds in industry. It is possible that the small opacities seen in the chest radiographs of some moulders and 'knock-out' men in foundries where moulding sands and parting powders have been replaced by zircon may be caused by zirconium rather than, or in addition to, iron (*see* 'siderosis').

Conclusion

Prolonged exposure to zirconium dusts may cause a 'benign' pneumoconiosis similar to siderosis but, at present, there is no evidence that it gives rise to granulomatous or fibrotic lung disease. The reaction to zirconium compounds in both man and animals, appears to be different from that which occurs in the case of beryllium compounds; delayed (Type IV) hypersensitivity does not seem to be involved.

Zirconium tetrachloride is referred to in Chapter 13, p. 472.

THE RARE EARTH METALS OR LANTHANIDES

These are placed into three categories: the *cerium, terbium* and *yttrium subgroups* which comprise *in toto* 14 rare earth elements whose atomic numbers range from 51 to 71. Cerium (atomic number 58) is the most abundant of these. They occur in a variety of minerals of which *monazite*, a rare-earth phosphate, and *bastnaesite*, a rare earth fluorocarbonate are the most important commercially. Monazite also contains up to 30 per cent thorium (atomic number 90), not itself a rare earth element, which is radioactive (*see* Chapter 14, p. 503).

Monazite occurs as a heavy, brown-black sand obtained from alluvial deposits in certain beaches by placer mining methods or by off-shore dredging. Conventional open cast mining is used for bastnaesite deposits. Milling, flotation and electromagnetic techniques are employed to produce pure sands from which the rare earth metals and thorium and yttrium are extracted. Australia, India and Brazil are the chief producers of monazite concentrates and the USA, the chief producer of bastnaesite concentrates.

Sources of exposure and uses

Some exposure to dust may occur during the mining, milling and refining processes but, at most stages, the minerals are either wet or in solution. The use of the cerium subgroup in some industries is more likely to give rise to dust.

Cerium (usually in the form of the dioxide) is employed as a mild abrasive for polishing lenses, mirrors and prisms; in the manufacture of fireworks, cigarette lighter 'flints'; for high temperature ceramics (such as crucibles); in light metal alloys; and, to increase light brilliance, as the nitrate, fluoride and oxide in the core of carbon arc rods. Because many of these processes are dry substantial amounts of rare-earth dust may be generated. The heat of an arc evaporates the salts which accumulate as fine dust on apparatus, on ledges and other objects in the work room. Benign pneumoconiosis attributed to cerium and other rare-earth elements has been reported in men who have worked in frequent contact with carbon arc lamps (Heuck and Hoschek, 1968) and in the preparation of cerium oxide (Nappée, Bobrie and Lambard, 1972). Unseparated rare-earth elements are also used for various 'misch-metal' alloys some of which, like lighter 'flints', are pyrophoric; the iron alloy, for example, is employed in the manufacture of luminous projectiles and tracer bullets. Latterly small amounts of europium and yttrium oxides of high purity have been employed as phosphors in colour television tubes and mercury vapour and fluorescent lamps.

Apart from its application in nuclear power reactors thorium is used in the manufacture of incandescent gas mantles and to harden and increase the strength and corrosion resistance of certain alloys. Thorium mining and the presence of radioactive thoron, daughters in certain mining operations is referred to in Chapter 14.

Pathology

In the early 1940s the late Dr L. U. Gardner (then Director of the Saranac Laboratory) suggested that small opacities in the chest radiographs of workmen in Ohio who had been exposed to dusts containing rare earth oxides and fluorides, were caused by the high atomic densities of the rare earth elements. Accordingly he initiated parallel experiments in guinea pigs with rare earths in which the ratios of oxides and fluorides were reversed. Intratracheal injection and inhalation techniques were used. The high oxide rare earths produced peribronchiolar and perivascular collections of dust with little or no evidence of fibrosis after 12 months but some small perivascular granulomas developed at the end of about 18 months. Most of the dust was transported to the hilar lymph nodes. The high fluoride rare earths resulted in regional bronchiolar strictures with localized emphysema but no fibrosis or granulomas (Schepers, Delahant and Redlin, 1955; Schepers, 1955a and b). More recently, neither cerium oxide nor cerium fluoride were found to cause lung fibrosis in guinea pigs following intratracheal injections (Hoschek, 1966). In another study the development of peribronchiolar and perivascular, macrophage-rich granulomas has been confirmed in some animals exposed to the inhalation of thorium-free rare-earth metals according to intensity and duration of exposure; but thorium-containing rare-earth metals caused lung fibrosis (Cain, Egner and Ruska, 1977). Inhalation of virtually pure gadolinium oxide (one of the rare-earth elements) with particle diameters of 0.1 to 0.5 μm does not cause fibrosis of the lungs in mice (Ball and Van Gelder, 1966). The level of acid and alkaline phosphatase activity is not altered in the lungs of rats exposed to monazite; which would seem to imply that this compound is inert in their lungs (Tandon *et al.*, 1977).

It is difficult to assess to what extent these observations are relevant to man. Overall, they suggest that the rare earths, in particular cerium, are not fibrogenic but whether or not granulomatous lesions occur is unknown. No pathological studies of human lungs appear to have been recorded.

Symptoms, signs and lung function

No symptoms, abnormal physical signs or alteration in lung physiology are attributable to these inhaled dusts.

Radiographic appearances

These consist of dense, discrete opacities similar to those of baritosis with increased density of the hilar shadows (Nappée, Bobrie and Lambard 1972) (*Figure 6.8*). The ILO/UC categories in the cases described by Heuck and Hoschel (1968) were 2 to 3q. The presence of thoron as ^{228}Th in their expired air or lungs (measured by the whole body counter) was regarded as confirmation that the opacities were caused by rare-earth elements. Few cases are on record so there is cause for regret that Gardner did not publish the findings in his Ohio work force.

Differential diagnosis

This is similar in all respects to other high-density dusts. Identification of relevant exposure by an informed occupational history is essential. In some cases the demonstration of thorium decay chain elements in exposed air or in the lungs may assist in diagnosis but the availability of this investigation is very limited. The diagnosis should be considered in cases in which high density opacities are not readily explicable.

Prognosis

No injurious effects of cerium and the related lanthanide salts are apparent in man but the co-existence of thorium (an α-particle emitter) and its decay chain products may be harmful (*see* Chapter 14). This risk may be encountered during extraction of the rare earths. Nothing appears to be known about possible clearance of radio-opacities after

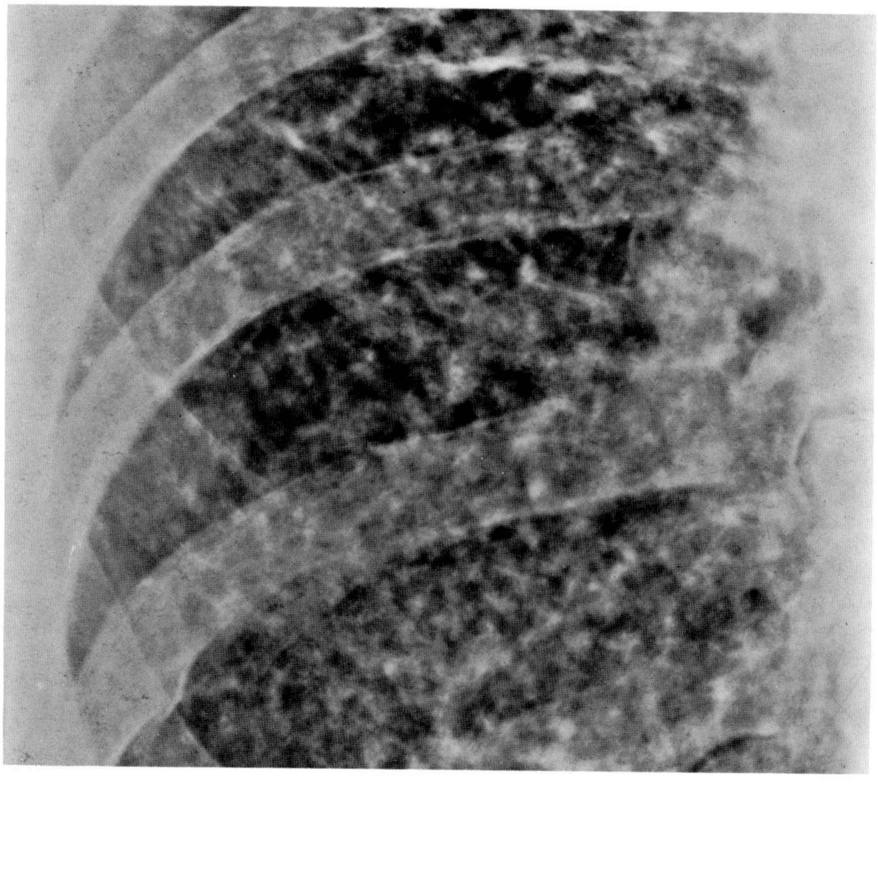

Figure 6.8 Appearances of benign pneumoconiosis in a worker exposed to rare earths, chiefly cerium dioxide, for 16 years

exposure has ceased, but none was evident in a case I observed 20 years after exposure had ceased.

Prevention

This depends on satisfactory dust control. The question of thorium is referred to in Chapter 14.

Awareness of the fact that an apparently benign pneumoconiosis may result from exposure to the salts of cerium and other lanthanides is of some importance in view of their increasing use in industry which may give rise to further cases in the future. In addition, thorium decay chain products may present a hazard during the extraction process of monazite.

CHROMITE

Chromite is the mineral ore of chromium, and it consists of chromium and iron oxides (Cr_2O_3FeO). The atomic numbers of chromium and iron are 24 and 26 respectively, but the effective atomic number of chromite is 22.

The world's largest producers of chromite are Zimbabwe, South Africa, Turkey and the USSR. In the Transvaal it occurs in association with pyroxenite, anorthosite and norite rocks and although there are occasional pegmatite veins which contain some quartz and alkaline feldspar these are few, and the amount of quartz in the mine dust is generally less than 1 per cent (Sluis-Cremer and du Toit, 1968).

The chest radiographs of miners who have been exposed to chromite mine dust for eight or more years may show small, discrete opacities similar to those of siderosis and increased opacity, but no enlargement, of the hilar shadows. There are no accompanying respiratory symptoms or signs (Sluis-Cremer and du Toit, 1968). No histological studies are available in these cases, but in view of the fact that chromite dust appears to cause only a minor cellular reaction and no fibrosis in the lungs of experimental animals (Goldstein, 1965; Worth and Schiller, 1955), Sluis-Cremer and du Toit (1968) consider the human lesions are benign and are not associated with fibrosis. However, histological examination of the lungs of three men who had worked in a chromate plant in which chromite was one of the three chromium compounds used, revealed large quantities of black pigment (identified as chromite) in the alveolar walls which were thickened, fibrotic and hyalinized (Mancuso and Hueper, 1951). But whether these changes were due to chromium rather than to some past inflammatory process or to other inhaled aerosols is uncertain.

From the available evidence, therefore, it appears that chromite dust is non-fibrogenic. In contrast to the apparent innocuousness of chromite, however, chromium salts may induce asthma (*see* Chapter 12), and chromic acid and chromates (hexavalent chromium compounds) are highly irritant to the respiratory tract; furthermore, an increased incidence of carcinoma of the lung is associated with exposure to chromates, but this has not been observed in chromite mine workers (Sluis-Cremer and du Toit, 1968) (*see* Chapter 14).

TITANIUM (ATOMIC NUMBER, 22)

Titanium dioxide (TiO_2) occurs in the form of the allotropes *rutile* and *anatase* in *ilmenite*, a mixed oxide of iron and titanium, found with magnetite or hematite in both rock and sand deposits. Because of its whiteness, high refractive index and light scattering qualities it is extensively used as a pigment for paints, paper, cosmetics, glass and ceramics, and as a mordant in dyeing; and it is an important constituent of a number of metal alloys, and of some 'hard metals' and welding rod coatings. Titanium metal, because of its high strength-weight ratio, resistance to corrosion and ability to withstand a very wide range of temperature, is widely used in the manufacture of high-speed aircraft, missiles, spacecraft and equipment for marine environments.

Sources of exposure

Exposure to significant amounts of titanium dioxide dust is unlikely to occur in mining of ilmenite rock or collection of ilmenite sands but is possible in processes using the oxide as a pigment and for the manufacture of barium titanate for electronic ceramics, and in the machining of titanium metal; and also from the dust collectors of exhaust ventilation systems employed in such industries. Because titanium is highly reactive with oxygen, nitrogen and carbon and no refractory material is able to resist it when in the molten state, it is fused in an enclosed consumable-arc furnace so that exposure of operatives to fume is improbable, though this could occur in the preparation of alloys in which titanium is used.

Two other types of exposure—which, though outside the context of this chapter are most conveniently referred to here—may occur. In the first sulphuric acid mist and sulphur trioxide are evolved during the process of extracting titanium dioxide from the ore by reaction with sulphuric acid. In the second titanium tetrachloride (an intermediary in the production of titanium metal) which is used as a mordant for the dyeing industry, as a pigment and for military smokes and sky writing has been recorded as causing acute lung disease (Lawson, 1961). It is highly corrosive and reacts violently with water to produce titanium particles, hydrochloric acid vapour and heat. Hydrochloric acid is probably released when unreacted titanium tetrachloride is inhaled due to hydrolysis in the humid conditions of the upper and lower respiratory airways. High concentrations of titanium tetrachloride may, therefore, cause acute rhinitis, tracheitis, bronchitis and pulmonary oedema.

Titanium tetrachloride is normally handled under inert conditions to avoid contact with oxygen and moisture in the air. In general, therefore, exposure of personnel is most unlikely to occur other than accidentally.

Pathology

In individuals previously exposed to titanium dioxide aggregations of carbon-like particles are present around respiratory bronchioles and in alveolar walls without microscopical evidence of fibrosis (Schmitz-Moorman, Horlein and Hanefield, 1964). Though a mild degree of alveolar fibrosis has been reported on occasions this has almost certainly been attributable to small amounts of associated quartz (Määtä and Arstila, 1975). Titanium particles can be demonstrated by electron microscopy and energy dispersive

X-ray analysis in the phagosomes of alveolar macrophages and macrophages in sputum and bronchial aspirations even two or three years after cessation of exposure; the viability of these cells is apparently unimpaired (Määtä and Arstila, 1975). Titanium dioxide particles are extremely birefringent and, therefore, show up brightly under crossed Nicol prisms.

The lack of fibrogenic potential in human lungs is confirmed in those of experimental animals (Christie, Mackay and Fisher, 1963; Dale, 1973); indeed, because of its inertness titanium dioxide is employed as a marker in experiments designed to study the effects of potentially noxious dusts and gases in animal lungs (Ferin and Leach, 1973 and 1976; Heppleston and Morris, 1965). However, titanium dioxide in the form of anatase is reported to be actively haemolytic to human erythrocytes *in vitro* whereas rutile is inert. This difference appears to be related to their crystal lattices. But inhalation of both anatase and rutile by rats does not result in increased proline hydroxylase levels which are raised in the initial stages of collagen fibrosis (Zitting and Skyttä, 1979). This indication of a lack of fibrogenicity of both allotypes agrees with Heppleston's (1971) finding that titanium dioxide does not induce fibroblasts to elaborate hydroxyproline (*see* Chapter 4).

Titanium can be identified in human and animal lungs by a histochemical method using tannic acid (De Vries and Meijer, 1968) as well as by electron microprobe techniques (Ferin, Coleman and Davis, 1976).

Widespread granulomatous lung disease in a worker who used titanium dioxide as an abrasive has been reported and regarded as due to titanium dioxide but, as the histology showed, this was a case of sarcoidosis. The fact that particles of the mineral were present in the lungs and the sarcoid lesions does not prove a causal relationship (Angebault *et al.*, 1979).

The features which follow acute severe exposure to titanium tetrachloride are those of pulmonary oedema with large amounts of proteinaceous fluid rich in fibrin, and swelling and hyperplasia of alveolar cells (Lawson, 1961).

Symptoms and physical signs

There are no subjective or objective abnormalities associated with titanium dioxide exposure. Some workers in the sulphuric acid extraction process complain of cough, shortness of breath and chest 'tightness', and wheezes may be heard on ausultation. These symptoms and signs appear to be due mainly, though not entirely, to exacerbation of the effects of smoking by the acid vapour (Daum *et al.*, 1977). No respiratory symptoms appear to result from prolonged exposure to low concentrations of titanium tetrachloride but all the signs of acute respiratory tract irritation or pulmonary oedema may follow heavy exposure.

Lung function

There are no abnormalities attributable to chronic exposure to titanium dioxide or titanium tetrachloride. Among workers in the acid extraction process a small proportion of non-smokers with more than 20 years' exposure have been found to have some evidence of airflow obstruction but, as might be expected, this was more widespread among smokers (Daum *et al.*, 1977).

Radiographic appearances

No evidence of pneumoconiosis has been observed in men extracting ilmenite sand (Uragoda and Pinto, 1972) but small discrete opacities similar to mild siderosis (*see* p. 116) have been recorded, especially where titanium dioxide is employed in the manufacture of pigments and 'hard metal' (*see* p. 464) (Schmitz-Moorman, Horlein and Hanefeld, 1964). The features of acute pulmonary oedema may follow acute exposure to titanium tetrachloride.

Diagnosis

The same principles apply as in the case of other benign pneumoconioses.

The effects of exposure to the sulphuric acid process or acute exposure to titanium hexachloride should be suspected from the work history.

Conclusion

The inhalation of titanium dioxide appears to be harmless whether or not there is radiographic evidence of its presence as a benign pneumoconiosis which is sometimes, but unhappily, referred to as 'titanosis' or 'titanicosis'. The rarity of reports of pneumoconiosis may be due—depending upon the process in question—to absence of titanium dioxide from the air or to dust particles being, in general, too large to reach alveolar level; or to dust concentrations or duration of exposure being too low for sufficient dust (the atomic number of which is only slightly in excess of that of calcium) to accumulate in the lungs to cause radio-opacities.

VANADIUM (ATOMIC NUMBER, 23)

Because vanadium pentoxide (V_2O_5) is capable of causing asthma and acute pulmonary disease, vanadium is considered in more detail in Chapter 13. The question to be clarified here is whether vanadium, which has an atomic number only slightly less than that of iron, causes a benign pneumoconiosis. The answer is that persistent discrete radiographic opacities related to exposure to metallic vanadium or vanadium pentoxide do not appear to have been described. This is probably due to the fact that vanadium moves rapidly from the lungs into the blood and is either excreted in the urine and faeces or deposited in other organs (Hudson, 1964; Sjöberg, 1950). Pure metallic vanadium dust is apparently harmless.

GENERAL CONCLUSIONS

The importance of inert dusts and fumes of high radiodensity is that they are not responsible for any symptoms, physiological impairment or progressive disease yet they may produce abnormal radiographic appearances (vanadium apparently excepted) which persist either permanently or for many years after the worker has left the relevant industry. It follows that whenever small discrete opacities of emphatic density are observed in the radiographs of a person with no other evidence of pulmonary disease industrial exposure to an inert radiodense dust should always be remembered and investigated.

In some cases the work processes in which these materials were used have been discontinued in recent years or are now carried out only on a small scale. Nevertheless, the chest radiograph may give clear evidence of past exposure years after it has ceased. Failure to recognize present or past exposure to one of these dusts as the cause of an abnormal chest radiograph will inevitably cause misdiagnosis with the possibility of irrelevant investigation and treatment.

INERT DUSTS OF LOW RADIODENSITY

Due to their low atomic numbers such dusts cause no evident radiographic abnormality but, when accompanied by free silica in the form of quartz, flint or chert, silicosis may result. In that case the appearances may be interpreted as due to the inert dust which is wrongly thought to be fibrogenic, or, if the work history is inadequate, to some unconnected disease process.

These dusts are included by the ACGIH among the 'nuisance particulates' which are not known to cause lung damage. Five examples will be briefly considered so that their negative place in the pathogenesis of pneumoconiosis may be recognized by contrast with the siliceous dusts with which they may be contaminated at some stage or another. They are: *limestone, marble, Portland cement, gypsum* and *silicon carbide.*

Carbon, which in general behaves as an inert dust of low radiodensity, is a special case and is discussed in Chapter 8.

Limestone

Limestones (*see* Chapter 2) generally contain small—usually minute—percentages of quartz and those containing more than about 15 to 20 per cent free silica are rare.

Industrial exposure to 'pure' limestone (that is, of less than 1 per cent quartz content) does not cause a fibrotic pneumoconiosis or abnormality of the chest radiograph even after many years' exposure (Collis, 1931; Davis and Nagelschmidt, 1956), and it has no systemic effect.

Chalk is similarly harmless.

However, when limestone contains flint or chert nodules or significant quantities of quartz grains there is a risk of silicosis. This may occur when siliceous limestone is quarried, crushed, milled, cut or polished (Doig, 1955).

Cement

Portland cement is manufactured on an enormous scale in large plants throughout the industrialized world, and production has been steadily increasing since 1961. The processes involved are often very dusty and, because they are sometimes wrongly regarded as causing fibrotic pneumoconiosis, must be briefly outlined.

There are three main groups of raw materials:

(1) *Calcareous:* limestone, marl and chalk.
(2) *Argillaceous:* shale, clay, marl, mudstone and, in some countries, volcanic rocks and schists.
(3) Gypsum.

Minor components are sand, quartzite and iron dusts.

The limestone must not contain too high a proportion of quartz but should this be deficient in the total mix, it is added in the form of sand, quartzite or sandstone.

The process most commonly used involves four stages:

(1) Raw materials are crushed in roll, jaw or gyratory crushers and then ground down to optimal size for chemical reaction. Grinding is done either dry in ball or roll mills, or wet in ball mills fed with water.
(2) The raw mix is blended to the required composition.
(3) It is then calcined at a temperature of about 1430 to 1650 °C, usually in rotary kilns, and appears at the far end of the kiln as clinker and is cooled. Calcination drives off moisture, breaks down carbonates to oxides and forms calcium silicates and aluminates so that negligible quantities of quartz remain.
(4) Clinker, to which about 5 per cent gypsum has been added, is then ground to a fine powder in ball or race mills. The gypsum controls the setting of the finished product.

Dust collected from grinding mills, crushers and conveyers is returned to the process. Although dust from the kiln stacks may contain some silicon dioxide in addition to other oxides, this is usually collected in electrostatic or mechanical precipitators and likewise returned to the process.

Certain types of blast furnace slag may be ground to produce Portland cement directly.

Clearly then, the chance of workers being exposed to significant quantities of free silica is small but, when such exposure does occur, it is in the preparatory stages of the process in those plants where quartz is added or siliceous clays or limestones are used.

The inhalation of cement dust by experimental animals causes neither acute nor chronic pathological changes (Baetjer, 1947). However, Einbrodt and Hentschel (1966) observed an uncommon situation in which dust recovered at the end of the process (in the packaging department) contained 5 per cent quartz and gave rise to atypical collagenous nodules when injected into the peritoneum of rats.

Surveys of large numbers of cement workers in many countries have revealed either no radiographic abnormalities or only an extremely low incidence of discrete opacities (Sayers, Dallavalle and Bloomfield, 1937; Gardner *et al.*, 1939; Sander, 1958; Jenny *et al.*, 1960). In a study of 2557 workers in Argentina, Vaccarezza (1950) did not find a single case of pneumoconiosis. But Hublet (1968) observed discrete opacities—mostly category 1q but also a few 2q (*see* Chapter 5)—in just over half of 478 men who had worked in a Belgian cement plant from five to 20 years. It is not clear what these appearances represented. However, silicotic-type nodules and conglomerate masses have been reported in men who worked at those stages in manufacture where quartz contamination was fairly high (Doerr, 1952; Prosperi and Barsi, 1957).

Conclusion

Cement dust does not cause a pneumoconiosis, but if more than 2 per cent 'free silica' is present as a contaminant, silicosis may occur after some years' exposure. This is most likely to apply in quarrying and milling of raw materials.

Nevertheless, the practical fact is that pneumoconiosis among cement workers is remarkably rare.

The lack of pathogenic effects of cement dust may also be attributed to its actively hygroscopic nature favouring flocculation of its particles so that the resulting aggregates are deposited very largely in the upper respiratory tract and mouth. Certainly rhinolithiasis has been a common annoyance to many workers in the industry.

Gypsum

Gypsum ($CaSO_4.2H_2O$: *see* Chapter 2), the crystalline massive deposits of which are known as *selenite,* has been used for some thousands of years as a building material (for example, as mortar between the blocks of the great pyramids and in Roman buildings) and this remains its major use today.

It occurs as a sedimentary deposit which originated as a saline residue precipitated during the evaporation of enclosed basins of sea water, and is commonly associated with shales, clays, marls, limestone and sandstone. Contamination by quartz is absent or very slight—rarely more than 1 to 2 per cent (Schepers and Durkan, 1955). However, contiguous beds of shale or siliceous limestone may contribute a variable quantity of quartz which may be encountered by gypsum miners when extending underground passages or sinking shafts, and by those engaged in crushing and calcining the raw material.

It is mined by opencast and underground methods, and is also quarried, the largest of the world's producers being the USA, Canada, France, the USSR, Spain, Italy and the UK.

First-stage crushing of the rock is usually done at the main processing plant by ball and hammer mills. Most of the gypsum produced is calcined and used in the preparation of various plasters and plaster boards for building purposes. Quartz is either absent or present in negligible amounts in the dust produced. Milled gypsum is extensively used as a retarder in Portland cement manufacture and also in agriculture as a soil conditioner. Calcined gypsum is employed for dental moulds and orthopaedic plasters; and there is a variety of other uses.

Gypsum does not cause lung fibrosis in experimental animals (Schepers, Durkan and Dellahant, 1955) but appears, rather, to inhibit the fibrogenic effects of quartz. Neither is pneumoconiosis or any other harmful effect caused in human lungs (Riddell, 1934), although cellular infiltration may be observed around the walls of some bronchioles (Schepers and Durkan, 1955). It is moderately birefringent.

In short, gypsum dust does not cause a pneumoconiosis. However, small discrete radiographic opacities, consistent with mild *silicosis* or *'mixed dust fibrosis'* (*see* Chapter 7) may be observed in men who have mined or crushed quartz-contaminated gypsum rock for many years. It is of interest that the lesions are usually of limited extent and show little tendency to progress.

Silicon carbide

Silicon carbide (SiC) is a universally used artificial abrasive of a hardness only slightly less than that of diamond. It is usually known by the trade name Carborundum, but sometimes by other names such as Crystolen and Carbolon. It is impervious to the action of acids, including hydrofluoric.

To produce silicon carbide high-grade silica sand and finely ground carbon (preferably in the form of petroleum coke), common salt and sawdust are fused in an electric furnace at a temperature of about 2400 °C. If the temperature is too high, silicon carbide decomposes, silica is volatilized and the carbon converted into graphite (Ladoo, 1960). At the end of the process silicon carbide crystals are surrounded by a variable amount of unreacted raw material. Fully-formed silicon carbide is then ground in crushers and mills, and impurities are removed.

It has long been used for abrasive wheels in place of the earlier, highly dangerous, sandstone wheels and is also employed as a refractory in the manufacture of boilers, forging and annealing furnaces and ceramic setter tiles.

Experimental animals exposed to high concentrations of silicon carbide dust do not develop lung fibrosis (Gardner, 1935; Holt, 1957) and, in general, it is remarkably inert. Neither is there any satisfactory evidence that it causes a pneumoconiosis in human lungs (Clark and Simmons, 1925; Miller and Sayers, 1934). Nonetheless, pneumoconiosis has been reported in workers engaged in the manufacture of Carborundum (Smith and Perina, 1948; Bruusgaard, 1949). But Bruusgaard's workers had been exposed to quartz dust from the raw material crushers, furnace residue and milling and sieving processes; those of Smith and Perina (who had significant radiographic evidence of a pneumoconiosis) had been previously exposed to other dust hazards.

There is no evidence to support the suggestion sometimes made that silicon carbide may liberate free silica or silicic acid in the lungs due to the action of tissue fluids.

Hence, although silicosis has occurred—and may still be observed—in men who have been exposed to quartz dust during the preparatory stages of the process or from furnace residue, silicon carbide dust does not cause pneumoconiosis. But the materials used to bond silicon carbide grains together contained, until recent years, variable quantities of flint, quartz, feldspar and ball and china clay, and silicosis has been recorded in men working in the bonding process (Posner, 1960). Latterly, bonding material has to a large extent been replaced by a flux (often called '*frit*') which consists of silicates, borates and oxides and is almost free of quartz or flint; or substituted by rubber, synthetic resins and organic materials.

It has been suggested (Posner, 1960) that particles of quartz and flint, or tridymite and cristobalite formed by the conversion effect of furnace temperatures of 2200 °C (*see* Chapter 2) may be released when grinding wheels are in use, but there does not seem to be any proof of this in fact.

Very recently the UK Atomic Energy Authority has developed self-bonded silicon carbide in which the grains themselves are bonded together by silicon carbide during manufacture. No additional substances are used and this new ceramic material is tougher and more resistant than the previous forms. It should find a wide application in industry and its dust will almost certainly have no fibrogenic potential.

It can be concluded that there is no evidence that exposure to silicon carbide dust gives rise to a pneumoconiosis, although pneumoconiosis, due to significant exposure to quartz or carbon dusts in the course of manufacture of silicon carbide grinding wheels may occur (*see* Chapter 7). And it must be remembered that the use of these grinding wheels on cast iron or steel (turning or grinding) may ultimately cause *siderosis* from attrition of the metal (Buckell *et al.*, 1946); or when employed for fettling metal castings moulded in siliceous sand, may give rise to silicosis or 'mixed dust fibrosis' (*see* Chapter 7).

Marble

Marble is a metamorphosed carbonate rock consisting predominantly of calcite ($CaCO_3$) and dolomite ($MgCO_3.CaCO_3$) or both (*see* Chapter 2), but some impurities in the form of talc, chlorite, non-fibrous tremolite, wollastonite (*see* p. 317), diopside (a pyroxene, $CaMgSi_2O_6$) and hematite may sometimes be present in amounts ranging from less than 1 per cent to about 50 per cent. However, it is important to note that commercially the term 'marble' is often used to refer to a variety of other rocks, including serpentines, which have an attractive appearance and will take a polish. Therefore, some stones described as marble may contain significant quantities of quartz so that it is important to know the correct identity of the stones worked by quarrymen, masons and artisans who have supposedly been occupied solely with marble. Conversely, stalagmitic marbles which are calcites with wavy bands similar to onyx are known commercially as 'onyx marbles', but true onyx—a banded chalcedony (microcrystalline silicon dioxide)—is, in fact, absent.

Marble proper is quarried by specialized techniques to produce good blocks of uniform quality which are subsequently cut and, for some purposes, polished. It is used for sculpture, various vessels, slabs and dimension stone, and is virtually pure (that is, more than 99 per cent) calcium carbonate or, occasionally, dolomite. Hence, it offers no risk of silicosis; but some harder varieties, such as are required for decorative flooring and stair treads, may contain a significant amount of quartz. Crushed (or milled) marble is used for the same purposes as crushed limestone.

Both calcite and dolomite are innocuous to the lungs but silicosis or a 'mixed dust fibrosis' (*see* Chapter 7) may result if the quartz content of the marble or pseudo-marble is significant.

It can be concluded, therefore, that pneumoconiosis does not occur in men working in occupations employing only true marble but may, of course, develop if quartz-containing pseudo-marbles or siliceous rocks of other types are also worked or quarried.

Other substances

Fibre glass, pumice, pumicite and perlite which are also apparently harmless are discussed in Chapter 9 because they are silicates.

REFERENCES

Abrasives (1971). *Ind. Minerals.* July, 12–13

Ampian, S. G. (1975). Zirconium and hafnium. *Mineral Facts & Problems Bull.* **667,** 1243–1259

Angebault, M., Berland, M., Parent, G., Bonniot, J-P. and Homasson, J. P. (1979). Toxicité pulmonaire du bioxyde de titane, risque lié au poncage des mastics. *Arch. mal. prof. Med. Trav.* **40,** 501–508

Arrigoni, A. (1933). La pneumoconiosi da bario. *Med. Lav.* **24,** 461–467

Baetjer, A. M. (1947). The effect of Portland cement dust on the lungs with special references to lobar pneumonia. *J. ind. Hyg. Toxicol.* **29,** 250–258

Ball, R. A. and Van Gelder, G. (1966). Chronic toxicity of gadolinium oxide for mice following exposure by inhalation. *Archs envir. Hlth* **13,** 601–608

Barnes, J. M. and Stoner, H. B. (1959). The toxicology of tin compounds. *Pharmac. Rev.* **11,** 211–231

Barrie, H. J. and Harding, H. E. (1947). Argyro-siderosis of lungs in silver finishers. *Br. J. ind. Med.* **4,** 225–229

Barták, F. and Tomečka, M. (1949). Stannosis (coniosis due to tin). *Proceedings of the Ninth International Congress of Industrial Medicine, London,* pp. 742–754. Bristol; Wright

Bech, A. O., Kipling, M. D. and Zundel, W. E. (1965). Emery pneumoconiosis. *Trans. Ass. ind. med. Offrs* **15,** 110–115

Boyd, J. T., Doll, R., Faulds, J. S. and Leiper, J. (1970). Cancer of the lung in iron ore (hematite) miners. *Br. J. ind. Med.* **27,** 97–105

Brown, J. R., Mastromatteo, E. and Horwood, J. (1963). Zirconium lactate and barium zirconate. *Am. ind. Hyg. Ass. J.* **24,** 131–136

Browne, R. C. (1955). Vanadium poisoning from gas turbines. *Br. J. ind. Med.* **12,** 57–59

Bruusgaard, A. (1949). Pneumoconiosis in silicon carbide workers. *Proceedings of the Ninth International Congress of Industrial Medicine, London,* pp. 676–680. Bristol; Wright

Buckell, M., Garrard, J., Jupe, M. H., McLaughlin, A. I. G. and Perry, K. M. A. (1946). The incidence of siderosis in iron turners and grinders. *Br. J. ind. Med.* **3,** 78–82

Cain, H., Egner, E. and Ruska, J. (1977). Deposits of rare earth metals in the lungs of man and in experimental animals. *Virchow's Arch. A. Anat. Histol.* **374,** 249–261

Cameron, J. D. (1970). (Group Medical Officer, Pilkington Bros Ltd.) Personal communication

Champeix, J. and Moreau, H. L. (1958). Observations récentes sur les pneumoconioses par terre d'ocre. *Archs Mal. prof. Méd. trav.* **19,** 564–573

Christie, H., Mackay, R. J. and Fisher, A. M. (1963). Pulmonary effects of inhalation of titanium dioxide by rats. *Am. ind. Hyg. Assoc. J.* **24,** 42–46

Clark, W. I. and Simmons, E. B. (1925). The dust hazard in the abrasive industry. *J. ind. Hyg.* **7,** 345–351

Cole, C. W. A., Davies, J. V. S. A., Kipling, M. D. and Ritchie, G. L. (1964). Stannosis in hearth tinners. *Br. J. ind. Med.* **21,** 235–241

Collins, R. S. (1972). Barium minerals. *Mineral Dossier No. 2.* Mineral Resources Consultative Committee. London; HMSO

Collis, E. L. (1931). Occupational dust disease. *Bull. Hyg.* **6,** 663–670

Cooper, D., Pendergrass, E. P., Vorwald, A. J., Maycok, R. L. and Brieger, M. (1968). Pneumoconiosis among workers in an antimony industry. *Am. J. Roentg.* **103,** 495–508

Cutter, H. C., Faller, W. W., Stocklen, J. B. and Wilson, W. L. (1949). Benign pneumoconiosis in a tin oxide recovery plant. *J. ind. Hyg. Toxicol.* **31,** 139–141

Dale, K. (1973). Early effects of quartz and titanium dioxide dust on pulmonary function and tissue. An experimental study on rabbits. *Scand. J. resp. Dis.* **54,** 168–184

Daum, S., Anderson, H. A., Lilis, R., Lorimer, W. V., Fischbein, S. A., Miller, A. and Selikoff, I. J. (1977). Pulmonary changes among titanium workers (abstract). *Proc. R. Soc. Med.* **70,** 31–32

Davis, S. B. and Nagelschmidt, G. (1956). A report on the absence of pneumoconiosis among workers in pure limestone. *Br. J. ind. Med.* **13,** 6–8

De Vries, G. and Meijer, A. E. F. H. (1968). Histochemical method for identification of titanium and iron oxides in pulmonary dust deposits. *Histochemie* **15,** 212–218

Doerr, W. (1952). Pneumokoniose durch Zementstaub. *Virchows Arch. path. Anat. Physiol.* **322,** 397–427

Doig, A. T. (1955). Disabling pneumoconiosis from limestone dust. *Br. J. ind. Med.* **12,** 206–216

Doig, A. T. (1976). Baritosis: a benign pneumoconiosis. *Thorax* **31,** 30–39

Doig, A. T. and McLaughlin, A. I. G. (1936). X-ray appearances of lungs of electric arc welders. *Lancet* **1,** 771–775

Doig, A. T. and McLaughlin, A. I. G. (1948). Clearing of X-ray shadows in welder's siderosis. *Lancet* **1,** 789–791

Doll, R. (1959). Occupational lung cancer, a review. *Br. J. ind. Med.* **16,** 181–190

Duggan, M. J., Soilleux, P. J., Strong, J. C. and Howell, D. M. (1970). The exposure of United Kingdom miners to radon. *Br. J. ind. Med.* **27,** 106–109

Dundon, C. C. and Hughes, J. P. (1950). Stannic oxide pneumoconiosis. *Am. J. Roentg.* **63,** 797–812

Einbrodt, H. J. and Hentschel, D. (1966). Tierexperimentelle Untersuchungen mit Arbeitsplatzstäuben ans einem Hüttenzememtwerk. *Int. Arch. Gewerbepath. Gewerbehyg.* **22,** 354–366

Epstein, W. L. (1967). Granulomatous hypersensitivity *Progr. Allergy* **11,** 36–88

Epstein, W. L., Skahen, J. R. and Krasnobrod, H. (1962). Granulomatous hypersensitivity to zirconium: Localization of allergen in tissue and its role in formation of epithelioid cells. *J. invest. Dermatol.* **38,** 223–232

Fairhall, L. T. and Hyslop, F. (1947). *The Toxicology of Antimony*. Suppl. to Publ. Hlth Rep. No. 195. US Treasury Dept

Faulds, J. S. and Stewart, M. J. (1956). Carcinoma of the lung in hematite miners. *J. Path. Bact.* **72,** 353–366

Ferin, J., Coleman, J. R. and Davis, S. (1976). Electron microprobe analysis of particle deposited in lungs. *Archs envir. Hlth* **31,** 113–115

Ferin, J. and Leach, L. J. (1973). The effect of SO_2 on lung clearance of TiO_2 particles in rats. *Am. ind. Hyg. Assoc. J.* **34,** 260–263

Ferin, J. and Leach, L. J. (1976). The effect of amosite and chrysotile asbestos on the clearance of TiO_2 particles from the lung. *Envir. Res.* **12,** 250–254

Fiori, E. (1926). Contributo alla clinica e alla radiologia delle pneumoconiosi rare. *Osp. magg.* **3,** 78–84

Fischer, H. W. and Zinnerman, G. R. (1969). Lung retention of stannic oxide. *Archs Path.* **88,** 259–264

Foá, V. (1967). La pneumoconiosi dei pulitori di oggetti metallici. *Medna Lav.* **58,** 588–602

Fogh, A., Frost, J. and Georg, J. (1969). Respiratory symptoms and pulmonary function in welders. *Ann. occup. Hyg.* **12,** 213–218

Fysh, D. (1977). Personal communication

Gardner, L. U. (1935). *Experimental Production of Silicosis*, US Publ. Hlth Rep. 50, pp. 695–702

Gardner, L. U., Durkan, T. M., Brumfield, D. M. and Sampson, H. L. (1939). Survey in seventeen cement plants of atmosphere dusts and their effects upon the lungs of twenty-two hundred employees. *J. ind. Hyg. Toxicol.* **21,** 279–318

Goldstein, B. (1965). Quoted by Sluis-Cremer, G. K. and du Toit, R. S. F. (1968)

Grant, M. M., Sorokin, S. P. and Brain, J. D. (1976). Lysosomal enzyme activities in pulmonary macrophages of rabbits breathing iron oxide. *Am. Rev. resp. Dis.* **113,** 101 (abstract)

Gregory, J. (1970). A survey of pneumoconiosis at a Sheffield steel factory. *Archs envir. Hlth* **20,** 385–399

Guest, L. (1976). Investigation into the endogenous iron content of human lungs by Mössbauer spectroscopy. *Ann. occup. hyg.* **19,** 49–62

Harding, H. E. (1948). The toxicology of zircon: preliminary report. *Br J. ind. Med.* **5,** 75–76

Harding, H. E. and Davies, T. A. L. (1952). The experimental production of radiographic shadows by the inhalation of industrial dusts. Part II. Zircon. *Br. J. ind. Med.* **9,** 70–73

Harding, H. E., Grant, J. L. A. and Davies, T. A. L. (1947). The experimental production of X-ray shadows in the lungs by inhalation of industrial dusts. I. Iron oxide. *Br. J. ind. Med.* **4,** 223–224

Heppleston, A. G. (1971). Observations on the mechanism of silicotic fibrogenesis. In *Inhaled Particles and Vapours 3*, edited by W. H. Walton, pp. 357–369. Old Woking, Surrey; Unwin Bros

Heppleston, A. G. and Morris, T. G. (1965). The progression of experimental silicosis. The influence of exposure to 'inert' dust. *Am J. Path.* **46,** 945–958

Heuck, F. and Hoschek, R. (1968). Cer-pneumoconiosis. *Am. J. Roentg.* **104,** 777–783

Holt, P. F. (1967). *Pneumoconiosis,* p. 177. London; Edward Arnold

Hoschek, R. (1966). Die biologische Wirkung von Seltenen Erden. Tieversuche mit intratrachealer Anwendung. *Zbl. Arb. Med.* **16,** 168–172

Hublet, P. (1968). Enquête relative au risque de pneumoconiose dans la fibrication des ciments de construction. *Arch. belg. Méd. soc.* **26,** 417–430

Hudson, T. G. E. (1964). *Vanadium. Toxicology and Biological Significance,* edited by E. Browning. Amsterdam, London and New York; Elsevier

Hunnicutt, T. N., Cracovaner, D. J. and Myles, J. T. (1964). Spirometric measurements in welders. *Archs envir. Hlth* **8,** 661–669

Huston, J., Wallach, D. P. and Cunningham, G. J. (1952). Pulmonary reaction to barium sulphate in rats. *Archs Path.* **54,** 430–438

Jenny, M., Battig, K., Horisberger, B., Havas, L. and Grandjean, E. (1960). Arbeitsmedizinische Intersuchung in Zementfabriken. *Schweiz. med. Wschr.* **90,** 705–709

Kang, K. Y., Bice, D., Hoffmann, E., D'Amato, R. and Salvaggio, J. (1977). Experimental studies of sensitization to beryllium, zirconium and aluminium compounds in the rabbit. *J. Allergy clin. Immunol.* **59,** 425–436

Karajovic, D. (1957). Pneumoconiosis in workers of an antimony smelting plant. *Proceedings of the 12th International Congress on Occupational Health, Helsinki,* Vol. 3, pp. 370–374

Karlish, A. J. (1962). Idiopathic pulmonary haemosiderosis with unusual features. *Proc. R. Soc. Med.* **55,** 223–225

Kleinfeld, M., Messite, J., Keoyman, O. and Shapiro, J. (1969). Welder's siderosis. *Archs envir. Hlth* **19,** 70–73

Klemic, H. (1975). Zirconium and hafnium minerals. In *Industrial Minerals and Rocks,* 4th edition, edited by S. J. Lefond *et al.* pp. 1275–1283. New York; Am. Inst. Mining, Metallurgical and Petroleum Engineers Inc.

Klučík, I., Juck, A. and Gruberová, J. (1962). Lesions of the respiratory tract and the lungs caused by antimony trioxide dust. *Prac. lek.* **14,** 363–368

Ladoo, R. B. (1960). Abrasives. In *Industrial Minerals and Rocks,* editor in Chief, J. L. Gillson, p. 18. New York; Am. Inst. Mining, Metal and Petrol Engineers

Lawson, J. J. (1961). The toxicity of titanium tetrachloride. *J. occup. Med.* **3,** 7–12

Lévi-Valensi, P., Drif, M., Dat, A. and Hadjadj, G. (1966). Á propos de 57 observations de barrytose pulmonaire (résultats et une equête systématique dans usine de baryte). *J. fr. Méd. Chir. thorac.* **20,** 443–454

Lewis, C. E. (1959). The biological effects of vanadium. *Archs ind. Hlth* **19,** 497–503

Määtä, K. and Arstila, A. W. (1975). Pulmonary deposits of titanium dioxide in cytologic and lung biopsy specimens. *Lab. invest.* **33,** 342–346

McCallum, R. I. (1963). The work of an occupational hygiene service in environmental control. *Ann. occup. Hyg.* **6,** 55–63

McCallum, R. I. (1967). Detection of antimony in process workers' lungs by X-radiation. *Trans. Soc. occup. Med.* **17,** 134–138

McCallum, R. I. (1977). Personal communication

McCallum, R. I., Day, M. J., Underhill, J. and Aird, E. G. A. (1971). Measurement of antimony oxide dust in human lungs *in vivo* by X-ray spectrophotometry. In *Inhaled Particles 3,* edited by W. H. Walton, pp. 611–618. London and Woking; Unwin

McCallum, R. I. and Leathart, G. L. (1975). Pneumoconiosis in zirconium process workers. September 1975 *XVIII International*

Congress on Occupational Health, Brighton, England

Mancuso, T. F. and Hueper, W. C. (1951). Occupational cancer and other health hazards in a chromatic plant: a medical appraisal. I. Lung cancer in chromatic workers. *Ind. Med. Surg.* **20,** 358–363

Mellissonos, J. C., Collet, A. and Daniel-Moussard, H. (1966). Étude expérimentale d'un émeri naturel des cyclades. *Int. Arch. Gewerbepath. Gewerbehyg.* **22,** 185

Miller, J. W. and Sayers, R. R. (1934). Physiological response of peritoneal tissue to dusts introduced as foreign bodies. *Publ. Hlth Rep., Wash.* **49,** 80–89

Morgan, W. K. C. and Kerr, H. D. (1963). Pathologic and physiologic studies of welder's siderosis. *Ann. intern. Med.* **58,** 293–304

Mosinger, M., Charpin, J., Rouyer, P., Luccioni, R., Dantin, F. and Dantin, B. (1968). Sur les siderose, sidero-scleroses et siderosilicoses. *Arch. Mal. prof.* **29,** 59–66

Nappée, J., Bobrie, J. and Lambard, D. (1972). Pneumoconiose au cérium. *Archs Mal. prof. Méd. trav.* **33,** 13–18

Oyanguren, H., Schüler, P., Cruz, E., Guijon, C., Maturana, V. and Valenzuela, A. (1957). Estanosis: neumoconiosis benigna debida a inhalacion de polvo y humo de estano. *Revta méd. Chile* **85,** 687–695

Pancheri, G. (1950). Su alcune forme di pneumoconiosi particolarmente studiate in Italia. *Medna lav.* **41,** 73–77

Pendergrass, E. P. and Pryde, A. W. (1948). Benign pneumoconiosis due to tin oxide. A case report with experimental investigation of the radiographic density of tin oxide dust. *J. ind. Hyg.* **30,** 119–123

Posner, E. (1960). Pneumoconiosis in makers of artificial grinding wheels, including a case of Caplan's syndrome. *Br. J. ind. Med.* **17,** 109–113

Prior, J. T., Cronk, G. A. and Ziegler, D. D. (1960). Pathological changes with the inhalation of sodium zirconium lactate. *Archs envir. Hlth* **1,** 297–300

Prosperi, G. and Barsi, C. (1957). Sulle pneumoconiosi dei lavatori del cemanto. *Rass. Med. Ind.* **26,** 16–24

Reed, C. E. (1956). Effects on the lung of industrial exposure to zirconium dust. *Archs ind. Hlth* **13,** 578–580

Renes, L. E. (1953). Antimony poisoning in industry. *Archs ind. Hyg.* **7,** 99–108

Riddell, A. R. (1934). Clinical investigation into the effects of gypsum dust. *Can. Publ. Hlth J.* **25,** 147–150

Robertson, A. J. (1960). Pneumoconiosis due to tin oxide. In *Industrial Pulmonary Diseases,* edited by E. J. King and C. M. Fletcher, pp. 168–184. London; Churchill

Robertson, A. J. and Whittaker, P. H. (1955). Radiological changes in pneumoconiosis due to tin oxide. *J. Fac. Radiol.* **6,** 224–233

Robertson, A. J., Rivers, D., Nagelschmidt, G. and Duncomb, P. (1961). Stannosis: Pneumoconiosis due to tin oxide. *Lancet* **1,** 1089–1095

Roche, A. D., Picard, D. and Vernhes, A. (1958). Silicosis in ocher workers: a clinical and anatomo-pathologic study. *Am. Rev. Tuberc.* **77,** 839–849

Roussel, J., Pernot, C., Schoumacher, P., Pernot, M. and Kessler, Y. (1964). Considérations statistiques sur le cancer bronchique du mineur de fer du bassin de Lorraine. *J. Radiol. Électrol.* **45,** 541–546

Rubin, L., Slepyan, A. H., Weber, L. F., Neuheuser, I. (1956). Granulomas of the axillas caused by deodorants. *J. Am. med. Ass.* **162,** 953–955

Safety in Mines Research (1963). *Safety in Miners Research Establishment Report for 1962,* p. 34. London; HMSO

Sander, O. A. (1958). Roentgen re-survey of cement workers. *Archs ind. Hlth* **17,** 96–103

Sayers, R. R., Dallavalle, J. M. and Bloomfield, S. G. (1937). *Occupational and Environmental Analysis of the Cement, Clay and Pottery Industries,* pp. 1–50. Public Hlth Rep. U.S. No. 238

Schepers, G. W. H. (1955a). The biological action of rare earths. I. *Archs ind. Hlth* **12,** 301–305

Schepers, G. W. H. (1955b). The biological action of rare earths II. *Archs ind. Hlth* **12,** 306–316

Schepers, G. W. H., Delahant, A. B. and Redlin, A. J. (1955). An experimental study of the effects of rare earths on animal lungs. *Archs ind. Hlth* **12,** 297–300

Schepers, G. W. H. and Durkan, T. M. (1955). Pathological study of the effects of inhaled gypsum dust on human beings. *Archs ind. Hlth* **12,** 209–217

Schepers, G. W. H., Durkan, T. M. and Delahant, A. B. (1955). The biological effect of calcined gypsum dust. An experimental study on animal lungs. *Archs ind. Hlth* **12,** 329–347

Schmitz-Moorman, P., Horlein, H. and Hanefeld, F. (1964). Lungenveranderungen bei titandioxyd staub exposition. *Beitr. Silikose forschung.* **80,** 1–17

Shelley, W. B. and Hurley, H. J. (1958). The allergic origin of zirconium deodorant granulomas. *Br. J. Derm.* **70,** 75–99

Shelley, W. B. and Hurley, H. J. (1971). The immune granuloma: late delayed hypersensitivity to zirconium and beryllium. In *Immunological Disease,* 2nd edition, edited by M. Samter, pp. 722–734. Boston; Little Brown & Co

Sjoberg, S. (1950). Vanadium pentoxide dust. *Acta med. scand.* Suppl. 238

Slater, D. (1974). Tin. *Mineral Dossier No 9.* Mineral Resources Consultative Committee. London; HMSO

Sluis-Cremer, G. K. and du Toit, R. S. F. (1968). Pneumoconiosis in chromite miners in South Africa. *Br. J. ind. Med.* **25,** 63–67

Smith, A. R. and Perina, A. E. (1948). Pneumoconiosis from synthetic abrasive materials. *Occup. Med.* **5,** 396–402

Spencer, G. E. and Wycoff, W. C. (1954). Benign tin oxide pneumoconiosis. *Archs ind. Hyg.* **10,** 295–297

Tandon, S. K., Gaur, J. S., Behari, J., Mathur, A. K. and Singh, G. B. (1977). Effect of monazite on body organs of rats. *Envir. resp.* **13,** 347–357

Teculescu, D. and Albu, A. (1973). Pulmonary function in workers inhaling iron oxide dust. *Int. Arch. Arbeitsmed.* **31,** 163–170

Turk, J. L., Badenoch-Jones, P. and Parker, D. (1978). Ultrastructural observations on epithelioid cell granulomas induced by zirconium in the guinea pig. *J. Path.* **124,** 45–49

Turk, J. L. and Parker, D. (1977). Sensitization with Cr, Ni and Zr salts and allergic type granuloma formation in the guinea pig. *J. invest. Derm.* **68,** 341–345

Uragoda, C. G. and Pinto, M. R. M. (1972). An investigation into the health of workers in an ilmenite extracting plant. *Med. J. Aust.* **1,** 167–169

Vaccarezza, R. A. (1950). *Higiene y Salubridad en la Industria del Cemento Portland. Su investigación en las Fábricas Argentinas.* Buenos Aires; Guillermo

Vorwald, A. J., Pratt, P. C., Durkan, T. M., Delahant, A. B. and Bailey, D. A. (1950). Siderosis—a benign pneumoconiosis due to the inhalation of iron dust. Part II: an experimental study of the pulmonary reaction following inhalation of dust generated by foundry cleaning room operations. *Ind. med. Surg.* **19,** 170–180

Waterhouse, D. F. (1951). Histochemical detection of barium and strontium. *Nature, Lond.* **167,** 358–359

Wende, E. (1956). Pneumokoniose bei Baryt und Lithopocarberten. *Arch. Gewerbepath. Gewerbehyg.* **15,** 171–185

Worth, G. and Schiller, E. (1955). Gesundheitsschädigungen durch Chrom und seine Verbindungen. *Arch. Gewerbepath. Gewerbehyg.* **13,** 673–686

Wynn-Williams, N. and Young, R. D. (1956). Idiopathic pulmonary haemosiderosis in an adult. *Thorax* **11,** 101–104

Zitting, A. and Skyttä, E. (1979). Biological activity of titanium dioxides. *Int. Arch. envir. Hlth* **43,** 93–97

7 Diseases due to Free Silica

It is sometimes suggested that lung disease due to various forms of free silica is now so uncommon as to be of little significance as an occupational hazard. And although it is true that, numerically, there has been a pronounced overall reduction in both the risk and prevalence of silicosis in Britain and most major industrial countries by comparison with the 1940s and earlier, it remains important for the following reasons.

(1) In a few industries the risk and prevalence of silicosis has fallen very little, or even increased as, for example, among granite workers in Austria, Sweden and Singapore (*see* Prevalence).
(2) As siliceous minerals are ubiquitous they may be encountered at any time in a multitude of work processes. A serious risk may exist if their presence is not recognized or if the fact that exposure to large concentrations of siliceous dust for a short period of time can cause rapid onset of disease is not understood. There is a particular possibility of this occurring in newly developing countries where there are areas of intensive industrial expansion.
(3) There is—and will be for some years to come—a 'survivor population' of unknown size with silicosis.
(4) The fact that silicosis is now comparatively uncommon increases the necessity for clinical vigilance to differentiate it promptly from other lung disorders.
(5) Silicosis, unlike other forms of pneumoconiosis, predisposes significantly to the development of pulmonary tuberculosis.

Disease types

Lung disease caused by free silica is of four different types which are best treated separately:

(1) Characteristic hyaline and collagenous nodular lesions due to dusts having a substantial content of quartz or flint. That is, the 'classic' or 'pure' form of *nodular silicosis*.
(2) Ill-defined, irregular, stellate fibrotic lesions due to the combined effect of dusts consisting of a mixture of free silica and an inert mineral—most commonly, iron oxide. This is referred to as *mixed dust fibrosis (Mischstaubpneumokoniosen)*.
(3) Predominantly DIPF (fibrosing 'alveolitis') often with a fairly well developed cellular component, caused by calcined diatomaceous earth—*diatomite pneumoconiosis*. Some cases in this group may exhibit similar microscopic features to those of a 'mixed dust fibrosis'.
(4) Alveolar lipoproteinosis with DIPF (fibrosing 'alveolitis'). Unlike the other three, disease in this group develops rapidly in weeks or months and can, therefore, reasonably be called '*acute silicosis*', although this term has sometimes been used to denote nodular silicosis of unusually quick development following heavy dust exposure.

'PURE' OR NODULAR SILICOSIS

This is nodular, hyaline fibrosis caused by free silica. It must be stressed that the term silicosis should be limited strictly to disease which is primarily due to free silica and not used, as is often the case, for coal pneumoconiosis and other types of pneumoconiosis the features of which are entirely different even if free silica may play some part in their pathogenesis (*see* Chapter 8). Accurate interpretation of some medical texts is impossible when this rule is not observed.

It should be pointed out that pure, or nearly pure, airborne free silica dust is hardly, if ever, encountered, as it is accompanied by variable amounts of other constituents. Strictly, therefore, all inhaled siliceous dusts are 'mixed'. 'Nodular silicosis' occurs when the proportion of free silica in the total dust is relatively high and 'mixed dust fibrosis', when the proportion is lower. Mixed dust fibrosis is also distinguished from nodular silicosis by different pathological and radiological features. When the quartz content of dust is unusually high the alveolar lipoproteinosis reaction is likely to occur.

Sources of exposure

'Free silica' dusts consist of quartz or flint, sometimes tridymite or cristobalite (or mixtures of any of these) and, rarely, of chert.

In Britain, flint is obtained mainly as a by-product of the quarrying of chalk for the cement industry (*see* Chapter 6). Flint nodules are separated, washed and then graded by hand; no risk is attached to this process. The best grade goes to the pottery industry for which the nodules are calcined at about 600 to 1100 °C and ground, usually in a ball-mill, during which a dust hazard may exist. Ground calcined flint is also used in mastic asphalt for roofing, making a finishing surface for timber and brickwork, and occasionally in the manufacture of refractory bricks. A silicosis risk may exist in these processes. The calcination of flint yields a small amount of cristobalite—about 5 per cent. *Flint clay* is not related to flint in any way and is a kaolinitic, non-plastic refractory clay.

Chert has a very limited use, chiefly for lining ball-mills and as a raw material in certain refractories (the second may offer some dust risk), but until recent years it was employed as an abrasive 'sand'-blasting agent for cleaning the stonework of buildings—potentially a most hazardous occupation.

The dust risk is usually evident (as in quarrying, drilling and tunnelling quartz-containing rocks) but may be unsuspected by those not conversant with the details of an industrial process. For example, quartz may be encountered during mining and crushing the harmless rock, gypsum (*see* Chapter 6) or during processing the montmorillonite clay, bentonite (Phibbs, Sundin and Mitchell, 1971).

Although the 'free silica' hazard has, in recent years, been greatly reduced or eliminated in major industrial countries, nevertheless, in some work places (often small) it still remains or has increased. As silicon dioxide is ubiquitous in Nature it is evident that it will always be available as a potential risk wherever there is an unsatisfactory standard of dust control and industrial hygiene, or where the risk is not recognized.

Only crystalline and cryptocrystalline (or microcrystalline) forms of silica are considered in this section, quartz and cristobalite being the most important members of the crystalline group, and flint and chert, and chalcedony, the most important of the cryptocrystalline group.

Mining, quarrying and tunnelling of siliceous rocks

Mining

During the mining of gold, tin, copper, platinum and mica, drilling, hewing, shovelling, crushing and the use of explosive charges are all productive of much dust. Wet rock drilling, introduced in 1897 but not widely used until about 1920 (Holman, 1947), is only partly successful in suppressing dust even when wetting agents are employed.

The major goldfields are in the Transvaal, the USSR, Canada, the USA and Australia. The ore usually occurs in quartz veins associated with granite masses.

The chief tin-producing countries of the world have been referred to already in Chapter 6. Tin ore is found in relation to rocks of the granite family.

Copper ores—*chalcopyrite, chalcocite* and *bornite* which may occur in association with igneous rocks, sandstone or shale—are mined in Chile, Zambia (where silicosis among the miners is on record; Paul, 1961), Zaire and the USA.

Mica which consists of a group of minerals—*muscovite, phlogopite, biotite, lepidolite, zinnwaldite, roscoelite* and *vermiculite* (*see also* Chapter 9)—is found in rocks of high quartz content (such as pegmatite veins) and these are a source of quartz dust during mining, crushing and milling; hence silicosis may result from any of these processes (Government of India Ministry of Labour, 1953; Thiruvengadam *et al.*, 1968). India and Brazil are the chief world producers of muscovite sheet mica; the Malagasy Republic has been the major source of phlogopite mica, a lesser producer being Mexico; and the USA is the largest producer of muscovite scrap and flake mica. The question of whether pure mica is capable of causing pulmonary fibrosis is discussed in Chapter 9.

Fluorspar (calcium fluorite, Ca F_2), which is worked by underground and open-cast mining methods, occurs in vertical veins or flat-lying masses in country rocks so that free silica, as well as other minerals (such as barytes), is often present. In the Derbyshire minefield (the most important in the UK), for example, microcrystalline quartz and chalcedony are widespread in the wall-rock, and the fluorspar itself may contain small siliceous nodules. Hence, 15 to 20 per cent SiO_2 may be found in the extracted ore which may require very fine grinding during beneficiation to remove it. The mineral has many uses: for example, in the manufacture of fluorine chemicals, glass fibre, mineral wool, pottery and microscope lenses; and as a flux in the manufacture of steel ceramics. Its required purity, therefore, varies: acid-grade fluorspar contains a maximum of 1 per cent SiO_2; ceramic-grade, up to 3 per cent; and metallurgical-grade, up to 12 per cent (Notholt and Highley, 1975). Hence, silicosis, may occur in fluorspar miners and grinders but, in the absence of quartz, fluorspar is apparently non-fibrogenic in the lungs of experimental animals (de Villiers and Gross, 1967; South African Medical Research Council, 1974).

Fireclays—a generic term used to refer to siliceous clays which constitute the seat-earths of some coal seams and also to a number of differently formed clays suited to various refractory purposes—are today chiefly extracted by open-cast methods. Prior to the Second World War, when there were more than 200 mines in the UK, extraction was almost exclusively by underground mining. In 1979 14 mines were still operating: in Scotland (which has a long history of fireclay mining as do most coal fields elsewhere), Yorkshire and Cumberland (Highley, 1980). Fireclays are also produced in many other countries—notably the USA, the Federal Republic of Germany and Japan. Typical coal measure fireclays have a highly variable composition consisting predominantly of disordered kaolinite, mica and quartz in varying proportions. The highest quality fireclays contain approximately 1.5 per cent free silica but those of lower quality may contain as much as 30 per cent. Hence, the mining and bagging of fireclays have caused silicosis in the past and remain a potential silica hazard. Most of the processing of fireclays in the manufacture of refractory goods, vitrified clay pipes, facing bricks and fireclay sanitary ware is in the wet or semi-wet state so that a silica risk is usually slight; only small quantities of fireclay are dried or ground.

Ball clays are similar in composition to fireclays but are less indurated and much more plastic.

Arenaceous shales are mined extensively by opencast methods, for the manufacture of heavy ceramic ware and for cement and light weight aggregates. Oil shales are also mined almost exclusively by opencast methods (though previously underground mining was not uncommon) for the extraction of crude oil in the USA, the USSR and Brazil but production in Scotland (Midlothian) and Sweden ceased in the 1960s due to operating costs. Thus, as the quartz content of these shales is usually substantial, their mining and processing has given rise to some cases of silicosis in the past and should still be counted as a potential, though uncommon, silica risk (Meiklejohn, 1956).

Tungsten, a metal of fundamental metallurgical importance (*see* Chapter 13) and application in the electronic, electrical and chemical industries, occurs as *wolframite* [(Fe Mn) WO_4] and *scheelite* (Ca WO_4) in fissures in association with granite, pegmatite and limestone. In England it is mined in Cornwall and Cumberland by cross-cutting from main shafts to metal-containing veins (Slater, 1973). Hence, variable amounts of quartz may be present in mine dust and silicosis has been reported.

Low grade iron ores, sometimes known as *taconite* in certain areas notably the Mesabi Range in Minnesota, which contain substantial quantities of free silica often in chalcedonic form as chert or as fine-grained quartz (although in some areas the amount of free silica is low) together with silicates, are now being extensively mined and processed as a source of iron. This would appear to be a potential silica risk, but no definite evidence of pneumoconiosis, adverse respiratory symptoms or ventilatory impairment was revealed in a recent survey of 249 men with 20 or more years mining or processing taconite ore (Clark *et al.*, 1980).

Sandstone or other siliceous sedimentary rocks may be encountered in some coal-mines during shaft sinking and the development of tunnels and roadways.

Quarrying

Granite quarrying The quartz content of granite varies from 10 to about 30 per cent. Quarrying is done with powered drills, wire belt saws fed with an abrasive slurry (usually aluminium oxide) and, in some quarries since the early 1950s, by a flame cutter in which the combustion of oxygen and fuel oil fed through a nozzle produces a flame with a temperature of over 2800 °C; a stream of water accompanies the flame and when it is directed against the rock, the rock disintegrates into fragments. The flame cutter produces a dust consisting of crystalline quartz particles, the concentration of which appears to be low (that is, less than 10 ppcf), and other particles less than 0.1 μm diameter which are apparently formed by vaporization of the granite (Burgess and Reist, 1969). The significance and possible effects of these submicron particles upon the lungs requires further study, but as they undoubtedly consist of 'fused silica' (quartz glass) owing to the high temperature they may be expected, like Aerosil particles, to have little fibrogenic potential (*see* p. 166).

Small quarries still rely on simple methods with little mechanization. Change to elaborate mechanization in large quarries has increased the concentration of dusts.

Sandstone quarrying This is carried on in many countries. In the UK quarries are worked in Cornwall, the Forest of Dean, Lancashire, Cumberland, Yorkshire and Scotland. The quartz content of the stone is always high. It is obtained by drilling and 'channelling' and, if hard, by the use of light blasting charges. It may be cut further and rough hewn in the quarry.

Slate quarrying Sericite (white mica) is the most abundant constituent of slates but the quartz content, though it varies widely, is usually in the range of 30 to 45 per cent by weight.

The chief slate-producing countries are the USA (Maine, Pennsylvania, Vermont and Virginia), the British Isles (North Wales—until recently the largest slate-producing area in the world—and Cornwall), and Tipperary and Cork in Southern Ireland, France and Germany. Welsh slate has a particularly high quartz content, especially that from Blaenau Ffestiniog.

The fact that the quartz content of slates is variable, and is low in some, probably explains the widely different prevalence of silicosis observed in this industry in different regions.

Exposure to dust occurs during quarrying, in the sawmills where the slate is cut into blocks, and during the splitting of blocks to specified thickness and size by hand or machine. Sawing and splitting are usually done at the quarry site. Slate may be still used for the manufacture of electric panels and switchboards, billiard and other table tops, and fireplaces. It is cut, trimmed and polished in the factory—activities which are also dusty. Production of slate pencils in Mandaur, India, has been reported to have caused severe silicosis (Jain *et al.*, 1977).

Production of commercial slate powders for use as fillers leads to some loss of free silica but their content is seldom less than 25 per cent.

Pumice and pumicite quarrying This and the subsequent refining processes which may be a source of exposure to free silica are referred to in Chapter 9.

Tunnelling

In civil engineering, cutting tunnels and excavation for a variety of purposes may be serious and often unexpected hazards, especially as ventilation is usually poor. Driving sewer tunnels (which may be called 'construction work'), digging graves in sandstone, and excavating deep foundations in sandstone for multistorey buildings (as, for example, in Sydney, New South Wales) have all caused silicosis, and are the sort of risks which can be easily overlooked.

Stone cutting, dressing, polishing, cleaning and monumental masonry

These stones (known as 'dimension stone' in the USA) include rough building stone, cut stone, ashlar, pavement flags, curbing and monumental stone. The most important materials for these, from the standpoint of silicosis, are sandstone and granite.

Quarried sandstone is cut by hand or machine, dressed, shaped and drilled for building and ornamental purposes, often in closed sheds, and until some 20 years ago (and rarely still) was fashioned into grindstones. Masons and their helpers who work the stone on benches (known as bankers) are likely to be exposed to high concentrations of dust when hygiene measures are inadequate. In some quarries the stone is crushed and sieved on site for road materials. This is a very dusty process although in the open air. Many men who worked Liverpool red sandstone during the building of the Anglican cathedral or in making graves developed serious silicosis.

Men restoring or cleaning sandstone buildings with powered tools may be exposed to high local concentrations of dust.

Quarried granite is cut to specified sizes by wire or gang saws (a gang saw employs steel shot and water), ground to a desired contour or profile, and polished. In large factories these procedures are highly mechanized and subjected to local and background exhaust ventilation, but in small firms mechanical methods may be limited. Fine cutting and finishing work is done with pneumatic hand tools. Designs and inscriptions are cut through stencils by abrasive blasting.

Where standards of local and general exhaust ventilation and enclosure are high—as in the Vermont granite industry (Hosey, Trasko and Ashe, 1957—the prevalence of silicosis has greatly decreased, but where these are lacking or deficient, it tends to be higher than in non-mechanized factories.

Monumental masons and curbstone dressers were, and occasionally still are, liable to be exposed to dust without protection. Power drilling, chiselling and hammering of floors and walls made of concrete reinforced with chips of flint or quartz-containing rock, if not recognized, remain an important, if limited, hazard.

Abrasives

Sandstone is now rarely used for the manufacture of grindstones, but such grindstones may still be found in use. Crushed sand, sandstone and quartzite have been used for metal polishes and scouring powders, and flint or quartz are crushed and graded to make sandpaper. Tripoli (*see* Chapter 2) is crushed and made into compositions for finishing and buffing metals, and ground rottenstone is used as a base for polishes.

Crushing and pulverizing these materials and mixing and sieving them during manufacture may give rise to a substantial dust hazard, but today the machinery is usually enclosed.

Although it has been known for 30 years or more that high concentrations of the dust of finely powdered quartz, quarzite rock or flint (so-called 'silica flour') used in the manufacture of abrasive soaps and scouring powders may cause rapidly progressive silicosis, their use in domestic scouring powders has only recently ceased in the UK but, apparently, may still continue elsewhere (Nelson *et al.*, 1978). Feldspar is often employed as a substitute.

Abrasive blasting

The principle of this technique consists of propelling abrasive grains at high velocity at a target by means of compressed air, water under pressure, or a controlled centrifugal force. The grains may be quartzose sands, flint or chert (*sandblasting*); but corundum, iron garnet [usually almadine, $Fe_3Al_2(SiO_4)_3$], zircon, a hard variety of barytes and silicon carbide, which do not cause silicosis, are also used. All are ground to specified grain size. Steel shot (*shot blasting*) has commonly replaced the siliceous grains for some years past, but is more costly, tends to be less hard and deteriorates when stored. Hence, sandblasting has by no means been eliminated from industry and is still extensively employed in the USA where, in the New Orleans area, its use has been greatly increased by the rapid development of off-shore oil drilling and shipbuilding. Both sandblasters and unprotected men working in their neighbourhood have developed silicosis (Ziskind *et al.*, 1976).

Sandblasting is used to clean metal castings and to remove 'burnt-on' moulding sand, in the preparation of metal surfaces for painting or enamelling, for cleaning building stone and concrete, and renovating stone veneer; for making inscriptions on memorial stones, and to etch glass and plastics.

If the size of the article to be blasted is suitable, the process can be enclosed and operated by remote control and, although this does not expose the operator to dust, significant concentrations of dust may be encountered when he enters the cabinet or cleans out detritus from the floor or trap beneath. When enclosure is not possible (for example, sandblasting ships or buildings) the operator must wear a special helmet supplied with uncontaminated air—preferably compressed air to prevent the entry of dust particles.

It should be remembered that even when non-siliceous abrasives are used to clean metal castings the dust produced from 'burnt-on' moulding sand may contain large amounts of quartz. Until recent times this was a notorious hazard and dangerous exposure may still be encountered.

Glass manufacture

Pure beach and river sands are employed to produce glass and, until the mid-1960s, sand of graded particle size was used in the form of a slurry to grind and polish plate glass. Subsequently the 'float glass process' (Pilkington, 1969) has largely replaced the previous techniques for manufacturing plate glass in most major glass industries in the UK and other countries. The earlier grinding and polishing methods, therefore, have now been abandoned by large companies but may still survive in small firms.

Fillers

Finely ground quartz-containing rock is used for some paints and as a filler in the rubber industry; Neuburg chalk (Neuburger Kieselkreide), which contains a high percentage of quartz (Schneider, 1966), is commonly used in Germany. Fillers employed in the manufacture of gramophone records from about 1908 to 1948 (when microgroove records were introduced) included powdered slate and rottenstone of about 10 μm or less particle size. This practice was discontinued in 1948 because of the need to reduce the signal–noise ratio in the new records (EMI, 1970).

Exposure is most likely to occur during the production of fillers but may exist to a variable degree during their use. An unusual example of this is the development of silicosis in Japanese woodworkers who used tonoko powder (which contains about 78 per cent silicon dioxide) to fill grains in wooden furniture (Kawakami, Sato and Takishima, 1977).

Foundry work

Free silica dust is produced in iron and steel foundries in the following ways:

(a) Moulding and core making
(b) Application of parting powders
(c) 'Knocking out' or 'shaking out' of castings
(d) Dressing, fettling and abrasive blasting of castings
(e) Contamination of foundry floors
(f) Maintenance and repair of refractory materials.

(a) A mould is normally made of highly refractory quartzose sand bonded with a clay (such as china clay or ball clay) and placed in a cast-iron or wooden box which splits into two or more parts. The sand is sufficiently plastic to take the 'pattern', or shape, of the casting to be made. If the casting is to be hollow a core of the desired shape is constructed from oil-bonded sand or plastic, and baked to impart strength. Core strength can also be increased by adding sodium silicate to the sand and passing carbon dioxide gas through it, but there are some technical drawbacks to this method.

Recent coremaking processes employ a phenolic resin and catalyst mixed into the sand. When heated by the molten metal ammonia, formaldehyde, phenol and carbon monoxide are released. A newer technique involves mixing a phenolic resin with an isocyanate in the sand and, when this is in the core box, passing triethylamine through it. These processes have to be subjected to strict hygiene control to prevent leaking of irritant and toxic gases after metal pouring (*see* Chapters 12 and 13).

When molten metal is poured in, the sand is subjected to a high temperature (about 1600 °C in the case of steel) and this is sufficient to convert some of the quartz to cristobalite, which is strongly fibrogenic (*see* Chapter 4). It may be re-used many times over for other moulds.

For a number of years some foundries have used zircon sands as a substitute for quartzose sands, but these have the disadvantage of being costly. Olivine sands are also used. Olivine consists of magnesium and ferrous orthosilicate and is non-fibrogenic in animals (*see* Chapter 9, p. 316).

(b) Some moulds require dusting with a 'parting powder' which gives increased resistance to thermal shock when the molten metal is run in. Powders of high free-silica content have been generally used for this purpose. Inevitably this was a dusty process and, in the UK, has been controlled since 1950 by the Foundries (Parting Materials) Special Regulations which forbid the use of materials having more than 3 per cent of silicon dioxide by weight of dry material. Replacement with olivine and zircon powders is now common.

(c) After the metal has cooled, the mould and core are separated—that is, 'knocked out' or 'shaken out'—from the casting. This can also be a very dusty job and a most important potential source of exposure. If the size of the cast is small enough it can be enclosed with the vibrating table which performs the task automatically, but large casts must be done by hand.

(d) Sand which is adherent, or burnt on to the casting, must be removed—a process known as 'fettling', 'roughing-off' or 'stripping'. Larger areas are chipped off by hammer and chisel; smaller areas are smoothed down with portable grinding wheels of Carborundum or emery which is another source of iron oxide dust. Some castings are finished by abrasive blasting (*see* p. 137). Small castings are cleaned in a revolving cylindrical mill which may contain steel balls (ball-mill) as an additional abrasive agency.

All knocking out and fettling operations are potentially very dusty and various methods of mechanization, enclosure and exhaust ventilation are now applied to eliminate or reduce the dust. In the UK both the 'knock out' and fettling processes are controlled by the Iron and Steel Foundries Regulations, 1953, and abrasive blasting specifically regulated by the Blasting (Casting and other Articles) Special Regulations, 1949.

Iron foundry fettling tends to produce a mixed dust consisting of different proportions of iron oxide and quartz which is an important cause of 'mixed dust fibrosis' described later in this chapter.

(e) At one time all foundries had earth floors and such floors are still occasionally to be found because they have the advantage that they can be dug up to make large moulds; their disadvantage, however, is that they become highly contaminated with siliceous dust which it is impossible to eradicate.

Conditions similar to those in iron and steel foundries may be met in some non-ferrous foundries, especially brass foundries, and in the UK are controlled by the precepts of the Joint Standard Committee in Safety Health and Welfare Conditions in Non-Ferrous Foundries (1957).

Ceramics

Ceramics may be defined as 'man-made articles which have been first shaped or moulded from a wide range of natural earths, minerals and rocks, and then permanently hardened by heat' (Adams, 1961).

The three main ceramic groups are defined and the essential features of Technical Ceramics and Structural Clay Products summarized in Chapter 2. Only *Pottery and Whiteware*—that is, bone china, porcelain and earthenware—and *Refractory Ceramics* are considered here. The manufacture of *Structural Clay Products*, the raw materials of which consist of argillaceous clays, does not normally present a 'silica risk'. But an exception to this exists in the case of some types of wall and fireplace tiles in which flint and ball clay are used and have caused, and may still cause, silicosis in men who manufacture and cut and trim them ('tile-slabbers').

Chinaware, porcelain, stoneware and earthenware

The raw materials for china ware ('bone china') are china clay, china stone (that is a granitic rock containing quartz and feldspar of which a high-quality form called 'Cornish Stone' is found in the UK near St Austell), and calcined animal bone; those for stoneware are similar apart from the bone, and some fireclay (a fine-grained equivalent of ganister) may be added. The ingredients for porcelain and vitreous china are china and ball clays, feldspar and quartz or flint; those for earthenware are china and ball clays, feldspar and flint but fireclay is added for some products such as sinks. The free silica content of china clay in the refined state necessary for the ceramic industry is 2 to 3 per cent; of ball clay, 5 to 25 per cent; and of natural red clay, about 30 per cent (HM Factory Inspectorate, 1959).

Briefly, the manufacturing processes are as follows. Non-plastic raw materials such as china stone, feldspar, fireclay, quartz and calcined flint are crushed and milled, and converted into a 'slip' by the addition of water. The plastic clay materials are also converted into a 'slip'. After the removal of contaminants the 'slips' are mixed, the mixture pumped through a press where most of the water is extruded and, if required in a plastic state for shaping, the contained air is expelled in a 'pug mill'. The final mixture is known as 'body'.

Crushing and milling calcined flint and quartz produces 'free silica' dust but the wet process does not. However, spillage and subsequent drying of non-plastic 'slip' and 'body' on benches, equipment, the floor and operatives' clothes can be a serious source of siliceous dust if the environmental conditions are not rigorously controlled by satisfactory standards of monitoring of airborne dust, local and general exhaust ventilation and special protective clothing worn by the operatives. Even so, the risk may not be wholly eliminated (*see* Prevention).

Next, 'body' is shaped on a revolving wheel (this is known as 'jollying' or 'jiggering') or pressed into the shapes desired by machine presses. If the shapes are complex, 'body' is liquefied and poured into a plaster-of-Paris (gypsum) mould ('slip-casting'), the mould allowed to dry before opening. Obviously, dried 'body' is a source of dust.

As china ware 'body' contains no flint it might be thought to offer no silicosis risk. However, silicosis has been observed in exposed workers (Posner, 1961) due, undoubtedly, to the high quartz content (about 30 per cent) of 'Cornish Stone'.

The rough surfaces and edges of the ware produced is fettled, usually by women, by applying small knives, abrasive rags and tow to the ware as it stands on a revolving wheel. This operation (known as 'towing') produces much dust and requires to be strictly controlled.

All shaped ware is then kiln fired between 900 and 1200 °C according to the type of ware (Adams, 1961). When removed from the kiln the ware is known as 'biscuit'. In the British pottery industry before about 1937 ware to be fired was placed in powdered flint for support in fireclay 'saggars'. This exposed kiln workers to high concentrations of 'free silica' dust and, consequently, there was a high prevalence of silicosis. Since that date, flint has been replaced by calcined alumina with the result that silicosis among these workers has been virtually eradicated (Posner and Kennedy, 1967).

Finally, 'biscuit' ware is glazed with liquid glaze and refired at from 1050 to 1400 °C. The glaze usually consists of feldspar, quartz, borax, sodium carbonate and zinc oxide; except for the pulverization of quartz during preparation and the drying of glaze spillage, it does not appear to offer any risk. When ware is decorated a third 'on glaze' firing at lower temperatures is required. Certain types of ceramics are fired at 1200 °C or more in order to produce in the ware a large concentration of cristobalite because this possesses a very high thermal expansion.

It should be noted that large numbers of women are employed in the pottery industry.

In the UK pottery manufacture is regulated by the Pottery (Health) Special Regulations, 1947, and the Pottery (Health and Welfare) Special Regulations, 1950.

In the USA, Finland and Denmark, wollastonite (*see* Chapter 2) is used as a substitute for flint, quartz sand, feldspar and china clay in 'body' and in 'glazes' with a consequent reduction in the potential silicosis hazard. For economic reasons of import costs and plant design it is little used in the UK other than in certain glazes and fluxes. Investigations into the possibility of synthesizing anhydrous calcium metasilicate are being conducted by the British Ceramic Research Association (Andrews, 1970).

Refractory ceramics

The most important group in the present context are referred to as *acid refractories*. These include lining bricks of various sorts, cements and different types of shaped ware. Bricks and cements are used in kilns, steel furnaces, ovens in gas-making plants, boiler houses and domestic hearths.

The raw materials—ganister or 'silica rock' (that is, quartzite sandstones, sands or grits) which have a very high quartz content—are crushed (usually in dry pans), milled, screened to desired size and mixed with a controlled quantity of water and, in some cases, with small amounts of paper-mill waste and 'milk of lime'. Power presses shape the resulting material into bricks, or it is made into shapes by hand or by the 'slip casting' method. The bricks and shapes are dried in ovens or on heated floors and then fired in a tunnel kiln at about 1450 °C. Before the bricks are fired they may be dusted with quartzite sand to prevent adherence, and this is afterwards retrieved, sieved and used again. With recurrent exposure to high temperatures a significant proportion of the quartz is transformed into cristobalite. In fact, most of the quartz in well-fired bricks is converted to cristobalite and tridymite.

The end-product is referred to as 'fireclay brick' when the raw material is ganister, and as 'silica brick' when it is 'silica rock'.

Obviously this process is capable of producing large concentrations of siliceous dust.

Kiln bricklayers and others who maintain and dismantle the refractory bricks of ovens, furnaces, kilns and retorts ('retort setting') are exposed to dust—which may contain up to 10 per cent cristobalite—from disintegrating bricks, and, in repair work, there may be an additional hazard in that the interstices of the bricks are often grouted with asbestos fibre mixed with water at the site, or with dry fibre or asbestos rope. This source of asbestos exposure is referred to in Chapter 9.

A coarse-grained quartzose sand with natural clay bonding is used to line the dams and runners of blast furnaces. These 'cast house' or 'runner' sands may be a source of dust.

Because, in the presence of small amounts of alkali, quartz converts to cristobalite at temperatures of about 1200 °C instead of about 1400 °C (*see* Chapter 2) cristobalite is the principal constituent of 'silica' refractories and may also be present in many pottery bodies. Moreover, in the temperature range 1150 to 1250 °C flint converts to cristobalite more readily than quartz and, in the presence of alkali (for example, chalk), cristobalite may be formed at a temperature as low as 950 °C. In view of the fact that cristobalite is apparently more fibrogenic than quartz (Chapter 4) it may enhance the severity of the resulting lung fibrosis. Calcined flint contains 5–10 per cent cristobalite.

Neutral refractories are made from chrome ore, aluminium oxides or sillimanite mixed with a small quantity of plastic clay and fired at temperatures of 1450 to 1650 °C. Under these circumstances aluminium oxides do not appear to offer any pneumoconiosis risk. Sillimanite is referred to in Chapter 9.

'Basic' refractories Refractory bricks and other materials are made from magnesium, chert-free dolomite and olivine rock, and they do not present any 'free silica' risk (*see* Chapter 9 for olivine minerals).

Boiler scaling

The tubes, flues and fireboxes of boilers require cleaning and scaling at regular intervals. Coal-fired boilers collect ash and concretions which consist of quartz (derived from roof and floor rock seams of coal-mines), carbon, iron, silicates and carbonates from coal combustion. The composition is variable but the relative amounts of quartz, iron and carbon in the dust influences the type of lung lesion which may be produced. This is referred to in the next section.

Cleaning is done with brushes, hammer and chisel, and compressed air jets in enclosed and restricted spaces so that dust concentrations are high.

Ash deposited in the gas passages, flues and smoke stacks of oil-fired boilers contains no quartz but occasionally has a high content of vanadium which is naturally present in large quantity in some oils—particularly Venezuelan oil (McTurk, Huis and Eckhardt, 1956) (*see* Chapter 6).

It should be noted that boiler scalers have often worked in close proximity to bricklayers dismantling and replacing refractory brick linings and may, therefore, have been exposed to quartz dust from this source. Furthermore, they may have been present during periodic relagging of boiler and neighbouring installations with asbestos insulating materials and even assisted the laggers.

Vitreous enamelling

Enamel consists of quartz, feldspar, metal oxides and carbonates in variable quantities. These ingredients are pulverized, mixed and then fused at temperatures up to 900 °C. Although the heat converts much of the quartz to silicates some remains unchanged. The resulting sinter (referred to as 'frit') is ground with water in a ball-mill and further quantities of the ingredients may be added. The mix is enamel. The process may be dusty. Enamel spraying in particular may present a hazard, especially when the inner surfaces of vessels are sprayed (Friberg and Öhman, 1957). Nowadays spraying is done in booths with special exhaust ventilation and the sprayer wears a respirator; nevertheless, the potential danger remains.

An additional risk is encountered when some enamelled objects are 'finished off' by sandblasting.

Manufacture of cultured quartz crystals

The huge demand for electronic grade quartz for resonators, transducers, laser technology, quartz thermometers, watches, and colour television circuits led to the production of cultured quartz crystals which has expanded more than three-fold since 1961. It is carried out in a few installations in the USA, the UK, Japan and the USSR using a hydrothermal system which simulates the natural geological process. Fragments of natural quartz crystal or high purity quartzite sand are used (Hale, 1975). The enclosed nature of the process, however, would seem to exclude a silica risk.

In concluding this section it should be pointed out that today circumstances in which dusts consist predominantly or wholly of free silica are likely to be few, though they still occur and are often unsuspected.

INCIDENCE AND PREVALENCE

Until the Second World War, silicosis was the most important and widespread form of pneumoconiosis. But since then, due mainly to substitution by other materials and hygienic measures, the incidence of new cases appears to have declined dramatically in the majority of industrial countries. But accurate statistics are rarely available as they are often based on compensation figures and, therefore, on selected cases; diagnostic criteria vary and, in some countries, coal pneumoconiosis is bracketed with 'silicosis'.

Furthermore, reliable information about the size of populations at risk is lacking.

As *Table 1.2* (p. 3) shows, the incidence of 'new' cases in the UK is low. In the USA, although the disease has been virtually eliminated from the Vermont granite (Hosey, Trasko and Ashe, 1957) and metal mining industries (Flinn *et al.*, 1963), there is reason to believe that the prevalence is not otherwise decreasing (Ayer, 1969). Some increase (often due to single industrial processes) has been reported in Bulgaria, Spain (WHO, 1968), Sweden (Ahlmark and Bruce, 1967) and Singapore (Khoo and Toh, 1968). In Finland there has been no change over a 30-year period ending in 1964, and it is anticipated that the annual number of new cases will rise in the next few years (Ahlman, 1968).

It is of interest that surveys of the granite industry in Cornwall and Devon in 1951 and 1961 (Hale and Sheers, 1963) showed little reduction in the silicosis risk and that Gründorfer and Raber (1970) found an increase among granite workers of lower Austria since 1958 due mainly to granite crushing for gravel production. Granite crushing is particularly hazardous when, as in Austria, it is a skilled and continuous occupation, but it is unlikely to be so when workers are casual and unskilled as, for example, they usually are in Sweden (Ahlmark, Bruce and Nyström, 1960) and the UK (Hale and Sheers, 1963).

Two surveys of monumental masons in Aberdeen disclosed a 10 per cent prevalence of silicosis in 1951 and 3 per cent in 1970, conglomerate lesions being present in 2 per cent of the former series but, absent in the latter (Lloyd Davies *et al.*, 1973). Discrete ('simple') pneumoconiosis, but no conglomerate ('massive') disease, was found in 1.6 per cent of 5684 workers in a recent survey of the British pottery industry (Fox *et al.*, 1975). However, it should be noted that the use of newly developed, powerful mechanical methods of excavating, tunnelling and quarrying and for dressing siliceous stones or concrete; or the addition of crushed or powdered quartz or flint to other materials in a variety of industrial processes may give rise to a serious, often unsuspected, silica hazard even if this only affects a small number of men. For example, silicosis—often in 'semi-acute' form—still appears to occur sporadically as a result of the use of 'silica flour' (*see* pp. 137 and 166) in the manufacture of abrasive soaps and cleansers, metal polishing compounds and autoclaved concrete blocks (Salam *et al.*, 1967; Nelson *et al.*, 1978; Zimmerman and Sinclair, 1977).

The ancient occupation of quarrying and fashioning sandstone grindstones in ill-ventilated pits and caves in northern Nigeria has resulted in a 39 per cent prevalence rate of silicosis (Warrell *et al.*, 1975), and the disease is also found in various stages among women in the Transkei District of South Africa who have used similar stones for many years to grind maize and corn (Palmer and Daynes, 1967). A recent survey of stone cutters in North India revealed a 35.2 per cent prevalence (Gupta *et al.*, 1972). These occupations are echoed by the ancient flint knapping industry in Brandon, Suffolk (UK) and the Meusnes district (Loir-et-Cher) in France in which flint nodules were split and shaped by hand with knapping and flaking hammers to produce bevelled flints about 1 × ¾ in in size for flint-lock guns (still used by 'black powder' enthusiasts) since the late seventeenth century. Though only small numbers of people were involved in the Brandon industry they suffered 'a terrible mortality from phthisis induced by flint dust generated in their work' and, at the turn of the century, 77.8 per cent of them died of 'phthisis' compared with 6.5 per cent of the general rural population in the area. Similar depredation occurred among the French knappers (Collis, 1915). Although no pathological details are known there is little doubt that silicosis was the disease in question. Dust counts of 1313 and 1192 particles (most of which were under 1 μm)/cm^3 of air were reported by Middleton (1930). Knapping in Brandon is now almost at an end but the trade is commemorated in the name and sign of a local inn (*Figure 7.1*).

An up-to-date report on workers in British mechanized iron foundries has shown that 'disabling' pneumoconiosis is now rare though there is a higher prevalence and rate of progression of pneumoconiosis (which, however, does not exceed Category 3 and was normally lower) in some occupations, notably fettlers, than in others (Joint Standing Committee on Health Safety and Welfare in Foundries, 1977).

In short, although the prevalence of silicosis has, in general, fallen significantly in the past 20 years it is still to be reckoned with in differential diagnosis and as a possible cause of respiratory disability.

Pathogenesis

The prevalence and severity of disease is chiefly determined by the intensity of exposure to free silica dust. For example, both are greater in sandstone than in granite workers because the quartz content of the former is significantly higher; and exposure to high concentrations in confined spaces over a short period—sometimes less than a year—may result in rapidly advancing and often fatal silicosis (Gardner, 1933; Bobear, Hanemann and Beven, 1962;

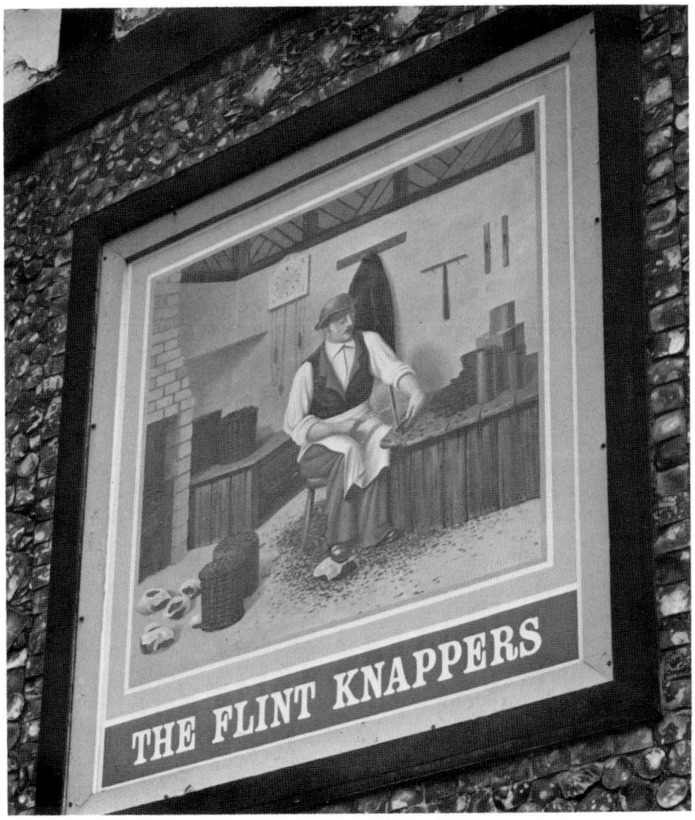

Figure 7.1 Inn sign at Brandon, Suffolk. Unworked flint nodules are seen on the floor to the left of the basket of finished gun-flints. The work place was poorly ventilated. Note the inn wall is constructed of flint nodules. (Reproduced by courtesy of the Managing Director of the Norwich Brewery, Limited)

Table 7.1 Prevalence of ANA in Relation to Radiographic Category in Silicosis of Sandblasters

Total number	*Small discrete nodules*		*Conglomerate lesions*					
			A		*B*		*C*	
	No	*%*	*No*	*%*	*No*	*%*	*No*	*%*
39	5/18	28	2/7	29	6/9	66	4/5	80
			X^2 P = 0.05					

Overall prevalence = 44% (17/39)
(Adapted with acknowledgement to Turner-Warwick *et al.*, 1977 and the Editor of *Ann. rheum. Dis.*)

Samimi, Weill and Ziskind, 1974). As pointed out on p. 66 experimental evidence suggests that cristobalite and tridymite are more fibrogenic than quartz, and observation of isolated cases in man tends to support this.

Silicosis appears to begin as a desquamative alveolitis (according, that is, to observations in baboons) and the evolution of the nodules consists of the formation and proliferation of collagenous fibrosis stimulated by the cytological events already discussed in Chapter 4, with subsequent hyalinization of the fibrous tissue. The possibility that lung reactive antibodies (*see* p. 61) might participate—at least in some cases—is suggested by the experimental observations that collagen is the primary antigen which reacts with lung antibodies (Burrell *et al.*, 1966) and that, *in vitro,* these antibodies stimulate macrophages to release a fibrogenic factor which prompts synthesis of collagen which, in turn, results in the production of more antigen (Lewis and Burrell, 1976). But, at present, there is no certainty that such events occur in man. And despite the fact that IgG and IgM have been recorded as occurring among, and bound to, the collagen fibres and fibrohyalin of human silicotic nodules (Pernis, 1968) Wagner and McCormick (1967) failed to identify the presence of RFs.

An unusually high prevalence of circulating ANAs related to increasing radiographic severity of disease has been demonstrated in sandblasters with silicosis (Jones *et al.,* 1976; Turner-Warwick *et al.,* 1977); and, although an increased prevalence of RFs was not found among African grindstone cutters with silicosis by Warrell *et al.* (1975), a slight increase has been observed in ceramic workers (Otto, 1969) and sandblasters with silicosis (*see Tables 4.3* and *7.1*). Certainly RF may be present, sometimes in high titre, in silicosis which exhibits sudden unexpected progression or enhanced activity in the absence of tuberculosis and irrespective of whether rheumatoid arthritis is present or not. The significance of these antibodies is uncertain but they may reflect the severity of macrophage destruction and release of the nuclear and other contents of these cells caused by free silica (*see* Chapter 4).

Other observations in men with silicosis caused by sand blasting have shown no reduction in total numbers of lymphocytes or the number of T and B cells in the peripheral blood and no impairment of delayed sensitivity to 'recall' antigens, such as PPD and *Candida* compared with control individuals. In addition, though there was no evident difference in *in vitro* responses of T cells to phytohaemagglutinin in the two groups, the responsiveness of these cells to low doses of conconavalin A was depressed in the silicotic group (Schuyler, Ziskind and Salvaggio, 1977). If, as has been suggested, this impairment indicates deficiency of suppressor T cells it could explain the development of auto-antibodies in silicosis and the occasional association of such autoimmune disorders as systemic sclerosis (*see* p. 157). But confirmation of this finding is needed.

The question as to whether a genetic influence may operate has been little investigated, but a survey of a large number of fluorspar miners and their families in Sardinia suggests that a predisposition for some persons to develop silicosis and for others to resist it may be genetically determined (Gedda *et al.,* 1964); and, indeed, a preliminary study of the HLA antigens in Caucasian men with silicosis indicates a decrease in B7 which could be linked to a greater propensity to silicosis by those who carry this antigen than those who do not (Gualde *et al.,* 1977). More detailed analysis of this important aspect of pathogenesis is awaited.

Pathology

Macroscopic appearances

The pulmonary pleura is usually thickened due to fibrosis and is often adherent to the parietal pleura especially over the upper lobes and in the vicinity of underlying conglomerate lesions. Thickening and symphysis may be extensive but only slight when there are no subpleural nodules.

Nodules are readily felt in the unopened lung and when it is cut are seen to vary from 2 to 6 mm in diameter, to have a whorled pattern (*Figure 7.2*) and to be grey-green to dark grey in colour. Similar lesions may be seen in the hilar nodes.

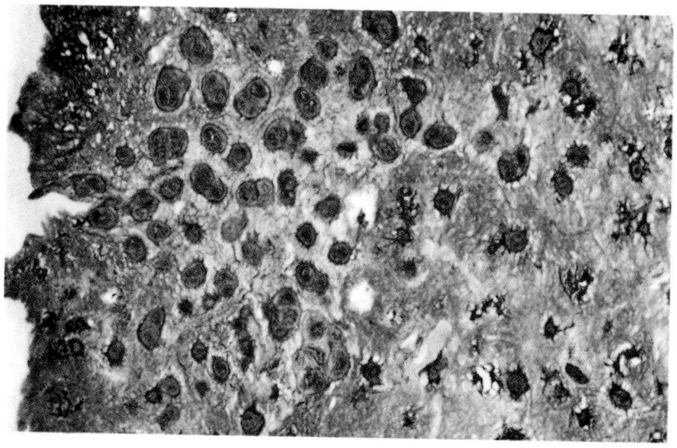

Figure 7.2 Natural size photograph of discrete silicotic nodules. Pigmentation is not uniform and a concentric pattern can be seen. There is no emphysema. (Whole lung section)

Both discrete nodules and conglomerations of nodules tend to be distributed more in the upper halves of the lungs than in the lower, and more in their posterior than anterior parts; but exceptions to this are seen. Rarely, they are largely confined to a narrow zone adjacent to the pulmonary pleura. When conglomerations of nodules (which may sometimes be large enough to occupy an upper lobe) are examined by reflected light, or in whole-lung section against transmitted light, they are clearly seen to consist of closely fused individual nodules (*Figure 7.3*).

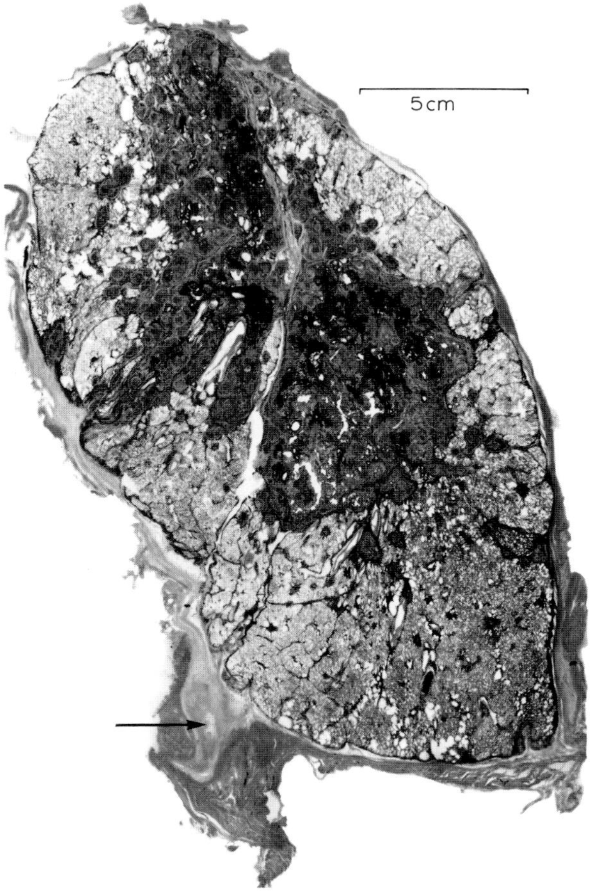

Figure 7.3 Conglomerate or massive silicosis. Matting of silicotic nodules many of which, with their whorled pattern, are still individually identifiable. Distribution is predominant in the upper parts of both lobes. Dense dust pigmentation is limited to a few areas and irregular (scar) emphysema is absent. Note widespread thickening of the pleura which is densely hyalinized in places (lighter areas) and there is a small zone of calcification (arrowed). (Whole sagittal section of left lung)

Unlike confluent coal pneumoconiosis (progressive massive fibrosis) conglomerate lesions only rarely develop cavities in the absence of tuberculosis. In some cases discrete nodules and conglomerations are found subpleurally and when the conglomerate lesions are calcified and fused to dense pleural fibrosis, the lung is locally encased; this is sometimes referred to as 'cuirasse' (armour plate). Occasionally, a large unilateral conglomerate nodular mass occurs with little other evidence of silicosis (Fiumicelli, Fiumicelli and Pagni, 1964).

The gross appearances of nodular silicosis are quite distinct from those of coal pneumoconiosis but silicotic lesions are sometimes found in the lungs of coal-miners who have done much drilling of siliceous rock seams (*see* Chapter 8).

Enlarged and fixed hilar and paratracheal lymph nodes occasionally cause distortion of the trachea, the main bronchi and branches of the pulmonary arteries near the hila (Pump, 1968), and similar pulmonary lymph nodes may restrict bronchial movements.

There appears to be a clear correlation between the amount of quartz/100 g of lymph node tissue and the degree of calcification, and the possibility of endocrine disturbances playing some part in pathogenesis has been raised (Einbrodt and Burilkov, 1972).

Microscopic appearances

Dust particles are found either in macrophages or in the naked state in the walls of alveoli—chiefly those of respiratory bronchioles—and collected in perivascular areas. Cell death, fibroblast proliferation and reticulin formation occurs. The walls of affected alveoli are thereby thickened, in some places sufficiently to obliterate neighbouring alveolar spaces. Collagenous fibrosis follows in a concentric arrangement. Subsequently, much of the collagen becomes 'hyalinized' and the resulting near-spherical nodules consist of concentrically arranged, or whorled zones of acellular hyaline which are enclosed by a moderately cellular collagenous capsule; the cells are macrophages (which often contain carbon particles) and plasma cells (*Figure 7.4*). Giant cells are not seen. Silicotic hyaline resembles amyloid in having a higher content of carbohydrate and phospholipids than other forms of hyaline, and is weakly birefringent.

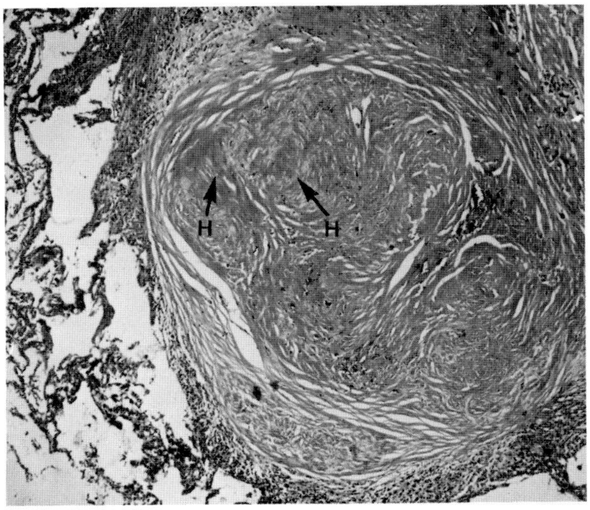

Figure 7.4 Microsection of a typical silicotic nodule showing the concentric ('onion skin') arrangement of collagen fibres, some of which are hyalinized (H), lack of dust pigmentation and the cellularity of the periphery. The lesion is clearly demarcated from adjacent lung tissue which is substantially normal. The appearances are those of a proliferation process. Compare with lesions of coal pneumoconiosis and asbestosis. (Original magnification × 55; H and E stain)

Silicotic nodules, by contrast with the lesions of coal pneumoconiosis (*see* Chapter 8), are 'proliferative' in that they contain an excess of collagen but little dust; indeed, the higher the quartz content of a dust the smaller the amount of dust required to produce a given severity of fibrosis (*see Figure 4.10*) (Nagelschmidt, 1965), and the longer quartz particles are retained in the lungs, the greater the fibrosis and the smaller the quantity necessary to cause fibrosis (Einbrodt, 1965). Continuous exposure to dust causes existing nodules to increase in size and new ones to form. But this progression may occur long after exposure has ceased and may be due either to a self-perpetuating tendency for quartz-containing macrophages to migrate and die in and around existing lesions (Heppleston, 1962) or to the intervention of a secondary immunological reaction. The distinguishing features between typical and 'rheumatoid' silicotic nodules are referred to in a later section in this chapter and between silicotic nodules, 'rheumatoid' coal nodules and tuberculous lesions in Chapter 8.

Silica content

The silica content of normal lungs with no exposure to industrial dusts has been found to be about 0.1 to 0.2 per cent of dried tissue and that of normal hilar lymph nodes to range from 0.23 to 0.6 per cent of dried tissue. The content of silicotic lungs is commonly about 2 to 3 per cent but may be as high as 20 per cent of the dried weight (Sweany, Porsche and Douglass, 1936; Fowweather, 1939) (*see Figure 4.10*.

Alveoli in proximity to silicotic nodules are usually of normal size; occasionally scar (irregular) emphysema is seen, but is exceptional and of slight order as the nodules are proliferative and expanding. Associated centrilobular emphysema is not seen.

Nodules tend to occur in clusters and may subsequently fuse into conglomerations of varying size. These conglomerations are not amorphous masses, for individual nodules do not wholly lose their identity. It is to be noted that calcification (which is sometimes pronounced) may occur in some nodules in the absence of tuberculosis or histoplasmosis, the insoluble calcium salts being deposited mainly in the central hyaline (Moreschi, Farina and Chiappinio, 1968). Central necrosis of conglomerate masses occasionally occurs in the absence of complicating tuberculosis apparently as a result of ischaemic changes.

Quartz particles can be demonstrated in variable amount in the central zone of the nodules and as a halo round their periphery by accurately orientated polarized light (*see* Appendix) or by dark ground microscopy after microincineration of the lesions, but they are absent from the collagenous capsule.

The growth of peribronchiolar silicotic nodules may narrow or obliterate these airways, and perivascular nodules may cause obstruction of lymphatics and arteritis with eventual obliteration of some vessels and destruction of their walls. Larger elastic arteries are rarely obstructed but may be compressed.

In the rare case in which silicosis develops rapidly from the start—sometimes following work with free silica in a finely divided state—and in which some additional unidentified determining factor (probably immunological) may play a part, the nodules are very numerous, small and lack the ordered, compact pattern of typical nodules (*Figure 7.5a*).

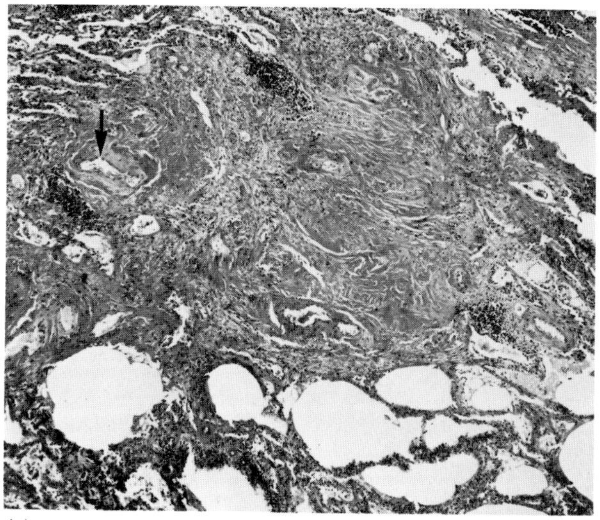

(*a*)

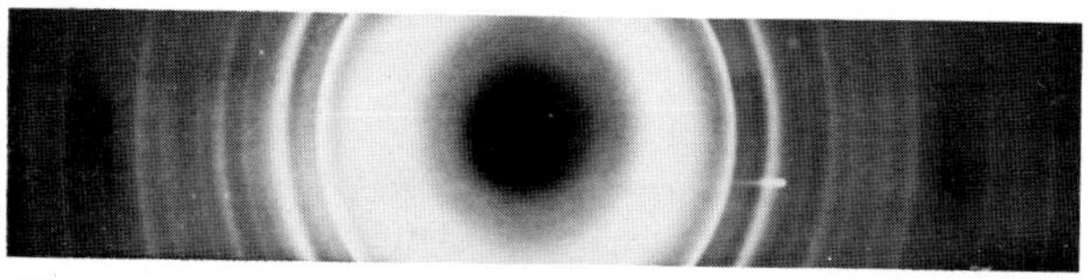

(*b*)

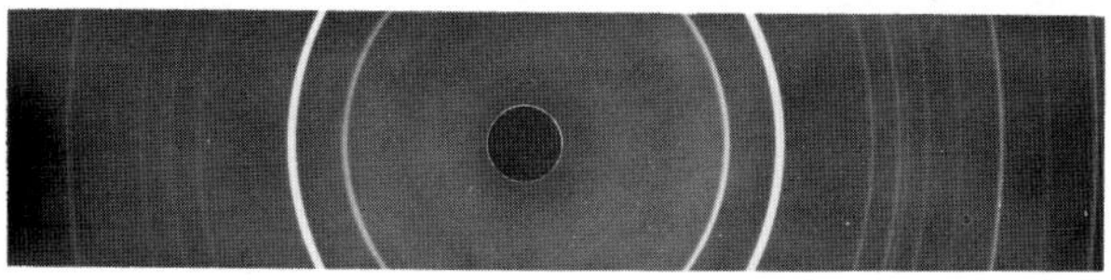

(*c*)

Figure 7.5 (a) Microsection of a representative lesion of rapidly developing atypical silicosis in a man exposed to high concentrations of uncalcined quartzite sands. There is only a suggestion of the ordered pattern which characterizes typical silicotic nodules and the fibrosis, which engulfs and artery (arrowed) and is partly hyalinized, extends in places into alveolar walls so that clear demarcation from normal lung is lacking. Numerous plasma cells were present adjacent to these lesions. Occasional typical silicotic nodules were also present elsewhere in the lungs. See Figure 7.14 *for radiographic features. (Original magnification × 55. H and E stain.) (b) X-ray diffraction of lung dust shows a strong quartz pattern. (Analysis by Dr F.D. Pooley, Cardiff.) (c) Standard quartz pattern*

Much of the dust reaching the lymphatics passes to the hilar lymph nodes, but some travels to the internal mammary nodes and to more distant extra-thoracic nodes, notably the supraclavicular, cervical and abdominal aortic groups. Particles gaining entry to the systemic blood stream may give rise to isolated nodules in the spleen (Belt, 1939) and liver (Lynch, 1942), but are too few to cause any functional damage; however, if calcified they may be radiographically visible.

Affected lymph nodes contain dense fibrosis or typical nodules with quartz particles. The capsular and peripheral regions of these nodes may calcify and resemble the shell of an egg. This change may appear early or late in relation to the evolution of the lung lesions, and may be present when silicotic lung disease is negligible. It has been suggested that this is due to an unusual propensity to deposit calcium salts (Chiesura, Terribile and Bardellini, 1968). There is no evidence that tuberculous infection is involved.

Tuberculosis

That silicosis predisposes to pulmonary tuberculosis has been established since the beginning of the century and in those days the majority of silicotics succumbed to it. In 1937 Gardner found evidence of co-existent tuberculosis in 65 to 75 per cent of silicotics from various industries. In recent years the rate has fallen dramatically in parallel with the general decline of tuberculosis but, nevertheless, it is still in excess of that in the general population. Bailey *et al.* (1974) observed ten cases (12 per cent), eight of whom died of silico-tuberculosis, in 83 New Orleans sandblasters. Predominant involvement of the lower lobes was unusually common. The more advanced the silicosis the greater the incidence of active tuberculosis is likely to be (Chatgidakis, 1963).

The enhancing effect of 'free silica' upon tuberculosis was demonstrated experimentally by Gardner (1929) by the reactivation of previously induced and healing tuberculous lesions in guinea-pig lungs after inhalation of a quartz aerosol, and by the production of tuberculous lesions in guinea pigs by a normally non-pathogenic strain of tubercle bacillus (R1) in the presence of quartz (Gardner, 1934). More recent experiments have confirmed the potentiating effect of quartz upon tuberculosis in guinea pigs (Policard *et al.*, 1967) and the demonstration that this occurs at macrophage level has been referred to already in Chapter 4.

'Rheumatoid' silicotic nodules

Nodules of larger than average size (that is, 3 to 5 mm diameter), frequently with light grey necrotic centres, may be found in the lungs of silicotic subjects in whom rheumatoid arthritis or circulating rheumatoid factor without arthritis were present in life. The association was noted by Clerens (1953) and Colinet (1953) in women exposed to a free silica hazard, and the pathology has been described in miners of siliceous rocks and others (Chatgidakis and Theron, 1961; Lamvik, 1963). To the naked eye the lesions look like tuberculous nodules and are easily misinterpreted as such, but acid-fast bacilli cannot be identified microscopically, nor can *M. tuberculosis* be isolated by culture or guinea-pig inoculation. In geographical areas where histoplasmosis is endemic this may be diagnosed in error but histoplasma cannot be identified in the nodules (Gough, 1959). Unlike the nodules of 'rheumatoid' coal pneumoconiosis, concentric black rings of deposited coal particles or other pigmented dust are either absent or feeble (*see Figure 7.16e* and Chapter 8). They are usually scattered discretely but are occasionally seen in conglomerations.

Microscopically, the lesions consist of an acidophilic, acellular necrotic centre in which there are the remains of collagen fibres, and at the periphery of the necrosis, fibroblasts are arranged in palisade form, although less prominently than in rheumatoid subcutaneous nodules. External to these is a zone of polymorphonuclear leucocytes and macrophages and there may be clefts containing cholesterol crystals. These are not seen in non-rheumatoid silicotic nodules. Outside this active zone are arranged normal reticulin and collagen fibres in various stages of maturation and numerous plasma cells, lymphocytes and fibroblasts, but no giant cells. Endarteritis, consisting mainly of plasma cells and lymphocytes, is found in close proximity to the lesions. When activity in the nodules has ceased they may, like 'pure' silicotic nodules, become calcified.

Eleven cases (2 per cent) of 'rheumatoid modified' silicotic nodules were found in 576 autopsies on European gold-miners studied at the Johannesburg Pneumoconiosis Research Unit (Chatgidakis and Theron, 1961). In general, however, the prevalence of 'rheumatoid silicosis' may be lower than this.

Clinical features

Symptoms

It is important to emphasize that there may be no symptoms even though the radiographic appearances may be surprisingly advanced.

Cough may develop as the disease advances and is of variable severity, mainly in the mornings but sometimes intermittently throughout the day and night. In the later stages there may be prolonged and distressing paroxysms due, possibly, to irritation of nerve receptors in the trachea and bronchi by silicotic lymph node masses.

Often there is no sputum or only a small quantity of mucoid appearance raised from time to time during the day. However, in advanced disease recurrent bronchial infections tend to occur and produce quite a large volume of purulent sputum. There is no haemoptysis in the absence of other complicating disease.

Unless there is accompanying chronic obstructive bronchitis or allergic asthma there is no wheeze, although some patients who have narrowing, distortion and fixity of the trachea and main bronchi caused by contiguous silicotic nodes may complain of stridor (*see* next section), especially during effort when there is increased velocity of air flow. This is an uncommon symptom.

Breathlessness occurs as the disease advances, first during pronounced effort and later with lesser degrees of effort; it is rarely complained of at rest unless other lung disease is present. The presence and severity of dyspnoea and impairment of lung function correlates poorly with radiographic appearances.

Chest pain is not a feature of silicosis.

General health is unimpaired unless tuberculosis or congestive heart failure supervenes. Haemoptysis and loss of weight may signal the presence of tuberculosis.

Physical signs

The general physical condition is good but deteriorates with the onset of congestive heart failure and in the presence of tuberculosis. Central cyanosis is absent unless there is complicating heart or lung disease, and dyspnoea at rest suggests disease other than silicosis.

Finger clubbing is not caused by silicosis and when observed is either of congenital type or evidence of other pathology.

The chest contour is usually normal but in advanced disease there may be localized flattening of one upper zone possibly with some degree of dorsal scoliosis. Expansion remains good and equal until a late stage of the disease when it may be somewhat diminished often on one side (where underlying fibrosis is greater) more than the other.

The trachea is sometimes displaced to one side either by silicotic hilar node masses or a large distorted conglomerate mass in an upper lobe. Occasionally, hard, non-tender, silicotic lymph nodes are palpable in the neck and supraclavicular fossae.

Percussion note is unaffected unless there are areas of unusually dense pleural fibrosis—chiefly in the upper zones.

Breath sounds are normal or reduced by pleural thickening, and inspiratory and expiratory stridor (of greater or lesser intensity) may be heard over the trachea and at the open mouth when there is excessive distortion of trachea or main bronchi; when this sign is present it is persistent.

Adventitious sounds are not heard in disease uncomplicated by chronic obstructive bronchitis or tuberculosis.

In the advanced stage of silicosis the signs of pulmonary heart disease may eventually develop with or without those of congestive heart failure.

Investigations

Lung function

In the early radiographic stages (ILO Category 2 to 3) impairment of any parameter of lung function is generally absent but in some cases slight reduction in VC and of arterial oxygen tension (on effort) may be observed. With more advanced disease, impairment is commonly present but often of a much less degree than the radiographic category might suggest. There is a decrease of TLC, VC, RV, FRC and compliance without evidence of airways obstruction and, in some cases, a slight reduction in gas transfer, although this is often remarkably little affected even in the presence of advanced disease. Oxygen desaturation is not present at rest or on moderate effort (300 kg.m/min) in the non-conglomerate stage of disease (Becklake, du Preez and Lutz, 1958), but may be observed on greater effort in some cases. As the disease progresses to massive conglomeration inequality of gas distribution and of ventilation–perfusion ratio occurs resulting in some impairment of Tl in addition to the volume changes mentioned. However, in a study of non-smoking men with non-conglomerate ('simple') silicosis Tl was not reduced and even in those with Category B and C conglomeration Kco was normal in most cases (Tećulescu and Stănescu, 1970). Ventilation–perfusion imbalance and arterial oxygen desaturation on effort are determined by the extent of arteritis as well as by silicotic fibrosis.

The best overall guide to the degree of respiratory disability in conglomerate disease is the ventilatory capacity.

There is nothing characteristic in the patterns of impaired function in silicosis.

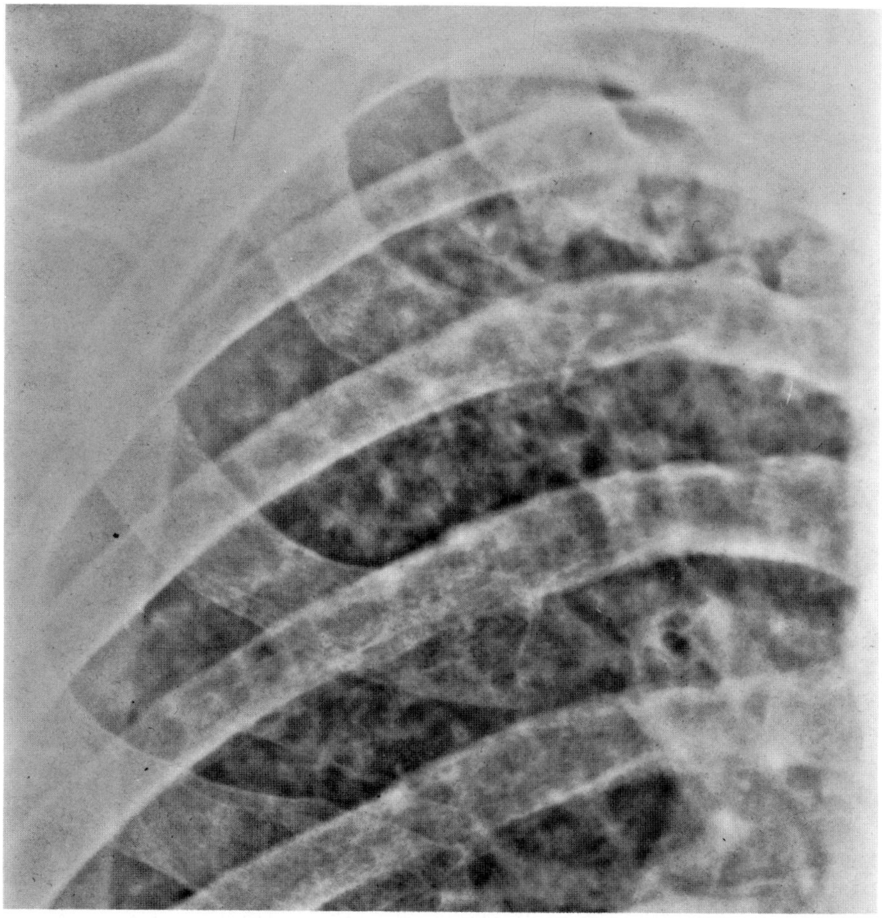

Figure 7.6 Discrete radiographic opacities of typical silicosis at an early stage. Category 'q' (Natural size)

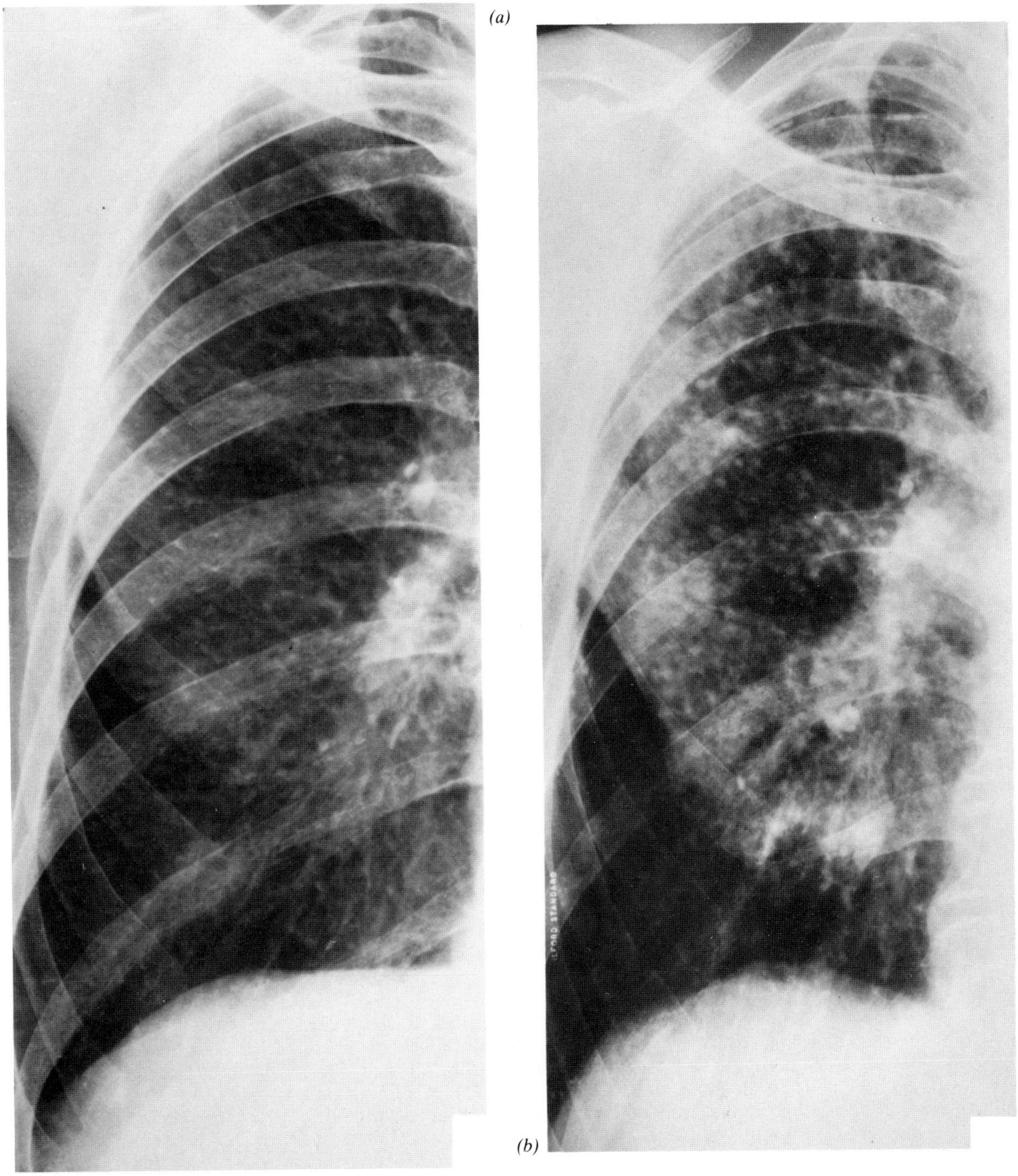

(a)

(b)

Figure 7.7(a) and (b) Progression of discrete 'nodules' of silicosis from low category 1q (1/0) to 2q (2/2) over 10 years (1958–1968). Slate quarry worker

Radiographic appearances

The earliest radiographic evidence of nodular silicosis consists of small discrete opacities of moderate radiodensity which appear in the upper halves of the lung fields and vary from 1 to 3 mm diameter (ILO Category 'p' and 'q') (*Figure 7.6*). It has been claimed, however, that linear opacities accompanying the normal vascular markings are the earliest evidence of silicosis but this is not generally accepted (Ashford and Enterline, 1966), and these appearances (of which it is difficult to be convinced) do not correlate with morbid anatomical evidence of silicosis.

There appears to be a clear relationship between total dust exposure and radiographic evidence of silicosis (Beadle, 1971).

As the disease advances, discrete opacities increase in number and size (ILO Category 'r') and occupy the lower as well as the other zones of the lung fields (*Figure 7.7*). In

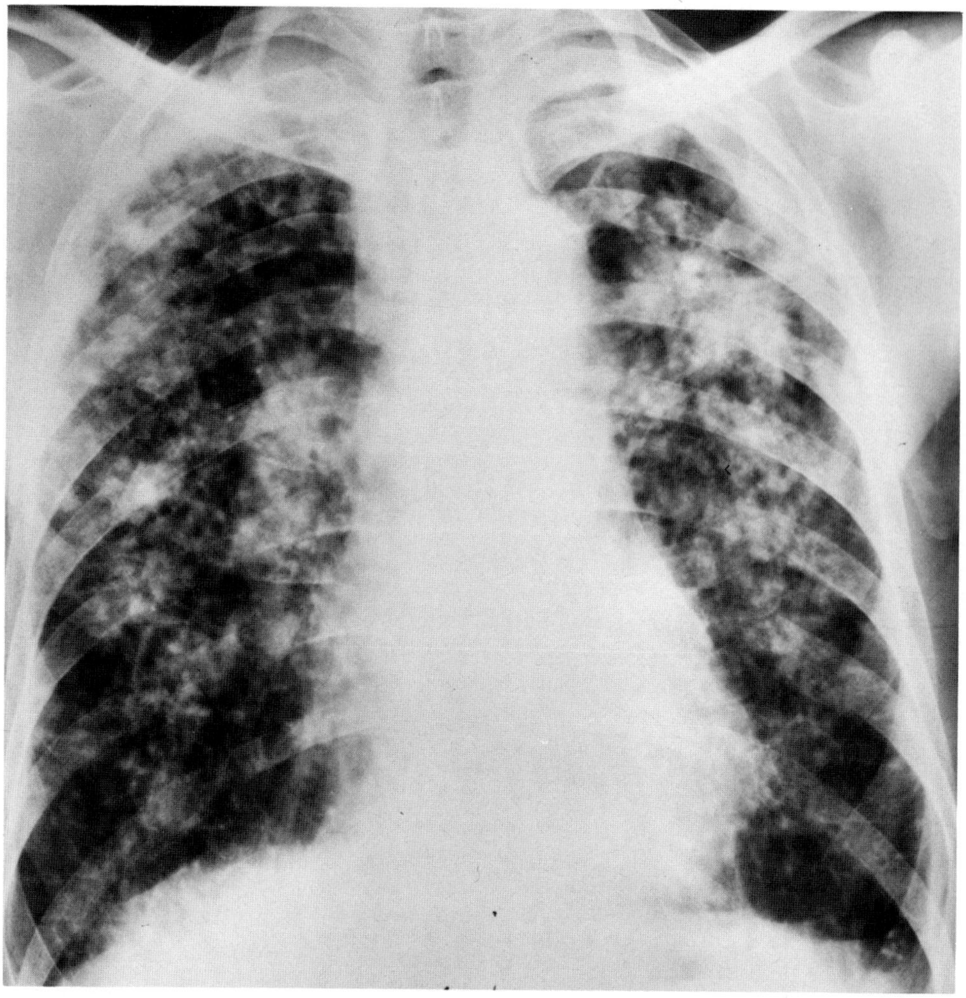

Figure 7.8 Moderately advanced silicosis with bilateral conglomeration. Note bilateral apical thickening of the pleura. Hilar node calcification is not evident. Foundry sandblaster for 16 years and fettler for five years

general they are roughly symmetrical in the two fields but are sometimes of disparate size and distribution. Small conglomerations (ILO Category A) may then appear—usually, but not always, in the upper zones—and subsequently develop into large, irregular and sometimes massive opacities which may occupy the greater part of both lung fields (*Figures 7.8* and *7.9*). Bullae may be seen in the vicinity of conglomerations and in some cases there may be significant bowing and distortion of the trachea (*Figure 7.9*). Cavity formation in the absence of complicating tuberculosis is uncommon. Rarely, unilateral conglomeration is present in the absence of other evidence of silicosis. The curious tendency for the silicotic masses in Lipari pumice workers to occupy the lower lung fields is referred to in Chapter 9.

Occasionally the discrete opacities are small and very dense and may closely resemble the appearances of the calcified nodules seen in some cases of 'rheumatoid' coal pneumoconiosis (*see* Chapter 8, p. 265) and in microlithiasis (*Figure 7.10*).

An important feature of some cases is evidence of lymph node calcification which is characterized by thin, very dense ring shadows around the nodes—so-called 'egg-shell' calcification (*Figures 7.11* and *7.12*). Nodes most commonly involved are those of the hilar and mediastinal groups but other intrathoracic nodes (for example, the internal mammary chain) and extrathoracic nodes (notably the supraclavicular, cervical and axillary groups and occasionally the intra-abdominal and inguinal groups) may also be affected (Polacheck and Pijanowski, 1960) (*Figure 7.13*). Curiously, there appears to be no correlation between the intensity of the calcification and the amount of silicosis or the presence of pulmonary tuberculosis (Chiesura, Terribile and Bardellini, 1968). Calcification may be prominent when there is little or no obvious lung involvement, or absent in the presence of advanced silicosis (*Figures 7.11* and *7.8*). Although not a pathognomonic sign—as it is seen occasionally in sarcoidosis, tuberculosis and histoplasmosis—predominantly peripheral calcification of hilar nodes is highly suggestive of silicosis or of exposure to some form of free silica.

Evidence of diffuse bilateral pleural fibrosis is present in many cases and in advanced disease may be extensive and partly calcified; occasionally calcified thickening occurs with little obvious lung disease (*Figures 7.8* and *7.13*).

The radiographic appearances of the rare cases of silicosis which develop exceptionally quickly (*see* Microscopic appearances) bear little resemblance to those of typical

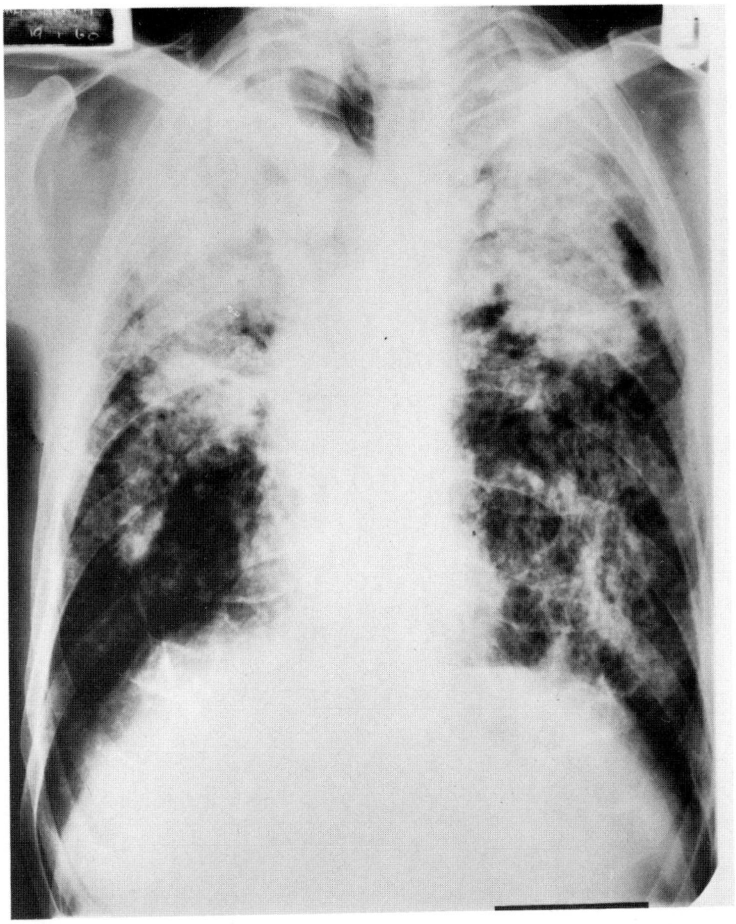

Figure 7.9 Massive silicotic conglomeration with bilateral upper zone pleural thickening and displacement of trachea to the right. Crusherman in granite quarry for 26 years

silicosis. Opacities are numerous, widespread, small and ill-defined, and spontaneous pneumothoraces are apt to occur (*Figure 7.14*).

Though the different patterns of behaviour of silicosis appear to be determined mainly by the amount of siliceous dust inhaled, idiosyncratic reaction, as stated already on p. 142, also seems to be involved. In general, sudden changes are most likely to be due to complicating tuberculosis but occasionally they are associated with rheumatoid disease. The typical appearances of Caplan-type necrobiotic nodules (*see* Chapter 8) are very uncommon, but have been reported (Chiesura, Bruguone and Mezzanotte, 1961; Gambini, Agnoletto and Magistretti, 1964; Lamvik, 1963) (*Figure 7.15*). Occasionally large, ill-defined opacities

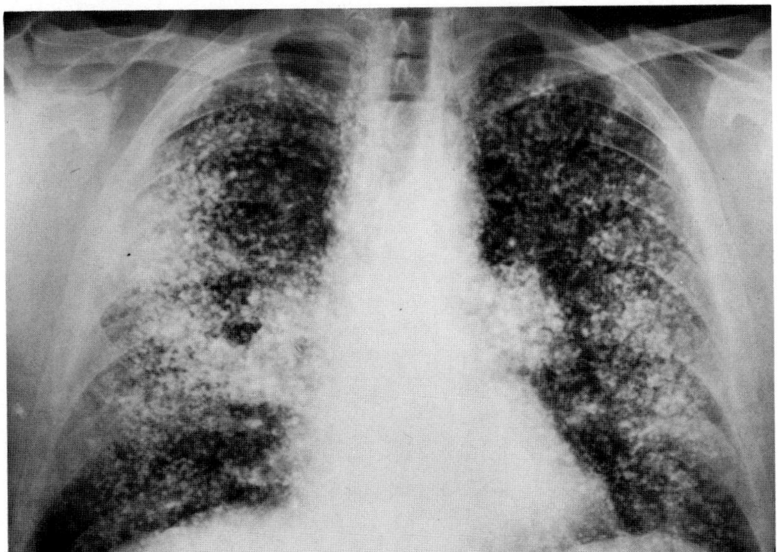

Figure 7.10 Multiple, dense, small opacities. Many of the nodules were calcified. Refractory brick worker for five years and granite quarry worker for three years

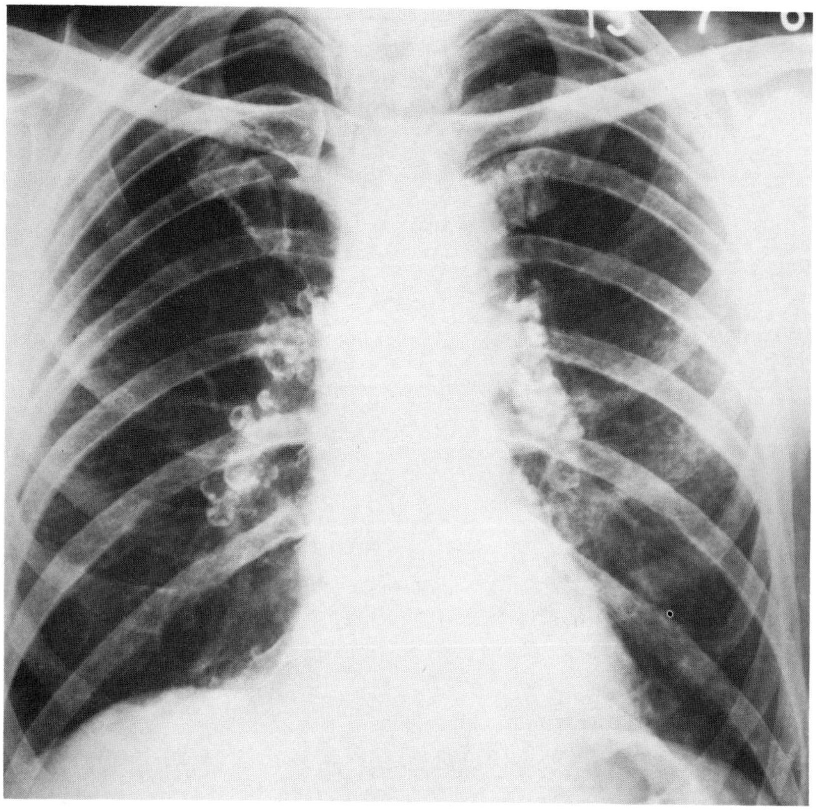

Figure 7.11 Bilateral hilar node, 'egg-shell' type calcification in a slate worker for 43 years. Note absence of evidence of intra-pulmonary disease and pleural thickening

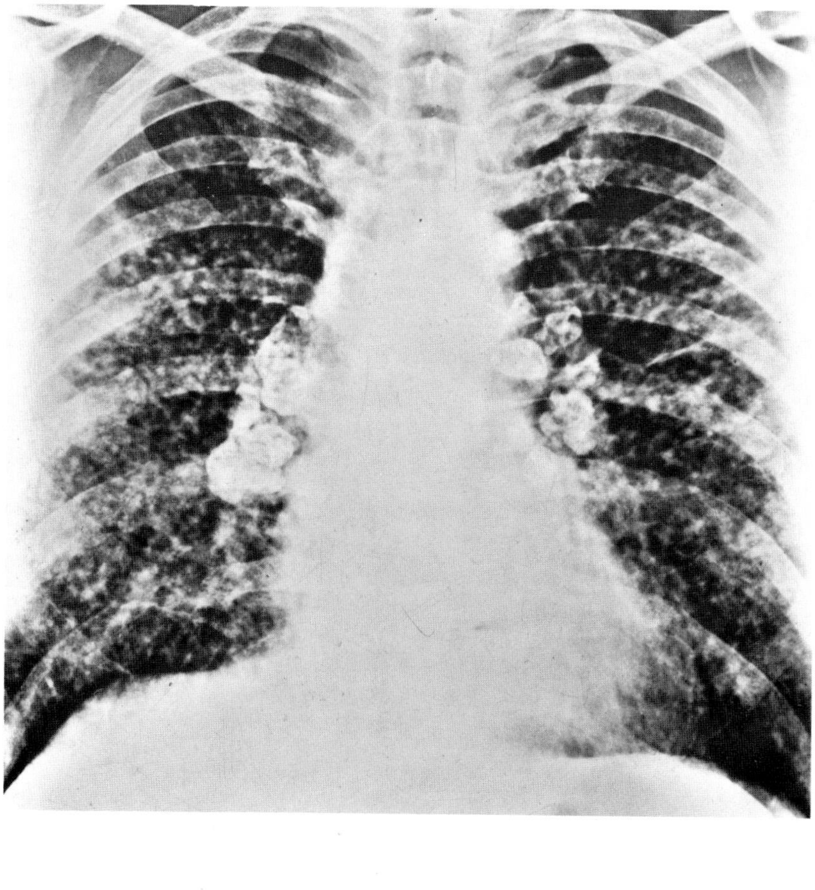

Figure 7.12 Gross egg-shell calcification of hilar nodes with category 3q discrete silicotic pulmonary lesions. Slate rock-man for 32 years, North Wales

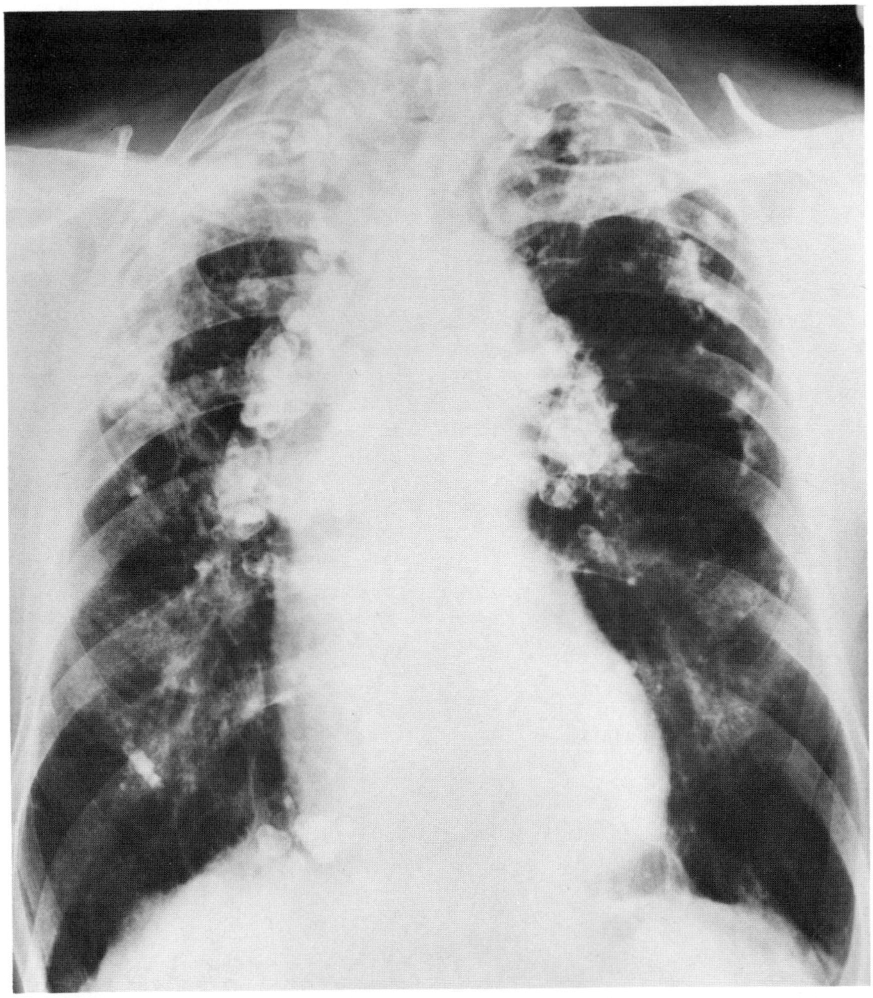

Figure 7.13 Extensive egg-shell calcification of the hilar, paratracheal, cervical (above the clavicles) and internal mammary nodes (right cardiophrenic angle). There is also bilateral irregular, pleural calcification in the upper zones and, to a lesser extent, in the middle zone but little evidence of intrapulmonary fibrosis. Kiln worker in silica brick works of 20 years

develop rapidly, exhibit vaccillant behaviour over subsequent years, and are sometimes associated with recurrent, transient pleural effusions in individuals with active rheumatoid arthritis or with high titres of circulating RF without overt arthropathy (*Figure 7.16*).

It is rarely necessary to use radiographic techniques other than PA, AP and lateral views for diagnosis, though tomography may be helpful in demonstrating silicotuberculous cavities. Bronchography may reveal bronchial distortion, filling defects and localized bronchiectasis in cases with conglomerate masses.

Bronchial arteriography demonstrates the presence of bronchial artery enlargement and bronchopulmonary shunts in areas of conglomerate masses but not in discrete nodular disease (Tada *et al.*, 1974).

Other investigations

Biopsy of lung tissue should not be required for diagnosis, although examination of a scalene lymph node may resolve occasional problematical cases by demonstrating silicotic nodules.

It is advisable to obtain samples of sputum for culture of *M. tuberculosis* periodically, for life, as tuberculosis may develop at any time.

Tests for circulating rheumatoid and antinuclear antibodies, when positive, suggest the possibility of an underlying immunological cause for suddenly advancing tuberculosis-negative silicosis.

Electrocardiography may be required in advanced cases to establish or refute the presence of cor pulmonale.

Investigations for sarcoidosis may be indicated on rare occasions to distinguish the two diseases (*see* next section).

The erythrocyte sedimentation rate is not raised in the absence of complicating tuberculosis or other disease.

Diagnosis

When a satisfactory occupational history is combined with good-quality radiographs, nodular silicosis should rarely be mistaken for other diseases. The chief cause of misdiagnosis is failure to recognize the 'silica' hazard of a past occupation, and the fact that the prevalence of silicosis is now low increases the possibility of this error.

An isolated conglomerate lesion (so-called 'silicoma') may be confused with bronchial carcinoma, especially in a first radiograph. Tomography may help in the distinction by revealing multiple small densities within a silicotic mass.

When silicotic lung lesions and hilar and pulmonary lymph nodes are calcified it is necessary to exclude:

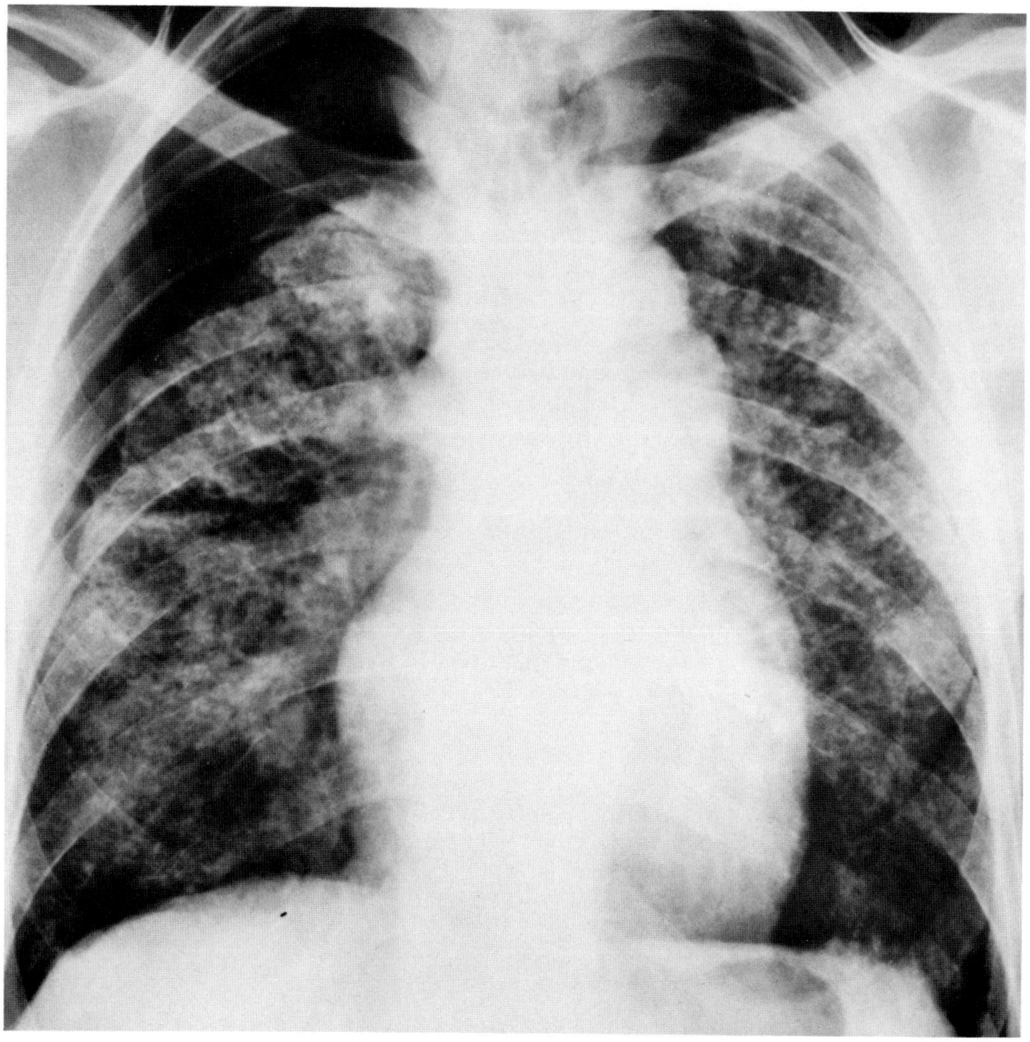

Figure 7.14 Film of case illustrated in Figure 7.5. *Opacities are numerous but small and indefinite unlike those caused by nodular silicosis. Bilateral pneumothoraces are present. The patient was in good health two years before death. Although there was no arthropathy latex fixation test was positive, circulating ANA present and serum IgG much increased. Thus, immunological activity may have featured in the development of this disease. (Radiograph by courtesy of Dr K. P. Goldman)*

(a) Tuberculosis
(b) Histoplasmosis
(c) Sarcoidosis. Confusion should rarely arise here but it has to be remembered that pulmonary and hilar node sarcoid lesions may calcify (Israel *et al.,* 1961; Scadding, 1967) and present a similar radiographic appearance, and non-calcified silicotic lesions in women (from past work in the pottery industry, for example) might initially be confused with sarcoidosis.
(d) Pulmonary alveolar microlithiasis. This rare disorder may occasionally be stimulated radiographically by silicosis when the lesions are very small and calcified (*Figure 7.10*).
(e) Calcified lung lesions as a sequela of chicken pox are usually few in number, small (about 2 to 3 mm diameter) and are not accompanied by the egg-shell sign of hilar node calcification.

Silicosis is unlikely to be confused with lung cancer but it may obscure the early signs of tumour development.

Complications

Tuberculosis and other infections

Silicosis is the only pneumoconiosis which predisposes to the development of tuberculosis. Although the incidence of tuberculosis in silicosis has fallen dramatically since the 1950s it is still the most common complication. It may occur at any stage in the evolution of silicosis, but is most likely in the fifth and later decades in association with a moderate to severe degree of silicosis (Chatgidakis, 1963; Jones, Owen and Corrado, 1967).

In the early stage of the tuberculous disease it is difficult or impossible to recognize any change in the established radiographic appearance of silicosis, and there may be no symptoms; a recently developed cough with scanty greenish sputum may, however, give a warning signal. Subsequently the characteristic symptoms develop, sometimes with haemoptysis. Rapid radiographic changes consistent with

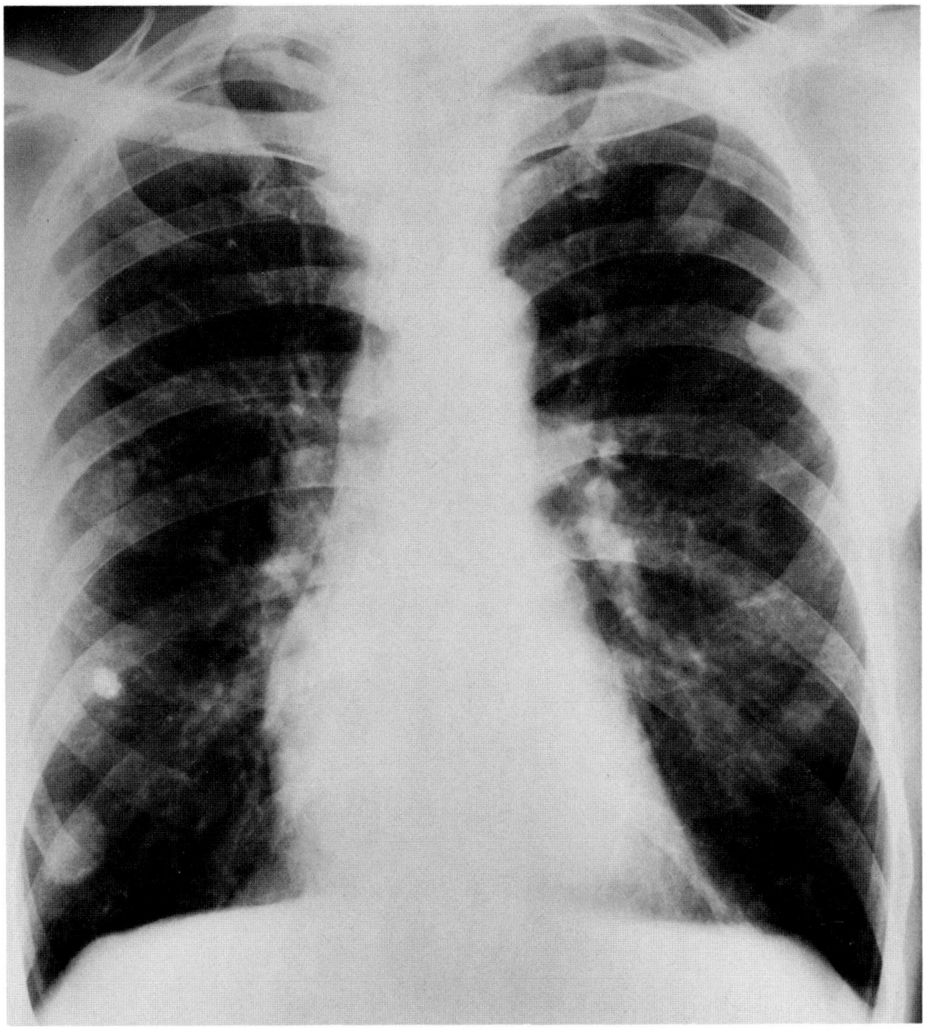

*Figure 7.15 Well circumscribed round opacities similar to those of Caplan's syndrome in coal workers (*see Figure 8.31*). Patient worked as a dipper in vitreous enamelling for seven years and crusher of reject pottery (containing free silica and china clay) for the manufacture of refractory enamel for ten years. Note cavity in lesion in left mid-zone and absence of discrete small nodules of silicosis. Rheumatoid arthritis developed 15 years before this film was taken. Circulating RF present. No evidence of tuberculosis. Lung biopsy confirmed rheumatoid nodules*

tuberculosis are then seen, possibly with evidence of cavitation. When the disease is of indolent nature, or after healing, scar emphysema with bullae may be detected radiographically in the areas of fibrosis.

Regular routine sputum cultures are, therefore, necessary in cases of silicosis and should be done immediately if rapid radiographic change—no matter how small—is observed.

It must be remembered, however, that photochromogenic and non-photochromogenic mycobacteria are sometimes isolated from the sputum of silicotic subjects (Schepers *et al.*, 1958). These organisms may occasionally be found in association with *M. tuberculosis* (Palmhert, Webster and Lens, 1968) and, in general, are probably not pathogenic, but *M. avium* (*see* Chapter 4) is a serious, if rare, complication and is poorly sensitive to antituberculous therapy; *M. kansasii* is also pathogenic. Infection by different 'opportunist' mycobacteria has been reported in 37 per cent of foundry workers with silicosis (Rosenzweig, 1967), and by *M. kansasii* in 11 per cent of silicotic sandblasters (Bailey *et al.*, 1974). The pathogenicity of these organisms is probably potentiated by quartz and other forms of free silica and the importance of distinguishing these organisms from *M. tuberculosis* is evident. Their prevalence is likely to vary according to geographical locality.

A residual tuberculous or ischaemic cavity in a conglomerate silicotic mass may be colonized by the *Aspergillus* species. The organism is usually *A. fumigatus;* occasionally, *A. niger, flavus* or *nidulans*. As a rule circulating precipitating antibodies to the relevant organisms are present but, in a few cases, are absent. The characteristic radiographic appearance of aspergilloma as a cavity containing a central density (due to a fungus ball) partly or wholly surrounded by a 'halo' of air may be seen and should alert the physician to the diagnosis. However, a proportion of such aspergillomata are first identified post mortem. Slight, recurrent haemoptysis is fairly common

(a)

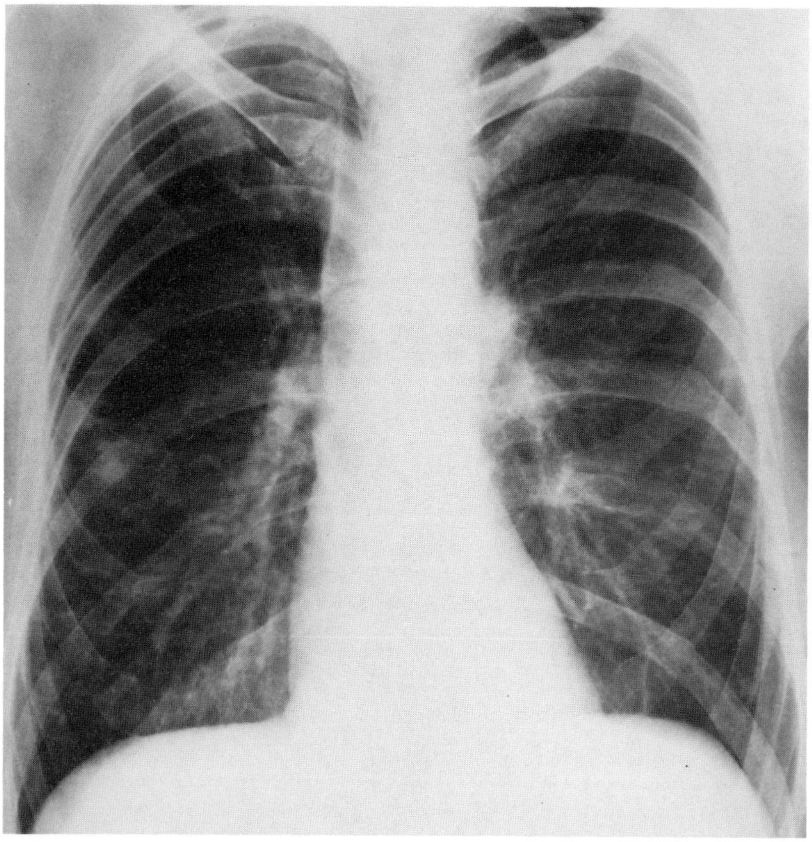

Figure 7.16(a) 1967: Single small opacity and slight pleural thickening right lower zone

(b)

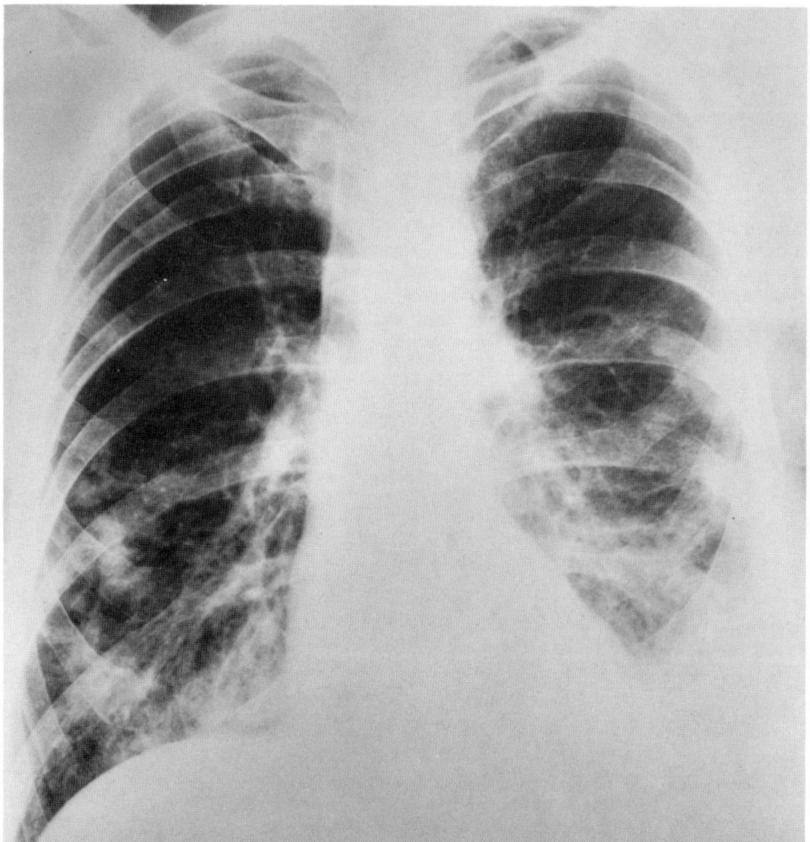

Figure 7.16(b) 1970: Multiple, ill-defined, dense opacities both middle and lower zones with pleural effusion on left

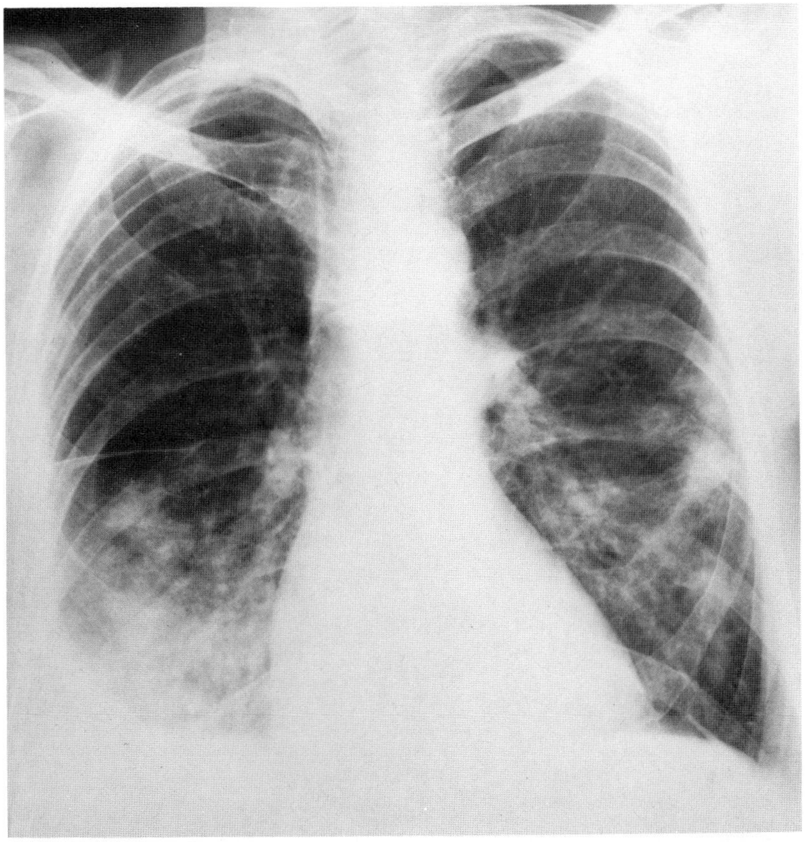

Figure 7.16(c) 1972: Some increase in size of lower zone opacities; right pleural effusion has now developed

(c)

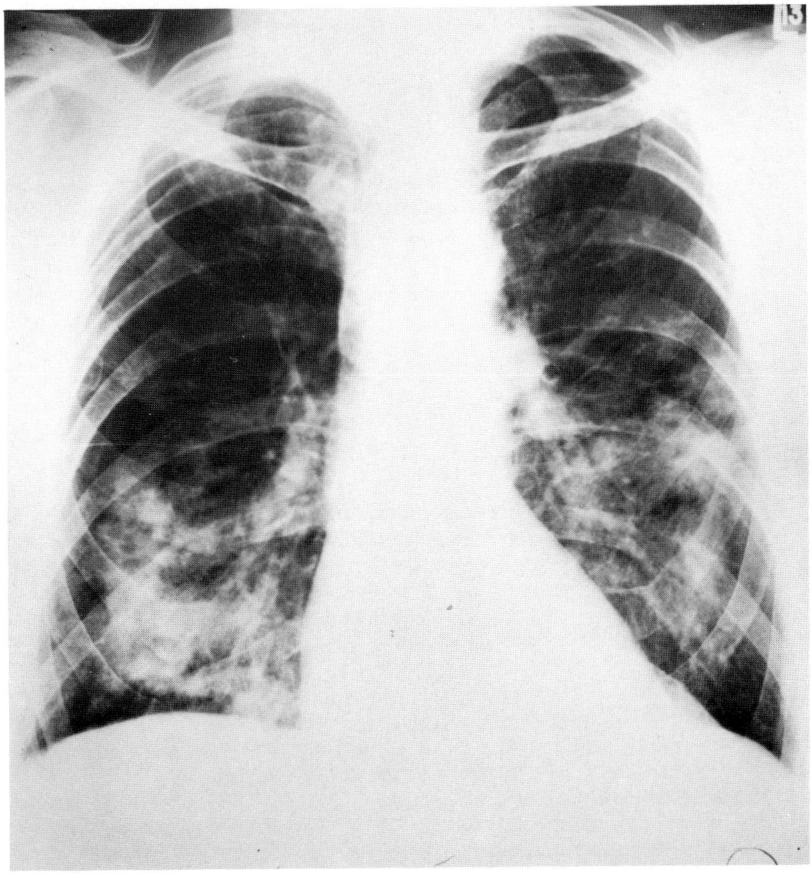

(d)

Figure 7.16(d) 1976: Further slight increase lung opacities but complete resolution of effusions. Note that the development, appearance and distribution of the lung opacities are unlike those of typical silicosis. Patient worked as a pottery caster and fettler for 36 years. Rheumatoid arthritis developed about 1962 and was progressive. Circulating RF consistently present in high titre. ANA: negative. No evidence of tuberculosis. Post mortem: bilateral diffuse thickening of the pulmonary pleura and well-circumscribed, grey coloured nodules with a faint concentric pattern in both lower lobes (7.16e)

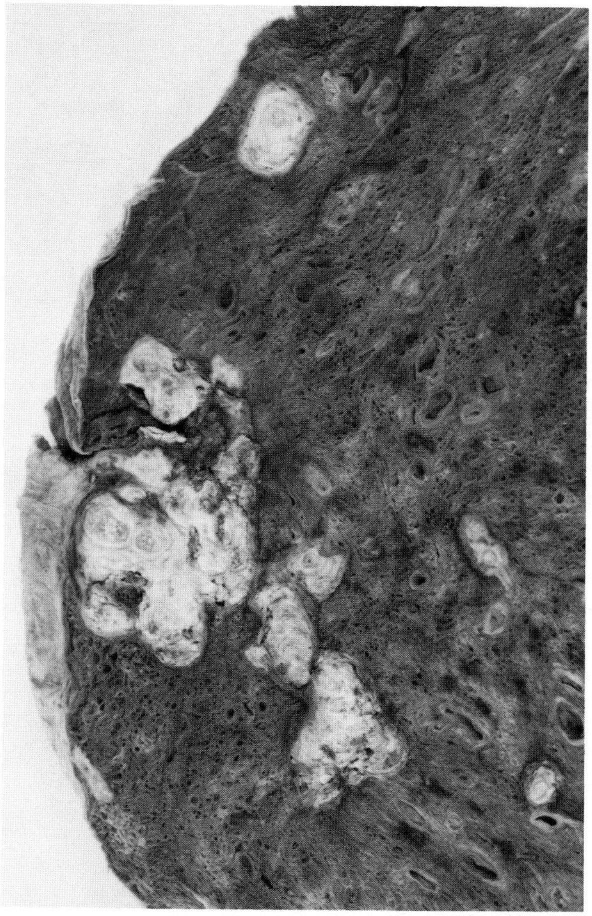

(e)

Figure 7.16(e) Note absence of typical silicotic nodules and slightness of dust pigmentation. Microscopy confirmed the presence of necrotic rheumatoid nodules and the absence of tuberculosis (see *Chapter 8)*

but, occasionally, may be massive and fatal. Therefore, haemoptysis in a silicotic patient may signal the presence of active tuberculosis, bronchial carcinoma or aspergilloma.

Pulmonary heart disease

This may develop in some cases of advanced conglomerate silicosis but right ventricular failure due to this cause (contrary to popular belief and many textbook descriptions) supervenes in only a small proportion, in whom, however, death is likely to occur in congestive heart failure. Co-existent and causally unrelated airflow obstruction may be an important contributory factor in some of these cases, and the likelihood of pulmonary heart disease causing death is significantly increased when there is complicating tuberculosis by contrast with silicosis alone (Becker and Chatgidakis, 1960).

Bronchitis

Episodes of acute and subacute bronchitis due to infection in deformed and rigid bronchi may occur in advanced stages of silicosis, but there is no correlation between chronic obstructive bronchitis, which is very largely associated with cigarette smoking, and silicosis and siliceous dusts (*see* Chapter 1). Inhalation of siliceous dust has not been clearly established as a cause of chronic obstructive bronchitis.

Emphysema

Although small areas of scar ('irregular') emphysema are occasionally observed around nodules and larger bullous areas of the same type of emphysema may be related to conglomerate lesions, emphysema is not a feature of silicosis. Centrilobular and panlobular types of emphysema may be present but are pathogenically unrelated to the silicosis.

Spontaneous pneumothorax

Spontaneous pneumothorax is an uncommon complication caused by the rupture of a bleb or bulla and the resulting pneumothorax is often localized due to the limitations imposed by pleural symphysis. For this reason it may be unsuspected unless detected fortuitously by radiography. Rarely, it may be bilateral and fatal (*Figure 7.14*).

Segmental and middle lobe collapse

Exceptionally, compression or occlusion of smaller bronchi by enlarged silicotic lymph nodes causes an area of lung collapse.

Rheumatoid syndrome

The progression of silicosis and the appearance of the lesions in the presence of rheumatoid arthritis or rheumatoid factor without rheumatoid arthritis has already been alluded to. They are important in that they may be mistaken for active tuberculous disease and, if pleural effusion occurs, carcinoma may be suspected.

Scleroderma (progressive systemic sclerosis)

Silicosis appears to be associated with an unusually high prevalence of scleroderma (systemic sclerosis). Byrom Bramwell, in 1914, first drew attention to this association in stonemasons but, since the late 1950s, there have been many reports of its occurrence in such workers as gold-miners, fluorspar miners, sand blasters and those involved in pottery and foundry processes (Bellini and Ghislandi, 1959; Carini and Lo Martire, 1965; Erasmus, 1960; Francia, Monarca and Cavallot, 1959; Gunther and Schuchhardt, 1970; Migueres *et al.*, 1966; Rodnan *et al.*, 1967; Ziskind *et al.*, 1976).

It has been suggested that the skin lesions are, in fact, pseudo-scleroderma because in almost all the reported cases Raynaud's phenomenon, microstomia and systemic involvement have been absent, and the skin disease is often localized (Jablońska, 1975). A 0.6 per cent incidence of scleroderma in silicotic individuals has been reported by Francia, Monarca and Cavallot (1959) who suggest that it adversely affects the course of the silicosis. If, in fact, this is not a chance association it may be that impairment of T lymphocyte function and consequent auto-antibodies production or a common anticollagen antibody against lung and skin are involved. Certainly there is an increased prevalence of circulating ANA in silicosis (*see* section on Pathogenesis, p. 142) and in scleroderma in which it may be as high as 90 per cent (Jayson, 1977). There is, however, no evidence that silicosis (or any other form of pneumoconiosis) provokes the onset of scleroderma, but, on the other hand, DIPF (fibrosing 'alveolitis') is a well recognized manifestation of systemic sclerosis (Campbell and LeRoy, 1975).

Carcinoma of the lung

Bronchial carcinoma occasionally occurs in silicotic lungs but there is no evidence of a causal relationship between it and silicosis or siliceous dusts; indeed, the incidence of lung cancer in miners with silicosis is significantly lower than in non-silicotic males (Miners Phthisis Medical Bureau, 1944; Rüttner and Heer, 1969).

The relationship of mine radioactivity to lung carcinoma is referred to in Chapter 14.

Neurological

Irreversible abductor paralysis of the left vocal cord is a rare sequel of involvement of the left recurrent laryngeal nerve in a mass of silicotic lymph nodes (Arnstein, 1941). Obviously, all other possible causes of paralysis must be excluded before this diagnosis is accepted.

Oesophageal compression

Oesophageal compression with dysphagia is another rare effect of large masses of silicotic lymph nodes (Longley, 1970).

Nephropathy

Renal lesions, which are claimed to be distinctive, have been attributed to heavy occupational exposure to free silica. They consist of thickening of glomerular capillary loops and basement membranes, increase in the numbers of mesangial and endothelial cells, periglomerular fibrosis and degenerative changes in the proximal convoluted tubules with deposition of electron-dense particles in cytosomes. Proteinuria and systemic hypertension have been ascribed to these changes (Saldanha, Rosen and Gonick, 1975). The loop of Henlé and distal convoluted tubules are apparently normal, as is their function, and mineral particles and silicotic nodules are absent. It has been suggested that auto-antibodies may be involved (Kolev, Doitschinov and Todorov, 1970). In a case of acute glomerulonephritis associated with silico-lipoproteinosis immunofluorescence demonstrated deposits of IgM and C3 component of complement in the mesangium and along the glomerular basement membrane but no antigen could be identified (Giles *et al.*, 1978). The silicon content of the renal tissue in these cases was much increased.

An endemic nephropathy with similar lesions in a Yugoslavian population has been attributed to the drinking water which has a high free silica content derived from rock erosion; and identical lesions consisting of periglomerular, peritubular and perivascular fibrosis have been produced in guinea pigs by adding 1 to 3 μm quartz particles to their drinking water for several months (Marković and Arambašić, 1971). But the underlying cause of this endemic 'Balkan nephropathy' (which appears to be concentrated in an area around the Danube in Jugoslavia, Bulgaria and Rumania) remains obscure (Leading article, 1977) though viral infection is considered to be likely in both natural and experimental disease (Apostolov, Spasić and Bojanić, 1975; Apostolov, 1977).

On present knowledge, therefore, it would be wrong, in clinical practice, to attribute renal disease in a patient with silicosis to silica exposure unless all other possible causes are excluded.

It is of interest, however, that in 1924 Gye and Purdey observed that glomerular damage and necrosis (primarily of the vascular endothelium) occurred in mice and rabbits after intravenous administration of silicic acid sol.

Prognosis

In general, it is unusual for normal life span to be shortened or for invalidism to be produced by uncomplicated silicosis although respiratory symptoms may be present. However, in a small proportion of cases, the disease progresses to severe respiratory disability and death often many years after the responsible industry has been left. In such cases—the prevalence of which is difficult to determine—the radiographic category may have been as low as 2q at the time of leaving. The likelihood of invalidism and death from pulmonary heart disease is increased by tuberculosis if this is not treated promptly and successfully, which, in the majority of cases, can be achieved (*see* next section).

The finding of rheumatoid arthritis or rheumatoid factor alone may signal impending progression of the disease. When chronic obstructive bronchitis or emphysema, or both, are present with large conglomerate silicotic masses or silicotuberculosis, serious invalidism and death from this cause are virtually inevitable.

Treatment

Prophylactic

Because it was shown that metallic aluminium dust is capable of preventing silicosis in experimental animals (Denny, Robson and Irwin, 1939), inhalation of aluminium aerosols by men with silicosis and those exposed to quartz dusts was advocated and widely employed from the early 1940s to the mid-1950s. Although it was claimed that development of silicosis and progression of existing silicosis was prevented this has not been substantiated, and there appears to have been no difference in the behaviour of the disease in treated and untreated groups (Kennedy, 1956). Experimental work in monkeys indicates that inhaled aluminium powder delays, but does not prevent, the appearance of silicotic lesions (Webster, 1968). There is the important additional feature that aluminium dust may itself be capable of causing diffuse interstitial fibrosis (*see* Chapter 13).

Therapeutic

There is at present no specific treatment available to halt the progress or cause resolution of human silicosis. As described in Chapter 4, PVPNO and related substances and polybetaine effectively prevent silicosis in experimental animals, but they are not suitable for use in man; for example, PVPNO is carcinogenic in animals and extremely slowly eliminated. However, it appears to be ineffective in preventing fibrosis due to coal–quartz mixtures (Weller, 1977). But, a related compound, poly-2-vinylpyridine-1-oxide, is apparently neither toxic nor carcinogenic, and is undergoing clinical trial (Schlipköter, 1970).

In theory agents capable of inhibiting or reversing cross-linking of collagen might be effective in preventing progression of silicosis. The one with most promise is β-amino-proprionitrile (BAPN) which has been shown to inhibit its progression in experimental animals (Levene, Bye and Saffrotti, 1968) and has been used successfully in controlling scar tissue in human surgery but, of course, it does not influence already established fibrosis. It is uncertain, therefore, that such an agent would be of value in clinical practice.

Corticosteroids do not influence or halt the progress of the disease and are obviously dangerous in the presence of unrecognized tuberculous disease. They may cause resolution of a complicating 'rheumatoid' pleural effusion but, again, a tuberculous cause must be excluded.

Appropriate treatment may be required for congestive heart failure or for co-existent acute or chronic obstructive bronchitis. Unproductive paroxysmal cough requires the use of an appropriate cough suppressant drug.

Treatment of silicotuberculosis

Treatment of complicating tuberculosis was shown to be effective if a satisfactory combination of antituberculous drugs is administered for a sufficient length of time (Keers, 1969), and this remains true for the more recently introduced drugs. Quiescence of disease is thereby achieved in the great majority of cases. The poor results reported in the 1950s appear to have been due to inadequate regimens. However, a few individuals with advanced cavitary silicotuberculosis may respond poorly, and the development of overall drug resistance greatly increases the likelihood of a fatal outcome.

Prevention

This depends upon the recognition of a 'free silica' hazard and upon a high standard of dust control and disposal which must be monitored by continual and random analysis of atmospheric dust in the work and 'background' areas. Whenever possible, a harmless material should be substituted.

The principles and methods of dust control are described in *Occupational Exposure to Crystalline Silica* by the US Department of Health, Education and Welfare (1974), in *The Prevention and Suppression of Dust in Mining, Tunnelling and Quarrying* by the ILO (1966) and, as they apply to the pottery industry, in *Health Conditions in the Ceramic Industry* (Davies, 1969).

New recommendations for the TLV for free silica have recently been made by the American National Institute of Occupational Safety and Health (Utidjian, 1975) but the evidence and assumptions upon which they were based are open to criticism (Morgan, 1975), and they do not distinguish between the various forms of free silica. Existing standards in the UK and various European countries are at present under review.

MIXED DUST FIBROSIS

The term 'mixed dust fibrosis', coined by Uehlinger (1946) and adopted by Harding, Gloyne and McLaughlin (1950), applies to lesions caused by crystalline silica (usually quartz or flint) and other dusts such as carbon, iron, kaolinite and feldspars inhaled simultaneously at the one process and not to those due to dusts from different processes at different times.

When the proportion of free silica to non-fibrogenic dust in the total dust inhaled is low, the typical nodular lesion of silicosis either does not occur or is infrequent, and irregular fibrotic lesions are produced. The commonest non-fibrogenic dusts are iron oxides.

Sources of exposure

Occupations in which 'mixed dust fibrosis' have occurred most commonly are casting, fettling and sand or shot-blasting in iron, steel and non-ferrous foundries; hematite mining, although in the UK this has caused a negligible amount of fibrotic pneumoconiosis since the 1930s owing to dust suppression measures (Bradshaw, Critchlow and Nagelschmidt, 1962); cleaning and scaling boilers; and electric arc welding and oxyacetylene cutting in foundries where there has also been some exposure to siliceous dusts from neighbouring operations in addition to iron fumes from welding or cutting.

'Mixed dust fibrosis' has been well documented as occurring in iron and steel foundry workers (Uehlinger, 1946; Harding, Gloyne and McLaughlin, 1950; Rüttner, 1954; McLaughlin and Harding, 1956), non-ferrous foundry workers (Harding and McLaughlin, 1955), boiler scalers (Harding and Massie, 1951), hematite miners (Stewart and Faulds, 1934) and ochre miners (*see* p. 114). It may also occur in potters in whom there may have been an additional exposure to feldspar, kaolinite and other dusts (*see* p. 138).

Mining of oil-shales for extraction of crude oil (*see* Chapter 2, p. 35) has been associated with pneumoconiosis of mild degree which consists, microscopically, of small lesions of 'mixed' dust fibrosis and also, occasionally, of calcification of hilar lymph nodes (Küng, 1979; Meiklejohn, 1956). Mining has been, or is, carried out chiefly by underground methods in the Scottish Lothians, USA, Brazil, Sweden and USSR. Operations in the Lothians (which commenced in the nineteenth century) and in Sweden ceased in the early 1960s having become uneconomic (Cameron and McAdam, 1978); but in the USA the rich deposits of the Green River formation of the Colorado plateau, estimated to be capable of producing 100 000 barrels of shale oil a day, are under active development (Costello, 1979). Although silicates, chiefly kaolinite, are predominant constituents of these shales their quartz content varies, according to site or location of origin, from some 3 to 8 per cent to almost 25 per cent in raw Green River shales and about 40 per cent in Estonian (USSR) shales; but the amount of quartz in mine air dust may be substantially lower (Küng, 1979; Weaver and Gibson, 1979). Meiklejohn (1956) warned that increased mechanization (introduced into the Lothian mines in the early 1950s) might increase the pneumoconiosis risk and this is potentially true of currently intensified oil shale mining in the USA and elsewhere, although the technology for effective dust control is available (Weaver and Gibson, 1979).

Pathogenesis

Lung dust in hematite-miners consists of hematite, quartz and mica, the quartz contributing 4 to 6 per cent of the total dust. This proportion of quartz resembles, but is rather more than, that in coal pneumoconiosis (Nagelschmidt, 1965), and, similarly to that pneumoconiosis, is not selectively concentrated in the PMF lesions. The more advanced the fibrosis the higher the quartz content (Faulds and Nagelschmidt, 1962). Hematite does not give a Prussian blue reaction but intracellular haemosiderin at the periphery of the lesions does (*see* Chapter 6, p. 115).

'Mixed dust fibrosis' appears to be due to modification of the effects of small quantities of 'free silica' (usually quartz) by the accompanying non-fibrogenic dusts. Animal experiments and observations in man have established that iron oxide inhibits or delays quartz-induced fibrosis in the lungs (Kettle, 1932; Gross, Westrick and McNerney, 1960; Reif, Landwehr and Bruckmann, 1963) and that, as hematite, it does not cause fibrosis (Byers and King, 1961). Iron hydroxide encountered by miners in the goethite iron ore mines in the Salzgitter district of the Federal German Republic appears to be even more effective in preventing fibrotic pneumoconiosis (Reichel, Bauer and Bruckmann, 1977).

According to McLaughlin (1957) the quartz content of the dust responsible for these lesions is under 10 per cent, but recent experimental work suggests that it may be appreciably higher than this (Goldstein and Rendall, 1970). If other factors play a part in pathogenesis they have not been identified. The incidence of complicating tuberculosis approaches that observed in nodular silicosis (Goldstein and Rendall, 1970) but there does not appear to be any evidence that it is involved in pathogenesis of the pneumoconiotic lesions.

The fibrogenic potential of combinations of quartz and kaolinite in animal lungs is referred to in Chapter 9, p. 312).

Coal pneumoconiosis in some respects resembles 'mixed dust fibrosis' but there are reasons for regarding it as a distinct entity (*see* Chapter 8).

Pathology

Macroscopic appearances

As in the case of nodular silicosis, the pulmonary pleura is often thickened to a variable degree and may be puckered where it overlies an intrapulmonary fibrotic mass. Distended bullae are sometimes present in these areas.

The cut surfaces of the lungs reveal irregular or stellate fibrous lesions which may vary in size from about 3 or 4 mm to confluent masses which may occupy the greater part of a lobe or lung. Characteristic, whorled, silicotic nodules are uncommonly seen either alone or within areas of fibrosis. Confluent lesions ('progressive massive fibrosis'—PMF) may be present, irregular in form, and often not limited by the anatomical boundaries of lobes or segments. In some cases of hematite-miners they are identical to the PMF lesions of coal pneumoconiosis (*see* Chapter 8), though of reddish colour, and do not resemble the conglomerate masses of silicotic nodules. Cavities are rarely seen unless there is complicating tuberculous or opportunist mycobacterial infection.

Both small and large lesions occur mainly in the upper halves and posterior zones of the lungs (but there are exceptions to this), and are rarely of similar size and distribution in the two lungs. Occasionally, only a few isolated lesions are present.

Grey-black pigment is intimately distributed through the lesions and in hematite lungs the fibrotic areas are, like the rest of the lungs, brick red in colour. Coal dust from mould facing materials is sometimes present in considerable quantity in foundry workers' lungs.

Microscopic appearances

Iron and quartz particles accumulate in alveolar walls adjacent to respiratory bronchioles and small arteries. In lesions in which there is no quartz there is no reaction other than a slight increase of reticulin fibres (siderosis) but when small quantities of quartz are present there is fibroblastic activity leading to peribronchiolar and perivascular collagen fibrosis which obliterates neighbouring alveoli and spreads, to a greater or lesser degree, farther into the lung. Reticulin and collagen fibres are arranged in both linear and radial fashion so that individual lesions are of irregular or stellate

('Medusa head') form and not concentrically nodular (*Figure 7.17*). Separate silicotic nodules may occur, however, in some cases and occasionally both types of lesion are seen together, but the nodular component is usually immature and hyaline changes are absent. PMF lesions consist of much dust which is mostly extracellular, and randomly arranged, often hyalinized, collagenous fibrosis; but in other cases the fibrosis has the whorled appearance of nodular silicosis.

Pulmonary arteries in the fibrotic areas may be engulfed by fibrous tissue and occluded or obliterated. In hematite mixed dust fibrosis there is a intense accumulation of iron-containing dust in and around pulmonary blood vessels but muscularized arteries are not evident. This is believed to imply an absence of constriction of the terminal regions of the arterial tree (Heath, Mooi and Smith, 1978).

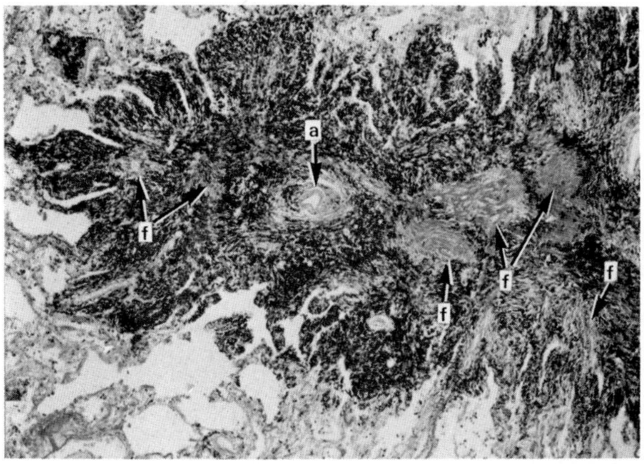

Figure 7.17 'Mixed dust fibrosis' in an iron foundry worker. 'Medusa head' formation with much dust and scattered, collagenous fibrosis some of which is unpigmented (f). The lesion surrounds an artery (a) and extends slightly into some alveolar walls though the adjacent lung is largely normal. (Original magnification × 55, H and E stain.) Compare with Figure 7.4

Scar (irregular) emphysema may be present around some 'mixed' lesions due to their concentration, and bullae with air-trapping may be found in relation to larger confluent masses. But scar emphysema is not a constant feature and in many cases it is absent or of very slight degree. Other types of emphysema which may be present are coincidental and not pathogenically related.

By contrast with nodular silicosis calcification does not occur in the 'mixed' lesions other than from healing of complicating tuberculosis.

Carbon, iron and other metallic dust particles are present in large quantity, and weakly, doubly refractile particles may suggest the presence of quartz. Siderosis often accompanies mixed dust fibrosis in iron foundry workers.

Clinical features

Symptoms, physical signs and lung function

The same considerations apply as in the case of nodular silicosis.

Radiographic appearances

When lesions in the lungs are small, the opacities they produce on the film may resemble those of discrete 'nodular' silicosis or coal pneumoconiosis; when larger, there are irregular opacities (usually in the upper and mid zones) which may be indistinguishable from those produced by fibrocaseous tuberculosis. As a rule, the well-demarcated opacities of discrete or conglomerate nodular silicosis are not observed. Calcification of lesions is not seen unless caused by quiescent tuberculosis, and 'egg-shell' calcification of hilar lymph nodes does not seem to occur (*Figure 7.18*).

In iron-foundry workers, hematite-miners and boiler-scalers numerous small radiodense opacities due to siderosis may also be present throughout the lung fields. In a survey of 1194 British foundry men small discrete opacities were observed in 34 per cent of fettlers and 14 per cent of foundry floor men but larger opacities indicative of conglomerate lesions were not seen (Lloyd Davis, 1971). It is likely that iron and, possibly, zircon dust contributed significantly to these appearances (*see* Chapter 6).

Diagnosis

The most difficult task is to distinguish radiographically between 'mixed dust fibrosis' and healed or active tuberculosis, but the presence of cavities favours active tuberculosis. However, when there is an appropriate occupational history and sputum cultures are positive for *M. tuberculosis*, it is virtually impossible to exclude the presence of co-existent 'mixed dust fibrosis'.

Occasionally, isolated lesions when seen radiographically for the first time may suggest collapse-consolidation or bronchial carcinoma.

Complications

These are similar to those already described for nodular silicosis in regard to tuberculosis and other infections, pulmonary heart disease, chronic bronchitis, emphysema and the 'rheumatoid' changes. Circumscribed 'rheumatoid-modified' nodules with naked-eye appearances of alternating concentric rings of black pigment and yellow-grey tissue, and the microscopic features described in Chapter 8 have been observed in a boiler scaler (Campbell, 1958) and an iron foundry worker (Caplan, Cowen and Gough, 1958); and consistent radiographic characteristics only have been recorded in a roof tile slabber (Hayes and Posner, 1960) and a worker in artificial grinding wheel manufacture (Posner, 1960).

Tuberculosis complicates 'mixed dust fibrosis' less often than it does in nodular silicosis, but is substantially more frequent than in the general population.

An increased incidence of cancer of the lung among hematite miners is referred to in Chapter 14.

Prognosis

This is much the same as in nodular silicosis but life expectancy is rarely shortened.

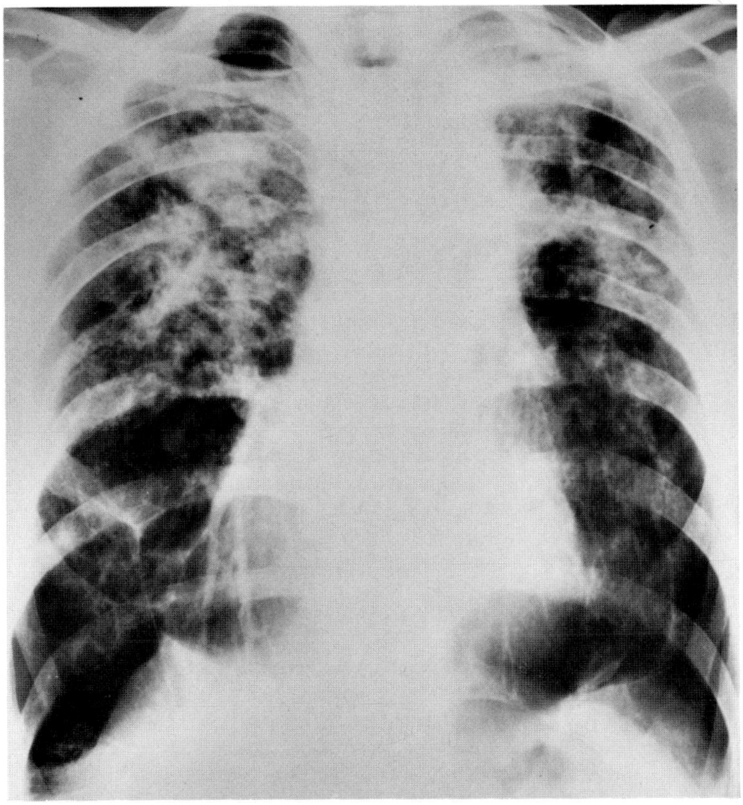

Figure 7.18 Moderately advanced mixed-dust fibrosis. Irregular massive opacities with very few discrete nodules in the rest of the lung fields. Extensive scar emphysema. Investigation for tuberculosis consistently negative

Treatment and prevention

The principles are exactly similar to those applying to nodular silicosis.

DIATOMITE PNEUMOCONIOSIS

Diatomite, a siliceous sedimentary rock—known also as diatomaceous earth and kieselguhr (*see* Chapter 2, p. 36)—consists mainly of the fossilized skeletons of a unicellular aquatic plant related to the algae and biologically dependent on silicon. *Diatomaceous silica,* an amorphous silicon dioxide, is its principal mineral component.

Origins

Commercially, the most important deposits occur in the USA (mainly in California, Nevada, Oregon and Washington), Mexico, South and East Africa, the Massif Central area of France, Denmark and Federal Germany. Although small quantities are produced in Cumberland and Northern Ireland the UK relies upon imported diatomite, mainly in the calcined form.

Mining and processing

Mining is done almost entirely by the opencast method and crude diatomite is transferred to the processing plant where it is crushed, screened, re-crushed and put into storage bins for blending into qualities appropriate to various uses. Natural moisture is removed by hot-air heaters at about 260 °C producing *natural dried diatomite.* It is then passed through a series of cyclones and separators to eliminate clays and other contaminants. Further processing may be done in the natural state but the greater part of the material is calcined. There are two different methods of calcination which were introduced in the 1920s. First, *straight calcination* in which natural diatomite is heated at approximately 816 to 1100 °C in a rotary kiln thereby removing organic matter, altering its structure and porosity, and converting some of it into cristobalite. Second, *flux calcination* in which caustic soda or sodium carbonate is added as a flux before the diatomite is fired in a kiln at 1100 °C or more resulting in the formation of tridymite. These differences in the phases of diatomite silica have important implications in relation to the development of pneumoconiosis (*see* Pathogenesis and pathology, this section; and Chapters 2 and 4).

Both natural and calcined forms are next milled, passed again through separators to remove grit and coarse kiln material, then to a cyclone 'classifier' where they are divided into fine (particles less than 10 μm size, mainly 0.5 to 2.2 μm) and coarse products which are stored in baghouse hoppers and finally bagged. Straight calcined diatomite is tan or pink coloured due to oxidation of iron, and flux calcined is white.

All these processes are potentially dusty but milling and bagging of calcined diatomite are the chief sources of a pneumoconiosis risk.

Processing diatomite is more advanced in the USA than elsewhere and world industrial demand, mainly of the calcined product, has greatly increased since the Second World War. Rigorous dust controls are now applied in the mines and processing plants.

Diatomite used in the UK is mostly imported in dried and straight or flux calcined forms from the USA, Denmark and other countries. There is only limited exploitation of domestic deposits: in Westmorland where straight calcined powders and granules are produced and in Northern Ireland which produces natural grades of dried diatomite; neither produce flux calcined diatomite.

Uses of diatomite

(1) Filtration is the most important. It is used in calcined form as a filter aid in liquid form, and in the manufacture of filters for inorganic and organic liquids; especially in wine, beer and fruit juice production, the manufacture of pharmaceutical liquids and antibiotics (such as penicillin and streptomycin), and in sugar refining. It has to a large extent replaced asbestos filters which were widely used for this purpose until recently. Berkfeld filters are made from diatomite.
(2) Heat and sound insulation. It is made into refractory bricks, moulded blocks, or used as a binder for pipe covering and insulating cement, for boilers, pipes, stills, furnaces and kilns, and was (and still is) frequently mixed with asbestos fibre for insulation cements.
(3) As a filler for plastics, rubber, paper, insecticides, paints, varnishes, linoleums, floor coverings, fertilizers and in special types of paper.
(4) As an adsorbent for industrial floor sweeping powders and chemical disinfectants.
(5) As a mild abrasive in silver, metal and motor car polishes, dental pastes and hand soaps.
(6) Other uses are as a carrier for catalysts, a pozzolanic component of certain cements and concrete, for various types of building materials (board, sheets, tiles, blocks and plasters), and in electrode coatings for welding. In the UK, English and Irish diatomite is used especially in cement manufacture for which purpose it is dried at a low temperature to remove organic matter such as peat and, hence, is unlikely to contain a significant amount of crystalline 'silica', if any.

Apart from processing, therefore, exposure to diatomite (usually in calcined form) may occur to a varying degree in the manufacture of these products and when mixed by hand for insulation. Maintenance work on processing plant is also a potential source of exposure.

Prevalence

This is an uncommon pneumoconiosis the severity of which appears to correlate with the cristobalite content of the dust and duration of exposure.

A survey in the diatomite processing industry in 1953–1954 showed that 25 per cent of 251 workers with more than 5 years' dust exposure, and nearly 50 per cent of 101 workers exposed to high concentrations of calcined dust had radiographic evidence of pneumoconiosis which, in the main indicated nodular and confluent lesions. The majority of these employees had been mill hands handling calcined material. There were no cases among the quarry workers (Cooper and Cralley, 1958).

Another radiographic survey of 869 diatomite workers revealed that of those who had been mill hands for more than five years 17 per cent had 'linear-nodular' ('simple') pneumoconiosis and 23.2 per cent larger confluent opacities (Oechsli, Jacobson and Brodeur, 1961).

Rigorous dust controls in quarrying and processing plants, however, have resulted in the virtual elimination of new cases. For example, by 1974 14 (3.3 per cent) of a work force of 428 men employed since 1853 in an American plant where these measures had been introduced in the mid-1950s had radiographic evidence of pneumoconiosis and this did not exceed ILO Category 1/1. Of 129 employees exposed before 1953 only two mill workers (2.6 per cent) had Category A opacities thought to indicate pneumoconiosis (Cooper and Jacobson, 1977).

There appears to be no information of the prevalence of pneumoconiosis among workers using calcined diatomite in the various manufacturing processes but the risk is probably low, although it is possible that some cases have passed unrecognized being interpreted as 'sputum-negative fibrotic tuberculosis' (*see Figure 7.21*).

Pathogenesis

The structural forms of silicon dioxide which may be found in diatomite has a crucial influence on its fibrogenic potential. Natural diatomite is non-crystalline (amorphous) and is associated with only minute quantities of quartz—less than 2 per cent in California, Nevada and Oregon (Cooper and Cralley, 1958)—and trace amounts of tridymite and cristobalite. When it is subjected to high temperature calcination, tridymite and cristobalite are formed at a rate related to the degree and duration of the applied heat (*see* Chapter 2); the cristobalite content may be about 21 per cent of the bag-house product (Cooper and Cralley, 1958). Flux calcination greatly facilitates the speed with which cristobalite is produced in the same temperature range as straight calcination (Bailey, 1947) in which case some 60 per cent cristobalite may be present in the bag-house product (Cooper and Cralley, 1958); and tridymite may also be present. *Figure 7.19* shows X-ray diffraction patterns of

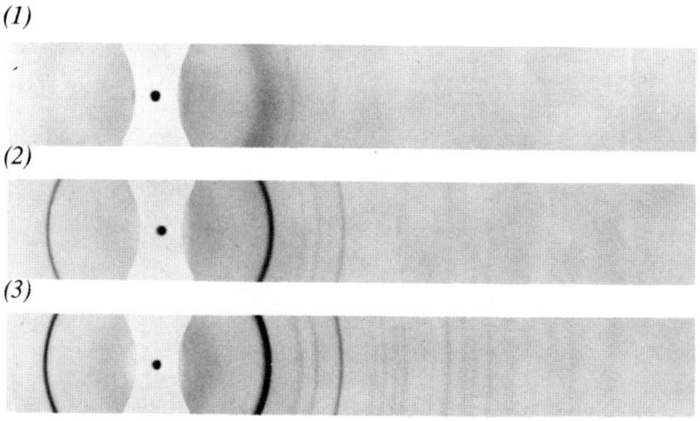

Figure 7.19 X-ray diffraction patterns of diatomite products. (1) Natural diatomite. The presence of the diffuse band and the absence of lines indicates that this is non-crystalline or amorphous. (2) Straight calcined diatomite. The distinct lines are characteristic of cristobalite. (3) Flux calcined diatomite. Lines are further increased in intensity. Disappearance of the diffuse bands indicates conversion of amorphous silicon dioxide to cristobalite. (Reproduced by courtesy of Dr W. D. Wagner et al. *(1968) and the Editor of the* American Industrial Hygiene Association Journal*)*

diatomite subjected to the different forms of calcination. The amount of cristobalite evolved is similar whether diatomite is of salt or fresh water origin (Cooper and Crally, 1958).

In experimental animals, natural diatomite causes infiltration of alveolar walls by macrophages, many of which contain dust particles, but no proliferation of connective tissue fibres (Tebbens and Beard, 1957); and in man there is no evidence that it causes lung fibrosis (Vigliani and Mottura, 1948; Luton *et al.,* 1956; Cooper and Cralley, 1958). By contrast, and as noted in Chapter 4, cristobalite and tridymite are more fibrogenic than quartz in experimental animals, and calcined diatomite has been shown to be fibrogenic in human lungs (Vorwald *et al.,* 1949). Uncalcined amorphous silicon dioxide is eliminated from the lungs more rapidly than either quartz or cristobalite (Klosterkötter and Einbrodt, 1965)—an indication of its lack of cytotoxicity.

The mean particle size of the final calcined product may be about 0.7 μm (Wagner *et al.,* 1968) which ensures penetration to the alveolar region.

It has been emphasized that any samples of supposedly 'amorphous silica' obtained for work-place analyses or experimental purposes must be shown by X-ray diffraction to be free of any crystalline silica contaminants or products modified by heat treatment if valid interpretations of data are to be made (Bell, Dunnom and Lott, 1978).

Macroscopic appearances

The pulmonary pleura is often thickened.

Areas of fine and coarse, grey coloured, diffuse interstitial fibrosis of both linear and stellate form are seen in lung slices, usually in the upper halves of the lungs, although the lower halves may be involved; and the subpleural region is a common site of selection. It may be of slight or extensive order. Confluent masses of fibrosis may also be present, again chiefly in the upper zones, and may contain ischaemic cavities. Characteristic whorled silicotic nodules and conglomerations are absent.

There may be scar emphysema sometimes with bullae (especially in relation to areas of subpleural fibrosis), but often there is no emphysema.

Microscopic appearances

Early lesions consist of collections of dust-containing macrophages in alveoli, alveolar walls and hilar lymph nodes with either no connective tissue reaction or with only a delicate reticulin proliferation (Carnes, 1954). As the lesions progress, diffuse collagen fibrosis occurs in the peribronchiolar and perivascular regions with much fibroblast activity and this extends into surrounding lung tissue as diffuse interstitial fibrosis producing thickening of alveolar walls and obliteration of adjacent alveolar spaces (*Figure 7.20*). The cellular element is often prominent and the lesions show some predilection for the subpleural zone (Spain, 1965).

Many dust particles which can be identified as fragmented diatoms may be seen in macrophages and fibrous tissue and rather stubby, pseudoasbestos bodies with rudimentary segmentation are sometimes observed (Nordmann, 1943). The birefringence of cristobalite is low. Characteristic silicotic lesions do not occur, but 'hyalinization' may be seen in some areas of fibrosis (Vorwald *et al.,* 1949; Dutra, 1965). In some cases both macroscopical and microscopical features are those of 'mixed dust fibrosis' associated, however, with fragments of diatoms.

The confluent masses consist of collagenous fibrosis—often unusually cellular—arranged in random fashion and showing little or no tendency to whorling. Necrosis may occur in them, sometimes with areas of calcification, due to ischaemic changes and in the absence of tuberculosis. Neighbouring blood vessels may be surrounded, and some obliterated, by fibrosis.

Scar emphysema may be related to the lesions but this is not a constant finding and it appears to occur chiefly in the form of small localized bullae in the vicinity of the subpleural fibrosis.

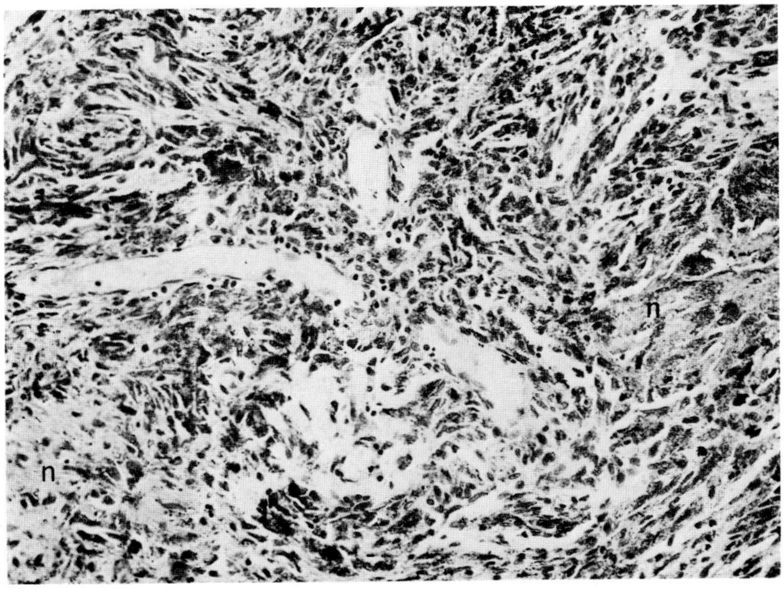

Figure 7.20 Pneumoconiosis due to calcined diatomite. This compact lesion consists of immature collagenous fibrosis which lacks the organized arrangement of typical silicotic nodules and is much more cellular. Areas of necrosis (n) are present. (Original magnification × 225. H and E stain. Section by courtesy of Dr F. R. Dutra, California)

Fibrotic lesions are also seen in the hilar lymph nodes. The quartz content of the lungs is low. In one study it was less than 2 per cent of the lungs by weight (Vorwald *et al.*, 1949).

Clinical features

Symptoms

In general, respiratory symptoms are uncommon. When they occur they consist of morning cough, which may be non-productive, and a mild to moderate degree of breathlessness on effort; rarely, in advanced cases, there is disabling dyspnoea. Haemoptysis does not seem to occur.

Physical signs

Finger clubbing is not a feature of the disease (Cooper and Cralley, 1958).

There may be no abnormal signs but in some cases breath sounds in the upper halves of the lungs may be of bronchial type accompanied by inspiratory crepitations which may also be heard over the lower lobe regions in some cases. Signs of spontaneous pneumothorax can sometimes be elicited. In advanced cases the signs of upper zone fibrosis with tracheal displacement may be present.

Evidence of congestive heart failure due to pulmonary heart disease appears to be rare.

Investigations

Lung function

Comprehensive studies have been done by Motley, Smart and Valero (1956) and Motley (1960). As in the case of other types of pneumoconiosis, abnormal values correlate poorly with radiographic appearances and good pulmonary function may be associated with faily extensive radiographic changes, but large confluent lesions are usually associated with abnormal function.

Maximum breathing capacity, timed FEV and FVC, may be slightly to moderately impaired, and arterial oxygen saturation often reduced in slight to moderate degree; RV is significantly increased and there may be some reduction in TLC and gas transfer (Tl). Uneven ventilation is present in some cases and, occasionally, there is pronounced airways obstruction.

Radiographic appearances

The earliest abnormality consists of linear or round ('nodular') opacities, or both ('linear-nodular'), in the upper and mid-zones of the lung fields and extending to their periphery. These appearances are sometimes fine and 'lace-like'. It is unusual for the discrete round opacities to exceed about 2 mm in diameter and they have low contrast with the surrounding tissues, rarely possessing the radiodensity of those due to nodular silicosis (Oechsli, Jacobson and Brodeur, 1961).

The opacities become more prominent as they coalesce and coalescent lesions, which are at first indistinct, later appear as well-circumscribed homogeneous densities (ILO Category B or C). These are mainly in the upper zones and usually bilateral and may exhibit evidence of contraction, distortion or cavities, but rarely calcification. Appearances consistent with DIPF may be seen in the lower zones, but have rarely been reported (*Figure 7.21*).

Enlargement or egg-shell calcification of hilar lymph nodes is not seen.

Other investigations

Apart from obtaining lung tissue for biopsy (which should rarely be necessary) there are none likely to give further assistance in establishing the diagnosis.

Diagnosis

This depends upon a history of an exposure of five or more years to calcined diatomite in processing or manufacture, and upon radiographic appearances.

Tuberculosis—active or quiescent—is the most important differential diagnosis.

Complications

There is an unusual tendency to spontaneous pneumothorax (Vigliani and Mottura, 1948; Smart and Anderson, 1952) although there is apparently no increased likelihood of tuberculosis. But when tuberculosis complicates diatomite pneumoconiosis it tends to pursue an indolent course (Smart and Anderson, 1952), and if cavities are present, antituberculous treatment may fail to prevent relentless progression of the disease (Spain, 1965).

Prognosis

Progression to the stage of advanced confluent masses may occur years after the worker has left the industry with the disease in an early stage.

Life expectancy appears rarely to be shortened and pulmonary heart disease is probably exceptional. Occasionally, however, rapidly progressive disease may occur and end in fatal cor pulmonale (Luton *et al.*, 1956); this has chiefly been associated with disease due to flux calcined diatomite.

Treatment

There is no treatment to prevent or reverse the course of the disease.

Prevention

A rigid programme of dust control (monitoring of local and atmospheric dust, enclosure systems where possible, exhaust ventilation, good housekeeping and use of respirators) is necessary in diatomite processing and the use of the calcined form in manufacture. These measures, as noted already, have been applied in the major processing plants in the USA since the mid-1950s with excellent results.

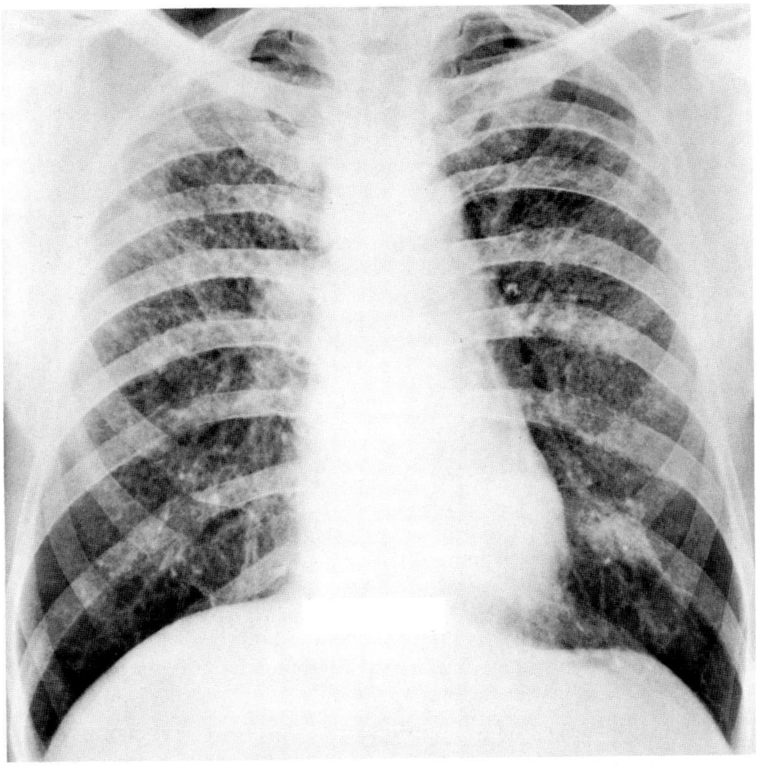

(a)

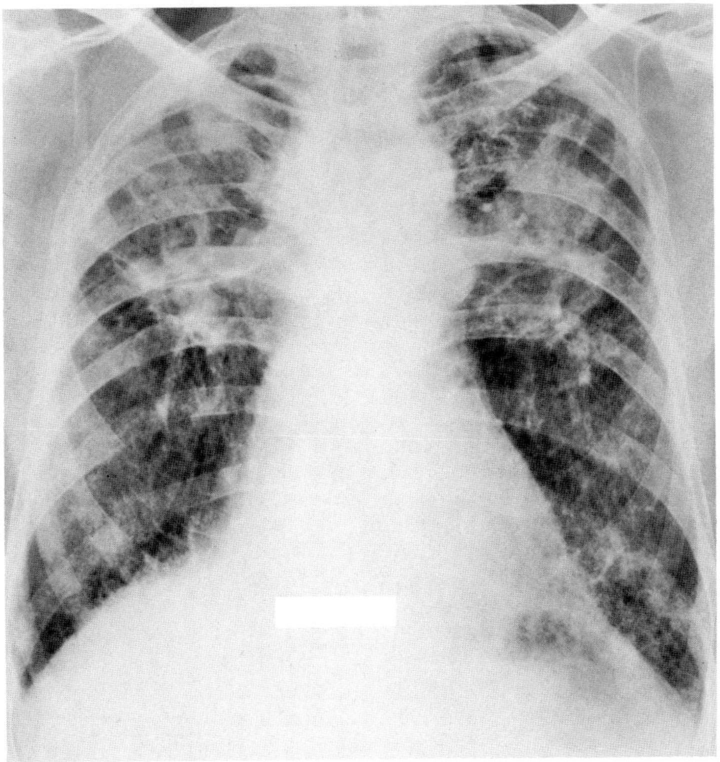

(b)

Figure 7.21 Diatomite pneumoconiosis in a man who spent 25 years in a processing mill with intermittent heavy exposure to flux calcined diatomite. He was removed from risk after the first film (a). The second film (b) was taken 10 years later. Tuberculin tests negative. No bacteriological evidence of tuberculosis. Note the appearances of diffuse interstitial fibrosis in the lower zones. (By courtesy of Dr W. Clark Cooper, Berkeley, Calif.)

SUBMICRON AMORPHOUS SILICON DIOXIDE (VITREOUS SILICA)

Before concluding this section some reference must also be made to submicron forms of amorphous silicon dioxide sometimes referred to as *synthetic silica, precipitated silica* and *colloidal silica*. These are now extensively used in industry: for example, as fillers for rubber, paints and paper; in cosmetics, inks, motor car polishes and electric light bulbs; as a diluent for insecticides and a carrying agent for catalysts. They are prepared by precipitation at high temperatures of sodium silicates (trade name Hi-Sil), hydrated calcium silicate (trade name Silene), or pure silicon tetrachloride (trade names Aerosil, Degussa or Dow Corning 'silica'). The content of non-crystalline silicon dioxide is about 99.8 per cent, and the crystalline and cryptocrystalline forms are absent. Particles are of uniform size and range from 5 to 40 nm (Volk, 1960). Neosyl, another hydrated silica precipitate, has a particle size of 100 to 200 nm but forms loose agglomerates of 1 to 10 μm diameter. Amorphous silica is also produced by vaporization of quartz in processes in the ferroalloy industries.

Potentially, the most dusty areas in the manufacture of the amorphous silicas are the furnace room, and the bagging and loading departments but in recent years these have been controlled by dust suppression measures. In ferrous and non-ferrous metallurgy the chief sources of amorphous silica are electric-arc furnaces, crucibles and ladles where it occurs either as fume or vapour. The tendency for fume particles to aggregate probably somewhat reduces their chances of penetrating to the lower respiratory tract.

Surveys of workers in the Hi-Sil, Silene and Aerosil processes, in which men were observed over periods of eight to 12 years, revealed no evidence of pneumoconiosis or harmful effects (Plunkett and De Witt, 1962; Volk, 1960). Similarly pneumoconiosis was not found in men who had worked some 25 years in the ferroalloy industry although 'clouds of flocculated particles' of precipitated silica were produced (Roberts, 1965). However, small amounts of quartz have been found in condensed furnace fume in the ferrosilicon industry but associated with only minimal evidence of pneumoconiosis (Swensson *et al.,* 1971). A report that 'amorphous silica dust' of 0.05 to 0.75 μm particle size originating from an electric-arc furnace in a metallurgical process in which quartz was vaporized at temperatures in excess of 2350 °C caused 'nodular', fibrotic pneumoconiosis can hardly be accepted in view of the fact that the dust from this plant—which was shown to provoke pulmonary fibrosis of similar severity to that of quartz in animals—was, as the authors themselves state, identified by the American National Institute of Occupational Safety and Health (NIOSH) as cristobalite with a layer of amorphous silica (Johnson, Lewis and Groth, 1973; Vitums, *et al.,* 1977). In the temperature range 900 to 1400 °C the crystallization of cristobalite from the amorphous silica in silicon metal furnaces and its further transformation to tridymite occurs more rapidly than with other forms of amorphous silica (Austrheim, 1977).

Experimental work in rats exposed to submicron amorphous silica particles—which are completely lacking in cytotoxicity to macrophages (Kessel, Monaco and Marchisio, 1963)—has demonstrated that they are eliminated from the lungs more rapidly than quartz although they are still detectable after a period of 12 months. The resulting lesions, which consist chiefly of macrophage accumulations and reticulin proliferation akin to the effect of an inert dust, regress as the 'silica' disappears from the lungs (Byers and Gage, 1961). A similar lack of significant collagenesis has also been observed in guinea pigs and rabbits (Schepers *et al.,* 1957a and b). However, it should be noted that some authors have claimed that submicron amorphous silica does cause fibrosis in animals (for example, Swensson, 1967; Zaidi, 1969) but in almost all of these reports indisputable evidence that the material administered was unadulterated has not been provided.

It is important, therefore, to recognize that some cristobalite (which, it will be recalled, is at least as fibrogenic as quartz) often survives temperatures above its melting point of 1723 °C so that its crystals may be present in the silica which results on cooling (*see* Chapter 2, p. 32); and indeed, the white powder deposited when silica condenses out of its gas phase may contain finely divided (microcrystalline) cristobalite in addition to micro-amorphous silica (Sosman, 1965). In short, any experimental or epidemiological study which purports to show that amorphous silica is, in its own right, fibrogenic must demonstrate beyond doubt that the material studied is in fact truly amorphous.

Hence, from critically appraised evidence to date it can be concluded that submicron amorphous silica does not cause pneumoconiosis in man, though cryptocrystalline silica which is sometimes associated with it may certainly do so.

'ACUTE' SILICOSIS

ALVEOLAR SILICO-LIPOPROTEINOSIS

By 'acute' silicosis is meant disease similar to idiopathic alveolar lipoproteinosis of rapid development following intense exposure to dusts of high free silica content. Mature silicotic nodules are either absent or few in number. This contrasts with rather less rapidly progressive nodular silicosis (referred to already) which is characterized by multiple small immature nodules.

The term 'alveolar lipoproteinosis' indicates the underlying pathology more accurately than 'alveolar proteinosis', and 'silico-lipoproteinosis' denotes the causal relationship.

Sources of exposure

Although there is evidence from mummified remains that this disorder occurred in Chilean metal ore miners in the sixteenth century (Munizaga *et al.,* 1975) attention was first drawn to it in workers in abrasive soap factories by Middleton in 1929 and subsequently by other authors (for example, McDonald, Piggott and Gilder, 1930; Chapman, 1932; Adler-Herzmark and Kapstein, 1937; Ritterhoff, 1941). Quartzite sand or sandstone were finely ground ('silica flour') and mixed with anhydrous sodium carbonate and soap resulting in exposure to both siliceous and alkaline dusts; workers in the packing department were exposed to the mixed dusts. Today quartz is not considered a suitable abrasive for household soap powders as its hardness damages enamels and glass. Nevertheless its use in domestic scouring powders has only recently ceased in the UK, and it is still used in non-domestic abrasive soaps.

However, exposure to high concentrations of quartz in the absence of alkalis occurs in various other and more important ways: notably, when tunnelling through rock of high quartz content (Gardner, 1933; Ashworth, 1970); when shovelling, loading and handling similar rock dusts in the holds of ships and other confined spaces, and when sand-blasting with quartzite sands (Gardner, 1933; Michel and Morris, 1964; Buechner and Ansari, 1969; Giles *et al.*, 1978). Features common to most of these activities are high concentrations of quartz or cristobalite, the particles of which are likely to be of predominantly small size, in confined spaces. Apparently sand is still frequently used in many countries for sandblasting in spite of recommendations that it should be substituted by non-siliceous abrasives (*see* Abrasive blasting, p. 137).

It is important to emphasize that although the types of exposure which cause this form of disease are often short (that is, weeks or months) they are intense and involve high concentrations of free silica. Casual contacts with low concentrations of siliceous dusts are unlikely to be hazardous to health.

Incidence

The disease is undoubtedly rare. Conditions which cause it have been uncommon and its incidence may have been underestimated because the clinical, radiographic and pathological characteristics which are so different from those of 'nodular silicosis' may have not been attributed to an occupational hazard. Moreover, it has, probably, often been diagnosed simply as tuberculosis which, in fact, is a common complication. Of 139 cases of alveolar lipoproteinosis reviewed by Davidson and McLeod (1969) ten had been exposed to free silica.

The pathological features are better outlined before those of pathogenesis.

Pathology

Macroscopic appearances

The pleura is usually thickened and adherent, but in some cases is free, and the lungs are voluminous, heavy and mostly airless. The hilar lymph nodes are often enlarged and a tenacious, mucinous material may be present in the large airways.

When the lungs are cut, there is grey-white consolidation interspersed by pink-red areas and DIPF which may be prominent in the upper halves of the lungs. A frothy (often blood-stained) or gelatinous fluid exudes from the cut surfaces. Silicotic nodules are either few and small or altogether absent.

Microscopic appearances

These are very variable and, as originally described some 40

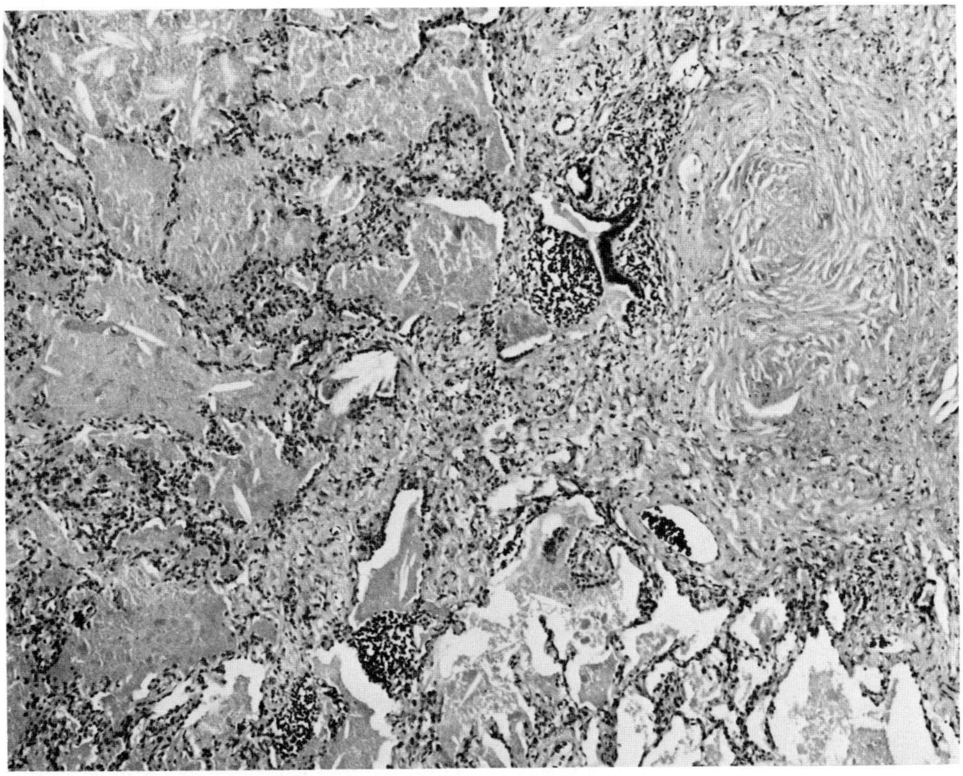

Figure 7.22 Alveolar silico-lipoproteinosis in a man who milled quartz for seven years. The majority of the alveolar spaces are filled with acellular, finely granular, eosinophilic, PAS-positive material with occasional cleft-like spaces. The alveolar walls are mostly normal in appearances but in places are thickened by mild infiltration of mononuclear cells and proliferation of reticulin (centre of field). There are also local aggregations of lymphocytes in the interstitium. On the right there are small, immature, but recognizable, silicotic nodules. (Original magnification × 40). (By courtesy of Dr J. M. Xipell and the Editor of Thorax*)*

years ago (McDonald, Piggott and Gilder, 1930; Chapman, 1932), may consist of areas of acellular fibrosis, sometimes with hyaline centres, around which there is an intense small-cell infiltration; alveolar walls are thickened by fibrous tissue and, in many places, alveolar spaces are filled by an acidophilic, high-protein alveolar fluid containing fine granules and many desquamated cells to which Mallory drew attention in 1934.

The early stage of the disease exhibits the features of endogenous lipid pneumonia (Costello *et al.*, 1975). Later some DIPF is present accompanied by infiltration of mononuclear and plasma cells and, in alveolar spaces, by desquamated cells and an abundant acidophilic, proteinaceous material which is strongly positive to the periodic acid Schiff (PAS) stain. The relative amounts and distribution of these entities vary from case to case. Silicotic nodules are usually absent, but, if present, are few in number and smaller and more immature than typical lesions (Hoffmann *et al.*, 1973; Roeslin *et al.*, 1980) (*Figure 7.22*); though exceptions to this in which there are moderate numbers of fairly mature nodules are on record (Suratt *et al.*, 1977). Widespread, irregular fibrosis is also seen in cases of prolonged survival. Hyalinized collagenous tissue and birefringent crystals may be found in the hilar lymph nodes (Xipell *et al.*, 1977).

Apart from the presence of occasional silicotic nodules and quartz crystals in the intra-alveolar material these features are identical with 'idiopathic' alveolar lipoproteinosis (Heppleston and Young, 1972; Rosen, Castleman and Liebow, 1958) in which the alveolar walls are usually, but not always, thickened by cellular infiltration, and the alveolar spaces filled with granular, strongly PAS-positive lipid and proteinaceous material (*Figure 4.7*, p. 69). The proteins are albumin and IgG apparently derived by transudation from serum proteins; indeed, serum proteins have been identified in bronchopulmonary lavage fluid from human alveolar lipoproteinosis (Hawkins, Savard and Ramirez-Rivera, 1967).

Electron microscopy reveals that the desquamated cells are predominantly Type II pneumocytes containing numerous osmiophilic lamellar inclusion bodies. Type I cells are scanty and fragmented. Many intra-alveolar macrophages contain lamellar bodies which probably originate from disrupted Type II cells, and these bodies are also free in the phospholipid material which possesses the hexagonal and parallel lamellated patterns already described in Chapter 4 (*Figure 4.8*, p. 69) and which is probably an excess of surfactant (Hoffmann *et al.*, 1973) Quartz crystals have been observed in supposedly Type II cells (Xipell *et al.*, 1977).

Pathogenesis

Because 'acute silicosis' was first identified in the abrasive soap industry, alkali (sodium carbonate) was considered to be a decisive pathogenic agent, and ingenious chemical theories suggesting that it exerted an enhancing effect on the fibrogenic potential of quartz were advanced, but these are invalidated by the fact that the same disease process occurs in the absence of exogenous alkali.

At least two conditions are thought to be necessary for the production of the disease:

(1) Exposure to high concentrations of quartz, cristobalite or tridymite dust.

(2) Small particle size. The disease is usually associated with exposure to finely divided quartz dust and is reproduced in animals by the inhalation of quartz (or cristobalite) particles less than 7 or 5 μm diameter (Corrin and King, 1969; Heppleston, Wright and Stewart, 1970) (*see* Chapter 4).

A third, speculative, immunological factor may, perhaps, be involved but remains to be identified (Gough, 1967).

The early changes of the experimental disease consist of a large influx of alveolar macrophages with swollen and vacuolated cytoplasm followed by production of PAS-positive intra-alveolar material in which there may be cholesterol crystals. There is some disagreement as to whether pronounced proliferation of Type II cells is an early key feature (Heppleston and Young, 1972; Corrin and King, 1970), but these cells appear to be the chief source of the phospholipid (surfactant) accumulation (Heppleston, Fletcher and Wyatt, 1974). The massive production of phospholipid and cell debris appears to isolate the quartz particles from macrophages thus preventing or reducing the formation of typical silicotic fibrosis. There is some evidence that alveolar clearance may be defective (Kuhn *et al.*, 1966). Macrophages obtained by bronchopulmonary lavage from cases of human idiopathic disease exhibit decreased viability in tissue culture and a reduced capacity to kill *Candida* organisms, though their phagocytic activity is unimpaired; suggesting that they are rendered defective by their abnormal environment. Monocytes from the peripheral blood, on the other hand, appear to function normally (Golde *et al.*, 1976).

Alveolar lipoproteinosis seems to be a non-specific, though characteristic, response to a variety of injurious agents in addition to free silica; it has been associated—though often circumstantially—with the inhalation of various dusts, both mineral and organic, and vapours (Davidson and McLeod, 1969), and in animals and man, with a number of different drugs (Hruban, 1976; Xipell *et al.*, 1977). But in many cases there is no identifiable cause.

Clinical features

Symptoms

These develop quickly over a period of a few weeks and usually within a year or two of first exposure to the responsible siliceous dust. Malaise, fatigue, loss of weight, cough and mucoid sputum, slight or recurrent haemoptysis, pleuritic type of chest pain, are complained of; but the chief symptom is rapidly progressive dyspnoea of sudden onset. In a proportion of cases, however, the onset is insidious and progression fairly slow.

Physical signs

The patient is usually dyspnoeic at rest and, in the later stages of the illness, orthopnoeic. The reason for this is that a large proportion of the lungs is involved by the disease process and it is possible, too, that reflex mechanisms (*see* Chapter 1) also play a part. Central cyanosis may be present together with fever ranging from 37.2 °C (99°F) to 40 °C (105°F).

There may be finger clubbing, impaired percussion note, and pleural rub. Breath sounds are either diminished or of bronchial type depending upon the degree of pleural thickening. Crepitations are usually heard over the greater part of the lung fields. In some cases, however, there are no abnormal signs.

Investigations

Lung function

Tests reveal a restrictive defect (Buechner and Ansari, 1969) with severe reduction of TLC, compliance and gas transfer, and consequent arterial oxygen desaturation. But these changes have no diagnositic significance.

Radiographic appearances

Early changes often consist of a diffuse haze in the lower zones of both lung fields (Pendergrass, 1958). Thereafter, appearances which may range from those of 'ground glass' type to a mixture of coarse linear and rounded opacities (similar to those of pulmonary oedema) appear rapidly throughout the lung fields. But, in other cases, there is a pattern of very small round opacities indicative of alveolar consolidation and resembling miliary tuberculosis distributed chiefly in the lower lung fields (*Figure 7.23*). Haziness of both fields, due to diffuse pleural thickening, may also be seen. In cases which take a protracted course a widespread pattern of irregular fibrosis, sometimes with 'honeycomb cysts', ultimately develops.

Other investigations

Sputum often contains strongly PAS-positive material and its differentiation from mucinous substances in other diseases by alcian blue, alcian green and mucicarmine stains is quick and simple, and, thus, a helpful diagnostic aid (Vidone *et al.*, 1966). Electron microscopy of sputum, though a more difficult procedure, may identify lamellar inclusion bodies (Costello *et al.*, 1975). It may be necessary to obtain lung tissue for biopsy to establish the diagnosis beyond doubt, but the discomfort and danger associated with thoracotomy and needle methods in patients with a very severe restrictive functional defect indicate that this should only be done if other methods fail. Sputum must be cultured for *M. tuberculosis* and 'opportunist' mycobacteria as soon as possible.

Diagnosis

If a detailed occupational history is not elicited, the diagnosis will in all probability be missed. Confusion may occur with pulmonary oedema, fibrosing 'alveolitis', sarcoidosis, tuberculosis and pneumonia of various types. It should also be borne in mind that alveolar silico-lipoproteinosis may occasionally develop in an individual with already established nodular silicosis or 'mixed dust fibrosis' following additional intense silica exposure.

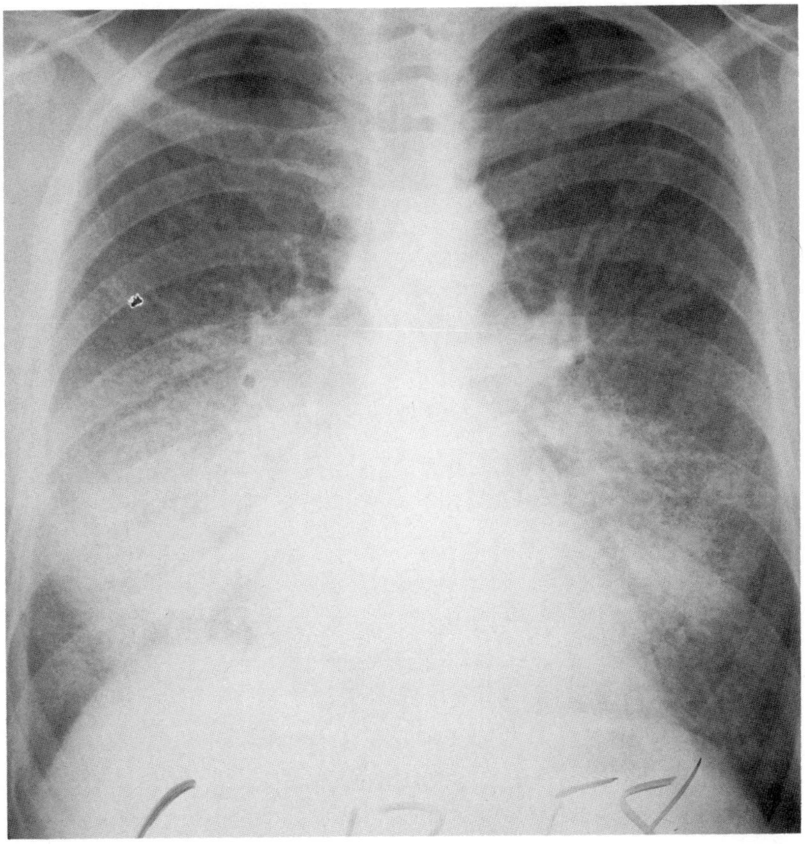

Figure 7.23 Radiographic appearances of acute silico-lipoproteinosis in a sandblaster exposed to high concentrations of quartzite sands (Courtesy of Dr H. A. Buechner and the Editor of Diseases of the Chest*)*

Complications

Tuberculosis and other pathogenic mycobacterial infections are especially apt to occur (Bailey *et al.*, 1974; Buechner and Ansari, 1969) due, no doubt, to the impaired activity of alveolar macrophages already referred to (p. 168); similarly fungous infection is also common and may be yet another distraction from the correct diagnosis. Spontaneous pneumothorax sometimes occurs. In some cases right heart failure supervenes.

It appears that acute glomerular nephritis which may be attributable to silicon toxicity is a rare complication (Giles *et al.*, 1978) (*see* p. 157).

Prognosis

Spontaneously occurring alveolar lipoproteinosis apparently resolves completely in the majority of cases but 'silica'-induced disease appears to be almost invariably fatal due to cardiorespiratory failure within about one year of development of the first symptoms. If the patient does recover some degree of intrapulmonary fibrosis will remain and may ultimately lead to death from pulmonary heart disease.

Treatment

If treatment is to succeed early diagnosis is imperative. Corticosteroids are ineffective and bronchopulmonary lavage with isotonic saline offers the best chance of recovery (Costello *et al.,* 1975; Ramirez-R. 1971) and, incidentally, electron microscopy of the lung washings will confirm the diagnosis. Prolonged daily inhalation of a trypsin aerosol also appears to be successful in idiopathic alveolar lipoproteinosis (Riker and Wolinsky, 1973) but its technical inconvenience and the possibility of its inflicting lung damage make it less attractive. Complicating mycobacterial, fungous or other pulmonary infections must be treated early and vigorously.

Prevention

The same principles as outlined for 'nodular silicosis' and diatomite pneumoconiosis apply. It is especially important that there should be an awareness of the dangers of high concentrations of quartz and cristobalite dust even over a short period of time.

REFERENCES

Adams, P. J. (1961). *Geology and Ceramics.* Department of Scientific and Industrial Research, Geological Survey and Museum. London; HMSO

Adler-Herzmark, J. and Kapstein, G. (1937). Weitere Untersuchungen über Silkos in Österreich. *Wien. med. Wschr,* **87,** 433–441

Ahlman, K. (1968). Silicosis in Finland. *Work Envir. Hlth* **4,** Suppl. 1

Ahlmark, A. and Bruce, T. (1967). The current pneumoconiosis situation in Sweden. *Scand. J. resp. Dis.* **48,** 181–188

Ahlmark, A., Bruce, T. and Nyström, A. (1960). *Silicosis and Other Pneumoconioses in Sweden.* Stockholm; Svenska Bokförlaget, London; Heinemann

Andrews, R. W. (1970). *Wollastonite.* Institute of Geological Sciences. London; HMSO

Apostolov, K. (1977). Personal communication

Apostolov, K., Spasić, P. and Bonjanić, N. (1975). Evidence of a viral aetiology in endemic (Balkan) nephropathy. *Lancet* **2,** 1271–1273

Arnstein, A. (1941). Non-industrial pneumoconiosis, pneumoconio-tuberculosis and tuberculosis of the mediastinal and bronchial lymph glands in old people. *Tubercle, Lond.* **22,** 281–295

Ashford, J. R. and Enterline, P. E. (1966). Radiological classification of pneumoconiosis. *Archs envir. Hlth* **12,** 314–330

Ashworth, T. G. (1970). Acute silico-proteinosis; case report in an African. *S. Afr. med. J.* **44,** 1214–1216

Austrheim, I. (1977). Cristobalite and tridymite crystallization in amorphous silica collected from the smoke from silicon metal furnaces. *Trans. J. Brit. Ceramic Soc.* **76,** 134–138

Ayer, H. E. (1969). The proposed ACGIH mass limits for quartz; review and evaluation. *Am. ind. Hyg. Ass. J.* **30,** 117–125

Bailey, D. A. (1947). Conversion of silica during ignition. *J. ind. Hyg. Toxicol.* **29,** 242–249

Bailey, W. C., Brown, M., Buechner, H. A., Weill, H., Ichinose, H. and Ziskind, M. (1974). Silico-mycobacterial disease in sandblasters. *Am. Rev. resp. Dis.* **110,** 115–125

Beadle, D. G. (1971). The relationship between the amount of dust breathed and the development of radiological signs of silicosis: and epidemiological study in South African gold miners. In *Inhaled Particles III,* edited by W. H. Walton, pp. 953–964. Old Woking, Surrey; Unwin Bros

Becker, R. J. P. and Chatgidakis, C. B. (1960). The heart in silicosis. *Proceedings of Pneumoconiosis Conference, Johannesburg, 1959,* edited by A. J. Orsenstein, pp. 205–216. London; Churchill

Becklake, M. R., du Preez, L. and Lutz, W. (1958). Lung function in the silicosis of the Witwatersrand gold mines. *Am. Rev. Tuberc. pulm. Dis.* **77,** 400–412

Bell, Jr, Z. G., Dunnom, D. D. and Lott, H. (1978). Basis for exposure standards for amorphous silica dusts. *Am. ind. Hyg. Ass. J.* **39,** 418–421

Bellini, F. and Ghislandi, E. (1959). Su due casi di silicosi e sclerodermia. *Med. Lav.* **50,** 63–70

Belt, T. H. (1939). Silicosis of the spleen: a study of the silicotic nodule. *J. Path. Bact.* **49,** 39–44

Bobear, J. B., Hanemann, S. J. and Beven, T. (1962). Silicosis in Louisiana: new or unrecognised hazard. *J. Louisiana State med. Soc.* **114,** 391–397

Bradshaw, F., Critchlow, A. and Nagelschmidt, G. (1962). A study of airborne dust in hematite mines in Cumberland. *Ann. occup. Hyg.* **4,** 265–273

Bramwell, B. (1914). Diffuse scleroderma: its frequency; its occurrence in stonemasons; its treatment by fibrinolysin-elevations of temperature due to fibrinolysin injection. *Edinb. med. J.* **12,** 387–401

Buechner, H. A. and Ansari, A. (1969). Acute silico-proteinosis. *Dis. Chest* **55,** 174–284

Burgess, W. A. and Reist, P. C. (1969). An industrial hygiene study of flame cutting in a granite quarry. *Am. ind. Hyg. Ass. J.* **30,** 107–112

Burrell, R., Esber, H. J., Hagadorn, J. E. and Andrews, C. E. (1966). Specificity of lung reactive antibodies in human serum. *Am. Rev. resp. Dis.* **94,** 743–750

Byers, P. D. and Gage, J. C. (1961). The toxicity of precipitated silica. *Br. J. ind. Med.* **18,** 295–302

Byers, P. D. and King, E. J. (1961). Experimental infective pneumoconiosis with *Mycobacterium tuberculosis* (var. *muris*) and hematite by inhalation and by injection. *J. Path. Bact.* **81,** 123–134

Cameron, I. B. and McAdam, A. D. (1978). *The Oil-Shales of the Lothians, Scotland: Present Resources and Former Workings* Report 78/28. Institute of Geological Sciences. HMSO; London

Campbell, J. A. (1958). A case of Caplan's syndrome in a boiler scaler. *Thorax* **13,** 177–180

Campbell, P. M. and LeRoy, E. C. (1975). Pathogenesis of systemic sclerosis: a vascular hypothesis. *Sem. Arthr. Rheum.* **4,** 351–368

Caplan, A., Cowen, E. D. H. and Gough, J. (1958). Rheumatoid pneumoconiosis in a foundry worker. *Thorax* **13,** 181–184

Carini, R. and Lo Martire, N. (1965). Sclerosi sistematica progressiva e silicosi pulmonare. *Med. Lav.* **56,** 708–715

Carnes, W. H. (1954). Quoted by Oechsli, Jacobson and Brodeur (1961) in Diatomite pneumoconiosis: roentgen characteristics and classification. *Am. J. Roentg.* **85,** 263–270

Chapman, E. M. (1932). Acute silicosis. *J. Am. med. Ass.* **98,** 1439–1441

Chatgidakis, C. F. (1963). Silicosis in South African white gold miners. *Med. Proc.* **9,** 383–392

Chatgidakis, C. F. and Theron, C. P. (1961). Rheumatoid pneumoconiosis (Caplan's syndrome). *Archs envir. Hlth* **2,** 397–408

Chiesura, P., Bruguone, F. and Mezzanotte, S. (1961). Due osservazioni di sindrome di Caplan in minatori di galleria. *Lav. Umano* **13,** 203–213

Chiesura, P., Terribile, P. M. and Bardellini, G. (1968). Le calcificazioni 'a guscio d'uovo nella silicosi: elementi tratti dall' osservazioni di 52 casi. *Minerva med., Roma* **59,** 5960–5968

Clark, T. C., Harrington, V. A., Asta, J., Morgan, W. K. C. and Sargent, E. N. (1980). Respiratory effects of exposure to dust in taconite mining and processing. *Am. Rev. resp. Dis.* **121,** 959–966

Clerens, J. (1953). Silicose pulmonaire et rheumatisme ou syndrome de Colinet-Caplan. *Arch. belges. med. Soc.* **11,** 336–342

Colinet, E. (1953). Polyarthritis chronique évolutive et silicose pulmonarie. *Acta physiother. Rheum. belg.* **8,** 37–41

Collis, E. L. (1915). Industrial pneumoconioses with special reference to dust-phthisis. *Public Hlth* **28,** 252–264

Cooper, W. C. and Cralley, L. J. (1958). *Pneumoconiosis in Diatomite Mining and Processing.* Publ. Hlth Serv. Publn No. 601. Washington; US Dept. Hlth Educ. and Welf.

Cooper, W. C. and Jacobson, G. (1977). A 21-year radiographic follow-up of workers in the diatomite industry. *J. occup. Med.* 563–566

Corrin, B. and King, E. (1969). Experimental endogenous lipid pneumonia and silicosis. *J. Path.* **97,** 325–330

Corrin, B. and King, E. (1970). Pathogenesis of experimental pulmonary alveolar proteinosis. *Thorax* **25,** 230–236

Costello, J. (1979). Morbidity and mortality study of shale oil workers in the United States. *Env. Hlth Perspect.* **30,** 205–208

Costello, J. F., Moriarty, D. C., Branthwaite, M. A., Turner-Warwick, M. and Corrin, B. (1975). Diagnosis and management of alveolar proteinosis: the role of electron microscopy. *Thorax* **30,** 121–132

Davidson, J. M. and MacLeod, W. M. (1969). Pulmonary alveolar proteinosis. *Br. J. Dis. Chest* **63,** 13–28

Davies, C. N. (Ed.) (1969). *Health Conditions in the Ceramics Industry,* pp. 101–170. Oxford; Pergamon

de Villiers, A. J. and Gross, P. (1967). The pulmonary response of rats to fluorspar and radiation. In *Inhaled Particles and Vapours II,* edited by G. N. Davies, pp. 135–140. Oxford; Pergamon Press

Denny, J. J., Robson, W. D. and Irwin, D. A. (1939). Prevention of silicosis by metallic aluminium. *Can. med. Ass. J.* **40,** 213–228

Dutra, F. R. (1965). Diatomaceous earth pneumoconiosis. *Archs envir. Hlth* **11,** 613–619

Einbrodt, H. J. (1965). Quantitative und qualitative Untersuchungen über die Staubretention in der menschlichen Lungen. *Beitr. Silkosforsch.* **87,** 1–105

Einbrodt, H. J. and Burilkov, T. (1972). Mineral dust content of the lung tissue and lymph nodes in egg-shell calcification. *Int. Arch. Arbèitsmed.* **30,** 223–236

EMI Records (Gramophone Co. Ltd.) (1970). Personal communication

Erasmus, L. D. (1960). Scleroderma in gold miners. *Proceedings of Pneumoconiosis Conference, Johannesburg,* edited by A. J. Orenstein, pp. 426–435. London; Churchill

Faulds, T. S. and Nagelschmidt, G. S. (1962). The dust in the lungs of hematite miners from Cumberland. *Ann. occup. Hyg.* **4,** 225–263

Fiumicelli, A., Fiumicelli, C. and Pagni, M. (1964). Contributo allo studio della silicosi massiva unilarale isolata. *Medna Lav.* **5,** 516–530

Flinn, R. H., Brinton, H. P., Doyle, H. N., Cralley, L. J., Harris, R. L., Westfield, J., Bird, J. H. and Berger, L. B. (1963). *Silicosis in the Metal Mining Industry. A Revaluation. 1958–1961.* Publ. Hlth Serv. Publn No. 1076. Washington; US Government Printing Office

Fowweather, F. S. (1939). Silicosis and the analyst. *Analyst* **64,** 779–787

Fox, A. J., Greenberg, M., Ritchie, G. L. and Barraclough, R. N. J. (1975). A survey of respiratory disease in the pottery industry. *Health and Safety Executive.* London; HMSO

Francia, A., Monarca, G. and Cavallot, A. (1959). Osservazioni clinico-roentzenologische sull' assazione silicosi-sclerodermia. *Med. Lav.* **50,** 523–540

Friberg, L. and Öhman, H. (1957). Silicosis hazards in enamelling. A medical technical and experimental study. *Br. J. ind. Med.* **14,** 85–91

Gambini, G., Agnoletto, A. and Magistretti, M. (1964). Tre casi di sindrome di Caplan. *Med. Lavaro.* **55,** 261–271

Gardner, L. U. (1929). Studies on experimental pneumonokoniosis, V. *Am. Rev. Tuberc.* **20,** 833–875

Gardner, L. U. (1933). Pathology of the so-called acute silicosis. *Am. J. Publ. Hlth* **23,** 1240–1249

Gardner, L. U. (1934). *Pathology, human and experimental,* edited by B. E. Kuechle. 1st Saranac Symposium on Silicosis. Trudeau Sch. Tuberc. Saranac Lake. New York

Gardner, L. U. (1937). *The significance of the silicotic problem,* edited by B. E. Kuechle. 3rd Saranac Symposium on silicosis. Trudeau Sch. Tuberc., Saranac Lake. New York

Gedda, L., Bolognesi, M., Bandino, R. and Brenci, G. (1964). Ricerche di genetica sulla silicosi die minatori della Sardegna. *Lavaro Um.* **16,** 555–562

Giles, R. D., Sturgill, B. C., Suratt, P. M. and Bolton, W. K. (1978). Massive proteinuria and acute renal failure in a patient with acute silicoproteinosis. *Am. J. med.* **64,** 336–342

Golde, D. W., Territo, M., Finley, T. N. and Cline, M. J. (1976). Defective lung macrophages in pulmonary alveolar proteinosis. *Ann. intern. Med.* **85,** 304–309

Goldstein, B. and Rendall, R. E. G. (1970). The relative toxicities of the main classes of minerals. In *Pneumoconiosis. Proceedings of he International Conference. J'burg. 1969,* edited by H. A. Shapiro, pp. 429–434. Capetown; Oxford University Press

Goldstein, B. and Webster, I. (1966). Intratracheal injection into rats of size-graded silica particles. *Br. J. ind. Med.* **23,** 71–74

Gough, J. (1959). Rheumatoid pneumoconiosis. *Bull. post Grad. Comm. Med. Univ. Sydney* **15,** 280–284

Gough, J. (1967). Silicosis and alveolar proteinosis. *Br. med. J.* **1,** 629

Government of India Ministry of Labour (1953). *Silicosis in Mica Mining in Bihar.* Office of the Chief Advisor Factories Report No. 3

Gross, P., Westrick, M. L. and McNerney, J. M. (1960). Experimental silicosis: the inhibitory effect of iron. *Dis. Chest* **37,** 35–41

Gründorfer, W. and Raber, A. (1970). Progressive silicosis in granite workers. *Br. J. ind. Med.* **27,** 110–120

Gualde, N., de Leobardy, J., Serizay, B. and Malinvand, G. (1977). HL-A and silicosis. *Am. Rev. resp. Dis.* **116,** 334–336

Gunther, G. and Schuchardt, E. (1970). Silikose und progressive sklerodermie. *Deutsch. med. Wschr.* **95,** 467–468

Gupta, S. P., Baja, A., Jain, A. L. and Vasudeva, Y. L. (1972). Clinical and radiological studies in silicosis: based on a study of the disease amongst stone cutters. *Indian. J. med. Res.* **60,** 1309–1315

Gye, W. E. and Purdey, W. J. (1924). The poisonous properties of colloidal silica. III. *Br. J. exp. Path.* **5,** 238–250

HM Factory Inspectorate (1959). *Industrial Health. A Survey of the Pottery Industry in Stoke-on-Trent.* London; HMSO

Hale, D. R. (1975). Electronic and optical uses. In *Industrial Minerals and Rocks,* 4th edition, edited by Stanley J. Lefond, pp. 205–224. American Institute of Mining, Metallurgical and Petroleum Engineers, Inc. New York

Hale, L. W. and Sheers, G. (1963). Silicosis in West Country granite workers. *Br. J. ind. Med.* **20,** 218–225

Harding, H. E. and McLaughlin, A. I. G. (1955). Pulmonary fibrosis in non-ferrous foundry workers. *Br. J. ind. Med.* **12,** 92–99

Harding, H. E. and Massie, A. P. (1951). Pneumoconiosis in boiler scalers. *Br. J. ind. Med.* **8,** 256–264

Harding, H. E., Gloyne, S. R. and McLaughlin, A. I. G. (1950). *Industrial Lung Diseases in Iron and Steel Foundry Workers,* edited by A. I. G. McLaughlin. London; HMSO

Hawkins, J. E., Savard, E. V. and Ramirez-Rivera, J. (1967). Pulmonary alveolar proteinosis. Origins of proteins in pulmonary washings. *Am. J. clin. Path.* **48,** 14–17

Hayes, D. S. and Posner, E. (1960). A case of Caplan's syndrome in a roof tile maker. *Tubercle, Lond.* **41,** 143–145

Heath, D., Mooi, W. and Smith, P. (1978). The pulmonary vasculature in hematite lung. *Br. J. Dis. Chest* **72,** 88–94

Heppleston, A. G. (1962). The disposal of dust in the lungs of silicotic rats. *Am. J. Path.* **40,** 493–506

Heppleston, A. G., Fletcher, K. and Wyatt, I. (1974). Change in the composition of lung lipids and the 'turnover' of dapalmitoyl lecithin in experimental alveolar lipo-proteinosis induced by inhaled quartz. *Br. J. exp. Path.* **55,** 384–395

Heppleston, A. G., Wright, N. A. and Stewart, J. A. (1970). Experimental alveolar lipo-proteinosis following the inhalation of silica. *J. Path.* **101,** 293–307

Heppleston, A. G. and Young, A. E. (1972). Alveolar lipoproteinosis: an ultrastructural comparison of the experimental and human forms. *J. Path.* 107–117

Highley, D. E. (1980). Personal communication

Holmann, A. T. (1947). Historical relationship of mining silicosis and rock removal. *Br. J. ind. Med.* **4,** 1–29

Hoffman, E. O., Lamberty, J., Pizzolato, P. and Coover, J. (1973). The ultrastructure of acute silicosis. *Arch. Path.* **96,** 104–107

Hosey, A. D., Trasko, V. M. and Ashe, H. B. (1957). *Control of Silicosis in the Vermont Granite Industry.* PHS Publ. No. 557. Washington, DC; US Dept of Hlth Educ. and Welfare

Hruban, Z. (1976). Pulmonary changes induced by ammophilic drugs. *Envir. Hlth Perspect.* **16,** 111–118

International Labour Office (1966). *The Prevention and Suppression of Dust in Mining. Tunnelling and Quarrying. Third International Report 1958–1962.* Geneva; ILO

Israel, H. L., Sones, M., Roy, R. L. and Stein, G. N. (1961). The occurrence of intrathoracic calcification in sarcoidosis. *Am. Rev. resp. Dis.* **84,** 1–11

Jabłońska, E. (1975). Scleroderma and pseudoscleroderma. Warsaw; Polish Medical Publishers, Pennsylvania, USA; Dowden, Hutchinson and Ross Inc.

Jain, S. M., Sepaha, G. C., Khare, K. C. and Dubey, V. S. (1977). Silicosis in slate pencil workers. *Chest* **71,** 423–426

Jayson, M. I. V. (1977). Collagen changes in the pathogenesis of systemic sclerosis. *Ann. rheum. Dis.* **36** (suppl) 26–28

Johnson, G. T., Lewis, T. R. and Groth, D. H. (1973). Evaluation of health hazard of amorphous silica-coated cristobalite following intratracheal injection in rats. US Dept. Hlth Educ. and Welfare. National Institute for Occupational Safety and Health. Cincinnati (SR-35)

Joint Standing Committee on Health Safety and Welfare in Foundries (1977). Some aspects of pneumoconiosis in a group of mechanised iron foundries. Health and Safety Executive. London; HMSO

Joint Standing Committee on Safety Health and Welfare Conditions in Non-ferrous Foundries (1957). Ministry of Labour and National Service. First Report. London; HMSO

Jones, J. G., Owen, T. E. and Corrado, H. A. (1967). Respiratory tuberculosis and pneumoconiosis in slate workers. *Br. J. Dis. Chest.* **61,** 138–143

Jones, R. N., Turner-Warwick, M., Ziskind, M. and Weill, H. (1976). High prevalence of antinuclear antibodies in sandblasters silicosis. *Am. Rev. resp. Dis.* **113,** 393–395

Kawakami, M., Sato, S. and Takishima, T. (1977). Silicosis in workers dealing with tonoko. *Chest* **75,** 635–639

Keers, R. Y. (1969). The treatment of silicotuberculosis. In *Health Conditions in the Ceramic Indistry,* edited by C. N. Davies, pp. 63–69. Oxford; Pergamon

Kennedy, M. C. S. (1956). Aluminium powder inhalations in the treatment of silicosis of pottery workers and pneumoconiosis of coal miners. *Br. J. ind. Med.* **13,** 85–99

Kessel, R. W. I., Monaco, L. and Marchisio, M. A. (1963). The specificity of the cytotoxic action of silica: a study *in vitro. Br. J. exp. Path.* **44,** 351–364

Kettle, E. H. (1932). The interstitial reactions caused by various dusts and their influence on tuberculous injections. *J. Path. Bact.* **35,** 395–405

Khoo, O. T. and Toh, K. K. (1968). Morbidity of silicosis in Singapore. *Singapore med. J.* **9,** 186–191

Klosterkötter, W. and Einbrodt, H. J. (1965). Quantitative tiexperimentelle Untersuchungen über den Abtransport von Staub aus den Lugen in die regionalen Lymphknoten. *Archs Hyg.* **149,** 367–384

Kolev, K., Doitschinov, D. and Todorov, D. (1970). Morphologic alterations in the kidneys by silicosis. *Med. Lav.* **61,** 205–210

Kuhn, C., Györkey, F., Levine, B. E. and Ramirez-Rivera, J. (1966). Pulmonary alveolar proteinosis: a study using enzyme histochemistry, electron microscopy and surface tension measurements. *Lab. Invest.* **15,** 492–509

Küng, V. A. (1979). Morphological investigations of fibrogenic action of Estonian oil shale dust. *Env. Hlth Perspect.* **30,** 153–156

Lamvik, J. (1963). Rheumatoid pneumoconiosis. *Acta Path. Microbiol. scand.* **57,** 169–174

Landwehr, M. (1963). Quoted by Reichel, Bauer and Bruckmann (1977)

Leading Article (1977). Balkan nephropathy. *Lancet* **1,** 683–684

Levene, C. I., Bye, I. and Saffiotti, U. (1968). The effect of beta-aminoproprionitrile on silicotic pulmonary fibrosis. *Br. J. exp. Path.* **49,** 152–158

Lewis, D. M. and Burrell, R. (1976). Induction of fibrogenesis by lung antibody-treated macrophages. *Br. J. ind. Med.* **33,** 25–28

Liebow, A. A. (1968). New concepts and entities in pulmonary disease. In *The Lung,* edited by Averill A. Liebow and David E. Smith, pp. 332–333. Baltimore; Williams and Wilkins

Lloyd Davies, T. A. (1971). Respiratory disease in foundry men. Report of a survey. London; HMSO

Lloyd Davies, T. A., Doig, A. T., Fox, A. J. and Greenberg, M. (1973). A radiographic survey of monumental masonry workers in Aberdeen. *Br. J. ind. Med.* **30,** 227–231

Longley, E. O. (1970). Oesophageal compression due to silicotic mediastinal lymph glands. *Trans. Soc. occup. Med.* **20,** 69

Luton, P., Champeix, J., Ravet, M. and Vallaud, A. (1956). Observations récentes sur la pneumoconiose parterre a diatomées. *Archs Mal. prof. Méd. trav.* **17,** 125–148

Lynch, K. M. (1942). Silicosis of systemic distribution. *Am. J. Path.* **18,** 313–321

McDonald, G., Piggott, A. P. and Gilder, F. W. (1930). Two cases of acute silicosis with a suggested theory of causation. *Lancet* **2,** 846–848

McLaughlin, A. I. G. (1957). Pneumoconiosis in foundry workers. *Br. J. Tuberc.* **51,** 297–309

McLaughlin, A. I. G. and Harding, H. E. (1956). Pneumoconiosis and other causes of death in iron and steel foundry workers. *Archs ind. Hlth* **14,** 350–378

McTurk, L. C., Huis, C. H. W. and Eckardt, R. E. (1956). Health hazards of vanadium containing residual oil ash. *Industr. Med. Surg.* **25,** 29–36

Mallory, T. B. (1934). Case records of the Massachusetts General Hospital, Case 20102. *New Engl. J. Med.* **210,** 551–554

Marković, B. L. and Arambašić, M. D. (1971). Experimental

chronic interstitial nephritis compared with endemic human nephropathy. *J. Path.* **103,** 35–40
Meiklejohn, A. (1956). 'Silicosis and other fibrotic pneumoconioses'. In *Industrial Medicine and Hygiene,* Vol. 3, p. 120. Edited by E.R.A. Merewether. London; Butterworths
Michel, R. D. and Morris, J. F. (1964). Acute silicosis. *Archs int. Med.* **113,** 850–855
Middleton, E. L. (1929). The present position of silicosis in industry in Britain. *Br. med. J.* **2,** 485–489
Middleton, E. L. (1930). Flint knapping. In *Silicosis.* Records of International Conference, Johannesburg, August, 1930, pp. 478–479. Geneva; International Labour Office
Miguères, J., Layssol, M., Moreau, G., Jover, A. and Tricoire, J. (1966). Sclérodermie pulmonaire et silicose du spath fluor associée rapports entre sclérodermie et silicose. *J. Fran. Med. Chir. Thorac* **20,** 603–618
Miners Phthisis Medical Bureau (1944). *Report upon the work of the MPMB for three years ended 31st July 1941.* Pretoria; Union of South Africa Government Printer
Moreschi, N., Farina, G. and Chiappinio, G. (1968). La silicosi pulmonaire calcificata. *Medna Lav.* **59,** 111–124
Morgan, W. K. C. (1975). The Walrus and the Carpenter or the silica criteria standard. Commentary. *J. occup. Med.* **17,** 782–783
Motley, H. L. (1960). Pulmonary function studies in diatomaceous earth workers. 2. A cross section survey of 98 workers on the job. *Ind. Med. Surg.* **24,** 370–378
Motley, H. L., Smart, R. H. and Valero, A. (1956). Pulmonary function studies in diatomaceous earth workers. 1. Ventilatory and blood gas exchange disturbance. *Archs ind. Hlth* **13,** 165–174
Munizaga, J., Allison, M. J., Gerszten, E. and Klurfeld, D. M. (1975). Pneumoconiosis in Chilean miners of the 16th century. *Bull. NY Acad. Med.* **51,** 1281–1293
Nagelschmidt, G. (1965). A study of lung dust in pneumoconiosis. *Am. ind. Hyg. Ass. J.* **26,** 1–7
Nelson, H. M., Rajhans, G. S., Morton, S. and Brown, J. R. (1978). Silica flour exposures in Ontario. *Am. ind. Hyg. Ass. J.* **39,** 261–269
Nordmann, M. (1943). Die Staublunge der Kieselgurarbelter. *Virchows Arch. path. Anat. Physiol.* **311,** 116–148
Notholt, A. J. G. and Highley, D. E. (1975). *Fluorspar.* Mineral Dossier No. 1. Mineral Resources Consultative Committee. London; HMSO
Oechsli, W. R., Jacobson, G. and Brodeur, A. E. (1961). Diatomite pneumoconiosis: roentgen characteristics and classification. *Am. J. Roentgen.* **85,** 263–270
Otto, H. (1969). Results of latex tests in 6,000 porcelain workers. In *Health Conditions in the Ceramic Industry,* edited by C. N. Davies, pp. 91–98. Oxford; Pergamon
Palmer, P. E. S. and Daynes, G. (1967). Transkei silicosis. *S. Afr. med. J.* **41,** 1182–1188
Palmhert, H., Webster, I. and Lens, C. (1968). Atypical mycobacteria and infections of the lung in the South Africa mining industry. *S. Afr. Pneumocon. Rev.* **3,** 6
Paul, R. (1961). Silicosis in Northern Rhodesian copper mines. *Archs envir. Hlth* **2,** 96–109
Pendergrass, E. P. (1958). *The Pneumoconiosis Problem,* pp. 95–97. Springfield; Thomas
Pernis, B. (1968). Silicosis. In *Textbook of Immunopathology.* Vol. 1, edited by P. A. Meischer and H. J. Muller-Eberhardt, pp. 293–301. New York and London; Grune and Stratton
Phibbs, B. R., Sundin, R. E. and Mitchell, R. S. (1971). Silicosis in Wyoming bentonite workers. *Am. Rev. resp. Dis.* **103,** 1–17
Pilkington, L. A. B. (1969). The float glass process. *Proc. R. Soc.* **314,** 1–25
Plunkett, E. R. and De Witt, B. J. (1962). Occupational exposure to Hi-Sil and Silene. *Archs envir. Hlth* **5,** 469–472
Polacheck, A. A. and Pijanowski, W. J. (1960). Extrathoracic egg-shell calcifications in silicosis. *Am. Rev. resp. Dis.* **82,** 714–720
Policard, A., Gernez-Rieux, C., Tacquet, A., Martin, J. C., Devulder, B. and Le Bouffant, L. (1967). Influence of pulmonary dust load on the development of experimental infection by *Mycobacteria kansasii. Nature, Lond.* **216,** 177–178
Posner, E. (1960). Pneumoconiosis in makers of artificial grinding wheels including a case of Caplan's Syndrome. *Br. J. ind. Med.* **17,** 109–113
Posner, E. (1961). Pneumoconiosis and tuberculosis in the North Staffordshire pottery industry. In *Symposium on Dust Control in the Pottery Industry,* pp. 5–18. Stoke; British Ceramic Research Assoc. Sec. Publ. 27
Posner, E. and Kennedy, M. C. S. (1967). A further study of china biscuit placers in Stoke-on-Trent. *Br. J. ind. Med.* **24,** 133–142
Pump, K. K. (1968). Studies in silicosis of the human lung. *Dis. Chest* **53,** 237–246
Ramirez-R., J. (1971). Alveolar proteinosis: importance of pulmonary lavage. *Am. J. resp. Dis.* **103,** 666–678
Reichel, G., Bauer, H-D. and Bruckmann, E. (1977). The action of quartz in the presence of iron hydroxides in the human lung. In *Inhaled Particles and Vapours IV,* edited by W. H. Walton, pp. 403–410. Oxford; Pergamon Press
Reif, E., Landwehr, M. and Bruckmann, E. (1963). Die Beeinflussung des Quartzstaub-granuloms durch Eisenerzstäube. In *Fortschritte der Staublungenforschung,* 1, pp. 427–439. Edited by Reichel, Bauer and Bruckmann
Riker, J. B. and Wolinsky, H. (1973). Trypsin aerosol treatment of pulmonary alveolar proteinosis. *Am. Rev. resp. Dis.* **108,** 108–113
Ritterhoff, R. J. (1941). Acute silicosis occurring in employees of abrasive soap powder industries. *Am. Rev. Tuberc.* **43,** 117–131
Roberts, W. C. (1965). The ferro-alloy industry: hazards of the alloys and semi-metallics. Part II. *J. occup. Med.* **7,** 71–77
Rodnan, G. P., Benedek, T. G., Medsger, T. A. and Cammarata, R. J. (1967). The association of progressive systemic sclerosis (scleroderma) with coal miner's pneumoconiosis and other forms of silicosis. *Ann. int. Med.* **66,** 323–334
Roeslin, N., Lassabe-Roth, C., Morand, G. and Batzenschlager, A. (1980). La silico-protéinose aiguë. *Arch. mal. prof.* **41,** 15–18
Rosen, S. H., Castleman, B. and Liebow, A. A. (1958). Pulmonary alveolar proteinosis. *New Engl. J. Med.* **258,** 1123–1142
Rosenzweig, D. Y. (1967). Silicosis complicated by a typical mycobacterial infection. In *Transactions of 26th VA-Armed Forces Pulmonary Disease Research Conference,* p. 47. Washington; United States Government Printing Office
Rüttner, J. R. (1954). Foundry worker's pneumoconiosis in Switzerland (anthra-silicosis). *Archs ind. Hyg.* **9,** 297–305
Rüttner, J. R. and Heer, H. R. (1969). Silicosis and lung cancer. *Schweiz. med. Wschr.* **99,** 245–249
Salam, M. S. A., El-Samra, G. H., El-Alamy, M. A. and Gomaa, T. (1967). Pulmonary manifestations in workers exposed to dusts of synthetic detergents and abrasive soaps. *Ann. occup. Hyg.* **10,** 105–112
Saldanha, L. F., Rosen, V. J. and Gonick, H. C. (1975). Silicon nephropathy. *Am. J. Med.* **59,** 95–103
Samimi, B., Weill, H. and Ziskind, M. (1974). Respirable silica dust exposure of sandblasters and associated workers in steel fabrication yards. *Archs envir. Hlth* **29,** 61–66
Scadding, J. G. (1967). *Sarcoidosis,* pp. 141–149. London; Eyre and Spottiswoode
Schepers, G. W. H., Durkan, T. M., Delahant, A. B., Creedon, F. T. and Redlin, A. J. (1957a). The biological action of Degussa submicron silica dust (Dow Corning silica), 1. *Archs ind. Hlth* **16,** 125–146
Schepers, G. W. H., Delahant, A. B., Schmidt, J. G., von Wecheln, J. C., Creedon, F. T. and Clark, R. W. (1957b). The biological action of Degussa submicron silica dust (Dow Corning silica), 3. *Archs ind. Hlth* **16,** 280–301
Schepers, G. W. H., Smart, R. H., Smith, C. R., Dworski, M. and Delahant, A. B. (1958). Fatal silicosis with complicating infection by an atypical acid fast photochromic bacillus. *Ind. Med. Surg.* **27,** 27–36
Schlipköter, H. W. (1970). Ätiologie und Pathogenese der Silikose sowie ihre kausale Beeinflussung. *Naturwissenschaften* **197,** 39–105

Schneider, H. (1966). Silikosegefahrrdung durch Neuburger Kieselkreide. *Int. Arch. Gewerbepath. Gewerbehyg.* **22,** 323–341

Schuyler, M., Ziskind, M. and Salvaggio, J. (1977). Cell-mediated immunity in silicosis. *Am. Rev. resp. Dis.* **116,** 147–151

Slater, D. (1973). *Tungsten.* Mineral Dossier No. 5. Mineral Resources Consultative Committee. London; HMSO

Smart, R. H. and Anderson, W. H. (1952). Pneumoconiosis due to diatomaceous earth. Clinical and X-ray aspects. *Ind. Med. Surg.* **21,** 509–518

Sosman, R. B. (1965). *The Phases of Silica.* New Jersey; Rutgers University Press

South African Medical Research Council (1974). Biological effects of South African minerals. *Nat. Res. Inst. occup. Dis. J'burg.* Fourth Annual Report p. 19

Spain, D. M. (1965). In Editorial to Diatomaceous earth pneumoconiosis by F. R. Dutra (1965). *Archs envir. Hlth* **11,** 619

Stewart, M. J. and Faulds, J. S. (1934). Pulmonary fibrosis in hematite miners. *J. Path. Bact.* **39,** 233–253

Suratt, P. M., Winn, W. C. Jr., Brody, A. R., Bolton, W. K. and Giles, R. D. (1977). Acute silicosis in tombstone sandblasters. *Am. Rev. resp. Dis.* **115,** 521–529

Sweany, H. C., Porsche, J. D. and Douglass, J. R. (1936). Chemical and pathological study of pneumoconiosis with special emphasis on silicosis and silico-tuberculosis. *Archs Path.* **22,** 593–633

Swensson, A. (1967). Tissue reaction to different types of amorphous silica. In *Inhaled Particles and Vapours II,* edited by C. N. Davies, pp. 95–102. Oxford; Pergamon Press

Swensson, A., Kvarnström, K., Bruce, T., Edling, N. P. G. and Glömme, J. (1971). Pneumoconiosis in ferrosilicon workers—a follow-up study. *J. occup. Med.* **13,** 427–432

Tada, S. Yasukochi, H., Shida, H., Chiyotani, K., Saito, K., Mishina, M. and Kozuka, Y. (1974). Bronchial arteriography in silicosis. *Am. J. Roent.* **120,** 810–814

Tebbens, B. D. and Beard, R. R. (1957). Experiments on diatomaceous earth pneumoconiosis. 1. Natural diatomaceous earth in guinea pigs. *Archs ind. Hlth* **16,** 55–63

Teculescu, D. B. and Stănescu, D. C. (1970). Carbon monoxide transfer factor for the lung in silicosis. *Scand. J. resp. Dis.* **51,** 150–159

Thiruvengadam, K. V., Anguli, V. C., Shetty, P., Sanibandam, S. and Kosairam, R. (1968). Silicosis in a mica-mine worker. *J. Indian med. Ass.* **51,** 248–250

Turner-Warwick, M., Cole, P., Weill, H., Jones, R. N. and Ziskind, M. (1977). Chemical fibrosis: the model of silica. *Ann. rheum. Dis.* **36,** (suppl), 47–50

Uehlinger, E. (1946). Übermischstaubpneumo-Koniosen. *Schweiz. Z. Path. Bakt.* **9,** 692–700

United States Department of Health, Education and Welfare (1974). Criteria for a recommended standard occupational exposure to crystalline silica. *National Institute for Occupational Safety and Health (NIOSH)* **75,** 120

Utidjian, H. M. D. (1975). Recommendations for a crystalline silica standard. Criteria documents. *J. occup. Med.* **17,** 775–781

Vidone, R. A., Hoffmann, L., Hukill, P. B., Nesbitt, K. A. and McMahon, F. J. (1966). The diagnosis of pulmonary alveolar proteinosis by sputum examination. *Dis. Chest* **49,** 326–332

Vigliani, E. C. and Mottura, G. (1948). Diatomaceous earth silicosis. *Br. J. ind. Med.* **5,** 148–160

Vitums, V. C., Edwards, M. J., Niles, N. R., Borman, J. O. and Lowry, R. D. (1977). Pulmonary fibrosis from amorphous silica dust, a product of silica vapour. *Archs envir. Hlth.* **32,** 62–68

Volk, H. (1960). The health of workers in plant making highly dispersed silica. *Archs envir. Hlth* **1,** 125–128

Vorwald, A. J., Durkan, T. M., Pratt, P. C. and Delahant, A. B. (1949). Diatomaceous earth pneumoconiosis. *Proc. IX Int. Congr. Ind. Med., Bristol,* pp. 726–741. Bristol; Wright

Wagner, J. C. and McCormick, J. N. (1967). Immunological investigations of coal workers' disease. *J. Roy. Coll. Phys. (Lond.)* **2,** 49–56

Wagner, W. D., Fraser, D. A., Wright, P. G., Dobrogorski, O. J. and Stokinger, H. E. (1968). Experimental evaluation of the threshold limit of cristobalite-calcined diatomaceous earth. *Am. ind. Hyg. Ass. J.* **19,** 211–221

Warrell, D. A., Harrison, B. D. W., Fawcett, I. W., Mohammed, Y., Mohammed, W. S., Pope, H. M. and Watkins, B. J. (1975). Silicosis among grindstone cutters in North Nigeria. *Thorax* **30,** 389–398

Weaver, N. K. and Gibson, R. L. (1979). The US oil shale industry: a health perspective. *Am. industr. Hyg. Assoc. J.* **40,** 460–467

Webster, I. (1968). Prevention of silicosis. *S. Afr. Pneumocon. Rev.* **4,** 11–12

Weller, W. (1977). Long-term test on rhesus monkeys for the PVNO-therapy of anthraco-silicosis. In *Inhaled Particles and Vapours IV,* edited by W. H. Walton, pp. 379–386. Oxford; Pergamon Press

World Health Organisation (1968). *Pneumoconiosis. Report on the Katowice Symposium, 1967,* pp. 29–31. Copenhagen; Regional Office for Europe

Xipell, J. M., Ham, K. N., Price, C. G. and Thomas, D. P. (1977). Acute silicoproteinosis. *Thorax* **32,** 104–111

Zaidi, S. H. (1969). Experimental pneumoconiosis pp. 113–117. Baltimore; The Johns Hopkins Press

Zimmerman, P. V. and Sinclair, R. A. (1977). Rapidly progressive fatal silicosis in a young man. *Med. J. Aust.* **2,** 704–706

Ziskind, M., Weill, H., Anderson, A. E., Samini, B., Neilson, A. and Waggenpack, C. (1976). Silicosis in shipyard sandblasters. *Envir. Res.* **11,** 237–243

8 Pneumoconiosis due to Coal and Carbon

This pneumoconiosis which may occur in workers in coal, graphite and other types of carbon is considered separately from silicosis because:

(1) the pathology is distinct from that of nodular silicosis;
(2) there is uncertainty as to what part quartz plays in pathogenesis;
(3) in some respects coal pneumoconiosis has been more extensively studied than silicosis.

Terminology

The Committee on Industrial Pulmonary Disease (Medical Research Council, 1942) proposed the term *coal-worker's pneumoconiosis* although, perhaps, 'coal pneumoconiosis' is adequate to the purpose. *Anthraco-silicosis* takes for granted that this pneumoconiosis is a form of silicosis but as this is uncertain it is best avoided. The recently current term, *black lung,* is uninformative and capable of including any of the 'pulmonary conditions which may be present in a coal-miner's chest' (Gross and de Treville, 1970); it should have no place in medical terminology.

The pathological appearances and behaviour of this pneumoconiosis are identical irrespective of whether it is due to exposure to coal, graphite or synthetic carbons. Since about 1948 in the UK the terms *simple pneumoconiosis, infective nodule, complicated* or *infective pneumoconiosis* and *progressive massive fibrosis* have been used to describe the various stages of the lesions. 'Simple pneumoconiosis' refers to small, discrete dust macules (*macula,* a stain or spot) or nodules not larger than about 5 mm in diameter which were believed to be uncomplicated by any other causative factor than the coal- or carbon-dust (Gough and Heppleston, 1960) in contrast to somewhat larger nodules previously thought to be associated with past infection, and the massive lesions consisting of dust and fibrosis which were considered to result from the 'complication' of a modified tuberculous process. The objection to these terms is that they are not simply descriptive but assume a mode of pathogenesis which is either unproven or not universally operative. 'Progressive massive fibrosis' (PMF) refers to larger confluent masses of dust and collagen fibrosis and is synonymous with 'complicated pneumoconiosis'. Although these lesions are not always continuously progressive and do not consist of solid collagenous masses (*see* p. 186) it is a useful and generally accepted term.

SOURCES OF EXPOSURE

COAL

The composition of coal and meaning of 'rank' of coal are briefly described in Chapter 2.

Coal-mining

The highest concentrations of dust have always occurred underground and mostly at the 'coal-face' (that is, a working place at the solid surface of a coal-seam which has separate intake and return roadways). In the UK coal was obtained by use of pick and shovel until the beginning of this century when machine-cutting methods were introduced and increasingly used over the following years. Hand-powered drills and cutters with water infusion to suppress dust also came into use during this period and in some collieries were employed until the early 1960s. In general, coal-getting has been almost completely mechanized since then. Men working at the coal-face have been known variously as coal-hewers, coal-getters and colliers.

A disadvantage of mechanical methods is that machines—unlike men—do not distinguish between rock intrusions and coal so that in some regions more quartz is contributed to the atmosphere than by hand-got methods.

Coal is loaded either manually or by mechanical means from the coal cutter on to a conveyor belt which carries it to a loading point, thence to be taken by a haulage system to the bottom of the pit shaft. From here it is lifted to the surface. As the coal-seam is developed, conveyers are dismantled and re-erected for re-positioning. Different types of haulage have been used: trucks ('tubs' or 'trams') drawn on a railway, previously by ponies, but now by diesel or electric locomotives, or by a continuous wire rope system powered by a stationary engine. Until the 1950s the point at which the conveyor discharged the coal into the trucks was extremely dusty.

Other work on the coal-face includes 'advancing' it and shot-firing to loosen the coal; this involves boring shot holes and placing and firing an explosive charge, although some new methods do not employ explosives.

Men who make new underground roadways ('developers'), increase the height of the 'roof' and erect supports ('rippers'), increase other roadway and airway dimensions ('dinters') or keep roadways in good repair ('repairers') are exposed to variable amounts of 'stone' dust as well as coal-dust. The composition of this varies according to the type of rock intrusion (*see* Chapter 2) but shale is usual and sandstone common. And so, drilling, shot firing and other work in these rocks may give rise to significant quantities of quartz-dust. Men working on the sinking of coal-mine shafts are particularly likely to have been exposed to the dust of quartz-bearing rocks.

In general, concentrations of dust are very low in haulage roadways and in the vicinity of the pit shaft bottom. The use of the 'long-wall' mining technique in Britain and European countries and the 'room-and-pillar' method in the USA gives rise to different dust conditions.

Since 1910 'stone dust' has been spread periodically along roadways and elsewhere in coal-mines to prevent coal-dust explosions, and shales, limestone and gypsum have been used. As shales have a high quartz content (Nagelschmidt and Godbert, 1951) and certain limestones may contain as much as 9 per cent (Beal, Griffin and Nagelschmidt, 1953), regulations to control the type of dust employed have been applied in the UK and the USA. Therefore, 'stone dusting' in the coal-mines of these countries is unlikely to have been a silicosis risk for 20 years or more.

Colliery surface work

Men who work as sorters on the 'screens' (that is conveyors carrying coal) remove shale and rock, and break and grade the coal. Dust concentrations are very low and ventilation is good.

Coal-trimming

This involves loading, stowing and levelling washed, dirt-free coal in the holds of ships or large stores. A mechanical loader deposits the coal into the hold, where the men shovel it into place. Dust concentrations in the holds are high. Pneumoconiosis in this occupation was first suspected by Collis and Gilchrist (1928) and later confirmed by Gough (1940).

Fly ash

This consists of particles in the form of microcrystals and microspheres engendered by coal-fired electric generating plants and blast furnaces (Fisher, Chang and Brummer, 1976). They are composed of silicates and oxides of aluminium, iron, calcium, sodium, titanium, magnesium and calcium including mullite and magnetite; and there is a small quantity of quartz altered or fused by the high temperatures. The ash may escape from effluent stacks or be collected in electrostatic precipitators ('hopper ash') from which it is extracted and pulverized for processing into light-weight aggregates, concrete and grouts or for use in ceramics.

Cytological studies indicate that the dust is not fibrogenic, and no lung disease has been observed in animals nor in man exposed to fly ash alone (Alarie *et al.*, 1975; Brummer and Schwarz, 1977; McFarland *et al.*, 1971; Raask and Schilling, 1980; Bonnell, Schilling and Massey, 1980). But there is conjecture that trace elements concentrated on the microcrystals might be toxic (Linton *et al.*, 1976).

ACTIVATED CARBON

Activated carbon is manufactured by subjecting lignites to a steam-activation process during which an original free silica content of up to 3 per cent is reduced to 0.12 per cent (Gross and Nau, 1967). It is used in industry primarily as an adsorbent.

GRAPHITE

Natural graphite, known also as plumbago, is elemental crystalline carbon mixed with a variety of mineral impurities. When the crystals are visible to the naked eye it is called 'flake' graphite; when they are small, or cryptocrystalline, it is known as 'amorphous' graphite. Amorphous graphite is the type most used in industry. Graphite is widely distributed geographically in igneous, sedimentary and metamorphic rocks; the most important commercial graphite occurs in metamorphic siliceous sediments, in veins of quartz–mica schists, feldspathic or micaceous quartzites and gneisses (as in Ceylon, Madagascar, Madras and Brazil). When mined, therefore, it contains variable quantities of quartz: 3.6 to 10 per cent 'free silica' has been reported in samples from Ceylon, Korea and South-West Africa (Harding and Oliver, 1949); about 11 per cent in samples from Italy (Parmeggiani, 1950); and 5.24 per cent in samples from Pennsylvania (Ladoo and Myers, 1951). Mica, iron oxides and other minerals may also be present.

Artificial graphite, by contrast, is almost pure crystalline carbon, made by subjecting coal or petroleum coke to a temperature of almost 3000 °C in an electric furnace. In contrast with natural graphite it contains negligible traces of free silica (Mantell, 1968). However, significant quantities of quartz and cristobalite are present in pyrolitic graphite (or retort carbon) because this is formed by deposition of carbon on the refractory brick surfaces of retorts, but its use is very limited. The manufacture of synthetic graphite was an extremely dusty process until after the Second World War.

Uses of graphite

(1) *Refractory ceramics and crucibles* Carbon is very resistant to thermal shock.

Natural flake graphite (usually from Ceylon and Madagascar) mixed with various proportions of bond clay and sand is used to make blast furnace hearths and linings, and, with the addition of china clay, to make crucibles and ladles for the chemical and non-ferrous metallurgical industries. The preparation of these materials and subsequent trimming of the products before firing was until recently (and in some instances may still be) a very dusty process. It is evident that there was the possibility of exposure to quartz dust as well as to graphite (*see* Pathology section). These ingredients have been replaced to a large extent by artificial graphite, bitumen and certain metals.

Natural graphite has many applications in rockets, missiles, furnaces and moulds.

(2) *Foundry facings* Pulverized natural graphite is mixed with sand, clay or talc to give a smooth surface to the mould sand before molten metal is added. It is important in the casting of bells.

(3) *Steel and cast iron manufacture* Flake graphite is used to increase the hardness and strength of the metal.

(4) *Pencils* Amorphous graphite of high purity is finely ground and mixed in varying proportions with clay. The wet mix is extruded through dies and fired. The famous mines in Borrowdale, Cumberland, which produce graphite for this purpose were started in the middle of the sixteenth century.

(5) *Lubricants* Either artificial or natural graphite of high purity is used after being ground to a fine powder and mixed with oil or employed without. There must be no abrasive impurities such as quartz.

(6) *Neutron moderators in atomic reactors* These are manufactured from large blocks of artificial graphite.

(7) *Electrodes* Carbon electrodes for electrolytic processes in the chemical and metallurgical industries are made from artificial graphite.

(8) *Electrotyping* High-purity natural graphite is used as a parting compound dusted on to wax moulds and re-applied after the print impression is taken. This was a very dusty process which has largely been replaced by other methods since the early 1950s. However, the use of graphite for this purpose was still recorded in 1968 (Mantell, 1968).

The use of pyrolytic graphite is virtually restricted to the manufacture of carbon brushes and metal alloys.

Graphite miners (notably in Ceylon) may develop pneumoconiosis after some 15 to 20 years in the industry (Dassanayake, 1948; Ranasinha and Uragoda, 1972). Grinding, mixing and bagging graphite for any of the processes just enumerated is a potential source of high concentrations of dust and, in some, of significant quantities of quartz; but today, dust control measures are usually applied, and in most large industries are very efficient. Pneumoconiosis both in discrete and PMF forms is well documented among natural graphite workers (Lochtkemper and Teleky, 1932; Faulkner, 1940; Dunner and Bagnall, 1949; Gloyne, Marshall and Hoyle, 1949; Parmeggiani, 1950; Jaffé, 1951; Haferland, 1957; Gaensler *et al.*, 1966), and it has also been recorded in workers in artificial graphite (Zahorski, 1961).

LAMP BLACK

Lamp black is the smoke of an unobstructed hydrocarbon flame deposited on the floors of condensing chambers. It is an amorphous carbon used mainly as a paint pigment and an oil-absorption agent. It contains no quartz.

CARBON BLACK

Carbon is liberated from flames produced by various methods from natural gas, petroleum distillates and residues, or mixed oil and gas; or by a non-flame, 'thermal' method using natural gas in a heated air-free chamber (Mantell, 1968). As refractory chambers are employed in some of these processes it is possible that a trace quantity of quartz or cristobalite might be present in the final product.

Some stages of the manufacturing process are likely to be dusty. This was especially so during the 1930s when, for example, a carbon black plant in Texas was visible a mile or so away due to the production of black dust; since then, however, the standard of dust control in this industry in the USA has been very high, but has lagged far behind in some plants in European countries, Japan, South America and India (Mantell, 1971). Collection and packaging of carbon black has always been a dusty and dirty job.

A particularly pure form of carbon black—known as acetylene black—is produced by thermal decomposition of acetylene.

Carbon black, unlike lamp black, is hard, brilliant and mainly crystalline.

Uses of carbon black

It is most extensively employed as a filler and colouring agent in rubber, plastics, gramophone records (in which it constitutes some 2 per cent of the ingredients) and printing inks; it is also used in paints and enamels, in the manufacture of carbon electrodes, and carbon paper, and as a filter aid, decolouring agent and clarifier.

Significant exposure to the dust has occurred mainly in the production of carbon black, while being emptied from bags, and weighed and mixed with other materials. Trimming and polishing carbon arc rods was also dusty. Pneumoconiosis due to carbon black has been recorded by a number of authors (Gärtner and Braus, 1951; Meiklejohn, 1957; Miller and Ramsden, 1961) although free silica is either completely absent or present in only trace amounts in most high grade carbons (Meiklejohn, 1957).

Carbon electrode manufacture

The materials used are either anthracite and coke or petroleum coke. Anthracite has been mostly employed in the UK and, after purification, it is virtually pure carbon as the quartz content is then of the order of only 0.20 to 0.84 per cent (Mantell, 1968). The materials are calcined, ground to size, mixed with pitch, pressed or extruded into appropriate shapes and then baked in a furnace. The electrodes—which may be very large—are finally drilled and threaded in a machining department. The first stages of this process were very dusty until about 1950 since when grinding plants have usually been totally enclosed, and

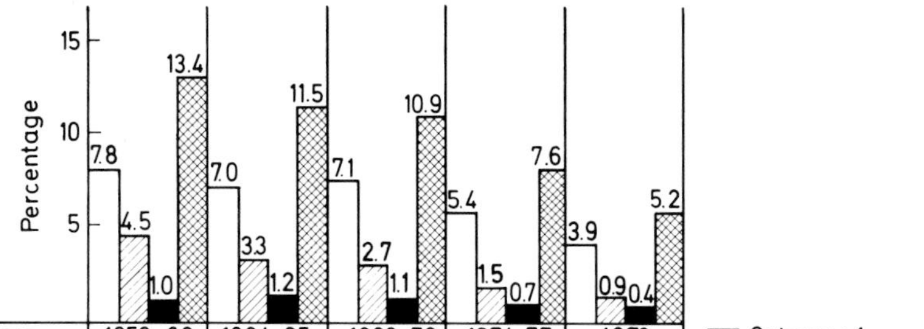

Years	1959-60	1964-65	1969-70	1974-77	1978
Collieries surveyed	259	180	118	244	54
Numbers of men	118 272	147 054	94 173	95 795	44 069

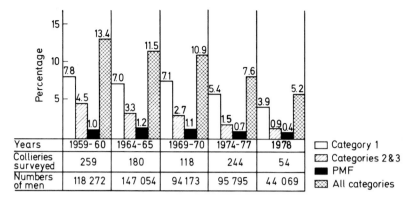

Figure 8.1 Prevalence of coal pneumoconiosis in the UK according to radiographic category. Rates per cent of working miners examined by the NCB Periodic X-ray Scheme. (Note: *The 1974–77 data are not strictly comparable with the earlier periods as some collieries surveyed in 1975 were originally surveyed in 1971, 1966 and 1961.) (Data from NCB Medical Service Annual Reports with permission)*

smoke and gases from the baking furnaces collected and scrubbed (Mantell, 1971). Although quartz is virtually absent (about 0.1 per cent), pneumoconiosis has been reported in workers in this industry (Watson *et al.*, 1959; Okutani, Shima and Sano, 1964; Foà, Grieco and Zedda, 1966). (*See* Pathogenesis.)

EPIDEMIOLOGY

PREVALENCE, INCIDENCE AND PROGRESSION

In the late 1940s the prevalence of coal pneumoconiosis in the UK was high due to a lack of adequate dust control measures over preceding years and a greatly increased production drive during the Second World War. However, a great reduction in the levels of airborne dust in the mines was achieved between those years and the early 1960s and, although the problems of dust control were exacerbated by increased mechanization at the coal face since 1965, much progress has been made in recent years so that conditions now meet current dust standards in all working areas (National Coal Board, 1977, 1980).

The British National Coal Board (NCB) introduced a five-yearly periodic X-ray schedule for all collieries in 1959 with two purposes in mind: to provide each examinee with the safeguard of regular chest radiographs; and to assess the effectiveness of dust suppression methods. By 1969 it was evident that a higher correlation exists between radiographic changes of pneumoconiosis and dust exposure when the *mass* of 'respirable' coal mine dust (size range 1 to 5 μm) is used as an index instead of the *number of particles* (in the same size range)/mm^3 of air previously employed (Jacobsen *et al.*, 1971). Hence, gravimetric sampling has been employed in British coal mines since 1970.

In Britain the prevalence of *all categories* of coal pneumoconiosis in working miners has fallen from 13.4 per cent in 1959–1960 to 5.2 per cent in 1978 due mainly to a more than 50 per cent reduction in 'simple' pneumoconiosis; and the prevalence of PMF in 1978 was 0.4 per cent (*Figure 8.1*). This trend, which is the result of increasingly effective dust control is also reflected in the numbers of cases first diagnosed by the Pneumoconiosis Medical Panels in the UK with the important proviso that these include ex-miners (*Figure 8.2*). The slight increase in 1975 was due largely, if not entirely, to the rallying of ex-miners by a new NCB compensation scheme. Overall prevalence is higher in older (that is, over 44 years of age) than in younger age groups, but has fallen in both over this period and, in South Wales where it has always been substantially higher than elsewhere, it has also shown an encouraging decline (National Coal Board, 1977, 1980).

A similar trend appears to have occurred in the USA where the recent prevalence of all categories is estimated to be 10.1 per cent and of PMF, 0.4 per cent (Morgan and Lapp, 1976); in Australia and West Germany, and probably

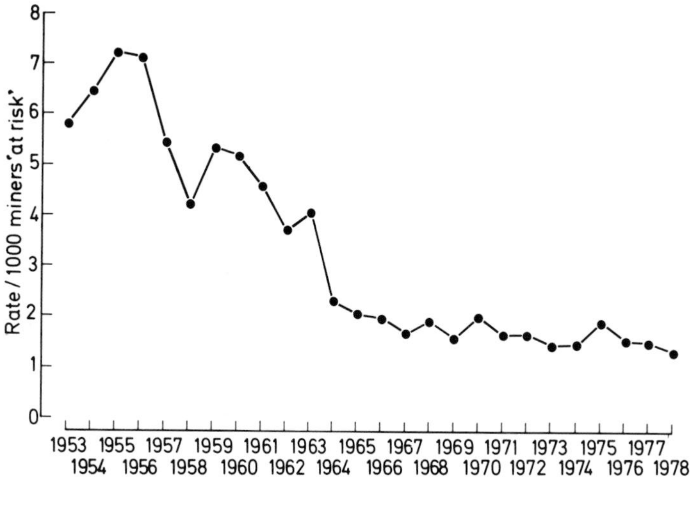

Figure 8.2 Trend in numbers of cases of pneumoconiosis in miners and ex-miners diagnosed for first time by the Pneumoconiosis Medical Panels (UK). (Note: *Value of denominator before 1960 underestimated, but net effect apparently small.) (Prepared by Dr M. Jacobsen from data produced in the NCB Medical Service Annual Reports and the NCB Mineworkers Pension Scheme Annual Reports. Reproduced with permission)*

in France and Belgium. However, it is not possible to make valid comparisons of prevalence between different countries because of differences in composition of coal-mine dust, working conditions and, of course, the technique and standard of radiographic surveys and other criteria (*see* Chapter 5, p. 107). There is some evidence that the rank of coal may influence pathogenesis and, therefore, prevalence but the possible importance of non-coal minerals—notably quartz—in mine dust remains controversial (Walton *et al.*, 1977).

The incidence or *attack rate* of 'simple' pneumoconiosis—that is, the number of men who develop pneumoconiosis per 1000 workers per year—is related chiefly to the mass of 'respirable' dust over the period of exposure (Walton *et al.*, 1977) which, in turn, correlates with the amount of coal and other mineral dust in the lungs (Rossiter, 1972a) (*see* p. 108 and *Figure 8.20*). Smoking habits do not, apparently, modify the attack rate of 'simple' pneumoconiosis (Jacobsen, Burns and Attfield, 1977). The attack rate of PMF is substantially greater in men with category 2 or 3 radiographs than in those with category 1 in whom it is very low (*see Figure 8.3*) (McLintock, Rae and Jacobsen, 1971),

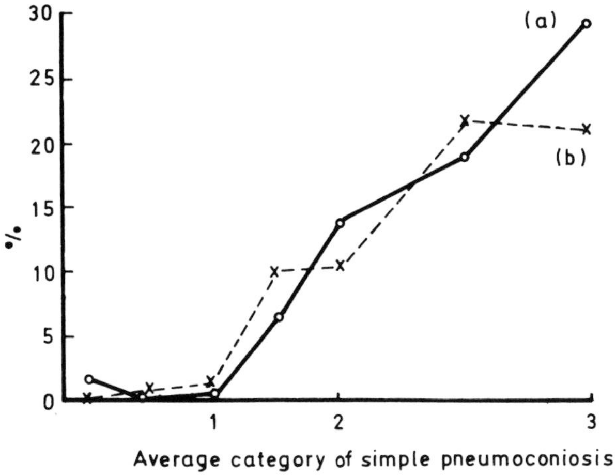

Figure 8.3 Attack rate of PMF over an eight-year period in relation to average category of 'simple' pneumoconiosis as defined by Cochrane (1962). (a) Cochrane's data; South Wales—eight-year period; (b) National Coal Board Periodic X-ray Scheme, Great Britain—five-year period, adjusted (linearly) to eight years. The Coal Board data, which are more recent than Cochrane's and cover most British collieries, show a substantially lower attack rate for average ILO Category 3. (By courtesy of Dr J. S. McLintock and colleagues and the Editor of Inhaled Particles **3**, *1971)*

and is highest in the South Wales and lowest in the Scottish coalfields. It is not influenced by expenditure of energy at work, smoking habits, body type or tuberculous infection (either exogenous or endogenous) (Cochrane, 1962). However, the 'rheumatoid' variant of coal pneumoconiosis is exceptional in that it develops most commonly in a category 0 or 1 'background'.

Progression of pneumoconiosis appears to be related to the category of the radiograph when a man is first seen (Jacobsen *et al.*, 1971). Recent analysis of the mean dust exposure of *individual* miners in 20 British collieries has confirmed the correlation between level of exposure and radiographic progression over a ten-year period. Calculations based on analysis of the mean dust concentrations over all coal faces in these collieries showed that, if the concentrations do not exceed 4.3 mg/m³ on average over a 35-year period, the probability of category 2 or higher developing should not exceed 3.4 per cent (Jacobsen, 1973 and 1975). This prediction formed the basis of the 'permitted dust levels' introduced in the British coal mines in 1975. A similar conclusion was reached in Germany by Reisner (1971). Recently this general correlation between exposure to coal-mine dust and 'simple' pneumoconiosis has been confirmed unequivocally though the long-term risks appear to have been underestimated by 1 to 2 percentage probability units in the earlier computation (Jacobsen, 1979) (*see Figure 8.4*).

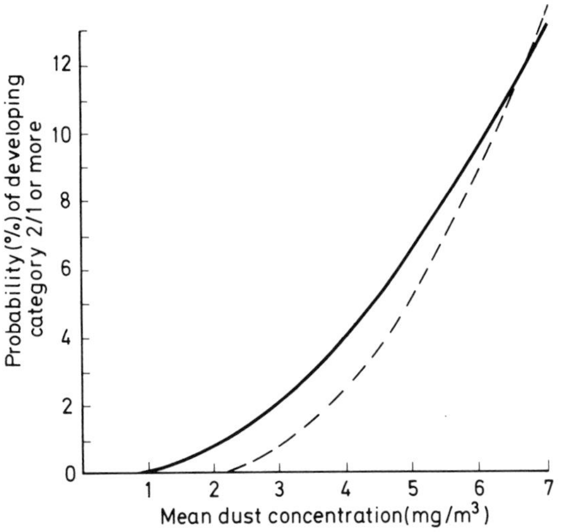

Figure 8.4 Estimates of probabilities of developing category 2 or more simple pneumoconiosis over an approximately 35-year working life at the coalface. ——— Based on average results from 2600 miners at ten British collieries, and taking a 35-year working life as equivalent approximately to 35 × 1740 working hours; 1978 study. --- Based on statistical extrapolation of radiological changes over ten years in 20 collieries. (By courtesy of Dr M. Jacobsen and the Institute of Occupational Medicine, Edinburgh)

The rate of progression of PMF is influenced chiefly by age; the younger the man with a category A radiograph the more likely is progression to occur, and this is also true if he leaves the mining industry. But 'rheumatoid' pneumoconiosis may progress unexpectedly and rapidly at any age (*see* p. 217).

MORTALITY

A recent detailed 20-year follow-up study of miners and ex-miners in South Wales (Rhondda Fach) has shown that those with 'simple' pneumoconiosis (categories 1, 2 and 3) and category A opacities survive as well as those with no evidence of pneumoconiosis (category 0) (Cochrane *et al.*, 1979). This confirms the findings of earlier surveys in Britain (Higgins *et al.*, 1968a; Cochrane, 1973; Cochrane and Moore, 1978) and in the USA where the life expectancy of miners as a whole is the same as that of the general population (Ortmeyer *et al.*, 1974). Interestingly, among Pennsylvanian miners with category B pneumoconiosis mortality is higher in those who worked in anthracite mines than in those in bituminous mines (Ortmeyer, Baier and Crawford, 1973). In 88 miners and ex-miners with category B or C pneumoconiosis who died in the quinquennium 1966–1970 the average age at death from all causes was 70 years, the range being 53 to 85 years (Parkes, 1972); and Rooke *et al.* (1979) found that the mean age of death among Lancashire miners with PMF was 72 years. In a group of 346 South Wales miners and ex-miners with category B or C pneumoconiosis death was attributable to the pneumoconiosis in about one-third of cases (Sadler, 1974).

It can be concluded that 'simple' pneumoconiosis does not curtail life expectancy, and advanced PMF affects mortality in only a minority of cases. The question of the mortality experience of miners with category p opacities only is discussed on p. 216.

PNEUMOCONIOSIS DUE TO 'NEARLY PURE' CARBON

This is very uncommon because the number of men exposed in various industries in the past was small and, in recent years, dust control has been in operation fairly generally. But it is likely that there are still some men surviving with substantial exposures in the past who have escaped diagnosis.

Details of prevalence are limited and not always reliable. Among 29 men in an English factory producing high grade carbon for the manufacture of arc lamp electrodes category 1 pneumoconiosis was present in three of them, category 2 in two and category 2A in one (Meiklejohn, 1957); and categories 1 to 3 p and q were found in 21 (6.7 per cent) of 308 Italian carbon electrode workers (Foà, Grieco and Zedda, 1966). Cocarla *et al.* (1976) reported a 20 per cent prevalence of pneumoconiosis—categories 1 and 2 p and q—in a group of Rumanian carbon black workers; and Wehr *et al.* (1975) recorded 'definite p-type opacities' in 9.6 per cent of 397 employees exposed to activated carbon. Though these reports are undoubtedly based on differing radiographic methodology at least they show that the categories of pneumoconiosis in recent years are uniformly low. However, PMF associated with carbon black and artificial graphite has been described in the past and is referred to in the section on Pathogenesis, p. 191. Apparently no new cases of pneumoconiosis have occurred in the American carbon electrode industry since the 1940s (Mantell, 1971), and a recent survey of carbon black workers in the UK and the USA has not revealed any harmful effects due to carbon dust (Crosbie *et al.*, 1979).

PATHOLOGY

Extrapulmonary appearances

The intercostal parietal pleura is often tattooed with black lines running parallel to the ribs due to coal dust in and around extrapleural perivascular lymphatic vessels. The pulmonary pleura is marbled blue-black by subpleural deposits of dust and is not thickened unless it overlies a

(*a*)

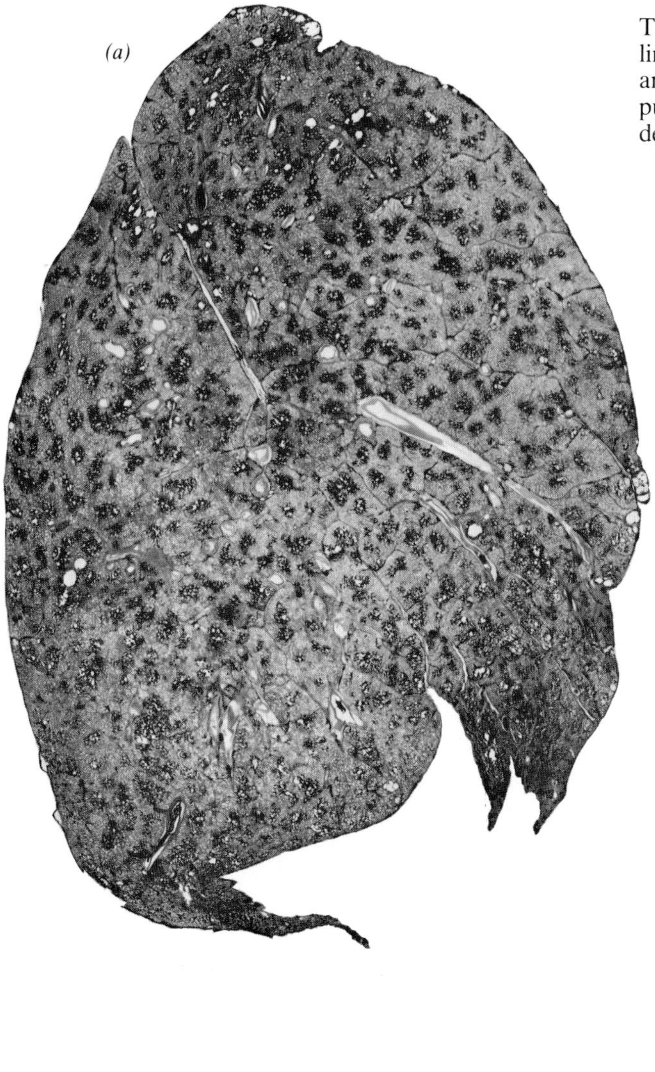

(*b*)

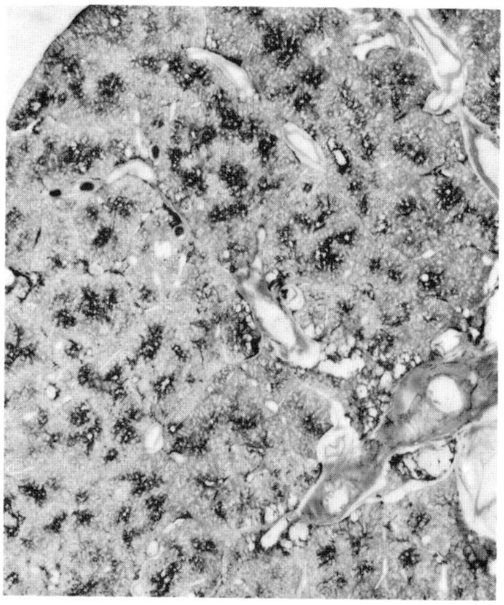

Figure 8.5 (a) Multiple coal macules (pigmentation) distributed fairly evenly in the lung. There is dust pigmentation of some interlobular septa. Very slight centrilobular emphysema is present in some areas (Paper-mounted section). (b) Coal dust macules without associated emphysema (Paper mounted section, natural size)

confluent mass of pneumoconiosis (PMF) in which case it may be fibrotic and puckered, occasionally in the form of a hyalinized plaque. Apart from this, pleural fibrosis should lead one to suspect the presence of some other disease process.

Hilar and mediastinal lymph nodes are densely black and may be slightly enlarged.

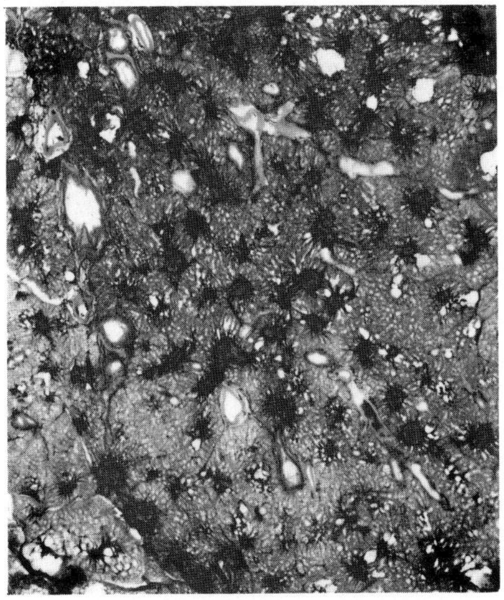

Figure 8.6 Coal nodules. They are indurated and more sharply demarcated than macules. Some nodules exhibit very slight scar (irregular) emphysema. (From paper-mounted lung section, natural size)

DISCRETE LESIONS ('SIMPLE' PNEUMOCONIOSIS)

Macroscopic appearances

When the lungs are cut through with a knife a variable number of black dust macules (ranging from few to very many) are seen and are commonly predominant in the upper halves of the lungs, but may be distributed symmetrically throughout (*Figure 8.5*). Between these lesions the lung tissue is frequently free of dust pigment. Some lungs are uniformly pigmented black so that individual macules are not discernible, but much of this pigment can usually be washed away by a stream of water to reveal the macules. The fact that diffuse and dense black staining is found in some cases but not in others, though in both instances pneumoconiotic lesions of similar severity may be present, is not readily explicable. Macules are not raised above or depressed below the cut surface and they yield no sense of induration to the touch. Interlobular septa and the subpleural region are commonly dust pigmented.

Black, indurated nodules, some 2 to 5 mm in diameter, which stand out from the cut surface and are readily palpable, may also be present—again in variable numbers—and are usually distributed in the upper parts of the upper and lower lobes; but in some cases nearly all the lesions are nodular and may be scattered throughout the lungs, dust macules being virtually absent (*Figure 8.6*). They may also occur in satellite groups around areas of PMF. Although many nodules are round (that is, of near spherical form) some are of stellate or irregularly linear shape. Nodules larger than 5 mm and less then 3 cm diameter have, as mentioned earlier, sometimes been referred to as 'infective nodules'.

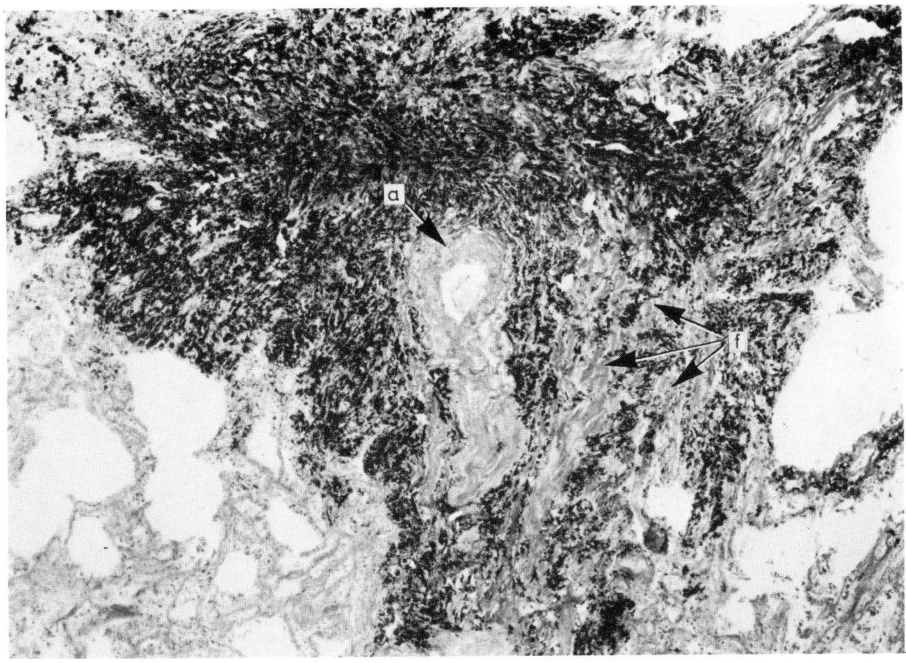

Figure 8.7 Coal nodule showing collagen fibres (f) arranged in irregular fashion, and a large quantity of coal-dust which is both intra- and extracellular. The appearances are in pronounced contrast with those of the typical silicotic nodule (see Figure 7.4)*. (a, artery; original magnification, × 55, reproduced at × 44; H and E stain)*

As the nodules are uniformly black they are readily distinguishable from typical silicotic nodules (*see Figure 7.2*) although 'rheumatoid' Caplan-type nodules may closely resemble silicotic lesions—a mistake that is often made. However, silicotic nodules or 'mixed dust fibrosis' are sometimes found together with coal or carbon nodules when there has been a significantly siliceous component in past coal-mine dust exposure.

As stated in Chapter 1, in many cases, emphysema of centrilobular type with holes more than 1 mm in diameter is present in a variable proportion of dust macules—'focal emphysema' of Gough (1947). This is discussed in more detail later. Emphysema is rarely associated with nodular lesions, but when it is, it is of scar (or 'irregular') type and of mild degree.

Microscopic appearances

Dust macules consist of intra- and extracellular dust particles concentrated mainly around or near respiratory bronchioles and their vessels, and in Lambert's canals. There is some proliferation of reticulin fibres, demonstrable by silver impregnation, which loosely enmeshes particles and cells. Collagenous fibrosis is absent. Dust-containing macrophages are present in great numbers in some alveolar spaces some of which may become completely filled and consolidated. Dust accumulations may also be found in the small aggregations of lymphoid tissue at the divisions of respiratory bronchioles and in the adventitia of accompanying arterioles which, however, otherwise remain intact; capillaries, on the other hand, are often obliterated (Wells, 1954a).

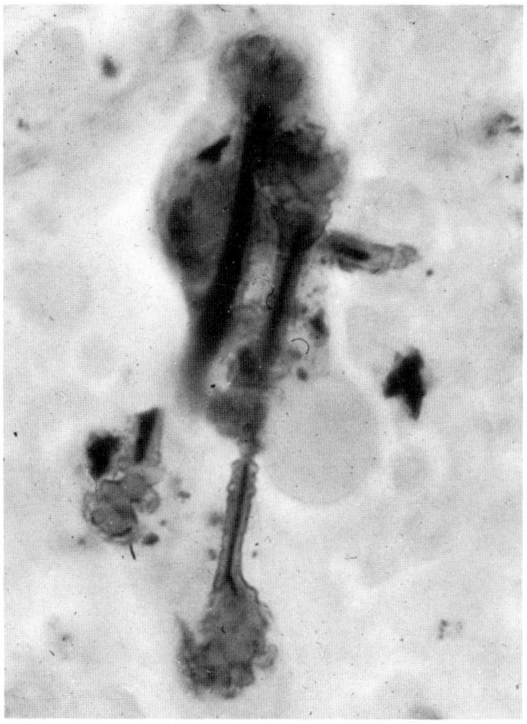

Figure 8.8 Coal bodies. These bear a superficial resemblance to asbestos bodies but, though their coating is golden coloured, it lacks definition, segmentation and their cores are densely black and usually splinter-like. Fragments of bodies may be seen. Graphite bodies are similar. (Original magnification × 500). Compare with Figure 9.2

Nodular lesions consist of much dust, macrophages and both collagen and reticulin fibres which run in random directions in contrast to the characteristic concentric arrangement of collagen in silicotic nodules (*Figure 8.7*). The proportion of reticulin to collagen is higher than in silicotic nodules. Some nodules assume a contracted stellate form and may then be surrounded by localized scar emphysema.

Vasculitis with foci of plasma cells and lymphocytes may be present around some nodules, and rheumatoid factor (IgM) has been found in coal nodules with no histological evidence of rheumatoid changes in seven of 35 cases (Wagner and McCormick, 1967). (*See* Pathogenesis.)

'Curious' bodies, known also as pseudo-asbestos or *coal bodies,* may be found in areas of dust concentration in both coal and graphite pneumoconiosis (Tylecote and Dunn, 1931; Williams, 1934; Town, 1968). They vary from 30 to 70 μm in length, are clubbed at both ends and their cores consist of black splinters of coal or carbon. Like asbestos bodies (*see* p. 239) their coating is golden yellow and gives a positive reaction to Perl's Prussian blue reagent, and their refractive index is similar (Gloyne, 1932–33). They are distinguished from asbestos bodies, however, in being coarser having a continuous, non-segmented coat and a black core (*Figure 8.8*). They are found only in a minority of cases in which they may be either numerous or scanty, and their presence is unrelated to the severity of pneumoconiosis. They have no known pathogenic significance and their mode of formation is not understood. Their importance lies in the fact that they are sometimes confused with asbestos bodies.

Centrilobular (proximal acinar) emphysema with dust ('focal emphysema')

Emphysema of 'distensive' centrilobular type is seen in some coal and carbon macules. Depending upon the level and plane of section, these lesions appear either as black cuffs of dust or pigment around dilated respiratory bronchioles or as 'rosettes' of similar proportions with small black centres surrounded by dilated, partly pigmented, alveolar walls. This has been regarded by Gough (1947) and Heppleston (1947, 1953) as a distinctive form of emphysema—'focal emphysema'—believed to result from the weakening of the muscular walls of those respiratory bronchioles in which dust has accumulated and which, in turn, causes them to dilate due to the traction effect of the negative transpulmonary pressure exerted during inspiration (Heppleston, 1968).

But the existence of 'focal emphysema' as distinct from 'distensive' centrilobular emphysema is not universally accepted (Reid, 1967; Heath, 1968). Some pathologists do not consider that these lesions are essentially different from those found in the general population apart from the presence of dust. Nonetheless, Heppleston (1968, 1972) believes that they are in fact distinguishable, although only by the use of three-dimensional microtechniques; and he points to a loss of smooth muscle in the affected respiratory bronchioles as causing a reduction in their elastic recoil and, hence, dilatation. Against this, however, Thurlbeck (1976) states that smooth muscle loss is not a distinctive pathological feature as it may also be seen in the inflamed walls

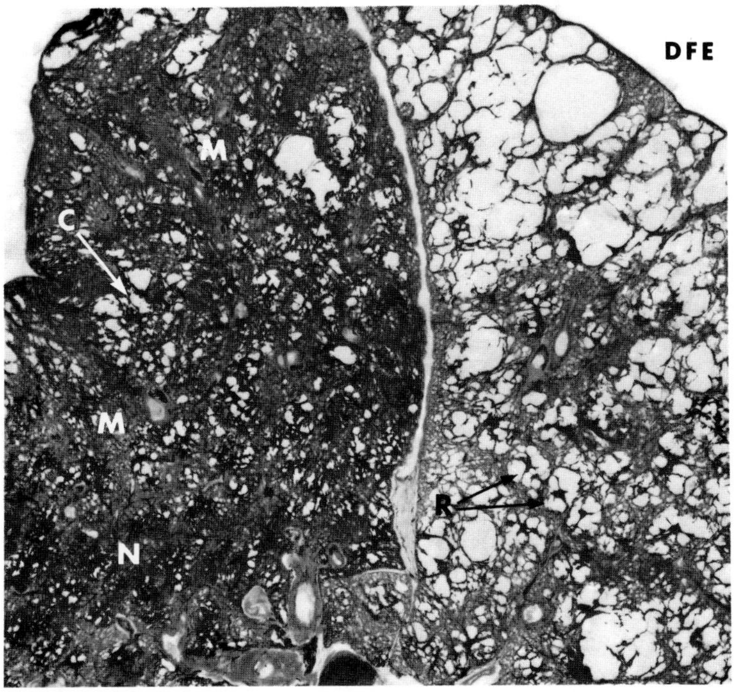

Figure 8.9 Apical region of upper and lower lobes showing coal macules (M) and nodules (N) without associated, mild dust-pigmented centrilobular emphysema (C), irregular emphysema around dust-pigmented scars forming 'rosette' patterns (R) and completely dust-free centrilobular emphysema in apex of lower lobe (DFE). (Paper-mounted section, natural size.) (See also Figure 1.8b)

of centrilobular emphysema without dust; and Macklem (1968) has argued that such loss is unlikely to result in diminution of elastic recoil. Although, 'focal emphysema' is usually considered to be of 'distensive' type, Gough (1968) believed that, in time, it may become 'destructive'.

There are other reasons for doubting that 'focal emphysema' is a unique form of emphysema (*Figures 8.5, 8.6* and *8.9*).

(1) Coal (or carbon) macules are frequently seen without attendant emphysema.
(2) In some cases a majority of macules may be emphysematous whereas, in others with an apparently similar amount of dust exposure, emphysema is negligible or absent.
(3) The dissecting microscope shows that dust may be present in only one segment of a dilated respiratory bronchiole while the remainder of its wall is dust-free. This does not suggest that the dilatation is caused by the dust.
(4) Coal nodules are not associated with 'focal emphysema' though there may be varying degrees (often slight) of scar, or irregular, emphysema.
(5) Macules with and without associated centrilobular emphysema, nodules without emphysema, and centrilobular emphysema without dust may all be seen in different areas of the same lung (*Figure 8.9*).
(6) There seems to be no reason to suppose that soot or pigment are the cause of distensive centrilobular ('focal') emphysema rather than that they have accumulated in pre-existing emphysematous lesions in preference to normal lung (Heard and Izukawa, 1963)—which is consistent with the aerodynamic behaviour of compact particles.

Dust may also be present in the walls of panlobular and paraseptal emphysema (*Figure 1.14*, p. 15) (Heard, 1969) but there is nothing to suggest that it is the causal agency.

To summarize

It is misleading to conclude that 'focal emphysema' is 'an integral part of the simple lesion of coal worker's pneumoconiosis' (Report of the Pneumoconiosis Committee of the College of American Pathologists, 1979) if one takes 'integral' to mean 'necessary to the completeness of the whole' (*Shorter Oxford English Dictionary*); for, on the one hand, distensive, dust-pigmented centrilobular emphysema is not always present in the lungs of coal or carbon workers and, on the other, it may be found in those of the general population. It is, of course, possible that a susceptibility to develop centrilobular emphysema may be exacerbated by the presence of coal (or carbon) dust (Davis *et al.*, 1979). Therefore, because the concept of 'focal emphysema' as a separate entity is controversial it might be preferable to substitute this term by 'centrilobular emphysema with dust' as a counterpart to 'centrilobular emphysema without dust'.

However, it must be emphasized that whatever the truth of the matter may be, it is of no importance in practice because centrilobular emphysema with dust does not cause any symptoms or physical signs and, although it has been suggested that it may be responsible for a slight reduction in gas transfer and arterial oxygen found in *some* cases of apparent 'simple' coal pneumoconiosis, this reduction is too small to be of clinical significance (*see* Lung function).

Emphysema in general

A post-mortem study in South Wales by Ryder *et al.* (1970) claimed to show that emphysema is much more common among coal-miners and ex-miners than among non-miners; that 'extensive emphysema' is more common in miners with pneumoconiosis; and that there is a close relationship between the amount and severity of emphysema and changes in FEV_1. However, the validity of these conclusions is questionable for a variety of reasons. As the authors took the unprecedented step of extending the term 'focal emphysema' to include the whole lobule when this was emphysematous and pigmented (panlobular emphysema) it is not surprising that they found nearly all emphysema in miners to be of 'focal' type. But it is unlikely that the miners studied were as representative of all miners as the control subjects were of the general population because the miners, unlike the controls, were drawn from a compensation population confined to one mining area (Rae, Muir and Jacobsen, 1970); and the fact that there was no age gradient for emphysema and FEV_1 levels is further evidence of bias in selection (Fletcher, 1970). In relating FEV_1 prior to death to amount of emphysema no account was taken of PMF nor of 'obstructive bronchitis' both of which may also affect this index (Gilson and Oldham, 1970).

In a later study the same authors concluded that 'simple' coal pneumoconiosis usually causes progressive impairment of ventilation which is not related to radiographic category but is due to emphysema which cannot be detected on the X-ray film (Lyons *et al.*, 1972). But this is also open to question because their conclusion that the emphysema is due to the pneumoconiosis is directly contradicted by their evidence: for, as their data showed no quantitative relationship between the severity of post-mortem emphysema and the amount of dust in the lungs—according to radiographic category—it is hardly possible to conclude that such emphysema is caused by coal dust (Fletcher, 1972a and b; Higgins, 1972; Oldham and Berry, 1972). And no physiological confirmation of this contention has been demonstrated in American coal-miners with all categories of 'simple' pneumoconiosis (Seaton, Lapp and Morgan, 1972a). Furthermore, there seems to be no simple relationship between the mass and composition of inhaled coal-mine dust and the extent of post-mortem emphysema (Davis *et al.*, 1979).

The following points are also worth noting: (1) Category 0 to 1 radiographs of coal-miners correlate post mortem with minimal 'simple' pneumoconiosis and often with a 'moderate or severe' degree of emphysema (Caplan, 1962), which is in agreement with the low mean dust content of the lungs in these cases (Rossiter *et al.*, 1967; Rossiter, 1972a); (2) Increasing category of 'simple' pneumoconiosis in coal workers is closely related to the dust content of the lungs (Rossiter, 1972b; Davis *et al.*, 1979); and (3) no correlation between the radiographic signs of dust retention, on the one hand, and widespread emphysema, on the other, was found in coal-miners by Caplan, Simon and Reid (1966).

A more recent post-mortem analysis of 500 coal-miners from 25 collieries in the UK has shown that age and smoking habit were associated with the development of 'overall emphysema' but that the presence of 'severe pneumoconiosis' (that is, PMF) was an important added factor. Preliminary statistical investigation of the results showed that smokers are prone to develop 'overall emphysema' because of their smoking habits but that when this is accounted for the lung dust content contributes more to emphysema levels in non-smokers than in the smokers, though the number of non-smokers with high dust levels in this analysis were few. However, it should be noted that this association of emphysema with age, smoking and lung dust was related only to the *presence* of emphysema and not to its type or extent (Davis *et al.*, 1979).

In short: there is no convincing evidence to support the view that disabling emphysema, other than irregular or scar

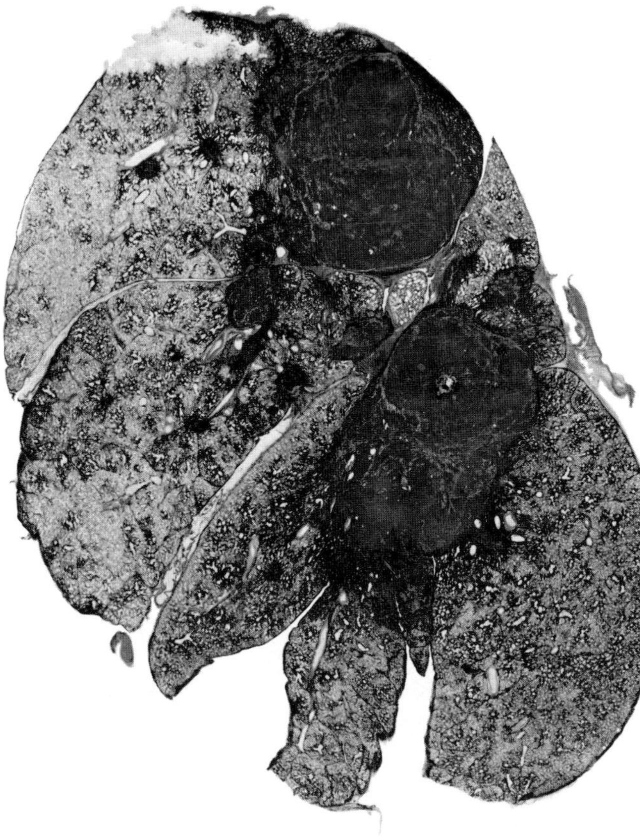

Figure 8.10 Advanced PMF in upper and lower lobes of right lung. The upper lobe mass is well-circumscribed whereas the lower is mostly ill-defined. Three large nodules are present in the middle lobe. Elsewhere there are multiple dust macules and a few small nodules

emphysema associated with some cases of PMF, is more common in coal-miners (or carbon workers) than in the population at large.

PROGRESSIVE MASSIVE FIBROSIS (PMF)

Macroscopic appearances

These black fibrotic masses usually favour the upper halves and posterior parts of the lungs but there are many exceptions to this. They may be found in the centre of the lung, in the base of a lower lobe, or in the lingula or middle lobe (*Figure 8.10*). They may be bilateral and roughly symmetrical in size and outline or, more commonly, of disparate shape, size and distribution in the two lungs. Sometimes only a single mass occurs. When a mass is near the periphery the overlying pulmonary pleura is often puckered and fibrotic and may be adherent to the parietal layer. A remarkable feature of these lesions is their variable conformation and the fact that they are frequently not confined by the anatomical boundaries of lobes, segments or septa. Therefore, when cut across they may be round, elliptical or linear in shape and so well circumscribed that they appear almost encapsulated and as if dropped into the lung which is neither distorted nor evidently compressed adjacently; but in other cases they are of irregular shape with poorly defined margins which extend in stellate fashion into the surrounding lung (*Figure 8.11*). Scar emphysema, sometimes with bullae, may surround some irregular masses, but is exceptional and does not occur in relation to circumscribed masses. Bullae may remain distended due to air-trapping after the lung has been removed from the chest.

A massive lesion or nodule has been arbitrarily defined as PMF when its diameter exceeds 3 cm (James, 1954) though the microscopical features are the same. The cut surface of the mass is commonly homogeneously black—occasionally there are grey areas—and is uniformly hard or rubbery. Some masses, however, contain black pultaceous necrotic material or fluid which may scintillate due to the presence of cholesterol crystals; and others are black, shaggy-walled cavities caused by the previous evacuation of the necrotic contents into a connecting airway. This necrosis is primarily of ischaemic origin (*see* next section, p. 186). After evacuation such cavities often refill with fluid of similar composition to blood plasma (Gernez-Rieux *et al.*, 1958). Exceptionally, small caseous or calcified areas which might suggest past tuberculosis are seen within a mass. A well-demarcated PMF may appear encapsulated but, in fact, there is no true capsule.

Coal or carbon PMF is readily distinguished from a silicotic conglomeration by the excess of black dust and by the absence of individually identifiable silicotic nodules with their distinctive whorled pattern in the aggregate. 'Simple' dust macules or nodules, or both, are usually present to a greater or lesser degree in the rest of the lung, but in rare

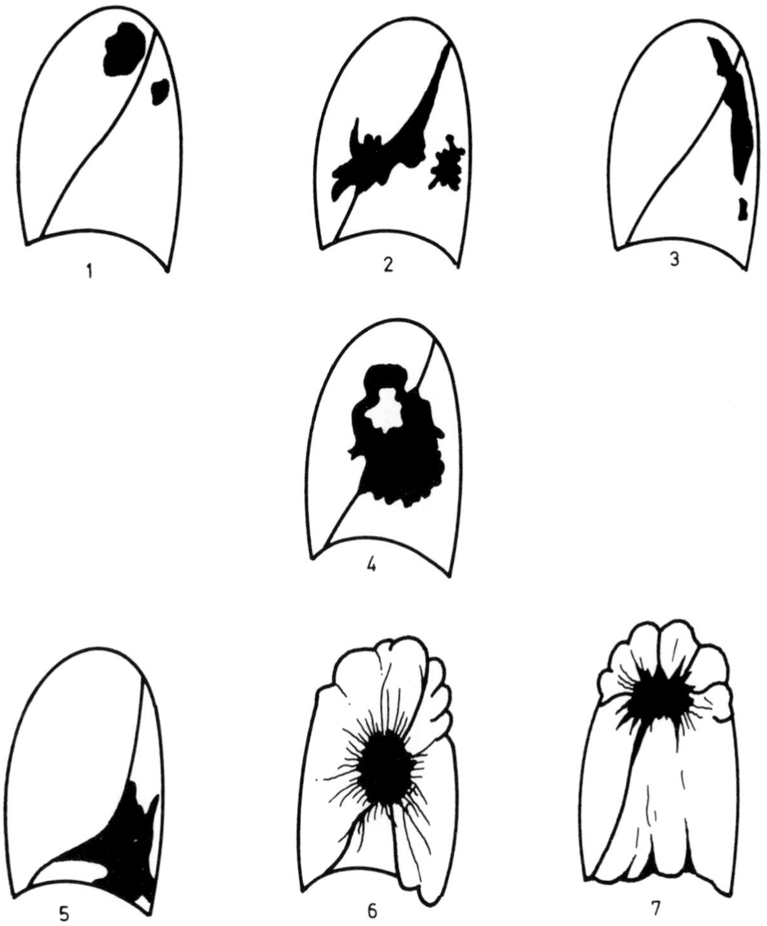

Figure 8.11 Diagram of the variable conformations of PMF which may be seen when the lung is cut in the sagittal plane. (1) Solid, well circumscribed mass without scar emphysema; (2) and (3) roughly linear and irregular masses. Often these do not respect lobar boundaries; (4) large, well circumscribed, cavitary central mass without scar emphysema. When bilateral, masses of this sort usually cause obliteration of many pulmonary artery branches, leading to cor pulmonale; (5) irregular contracted mass in the uncommon location of the lower lobe; (6) contracted irregular central mass with scar emphysema; (7) contracted irregular mass in upper part of lung with severe scar and bullous emphysema

cases they are virtually absent. In the case of graphite or other forms of carbon the lungs are often intensely and uniformly black-pigmented.

If there has been past exposure to fairly high concentrations of quartz as well as to coal or carbon dust typical—but sometimes immature—silicotic nodules or areas of 'mixed dust fibrosis' (*see* Chapter 7) may be present in addition to the coal or carbon lesions, and there may be egg-shell calcification of the hilar lymph nodes. This is seen particularly in coal-miners who have done much rock drilling in shaft sinking or road developing or repairing, or who worked in collieries with heavily faulted ground. Indeed, in some mining areas, silicotic nodules—both discrete and conglomerate—may predominate, there being only very little characteristic coal pneumoconiosis; for example, in the UK, the Wigan area of Lancashire (Spink and Nagelschmidt, 1963) and the West Cumberland area (Faulds, King and Nagelschmidt, 1959). Silicotic nodules have also been observed with carbon pneumoconiosis in men who worked with natural graphite in the manufacture of carbon refractories (Gloyne, Marshall and Hoyle, 1949).

Hilar lymph nodes are usually black, firm and slightly enlarged.

Microscopic appearances

The structure of PMF is identical to that of coal nodules and consists of a large quantity of coal (or carbon) dust, lymphocytes, dust-laden macrophages and dense bundles of reticulin and collagen fibres some of which are hyalinized. Bronchioles are usually annihilated but remnants of small pulmonary arteries and arterioles may be found in which there is progressive invasion by dust-bearing fibrous tissue from adventitia to intima to the point of obliteration; at this stage fragments of elastic lamina (revealed by elastic tissue stains) are the only evidence that these vessels existed (Wells, 1954a). At the periphery of PMF, arteries are partly or completely obstructed by endarteritis and the bigger the mass, the larger and more proximal are the arteries involved. Thrombosis may occur in these arteries and spread in retrograde fashion sometimes as far as the main pulmonary artery branches (Wells, 1954b), but embolism from this source is rare. Arterial obstruction may cause ischaemic colliquative necrosis within the mass and if a bronchus is eroded the necrotic material is expelled in the sputum resulting in cavitation as already described. Similar changes may be found in the small arteries around coal nodules and in pneumoconiosis due to graphite (Pendergrass *et al.*, 1968).

In some cases plasma cells are very prominent in endarteritis adjacent to PMF and immunofluorescent techniques have demonstrated that rheumatoid factor (IgM) is present in these cells (Wagner and McCormick, 1967) even though the masses show none of the features of 'rheumatoid' coal nodules (*see* next section). In addition, rheumatoid factor has been found in aggregations of plasma cells and in subcapsular follicles in hilar lymph nodes in these cases (Wagner and McCormick, 1967). This suggests the possibility of immune reactivity being involved in the pathogenesis of some PMF lesions. In others, caseous areas with the histological characteristics of tuberculosis are present and may yield tubercle bacilli on culture; but such cases are exceptional.

Occasionally typical or immature silicotic lesions may be found in a mass, but the amount of collagen in PMF is substantially less than in silicotic conglomerations. Recent analysis of PMF lesions indicates that while collagen is present in the peripheral zone it is replaced near and at the centre by another insoluble protein (or proteins) which appears to be stabilized by some form of cross-linking. One-third of the weight of these masses is attributed to this protein complex and the remaining two-thirds to approximately equal amounts of mineral dusts and calcium phosphate (Wagner *et al.*, 1975). Interestingly, the collagen elaborated in PMF appears to be of similar type to that in the hyaline pleural plaques which may be associated with asbestos exposure (*see* Chapter 9); in both it is typical of collagen produced in response to injury or irritation, and there is a similar propensity to calcification (Wusteman, Gold and Wagner, 1972). But whereas the collagen content of PMF is not greater than about 30 per cent that of plaques is about 90 per cent (Wagner, 1972).

'RHEUMATOID' COAL PNEUMOCONIOSIS

Following the first clear description by Caplan (1953) this is commonly referred to as a *clinical* syndrome. Strictly, *Caplan's syndrome* consists of multiple large (0.5 to 5 cm diameter), round radiographic opacities frequently associated with evidence of cavity formation or calcification, and usually unaccompanied by the small opacities of 'simple' pneumoconiosis, in coal-miners with rheumatoid arthritis; the lesions causing the opacities having gross and microscopical features unlike those of coal pneumoconiosis (Gough, Rivers and Seal, 1955). Its existence as a distinct entity has since been widely confirmed and the concept extended beyond the original syndromal confines to include the occurrence of similar, as well as less distinctive and pleomorphic, opacities in the absence of rheumatoid arthritis but associated with circulating rheumatoid factor (Caplan, Payne and Withey, 1962). The typical radiographic appearances are completely unlike those of 'non-rheumatoid' pneumoconiosis in character and behaviour in time, and the variant forms of 'rheumatoid' pneumoconiosis are usually different (*see* section on Radiographic Appearances). Rheumatoid arthritis may precede or occur after the appearance of lung lesions by a number of years, and in some cases never develops. There is no evident relationship between severity of rheumatoid arthritis when present and the amount of rheumatoid pneumoconiosis.

It is difficult to assess prevalence (which rests chiefly on clinical and not on pathological observations) with any accuracy because, owing to its diverse radiographic appearances (*see* p. 201), 'rheumatoid' coal pneumoconiosis has been, and is, often unrecognized; because many individuals have been followed for too short a time for its development to be observed; and because of varying reliability of tests for rheumatoid factor. Most commonly it has been expressed in terms of the number of cases occurring in coal-mining populations. Lindars and Davies (1967) found that the prevalence among 21 557 miners with and without pneumoconiosis from the East Midlands collieries of Britain was 0.26 per cent but among those with pneumoconiosis it lay between 2.3 and 6.2 per cent—a similar range, in fact, to that of the prevalence of circulating rheumatoid factor in European populations (*see* p. 61). Among 896 Welsh miners with pneumoconiosis there were 20 (2.2 per cent) with rheumatoid pneumoconiosis (Miall *et al.*, 1953). Up to the end of 1966 the total number of cases of Caplan's syndrome said to have been reported internationally was 251 (Niedobitek, 1969) but some were doubtful or wrongly diagnosed, and when these were excluded only three authentic cases appeared to have been recorded in the USA. By 1972 only two more cases seem to have been added in the USA (Benedek, 1973). Whether this extraordinary rarity of rheumatoid coal pneumoconiosis in the USA is due to cases going unrecognized or unreported, or to some other reason, remains to be discovered. It is possible that, pathologically, some cases are misdiagnosed as 'silicosis'.

Conversely, when 'rheumatoid' pneumoconiosis has been sought radiographically in coal-miners with rheumatoid arthritis two cases were reported among 190 Ruhr miners though the prevalence of apparently 'ordinary' PMF was significantly higher than in men without rheumatoid arthritis (Petry, 1954) (but as the range of radiographic appearances was not recognized at the time it is likely that some cases were missed); and, surprisingly, no cases were identified among 100 Pennsylvanian miners with rheumatoid arthritis and there was no increase in pneumoconiosis prevalence (Benedek, Zawadski and Medsger, 1976). It is, of course, true that in some miners and ex-miners with rheumatoid arthritis pneumoconiosis has no 'rheumatoid' features, and in others no radiographic evidence of pneumoconiosis ever develops.

Nothing appears to be known of the prevalence in graphite and other carbon workers.

Macroscopic appearances

The pulmonary pleura is thickened in a proportion of cases, often more on one side than the other. Individual nodules vary from about 0.3 to 3.0 cm diameter but may be grouped

(*a*)

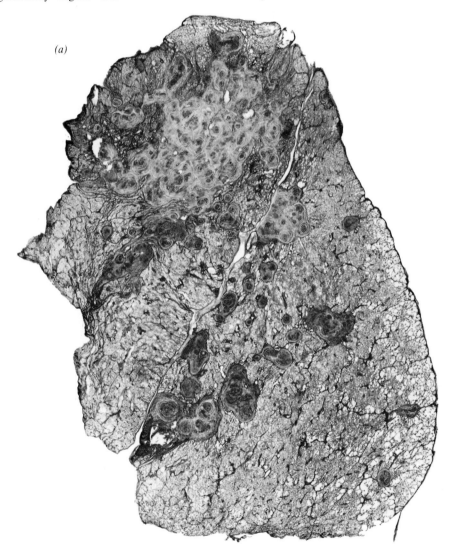

Figure 8.12(a) Multiple necrobiotic (Caplan) nodules many of which are matted together though they retain their identity. Their concentric pattern is clearly visible. Note the absence of 'non-rheumatoid' pneumoconiosis

(b)

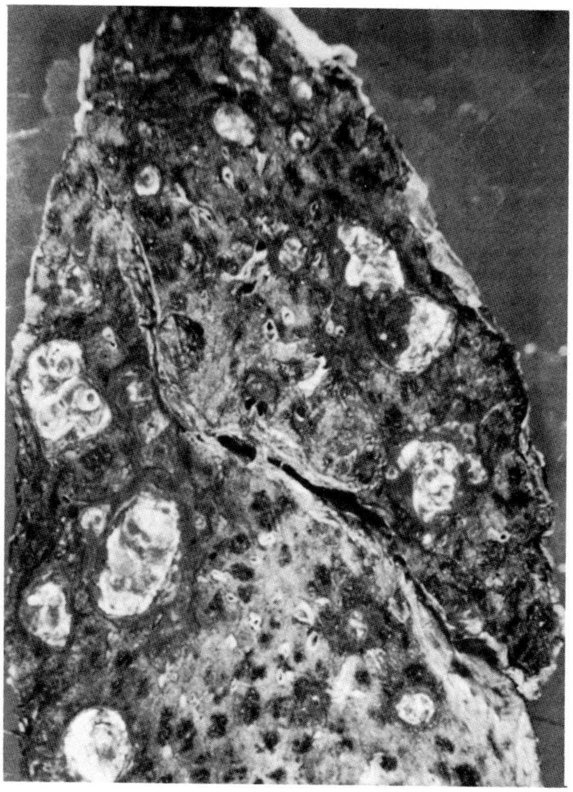

Figure 8.12(b) Large, well circumscribed and encapsulated necrobiotic (Caplan) nodules. Discrete, 'non-rheumatoid' coal nodules are also scattered in the lung; these are not often so numerous in 'rheumatoid' coal pneumoconiosis as in this case. (Approximately three-quarters natural size; courtesy, Dr R. M. E. Seal)

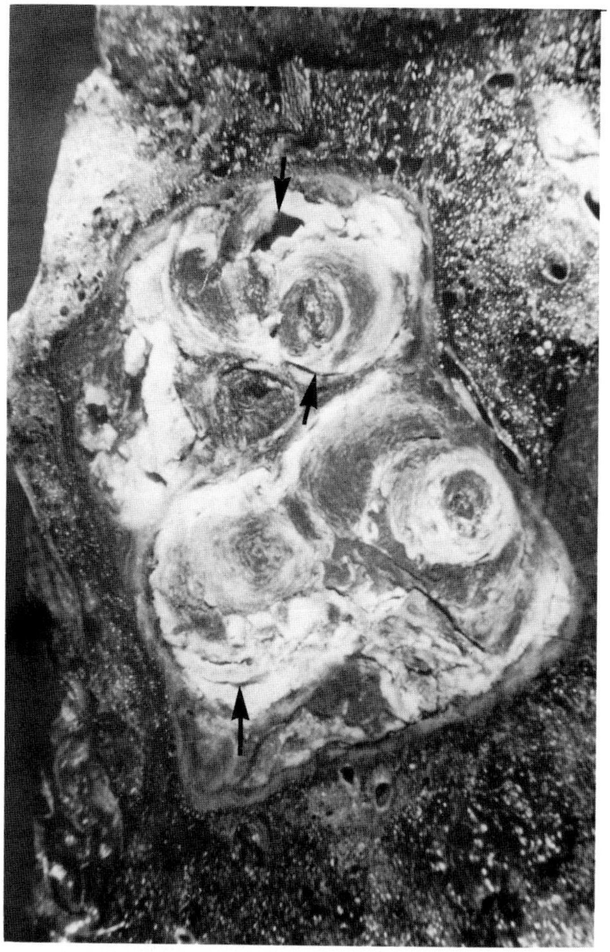

Figure 8.13 Collection of necrobiotic nodules in apex of the lower lobe in Figure 8.12(b). *Note clefts (arrowed) and circular zones of dust. (Magnification × 2.75 approx; courtesy of Dr R. M. E. Seal)*

into aggregates up to some 5 cm overall diameter (*Figure 8.12*), and are scattered irregularly in any part of the lungs though with some propensity for the periphery and upper zones. Rarely only a single large nodule may be present. The cut surface of the nodules has a distinctive concentric arrangement of alternating black and grey-white to yellow rings due respectively to laminated collections of dust and necrotic collagen (*Figure 8.13*). Liquefaction in the lighter areas may appear as clefts and may contain collections of cholesterol crystals (*Figure 8.13*). Indeed, whole nodules may become necrotic and, if connected with airways, discharge their contents into them leaving small cavities which subsequently close in most cases (*Figure 8.14*); but if their contents are not discharged they may calcify. These typical features, however, are by no means always seen and in some cases the nodules are uniformly small (that is, less than about 1 cm) perhaps with an occasional larger nodule, are either scattered or clustered into composite groups, and may be calcified. In these circumstances they may bear a close resemblance to silicotic nodules (*Figure 8.15*). Inspection of a 'rheumatoid' coal nodule with a hand lens helps to distinguish its features from those of a silicotic nodule, but microscopy may be required for confirmation.

General dust pigmentation is slight and ordinary coal macules and nodules are often absent or fairly few in number in most of these cases; but occasionally, isolated Caplan nodules are seen in lungs with otherwise typical non-rheumatoid, 'simple' pneumoconiosis and PMF

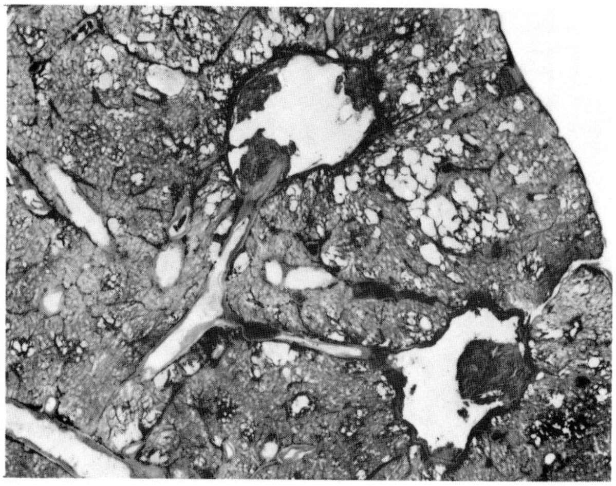

Figure 8.14 Cavitary Caplan nodules adjacent to small bronchi. Contents expelled into airways. Collier with active rheumatoid arthritis, DAT 1: 128. Note scarcity of ordinary lesions of coal pneumoconiosis. (From paper-mounted lung section, natural size). (See Figure 8.31(b))

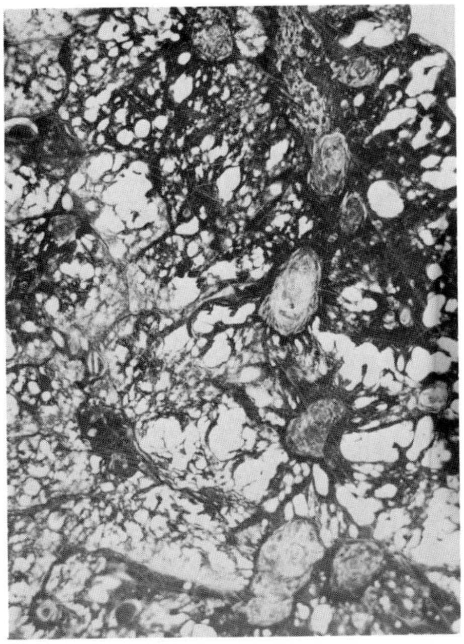

Figure 8.15 Small 'rheumatoid' coal nodules resembling silicotic nodules. (From paper-mounted lung section, natural size). Microscopical confirmation

indicating that the 'rheumatoid' process does not necessarily involve all lesions (*Figure 8.38*).

Microscopic appearances (*Figure 8.16*)

The centres of most of the nodules consist of necrotic tissue in which there are no surviving cells and which stains pink with haematoxylin and eosin; its collagen content is variable. A blue-staining area of cellular infiltration surrounds this zone and in some instances forms a complete circle and in others a segment only, depending upon the plane of section; the cells are macrophages, polymorphonuclear leucocytes, fibroblasts and occasionally, multinucleated giant cells. More peripherally there are circumferentially arranged collagen fibres, fibroblasts and numerous plasma cells. Fibroblasts adjacent to the necrotic area are often grouped in palisade formation though not so strikingly as in subcutaneous rheumatoid nodules. Special stains for 'fibrinoid' are not helpful (Gough, Rivers and Seal, 1955). By contrast with silicotic nodules, clefts containing cholesterol crystals are often present. During periods of activity, dust-containing macrophages migrate into the lesions and later disrupt and discharge their dust load which remains distributed in concentric rings which alternate with the other changes. Necrosis in these active zones is the cause of the segmental clefts. Numerous plasma cells and lymphocytes are an important feature in the collagenous zones.

Arteries around the nodules exhibit endarteritis in which plasma cells are significantly more predominant than in 'non-rheumatoid' pneumoconiosis; IgM is present in their walls (Wagner and McCormick, 1967) and in the cells (Wagner, 1971), and 7S γ-globulin (presumably IgG) has been observed near the centres and in the outer collagenous zones of the nodules (Pernis *et al.*, 1965).

When activity in the nodule has ceased the necrotic areas tend to calcify in which case the multiple concentric rings of dust are the only remaining evidence suggestive of their 'rheumatoid' origin. In those cases where the nodules are small (4–5 mm diameter) and numerous, their microscopical features are similar to those of larger nodules.

Unlike Caplan nodules, rheumatoid necrobiotic nodules, which are not associated with occupational exposure, do not have an annular dust pattern.

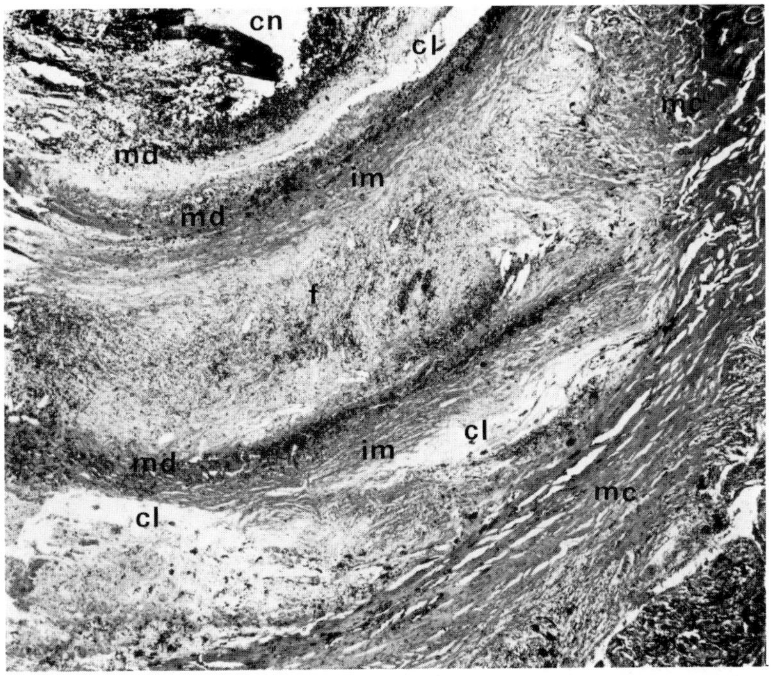

Figure 8.16 Microsection of a necrobiotic (Caplan) nodule showing characteristic concentric zones. (cn) Central area of necrosis; (md) zones of macrophages infiltration and coal dust; (f) zone of fibroblasts and other cells; (im) immature collagen; (cl) clefts which contain cholesterol crystals; (mc) mature collagen with cellular infiltration at the periphery. (Original magnification × 45. Martius scarlet blue stain: Collagen—blue; fibrin—red; nuclei—blue-black). Coal face worker for 18 years. Rheumatoid arthritis; DAT 1:1024

Bacteriology

Tubercle bacilli cannot be isolated by culture or guinea-pig inoculation from the lesions.

Distinguishing features

'Rheumatoid' coal nodules, clearly, are distinct from the typical nodules of coal pneumoconiosis or silicosis, and they show evidence of immunological reactivity. The features which distinguish between Caplan necrobiotic nodules, typical silicosis and tuberculosis may be summarized as follows.

Gross appearances

Caplan nodules are generally discrete, up to 3 cm diameter but may be larger, and are sometimes formed into composite groups. They are distributed at random in the lungs. There is a clear-cut concentric ring pattern of dust in nodules sectioned through or near their centres, and necrosis cavitary is fairly common in one or more lesions.

Typical silicotic nodules may also be discrete but, as a rule, are smaller than Caplan nodules and tend to occupy the upper halves of the lungs. Conglomerations of nodules are usually more closely matted than composite Caplan nodules. Concentric rings of dust are either absent or very poorly defined but occasionally the gross appearances may be identical. Central necrosis is rare (*see* Chapter 7). The occupational history should point to silicosis.

Tuberculous lesions are not defined or circumscribed like Caplan nodules and tend to agglomerate in irregular form and occupy the upper parts of the lungs. Dust rings are rarely present and caseation is often evident.

Microscopic appearances

These and the bacteriological findings are shown in *Table 8.1*.

Differentiation on histological grounds alone may present some difficulty at times but the correct diagnosis of 'rheumatoid' pneumoconiosis can be made in almost all cases by gross inspection of the lesions—possibly with the aid of a hand-lens—by an experienced observer.

DIFFUSE INTERSTITIAL PULMONARY FIBROSIS

Diffuse interstitial pulmonary fibrosis (DIPF)—often with honeycomb cysts—is sometimes found in association with coal pneumoconiosis and has also been observed with graphite pneumoconiosis (Gaensler *et al.*, 1966; Pendergrass *et al.*, 1968). The fibrotic areas are commonly

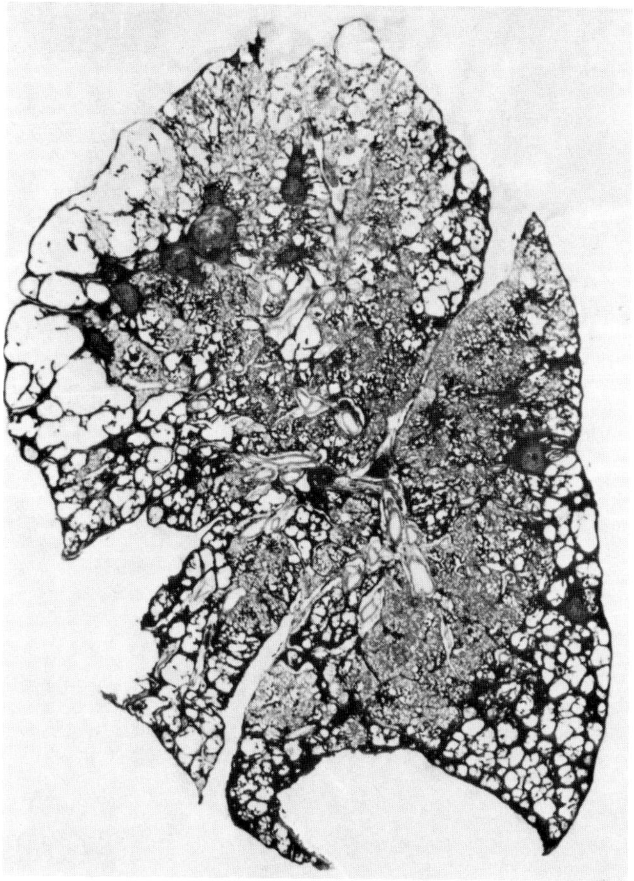

Figure 8.17 Extensive DIPF of right lung with coarse cyst formation ('honeycombing') in all lobes. Typical Caplan necrobiotic nodules in upper and lower lobes. The areas of DIPF (which are sharply demarcated from adjacent unaffected lung) are intensely pigmented with dust. Pigmentation in other areas is slight. Coal-miner with rheumatoid arthritis. Compare with Figure 4.15

Table 8.1

	Nodules of coal pneumoconiosis	*Caplan nodules*	*Typical silicotic nodules*	*Tuberculosis and dust*
Dust lamination	–	+ + +	–	+
Palisading of fibroblasts	–	+	–	+
Cholesterol crystal spaces	–	+ +	–	+
Central necrosis	–	+ +	+ (rare)	+ +
Calcification	+ (rare)	+ +	+	+ +
Excess of peripheral lymphocytes and plasma cells	+ (occ.)*	+ + +	–	+
M. tuberculosis (culture or guinea-pig inoculation)	–	–	–	+ +

*Occasional

deeply dust pigmented (*Figure 4.15*) but in some cases they are free of pigment (*Figure 8.16*). Usually they are predominant in the subpleural zones of the lower lobes but may be widespread in all lobes. Occasionally Caplan nodules are also present and in such cases circulating rheumatoid factor, with or without rheumatoid arthritis, is invariably found (*Figure 8.17*).

In addition to causing irregular opacities on the chest radiograph diffuse interstitial fibrosis and coal dust together may also cause p type opacities. The question of pathogenesis is discussed on p. 194 and more generally in Chapter 4.

PATHOGENESIS

The complex and incompletely solved problem of the pathogenesis of coal pneumoconiosis—already referred to in Chapter 4—can be reviewed only briefly.

From what has been said earlier the quartz content of coal-mine dust may range from negligible to high, depending upon the geological horizons of the mines and the occupation of the miners but, in general, it tends to be low. Similarly, the quartz content of natural graphite varies considerably (*see* p. 176), but that of artificial graphite and carbon black is less than 0.4 per cent.

Dust content of the lungs

The total amount of dust in the lungs with coal pneumoconiosis is greatly in excess of that found in lungs with nodular silicosis and it consists mainly of coal, but non-coal minerals and a small amount of quartz are also present (*see Figure 4.10*).

The mean size of coal particles recovered from the lungs has been referred to in Chapter 3.

Rank of coal

The rank of coal (*see* Chapter 2) does not influence the gross or microscopical features of coal pneumoconiosis which are identical in the UK and the USA (Heppleston, 1951) and elsewhere. But high-rank coals—chiefly anthracite—are associated with a greater prevalence of pneumoconiosis than low rank coals (Hicks *et al.*, 1961; Morgan, 1968; Morgan *et al.*, 1973; Reisner and Robock, 1977). Furthermore, the composition of lung dust varies with rank: the higher the rank, the higher the coal content and the lower the content of quartz and other minerals (Bergmann and Casswell, 1972; Davis *et al.*, 1979). The demonstration by Jacobsen *et al.* (1971) that the effects attributed to rank correlate better with the mass concentration of respiratory dust as a single index of the pneumoconiosis hazard is consistent with the possibility that high-rank coals may be fragmented more readily than low-rank coals thus yielding a greater mass concentration of small 'respirable' particles (that is, less than 5 μm). Indeed, *experimentally*, the long-term clearance and lymphatic removal is better for low rank than high-rank coals and, in this, the concentration of dust and duration of exposure experienced by the animals appear to be the important factors. Retention of dust in the lungs is consistently less with prolonged exposure to low-rank than to high-rank coal. This is analogous to the lower prevalence of pneumoconiosis in miners from low-rank than from high-rank collieries (Heppleston, Civil and Critchlow, 1971; Civil, Heppleston and Casswell, 1975).

Hence, the quantity and rate of accumulation of coal dust in the lungs appears to be a most important factor in pathogenesis—possibly more so than chemical composition.

Effect of quartz

Coal and carbon themselves are not cytotoxic (*see* Chapter 4) and they behave as inert dusts causing only mild reticulin proliferation in the lungs of experimental animals; but coal dust and 0.2 per cent quartz are cytotoxic to guinea-pig macrophages (Robock and Klosterkötter, 1971). Ross *et al.* (1962) found that when coal and quartz mixtures were inhaled by rats definite collagenous fibrosis occurred only when the quartz content was about 20 per cent, but collagen formation was observed by Martin *et al.* (1972) after 18 months in rats which had inhaled a mixture with 5 per cent quartz. However, after inhalation of a mixture containing 2 per cent quartz, no fibrosis was observed (King *et al.*, 1958). Fibrogenesis caused by large concentrations of quartz in animals is substantially reduced by the presence of coal dust, and with lower concentrations (3 per cent), is reduced even more. But an apparent reduction of fibrogenic effect due to mixed dust in animals by the administration of PVPNO (*see* Chapter 4) has been interpreted as confirming that this effect is due to quartz (Schlipköter *et al.*, 1971). And there is suggestive evidence of preferential retention of non-coal minerals, especially quartz, in lungs of miners with the more advanced stages of pneumoconiosis (Davis, Ottery and Le Roux, 1977) (*see* next section).

The implication of these studies, therefore, seems to be that even a small quantity of quartz, though muted in its effects by coal and other dusts, may influence the pathogenesis of coal pneumoconiosis.

This interpretation, however, is contradicted by a number of observations in human beings. The attack rate of PMF in British coal miners is associated with a higher mean dust exposure than that experienced by men without PMF, but not with higher concentrations of quartz (McLintock, Rae and Jacobsen, 1971). Coal trimmers (*see* p. 176) working with washed clean coal developed typical coal pneumoconiosis (Gough, 1940). Both 'simple' pneumoconiosis and PMF have occurred in men exposed to carbon black (Miller and Ramsden, 1961; Lister and Wimborne, 1972), artificial or quartz-free graphite (Rüttner, Bovet and Aufdermaur, 1952; Zahorski, 1961; Gaensler *et al.*, 1966; Pendergrass *et al.*, 1967; Town, 1968), and coal and coke mixtures used in carbon electrode manufacture (Otto and Einbrodt, 1958; Watson *et al.*, 1959; Foà, Grieco and Zedda, 1966). In each instance quartz was either absent or of negligible amount—that is, less than 1 per cent. And the absence of chemically identifiable quartz in the lungs in such cases implies that it is unlikely to have been an essential pathogenic factor. The quartz content compared to total dust concentration in lungs with 'simple' coal pneumoconiosis and all grades of PMF has been observed to be similarly low in all, ranging from 2 to 4 per cent (Rivers *et al.*, 1960; Nagelschmidt, 1965; Sweet, Crouse and Crable, 1974) in contrast to some 20 per cent of total dust in nodular silicosis (Nagelschmidt, 1960).

Experimentally, Policard *et al.* (1967) found that the effect on the lungs of rats of samples of coal dust with a quartz content varying from 0 to 4.9 per cent from 13 French collieries was inhibited by the aluminium silicate clays—kaolin, illite and montmorillonite—which were also present. This, the authors believe, virtually exonerates quartz from playing a significant role in the development of coal pneumoconiosis. And Weller's (1977) observation that the administration of PVPNO to monkeys after prolonged inhalation of a coal–quartz mixture did not cause regression of pneumoconiosis nor prevent its progression—contrary to the conclusion of Schlipköter *et al.* (1971) referred to already—can also be interpreted as indicating that the effect of quartz is insignificant. It is interesting, therefore, that the cytotoxicity of coal dust *in vitro* has been found to be related to its rank and total dust content whereas the role of quartz was enigmatic (Gormley *et al.*, 1979).

Conclusion

It must be emphasized that consideration of the 'silica controversy' is not an academic exercise because it has a practical bearing upon the most suitable index of dust hazard for use in coal mines. This is exemplified by recent epidemiological analyses in British mines which indicate that an apparent increase in the prevalence of pneumoconiosis with increasing quartz exposure is reversed in the presence of high clay mineral exposure, and that mass concentration of 'respirable' dust unadjusted for composition is the most suitable index when the quartz content does not exceed 7.5 per cent (Walton *et al.*, 1977). Indeed, there is good evidence that quartz exposures which amount to *less* than 10 per cent of mixed coal-mine dust do not affect the probability of developing pneumoconiosis (Jacobsen, 1979) (*see* section on Prevention, p. 223).

Trace metals and organic constituents

The lungs of miners of bituminous coal in West Virginia have been found to contain higher concentrations of trace metals than those of the general population but there was no correlation between severity of pneumoconiosis and chromium, copper, iron, manganese, nickel, titanium or zinc (Sweet, Crouse and Crable, 1974). However, Sorenson, Kober and Petering (1974) reported a higher content of copper, iron, nickel, lead and zinc in the lungs of bituminous miners in Pennsylvania with a high prevalence of pneumoconiosis compared with miners of similar coal with a low incidence of pneumoconiosis in Utah; and they suggested that certain trace metals in coal might play a role in the pathogenesis of coal pneumoconiosis.

The aliphatic and aromatic hydrocarbons which may be present in coal can be leached out by biological fluids and, according to Harington (1972), should be considered as possible factors in pathogenesis. Small amounts of organic humic and fulvic acids, which have the capacity to bind trace metals, are, apparently, more prevalent in some coals than in others, and it has been postulated that they may be slowly leached out in the lungs and exert a harmful effect by interfering, for example, with metal-dependent enzymes (Kober *et al.*, 1976).

However, a pathogenic relationship between these factors and coal pneumoconiosis is conjectural and would seem to be unlikely, but further investigation is clearly necessary. It has already been pointed out (Chapter 2, p. 36) that potentially immunogenic organic matter is unlikely to survive in coals.

PROGRESSIVE MASSIVE FIBROSIS

Five possible factors in the genesis of these lesions must be considered.

(1) *Local concentration of quartz* Higher concentrations of quartz in some parts of the lungs than in others with consequent local increase in fibrogenesis have often been postulated and, although not supported by studies such as those referred to in the last section (Nagelschmidt, 1965; Sweet, Crouse and Crable, 1974), this was reported in a small number of PMF lesions by Vyskočil, Tůma and Macek (1970). However, though Davis, Ottery and Le Roux (1977) found an apparent preferential retention of quartz and other non-coal minerals in lungs with more advanced PMF, some PMF lesions had a very low quartz content. And, while the total dust concentrations in these lesions was two or three times higher than in the rest of the lungs its composition was the same. Hence, it appears improbable that quartz accumulation can be the only, or primary, cause of these lesions. And, as already stated, they occur in the absence, or near absence, of quartz.

(2) *Total lung dust* It is well established, as previously cited evidence shows (*see* section on Epidemiology), that the overall mass of respirable dust is the most significant variable in the progression of coal pneumoconiosis which suggests that, in some unknown way, its accumulation triggers fibrogenesis. There is evidence that PMF cases from high-rank collieries have been exposed to more dust than those from low-rank collieries; and, since high-rank coals have a low proportion of non-coal minerals (quartz, kaolinite and mica) and low-rank coals have a much higher proportion, coal rank affects the composition of dust deposited in the lungs. Furthermore, the compositional difference is increased by selective accumulation of non-coal minerals in men from low-rank collieries. Hence, PMF develops in lungs with a wide range of dust mass and composition. A possible, and likely, explanation of this fact is that there is a critical mass-composition relationship for any individual at which PMF will tend to develop, and that the mass required for this will be less as the percentage of non-coal minerals is increased (Davis *et al.*, 1979). These findings, incidently, provide further evidence that quartz is unlikely to be an essential factor in the development of PMF.

PMF may develop and progress in the absence of continuing dust exposure, often years later, which raises the possibility of intervention by some other factor. The observation that serum proteins are absorbed onto coal particles (irrespective of coal rank) in amounts which are sufficient to hold large quantities of protein in the lungs, however, adds weight to the total lung dust hypothesis (Jones, Edwards and Wagner, 1972). But, how, and why the PMF process is localized and why it has a predilection for certain sites remains unanswered.

(3) *Tuberculosis* An alleged modification of tuberculous disease by coal dust held a dominant place for years. James (1954) reported that evidence of tuberculosis was present in 40 per cent of 454 cases of confluent masses at autopsy, culture or guinea-pig inoculation being positive in 36 per cent. Rivers *et al.* (1957) also cultured tubercle bacilli from 35 per cent of cases of PMF. However, during

pathogenesis, though due to a multiplicity of factors, is immunological in many cases (*see* Chapter 4). In some instances the fibrosis may represent the end-stage of extrinsic allergic 'alveolitis' (*see* Chapter 11) especially as many British miners are devoted to pigeon fancying and racing, and breeding budgerigars; and those who, until recent years, looked after haulage ponies underground necessarily handled hay and straw. A probable case of chronic disease in a colliery underground stable man is on record (National Coal Board, 1977). However, it is important to note that organic allergens with the potential to cause the allergic 'alveolitis' are almost certainly absent from coal itself (*see* Chapter 2, p. 36). Acute extrinsic allergic 'alveolitis' seems rarely to have been recognized in coal-miners.

CLINICAL FEATURES

SYMPTOMS

'Simple' pneumoconiosis is symptomless. When cough, sputum, wheeze or breathlessness are complained of they are due to coincidental lung disease—most frequently, in the UK, chronic obstructive bronchitis. Among British coal miners smoking has been found to be the chief factor contributing to respiratory symptoms (Ashford *et al.*, 1970).

There is little correlation between radiographic category of PMF and respiratory symptoms. Category A lesions cause no symptoms and larger masses may be associated with either no symptoms or with symptoms ranging from the trivial to very severe respiratory disability. The reasons for this variability are referred to in the section on Lung function. Dyspnoea in coal-miners with no radiographic evidence of pneumoconiosis is due to unrelated non-occupational disease. The question of chronic bronchitis is discussed in Chapter 1.

There is usually no sputum associated with PMF if the subject is a non-smoker; when there is, it is generally of small volume but may be large if there is infection in distorted and dilated bronchi in proximity to a mass of PMF. It is commonly gelatinous and grey coloured (due to small quantities of coal- or carbon-dust), but may become much darker during chest infection which causes increased elimination of coal-dust even years after the man has ceased to be exposed to dust. In the absence of active tuberculosis (or other causes) haemoptysis is rare in cases of PMF but is not uncommon—although consisting of little more than staining of the sputum with blood—in cases of 'rheumatoid' pneumoconiosis; this, in association with the radiographic appearance of cavities (*see* Radiographic appearances), may compound a mistaken diagnosis of 'sputum negative' tuberculosis. Large haemoptysis is very rare. Jet-black sputum is produced by the occasional rupture of PMF with ischaemic necrosis into a bronchus; it may be large in amount, suddenly raised by distressing paroxysmal coughing and may continue in smaller amounts for some days. It consists of mucus containing large quantities of coal (or carbon) dust with cholesterol crystals and, occasionally, small amounts of blood.

Cough is, in general, related to cigarette smoking and the quantity or viscidity of the sputum. But in some cases of large PMF lesions cough may be frequent, severe and paroxysmal although productive of a negligible amount of sputum, and is often provoked by effort. The reason for this is uncertain: it may be related to 'irritation' of the trachea and main bronchi by large adjacent masses.

Men with PMF uncomplicated by severe scar emphysema or chronic airways obstruction rarely complain of breathlessness at rest but may do during or after effort.

Pain in the chest is sometimes complained of and is usually mild and transient; it appears to arise from thoracic muscular 'strains' but rarely may be due to cough fracture of the ribs.

PHYSICAL SIGNS

There are no characteristic abnormal physical signs of coal or carbon pneumoconiosis.

Finger clubbing is not a feature of either 'simple' pneumoconiosis or PMF. The author found only seven cases of undisputed clubbing in 252 men with Category B or C lesions (3 per cent). But it is often present in men whose radiographs also indicate the presence of DIPF (fibrosing 'alveolitis').

Central cyanosis is not seen in the absence of airways obstruction of 'blue bloater' type or unrelated heart disease.

'Simple' pneumoconiosis and many cases of PMF (even Category C) cause no abnormal signs. But impaired breath sounds and expiratory wheezes are found when massive lesions are associated with severe scar emphysema. Wheezes and rhonchi are more commonly due to coincidental chronic obstructive bronchitis. The trachea is occasionally drawn to one side on which the upper chest wall may be slightly flattened and limited in expansion due to an underlying large, contractile mass of PMF. Inspiratory and expiratory stridor caused by distortion of large airways may be heard at the mouth in such cases. In some men with 'irregular' or category p radiographic opacities persistent inspiratory crepitations may be heard at the bases of the lungs.

Rheumatoid arthritis and subcutaneous rheumatoid nodules should be looked for. The signs of pleural effusion may occasionally be present and may mark the onset or exacerbation of rheumatoid disease.

Large, bilateral PMF lesions may be accompanied by signs of pulmonary heart disease and, ultimately, congestive failure.

INVESTIGATIONS

LUNG FUNCTION

There are no abnormal physiological patterns which are characteristic of coal or carbon pneumoconiosis and so lung function tests are of no help in establishing the diagnosis.

Ventilatory function does not decline with increasing radiographic category of 'simple' pneumoconiosis (*Figure 8.20*) (Cochrane and Higgins, 1961; Morgan *et al.*, 1974); and, though Rogan *et al.* (1961) observed a slight reduction in FEV_1, this was not significant when age was taken into account. Neither is there any reduction in Category A cases. An apparently anomalous relationship between duration of exposure to coal-mine dust and reduction in FEV_1 and FEF is discussed in Chapter 1, Chronic bronchitis. By contrast, category B and C PMF is associated with variable but significant impairment of FEV_1, FVC and FEV_1/FVC,

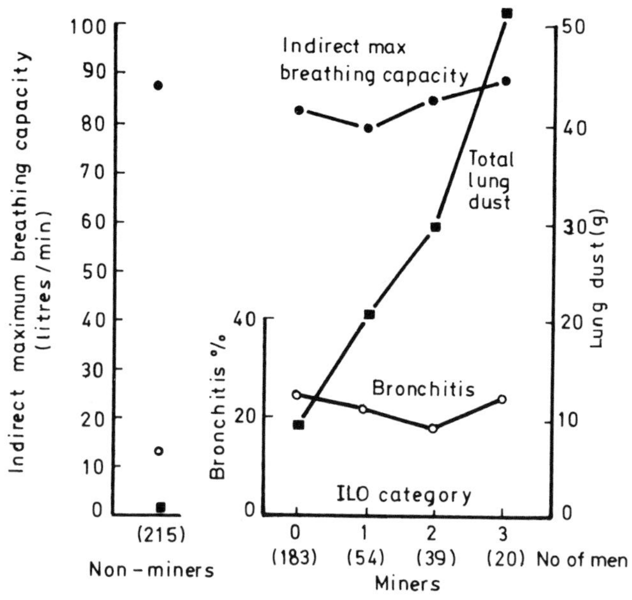

Figure 8.20 Showing the relationship of indirect maximum breathing capacity, prevalence of bronchitis, radiographic category and estimated lung dust in three samples of men aged 55 to 64 years. (By courtesy of Dr J. C. Gilson and the Hon. Editors of the Proceedings of the Royal Society of Medicine*)*

although in some cases—usually non-smokers—they are all well preserved.

Closing volume and closing capacity are not significantly different in miners with and without 'simple' pneumoconiosis (Lapp *et al.*, 1976).

No relationship between category of 'simple' pneumoconiosis and physiologically determined RV and TLC was found by Gilson and Hugh-Jones (1955) but, using Barnhard's radiographic method, Morgan *et al.* (1972) reported some increase in both with increasing category in miners without airflow obstruction. But as various factors other than pneumoconiosis may have caused the divergence between predicted and observed results physiological verification is needed.

Static compliance is not affected by 'simple' pneumoconiosis (Seaton, Lapp and Morgan, 1972a), and such changes as have been observed in frequency dependent dynamic compliance—a test tedious to perform and productive of results of uncertain significance—are, on present evidence, uninformative (Morgan, Lapp and Morgan, 1974).

Gas transfer (Tl) is not reduced in Category q and r 'simple' pneumoconiosis but may be to a slight degree in some category p cases (Cotes *et al.*, 1971; Englert and de Coster, 1965; Frans, Veriter and Brasseur, 1975). Seaton, Lapp and Morgan (1972a) confirmed this and also the fact that there is no difference in FEV_1, FVC, FEV_1/FVC, lung volumes and lung mechanics between category p and q cases. However, a gas transfer defect has not been observed by all investigators (Pivoteau and DeChoux, 1972) and, when measured by the steady state method at rest and during exercise in working miners with 'simple' pneumoconiosis, Tl has been found to be normal in non-smokers irrespective of age and years spent underground, but reduced among smokers regardless of the duration of their exposure to dust (Kibelstis, 1973). When Tl is impaired the reduction is minimal and its percentage increase on exercise, normal (Frans, Veriter and Brasseur, 1975).

The alveolar–arterial oxygen (A-a)P_{O_2} gradient may be increased and arterial oxygen tension slightly reduced at rest in 'simple' pneumoconiosis especially category p cases, though tending to correct on effort; but the changes are minimal in miners who do not smoke (Frans *et al.*, 1975; Lapp and Seaton, 1971; Pivoteau and DeChoux, 1972). It has been suggested that the underlying cause of these changes may be some diminution of the pulmonary capillary bed (Lapp and Seaton, 1971), but lung photoscanning techniques indicate that the vascular bed is normal in almost all cases of 'simple' coal pneumoconiosis (Seaton, Lapp and Chang, 1971).

As category p opacities have attracted some interest the following points are worth noting.

(1) There is much more difficulty in relegating abnormal radiographic appearances accurately to the p category than to the q and r categories, and this is particularly influenced by X-ray technique (*see* Chapter 5).
(2) It cannot be taken for granted that the pneumoconiosis is responsible for the minimal physiological changes. Indeed, in a fair proportion of individuals with category p radiographs during life the chief abnormalities in the lungs post mortem are fine DIPF or generalized dust-pigmented panlobular emphysema (*Figure 8.21*) (Parkes, 1972) (*see also* Chapter 5). Some support for the contention, suggested in the first edition of this book, that increased air-space size—a potentially effective contrast medium in dust pigmented lungs—may be a contributory factor in some cases has been furnished by Lyons *et al.* (1974) and by the demonstration of a longer period of residence of inhaled 0.5 μm particles in the lung parenchyma in category p compared with category q and o cases and with normal non-miners (Hanskinson, Palmes and Lapp, 1979), and by the finding of more 'overall emphysema' in these cases than in category q and r cases (Davis *et al.*, 1979). There is also a larger physiological dead space relative to tidal volume in these cases and

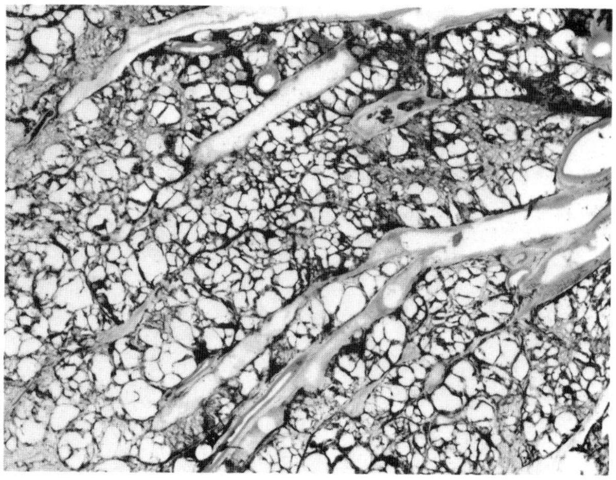

Figure 8.21 Coal dust-pigmented emphysema which was almost uniform throughout both lungs. No fibrotic nodules in any part of either lung. Radiographic category 3p. (Paper-mounted section)

there may be some increase in ventilation during maximal exercise (Cotes and Field, 1972).

(3) The physiological abnormalities are very small and are not associated with respiratory symptoms or with any reduction of capacity for heavy work (Lavenne, 1968, 1970).

Thus, 'simple' pneumoconiosis does not cause any significant reduction in Tl, and the observations in category p cases—though of academic interest and requiring longitudinal investigation—have no practical significance.

Pulmonary artery pressure is not increased in subjects with 'simple' pneumoconiosis but no airflow obstruction (Krémer and Lavenne, 1966; Navrátil, Widmisky and Kasalicky, 1968).

In PMF there is wide variation in the pattern and severity of impaired function which correlates very poorly with the radiographic appearances. It is determined variously by the size and anatomical site of the masses, the amount of associated vasculitis and the presence or absence of scar (irregular) or panlobular emphysema and chronic obstructive bronchitis. Total lung capacity and vital capacity are usually reduced and residual volume increased, both as an absolute value and as a percentage of total lung capacity; ventilatory capacity may be reduced and, in some cases, there is irreversible airways obstruction. Compliance may be reduced but not to the extent commonly observed in asbestosis. The ventilation–perfusion ratio is impaired to a greater or lesser degree and Tl is reduced so that, in a proportion of cases, there is hypoxaemia on effort. In category B and C cases, in which airflow obstruction is fairly common, (A-a)P_{O_2} may be increased at rest and increase further on exercise (Morgan and Lapp, 1976). The presence of a significant reduction in the vascular bed by large, central masses and associated arteritis is chiefly responsible for these changes, and is reflected in 'avascular zones' in the regions of the masses in lung perfusion scans (Seaton, Lapp and Chang, 1971) and in pulmonary hypertension in a proportion of cases (Navrátil, Widmisky and Kasalicky, 1968). Ventilation on effort may be normal or increased. Reduction in ventilatory capacity is one of the best simple guides to the severity of disability in men with PMF.

Typical 'rheumatoid' coal pneumoconiosis of Caplan type (1953) is usually associated with remarkably little, if any, impairment of lung function presumably because only a small amount of lung tissue is involved and scar (irregular) emphysema is absent. This is confirmed by comparison of the values of FEV_1, FVC and RV/TLC ratio in Caplan's syndrome with those in non-rheumatoid PMF when differences in age, years worked underground, smoking habits and radiographic category are allowed for (Constantinidis *et al.*, 1978). But atypical cases with confluent lesions exhibit the functional changes just described in varying degree.

To summarize

(1) Impairment of lung function may be pronounced in some cases of category B and C pneumoconiosis but in others of similar category, is remarkably slight. The degree of respiratory disability is determined largely by ventilatory capacity which may be improved by therapeutic measures to relieve airflow obstruction.

(2) In 'simple' pneumoconiosis all the indices are within normal range unless there is other accompanying disease (in particular, chronic non-specific lung disease), and such changes as have been reported are minimal and insufficient to cause breathlessness (Cotes, 1979).

RADIOGRAPHIC APPEARANCES

Ordinary (or usual) pneumoconiosis

The earliest abnormal appearances consist of a few small, ill-defined opacities which can be distinguished from vascular shadows in the outer third of the lung fields and are seen mainly in the upper and middle zones. Subsequently they are better defined and more widely distributed.

The opacity size of discrete ('simple') pneumoconiosis most commonly seen is category q (m); category r (n) is less common, and category p (the interpretation of which it is often difficult to be confident) is most uncommon—if not rare (*see* Chapter 5). Opacities of different category may be present in the one film but one category is usually predominant, and this is the category quoted. The good correlation which exists between the profusion of opacities (categories 1 to 3) and the lesions found in the lungs post mortem is referred to in Chapter 5, and the clear relationship to total content of lung dust is shown in *Figure 8.20.* It has been computed that the relative contributions of coal and other minerals to the radiographic score of 'simple' pneumoconiosis is 1:3.8 which is similar to the X-ray mass absorption coefficients of these two fractions (Rossiter, 1972c) (*see* p. 108, Chapter 5); in particular, the iron content of the lungs is especially well correlated with category (Bergman and Caswell, 1972; Rossiter, 1972c). There is, in general, a good correlation between overall lung dust content and the category of radiographic profusion (Davis *et al.*, 1979).

The opacities of 'simple' pneumoconiosis tend to be distributed in the upper halves of the lung fields until the category 3 stage is reached when the whole of the lung fields are more or less equally involved. PMF opacities—which, arbitrarily, are those larger than 1 cm in diameter (*see Table 5.3*) in contrast to the pathological criterion (*see* p. 185)—are also more commonly seen in the upper than in the lower halves of the lung fields. They may be unilateral or bilateral, and, if the latter, are distributed roughly symmetrically or asymmetrically (*Figures 5.10, 5.11* and *8.22*). In a minority of cases, however, they are confined to the lower lung fields (*Figure 8.23a* and *b*). An opacity caused by a single lesions may be obscured by the heart shadow on the standard PA film and is only clearly seen in lateral or oblique radiographs. Normally there is a 'background' of category 2 or 3 'simple' pneumoconiosis with PMF but in a few cases this is absent.

PMF opacities vary greatly in shape as well as in size. They may be round, ovoid, sausage-like or linear in outline, and, as a rule, are well demarcated from the adjacent lung. An example of the unusual configurations which are sometimes seen is shown in *Figure 8.24* (cf. *Figure 8.11*). Occasionally linear markings radiate from the PMF into the lung field and may reach the chest wall (*Figures 8.22c* and *8.25*). The development of a cavity within a PMF lesion is indicated by a well-defined, circumscribed translucency (*Figures 8.26a* and *b*) in which there may be evidence of fluid. In most cases the cavity vanishes sooner or later and

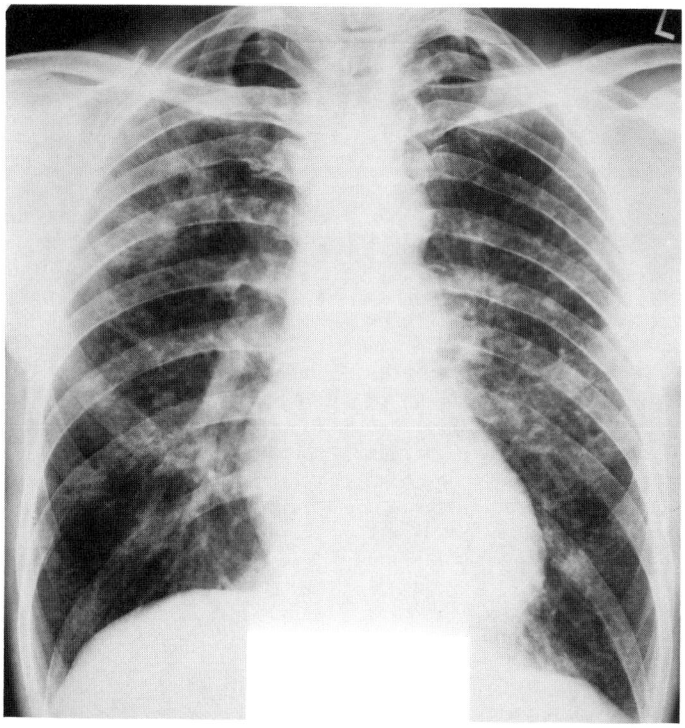

Figure 8.22(a) 1959

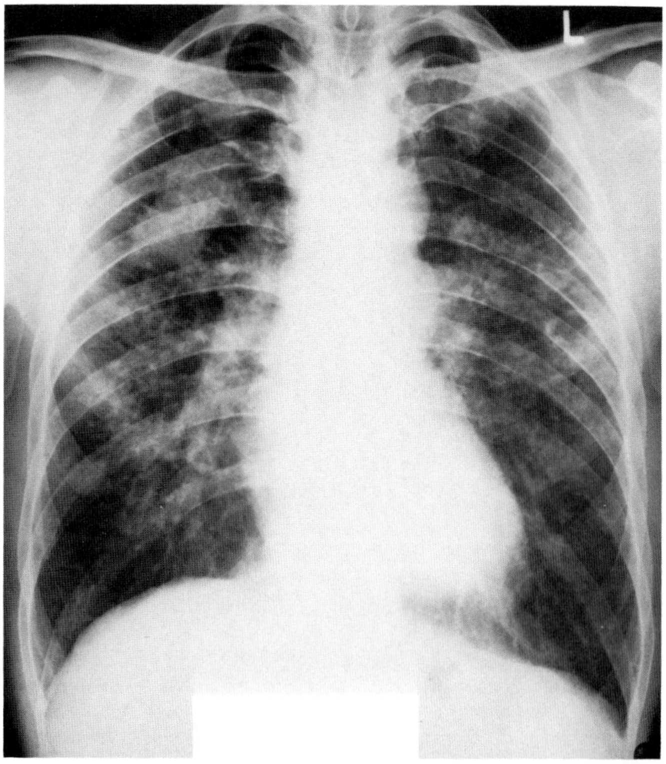

Figure 8.22(b) 1965

Figure 8.22(c) 1976

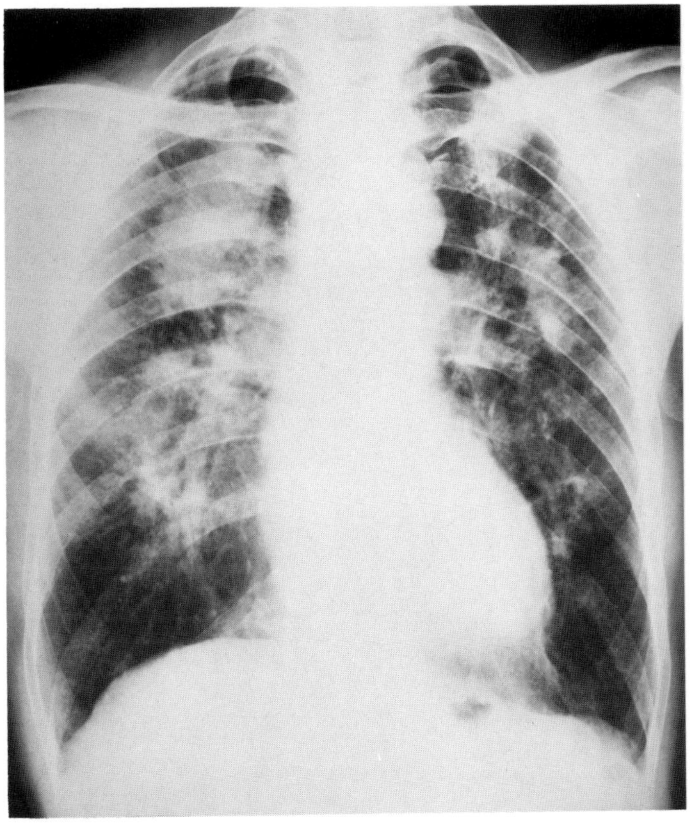

Figure 8.22 Radiographs showing progression of coal pneumoconiosis in a miner who worked 16 years at the coal face and left the mines in 1960. The 1959 film (a) shows early confluence in the right upper zone (Category 2qA). Both the 1965 (b) and 1976 (c) are Category 2qB. In 1976 the PMF opacity is well circumscribed: note the presence of linear opacities radiating from the PMF opacities. It is of interest that circulating RF (DAT 1:128) and ANA were present in 1976 but there were no rheumatic symptoms and no clinical arthropathy

appearances return wholly or partly to the *status quo*. An occasional feature of PMF is a dense peripheral arc or rim at its lower pole which represents calcification. This may be a sequel to accumulation of fluid in a previous cavity (*Figure 8.27*) and, though probably not pathognomonic, the appearance is rarely seen in other diseases. Evidence of dense calcification within the lesion is also sometimes seen (*Figure 8.28*). PMF of irregular stellate outline is often associated with the signs of bullous emphysema, distortion of the lung, and shift of the trachea and mediastinum to the affected side. Sometimes a mass alters position over a period of years due mainly to hyperinflation of adjacent emphysematous lung when its appearances could be mistaken for a tumour (*Figures 8.29a* and *b*).

The signs of 'eggshell' calcification of hilar lymph nodes, similar to those which may occur in silicosis (*see* Chapter 7), are present in a small proportion of cases of coal and natural graphite pneumoconiosis. According to Jacobson *et al.* (1967) they are more often found with PMF than with 'simple' pneumoconiosis and my experience agrees with this (*Figure 8.30*). These appearances are related to past exposure to dust from siliceous rocks in shaft sinking or maintaining colliery roads and airways, or to the quartz of natural graphite.

Multiple short Kerley's B lines are present in some cases of higher category 'simple' pneumoconiosis and PMF (Trapnell, 1964) due to the accumulation of dust in peripheral interlobular septa. When these occur in the lower lung fields they may be mistaken as evidence of DIPF (*see* p. 109 and *Figure 8.25*). Other fine irregular opacities (usually category 's') are sometimes seen, again mainly in the lower lung fields, and may be associated with reduced mean FEV_1, FEV_1/FVC, increased mean RV and TLC, cigarette smoking and years spent underground (Amandus *et al.*, 1976; Lyons *et al.*, 1974). It is probable that these opacities are also explained by increased radiodensity contrast of dust-containing lung and air spaces of abnormal size (*see* p. 196). Hence, interlobular dust accumulation and increased dust-air X-ray contrast appear to be the commonest causes of irregular opacities in coal pneumoconiosis, and may be contributed to by smoking (Weiss, 1969). This would seem to be confirmed by the demonstration by Davis *et al.* (1979) of a significant association of irregular opacities with 'overall emphysema' compared with category 0 cases. Occasionally, however, the unmistakable features of DIPF with 'honeycomb' cysts are seen and have also been observed in graphite pneumoconiosis (Gaensler *et al.*, 1966; Pendergrass *et al.*, 1968).

(a)

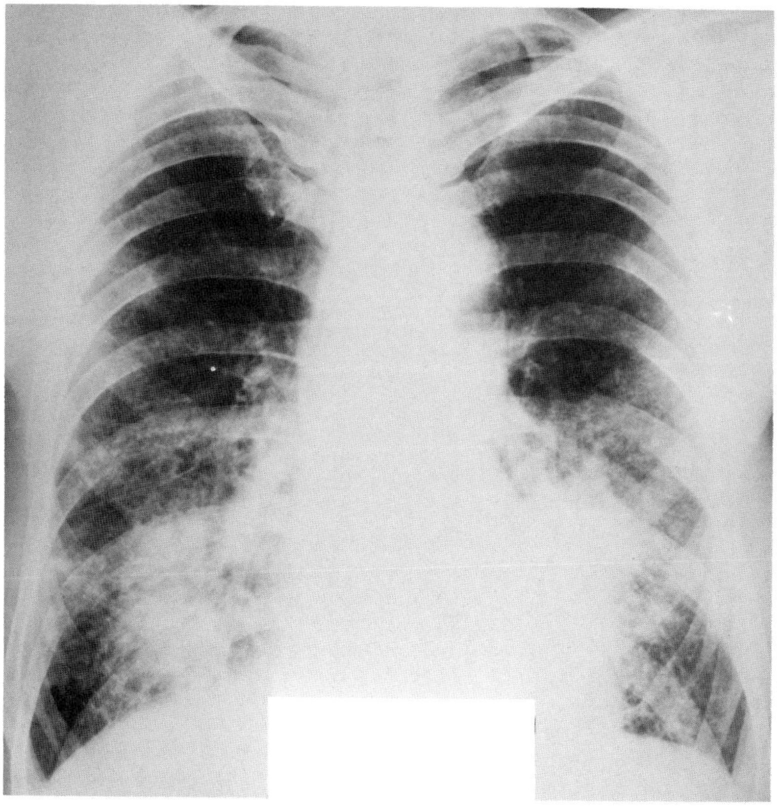

(b)

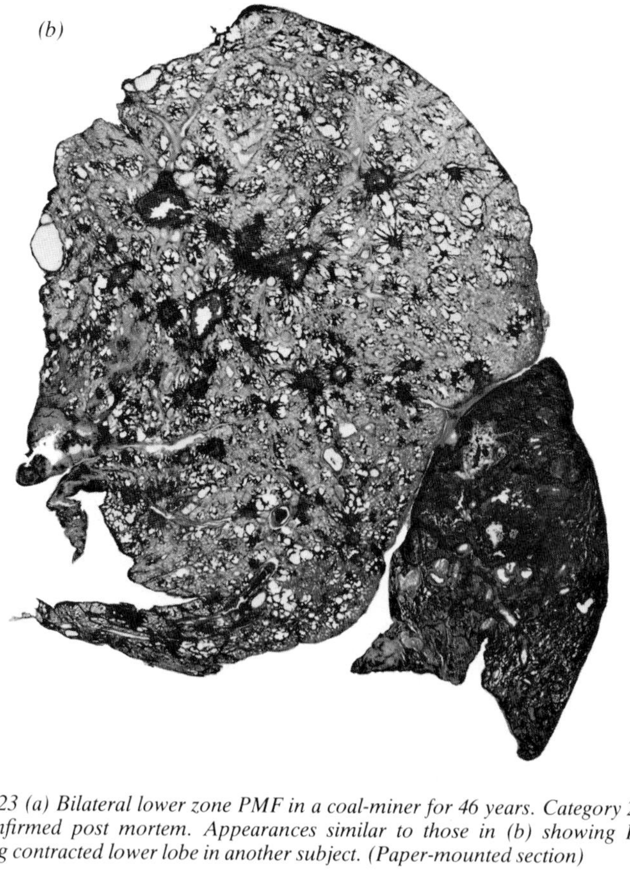

Figure 8.23 (a) Bilateral lower zone PMF in a coal-miner for 46 years. Category 2qB. PMF confirmed post mortem. Appearances similar to those in (b) showing PMF occupying contracted lower lobe in another subject. (Paper-mounted section)

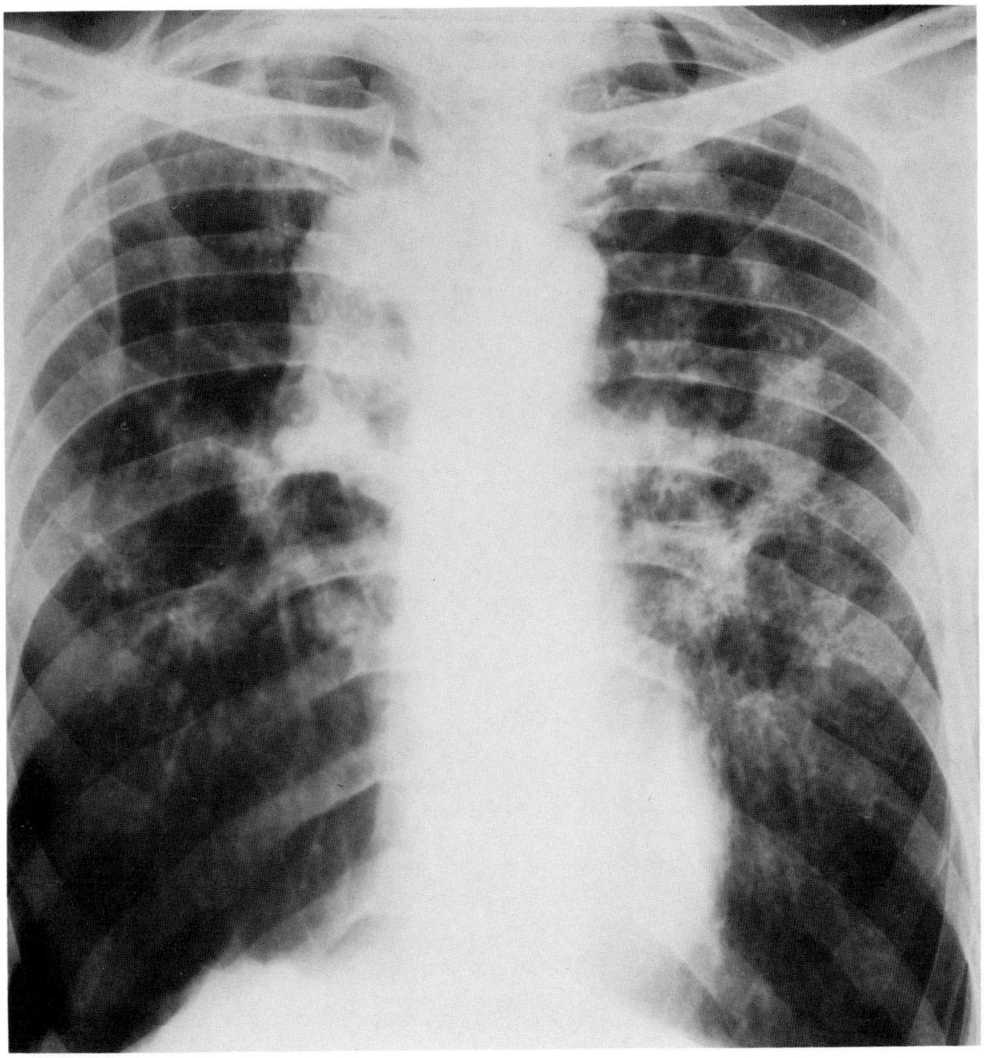

Figure 8.24 Coal PMF of bizarre appearance in left lung field. PMF close to mediastinum on the right. Autopsy confirmation. (See Figure 8.11)

Many of these are probably related to rheumatoid disease (*see Figure 8.42*). It is perhaps relevant to point out that a widely held early opinion that 'the outstanding feature of coal pneumoconiosis is reticulation' (Hart and Aslett, 1942) (*see* Chapter 5, p. 97) is incorrect and may have been due to the technical quality of radiographs over 30 years ago.

Photoscanning of the lung fields after intravenous injection of albumin-^{131}I correlates well with the vascular pathology. The vascular bed is normal in 'simple' pneumoconiosis except in the case of larger 'nodular' opacities when small avascular areas are revealed. Avascular zones of varying extent are found in and around all PMF lesions.

'Rheumatoid' pneumoconiosis

It has already been noted (p. 186) that the radiographical as well as the pathological features of this variant of the disease differ from those of ordinary coal pneumoconiosis both in appearances and behaviour. The X-ray changes which may occur vary widely and can be enumerated as follows:

(1) 'Classic' Caplan-type opacities.
(2) Scanty, large round opacities.
(3) Mixed, small and large round and irregular opacities.
(4) Scanty, small round opacities.
(5) Multiple, small round opacities.
(6) One or other of these in association with pneumoconiosis of ordinary or usual appearance.
(7) Sudden development of widespread 'woolly' opacities.

Caplan-type opacities (Caplan, 1953)

Typically these are round, fairly dense, vary from about 0.5 to 3.0 cm in diameter (occasionally up to 5 cm) and correspond to the discrete nodules or matted groups of nodules described earlier. They are usually moderate in number and are scattered irregularly in the lung fields. The density of individual opacities is variable and rarely completely homogeneous. Evidence of calcification within the lesions is fairly common. Ring shadows due to excavation of some nodules are common and, in some, there are signs of fluid.

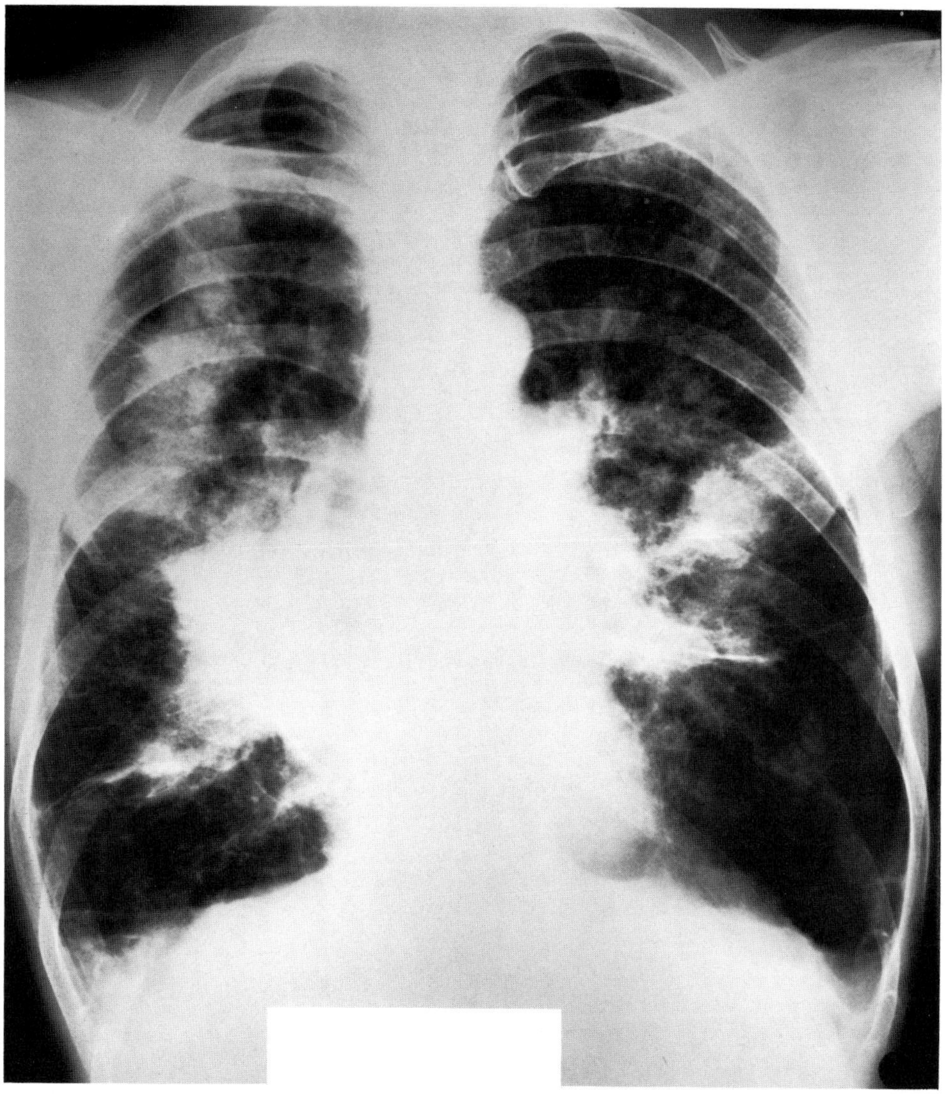

Figure 8.25 PMF with prominent linear projections, Kerley's B lines and emphysema of the lower zones. $FEV_1 = 0.71$; $FVC = 1.41$. Coal-miner for 11 years up to 1945

Subsequently these ring shadows either disappear leaving little or no trace or resume their original appearance (*Figure 8.31*). Disappearance of re-existing opacities and development of new ones in different locations is usual. Appearances may change in a period of months or remain unaltered for years after which erratic behaviour may resume, sometimes during an exacerbation or first evidences of arthropathy. The superimposition effect of a number of nodules in the X-ray beam may, exceptionally, give the appearances of large lobulated masses (*Figure 8.32*).

Unlike most cases of ordinary PMF there is, as a rule, no 'background' of 'simple' pneumoconiosis, but exceptions to this occur (*see Figure 8.38*).

Scanty, large round opacities

These are identical in appearance and behaviour to 'classic' Caplan opacities but are not more than about four in number. Occasionally only one opacity is evident (*Figure 8.33*).

Mixed, small and large round and irregular opacities

These are of widely disparate size but the majority range from less than 0.5 cm to about 1 cm in diameter and only a few are larger. Often they exhibit a less well-defined or woollier appearance than those of 'classic' Caplan type. In other respects their development and behaviour of these lesions are similar to the 'classic' nodules though they are especially prone to calcification (*Figure 8.34*). In some cases their distribution is chiefly peripheral, sometimes with signs of related diffuse pleural thickening (*Figure 8.35*). In others, they are clustered into one or two zones of the lung fields.

(a) (b)

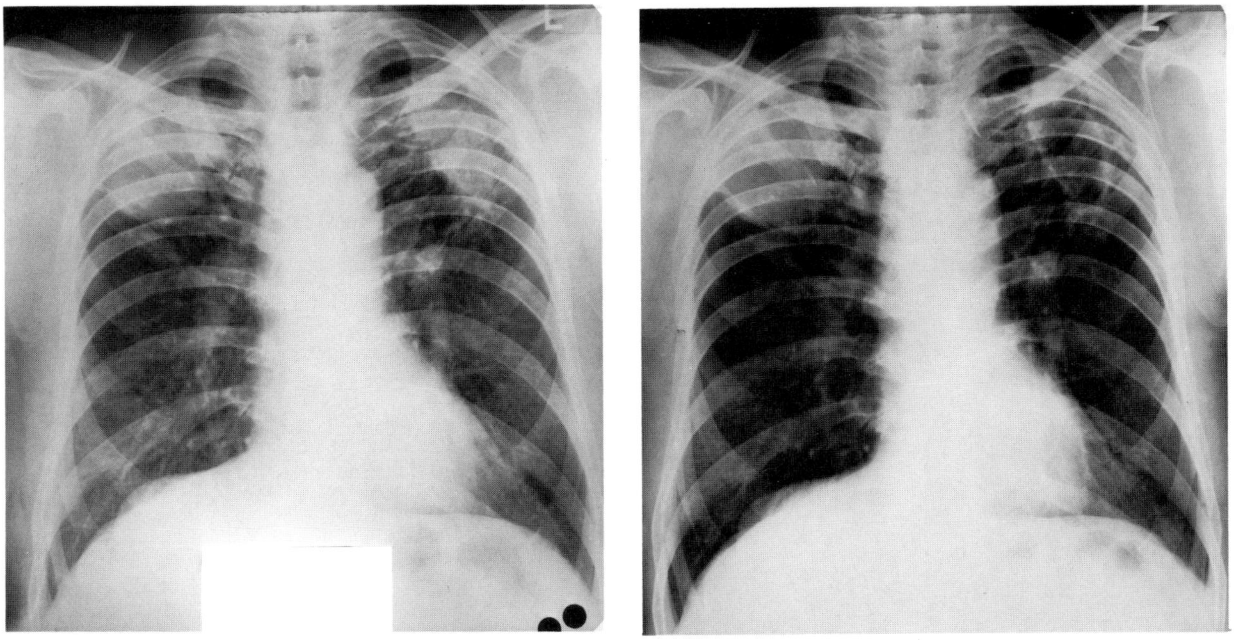

Figure 8.26 (a) and (b). Development of ischaemic cavity in upper lobe PMF within 12 months associated with episodes of paroxysmal cough and jet-black sputum. Such cavities are prone to secondary fungous infection. (See Figure 8.46)

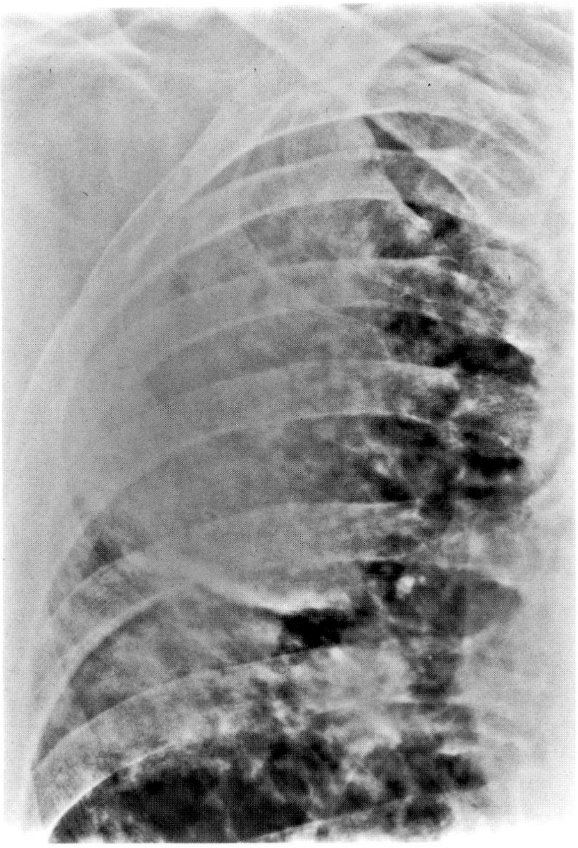

Figure 8.27 Dense opaque rim to lower pole of PMF which frequently represents a zone of calcification. A helpful sign in differentiating PMF from carcinoma

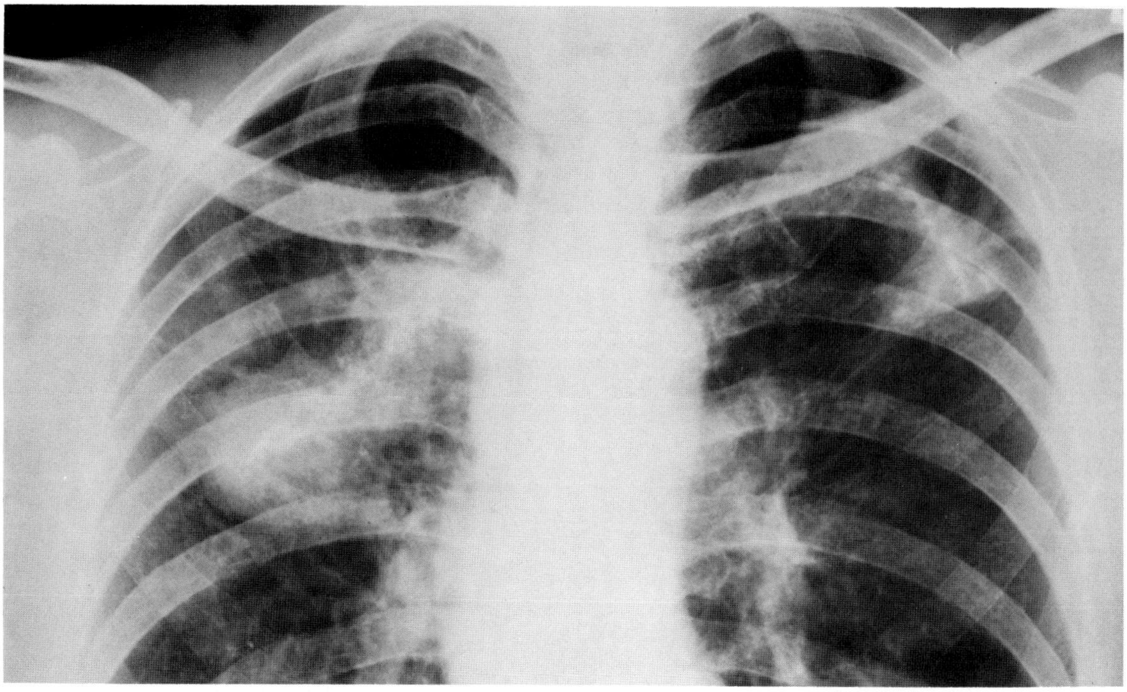

Figure 8.28 Central calcification in PMF. No evidence of tuberculosis at any time. Calcification confirmed post mortem

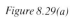

Figure 8.29(a)

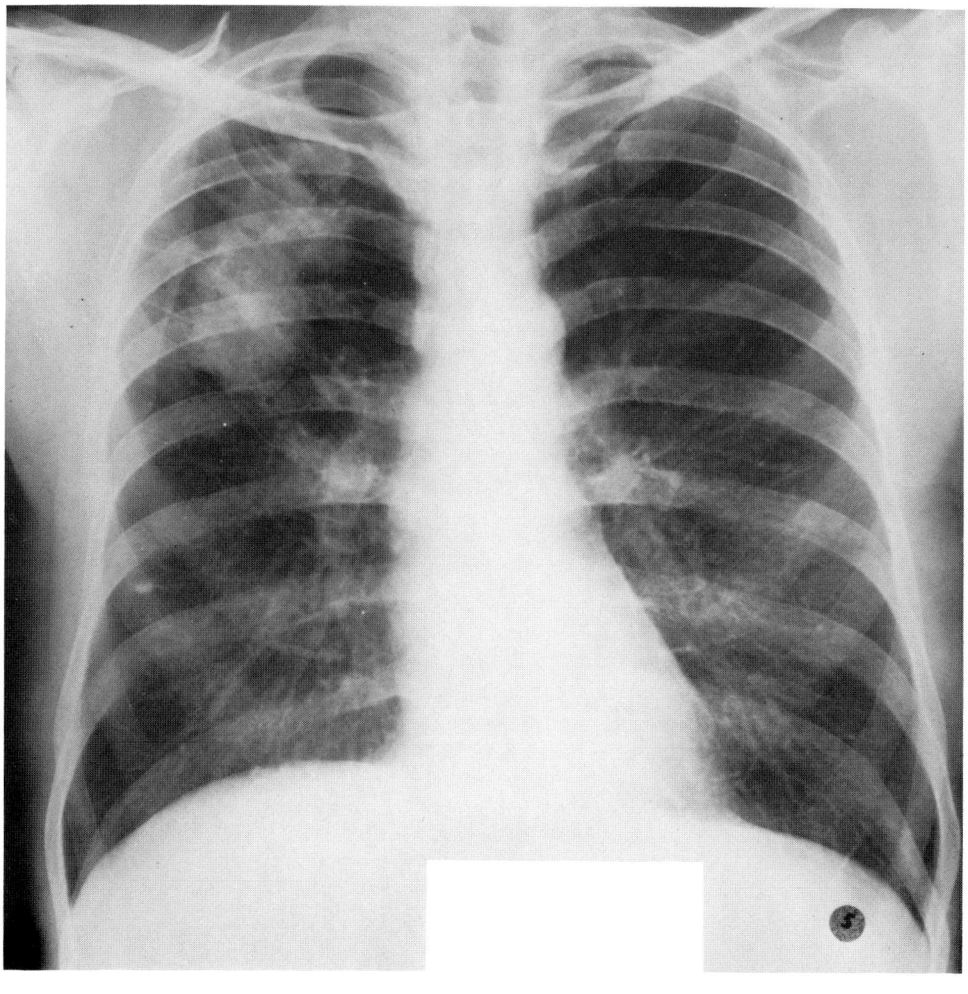

Figure 8.29(b)

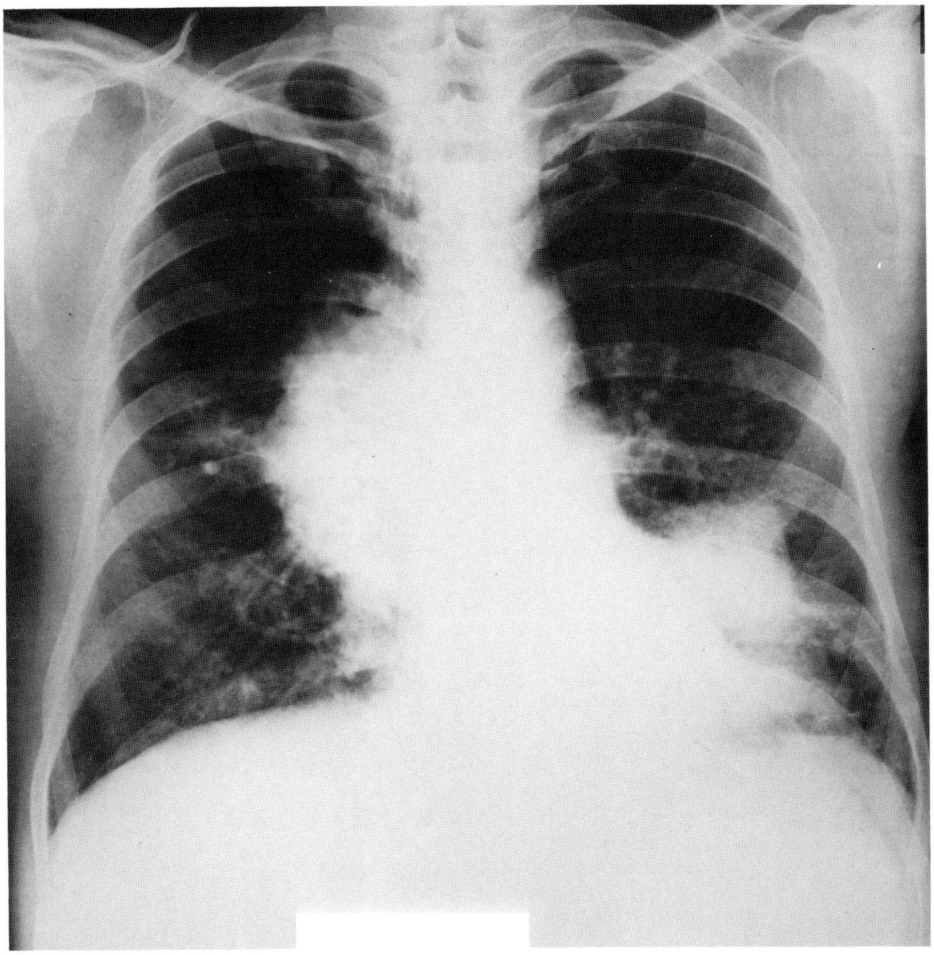

Figure 8.29 (a) Right upper zone PMF with very few accompanying discrete opacities. (b) Twenty years later PMF is larger well-circumscribed and has shifted to the right hilar region. Another PMF is now present in the left lung. There is severe hyperinflation—lung markings absent in upper half of lung fields. Seen in isolation the appearances of both lungs might be mistaken for other pathology. Note linear opacities radiating from PMF in (a)

Scanty, small round opacities

Opacities of this type, which are few in number, do not, on the whole, vary greatly in size. They may be grouped together in one lung field or scattered in both fields (*Figures 8.36* and *8.37*).

Multiple, small round opacities

As a rule these are more or less similar in size and usually widely scattered although some clustering may be seen.

Occurrence of one or other of the foregoing with pneumoconiosis of ordinary type

In these cases—which seem to be rare—the appearances of ordinary discrete ('simple') pneumoconiosis or PMF have been present for years when additional changes consistent with rheumatoid pneumoconiosis develop within a short period of time sometimes in relation to the onset or exacerbation of rheumatoid arthritis (*Figures 8.38* and *8.39*).

Sudden development of widespread 'woolly' opacities

This is another rare phenomenon in which bilateral opacities appear and progress with extraordinary rapidity and become widespread. The disease may be fatal within two to three years and can reasonably be described as acute 'rheumatoid' coal pneumoconiosis (*Figure 8.40*).

Of the first five of these variants the mixed and small nodular types are probably the most common, with the 'classic' Caplan type next and the scanty large type least common. Occasionally, however, one type changes into another. The last two are rare.

Important additional features which may develop in any of the first six variants are:

(1) Calcification of some or all of the lesions (*Figure 8.34*).
(2) Signs of pleural effusion—a recognized complication of rheumatoid disease (Ward, 1961; Walker and Wright,

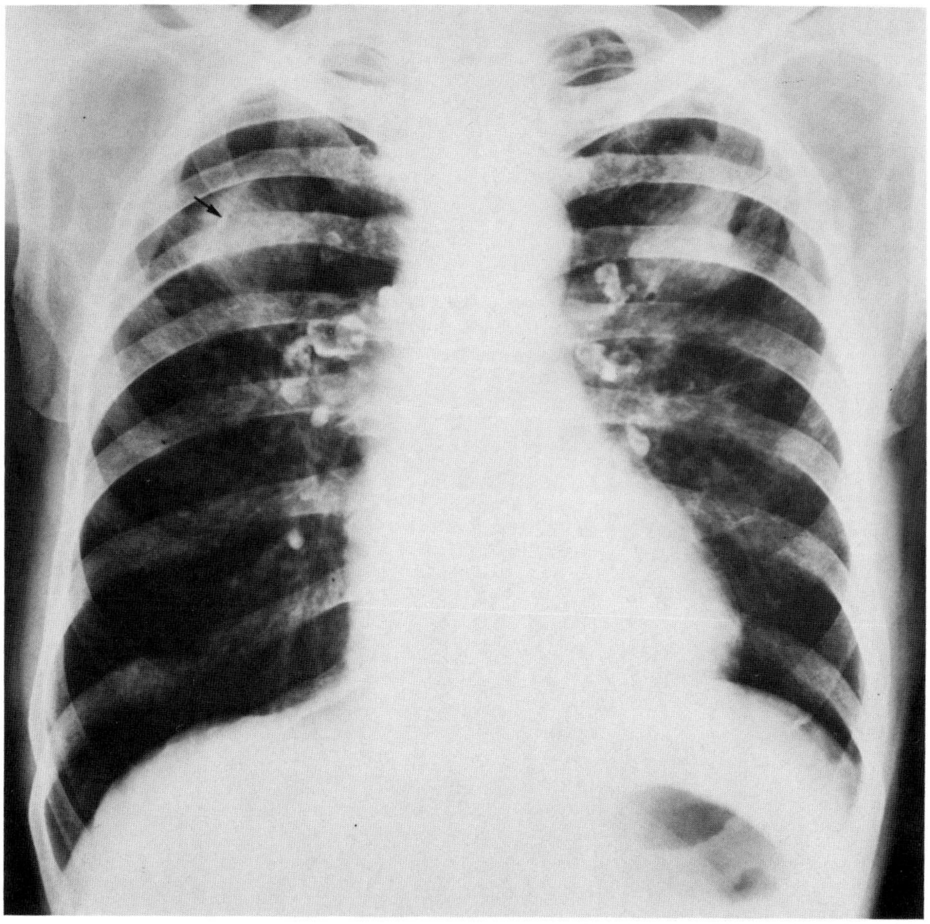

Figure 8.30 Calcification (arrowed) in coal PMF. This sign, which sometimes requires tomography for demonstration, is helpful in distinguishing PMF from circumscribed bronchial carcinoma. Eggshell calcification of the hilar lymph nodes is also present. Case of a collier for 30 years some of which time was spent rock-drilling in drifts

1967) first remarked upon by Fuller in 1860. Effusion may be single or recurrent on the same or opposite sides. Its development does not correlate with the amount of intrapulmonary disease (*Figure 8.37*).

(3) Diffuse interstitial pulmonary fibrosis (*Figure 8.17* and *8.33*).

It should be noted that a coal-miner with rheumatoid arthritis, even of severe degree, may show no evidence of 'rheumatoid' pneumoconiosis. Nonetheless, continued observation of such cases is essential as the possibility of its developing subsequently is always present even in old age (*Figure 8.33*). Similarly, the appearances of 'simple' coal pneumoconiosis may remain unchanged for many years in a man with active rheumatoid arthritis, and 'rheumatoid' pneumoconiosis may never develop.

Evidently, there is some overlap of 'rheumatoid' and ordinary pneumoconiosis both radiographically and immunologically. The range of the X-ray appearances of 'rheumatoid' pneumoconiosis compared with ordinary PMF and their possible relationship to the levels of dust exposure and immunological activity is summarized diagrammatically in *Figure 8.41*.

BACTERIOLOGY

When the radiograph shows a cavitary PMF or opacities of recent development, sputum should be cultured for tubercle bacilli and opportunist mycobacteria. Tubercle bacilli are very rarely recovered from the 'rheumatoid' cases whether or not the lesions are excavated.

IMMUNOLOGY

Rheumatoid factor

DAT is positive in almost all cases of 'rheumatoid' pneumoconiosis often in high titre whether or not there is accompanying arthritis, but variations in titre may be observed over a period of time. The latex fixation test is less consistently positive. The occasional sero-negative case usually proves to be positive subsequently if tests are repeated over a period of months.

Circulating rheumatoid factor (DAT) has also been shown to be present in 6 per cent of British coal-miners with 'simple' pneumoconiosis and in 18 per cent of those with

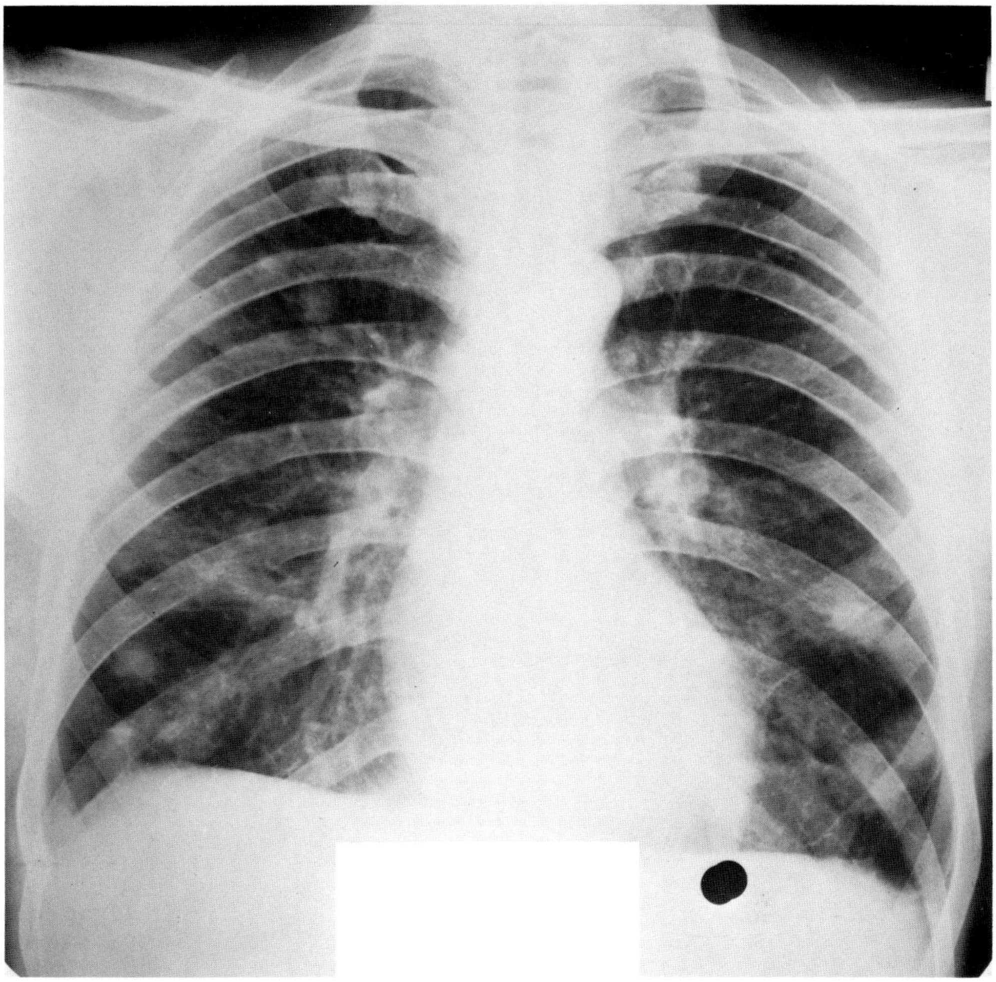

Figure 8.31 (a) 1957

category C PMF (Soutar, Turner-Warwick and Parkes, 1974) (*see Table 8.2*); and Benedek, Zawadzki and Medsger (1976) found a slight but signficant increase of positive latex fixation titres in American miners which, however, was not related to category. But Lippmann *et al.* (1973), also using a latex test in American miners, found no increase in any category. If a carefully standardized DAT technique is used (*see* Chapter 4, p. 61) circulating rheumatoid factor is more likely to be present in individuals with higher categories of pneumoconiosis than in the general population—at least among British miners. However, this has no diagnostic significance.

Antinuclear antibody

Circulating antinuclear antibody is also present more often in miners with pneumoconiosis than in the general population, especially in those with PMF—more so than rheumatoid factor (Kang *et al.*, 1973; Lippmann *et al.*, 1973;

Table 8.2 Presence of ANA and RF in the 109 British Coal-Miners According to Category of Pneumoconiosis

	Category of pneumoconiosis				
	Simple	*Progressive massive fibrosis*			*Total*
		A	*B*	*C*	
No. of men:	32	28	38	11	109
No. (%) with ANA	3 (9)	4 (14)	9 (24)	3 (27)	19 (17)
No. (%) with RF	2 (6)	1 (4)	6 (16)	2 (18)	11 (10)
No. (%) with ANA or RF or both	4 (13)	5 (18)	12 (32)	5 (45)	26 (24)

χ^2 trend for ANA in all categories = 3.32, P = 0.07; for RF, not significant; for ANA and RF together = 6.6, P = 0.01. (Courtesy of the Editor, *Br. med. J.*)

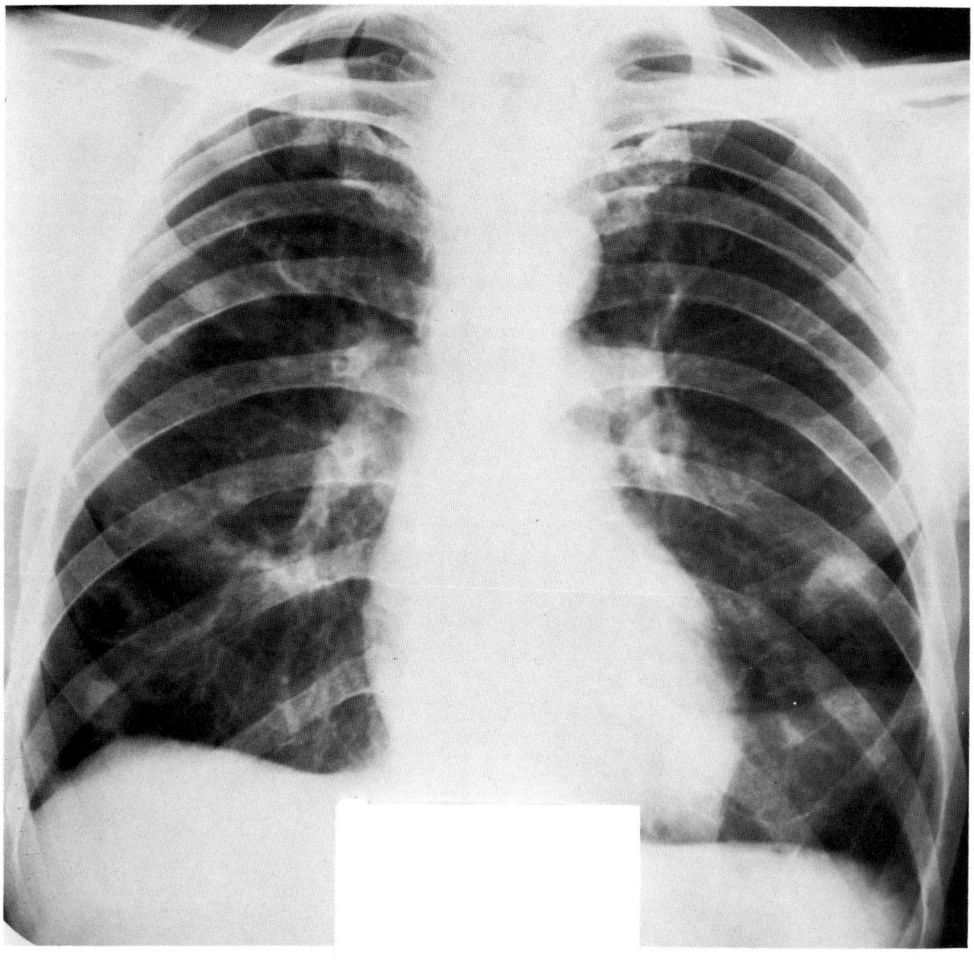

Figure 8.31 (b) 1958

Soutar, Turner-Warwick and Parkes, 1974) (*Table 8.2*). The prevalence trend is similar to, but much weaker than that in nodular silicosis (*Table 7.1*). Again, this has no diagnostic significance. It is interesting that the prevalence of ANA is reported to be significantly higher in anthracite than in bituminous miners with PMF (Lippmann *et al.* 1973).

The trend of an increased prevalence of auto-antibodies in the higher categories of pneumoconiosis is most pronounced when circulating rheumatoid factor and anti-nuclear antibody are found together (Soutar, Turner-Warwick and Parkes, 1974) (*see Table 8.2*).

When DIPF and pneumoconiosis co-exist both antibodies are often present.

Serum immunoglobulins

Increased IgA concentrations were noted by Lewis, Lapp and Burrell (1971) in miners with 'simple' pneumoconiosis or PMF. And levels of IgA, IgG, C3 component of complement and α-1 antitrypsin are apparently significantly higher in anthracite compared with bituminous miners with PMF, but not in those with lower categories of pneumoconiosis. Furthermore, serum IgA, IgG, C3 and α-1 antitrypsin are significantly higher in Caplan's syndrome, PMF and (α-1 antitrypsin excepted) 'simple' pneumoconiosis than in a control population. These observations may suggest selective stimulation of immunoglobulin systems by coal-mine dusts (Hahon, Morgan and Petersen, 1980).

Antireticulin and anticollagen antibodies (*see* Chapter 4, p. 64)

Although there is evidence that antibodies reactive with reticulin and collagen may occur in experimental coal pneumoconiosis (Burrell, 1972) they do not seem to have been demonstrated so far in the human disease.

Peripheral blood lymphocytes

Preliminary investigation has indicated some impairment of activity of both T and B cell systems in the higher categories of pneumoconiosis but this requires confirmation (Dauber,

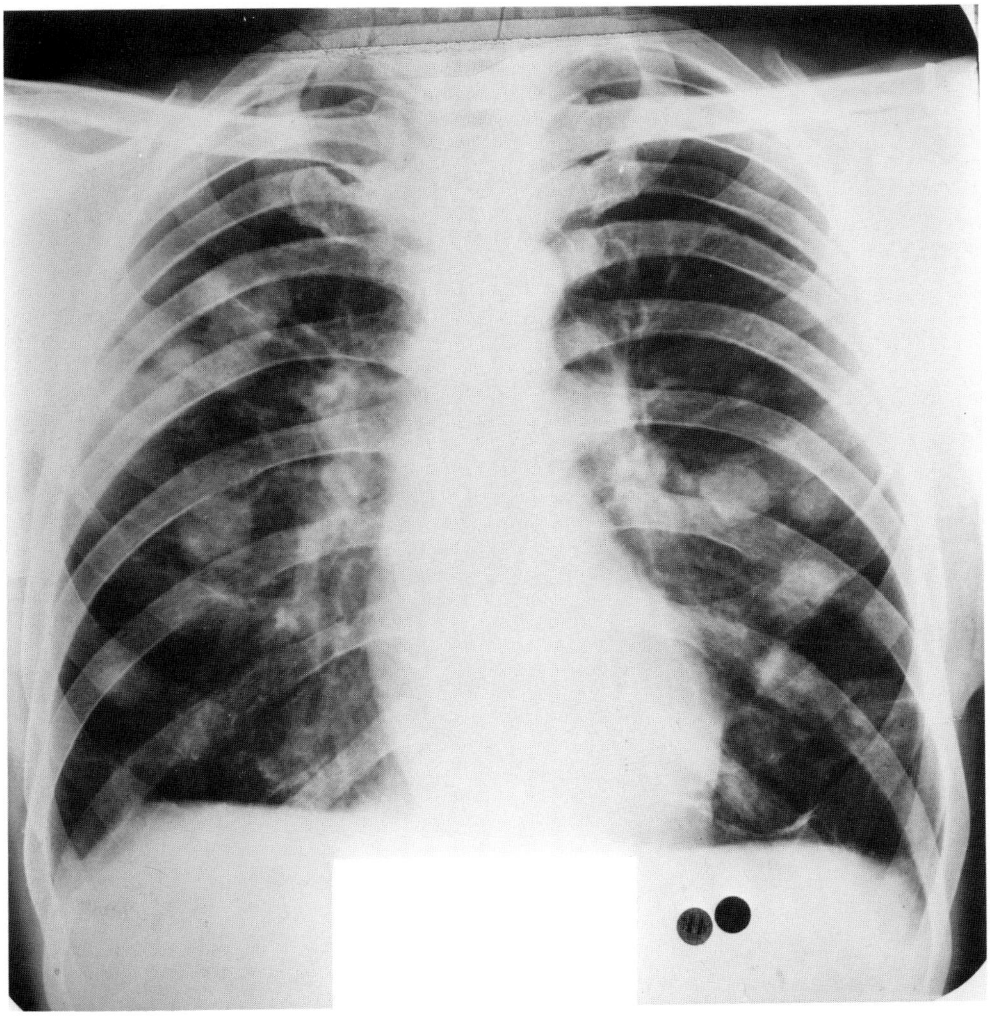

Figure 8.31 (c) 1964

Finn and Daniele, 1976). Reduction in activity of suppressor T cells, however, might explain the presence of the auto-antibodies (*see also* similar findings in silicosis, p. 142).

HAEMATOLOGY

Mild normochromic or slightly hypochromic anaemia is fairly common among coal-miners with PMF in South Wales and haemodilution due to expanded plasma volume appears to be an important determining factor (Chan, 1969b) in addition to low serum iron already referred to. The cause is unknown.

OTHER INVESTIGATIONS

Electrocardiography may be indicated to verify the presence of right ventricular strain and pulmonary hypertension in PMF cases. But this is not normally observed until FEV_1 is reduced to about 1.0 l or less.

DIAGNOSIS

Occupational and medical histories and the radiographic appearances together provide the diagnosis. The presence of blue-black, coal tattoo marks in the skin of the hands, forearms, face and torso is additional evidence of past coal mining, and is a valuable sign in men who have been away from the industry for years and in whom the relevant history has been missed or is unobtainable. Lung biopsy is never indicated except to exclude other pathology.

Occasionally the radiographic appearances of miliary tuberculosis, sarcoidosis or connective tissue diseases such as polyarteritis nodosa and systemic lupus erythematosus may resemble 'simple' pneumoconiosis although the quality of the opacities is different and the patient, in most cases, is ill. For a reminder of the causes of small discrete opacities *see Table 5.2*. Opacities caused by the 'benign' pneumoconioses are denser and, as a rule, more widely scattered in the lung fields than those of 'simple' pneumoconiosis (*see* Chapter 6).

It should be remembered that coal pneumoconiosis and some other type of pneumoconiosis may co-exist—asbestosis, for example (*see* Chapter 9).

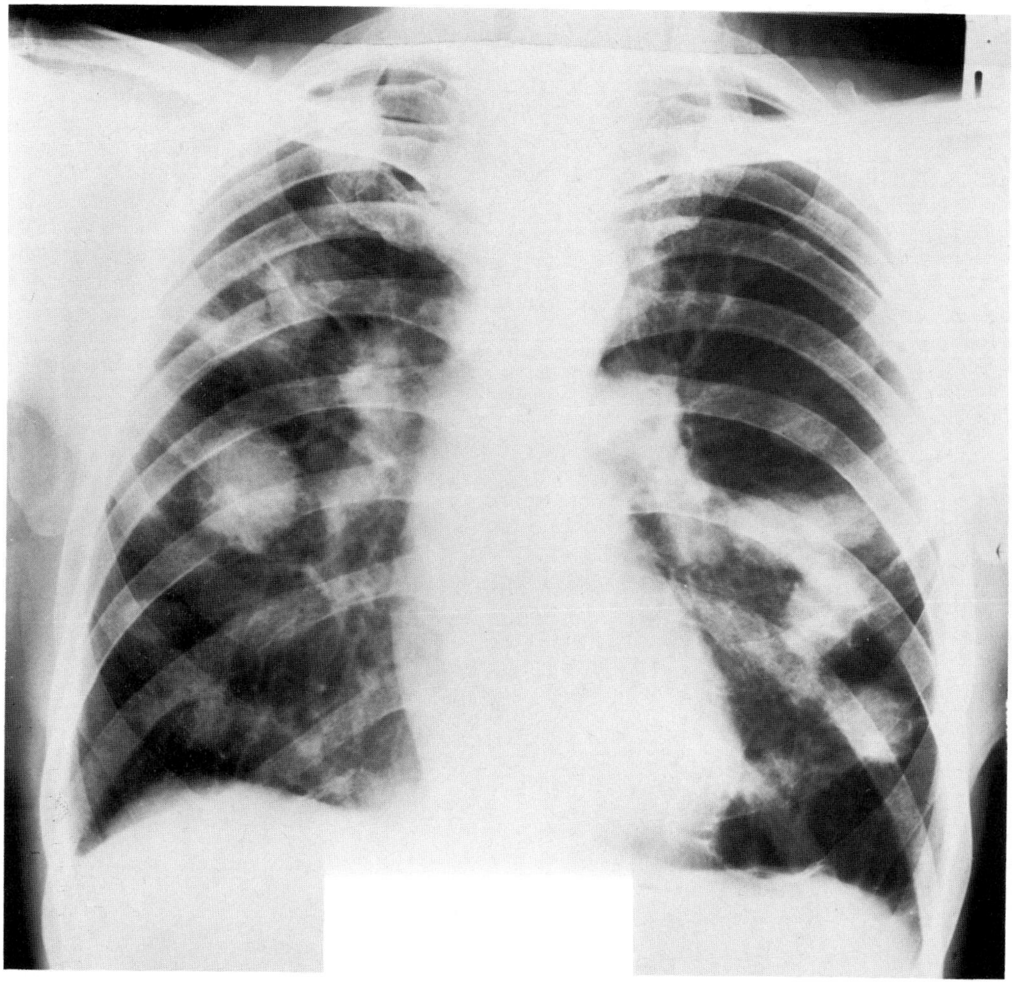

Figure 8.31 (d) 1970

*Figure 8.31 Typical appearances and development of 'classic' Caplan-type necrobiotic nodules (microscopically confirmed) in a coal-miner at the coal face for 20 years. Mild rheumatoid arthritis. A background of discrete ('simple') pneumoconiotic lesions is absent throughout. Note that most of the lesions in the right lung in 1958 are cavitary (*see Figure 8.14*) and that there is a curiously shaped large opacity in the left lower zone due to confluence of necrobiotic nodules which, in 1964, has disappeared. The disease presented with small haemoptyses and was initially diagnosed as multiple metastasis of carcinoma or tuberculomas. Cultures for* M. tuberculosis *consistently negative*

Rarely, widespread DIPF in coal-miners is confused with pneumoconiosis. However, the irregularity of the opacities and the frequent presence of a 'cystic' or 'honeycomb' pattern should prevent this mistake (*Figure 8.42*). In some of these cases, when the lungs are examined, the fibrosis is deeply pigmented with coal dust, in others it is dust-free (*see Figures 4.14* and *4.15*). In the former instance this suggests that the fibrosis developed during the period of dust exposure, and, in the latter, that it may have occurred after exposure had ceased. (*See* section on Diffuse Interstitial Pulmonary Fibrosis and Fibrosing 'Alveolitis', Chapter 4.)

A close resemblance between PMF opacities and those caused by other disease may sometimes give rise to difficulty or errors in diagnosis in either direction.

TUBERCULOSIS

Large fibrocaseous tuberculous lesions and PMF may be mistaken for each other especially in the presence of category 2 or 3 'simple' pneumoconiosis. In the former case the patient is unwell, his sputum usually yields tubercle bacilli, and antituberculous treatment causes complete or partial resolution of the radiographic appearances. In the latter case, the man is in good health even if complaining of some respiratory disability. PMF with ischaemic cavity formation is frequently mistaken for active tuberculous disease but there is a history of coughing up jet-black sputum from which tubercle bacilli cannot be isolated. When active tuberculosis and coal pneumoconiosis with PMF co-exist the extent of the pneumoconiosis can only be judged when antituberculous treatment has achieved maximal resolution of the tuberculosis.

Tuberculous bronchial 'abcesses' (Clegg, 1953)—now rare—cause fairly dense round radiographic opacities 1 to 2 cm in diameter which are identical in appearances to typical Caplan lesions but are usually few in number, and tubercle bacilli may be cultured from the sputum. Rheumatoid arthritis and circulating RF are absent.

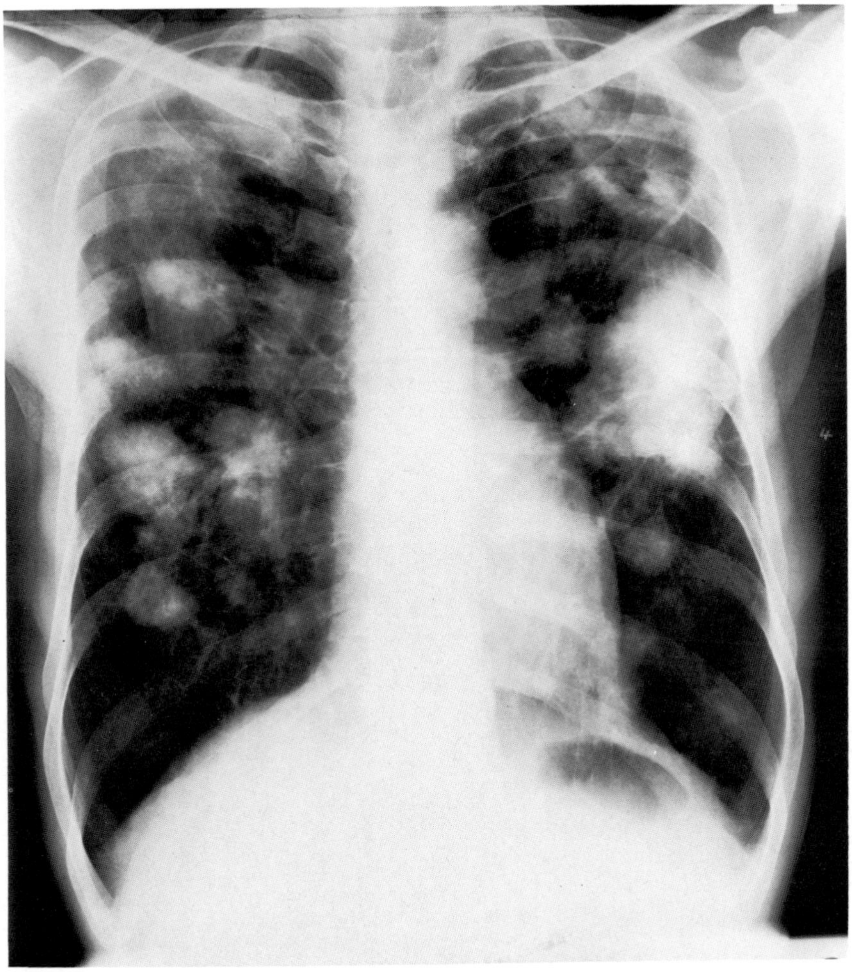

Figure 8.32(a)

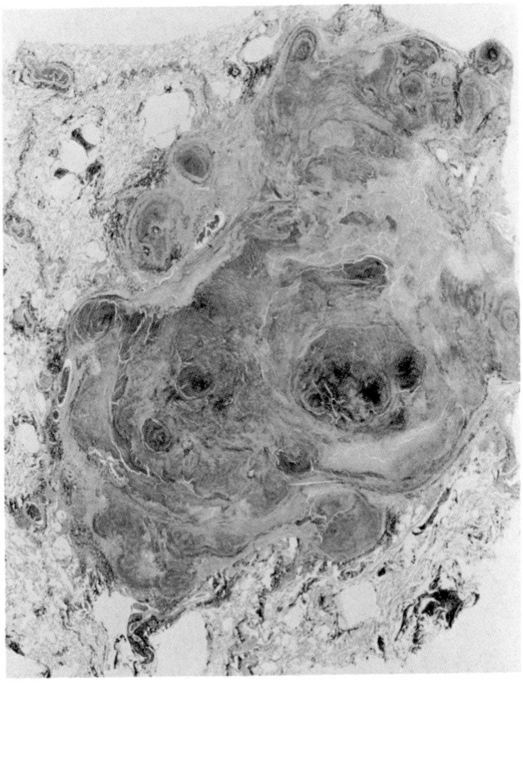

Figure 8.32(b)

Figure 8.32(c)

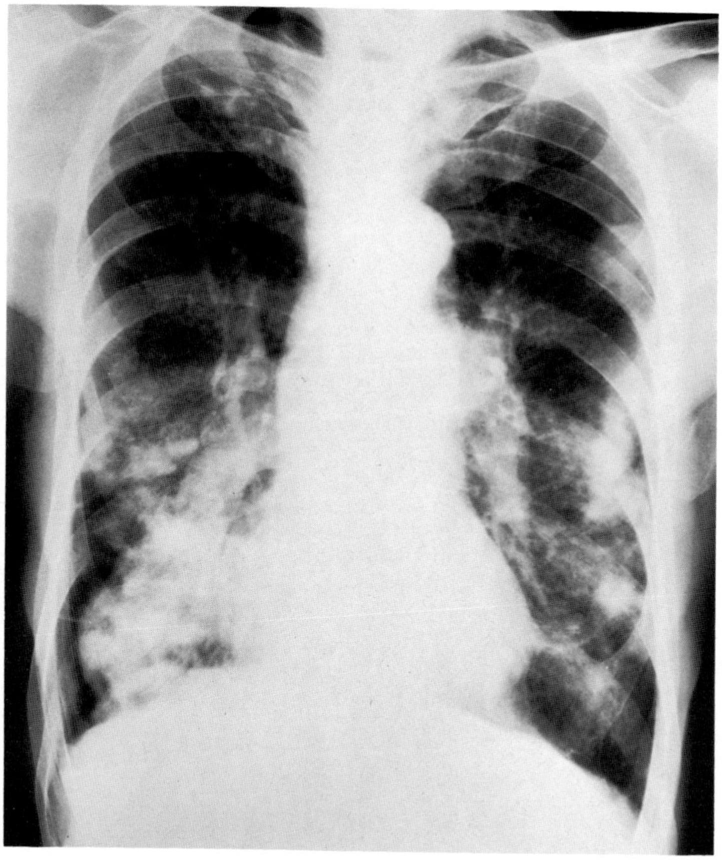

Figure 8.32 Two examples of multiple large opacities caused by rheumatoid coal pneumoconiosis. In both cases pulmonary metastasis was mistakenly diagnosed many years after the men had left the coal mines. (a) Note the cavitary lesion in the left upper zone. Severe rheumatoid arthritis, sputum consistently negative for M. tuberculosis. *Post mortem: discrete masses of matted nodules present in both lungs. (b) This section shows typical agglomeration of nodules—a common feature of rheumatoid pneumoconiosis—and, although the amount of coal dust accumulation is slight, a number of thin, 'tidal' circles, crescents and arcs of dust are clearly visible. Microscopical appearances characteristic and acid fast bacilli absent. (Magnification, approximately × 2. H and E stain). (c) The appearances in the right lower zone are unusual but post mortem the lesions were grossly and microscopically characteristic*

'RHEUMATOID' PNEUMOCONIOSIS

A diagnostic feature of many of these cases, if serial radiographs are available is the appearance of lesions within a few months and the equally rapid disappearance of some of them with or without evidence of cavity formation. In the absence of earlier films a history of past coal mining and the presence of rheumatoid arthritis or circulating rheumatoid factor should suggest the diagnosis. When, however, the lesions are few and contain cavities or are small and clustered they are particularly likely to be diagnosed as tuberculous even when no tubercle bacilli are cultured from the sputum; and, when they are small, scattered and apparently calcified they may be interpreted as calcified silicotic nodules or healed lesions of tuberculosis, histoplasmosis or pulmonary chicken pox. Lesions which are neither cavitary nor calcified may be mistaken for secondary tumour deposits (from carcinoma of the prostate and kidney especially), although tumour opacities usually have a more homogeneous appearance. Rare disorders which may simulate rheumatoid pneumoconiosis of mixed type in appearance and speed of development are nodular sarcoidosis, Wegener's granuloma and multiple nodular pulmonary amyloidosis (Lee and Johnson, 1975). The appearance of acute blastomycosis may imitate typical Caplan-type lesions fairly closely (*see* Chapter 11).

The usual absence of a 'background' of 'simple' pneumoconiosis is of limited value as an additional pointer to 'rheumatoid' pneumoconiosis because the latter is sometimes associated with ordinary PMF (*Figure 8.39*).

Sputum cultures are consistently negative for *M. tuberculosis,* and large haemoptysis is strongly against 'rheumatoid' pneumoconiosis. In many cases there is a family history of rheumatoid disease.

The pathological diagnosis is discussed on p. 190.

CARCINOMA OF LUNG

It is obviously important to distinguish between PMF and bronchial carcinoma radiographically and this is possible in most cases. But difficulty may arise when a patient is seen

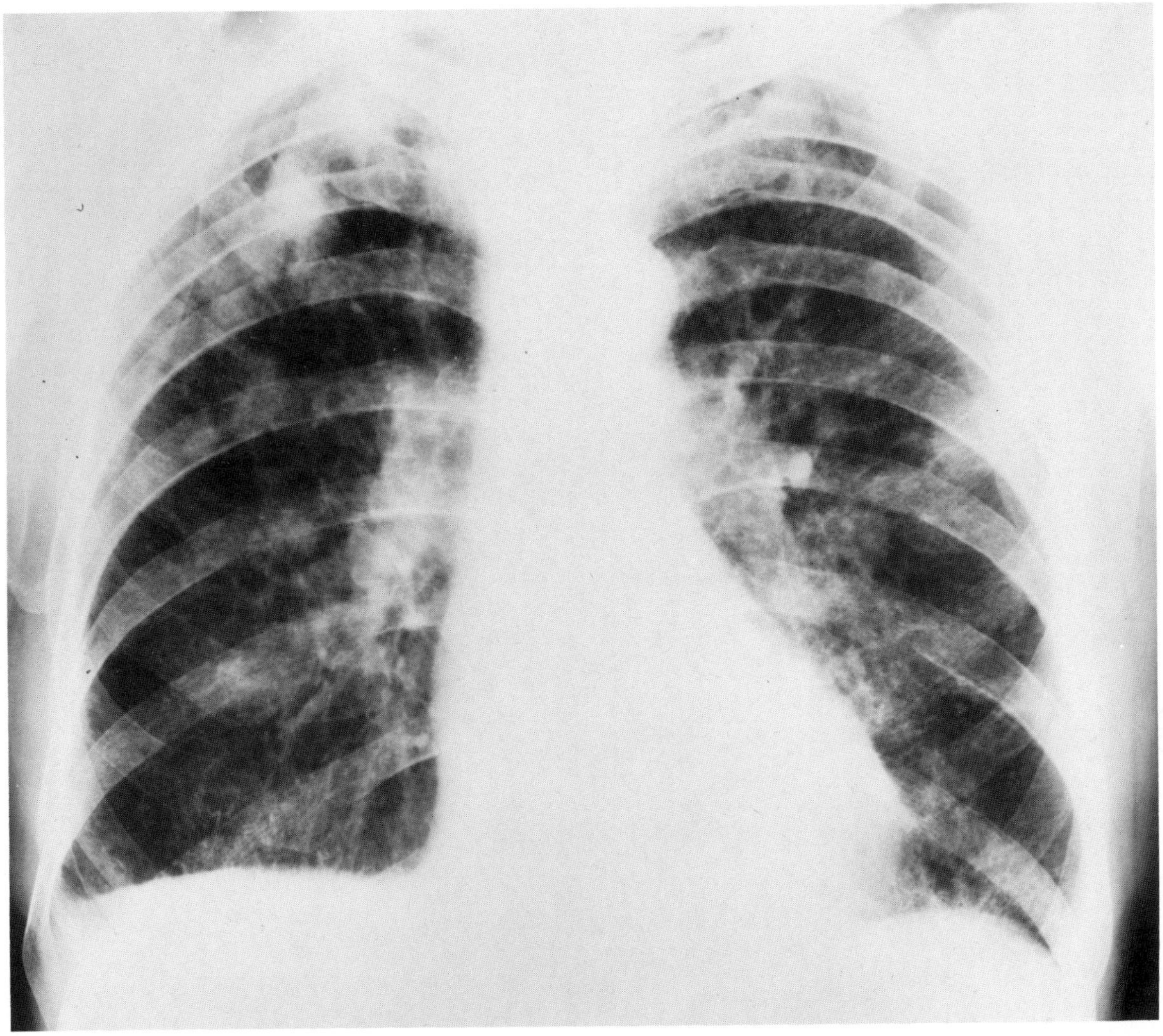

Figure 8.33 Appearances unlike those of the 'classic' Caplan syndrome. They developed simultaneously with the abrupt onset of rheumatoid arthritis and multiple large subcutaneous nodules at the age of 65 in a coal-miner 35 years underground. Irregular opacities which became evident three years later are also present in both lower zones. Circulating RF present in high titres. Cultures for M. tuberculosis *consistently negative. Post mortem: a few typical, Caplan-type necrobiotic nodules in the upper lobes and DIPF with small 'honeycomb' cysts in the lower lobes, both types of lesion confirmed microscopically*

for the first time or after the lapse of a number of years when the evolution of the opacities in question is not known (*Figure 8.43*). Features, referred to earlier, which may be helpful in distinguishing PMF are variable radiodensity of the opacities, linear markings at its periphery and evidence of calcification within the lesion (*Figures 8.25, 8.27* and *8.28*). However, spiculation or scalloping of the periphery of a mass may be seen both in PMF and peripheral carcinoma though the latter lacks the other features of PMF. Calcification is rare in carcinomas and almost never demonstrable during life, and, although it may be seen in benign adenomas and hamartomas it does not display the pattern illustrated in *Figures 8.27* and *8.28*. Tomography may clarify these features. A cavitary lesion may be difficult or impossible to differentiate but in the case of PMF there is usually a recent history of expectoration of jet-black sputum, often over a number of consecutive days (*Figure 8.26b*).

If earlier films are available they should *always* be obtained for comparison whenever there is uncertainty about the nature of the lesion. On the one hand, an opacity which is seen to appear and enlarge rapidly in a film series is most likely to represent carcinoma; whereas, on the other hand, one which results from the aggregation of earlier small opacities is probably due to PMF.

If a 'rheumatoid' pneumoconiosis lesion increases in size over a short period of time in a man with rheumatoid arthritis it may be mistaken for carcinoma with hypertrophic pulmonary osteoarthropathy if care is not taken to distinguish the two arthropathies. In the case of a single nodule of 'rheumatoid' pneumoconiosis it may be impossible to reach the diagnosis without thoracotomy and biopsy. Otherwise this method of investigation should rarely be necessary.

Bronchoscopy is not always helpful in differential diagnosis but bronchography, in cases of PMF, shows that

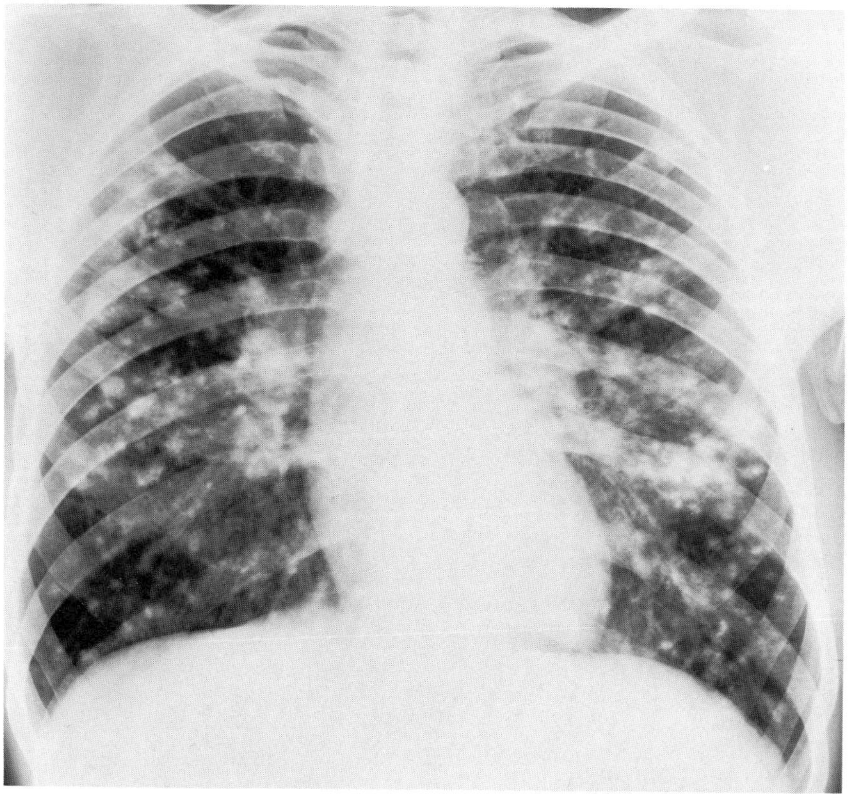

Figure 8.34 Rheumatoid coal pneumoconiosis with small and large ('mixed') opacities resembling silicosis. Calcification of some lesions apparent five years after development of rheumatoid arthritis. DAT titres consistently high (1:256 or more). Coal-miner for 45 years. Family history of rheumatoid arthritis

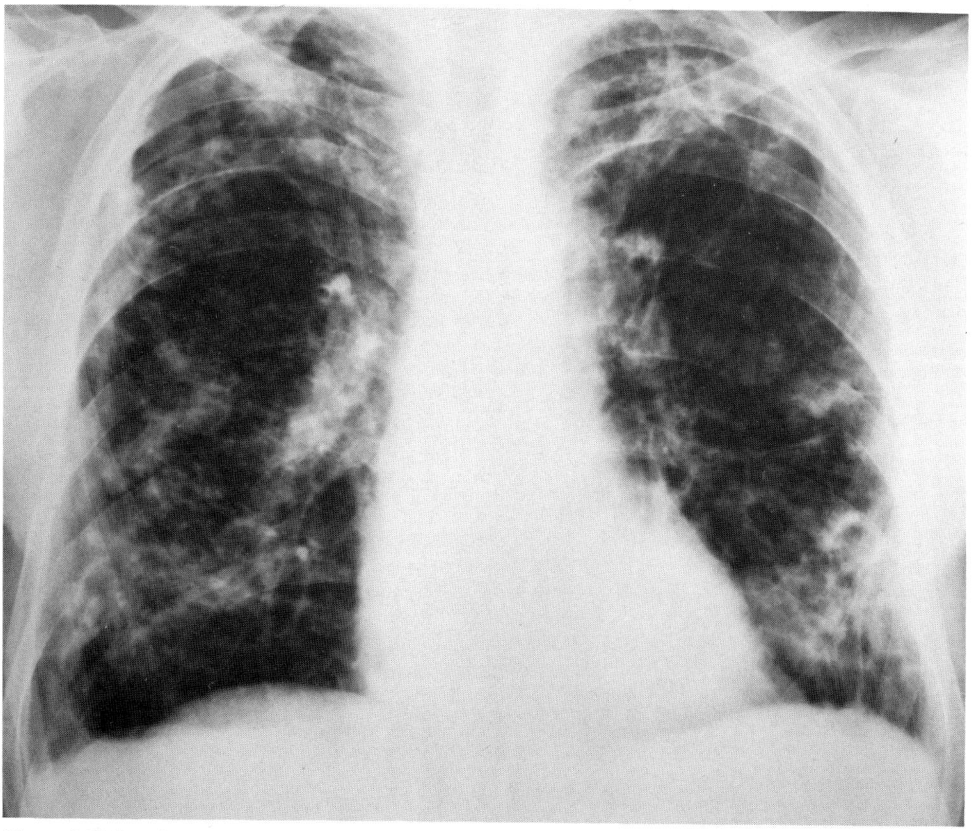

Figure 8.35 Peripheral 'mixed' type of rheumatoid pneumoconiosis in a man exposed to coal and graphite dust. Cavities are present in some lesions and there is some pleural thickening. Severe rheumatoid arthritis with numerous subcutaneous nodules. DAT titres 1:64 or higher, ANAs absent. Post mortem: moderate diffuse thickening of pulmonary pleura and many typical Caplan necrobiotic nodules, some containing cavities, within 2 to 3 cm of the pleura; rheumatoid vasculitis widespread in the lungs and elsewhere. No evidence of tuberculosis

(a) (b)

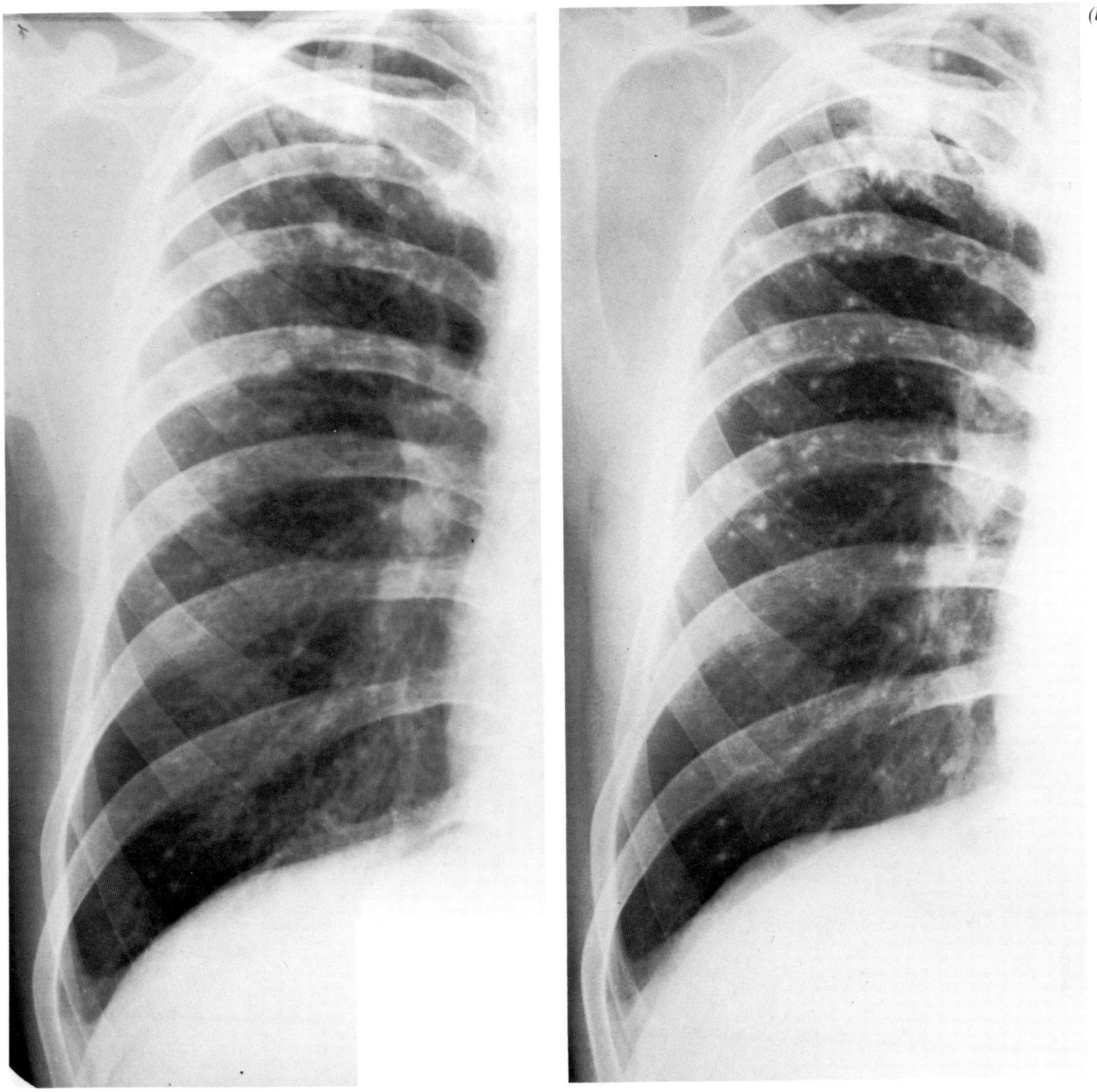

Figure 8.36(a) and (b) Small round lesions of rheumatoid coal pneumoconiosis many of which have subsequently calcified. Time between films (a) and (b) is 15 years. Coal-miner for 15 years. Moderately severe rheumatoid arthritis; DAT 1:256. Sputum cultures for M. tuberculosis, *negative*

bronchi adjacent to the mass, though distorted and displaced, are not occluded; whereas in peripheral carcinoma of the lung they are often abruptly occluded or gradually narrowed to the point of disappearance ('rat tail'sign) (Goldman, 1965a).

Occasionally metastatic tumours in the lungs may simulate PMF very closely but the opacities are usually sharply circumscribed and of uniform density (*Figure 8.44*).

EXOGENOUS LIPOID PNEUMONIA

An uncommon simulator of both 'simple' pneumoconiosis and PMF. It is discussed in more detail in Chapter 11 (pp. 395–398), but an example, due probably to aspiration of medicinal liquid paraffin and misinterpreted as PMF, is shown in *Figure 8.45* (cf. *Figure 8.23a*).

PROGNOSIS AND COMPLICATIONS

The influence of the radiographic category of 'simple' pneumoconiosis on the development of PMF, and the effect of PMF on life expectancy are discussed in the section on Epidemiology. On occasion PMF may, after many years of apparent inactivity, progress to considerable size in the

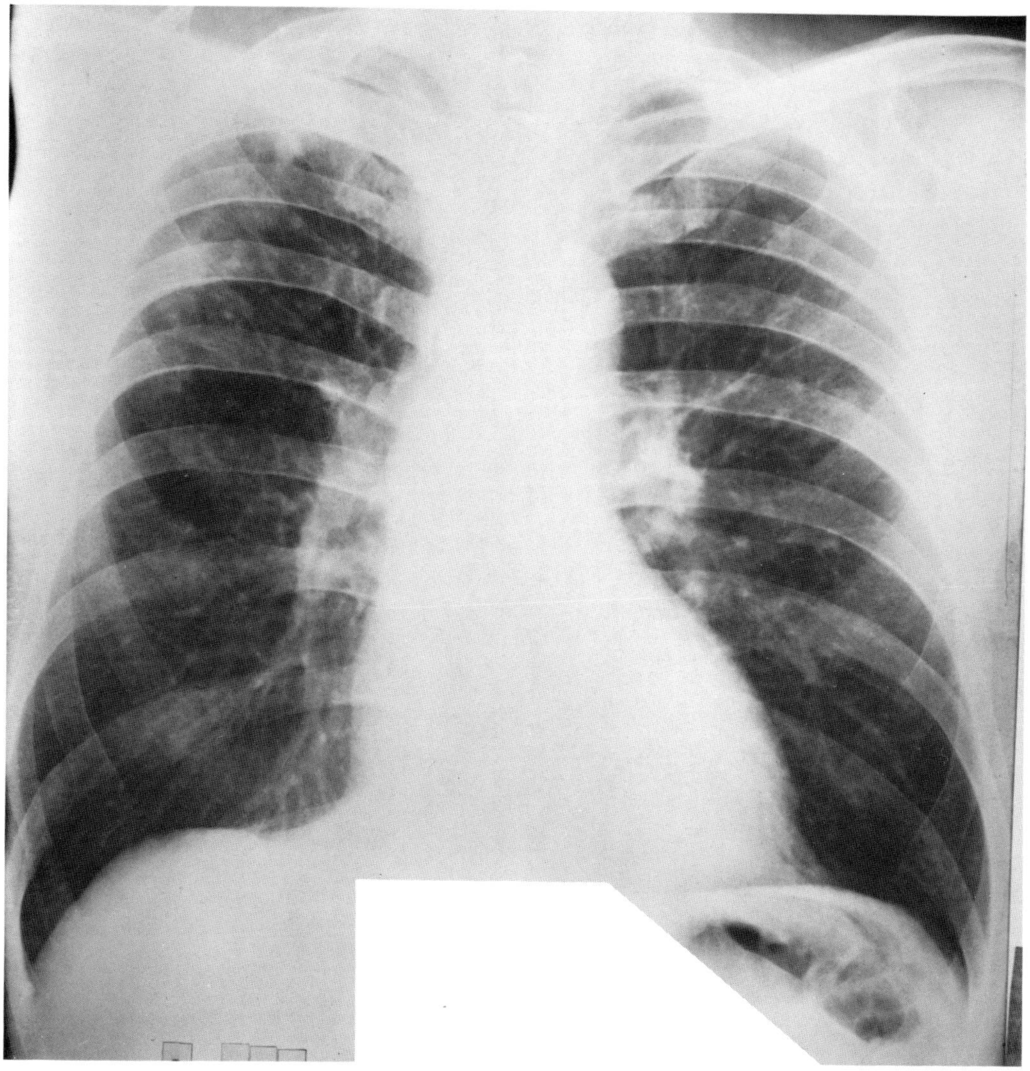

Figure 8.37 (a) 1970

elderly due, possibly, to immunological activity. Prognosis is not worsened by the presence of ischaemic cavities unless they are infected by pathogenic 'opportunist' mycobacteria (*see later*). In view of the apparent association of a mild reduction of Tl or of the presence of emphysema in some category p cases, in comparison with category q and r cases (*see* p. 196), it is important to note that the mortality rate in Welsh miners and ex-miners with punctiform opacities is, if anything, lower than in those with other categories of pneumoconiosis (Waters, Cochrane and Moore, 1974).

PULMONARY HEART DISEASE

Pulmonary heart disease is not caused by 'simple' pneumoconiosis and it occurs in only a small proportion of PMF cases, but is likely to do so when the masses are large, central and bilateral; or when there is concomitant severe chronic airflow obstruction or bronchopneumonia.

TUBERCULOSIS AND OTHER INFECTIONS

If tuberculosis develops in the presence of PMF, permanent decline in ventilatory capacity may occur in some cases in spite of effective antituberculous treatment. Antituberculous treatment has been reported to be less effective in men with coal pneumoconiosis than in men with tuberculosis only (Medical Research Council/Miner's Chest Diseases Treatment Centre, 1963), but there is reason to believe that this was due to irregularity of treatment (Annotation, 1967), and at least one other study has shown satisfactory results (Ramsey and Pines, 1963). More recent experience confirms this.

Opportunist mycobacteria are apt to establish themselves in lungs with PMF especially if there is an ischaemic cavity (Marks, 1970). This is discussed in Chapter 4, p. 72. In addition to the organisms referred to there *M. peregrinum* has also been recorded (Ball *et al.*, 1969).

Infestation of ischaemic cavities by the *Aspergillus* sp. may sometimes occur, the circumstances and clinical

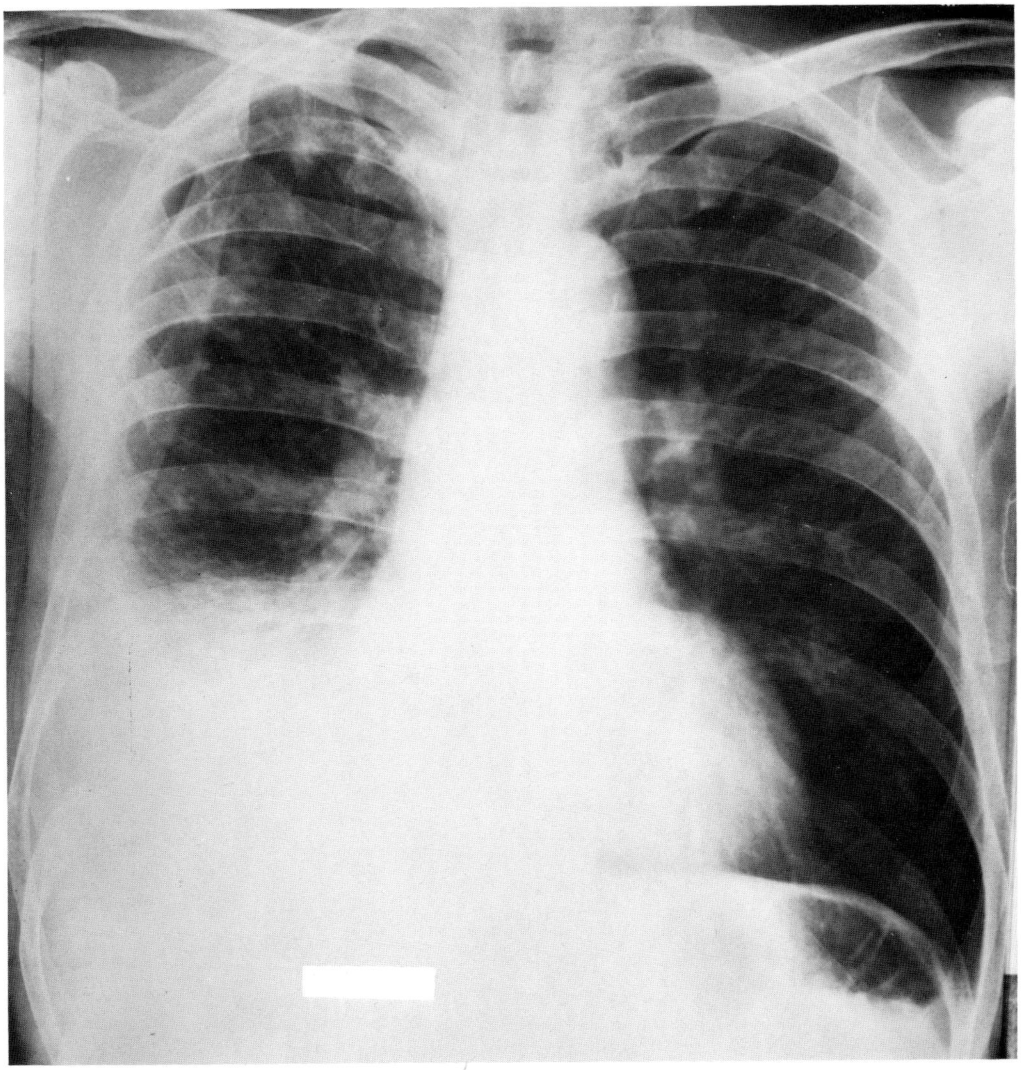

Figure 8.37 (b) 1971

features of which are identical to those described in Chapter 7, p. 153 (*Figure 8.46*).

'RHEUMATOID' PNEUMOCONIOSIS

As described already this behaves erratically and may progress suddenly in a short time but it rarely threatens life and only occasionally causes significant respiratory disability. However, the highly exceptional case in which the course of the disease is acute and the patient seriously ill may end fatally within two to three years. The occasional development of pleural effusion (which may be recurrent) is generally due to the rheumatoid process though other causes, especially neoplasia, must be excluded. 'Rheumatoid' effusions often have an unusually low glucose content. Rupture of a peripheral nodule through the pulmonary pleura may also result in spontaneous pneumothorax, hydro-pneumothorax, pyo-pneumothorax or, occasionally, bronchopleural fistula.

CHRONIC BRONCHITIS

This topic is discussed in Chapter 1 (pp. 17–22).

CARCINOMA OF THE LUNG

There is no evidence of a causal relationship between coal pneumoconiosis and carcinoma of the lung (Rooke *et al.*, 1979). The death rate due to this tumour is lower in British and American coal-miners than in non-miners of comparable age (Costello, Ortmeyer and Morgan, 1974; Kennaway and Kennaway, 1947; Goldman, 1965b; Liddell, 1973; Registrar General, 1958); and there is a lower post-mortem incidence of the growth in Welsh miners with pneumoconiosis than in age-matched non-miners from the same area (James, 1955). Furthermore, the survival time of men with this tumour is longer in those with category 2 or 3 'simple' pneumoconiosis than in those with category 0 (Goldman, 1965c). This lower rate of lung cancer, which is

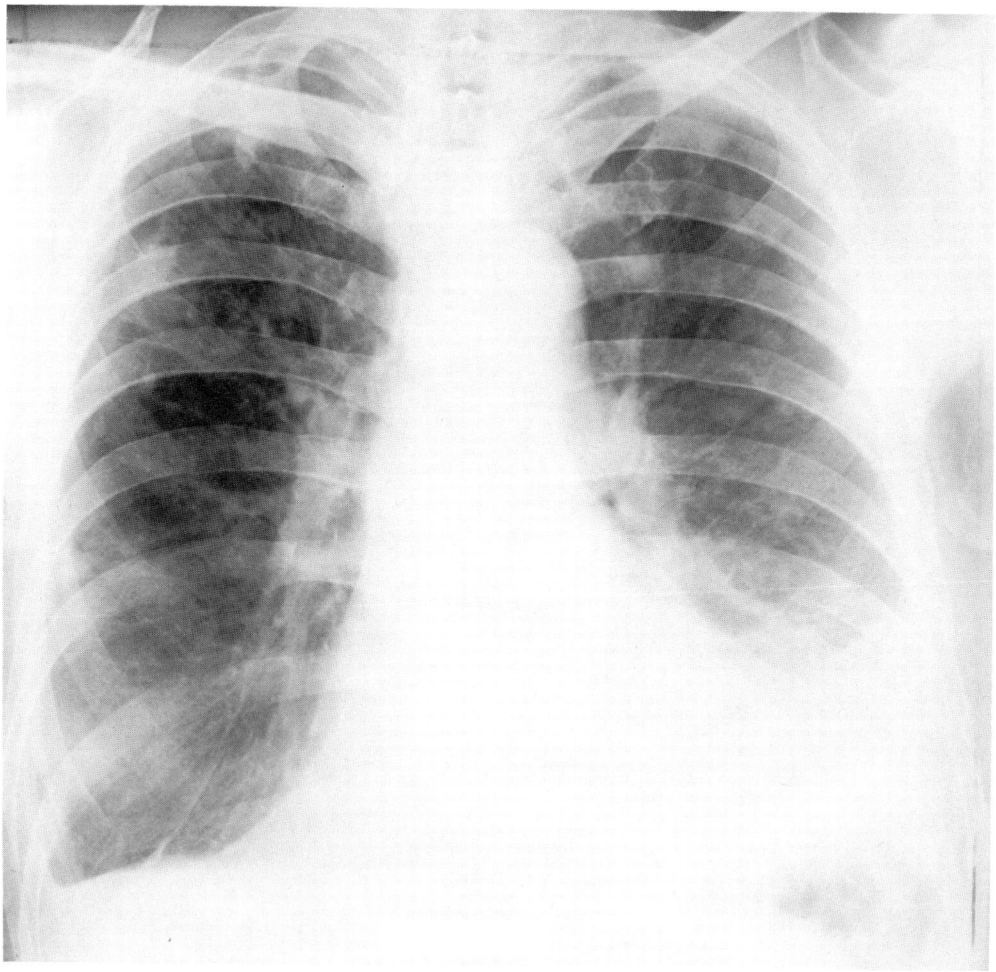

Figure 8.37 (c) 1972

Figure 8.37 Scanty, small opacities of rheumatoid coal pneumoconiosis in upper zones of both lungs and recurrent transient pleural effusions. (a) 1970; (b) 1971; (c) 1972. Moderately severe rheumatoid arthritis of rapid development in 1970 at age of 59; DAT onsistently positive (range 1:16 to 1:1024); ANA positive. No evidence of tuberculosis or cause of pleural effusion other than rheumatoid disease. Post mortem: moderate thickening of pulmonary pleura; a few dust macules and small coal pneumoconiosis nodules (2 mm diameter) and several subpleural, Caplan necrobiotic nodules up to 1 cm diameter in both lungs (confirmed microscopically). Coal-miner 26 years

not adequately explained by differences in smoking habits as miners—in Britain at any rate—do not appear to smoke less than non-miners (Jacobsen, 1977; Rooke *et al.*, 1978), seems to be a specific effect of occupation. However, an apparent excess of lung cancer has been reported in coal-miners with pneumoconiosis compared with non-miners in the Wyoming Valley of Pennsylvania which might be related to a higher than normal background of ionizing radiation from black shales associated with the coal measures in this region due to local uranium deposits (Myers, 1967; Scarano, Fadali and Lemole, 1972). It should be noted that in Myers' report miners and non-miners were not matched for age or smoking habits and, in that of Scarano *et al.*, only the ages of the cancer patients were recorded and not those of all the miners and non-miners in the survey. The question of ionizing radiation in coal and other mines is discussed in Chapter 14.

ISCHAEMIC HEART DISEASE

Higgins *et al.* (1969) found no difference in prevalence of chest pain and electrocardiographic abnormalities between miners, ex-miners and non-miners in an American mining community. The standard mortality ratio of working miners for ischaemic heart disease in Britain and the USA is lower than that of the general population except for maintenance workers in whom it is slightly increased; and in non-working miners it is similar to that of the general population (Costello, Ortmeyer, and Morgan, 1975; Higgins *et al.*, 1969; Liddell, 1973).

It is occasionally postulated that chronic hypoxaemia associated with some cases of advanced PMF—as with many other types of advanced lung disease—predisposes to myocardial infarction. But all the evidence is against this. The incidence of myocardial infarction and the death rate

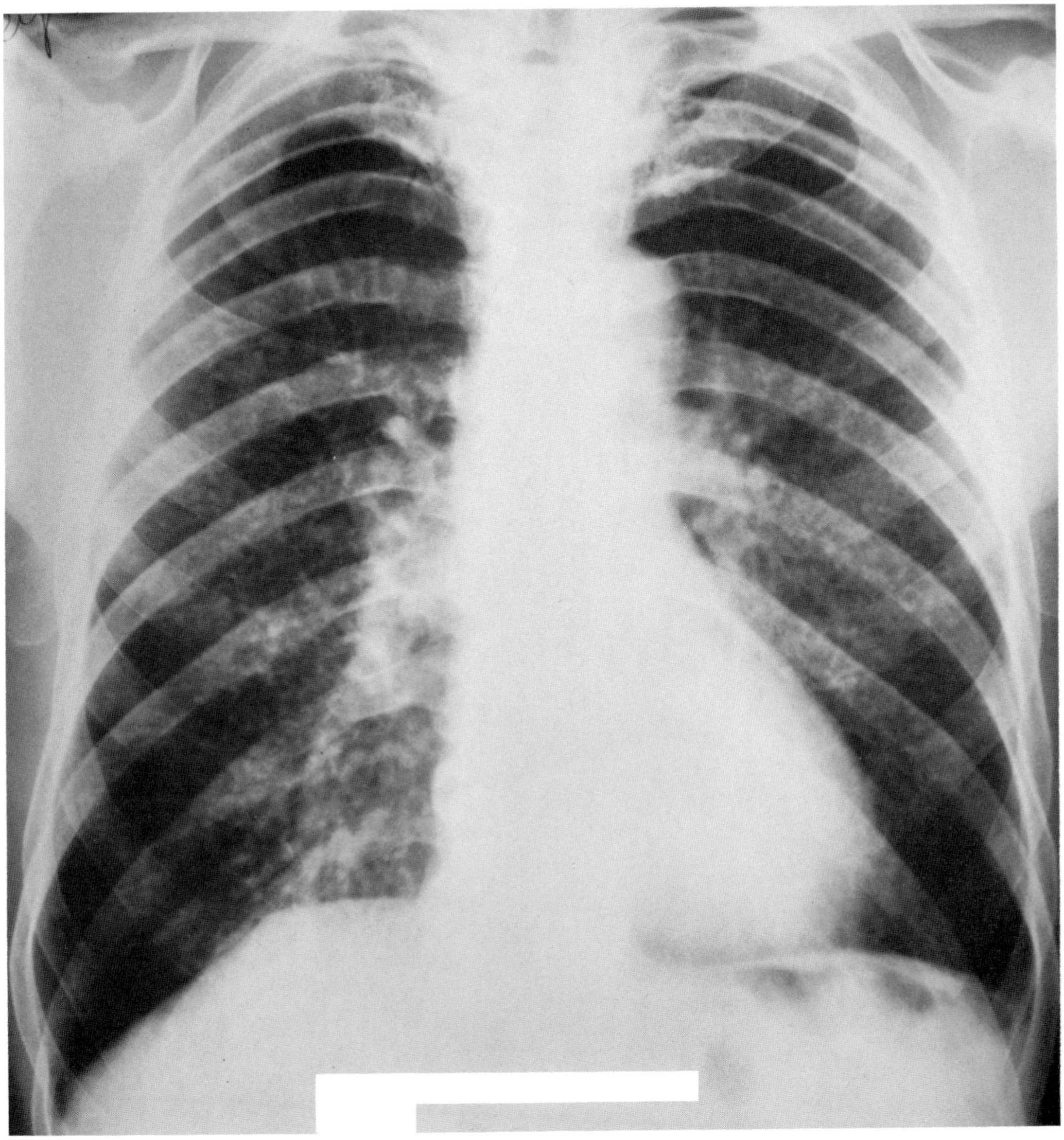

Figure 8.38 (a) 1967

from ischaemic heart disease are, in fact, lower than average in PMF and chronic respiratory insufficiency (Lindars *et al.*, 1972; Mitchell, Walker and Maisel, 1968; Nonkin *et al.*, 1964; Samad and Noehren, 1965; Sanders, 1970; Cochrane *et al.*, 1979). Chronic hypoxaemia appears rather to exert a protective than a precipitating effect. It causes dilatation and increased interarterial anastomoses of the coronary arteries (Keele and Neil, 1971; Zoll, Wessler and Schesingler, 1951) and coronary artery blood flow is not reduced in patients with emphysema and cor pulmonale (Rose and Hoffman, 1956). On the contrary, vascularization of the myocardium is greatly increased down to capillary level in people living in chronic hypoxia at high altitudes compared with those at sea level (Heath and Williams, 1981); and a significant serial decline in mortality from ischaemic heart disease, which is not due to racial differences, has been observed in men residing at increasingly high altitudes (Mortimer, Monson and MacMahon, 1977). Furthermore, the risk of severe cardiac arrhythmia is not, apparently, increased by chronic hypoxia (Parkes, Phillips and Williamson, 1976).

It can reasonably be concluded, therefore, that neither coal pneumoconiosis nor any other fibrotic occupational lung disease increase the likelihood of myocardial infarction or of sudden death due to its effects.

SCLERODERMA

Although scleroderma is reported to occur with unusual frequency in coal-miners as well as in men with silicosis (Rodnan *et al.*, 1967) (*see* Chapter 7, p. 157) there is no obvious association with radiographic evidence of pneumoconiosis. No cases appear to have been identified in

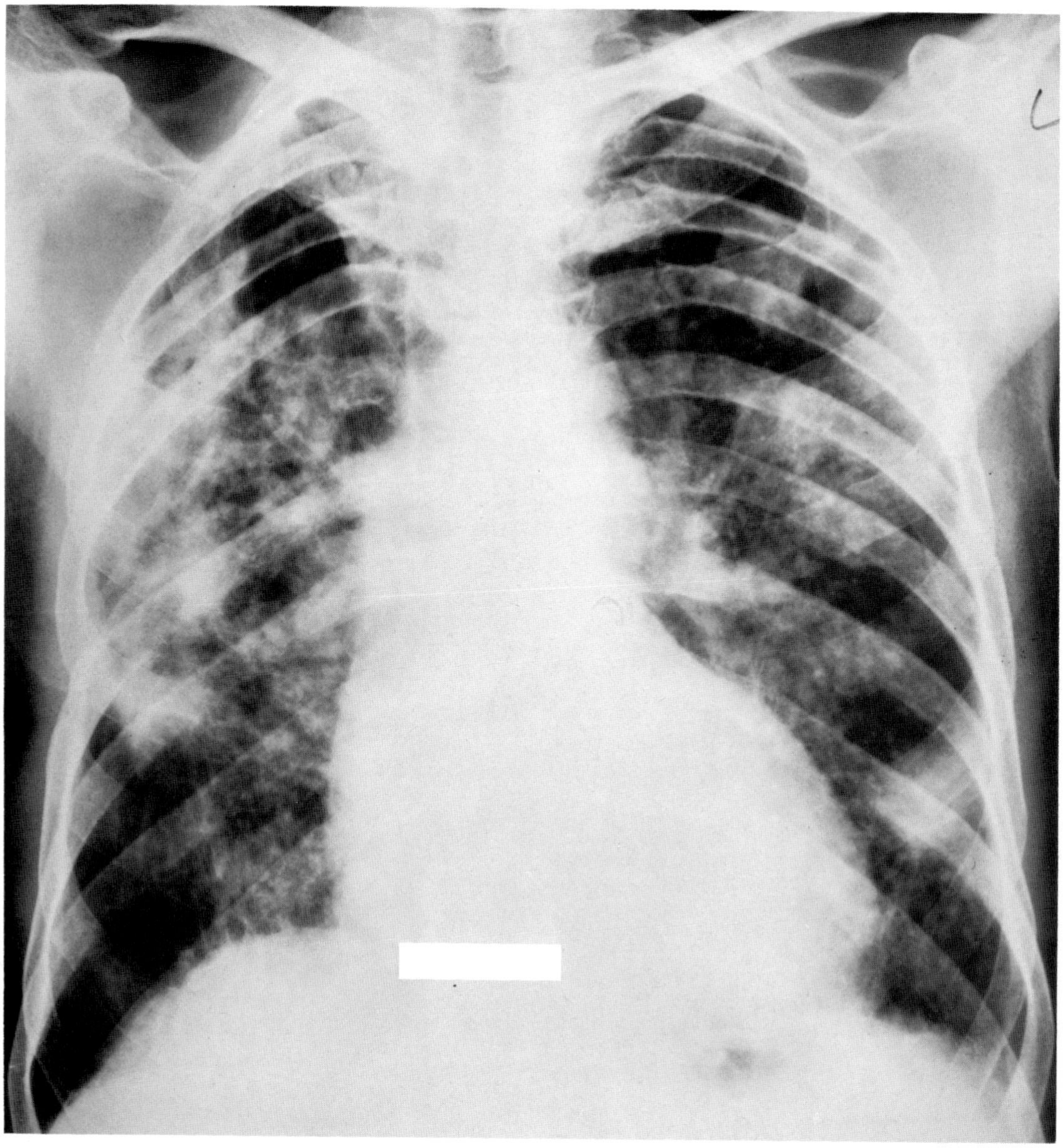

Figure 8.38 (b) 1972

British coal-miners (Rogan, 1960), and this has been my own experience.

MISCELLANEOUS

PMF is not a cause of fatal haemoptysis but intermittent blood streaking of sputum may occur from time to time. Copious jet-black sputum due to rupture of the contents of a cavitary PMF into an airway, though alarming, is usually harmless, and permanent aspiration sequelae do not appear to have been reported.

Proximal retrograde spread of a pulmonary artery thrombus adjacent to a PMF lesion (*see* p. 186) may occasionally lead to embolism and consequent pulmonary infarction, but this is rarely fatal.

Other complications, remarkable for their rarity, are spontaneous pneumothorax (which is often partial) and permanent dysphonia due to paralysis of the left recurrent laryngeal nerve from involvement by PMF in the upper part of the left lung near the hilum.

Finally, it should be emphasized that life expectancy in PMF cases today is much better than is commonly supposed and is normal in the majority.

The question as to whether oxides of nitrogen from shot firing, and other sources, in coal mines has any permanent effect on miner's lungs is discussed in Chapter 13.

TREATMENT

No treatment affects the pneumoconiosis, but treatment is required for chronic obstructive bronchitis, cor pulmonale

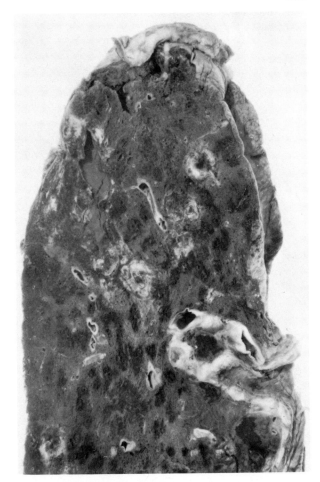

Figure 8.38 (c)

Figure 8.38 (a) Category 2q discrete ('simple') pneumoconiosis established about 12 years in a graphite worker of 24 years with subsequent fairly rapid development of bilateral rounded and irregular opacities (b) which distantly resemble 'classic' Caplan syndrome appearances. Absence of right 6th rib due to thoracotomy for wrongly suspected carcinoma. Biopsy: necrobiotic nodules with prominent palisading of fibroblasts but no tumour. Recurrent joint pains but no clinical arthropathy. Post mortem two years later: multiple black nodules of non-rheumatoid pneumoconiosis (up to 4 mm diameter) with several typical Caplan-type necrobiotic nodules up to 2 cm diameter (some with cavities) in both lungs. (c) Slice of unperfused left lung shows these features (main bronchus and pulmonary artery on the right). Microscopy: typical appearances of rheumatoid pneumoconiosis; numerous graphite bodies; no evidence of growth or tuberculosis

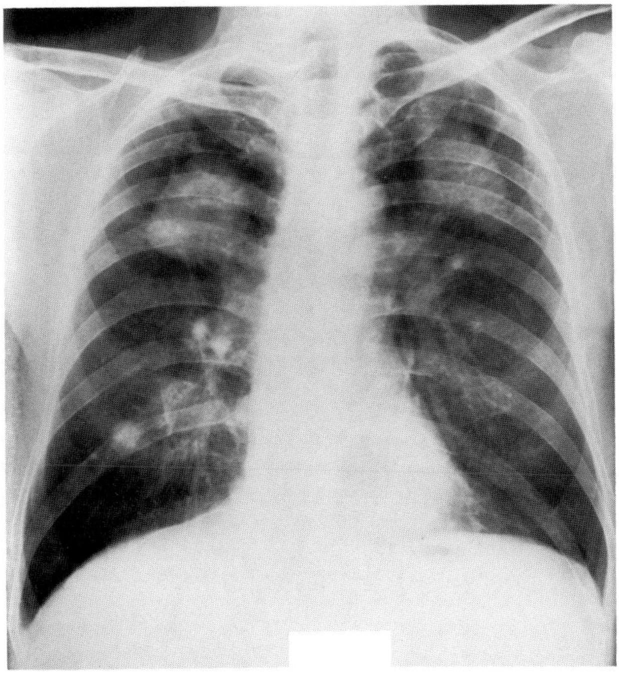

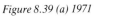

Figure 8.39 (a) 1971

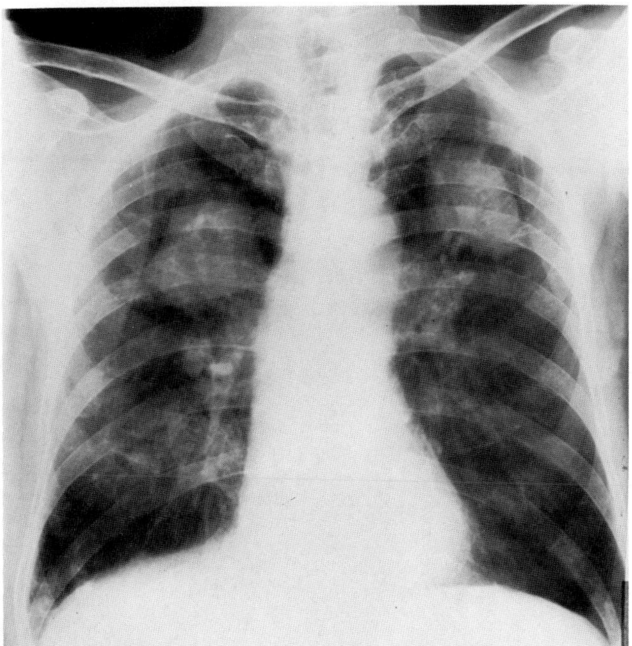

Figure 8.39 (b) March, 1977

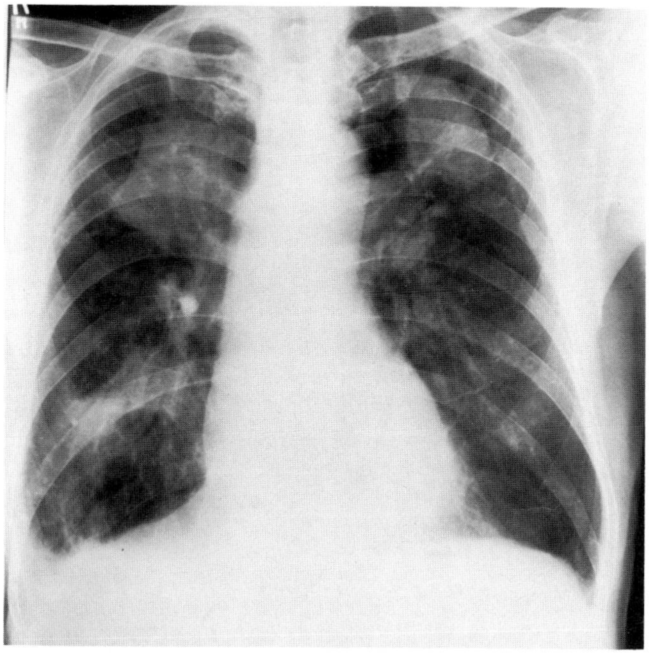

Figure 8.39 (c) November, 1977

Figure 8.39 (a) Bilateral 'conventional' PMF present for years when small right middle and lower zone opacities appeared in 1968; neoplasm suspected (1971). (b) Appearances unchanged for about six years after which the lesions have virtually disappeared (March, 1977). (c) Reappearance of lower zone lesion, now increased in size, and right basal pleural effusion (November, 1977). Rheumatoid arthritis developed suddenly in 1973. Latex test, positive 4 plus; DAT 1:1024. Post mortem: rheumatoid necrobiotic nodules confined to right lower lobe; no evidence of neoplasm or tuberculosis. Microscopical confirmation. Coal-miner for 29 years

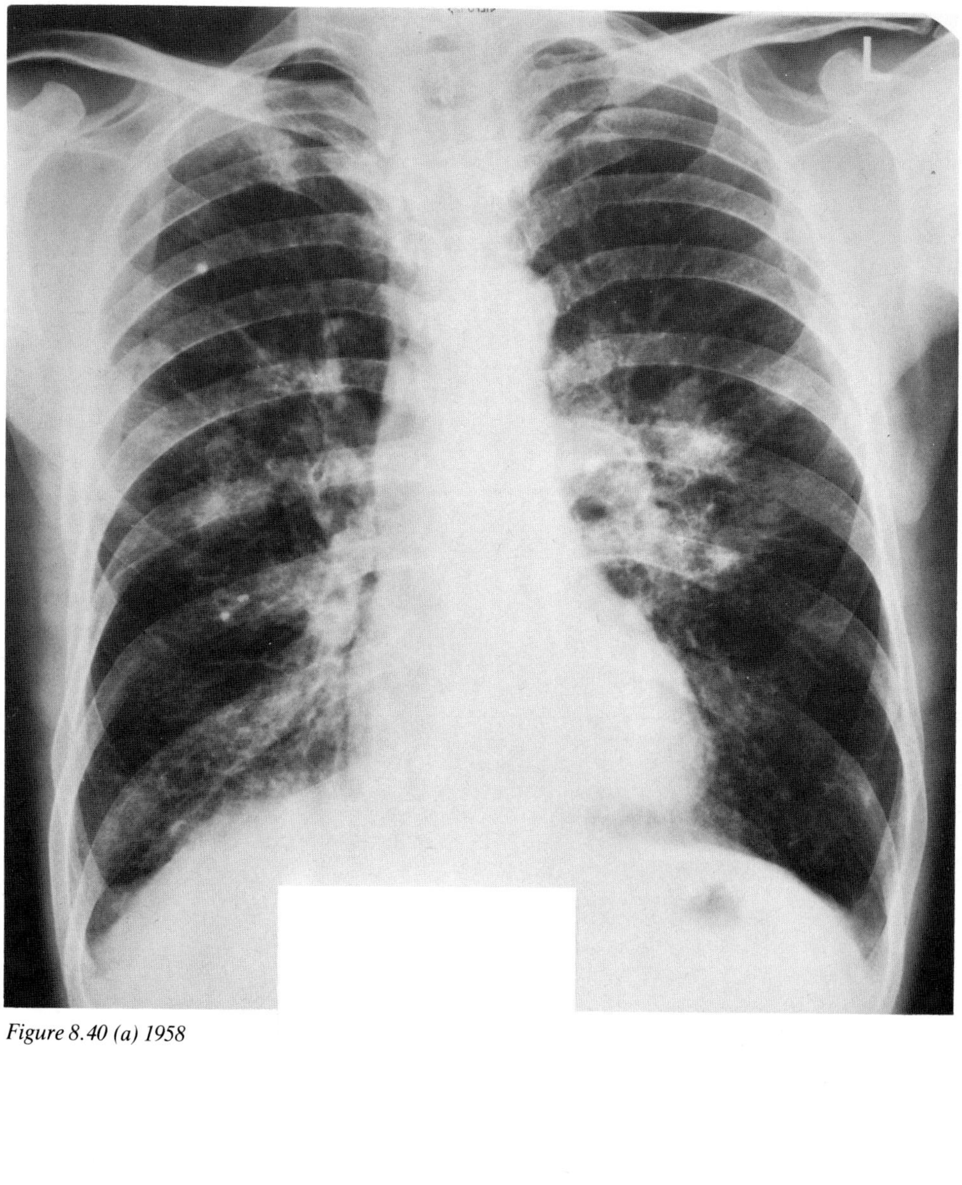

Figure 8.40 (a) 1958

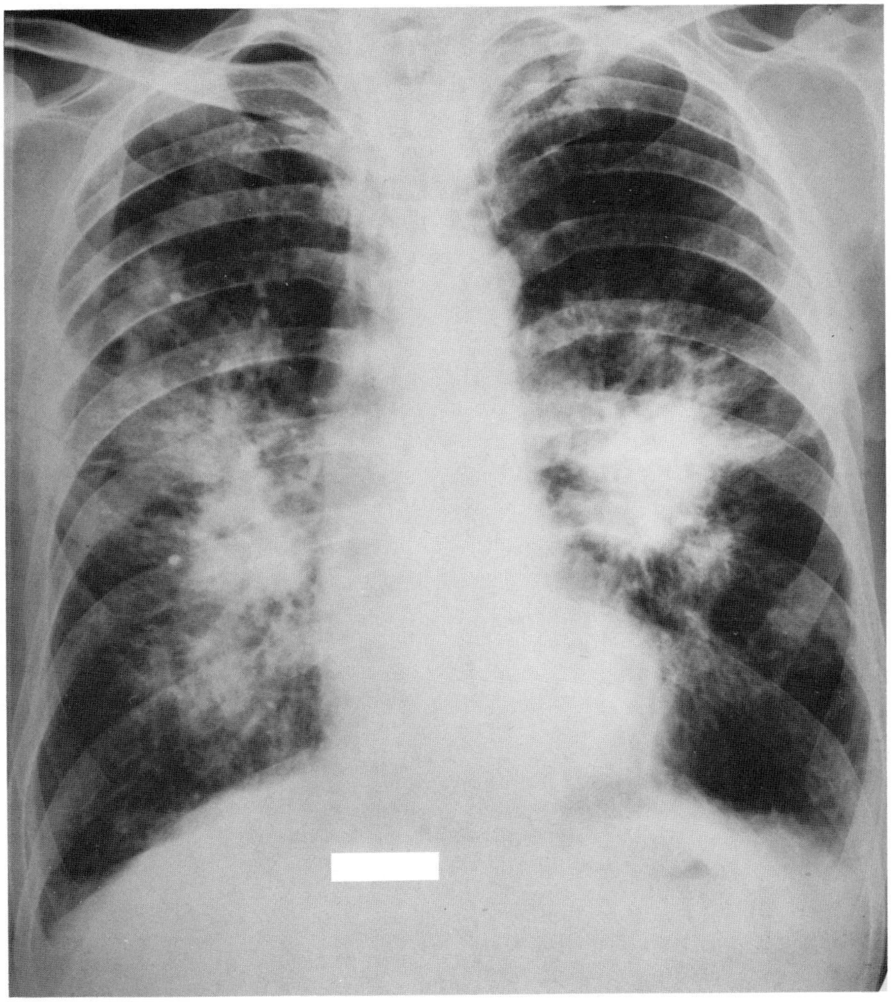

Figure 8.40(b) January, 1960

or tuberculosis. In cases where sudden expectoration of large amounts of black sputum has occurred from excavated PMF, reassurance and mild sedation is indicated. Reassurance is also necessary when haemoptysis occurs in cases of 'rheumatoid' pneumoconiosis or ordinary PMF—provided that other causes have been confidently excluded.

Complicating tuberculosis is treated as outlined in Chapter 7. Although the results are as good as those in the general population in most PMF cases, there are occasional exceptions in which recurrent relapse occurs due, possibly, to partial incarceration of the tuberculous process in a PMF lesion.

In the event of infection by opportunist mycobacteria the organism must be carefully typed and tested against as many drugs as possible before treatment is started. Photochromogenic organisms often respond well to a regime of standard doses of drugs used in the treatment of tuberculosis. The non-chromogen, *M. avium,* responds poorly to treatment with any drug.

There is no evidence that 'rheumatoid' pneumoconiosis is influenced in any way by corticosteroids but they should be tried in the rare case of fulminant progressive disease. Neither, apparently, does penicillamine have any effect.

Respiratory infections in patients with advanced PMF must always be treated promptly and adequately in order to prevent the development or worsening of congestive heart failure.

PREVENTION

In the UK this rests on three principles:

(1) 'Permitted' dust levels.
(2) Control of dust production and regular dust measurements.
(3) Medical supervision.

'PERMITTED' DUST LEVELS

These were introduced by the National Coal Board (NCB) as 'approved dust conditions' in 1949 and were originally based on concentrations of 'respirable dust' measured in terms of the *number* of compact particles 1 to 5 $\mu m/mm^3$. Since 1969, however, dust levels have been determined in

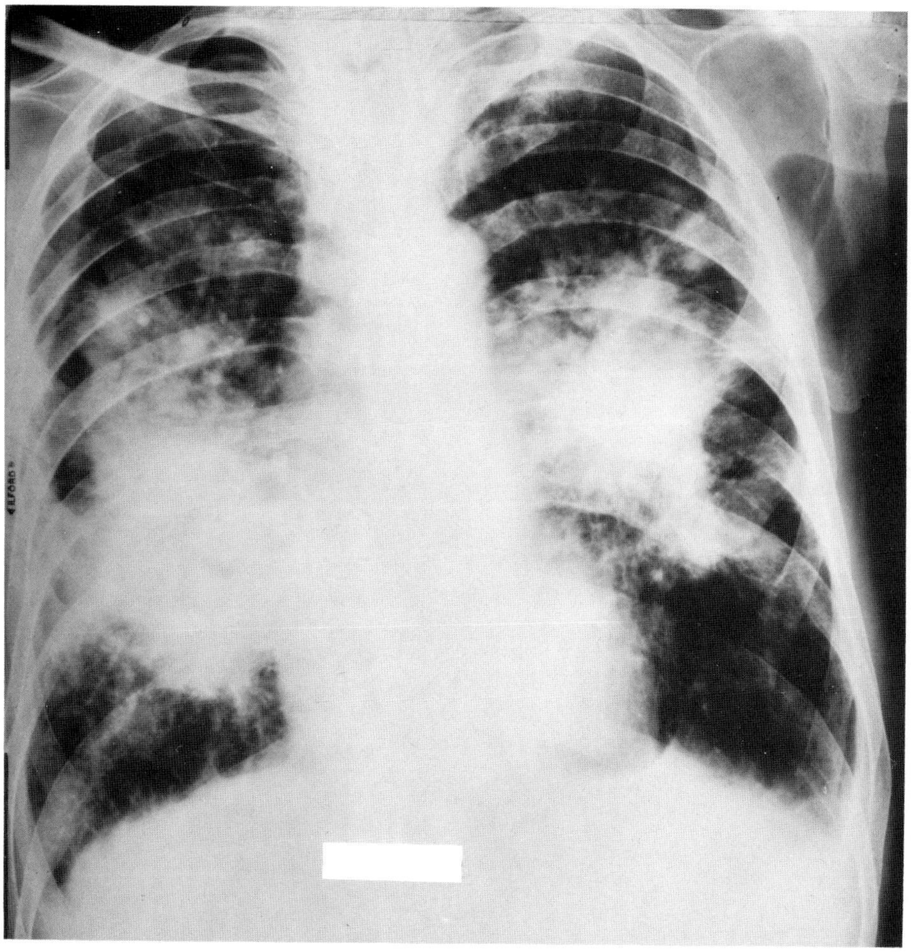

Figure 8.40 (c) November, 1960

Figure 8.40 Dramatically fast development of rheumatoid coal pneumoconiosis with radiographic features atypical of this syndrome. Coal-miner aged 60, 40 years underground (a) 1958. Abrupt onset of severe polyarthropathy at this time. DAT 1:1024. (b) January, 1960. Crippled by arthritis. (c) November, 1960. Advanced bilateral lung disease. Post mortem: large, grey-black masses with necrotic cavities in both lungs. Microscopically, typical rheumatoid nodules in these lesions

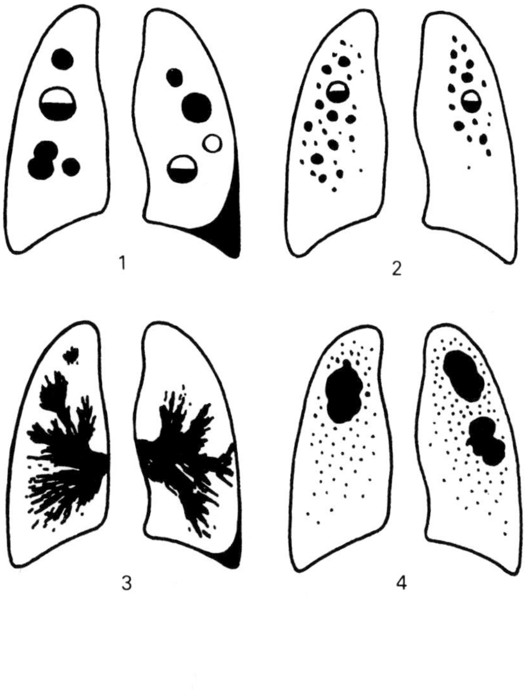

Figure 8.41 Possible relationships of the relative intensities of dust exposure and immunological activity to the range of radiographic appearances in coal pneumoconiosis. (1) Low dust, high immunoactivity. 'Classic' Caplan necrobiotic nodules. (2) Intermediate dust, intermediate immunoactivity. Mixed small and large round lesions of rheumatoid pneumoconiosis, and uniform, small round opacities. (3) High dust, high immunoactivity. 'Acute' rheumatoid pneumoconiosis, (rare). (4) High dust, absent or low immunity. Ordinary ('conventional') PMF and 'simple' pneumoconiosis

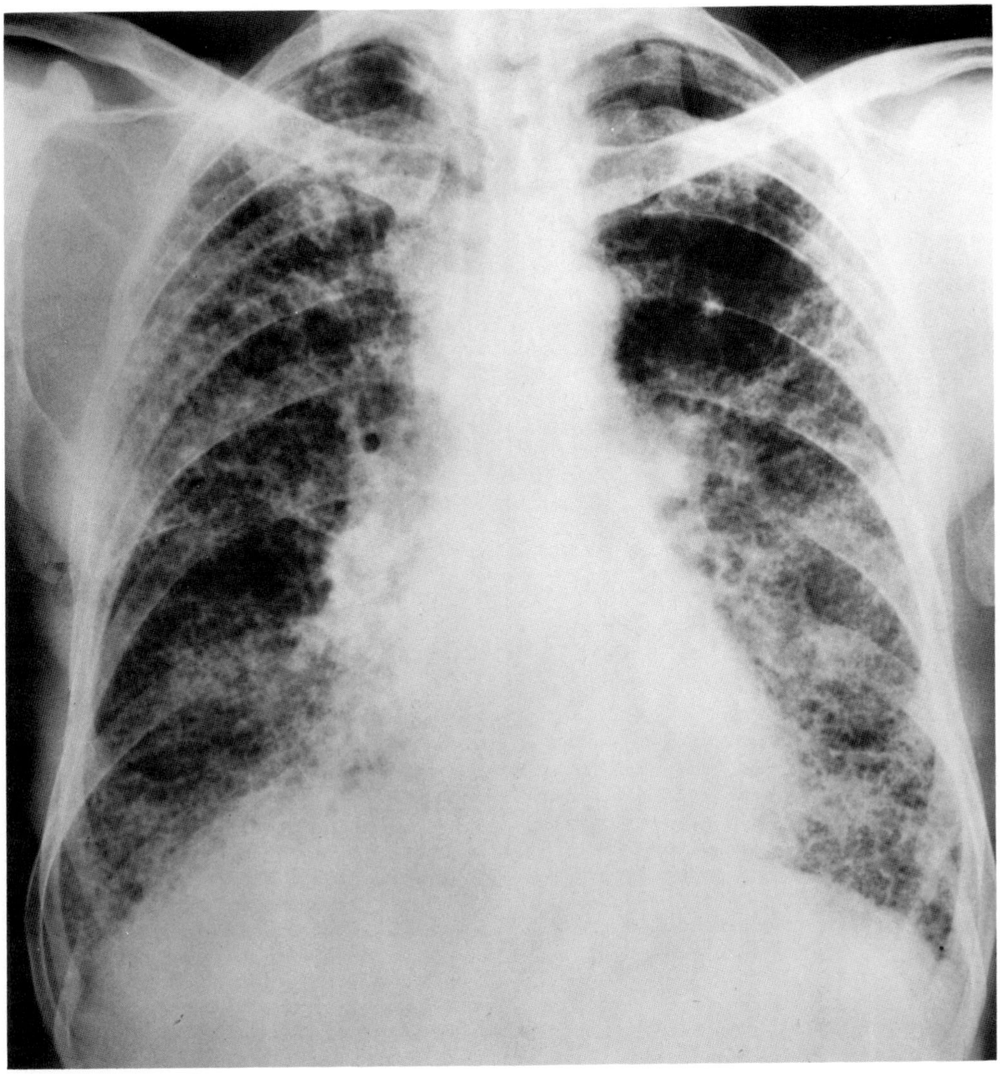

Figure 8.42 Appearances of widespread DIPF with multiple cysts wrongly diagnosed during life as coal pneumoconiosis. See Figure 4.15 *for section of right lung; note the absence of pneumoconiosis. Collier, 20 years. Rheumatoid arthritis, 20 years. Diagnosis: rheumatoid lung*

terms of *mass concentration* as this has proved to be a better index of the risk of developing pneumoconiosis (Jacobsen *et al.*, 1971). The current method of collecting and evaluating dust samples is laid down by the Coal Mines (Respirable Dust) Regulations, 1975. Compact particles from 1 to 7 μm diameter are collected by stationary, standard four-channel, size-selective, gravimetric elutriators (NCB/MRE Type 113 A—Dunmore, Hamilton and Smith, 1964) situated in specified working places.

Three permitted levels are prescribed by a 1978 amendment to the 1975 Regulations with regard to various locations underground and are based on a standard attainable in mines by the use of available measures of dust control.

(a) 7 mg/m³ of air for operations at longwall coal faces.
(b) 3 mg/m³ for operations in drivages and headings where the average quartz content exceeds 0.45 mg/m³.
(c) 5 mg/m³ for operations in other localities.

Before the 1978 amendment an 8 mg/m³ level had been selected for longwall face operations. This is equivalent to an average working shift exposure of 4.3 mg/m³ when allowance is made for travelling time to and from the coal face, differing concentrations of dust along and near an individual face and between different faces, and the fact that sampling is done at a fixed distance away from the face. It will be recalled that a mean dust concentration which does not exceed 4.3 mg/m³ over 35 years carries a small pneumoconiosis risk (*see* p. 179). The current 5 mg/m³ level for work in 'other localities' was preceded by a 6 mg/m³ level which is also equivalent to the basic 4.3 mg/m³ average but was set lower than the 8 mg/m³ level because sampling is taken nearer the miner's breathing zone.

CONTROL OF DUST PRODUCTION

This is achieved by special attention to mining techniques

(a) (b)

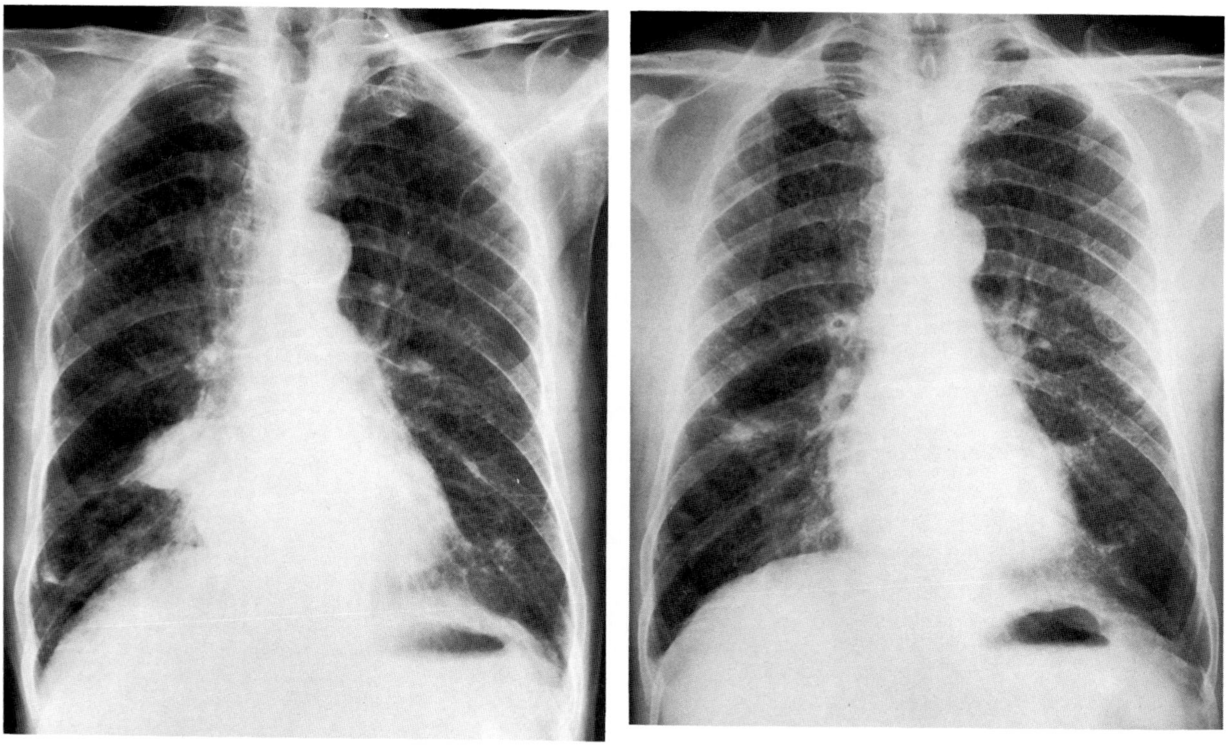

Figure 8.43 (a) and (b) Coal-miner for 36 years. (a) 1973. Right lower zone opacity interpreted first as encysted effusion of lesser fissure and later as carcinoma. Comparison with the earlier film (b) (1958) would have prevented this difficulty. Post mortem: moderate numbers of small coal nodules (about 2 mm diameter) and PMF 4.5 × 3.0 × 3.0 cm in right lower lobe. No evidence of neoplasm

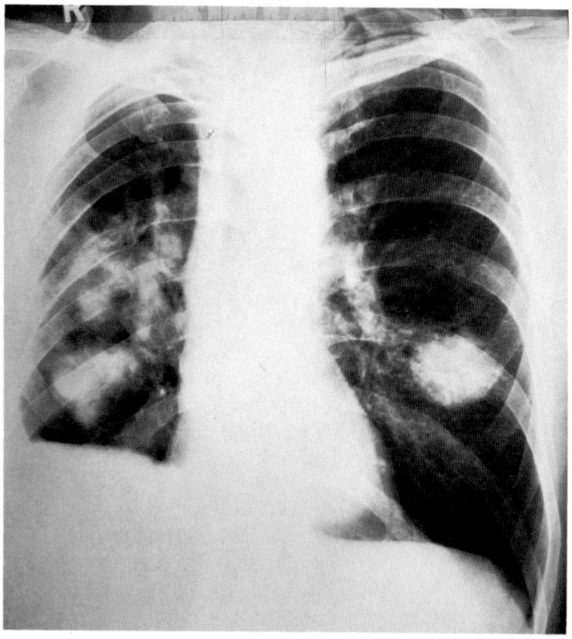

Figure 8.44 Secondary pulmonary tumour deposits resembling PMF and initially diagnosed as such. Post mortem: adenocarcinoma in both lungs; very occasional small coal nodules but no PMF. Coal-miner eight years

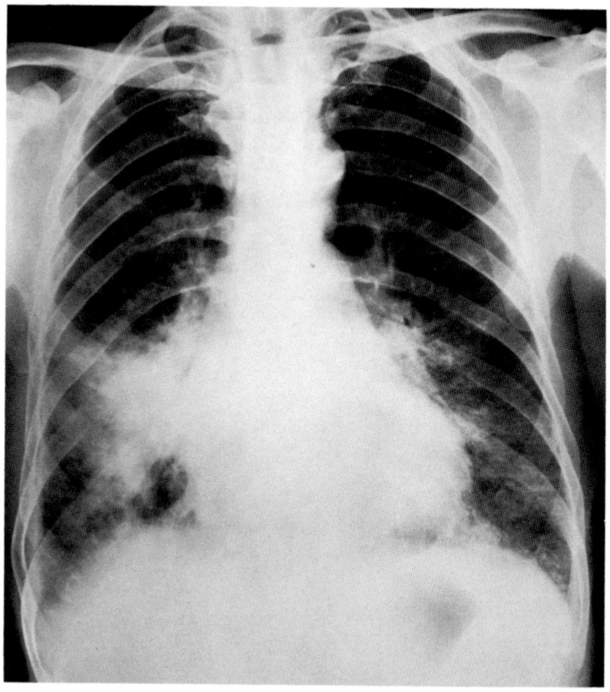

Figure 8.45 Lipoid pneumonia (paraffinoma) resembling, and diagnosed as, lower zone PMF in an aged ex-coal-miner addicted to medicinal paraffin oil. Radiographic appearances unchanged for a few years before death. Post mortem: moderate numbers of dust macules and occasional small coal pneumoconiosis nodules but no PMF; mass in right lower lobe thought, naked eye, to be a carcinoma but frozen and H and E microsections demonstrated lipoid pneumonia. (Compare with Figure 8.23(a)*)*

(a)

(b)

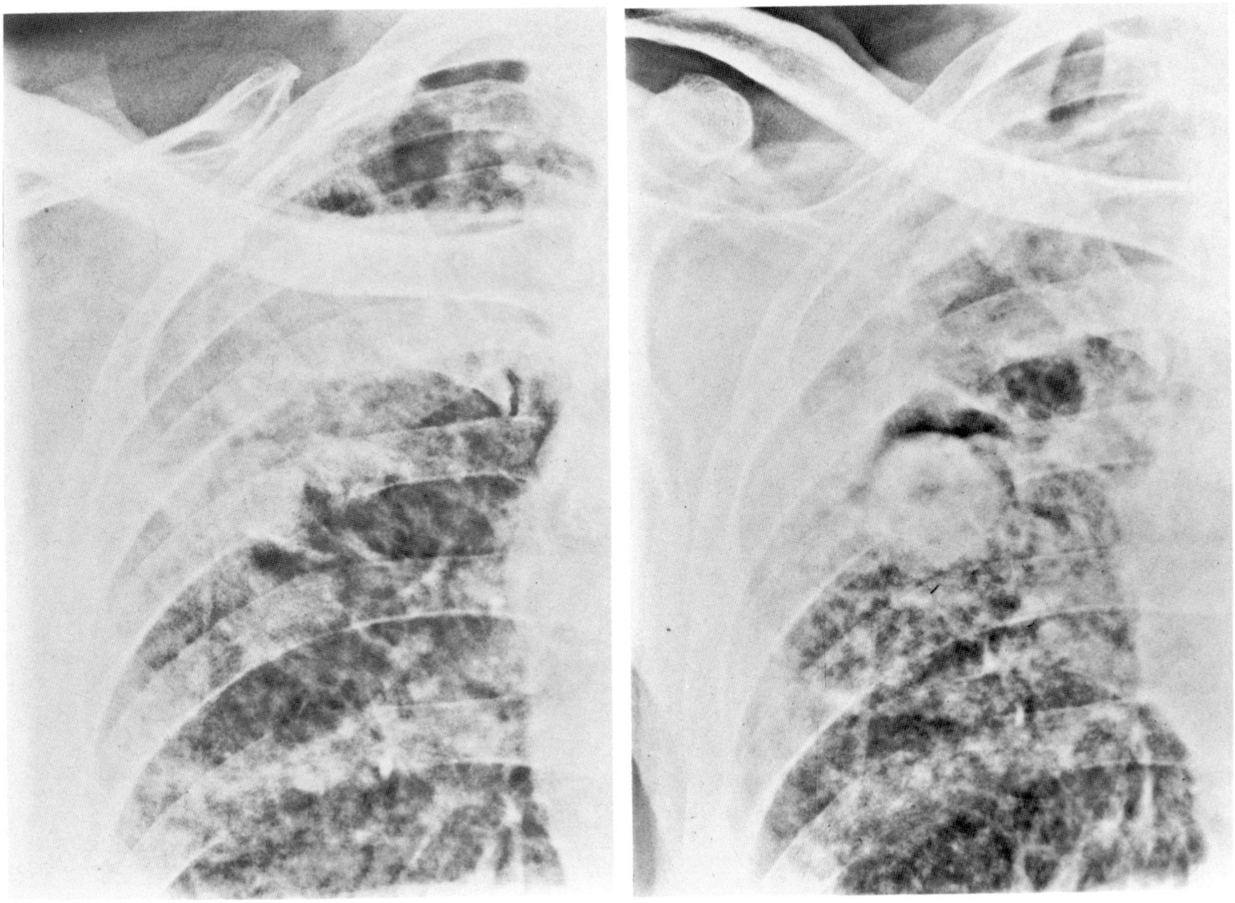

Figure 8.46 (a) Ill-defined PMF in coal-miner for 21 years. (b) Subsequent development of typical appearances of a mycetoma in an ischaemic cavity. Aspergillus fumigatus *isolated*

and the designing of equipment to give rise to a minimum of dust.

MEDICAL SUPERVISION

The 1975 Regulations require medical examination and a chest radiograph of all new entrants. These facilities and lung function testing are also offered on a voluntary basis at approximately two-yearly intervals to all mine workers, and at other times to men under 35 years of age with chest radiographs believed to show Category 1 changes, and to older men with pneumoconiosis showing rapid progression.

STONE DUSTING TO PREVENT COAL-DUST EXPLOSIONS (UK)

Pulverized limestone is used. It must satisfy the requirements that it shall not contain more than 5 per cent total silica of which free silica is not more than 3 per cent.

Shale dust has not been used since the early 1950s because of high quartz content.

COAL-MINE DUST STANDARDS IN THE USA

The present coal-mine dust standard is 2 mg/m^3 for an eight hour working shift. Dust is collected by personally carried AEC cyclone samplers. To compare measurements made by these instruments with those of the NCB/MRE elutriator they must be multiplied by a factor of 1.6; hence, by British Standards 2 mg/m^3 becomes 3 mg/m^3.

Anti-explosion rock dusts can be pulverized limestone, marble, anhydrite, shale and adobe, but limestone is preferred; they should not contain more than 'a total of 5 per cent free and combined silica (SiO_2)' (Bureau of Mines, 1960).

REFERENCES

Alarie, Y. C., Krumm, A. A., Busey, W. M., Ulrich, C. E. and Kantz II, R. I. (1975). Long-term exposure to sulfur dioxide, sulfuric acid mist, fly ash and their mixtures. *Archs envir. Hlth* **30,** 254–262

Amandus, H. E., Lapp, N. L., Jacobson, G. and Reger, R. B. (1976). Significance of irregular small opacities in radiographs of coalminers in the USA. *Br. J. ind. Med.* **33,** 13–17

Annotation (1967). Tuberculosis and pneumoconiosis. *Lancet* **2,** 410

Ashford, J. R., Morgan, D. D., Rae, S. and Sowden, R. R. (1970). Respiratory symptoms in British coal miners. *Am. Rev. resp. Dis.* **102,** 370–381

Ball, J. D., Berry, G., Clarke, W. G., Gilson, J. C. and Thomas, J. (1969). A controlled trial of anti-tuberculosis chemotherapy in early complicated pneumoconiosis of coal workers. *Thorax* **24,** 399–406

Beal, A. J., Griffin, O. G. and Nagelschmidt, G. (1953). *The Health Hazard of Limestone and Gypsum used for Stone Dusting in Coal Mines.* Safety in Mines Research Establishment, Ministry of Fuel and Power. Res. Rep. No. 72

Benedek, T. G. (1973). Rheumatoid pneumoconiosis. *Am. J. Med.* **55,** 515–524

Benedek, T. G., Zawadzki, Z. A. and Medsger, Jr. T. A. (1976). Serum immunoglobulins, rheumatoid factor, and pneumoconiosis in miners with rheumatoid arthritis. *Arth. Rheum.* **19,** 731–736

Bergman, I. and Casswell, C. (1972). Lung dust and lung iron contents of coal workers in different coalfields in Great Britain. *Br. J. ind. Med.* **29,** 160–168

Bonnell, J. A., Schilling, C. J. and Massey, P. M. O. (1980). Clinical and experimental studies of the effects of pulverized fuel ash—a review. *Ann. occup. Hyg.* **23,** 159–164

Brummer, M. E. G. and Schwartz, L. W. (1977). Pulmonary responses to prolonged fly ash exposure. Rat exposure followed by a recovery period. *Am. Rev. resp. Dis.* **115,** 203 (abstract)

Bureau of Mines (1960). *American Practice for Rock Dusting Underground Bituminous-coal and Lignite Mines to Prevent Coal Dust Explosions.* (ASA Standard M13. 1–1960, UDC 622. 81.) US Department of the Interior

Burrell, R. (1972). Immunological aspects of coal workers' pneumoconiosis. *Ann. N.Y. Acad. Sci.* **200,** 94–105

Caplan, A. (1953). Certain unusual radiological appearances in the chest of coal miners suffering rheumatoid arthritis. *Thorax* **8,** 29–37

Caplan, A. (1962). Correlation of radiological category with lung pathology in coal-workers' pneumoconiosis. *Br. J. ind. Med.* **19,** 171–179

Caplan, A., Payne, R. B. and Withey, J. L. (1962). A broader concept of Caplan's syndrome related to rheumatoid factors. *Thorax* **17,** 205–212

Caplan, A., Simon, G. and Reid, L. (1966). The radiological diagnosis of widespread emphysema and categories of simple pneumoconiosis. *Clin. Radiol.* **17,** 68–70

Cate, C. C. and Burrell, R. (1974). Lung antigen induced cell mediated immune injury in chronic respiratory disease. *Am. Rev. resp. Dis.* **109,** 114–123

Chan, B. W. B. (1969a). Serum iron and iron kinetics in coal workers with complicated pneumoconiosis. *Br. J. ind. Med.* **26,** 65–70

Chan, B. W. B. (1969b). Haemodilution as a cause of anaemia in coal workers. *Br. J. ind. Med.* **26,** 237–239

Civil, G. W., Heppleston, A. G. and Casswell, C. (1975). The influence of exposure duration and intermittency upon the pulmonary retention and elimination of dusts from high and low rank coal mines. *Ann. occup. Hyg.* **17,** 173–185

Clegg, J. W. (1953). Ulcero-caseous tuberculous bronchitis. *Thorax* **8,** 167–179

Cocarla, A., Cornea, G., Dengel, H., Gabor, S., Milea, M. and Papilian, V. V. (1976). Pneumoconiose au noir de fumée. *Int. Arch. occup. envir. Hlth* **36,** 217–218

Cochrane, A. L. (1962). The attack rate of progressive massive fibrosis. *Br. J. ind. Med.* **19,** 52–64

Cochrane, A. L. (1973). Relation between radiographic categories of coalworkers' pneumoconiosis and expectation of life. *Br. med. J.* **1,** 532–534

Cochrane, A. L., Cox, J. G. and Jarman, T. F. (1952). Pulmonary tuberculosis in the Rhondda Fach. *Br. med. J.* **2,** 843–853

Cochrane, A. L., Haley, T. J. L., Moore, F. and Hole, D. (1979). The mortality of men in the Rhondda Fach, 1950–1970. *Br. J. ind. Med.* **36,** 15–22

Cochrane, A. L. and Higgins, I. T. T. (1961). Pulmonary ventilatory functions of coal miners in various areas in relation to the X-ray category of pneumoconiosis. *Br. J. prev. Soc. Med.* **15,** 1–11

Cochrane, A. L. and Moore, F. (1978). Preliminary results of a twenty-year follow-up of a random sample of an industrial town. *Br. med. J.* **1,** 411–412

Collis, E. L. and Gilchrist, J. C. (1928). Effects of dust on coal trimmers. *J. ind. Hyg. Toxicol.* **10,** 101–109

Constantinidis, K., Musk, A. W., Jenkins, J. P. R. and Berry, G. (1978). Pulmonary function in coal workers with Caplan's syndrome and non-rheumatoid complicated pneumoconiosis. *Thorax* **33,** 764–768

Costello, J., Ortmeyer, C. E. and Morgan, W. K. C. (1974). Mortality from lung cancer in US coal miners. *Am. J. publ. Hlth* **64,** 222–224

Costello, J., Ortmeyer, C. E. and Morgan, W. K. C. (1975). Mortality from heart disease in coal mines. *Chest* **67,** 417–421

Cotes, J. E. (1979). *Lung Function*, 4th edition. Oxford; Blackwell

Cotes, J. E. and Field, G. B. (1972). Lung gas exchange in simple pneumoconiosis of coal workers. *Br. J. ind. Med.* **29,** 268–273

Cotes, J. E., Deivanayagam, C. N., Field, G. B. and Billiet, L. (1971). Relation between types of simple pneumoconiosis (p or m) and lung function. In *Inhaled Particles, 3* edited by W. H. Walton, pp. 633–641. Woking; Unwin

Crosbie, W. A., Cox, R. A. F., Leblanc, J. V. and Cooper, D. (1979). Survey of respiratory disease in carbon black workers in the UK and USA. *Am. Rev. resp. Dis.* **119,** 209 (Suppl.)

Dassanayake, W. L. P. (1948). The health of plumbago workers in Ceylon. *Br. J. ind. Med.* **5,** 141–147

Dauber, J. H., Finn, D. R. and Daniele, R. P. (1976). Immunologic abnormalities in anthrosilicosis. *Am. Rev. resp. Dis.* **113,** 94 (abstract)

Davies, D. and Lindars, D. C. (1968). Rheumatoid pneumoconiosis. *Am. Rev. resp. Dis.* **97,** 617–629

Davis, J. M. G., Chapman, J., Collings, P., Douglas, A. N., Fernie, J., Lamb, D., Ottery, J. and Ruckley, A. (1979). Autopsy study of coalminers' lungs. *Inst. occup. Med. Edinb.* Report No. TM/79/9 (Eur. P27)

Davis, J. M. G., Ottery, J. and Le Roux, A. (1977). The effect of quartz and other non-coal dusts in coal workers' pneumoconiosis. Part II Lung autopsy study. In *Inhaled Particles IV,* edited by W. H. Walton, pp. 691–700. Oxford; Pergamon Press

Dunmore, J. H., Hamilton, R. J. and Smith, D. S. G. (1964). An instrument for the sampling of respirable dust for subsequent gravimetric assessment. *J. scient. Instrum.* **41,** 669–672

Dunner, L. and Bagnall, D. J. T. (1949). Pneumoconiosis in graphite workers. *Br. J. Radiol.* **22,** 573–579

Englert, M. and De Coster, A. (1965). La capacité de diffusion pulmonaire dans l'anthrasilicose micronodulaire. *J. fr. Med. Chir. thorac.* **19,** 159–173

Faulds, J. S., King, E. J. and Nagelschmidt, G. (1959). The dust content of the lungs of coal workers from Cumberland. *Br. J. ind. Med.* **16,** 43–50

Faulkner, W. B. (1940). Bilateral pulmonary abscess secondary to pneumokoniosis. *Dis. Chest* **6,** 306–307

Fisher, G. L., Chang, D. P. Y. and Brummer, M. (1976). Fly ash collected from electrostatic structures and the mystery of the spheres. *Science* **192,** 553–555

Fletcher, C. M. (1970). Correspondence. *Br. med. J.* **4,** 176

Fletcher, C. M. (1972a). Correspondence. *Br. med. J.* **2,** 353

Fletcher, C. M. (1972b). Correspondence. *Br. med. J.* **3,** 116

Foà, V., Grieco, A. and Zedda, S. (1966). Indagine clinica-radiologica sull'incidenza della pneumoconiosi fra gli operai adetti alla fabricazione di carbon. *Med. Lav.* **57,** 684–695

Frans, A., Veriter, C. and Brasseur, L. (1975). Pulmonary diffusing capacity for carbon monoxide in simple coal workers' pneumoconiosis. *Bull. physiopath. resp.* **11,** 479–502

Frans, A., Veriter, C., Gerin-Portier, N. and Brasseur, L. (1975). Blood gases in simple coal workers' pneumoconiosis. *Bull. physiopath. resp.* **11,** 503–526

Fritze, E., Gundel, E., Ludwig, E., Muller, G., Muller, H. O. and Petersen, B. (1969). Die gesundheitliche Situation van Bergar beitern einer Kohlenzeche. *Dt. med. Wschr.* **94,** 362–367

Fuller, H. W. (1860). *On Rheumatism, Rheumatic Gout and*

Sciatica, their Pathology, Symptoms and Treatment, 3rd edition pp. 305–326. London; Churchill

Gaensler, E. A., Cadigan, J. B., Sasahara, A. A., Fox, E. O. and MacMahon, H. E. (1966). Graphite pneumoconiosis of electrotypers. *Am. J. Med.* **41,** 864–882

Gärtner, K. and Braus, F. W. (1951). Untersuchungen zur Frage der Russlunge und zur Schädlichkeit des reinen Kohlenstanbanteiles im Staub der Kohlenbergwerke. *Med. Welt.* **20,** 253–256

Gernez-Rieux, C., Balgaires, E., Fournier, P. and Voisin, C. (1958). Une manifestation souvent méconus de la pneumoconiose des mineurs: La liquéfaction aseptique des formations pseudatumorales. *Sem. Hôp. Paris* **34,** 1081–1089

Gernez-Rieux, C., Tacquet, A., Devulder, B., Voisin, C., Tonnel, A. and Aerts, C. (1972). Experimental study of interactions between pneumoconioses and mycobacterial infections. *Ann. N.Y. Acad. Sci.* **200,** 106–126

Gilson, J. C. and Hugh-Jones, P. (1955). Lung function in coal workers' pneumoconiosis. Spec. Rep. Ser. No. 290. *Medical Research Council.* London; HMSO

Gilson, J. C. and Oldham, P. D. (1970). Correspondence. *Br. med. J.* **4,** 305

Gloyne, S. R. (1932–33). The morbid anatomy and histology of asbestos. *Tubercle (Edin.)* **14,** 445–451; 493–497; 550–558

Gloyne, S. R., Marshall, G. and Hoyle, C. (1949). Pneumoconiosis due to graphite dust. *Thorax* **4,** 32–38

Goldman, K. P. (1965a). The diagnosis of lung cancer in coal miners with pneumoconiosis. *Br. J. Dis. Chest* **59,** 141–147

Goldman, K. P. (1965b). Mortality of coal-miners from carcinoma of the lung. *Br. J. ind. Med.* **22,** 72–77

Goldman, K. P. (1965c). Prognosis of coal miners with cancer of the lung. *Thorax* **20,** 170–174

Gormley, I. P., Collings, P., Davis, J. M. G. and Ottery, J. (1979). An investigation into the cytotoxicity of respirable dusts from British collieries. *Br. J. exp. Path.* **60,** 526–536

Gough, J. (1940). Pneumoconiosis in coal trimmers. *J. Path. Bact.* **51,** 277–285

Gough, J. (1947). Pneumoconiosis in coal workers in Wales. *Occup. Med.* **4,** 86–97

Gough, J. (1968). The pathogenesis of emphysema. In *The Lung,* edited by A. A. Liebow and D. E. Smith, pp. 109–133. Baltimore; Williams and Wilkins

Gough, J. and Heppleston, A. G. (1960). The pathology of the pneumoconioses. In *Industrial Pulmonary Diseases,* edited by E. J. King and C. M. Fletcher, pp. 23–36. London; Churchill

Gough, J., Rivers, D. and Seal, R. M. E. (1955). Pathological studies of modified pneumoconiosis in coal-miners with rheumatoid arthritis (Caplan's syndrome). *Thorax* **10,** 9–18

Gross, P. and de Treville, R. T. P. (1970). Black lungs. *Archs envir. Hlth* **20,** 450–451

Gross, P. and Nau, C. A. (1967). Lignite and the derived steam-activated carbon. *Archs envir. Hlth* **14,** 450–460

Haferland, W. (1957). Graphitstaublunge und Silikose. *Arch. Gewerbepath. Gewerbehyg.* **16,** 53–62

Hahon, N., Morgan, W. K. C. and Petersen, M. (1980). Serum immunoglobulin levels in coal workers' pneumoconiosis. *Ann. occup. Hyg.* **23,** 165–174

Hankinson, J. L., Palmes, E. D. and Lapp, N. L. (1979). Pulmonary air space size in coal miners. *Am. Rev. resp. Dis.* **119,** 391–397

Harding, H. E. and Oliver, G. B. (1949). Changes in the lungs produced by natural graphite. *Br. J. ind. Med.* **6,** 91–99

Harington, J. S. (1972). Investigative techniques in the laboratory study of coal workers' pneumoconiosis: recent advances at the cellular level. *Ann. N.Y. Acad. Sci.* **200,** 816–834

Hart, P. D'A. and Aslett, E. A. (1942). Chronic pulmonary disease in South Wales and miners. Part I. Section B. *Med. Res. Counc. Spec. Rep. Ser. No. 243.* London; HMSO

Hart, J. T., Cochrane, A. L. and Higgins, I. T. T. (1963). Tuberculin sensitivity in coal worker's pneumoconiosis. *Tubercle, Lond.* **44,** 141–152

Heard, B. E. (1969). *Pathology of Chronic Bronchitis and Emphysema.* London; Churchill

Heard, B. E. and Izukawa, T. (1963). Dust pigmentation of the lungs and emphysema in Londoners. In *Fortschritte Staublungenforschung,* edited by H. Reploh and W. Klosterkötter, pp. 249–255. Dinslaken; Niederrheinische Druckerie

Heath, D. (1968). In *Form and Function in the Human Lung,* edited by G. Cumming and L. B. Hunt, p. 35. Edinburgh and London; Livingstone

Heath, D. and Williams, D. R. (1981). *Man at High Altitude,* 2nd edn, pp. 189–191. Edinburgh, London and New York; Churchill Livingstone

Heise, E. R., Major, P. C., Mentnech, S. H., Parrish, E. J., Jordan, A. L. and Morgan, W. K. C. (1977). Predominance of histocompatibility antigens W18 and HL-A1 in miners resistant to complicated coalworkers' pneumoconiosis. In *Inhaled Particles* IV, edited by W. H. Walton, pp. 495–505. Oxford; Pergamon Press

Heise, E. R., Mentnech, M. S., Olenchock, S. A., Kutz, S. A., Morgan, W. K. C., Merchant, J. A. and Major, P. C. (1979). HLA-A1 and coal workers' pneumoconiosis. *Am. Rev. resp. Dis.* **119,** 903–908

Hendriks, C. A. M. and Bleiker, M. A. (1964). Tuberculin sensitivity in coal miners with pneumoconiosis. *Tubercle, Lond.* **45,** 379–383

Heppleston, A. G. (1947). The essential lesion of pneumoconiosis in Welsh coal workers. *J. Path. Bact.* **59,** 453–460

Heppleston, A. G. (1951). Coal worker's pneumoconiosis. *Archs ind. Hyg.* **4,** 270–288

Heppleston, A. G. (1953). The pathological anatomy of simple pneumoconiosis in coal miners. *J. Path. Bact.* **66,** 235–246

Heppleston, A. G. (1968). In *Form and Function in the Human Lung,* edited by G. Cumming and L. B. Hunt, pp. 35–36. Edinburgh and London; Livingstone

Heppleston, A. G. (1972). The pathological recognition and pathogenesis of emphysema and fibrocystic disease of the lung with special reference to coal workers. *Ann. N.Y. Acad. Sci.* **200,** 347–369

Heppleston, A. G., Civil, G. W. and Critchlow, A. (1971). The effects of duration and intermittency of exposure on the elimination of high and low rank coal dusts. In *Inhaled Particles, III,* edited by W. H. Walton, pp. 261–270. Woking; Unwin

Hicks, D., Fay, J. W. J., Ashford, J. R. and Rae, S. (1961). *The Relation between Pneumoconiosis and Environmental Conditions.* London; National Coal Board

Higgins, I. T. T. (1972). Correspondence. *Br. med. J.* **2,** 713

Higgins, I. T. T., Gilson, J. C., Ferris, B. G., Waters, W. E., Campbell, H. and Higgins, M. W. (1968a). IV Chronic respiratory disease in an industrial town; a nine-year follow-up study. Preliminary report. *Am. J. publ. Hlth* **58,** 1667–1676

Higgins, I. T. T., Higgins, M. W., Lockshin, M. D. and Canale, N. (1968b). Chronic respiratory disease in mining communities in Marion County, West Virginia. *Br. J. ind. Med.* **25,** 165–175

Higgins, I. T. T., Higgins, M. W., Lockshin, M. D. and Canale, N. (1969). Coronary disease in mining communities in Marion County, West Virginia. *J. chron. Dis.* **22,** 165–179

Hutchinson, J. E. M. (1966). Twins with coal-workers' pneumoconiosis. *Br. J. ind. Med.* **23,** 240–244

Jacobsen, M. (1973). Progession of coal workers' pneumoconiosis in Britain in relation to environmental conditions underground. *Proceedings Conference on Technical Measures of Dust Prevention and Suppression in Mines,* pp. 77–93. Luxembourg; Commission of the European Communities

Jacobsen, M. (1975). Effects of some approximations in analysis of radiological response to coal mine dust exposure. *Recent Advances on the Assessment of the Health Effects of Environmental Pollution* Volume I, pp. 211–228. Luxembourg; Commission of the European Communities

Jacobsen, M. (1977). Discussion. In *Inhaled Particles IV,* Vol. 2, edited by W. H. Walton, p. 772. Oxford; Pergamon Press

Jacobsen, M. (1979). Dust exposure and pneumoconiosis at 10 British coal mines. Paper presented at the ILO Vth International Conference on Pneumoconiosis, Caracas, 1978

Jacobsen, M., Burns, J. and Attfield, M. D. (1977). Smoking and coalworkers' simple pneumoconiosis. In *Inhaled Particles IV*. Vol. 2, edited by W. H. Walton, pp. 759–771. Oxford; Pergamon Press

Jacobsen, M., Rae, S., Walton, W. H. and Rogan, J. M. (1971). The relation between pneumoconiosis and dust-exposure in British coal mines. In *Inhaled Particles III*, edited by W. H. Walton, pp. 903–917. Woking; Unwin

Jacobson, G., Felson, B., Pendergrass, E. P., Flinn, R. H. and Lainhart, W. S. (1967). Eggshell calcification in coal and metal miners. *Semin. Roentgenol.* **2,** 276–281

Jaffé, F. A. (1951). Graphite pneumoconiosis. *Am. J. Path.* **17,** 909–923

James, W. R. L. (1954). The relationship of tuberculosis to the development of massive pneumokoniosis in coal workers. *Br. J. Tuberc.* **48,** 89–101

James, W. R. L. (1955). Primary lung cancer in South Wales coal miners with pneumoconiosis. *Br. J. ind. Med.* **12,** 87–91

Jones, B. M., Edwards, J. H. and Wagner, J. C. (1972). Absorption of serum proteins by inorganic dusts. *Br. J. ind. Med.* **29,** 287–292

Kang, K. Y., Yagura, T., Sara, Y., Yokoyama, K. and Yamamura, Y. (1973). Antinuclear factor in pneumoconiosis and idiopathic pulmonary fibrosis. *Med. J. Osaka Univ.* **23,** 249–256

Keele, C. A. and Neil, E. (1971). *Samson Wright's Applied Physiology*. 12th edition, p. 141. London; Oxford University Press

Kibelstis, J. A. (1973). Diffusing capacity in bituminous coal mines. *Chest* **63,** 501–504

Kennaway, E. L. and Kennaway, N. M. (1947). A further study of the incidence of cancer of the lung and larynx. *Br. J. Cancer* **1,** 260–298

Kilpatrick, G. S., Heppleston, A. G. and Fletcher, C. M. (1954). Cavitation in the massive fibrosis of coal workers' pneumoconiosis. *Thorax* **9,** 260–272

King, E. J., Zaidi, S. H., Harrison, C. V. and Nagelschmidt, G. (1958). The tissue reaction of the lungs of rats after the inhalation of coal dust containing 2% of quartz. *Br. J. ind. Med.* **15,** 172–177

Kober, T. E., Sorenson, J. R. L., Menden, E. E. and Petering, H. G. (1976). Some natural products from two soft coals. Their removal, metal-binding and enzyme inhibitory activity. *Archs envir. Hlth* **31** 182–188

Krémer, R. and Lavenne, F. (1966). La circulation pulmonaire dans les pneumoconioses. *Poumon. Couer,* **22,** 767–791

Ladoo, R. B. and Myers, W. M. (1951). *Non-metallic Minerals,* p. 250. New York and London; McGraw-Hill

Lapp, N. L., Block, J., Boehlecke, B., Lippmann, M., Morgan, W. K. C. and Reger, R. B. (1976). Closing volume in coal miners. *Am. Rev. resp. Dis.* **113,** 155–161

Lapp, N. L. R. and Seaton, A. (1971). Pulmonary function. In *Pulmonary Reactions to Coal Dust,* edited by M. M. Key, L. E. Kerr, and M. Bundy, pp. 153–177. New York and London; Academic Press

Lavenne, F. (1968). Assessment of lung function in silicosis and mixed dust pneumoconiosis. In *Pneumoconiosis.* Report in the 1967 Katowice Symposium. EURO 0379. Copenhagen; WHO

Lavenne, F. (1970). Discussion. In *Pneumoconiosis. Proceedings of the International Conference, J'burg, 1969,* edited by H. A. Shapiro, p. 521. Cape Town; Oxford University Press

Lee, S. C. and Johnson, H. A. (1975). Multiple nodular amyloidosis. *Thorax* **30,** 178–185

Lewis, D. M., Lapp, N. L. and Burrell, R. (1971). Quantitation of secretory IgA in chronic pulmonary disease with particular reference to coal workers' pneumoconiosis. In *Inhaled Particles III,* edited by W. H. Walton, pp. 579–586. Woking; Unwin

Liddell, F. D. K. (1973). Mortality of British coal miners in 1961. *Br. J. ind. Med.* **30,** 15–24

Lindars, D. C. and Davies, D. (1967). Rheumatoid pneumoconiosis. A study in colliery populations in the East Midlands coalfield. *Thorax* **22,** 525–532

Lindars, D. C., Rooke, G. B., Dempsey, A. N. and Ward, F. G. (1972). Pneumoconiosis and death from coronary heart disease. *J. Path.* **108,** 249–259

Linton, R. W., Loh, A., Natusch, C. A., Evans, Jr. C. A. and Williams, P. (1976). Surface predominance of trace elements in airborne particles. *Science* **191,** 852–854

Lippmann, M., Eckert, H. L., Hahon, N. and Morgan, W. K. C. (1973). Circulating antinuclear and rheumatoid factors in coal mines. *Ann. intern. Med.* **79,** 807–811

Lister, W. B. and Wimborne, D. (1972). Carbon pneumoconiosis in a synthetic graphite worker. *Br. J. ind. Med.* **29,** 108–110

Lochtkemper, I. and Teleky, L. (1932). Studien über Staublunge; die Staublunge in einzelnen besonderin Betrieben und bei besonderen Arbeiten. *Arch. Gewerbepath. Gewerbehyg.* **3,** 600–672

Locke, G. B. (1963). Rheumatoid lung. *Clin. Radiol.* **14,** 43–53

Lyons, J. P., Ryder, R. C., Campbell, H., Clarke, W. G. and Gough, J. (1974). Significance of irregular opacities in the radiology of coal workers' pneumoconiosis. *Br. J. ind. Med.* **31,** 36–44

Lyons, J. P., Ryder, R., Campbell, H. and Gough, J. (1972). Pulmonary disability in coal workers' pneumoconiosis. *Br. med. J.* **1,** 713–716

McCallum, R. I. (1961). Treatment of progressive massive fibrosis in coal miners. *Proceedings XIII International Congress on Occupational Health, New York,* 741–745

McCormick, J. N. (1972). Quoted by Jones, B. M., Edwards, J. H. and Wagner, J. C. (1972)

McFarland, H. N., Ulrich, C. E., Martin, A., Krumm, A., Busey, W. M. and Alarie, Y. (1971). Chronic exposure of cynamolgus monkeys to fly ash. In *Inhaled Particles and Vapours III,* edited by W. H. Walton, pp. 313–326. Old Woking, Surrey; Unwin Bros

McLintock, J. S., Rae, S. and Jacobsen, M. (1971). The attack rate of progressive massive fibrosis in British coal miners. In *Inhaled Particles, III,* edited by W. H. Walton, pp. 933–950. Woking; Unwin

Macklem, P. T. (1968). Discussion of Session One. In *Form and Function in the Human Lung,* edited by G. Cumming and L. B. Hunt, pp. 33–34. Edinburgh and London; Livingstone

Mantell, C. L. (1968). *Carbon and Graphite Handbook.* New York and London; Wiley

Mantell, C. L. (1971). Personal communication

Marks, J. (1961). Infective pneumoconiosis due to anonymous mycobacteria. *Br. med. J.* **2,** 1332

Marks, J. (1970). New mycobacteria. *Hlth Trends* **3,** 68–69

Martin, J. C., Daniel-Moussard, H., Le Bouffant and Policard, A. (1972). The role of quartz in the development of coal workers' pneumoconiosis. *Ann. N.Y. Acad. Sci.* **200,** 127–141

Medical Research Council (1942). *Report by the Committee on Industrial Pulmonary Disease.* S.R.S. 243, p. 11. London; HMSO

Medical Research Council/Miners Treatment Centre (1963). Chemotherapy of pulmonary tuberculosis with pneumoconiosis. *Tubercle, Lond.,* **44,** 47–70

Meiklejohn, A. (1957). Carbon and pneumoconiosis. *XII International Congress on Occupational Health, Helsinki.* **31,** 335–337

Miall, W. E. (1955). Rheumatoid arthritis in Wales. An epidemiological study of a Welsh mining community. *Am. rheum. Dis.* **14,** 150–158

Miall, W. E., Caplan, A., Cochrane, A. L., Kilpatrick, G. S. and Oldham, P. D. (1953). An epidemiological study of rheumatoid arthritis associated with characteristic chest X-ray appearances in coal miners. *Br. med. J.* **2,** 1231–1236

Miller, A. A. and Ramsden, F. (1961). Carbon pneumoconiosis. *Br. J. ind. Med.* **18,** 103–113

Mitchell, R. S., Walker, S. H. and Maisel, J. C. (1968). The causes of death in chronic airway obstruction. II. Myocardial infarction. *Am. Rev. resp. Dis.* **98,** 611–612

Morgan, W. K. C. (1968). The prevalence coal workers' pneumoconiosis. *Am. Rev. resp. Dis.* **98,** 306–310

Morgan, W. K. C., Burgess, D. B., Jacobsen, G., O'Brien, J., Pendergrass, E. P., Reger, R. B. and Shoub, E. P. (1973). The prevalence of coal workers' pneumoconiosis in US coal mines. *Archs envir. Hlth* **27,** 221–226

Morgan, W. K. C., Handelsman, L., Kibelstis, J., Lapp, N. L. and Reger, R. B. (1974). Ventilatory capacity and lung volumes of US coal miners. *Archs envir. Hlth* **28,** 182–189

Morgan, W. K. C. and Lapp, N. L. (1976). Resiratory disease in coal miners. *Am. Rev. resp. Dis.* **113,** 531–559

Morgan, W. K. C., Lapp, N. L. and Morgan, E. J. (1974). The early detection of occupational lung disease. *Br. J. Dis. Chest* **68,** 75–85

Morgan, W. K. C., Seaton, A., Burgess, D. B., Lapp, N. L. and Reger, R. B. (1972). Lung volumes in working coal workers. *Ann. N.Y. Acad. Sci.* **200,** 478–493

Mortimer, E. A., Monson, R. R. and MacMahon, B. (1977). Reduction in mortality from coronary heart disease in men residing at high altitude. *New Engl. J. Med.* **296,** 581–585

Myers, C. F. (1967). Anthracosilicosis and bronchogenic carcinoma. *Dis. Chest* **52,** 800–805

Nagelschmidt, G. (1960). The relation between lung dust and lung pathology in pneumoconiosis. *Br. J. ind. Med.* **17,** 247–259

Nagelschmidt, G. (1965). The study of lung dust in pneumoconiosis. *Am. ind. Hyg. Assoc. J.* **26,** 1–7

Nagelschmidt, G. and Godbert, A. L. (1951). *The Health Hazard of Shales used for Stone Dusting.* Safety in Mines Res. Estab., Min. of Fuel and Power, Res. Rep. No. 19

National Coal Board (1969). *Aproved Conditions for Airborne Dust.* F 4040. London; NCB

National Coal Board (1971). *Medical Service and Medical Research: Annual Report 1969–1970.* London; NCB

National Coal Board (1972). *Medical Service and Medical Research: Annual Report 1970–1971.* London; NCB

National Coal Board (1977). *Medical Service Annual Report 1975–76.* London; NCB

National Coal Board (1980). *Medical Service Annual Report 1978–79.* London; NCB

Navrátil, M., Widmisky, J. and Kasalicky, J. (1968). Relationships of pulmonary haemodynamics and ventilation and distribution in silicosis. *Bull. physiopath. resp. (Nancy)* **4,** 349–359

Niedobitek, F. (1969). Zur morphologie und pathogenese dis Caplan-Syndroms. *Z. Rheumaforsch.* **28,** 175–191

Nonkin, P. M., Dick, M. M., Baum, G. L. and Gables, C. (1964). Myocardial infarction in respiratory insufficiency. *Archs intern. Med.* **113,** 42–45

Noonan, C. D., Taylor, F. B. Jr. and Engleman, E. P. (1963). Nodular rheumatoid disease of the lung with cavitation. *Arth. Rheum.* **6,** 232–240

Okutani, H., Shima, S. and Sano, T. (1964). Graphite pneumoconiosis in carbon electrode makers. In *XIV International Congress of Occupational Health, 1963.* Vol. 2. (Int. Congr. Series No. 62). pp. 626–632. Amsterdam; Excerpta Medica

Oldham, P. D. and Berry, G. (1972). Correspondence. *Br. med. J.* **2,** 292–293

Ortmeyer, C. E., Baier, E. J. and Crawford, G. M.Jr (1973). Life expectancy of Pennsylvania coal miners compensated for disability. *Archs envir. Hlth* **27,** 227–230

Ortmeyer, C. E., Costello, J., Morgan, W. K. C., Swecker, S. and Petersen, M. (1974). The mortality of Appalachian coal miners 1963–71. *Archs envir. Hlth* **29,** 67–72

Otto, H. and Einbrodt, H. J. (1958). Lugenstaubanalyse bei Anthracose und ihre versicherung-srechtliche Bedeutung. *Frankf. Z. Path.* **69,** 404–415

Parkes, W. R. (1972). Unpublished observations

Parkes, W. R., Phillips, T. and Williamson, R. G. B. (1976). Coronary artery disease and coal workers' pneumoconiosis. *Br. med. J.* **2,** 1319–1320

Parmeggiani, L. (1950). Graphite pneumoconiosis. *Br. J. ind. Med.* **7,** 42–45

Payne, R. B. (1963). *Rheumatoid Pneumoconiosis.* Thesis for Degree of Doctor of Medicine to the University of South Wales and Monmouthshire, Cardiff

Pendergrass, E. P., Vorwald, A. J., Mishkin, M. M., Whildin, J. G. and Werley, C. W. (1967). Observations on workers in the graphite industry. Part 1. *Med. Radiogr Photogr.* **43,** 70–99

Pendergrass, E. P., Vorwald, A. J., Mishkin, M. M., Whildin, J. G. and Werley, C. W. (1968). Observations on workers in the graphite industry. Part 2. *Med. Radiogr. Photogr.* **44,** 1–17

Pernis, B., Chiappino, G., Gilson, J. C., Wagner, J. C., Caplan, A. and Vigliani, E. C. (1965). Studies on Caplan's nodules by means of immunofluorescence. *Beitr. Silkosforsch. Bd.* **6,** 339–341

Petry, H. (1954). Silicose und polyarthritis. *Arch. Gewerbepath.* **13,** 221–236

Pivoteau, C. and Dechoux, J. (1972). Le retentissement des pneumoconioses à opacités fines de mineurs de charbon sans tombes ventilatoires. *Resp.* **29,** 161–172

Policard, A., Letort, M., Charbonnier, J., Martin, J. and Daniel-Moussard, H. (1967). Recherches sur les interactions charbon-quartz dans le développement des pneumoconioses des houlleurs. *Archs Mal. prof. Méd. trav.* **28,** 589–594

Raask, E. and Schilling, C. J. (1980). Research findings on the toxicity of quartz particles relevant to pulverized fuel ash. *Ann. occup. Hyg.* **23,** 147–157

Rae, S., Muir, D. C. F. and Jacobsen, M. (1970). Coal workers' pneumoconiosis. (Correspondence.) *Br. med. J.* **3,** 769

Ramsey, J. H. R. and Pines, A. (1963). The late results of chemotherapy in pneumoconiosis complicated by tuberculosis. *Tubercle, Lond.* **44,** 476–479

Ranasinha, K. W. and Uragoda, C. G. (1972). Graphite pneumoconiosis. *Br. J. ind. Med.* **29,** 178–183

Registrar General (1958). The Registrar General's Decennial Supplement, England and Wales 1951. *Occupational Mortality.* Part II Volume 1 commentary. London; HMSO

Reisner, M. T. R. (1971). Results of epidemiological studies of pneumoconioses in West German coal mines. In *Inhaled Particles III,* edited by W. H. Walton, pp. 921–929. Old Woking, Surrey; Unwin Bros Ltd

Reisner, M. T. R. and Robock, K. (1977). Results of epidemiological, mineralogical and cytological studies on the pathogenicity of coalmine dusts. In *Inhaled Particles IV,* edited by W. H. Walton, p. 703–715. Oxford; Pergamon Press

Reid, L. (1967). *The Pathology of Emphysema,* London; Lloyd-Luke

Report of the Pneumoconiosis Committee of the College of American Pathologists to the National Institute for Occupational Safety and Health (1979). Pathology Standards for Coal Workers' Pneumoconiosis. Kleinerman, J. (Chairman). *Arch. Path. Lab. Med.* **103,** 375–432

Rivers, D., James, W. R. L., Davies, D. G. and Thomson, S. (1957). The prevalence of tuberculosis at necropsy in massive fibrosis of coal workers. *Br. J. ind. Med.* **14,** 39–42

Rivers, D., Wise, M. E., King, E. J. and Nagelschmidt, G. (1960). Dust content, radiology and pathology in simple pneumoconiosis of coal workers. *Br. J. ind. Med.* **17,** 87–108

Robock, K. and Klosterkötter, W. (1971). The cytotoxic action of semi-conductor properties of mine dusts. In *Inhaled Particles III,* edited by W. H. Walton, pp. 453–460. Old Woking, Surrey; Unwin Bros Ltd

Rodnan, G. P., Benedek, T. G., Medsger, T. A. and Cammarata, R. J. (1967). The association of progressive systemic sclerosis (scleroderma) with coal miners' pneumoconiosis and other forms of silicosis. *Ann. intern. Med.* **66,** 323–334

Rogan, J. M. (1960). Discussion. *Proc. Pneumoc. Conf. Johannesburg.* Edited by A. J. Orenstein, p 434. London; Churchill

Rogan, J. M., Ashford, J. R., Chapman, P. J., Duffield, D. P., Fay, J. W. J. and Rae, S. (1961). Pneumoconiosis and respiratory symptoms in miners at eight collieries. *Br. med. J.* **1,** 1337–1342

Rooke, G. B., Ward, F. G., Dempsey, A. N., Dowler, J. B. and Whitaker, C. J. (1979). Carcinoma of the lung in Lancashire coal miners. *Thorax* **34,** 229–233

Rose, L. B. and Hoffman, D. L. (1956). The coronary blood flow in pulmonary emphysema and cor pulmonale. *Circ. Res.* **4,** 130–132

Ross, H. F., King, E. J., Yoganathan, M. and Nagelschmidt, G. (1962). Inhalation experiment with coal dust containing 5%,

10%, 20% and 40% quartz: tissue reactions in the lungs of rats. *Ann. occup. Hyg.* **5,** 149–161
Rossiter, C. E. (1972a). Relation between content and composition of coal worker's lungs and radiological appearances. *Br. J. ind. Med.* **29,** 31–44
Rossiter, C. E. (1972b). Evidence of dose-response relation in pneumoconiosis. *Trans. Soc. occup. Med.* **22,** 83–97
Rossiter, C. E. (1972c). Relation of lung dust content to radiological changes in coal workers. *Ann. N.Y. Acad. Sci.* **200,** 465–477
Rossiter, C. E., Rivers, D., Bergman, I., Caswell, C. and Nagelschmidt, G. (1967). Dust content, radiology and pathology in simple pneumoconiosis of coal workers. In *Inhaled Particels and Vapours, II,* edited by C. N. Davies, pp. 419–434. Oxford; Pergamon
Rüttner, J. R., Bovet, P. and Aufdermaur, M. (1952). Graphit, Caborund, Staublunge. *Dt. med. Wschr.* **77,** 1413–1415
Ryder, R., Lyons, J. P., Campbell, H. and Gough, J. (1970). Emphysema in coal workers' pneumoconiosis. *Br. med. J.* **3,** 481–487
Sadler, R. L. (1974). Attributability of death to pneumoconiosis in beneficiaries. *Thorax* **29,** 699–702
Samad, I. A. and Noehren, T. H. (1965). Myocardial infarction in pulmonary emphysema. *Dis. Chest* **47,** 26–29
Sanders, W. L. (1970). Heart disease and pneumoconiosis. *Thorax* **25,** 223–225
Scarano, D., Fadali, A. M. A. and Lemole, G. M. (1972). Carcinoma of the lung and anthracosilicosis. *Chest* **62,** 251–254
Schlipköter, H. W., Hilscher, W., Pott, F. and Beck, E. G. (1971). Investigations into the aetiology of coal workers' pneumoconiosis, with the use of PVN-oxide. In *Inhaled Particles, III,* edited by W. H. Walton, pp. 379–389. Woking; Unwin
Seaton, A., Lapp, N. L. and Chang, C. H. J. (1971). Lung scanning in coal workers' pneumoconiosis. *Am. J. resp. Dis.* **103,** 338–349
Seaton, A., Lapp, N. L. and Morgan, W. K. C. (1972a). The relationship of pulmonary impairment in simple coal pneumoconiosis to type of radiographic opacity. *Br. J. ind. Med.* **29,** 50–55
Seaton, A., Lapp, N. L. and Morgan, W. K. C. (1972b). Lung mechanics and frequency dependence compliance in coal miners. *J. clin. Invest.* **51,** 1203–1211
Sorenson, J. R. J., Kober, T. E. and Petering, H. G. (1974). The concentration of Cd, Cu, Fe, Ni, Pb and Zn in bituminous coals from mines with differing incidences of coal workers' pneumoconiosis. *Am. ind. Hyg. Assoc. J.* **25,** 93–98
Soutar, C. A., Coutts, I., Parkes, W. R., Dodi, I. A., Gauld, S., Caśtro, J. E. and Turner-Warwick, M. (1980). Histocompatibility antigens in coal miners with pneumoconiosis (To be published)
Soutar, C. A., Turner-Warwick, M. and Parkes, W. R. (1974). Circulating antinuclear antibody and rheumatoid factor in coal pneumoconiosis. *Br. med. J.* **3,** 145–147
Spink, R. and Nagelschmidt, G. (1963). Dust and fibrosis in the lungs of coal workers from the Wigan area of Lancashire. *Br. J. ind. Med.* **20,** 118–123
Sweet, D. V., Crouse, W. E. and Crable, J. V. (1974). The relationship of total dust, free silica, and trace metal concentrations to the occupational respiratory disease of bituminous coal miners. *Am. ind. Hyg. Assoc. J.* **35,** 479–488
Thurlbeck, W. M. (1976). Chronic airflow obstruction in lung disease. Volume 5. *Major Problems in Pathology,* edited by James L. Bennington. Philadelphia; W. B. Saunders Company
Town, J. D. (1968). Pseudoasbestos bodies and asteroid giant cells in a patient with graphite pneumoconiosis. *Can. med. Ass. J.* **98,** 100–104
Trapnell, D. H. (1964). Septal lines in pneumoconiosis. *Br. J. Radiol.* **37,** 805–810
Tylecote, F. E. and Dunn, J. S. (1931). Case of asbestos-like bodies in the lungs of a coal miner who had never worked in asbestos. *Lancet* **2,** 632–633
Vyskočil, J., Tůma, J. and Macek, M. (1970). Relationships between morphological changes and content of silica and hydroxyproline in bronchi and lungs of coal miners. *Int. Arch. Arbeitsmed.* **26,** 157–166
Wagner, J. C. (1970). Complicated coal workers' pneumoconiosis. In *Pneumoconiosis. Proceedings of International Conference, Johannesburg 1969,* edited by H. A. Shapiro, pp. 306–308. Cape Town; Oxford University Press
Wagner, J. C. (1972). Etiological factors in complicated coal workers' pneumoconiosis. *Ann. N.Y. Acad. Sci.* **200,** 401–404
Wagner, J. C. and McCormick, J. N. (1967). Immunological investigations in coal workers' disease. *J. R. Coll. Physns, London.* **2,** 49–56
Wagner, J. C., Wusteman, F. S., Edwards, J. H. and Hill, R. J. (1975). The composition of massive lesions in coal miners. *Thorax* **30,** 382–388
Wagner, M. M. F. and Darke, C. (1979). HLA-A and B antigen frequencies in Welsh coal workers with pneumoconiosis and Caplan's syndrome. *Tissue Antigens* **14,** 165–168
Walker, W. C. and Wright, V. (1967). Rheumatoid pleuritis. *Ann. rheum. Dis.* **26,** 467–474
Walton, W. H., Dodgson, J., Haddon, G. G. and Jacobson, M. (1977). The effect of quartz and other non-coal dusts in coal workers' pneumoconiosis. Part I: Epidemiological studies. In *Inhaled Particles IV,* edited by W. H. Walton, pp. 669–700. Oxford; Pergamon Press
Ward, R. (1961). Pleural effusion and rheumatoid disease. *Lancet* **2,** 1336–1338
Waters, W. E., Cochrane, A. L. and Moore, F. (1974). Mortality in punctiform type of coal workers' pneumoconiosis. *Br. J. ind. Med.* **31,** 196–200
Watson, A. J., Black, J., Doig, A. T. and Nagelschmidt, G. (1959). Pneumoconiosis in carbon electrode markers. *Br. J. ind. Med.* **16,** 274–285
Wehr, K. L., Johanson, W. G., Chapman, J. S. and Pierce, A. K. (1975). Pneumoconiosis among activated carbon workers. *Archs envir. Hlth.* **30,** 578–582
Weinstein, I. M. (1959). A correlative study of the erythrokinetics and disturbances of iron metabolism associated with the anaemia of rheumatoid arthritis. *Blood* **14,** 950–966
Weiss, W. (1969). Cigarette smoking and diffuse pulmonary fibrosis. *Am. Rev. resp. Dis.* **99,** 67–72
Weller, W. (1977). Long-term test on Rhesus monkeys for the PVPNO therapy of arthracosilicosis. In *Inhaled Particles IV,* edited by W. H. Walton, pp. 379–386. Oxford; Pergamon Press
Wells, A. L. (1954a). Pulmonary vascular changes in coalworkers' pneumoconiosis. *J. Path. Bact.* **68,** 573–587
Wells, A. L. (1954b). Cor pulmonale in coal worker's pneumoconiosis. *Br. Heart J.* **16,** 74–78
Williams, E. (1934). 'Curious bodies' found in the lungs of coal workers. *Lancet* **2,** 541–542
Wusteman, F. S., Gold, C. and Wagner, J. C. (1972). Glycosaminoglycans and calcification in the lesions of progressive massive fibrosis and pleural plaques. *Am. Rev. resp. Dis.* **106,** 116–120
Zahorski, W. (1961). Pneumoconiosis dans l'industrie du graphite artificial. *Proceedings XIII International Congress on Occupational Health, New York,* pp. 828–832
Zoll, P. M., Wessler, S. and Schlesinger, M. J. (1951). Interarterial coronary anastomoses in the human heart with particular reference to anaemia and relative cardiac anoxia. *Circulation* **4,** 797–815

9 Silicates and Lung Disease

Silicates (defined in Chapter 2) both of natural or synthetic origin, may be of fibrous or of tabular, equant, prismatic and acicular (needle-like) crystalline habits. As some natural silicates are capable of causing serious disease— notably the asbestos group— whereas others cause no evident clinical disease and are experimentally inert, the general, but uninformative, term *silicatosis* is better not used.

ASBESTOS-RELATED DISORDERS

The association of asbestos minerals with disease can be placed in two broad categories.

(1) *Disorders proved to be related to asbestos exposure*
- (a) Hyaline plaques of parietal pleura.
- (b) Diffuse interstitial pulmonary fibrosis (DIPF), that is asbestosis.
- (c) Carcinoma of lung associated with asbestosis.
- (d) Malignant mesothelioma of pleura and peritoneum.
- (e) Skin corns.

(2) *Disorders which may be related to asbestos exposure*
- (a) Benign pleural effusion and diffuse thickening.
- (b) Carcinoma of lung in the absence of asbestosis.
- (c) Carcinoma of larynx.
- (d) Other forms of neoplasia.

The terminology employed for such widely disparate disorders should be free of any ambiguity. Cooke (1924) named the diffuse intrapulmonary fibrosis '*asbestosis*' by analogy with 'silicosis', and the term was restricted to this sense until recent times. Lately, however, there has been an unfortunate tendency to use it indiscriminately for other asbestos-related disorders. To safeguard against avoidable confusion, therefore, this term should be confined to its original sense: that of a *fibrotic pneumoconiosis*. It is confusing, and imprecise to refer to the other disorders, including plaques of the parietal pleura which is not 'lung', as 'asbestosis' (*see* Definition of pneumoconiosis, p. 1).

The estimated number of asbestos workers, 'at risk' in the UK in 1958 was 18 700, in 1967, 20 000 and in 1970, 30 000. But the figures do not include the unknown number of persons working regularly or intermittently in the vicinity of asbestos operations. In the USA the estimated number of 'exposed workers' was 1 600 000 in 1975 (National Cancer Institute, 1975).

CLASSIFICATION AND CHARACTERISTICS OF ASBESTOS MINERALS

Asbestos (α+σβετοσ, unquenchable) is a collective term for some of the metamorphic fibrous, mineral silicates of the *serpentine* and *amphibole* groups (*see* Chapter 2). They have different genetic, physical and chemical properties, but share in common a fibrous form or habit.

The importance of strict adherence to mineralogical terms in regard to the asbestos minerals is referred to briefly in Chapter 2, p. 38. But it is also essential that the sense in which the term 'fibre' is used should always be stated clearly and unambiguously because the length-to-breadth, or *aspect*, ratios which distinguish fibres from other crystal habits have not been precisely defined. In general, mineralogists have taken a particle with a length-to-breadth ratio of 10:1 or more (to which the term 'acicular' could hardly apply) to be a 'fibre'. If it is assumed that the average width of the fundamental fibrils of asbestos is 100 nm (the range lies between 20 and 200 nm) then a fibril 1 mm in length has an aspect ratio of 1000:1; one 10 μm in length, a ratio of 100:1; and one 1 μm in length, a ratio of 10:1. Although some very short fibres are present in natural, untreated asbestos the majority have aspect ratios around 100:1 or more. In milled asbestos most of the particles (some of which are cleavage fragments and not fibres) have aspect ratios which range from 5:1 to 20:1 or more and, in the case of chrysotile, mostly greater than 50:1. But for

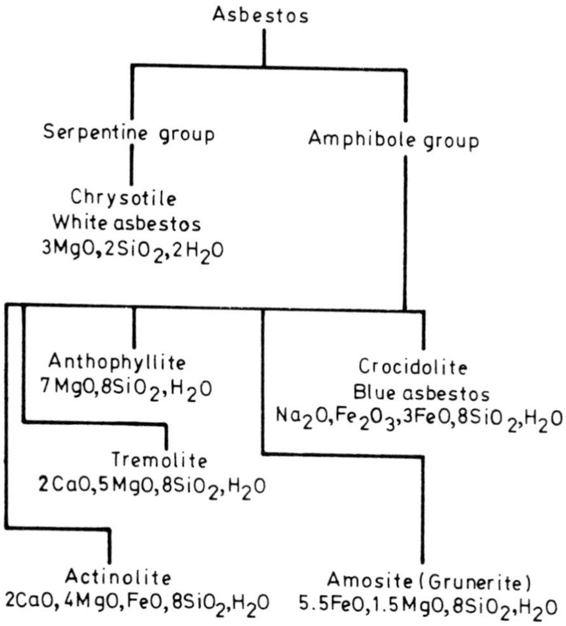

milled non-asbestos amphiboles the ratio of the majority of particles (most of which are cleavage fragments) is less than 3:1 (Campbell, 1978; Zussman, 1979). Unfortunately, in recent years a 'fibre' has been arbitrarily defined in medical, environmental and other non-mineralogical literature as a mineral particle 'the length of which is at least three times greater than its diameter'. The definition given by the US Occupational Safety and Health Administration (1974) is referred to in Chapter 3, p. 46.

Departure from generally accepted mineralogical terminology may result in all amphiboles and a number of other minerals being included in the term 'asbestos'; and, by defining a 'fibre' as a mineral particle having an aspect diameter of 3:1 or more all acicular, prismatic cleavage fragments become 'fibres' and, by implication, all amphibole 'fibres' thus become 'asbestos'. And although acicular fragments or particles are not fibres, are not composed of fibrils and are not flexible they may be indistinguishable from asbestos fibres on routine electron microscopy. Furthermore, the use of the term 'asbestiform' to describe a mineral which may on occasion occur as 'asbestos' and produce 'fibres' (according to the 3:1 criterion) when crushed is misleading. Examples of this are tremolite (*see* p. 297) and nephrite (an actinolite-tremolite or Greenstone jade) which, as a result of altered terminology, become 'asbestiform' minerals and their acicular fragments, 'asbestos-like fibres'. Such alterations in definition may result in the false conclusion that if all amphiboles are 'asbestiform' and their fragments 'asbestos-like' then 'asbestos' will be ubiquitous in most minerals and rocks and, thus, present in many non-asbestos materials used in industry (Zoltai, 1978, 1979). Anthophyllite, tremolite and actinolite, which are all rock-forming amphiboles, occur in prismatic, monoclinic, crystalline form far more commonly than in fibrous form.

The foregoing considerations are essential to the interpretation of reported pathological, epidemiological and animal studies, and possible health hazards. Zussman (1979) has suggested that the boundary between the aspect ratios of asbestos minerals and non-asbestos amphiboles should be at least 10:1.

Economically and technically the most important forms of asbestos are chrysotile, crocidolite, and amosite (grunerite). Anthophyllite, actinolite and tremolite have little commercial value owing to their limited availability and low tensile strength. *Asbestine* is the term loosely applied to various grades of talc some of which contain substantial amounts of tremolite and anthophyllite (*see* pp. 39 and 298).

Chrysotile is mined extensively in Canada in the Provinces of Quebec, Ontario and British Columbia chiefly by open cast methods and, to a lesser degree, by underground mining. It is also mined in South Africa and Zimbabwe, in Russia, China and, to a limited extent, in Italy, Cyprus and the USA. The production of amphiboles is almost entirely confined to South Africa. Crocidolite occurs in isolation in North Cape Province ('Cape Blue asbestos') and amosite in the Eastern Transvaal. But smaller deposits of crocidolite, which are noteworthy for their close association with amosite, are exploited in the Malips River area of the Eastern Transvaal ('Transvaal Blue asbestos') and veins of both amphiboles are often found in the same reef (Hodgson, 1977). This is probably significant in some instances of disease which have been attributed to amosite exposure only (*see* p. 286).

Since the introduction of the asbestos minerals into modern industry in 1878 their production and consumption

Table 9.1 World Production of Asbestos

Year	*Chrysotile*	*Crocidolite*	*Amosite*	*Anthophyllite*	*Total*
1920	184 100	2801	727	Nil	187 628
1950	928 500	28 500	37 850	11 350	1 006 000
1977	4 961 000	178 000	60 000	2000	5 223 000
Countries of origin	Canada USA South Africa Europe USSR China	South Africa	South Africa	Finland South Africa	

*All the figures indicate metric tonnes

(Information on the Russian contribution to World Production is incomplete but by 1950 is computed to be approximately one-third of the total)

[By courtesy of Cape Industries, Ltd.]

have grown to enormous proportions (*see Table 9.1*). Because crocidolite has been particularly associated with malignant mesothelioma stringent regulations have virtually banned its use in the UK since 1970 but in Western Europe, the USA and Japan imports have continued to increase. It is of interest that there appear to be no records showing that crocidolite was ever imported to Southern Ireland where the estimated total consumption of chrysotile and amosite in 1952 was 2884 metric tonnes and in 1973, 6611 metric tonnes. Imports of amosite to the UK have fallen gradually from 26 944 metric tonnes (the highest in the 1960s) to 10 139 metric tonnes in 1977 (Asbestos Information Committee, 1975 and 1978).

Chrysotile fibres are long, white, soft, flexible and often curly but there is some variation in these physical features in fibre from different regions. Crocidolite and amosite fibres are blue and brown respectively, shorter than those of chrysotile, stiff and straight; in addition, amosite is more brittle and has less tensile strength than the other two (*see Figure 9.1*). Tremolite looks fibrous but is brittle and tends to break down into 'chunky' fragments.

The physical properties which make the asbestos minerals invaluable are fire resistance, poor conduction of heat and sound; the facility with which chrysotile, and to a lesser extent crocidolite, can be woven into fabrics; resistance to acids and chemicals (except for chrysotile); electrical resistance, and mechanical strength.

Asbestos fibres, even as single fibres of 'submicroscopic' size, from the environment or the lungs can be accurately identified and analysed by means of standard transmission electron microscopy fitted with energy dispersive X-ray analytical equipment (Pooley, 1975).

It is sometimes said that asbestos is indestructible, but this is not correct. It is true, in general, that the various asbestos types possess good resistance to weathering and to heat but at certain temperatures all decompose. Chrysotile breaks down to forsterite (an anhydrous silicate, Mg_2SiO_4) and silicon dioxide (SiO_2) between 800 and 850 °C; crocidolite breaks down between 800 and 900 °C; amosite, between 600 and 900 °C; and anthophyllite, between 850 and 1000 °C (Hodgson, 1966). Hence, under industrial and other conditions which generate high temperatures, decomposition will occur. Forsterite is not known to have any harmful effects (*see* p. 316).

Uses of asbestos and sources of exposure

Uses

It is impossible to enumerate all past and present uses: for chrysotile alone these were already extensive in the 1930s (Ross, 1931) and, for all forms of asbestos, have more recently been estimated to be over a thousand (Hendry, 1965).

The manufacture of *asbestos-cement products* consumes the greatest quantity of asbestos fibre; these products consist of tiles, corrugated roofing, gutters, water and drain pipes, chimneys, pressure piping and flat sheets. The fibre, which is mainly chrysotile, acts as a reinforcing agent. Fibre is milled to appropriate size mixed with cement as a slurry and then passed on to a conveyer to make sheeting, or into moulds for making pipes and other shapes. Water is then extruded and the product air-cured for some 28 days. Sheeting and pipe sections require cutting to desired size specifications. In the UK the quartz content of the cement mixture is negligible but in the USA it may average about 18 per cent and present a silicosis risk.

The *floor tiling industry* takes the next largest quantity of chrysotile. Some 10 to 30 per cent of short fibre acts as a reinforcing agent and filler in asphalt floorings and with organic resins for vinyl tiles. In the manufacture of tiles, fibre is added to the mix in controlled amounts from a hopper, pressed into sheet form, calendered and cut to required size and shape. Asbestos–asphalt mixtures have been suggested as road surfacing material.

Fibre is used widely for *insulation and fireproofing*. Low-density asbestos-cement products are made in sections for pipe and boiler covering; amosite mixed with calcium silicate or light-weight magnesia has similar use as well as an important place for lining ships' bulkheads. Until the late 1960s laggers mixed chrysotile or amosite and, occasionally, crocidolite with water by hand and applied the mixture after stripping away pre-existing lagging—an unavoidably dusty job. Insulation, fireproofing and soundproofing is also done by spraying a fibre mixture (chrysotile or amosite with inorganic binders in water) on to walls, ceilings, girders and spandrils of buildings, and ships' bulkheads. Crocidolite has also been used for the same purpose. This technique has been extensively used in shipbuilding and repair since the middle of the Second World War.

Asbestos textiles employ chrysotile, crocidolite to a lesser extent, and sometimes both together; but crocidolite has not been used in the UK since 1970. Other types of fibre are unsuitable. Fibre freed of extraneous matter is mixed with cotton, hemp or man-made fibre; then carded, spun, woven, braided or plaited, and calendered. Until recent times these were dry and potentially dusty processes (though, in many cases, well protected by exhaust ventilation) but now they are wet. Fibre is first blended in a slurry and then extruded into a coagulant to form tough, wet strands which are conveyed to the spinning or other machines. The process continues in the wet state so that dust emission is eliminated. Carding is now usually done by an enclosed wet dispersion process. Asbestos textiles have a wide range of uses: for fire-protective clothing, gloves, hoods and leggings, fire barriers, blankets and safety curtains, conveyer belts, brake and clutch linings, wicks for oil heaters and lamps, ropes, flexible tubings, and packings for groutings, autoclaves, ovens and the like. Fire-protective clothing consists of chrysotile only and since the mid-1960s has been sealed by an 'aluminized' coating; this prevents any release of fibre, increases heat resistance and renders it lighter to wear.

Chrysotile is the main constituent (about 80 per cent) of *asbestos paper products* which include millboard, insulating papers, engine gaskets, roofing felts, wall coverings, soldering pads, cooking mats and flooring felt.

Another very important application of chrysotile is in *friction materials*—most notably brake linings and clutch facings—which consist of about 60 per cent of fibre in combination with phenolic resins, polymers, graphite, barytes, metals and pigments.

Chrysotile 'floats' are used in paints and welding rods and to re-inforce thermosetting and polypropylene plastics. Machining and grinding asbestos-reinforced plastics may release a small amount of fibre. Chrysotile 'flock' has an extensive application in filters for wines, beers, drugs and other fluids.

A limited use of crocidolite (but important from the point of view of disease potential) was in the manufacture of respirator filters—especially gas masks during the Second World War. Chrysotile has found unusual uses as 'snow' in motion picture production, for Christmas decoration, and for the manufacture of Santa Claus whiskers (Ross, 1931). It has also been incorporated into the filter tips of cigarettes in the USA but not, as far as is known, in Britain (Tobacco Research Council, 1970).

Anthophyllite has a much more restricted application, being used as a filler in rubber and plastics. However, it has the oldest history having been employed in the making of cooking pottery in Finland since about 2500 BC (Noro, 1968). Of least importance are actinolite (which is rare) and fibrous tremolite, but they find some use as fillers and filter materials.

Although it is possible to substitute other materials for asbestos in some products, for many—especially those for safety purposes—the asbestos minerals are irreplaceable; and their importance is likely to increase in the future where, for example, large quantities of low cost structural materials are required.

Sources of exposure

The asbestos risk is low in opencast mining of chrysotile and, as the serpentine rocks in which it occurs contain no quartz, there is no risk of silicosis.

Amphibole asbestos is obtained mainly by underground methods which involve drilling, blasting and shovelling. The related rocks (banded ironstones) contain significant amounts of quartz. Dust is controlled by 'wetting down' methods. The asbestosis risk is low but silicosis may occur. Although pure fibre was present in the final milling process in a crocidolite mine (closed in 1966) in Western Australia, quartz was also present in dust from the crushers and shakers, and in the early stages of milling. Under such conditions asbestosis and silicosis may occur together (McNulty, 1968).

Gangue from the mines ('cobs') may contain 90 per cent or more rock and less than 10 per cent asbestos. Long fibre is extracted by 'hand-cobbing', that is, gentle hammering to dislodge attached rock; otherwise the bulk of the gangue is crushed, screened, sieved and air-lifted. In this way seven grades of milled fibre ranging from that suitable for textiles to that appropriate for cements, roof coatings, floor tiles, plastics and other filler purposes are produced. These were dusty processes until the late 1940s but application of wet methods or total enclosure have since effectively eliminated pollution of the working environment by milling plants at the mine and by 'fiberizing' processes in the factory.

Bagging of fibre was commonly a dusty operation until the 1960s when the introduction of pressure-packing of all fibre types in 'leak-proof' bags of polythene-lined hessian or woven polythene was introduced. Previously bags consisted of hessian only and were readily damaged in transit resulting in substantial leakage of fibre. Hence, dockers working in the holds of ships and in dock-side warehouses were intermittently exposed to a dust hazard and, to a lesser degree, so were truck drivers and loaders. The transport of bags in sealed containers has eliminated this risk at all stages. Regulations in the UK which enforce these measures are referred to on p. 296.

Mixing fibre for manufacturing processes has been, and exceptionally may still be, productive of much dust. The application of insulation and lagging materials (in which the fibre was often loosely-bound crocidolite) was also a dusty process until the late 1960s, since when little or no asbestos has been used in these products. So far as is known no crocidolite fibre has been imported into the UK for industrial purposes since 1970. The dismantling of old lagging produces large amounts of dust unless special precautions are taken. Men who built and maintained steam locomotives were often exposed to asbestos lagging materials. Spraying fibre on walls, ceilings and the like is a potential source of high local concentrations of airborne fibre. Spraying deckheads and bulkheads, lagging and stripping operations, and sweeping up of debris in the confined spaces of ships and submarines have, in the past, all been especially culpable; and, in many instances, dust was dispersed for considerable distances from its source (Harries, 1976). As might be expected shipbreaking is a potential source of high concentrations of dust.

Power drilling and sawing of asbestos boarding with high-speed tools produces significant quantities of fibre-containing dust but much of the fibre is captive in cement fragments and of 'non-respirable' dimensions, though some fibres—most of which are shorter than 5 μm—may escape (Nicholson, 1976). There is no risk when these operations are carried out with slow running tools and handsaws in the open air or in well-ventilated areas, and special precautions are not necessary. However, continuous runs with power tools, particularly in confined spaces, may produce hazardous dust levels close to the operator's face and extraction equipment (preferably attached to the tool) is required (Asbestos International Association, 1979). It is of interest that a woman who was reported during her life to have asbestosis as a result of helping her husband build a hut in the 1940s, for which he hand-sawed asbestos cement sheets, was found when she died in 1972 to have no evidence of asbestosis or of asbestos exposure but chronic fibro-caseous tuberculosis (Elmes, 1966, 1974).

Abrasive sanding and grinding of asbestos boards is always dusty and requires exhaust ventilation.

Filing and grinding brake linings may release some chrysotile fibres but the amount of free fibre in brake drums is rarely greater than 1 per cent of the total wear products (Hickish and Knight, 1970; Lynch, 1968). The high flash temperatures generated during braking exceed those at which chrysotile is decomposed (Carroll, 1962) (*see* p. 235) so that the asbestos content of brake emissions is usually substantially lower than 1 per cent (Lynch, 1968; Speil and Leinewerber, 1969; Hatch, 1970); indeed the overall average is often as low as 0.07 per cent (Anderson *et al.*, 1973; Jacko, Du Charme and Somers, 1973). However, Rohl *et al.* (1977) demonstrated the presence of minute chrysotile 'fibres' (invisible by light microscopy) in brake drum dust, and a low level of airborne fibre in the breathing zone of garage mechanics. But there is good reason to believe that these particles are probably harmless as almost all were shorter than 0.4 μm (*see* p. 73, Chapter 4, and p. 254, this Chapter). A recent German investigation indicates that the risk from these processes is slight (Fortschungbericht Asbest, 1978). Nevertheless, special precautions should be taken during brake maintenance and the flushing of drums with compressed air (Knight and Hickish, 1970). But it should be noted that for a short period during and after the Second World War crocidolite was employed in the manufacture of special brake blocks in the UK with subsequent development of cases of malignant mesothelioma (*see* p. 294).

Asbestos textile industries and insulation processes, therefore, offered the greatest asbestos risk until recent years and mining of asbestos, the least.

Unexpected sources of past exposure include the operation of machines for twisting asbestos string round welding rods (a dusty job often done by women in the 1930s) and the use of asbestos rope or fibre, either dry or wet, to grout bricks in furnaces and kilns; and, in the USA, the manufacture of cigarette filters containing crocidolite. Because furnace and kiln workers and some insulation workers in ships who use asbestos materials as well as refractory bricks for lining boilers are often known as 'brick layers' their exposure to asbestos may not be suspected. Demolition workers, too, may have been exposed intermittently to an asbestos hazard when breaking up old lagging and other types of insulation. It should be noted, incidently, that there is no risk to arc welders using equipment with asbestos-coated electrodes as the temperatures generated by the arcs are greatly in excess of those which cause decomposition of all types of fibre (*see* p. 235).

Men cleaning and maintaining exhaust ventilation ducts and dust disposal units in asbestos processing factories may be exposed to high concentrations of dust; and laundry workers may have been potentially at risk from asbestos used in lining rollers and ironing machines, and for insulation. Small numbers of chrysotile fibres may be released from old and worn fire protective garments (Bamber and Butterworth, 1970; Lumley, 1971), but 'aluminized' coating of more recent garments prevents this completely.

'Para-occupational' sources

During work done by others in their vicinity, workmen who themselves have never used asbestos materials may have been exposed to it intermittently in varying degree over many years. Important examples, of such 'indirect' exposure are maintenance fitters and electricians in asbestos-processing factories; stokers, fitters and others in boiler houses, power stations, and ships around whom insulation operations involving stripping, lagging and spraying have been carried out; and plumbers, welders and carpenters who may have been in proximity to insulation being applied often in the form of spraying.

Non-industrial

Residents in the immediate vicinity of asbestos-mines and dumps or processing factories from which exhaust effluent carrying the dust was discharged into the outside air may have been exposed to significant atmospheric contamination. In general, this latter practice is long past in Britain although it continued well into the 1950s in some European countries. Air samples taken recently from the vicinity of a textile factory in Britain and examined by a sensitive X-ray diffraction technique were not found to contain chrysotile asbestos (Rickards and Badami, 1971), though the authors did not state whether or not sampling coincided with peak production in the factory. Attention has also been drawn to a past potential hazard to housewives who laundered their husbands' dust-contaminated overalls in the home (Newhouse and Thompson, 1965), although it has to be remembered that, prior to and during the Second World War women often worked in the asbestos industry themselves before marriage—a point which has sometimes been overlooked.

In view of public anxiety about asbestos materials it should be noted that environmental exposure in the home and elsewhere from products in which fibre is captive is highly improbable. Such products include floor tiles, partitions, ceiling panels, roofing, pipes and installed thermal and acoustic insulations (Walther, 1970). However, vinyl-asbestos floor tiles may be a source of minor exposure during installation and sanding (Murphy *et al.*, 1971a). If sprayed-asbestos insulation is not protected from damage by efficient sealing it may become friable so that fragments fall on the floor, ledges and elsewhere where they may collect and thus become a possible source of low level exposure (Lumley, Harries and O'Kelley, 1971).

Asbestos is also used in many domestic appliances such as electric toasters, iron rests, cooker door-seals, boilers, hair-driers and the like. But the amount of fibre released is non-existent or minute. Heavy routine use of new electric toasters and portable hair-driers and repeated opening and shutting of oven doors with both good and worn seals have been shown to release either no fibres at all or minute numbers ranging from 0.01 to 0.18 fibres/ml and, in the majority of samples, less than 0.08 fibres/ml (Asbestos Research Council, 1976).

The use of chrysotile sheets for filtration of beers, wines and drugs yields, on average, 10^{-8}g fibre/litre of fluid and is not known to have any harmful effects (Asbestos Information Committee, 1976). Fear is sometimes expressed that pollution of urban air by fibre released by braking vehicles may endanger public health. When levels of fibres in the air have been analysed, however, they have been found to be at least 1000 times less than the TLV for industry (Asbestos Information Committee, 1976). Sampling of environmental air in Paris revealed an average concentration of chrysotile and amphiboles of 0.5 ng/m^3 (Sébastien *et al.*, 1976). Chrysotile was found in low levels (only a few ng/m^3 of air) in 49 American cities and in somewhat higher levels in New York City during the period when asbestos spraying of 'sky-scraper buildings' was permitted. It is improbable, however, that such minute concentrations of asbestos as observed in these surveys offer a danger to public health.

Perspective

It is important to emphasize that substantial exposure to asbestos minerals is necessary to cause asbestos-related disorders; that is, the cumulative dose of asbestos is a vital determining factor. This relationship is strongest in the case of asbestosis but somewhat weaker, though nonetheless evident, in the case of malignant mesothelioma and parietal pleural plaques (*see* appropriate Pathogenesis sections). Hence, while the potential hazard of asbestos in industry is clear and it is imperative that strict hygiene control is applied to the manufacture and use of asbestos products, there is no reason to believe that casual contact with asbestos fibre, handling of the numerous available asbestos-containing products, sailing in asbestos-treated ships or living and working in buildings with asbestos-containing insulation and appliances offer any risk of disease. Occasional reports to the contrary are infrequently found to have any scientific foundation when critically examined and alarmist statements based on supposition or inadequate evidence are wholly unjustifiable. But, of course, physicians and medical scientists must be unceasingly vigilant concerning this aspect of public health.

It is unfortunate that in recent years sensational and misleading television and radio programmes and newspaper articles on the subject have been, and remain, a source of anxiety to asbestos workers and their families; an anxiety which is heightened if 'asbestosis' is diagnosed. Referring to such television features a leading article in the *British Medical Journal* (1978a) gave this sober advice which applies equally to other forms of communication: 'The test to be applied should be objective: is the programme likely to confuse, worry or misinform patients?' It is imperative, therefore, that the clinician should have an accurate and balanced knowledge of the degree of risk which may have been involved in past occupations or may exist in the present and of the relevance (or otherwise) of any associated respiratory disorder so that he may give appropriate advice and confidence to his patient (or healthy worker) and family.

AERODYNAMIC BEHAVIOUR OF ASBESTOS FIBRES

The aerodynamic behaviour of fibrous particles is, as pointed out in Chapter 3, determined differently from that of compact particles. This is important not only in explaining the degree to which fibres penetrate to the depth of the lungs but also in the design of dust sampling instruments.

The 'free falling speed' (*see* Chapter 3) of fibres is determined by the square of their diameter and is little influenced by their length. Hence, a fibre with a length of 200 μm or more and a diameter of about 3 μm has the same 'free falling speed' as a unit density spherical particle of 10 μm diameter; that is, the fibre has an 'equivalent (aerodynamic) diameter' of 10 μm (Timbrell, 1965). Fibres with a diameter of less than 3 μm will tend to escape *sedimentation* and *inertial impaction* suffered by those with a greater 'free falling speed' and so penetrate to the level of respiratory bronchioles (Timbrell, 1970), although many very long fibres are captured by nasal hairs. The greater the length of a fibre the more likely it is to suffer *interception* by the decreasing diameter of peripheral airways (Timbrell, Pooley and Wagner, 1970). Furthermore, the flexural modulus—or degree of *harshness*—of fibres appears to be of particular significance. Most amphiboles are harsh and stiff even when extremely fine but most chrysotile fibres are soft, or semi-harsh, and curly (*Figure 9.1*); harsh chrysotile fibres (which are relatively rigid) have little commercial use (Speil and Leineweber, 1969). The curling of long soft chrysotile fibres renders them more liable than rigid amphibole fibres to interception higher up the small airways (Timbrell, 1970). This effect may ensure that more chrysotile fibres are intercepted on the ciliary 'escalator' than pass deeply into the non-ciliated region, whereas more amphibole fibres (such as crocidolite) penetrate beyond the reach of ciliary clearance. But as both short and long chrysotile fibres possess the same radii of curvature short fibres, having short arcs, are virtually straight and thus behave aerodynamically like amphibole fibres and are equally capable of reaching the periphery of the lung (Timbrell, 1973). However, due to the selectivity of the lungs the relative concentrations of chrysotile and

(a)

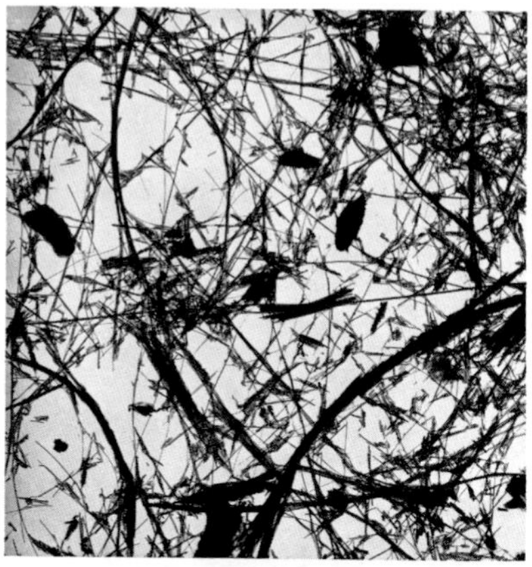

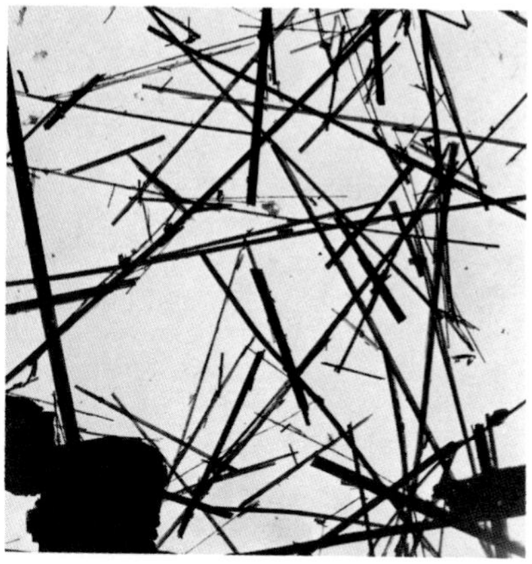

(b)

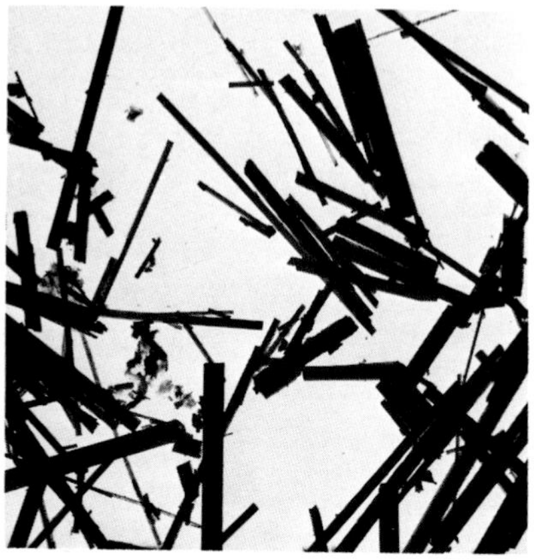

(c)

(d)

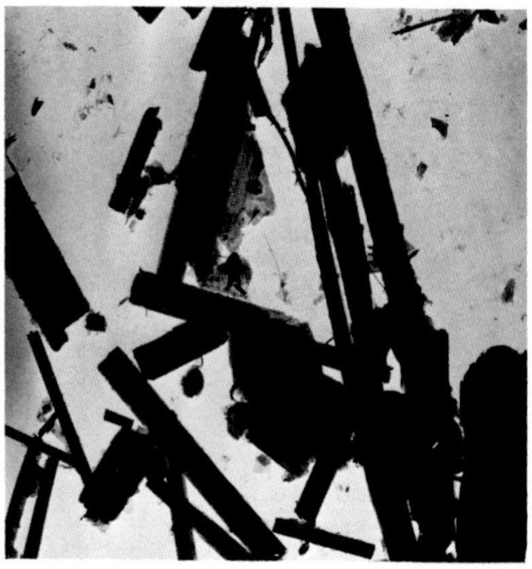

Figure 9.1 Electron micrographs showing characteristics of the four important asbestos fibre types: (a) chrysotile; (b) crocidolite; (c) amosite; (d) anthophyllite. (Original magnification × 4500 reproduced at quarter scale. By courtesy of Dr F. D. Pooley)

amphiboles are not representative of the dusts to which the individual was exposed.

Fibres found in the alveolar regions of the lungs are less than 3 μm in diameter, their mean diameter being usually less than 1 μm (Timbrell, Pooley and Wagner, 1970). It appears that the longest fibres tend to be found in the respiratory bronchioles and alveolar ducts, and short fibres deeper in the acini (Timbrell, Pooley and Wagner, 1970). Some fibres—or fibrils—are beyond the resolution of the optical microscope and their diameter may be as small as 0.010 μm (Timbrell, Pooley and Wagner, 1970). To what extent the difference in aerodynamic behaviour determines pathogenesis remains to be clarified but long fibres in and beyond respiratory bronchioles are probably mainly, if not exclusively, responsible for the DIPF of asbestosis (*see* Chapter 4 and p. 254).

The demonstration by Timbrell (1975) that asbestos fibres of respiratory size can be aligned in magnetic fields and, under these conditions, possess distinctive light scattering patterns when illuminated by a laser beam is a great advance in the estimation of fibres in air samples and in dust recovered from human and animal lungs, in providing indices of fibre size, and in aiding identification of the geographical origin of asbestos.

Because of earlier difficulties in comparing experimental results obtained by different laboratories due to differences in the type and quality of asbestos materials used, standard UICC reference samples of chrysotile and the amphiboles have been prepared for international use since the late 1960s (Timbrell and Rendall, 1971/2) and should be specified in all reported studies.

ASBESTOS BODIES (COATED ASBESTOS FIBRES)

The first clear description of these bodies was by Marchand in Leipzig in 1907 though he did not associate them with asbestos fibres or exposure. They have been found in the lungs following as little as two months' occupational exposure to asbestos (Simson and Strachen, 1930). They are long structures, 20 to 150 μm in length and 3 to 5 μm in diameter, golden yellow or brown in colour, each of which consists of an asbestos fibre wholly or partly coated with layers of iron-containing protein. This coat, which stains blue with Perl's reagent, is usually segmented giving a 'string of beads' appearance and both ends of the 'body' are bulbous or swollen. Some bodies, however, show little segmentation. Ultimately they disintegrate and various stages of degeneration down to beaded fragments in phagocytes and extracellular dark brown segmented granular fragments are seen (*Figure 9.2*). Electron microscopy indicates that uncoated fibres greatly outnumber asbestos bodies and may be found in their

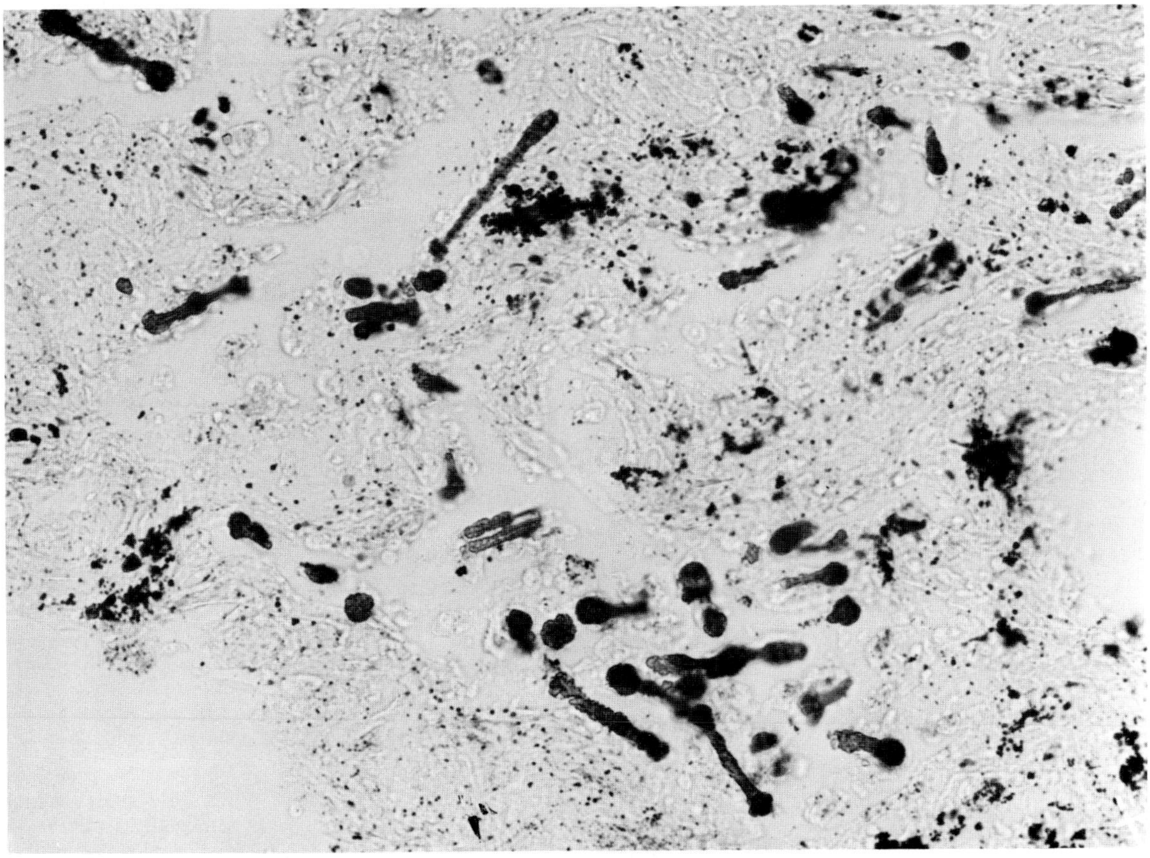

Figure 9.2 Asbestos ('ferruginous') bodies in an unstained 30 μm section of lung with asbestosis. There are long segmented bodies with clubbed ends and others which are shorter and stumpy. Fragments of bodies are scattered throughout the field in the centre of which a short, partly coated fibre is seen. A few small aggregations of carbon particles are also present. Compare these bodies with coal and graphite bodies which have thick, black cores (Figure 8.7)

absence (Langer *et al.*, 1971; Pooley *et al.*, 1970; Ashcroft and Heppleston, 1973). In advanced asbestosis several million fibres may be recovered from 1 g of dried lung tissue (*see* Diagnosis, p. 265). Bodies may form on all types of asbestos fibres though only occasionally on chrysotile (Pooley, 1972). This seems to be explained by the fact that chrysotile is cleared from the lungs more rapidly than the amphiboles, tends to split into fibrils and, because its magnesium readily leaches out, probably breaks up and dissolves. But short fibres are sometimes coated (Langer, Rubin and Selikoff, 1970). In general, bodies form on asbestos fibres longer than about 40 μm and rarely on those less than 10 μm; in other words, the longer the fibre the more likely it is to be coated (Morgan and Holmes, 1980).

In asbestosis asbestos bodies and uncoated fibres are found singly or in groups in association with carbon-laden macrophages in and adjacent to the fibrosis in the walls of respiratory bronchioles (Heard and Williams, 1961). In these circumstances the bodies are, on the whole, found with little difficulty by light microscopy, thus indicating occupational exposure. Asbestos bodies are not found in malignant mesothelioma tissue but short or fragmented bodies have been identified in parietal pleural plaques (Sébastien *et al.*, 1977).

For routine purposes coated fibres can be demonstrated by light microscopy of slides on to which fluid expressed from the base of the lung is placed either directly or after concentration by centrifuge, and is unstained (Whitwell and Rawcliffe, 1971). However, they are more readily identified in unstained 30 μm sections of lung. Using either phase contrast or electron microscopy there appears to be a rough quantitative relationship between the number of coated and uncoated fibres present; the ratio of coated fibres counted by light microscopy to uncoated fibres counted by electron microscopy may range from 1:50 to 1:400 (Ashcroft and Heppleston, 1973; Fondmiare and Desbordes, 1974). Thus, counts of coated fibres made by light microscopy are a valuable routine index of the intensity of asbestos exposure and the uncoated fibre content of the lungs. Identification of fibres in lung tissue is facilitated by potassium hydroxide digestion (Gold, 1967) or by ashing techniques. Stricter methods and standards which are necessary for research purposes are described by Pooley (1973a). (*See* Addendum, p. 332.)

Asbestos bodies can also be detected in the sputum by dissolving the specimen with 4 per cent of sodium hydroxide and examining the centrifuge deposit by direct or phase contrast microscopy. Bodies in swallowed sputum are resistant to gastro-intestinal enzymes and so may be found in the faeces (Gloyne, 1931). Uncoated fibres can be identified by light and electron microscopy in bronchopulmonary lavage fluid and their numbers increase with the duration of asbestos exposure but decrease with the length of time since exposure ceased. The average length of the fibres isolated—which is similar in sputum and lavage fluid—is shorter than those found in the lung tissue of individuals with identical exposures (Bignon *et al.*, 1978a) (*see* p. 254).

In one study asbestos bodies were present in the sputum, or bronchial aspiration in 57 per cent of individuals with 'heavy' occupational exposure to asbestos, 18 per cent of those with 'light' exposure and in none with no exposure. There was no correlation between the number of bodies in the sputum and the duration of exposure but there was with the number of bodies present in surgical specimens of the lung (Bignon *et al.*, 1973). One body found in the sputum is said to correspond to 1000 bodies/cm^3 of lung (Sébastien *et al.*, 1973).

It must be stressed, however, that the finding of asbestos bodies in the sputum does not prove the presence of asbestosis nor of any other asbestos-induced disease but signifies only past exposure to asbestos; equally, failure to find them does not exclude the possibility of asbestos-related disease.

In experimental animals the formation of asbestos bodies has been shown to involve partial phagocytosis of a fibre by alveolar macrophages, accumulation of endogenous iron (ferritin) within the cells and compaction of iron on to the fibres which appear to be coated with a hyaline layer containing acid mucopolysaccharides (Davis, 1965; Governa and Rosanda, 1972; Suzuki and Churg, 1969). Coating increases with time. A similar process may occur in man. Unlike uncoated fibres asbestos bodies lack fibrogenic potential (Vorwald, Durkan and Pratt, 1951).

Specificity of asbestos bodies

'Curious', or pseudo-asbestos, bodies which are often found in lungs with coal or graphite pneumoconiosis have already been alluded to in Chapter 8. Although these may be segmented, are golden yellow and give a positive Prussian blue reaction they are differentiated by the fact that they have a black core and are usually shorter and thicker than asbestos bodies. However, bodies which are indistinguishable may sometimes be found in the lungs of talc workers with or without 'talc' pneumoconiosis and are probably due to fibres of tremolite or possibly, anthophyllite, which may be present in some forms of 'talc' (*see* Talc pneumoconiosis).

Asbestos bodies, or bodies which are closely similar, have been found at autopsy in the lung fluid of 20 to 48 per cent of adults in urban areas with no known exposure to asbestos (Thomson, Kaschula and McDonald, 1963; Cauna, Totten and Gross, 1965; Anjilvel and Thurlbeck, 1966), but their numbers are small by comparison with the quantity found in cases of asbestosis. Intensive searching has demonstrated 'bodies' in almost 100 per cent of city dwellers (Utidjian, Gross and de Treville, 1968). Sections of lung tissue of individuals who died in London between 1936 and 1966 showed that the prevalence of occasional bodies rose from zero in 1936 to 20 per cent in 1966, and that this increase correlated with the cumulative total of asbestos imported into Britain from 1910 onwards (Um, 1970). In the East End of London during the period 1965 to 1966 the prevalence was 42 per cent in men and 30 per cent in women (Doniach, Swettenham and Hathorn, 1975). A similar study in New York, however, showed that the prevalence altered little between 1934 and 1967, being between 53 and 60 per cent (Selikoff and Hammond, 1970), although in lung blocks at the Sinai Hospital in Baltimore it is reported to have risen from 40.9 per cent in 1940–49 to 91.1 per cent in 1970–72 (Bhagavan and Koss, 1976).

Some authorities have doubted that these bodies always contain asbestos fibres pointing out that similar bodies form on filamentous ceramic aluminium silicate fibres, sheet silicates and fine glass fibres under experimental conditions, and that many non-asbestos minerals of fibrous habit are present in the environment (Gross, Cralley and de Treville, 1967; Cralley *et al.*, 1968; Gross, de Treville and Haller, 1969; Wright, 1969; Davis, Gross and de Treville, 1970;

Churg, Warnock and Green, 1979). Thus, the term '*ferruginous bodies*' has been suggested as preferable to 'asbestos bodies' (Gross, Cralley and de Treville, 1967). However, electron microprobe analysis indicates that most of these bodies found in the lungs of the general population contain amphiboles—usually crocidolite or amosite (Warnock and Churg, 1980).

Hence, in spite of this apparent uncertainty and the fact that the nature of the core can only be established indisputably by specialized mineral analysis (*see* Appendix, p. 509)—techniques limited to research laboratories—three practical points can reasonably be made when at least three 30 μm sections from a lower lobe are examined by the optical microscope:

(1) Bodies in which cores are either not apparent or are thin and translucent, and which have golden coloured beading and swollen or globular ends staining blue with Perl's reagent are most probably asbestos bodies.
(2) Their presence in large numbers (that is, easily found) and often in clumps indicates occupational exposure to asbestos but *does not necessarily* establish that coincident intrapulmonary fibrosis has been caused by it (*see* Chapter 4, p. 82).
(3) When only occasional bodies are found after an extensive search past occupational exposure to airborne asbestos is improbable and the lung burden of uncoated fibres is proportionally small.
(4) Ferruginous bodies found in the lungs of city dwellers with no occupational exposure to asbestos are, in many if not most cases, probably formed on amphibole fibres.

DISORDERS PROVED TO BE RELATED TO ASBESTOS EXPOSURE

HYALINE PLAQUES OF THE PARIETAL PLEURA

These are bilateral, discrete, circumscribed, well demarcated, raised areas of fibrosis (often partially calcified) on the inner surface of the rib cage. They are unrelated to past inflammatory disease, haemothorax or trauma. Asbestos exposure has been regarded as a cause of bilateral pleural calcification since the end of the 1940s (Cartier, 1949; Lynch and Cannon, 1948) and, in general, this has been confirmed in the UK, the USA, Canada, Finland and Bulgaria. But identical appearances are also observed in the absence of evident asbestos exposure (*see* Pathogenesis, p. 246).

Prevalence

The reported prevalence of plaques (which are distinct from fibrosis of the pulmonary pleura) varies widely according to a number of factors: (1) whether in occupationally or environmentally exposed populations; (2) whether derived from post mortem or radiographic evidence; (3) the methodological standards of radiographic studies; and (4) whether calcified or non-calcified plaques only are reported.

Radiographic surveys have shown an overall prevalence of about 5 per cent for calcified plaques in asbestos factory workers in London, Dresden, Bulgaria and Czechoslovakia; from 14 to 39 per cent in insulation workers in the UK, Denmark and the USA (Jones and Sheers, 1973), and from 5 to 17 per cent for calcified and non-calcified plaques in shipyard workers in the UK and the USA (Edge, 1976; Ferris *et al.*, 1971; Harries *et al.*, 1972; Langlands, Wallace and Simpson, 1971).

Pleural plaques have also been observed radiographically in South African crocidolite and amosite miners, Canadian and Italian chrysotile miners (Jones and Sheers, 1973) and anthophyllite miners (Kiviluoto and Meurman, 1969; Raunio, 1966); and in a small proportion of people who lived in the vicinity of asbestos mines and factories, and among relatives of exposed workers (Jones and Sheers, 1973). By contrast, in a survey of 3868 radiographs of individuals aged 40 years and older attending chest clinics in the Birmingham area (UK) there was no evident association between pleural shadowing, with or without calcification, and asbestos exposure (British Thoracic and Tuberculosis Association/MRC Pneumoconiosis Unit, 1972).

At autopsy an overall prevalence of plaques of 39.3 per cent was found in two urban populations (one of which was an anthophyllite mining community) in Finland with asbestos bodies in the lungs of 57.6 per cent (Meurman, 1966). They were present in 11.2 per cent of 134 consecutive cases in London and 12.3 per cent of 334 cases in Glasgow with asbestos bodies evident in the lungs of those with plaques (Hourihane, Lessof and Richardson, 1966; Roberts, 1971). However, in 198 randomized autopsies in Copenhagen in which hyaline plaques were present in 66 (33 per cent) asbestos bodies were found in only 14; but the technique for their detection may not have been adequate (Francis *et al.*, 1977). Hence, evidence of asbestos exposure is not apparent in all cases of pleural plaques.

As both hyaline and calcified plaques must be sufficiently dense to be visible on the standard chest radiograph their prevalence in radiographic surveys is lower than in post-mortem surveys. Only 15 per cent of the cases of plaques observed post mortem by Hourihane, Lessof and Richardson (1966) were detected during life.

From radiographic evidence prevalence seems to be related to intensity of exposure to asbestos. For example, in a naval dockyard 28 per cent of the men with continuous exposure were found to have pleural thickening compared to 1.9 per cent among those slightly and intermittently exposed (Sheers and Templeton, 1968). A similar relationship was observed in 150 cases of pleural calcification among 1117 New York insulation workers (Selikoff, 1965). In Belfast insulation workers the frequency of both pulmonary and pleural abnormality increased from 13 per cent of those who worked less than 10 years to 85 per cent in those who had worked 30 years or more (Langlands, Wallace and Simpson, 1971). Analysis of measured dust exposure in relation to radiographic appearances, however, indicates that, given a certain minimum initial exposure, the development of pleural calcification is related to age (Rossiter *et al.*, 1972). In general, about 20 years from first exposure is required before calcification can be identified (Selikoff, 1965). Thus, plaques are more common in individuals over 40 years of age than those under, but occasionally cases have been encountered in young people with environmental exposure in childhood.

Of particular importance is the fact that bilateral calcified or hyaline plaques and asbestosis (intrapulmonary fibrosis) do not necessarily occur in conjunction. The post-mortem study of 56 cases of pleural plaques by Hourihane, Lessof and Richards (1966) showed microscopic evidence of asbestosis in only 24 cases (43 per cent) although asbestos bodies were present in the lungs of all. A similar observation was made by Cartier (1965) who found microscopical asbestosis in 29 per cent of pleural plaque cases. In one radiographic study of asbestos workers with hyaline plaques evidence of asbestosis was detectable in 46 per cent (Navrátil and Dobiáš, 1973). My own experience indicates a corresponding lack of correlation between the presence of plaques and evidence of asbestosis both pathologically and clinically. Implications of this interesting situation are discussed further under Pathogenesis.

In short, bilateral pleural plaques are most commonly associated with past occupational exposure to asbestos, less often with neighbourhood exposure near asbestos mines, mills and factories, and most infrequently in the absence of identifiable exposure.

Pathology

Macroscopic appearances

Hyaline plaques are entirely distinct from *diffuse* fibrosis of the pulmonary and parietal pleura which is a common accompaniment of asbestosis.

The lesions are bilateral, though not always of equal degree, and consist of elevated areas of hyaline fibrosis, a few mm to 1 cm thick, which are well circumscribed, of irregular shape with a smooth, polished, slightly convex, ivory-coloured surface which resembles articular cartilage.

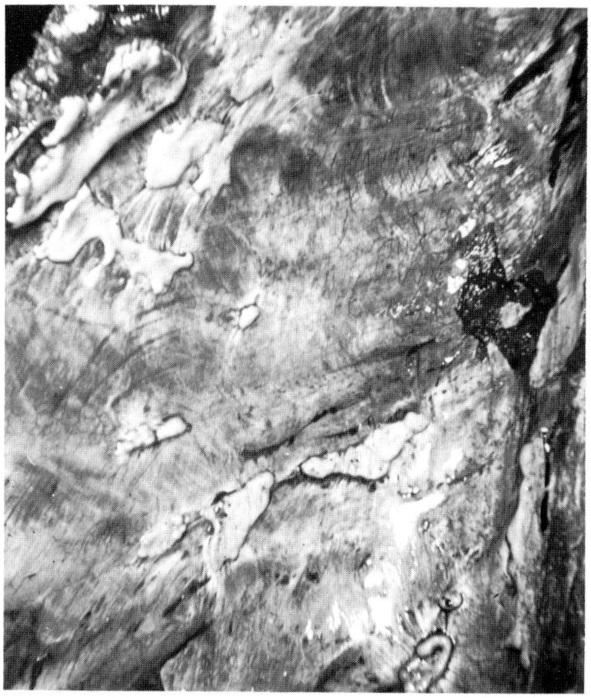

Figure 9.3 Post-mortem appearances of hyaline plaques of the parietal pleura (sternum to left, paravertebral gutter to right). They are flat, irregular in outline, sharply demarcated, smooth, shiny and raised a few millimetres above the adjacent pleural surface. The substernal and paravertebral lesions are elongated in the vertical axis; the contour of some of the others is roughly parallel with the ribs. (Photograph from colour transparency)

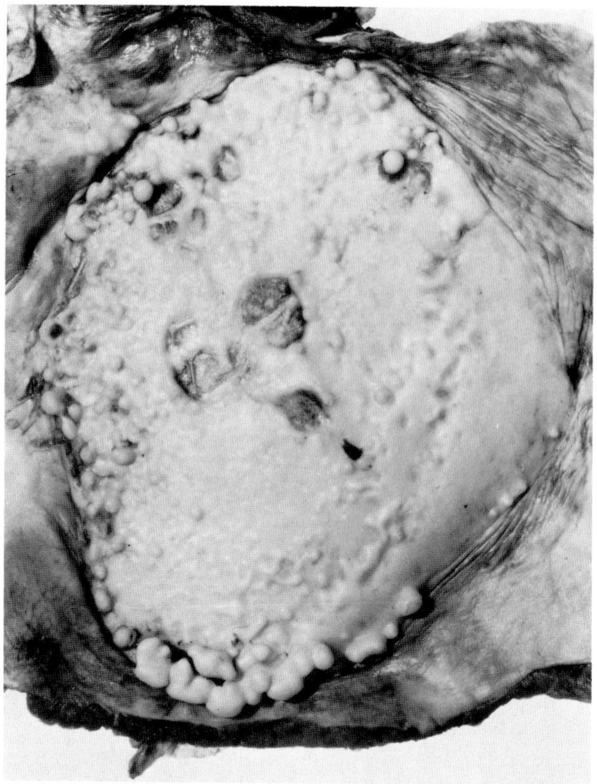

*Figure 9.4 Hyaline plaque over the central tendon of the diaphragm. It is sharply circumscribed, raised above the surface and exhibits both flat and nodular features. On section it was substantially calcified. These lesions (which are invariably bilateral) seen end-on in standard chest radiographs produce densely radio-opaque arcs (*see Figure 9.9*)*

Some are multinodular (the nodules having a mamillated appearance) and others consist of a combination of both forms (*Figures 9.3* and *9.4*). When removed they can be bent like leather. They are distributed irregularly on the inner surface of the rib cage (very rarely in the pulmonary pleura) chiefly in the mid zones anteriorly, laterally and posteriorly—but by no means equally—and tend to follow rib lines, although they are often spread at right angles across one or more intercostal spaces. When very advanced they fuse into large cuirass-like sheets. Their other common locations are along the paravertebral gutters and over the central tendons of the diaphragm. However, they do not occur at the thoracic apices, in the costophrenic sulci or in the mediastinum but are sometimes found in the pleura over the left cardiac border. Irregular areas of calcification of greater or lesser extent are frequently present in the plaques. Fusion of plaques with the pulmonary pleura rarely occurs so that the lungs move over them unimpeded during respiration; and neither is there fusion with the parietal pericardium. Any adhesions which may be present are in areas away from the plaques and only exceptionally are they involved in widespread pleural symphysis.

A proportion of plaques found post mortem or at thoracotomy are not sufficiently radio-opaque to be identified on the standard chest radiograph.

Plaque formation does not appear to occur in the parietal pericardium and is not, therefore, a cause of constrictive pericarditis. Neither are they seen in the peritoneum.

Microscopic appearances

Plaques consist almost entirely of avascular, acellular, laminated collagen fibres arranged parallel to the surface, with hyaline changes, but a few spindle-shaped fibroblasts may be found between the fibres. The appearances resemble 'basket-weave', but in the mamillary nodules the arrangement is concentric like the rings of an onion. In some plaques the fibres stain predominantly for elastic tissue rather than collagen and may be 'pseudo-elastic fibres' due to changes in the composition of collagen (Roberts, 1971). Dystrophic calcification is present in central areas where collagen has undergone degeneration. The surface is usually accellular but, at an early stage of development, appears to be covered by a mesothelial cell lining (Thomson, 1970). The deepest (that is, external) parts show fibroblastic activity with collections of lymphocytes and plasma cells, and there is some vascularity. This indicates that plaques are, in fact, of *extrapleural* rather than pleural origin (Hinson, 1973; Thomson, 1970) (*Figure* 9.5).

(*a*)

(*b*)

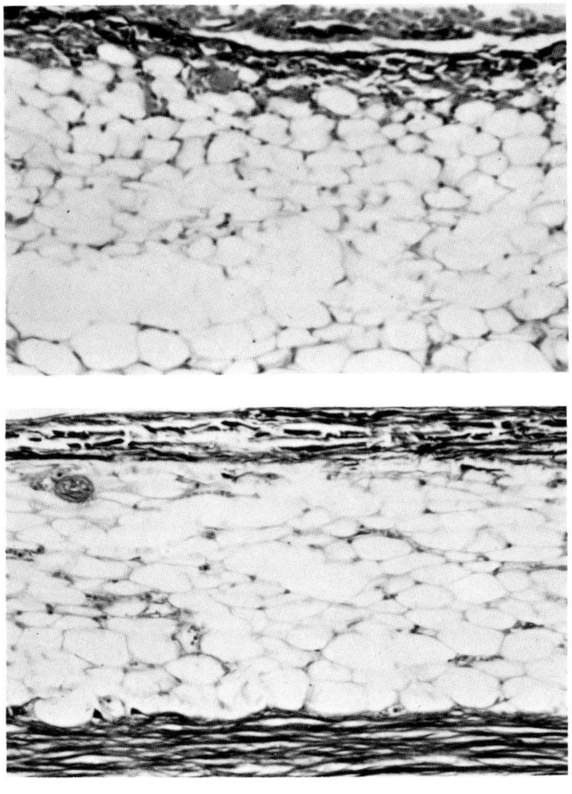

Figure 9.5 (a) Normal parietal pleura with some cellular exudate on surface. (b) Part of a hyaline plaque is seen external *to vascularized extrapleural tissue at bottom of the field. (Original magnification × 80)*

Asbestos or 'ferruginous' bodies can be identified in the lungs of most, but not all, cases and, although these are not visible in plaques by optical microscopy, occasional uncoated fibres may be seen (Thomson, 1970). However, with special chemical extraction techniques electron microscopy has demonstrated the presence of fragments of bodies, bodies shorter than those found in the lungs, and minute submicron fibres of amphiboles and chrysotile within plaques. Chrysotile tended to be concentrated in calcified areas (Le Bouffant *et al.,* 1973; Sébastien *et al.,* 1977). In this respect it is interesting that, in culture, mesothelial cells from the parietal pleura of the rat have been found to engage in phagocytosis of chrysotile fibres shorter than 4 μm (Jaurand *et al.,* 1979). It remains to be seen whether similar events are relevant in human disease.

In about half the cases both macroscopic and microscopic evidence of asbestosis (intrapulmonary fibrosis) is absent.

Pathogenesis

There is little doubt that bilateral pleural plaques are associated with exposure to all types of asbestos, especially anthophyllite; but the questions as to whether there may be some other causal agency, why the lesions are virtually confined to the parietal pleura and are irregular in shape, and why plaques and asbestosis so often occur independently remain to be answered.

Calcified plaques have been observed in individuals in agricultural communities with no known exposure to asbestos (Zolov, Burilkov and Babadjov, 1967; Navrátil, Morávkova and Trippe, 1978) and, in one such community in Czechoslovakia, they were also encountered in cattle in the same area (Rous and Studený, 1970). It is of particular interest, too, that in the Canadian (Quebec) chrysotile mining complex calcified plaques were found to be very common in workers in four mines, rare in those in four other mines and absent among men in yet another and largest mine which is not far distant from the rest (Cartier, 1965). These observations raise the possibility that asbestos may not be the causal agent. A recent study of 15 689 men in the Quebec industry in fact suggests that pleural calcification is related to some characteristic of airborne dust or a mineral closely associated with chrysotile, but as yet unidentified, in some mines (Thetford) but not in others (Gibbs, 1979). And an association of the non-asbestos mineral zeolite with calcified pleural plaques is referred to on p. 318.

On the other hand, in a tobacco-growing region of Bulgaria where pleural plaques are endemic among the human population, soil samples demonstrated the presence of small amounts of anthophyllite, tremolite and sepiolite (*see* p. 314) derived from out-cropping rocks (Burilkov and Michailova, 1970). Thus, although it is true that advanced techniques for identifying mineral fibres in the lungs have not been used in all reported studies and that chrysotile has been identified in plaques, it seems likely that these lesions are not due exclusively to asbestos minerals.

But assuming that asbestos minerals are responsible for most pleural plaques it is not clear by what route they reach the parietal pleura. It has been suggested that sharp fibres in the lungs penetrate the pulmonary pleura during respiration and pass directly into the parietal layer, possibly causing traumatic micro-haemorrhages and fibrin deposition (Thomson, 1970; Heard and Williams, 1961). Although, this hypothesis is compatible with plaques being sited predominantly where respiratory excursions are greatest it is unlikely as plaque formation is not preceded by episodes of inflammatory disease or fibrinous exudates (Meurman, 1968), adhesions between plaques and the pulmonary pleura are absent and, as already stated, they apparently originate on the external aspect of the parietal pleura. It is possible that they may gain access via lymphatic vessels. Fibres which are too long to be taken up by a single macrophage and are poorly cleared from the lungs are largely responsible for intrapulmonary fibrosis (asbestosis), whereas small fibres which are completely engulfed are carried either to the ciliary 'escalator' or into the lymphatic system (*see* Chapter 4). In fact, the mean length of fibres found in the lungs and pulmonary pleura has been shown to be greater than those in the parietal pleura (Le Bouffant *et al.*, 1976). Hence, fibres which reach the superior and inferior tracheobronchial lymph nodes may pass via the anterior broncho-mediastinal lymphatic vessels to the retrosternal lymph nodes and via the posterior vessels to the internal intercostal lymph nodes, and from these sites gain

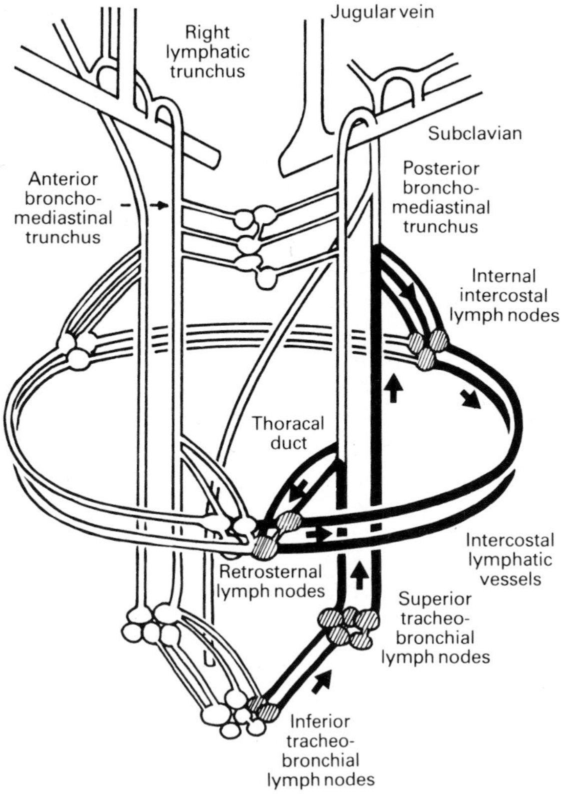

Figure 9.6 Diagram of the thoracic lymphatic system. The hypothetical routes by which dust particles may be transported is shown by black vessels and arrows. (Adapted with permission of the authors and the Editor of Chest *from Taskinen* et al., *1973)*

direct access to the intercostal lymphatic vessels which run along the upper and lower margins of the intercostal spaces on the outer surface of the pleura (von Hayek, 1960). Although this entails passage through valves against the direction of normal flow it is evidently possible as coal dust can be demonstrated in these vessels in cases of coal pneumoconiosis (Taskinen, Ahlman and Wiikeri, 1973) and may be due to a 'suction pump' action during inspiration (*Figure 9.6*). A similar process could operate in the network of lymphatic vessels in the diaphragm. Furthermore, the blood supply of the two pleural layers is different.

The common inverse relationship between asbestosis and pleural plaques might be explained by such differential distribution of fibres of different mean lengths, but there is an obvious objection: if short fibres (< 15 μm) are not fibrogenic in the lungs why should they be so in the parietal pleura? Do genetic or immunological factors (or both) influence events? It is important to establish whether there is any significant difference in HLA antigens in individuals with plaques only, asbestosis only or both together which might determine different levels of susceptibility or resistance to these processes. The presence of lymphocytes on the external surface of plaques suggests the possibility of cell-mediated immunological activity. There is also *in vitro* evidence that all four asbestos fibre types are capable of activating both the classic and alternative complement pathways (*see* section on Pathogenesis of asbestosis) which may provoke polymorphonuclear leucocytes to produce tissue-damaging enzymes, and macrophages to release a fibrogenic factor (*see* Chapter 4). Although there is an increased prevalence of circulating ANA and RF in asbestosis preliminary observations suggest that this is not true of plaques alone (Stansfield and Edge, 1974).

Clinical features

Whether calcified or not pleural plaques alone are symptomless as they do not hinder the normal respiratory excursions of the lungs; hence, dyspnoea, chest pain, abnormal physical signs, and impairment of lung function are absent (Leathart, 1968; Lumley, 1977). In the absence of accompanying radiographic evidence of diffuse intrapulmonary fibrosis (asbestosis), regional lung function is normal (*see* p. 256). Exceptionally, however, when they are very extensive, widely calcified and cuirass-like there may be some restriction in movement of the chest wall with a mild degree of breathlessness on effort and restriction of ventilation: a severe restrictive defect is highly exceptional.

Radiographic appearances

Plaques are not visible radiographically until the thickness of their fibrous tissue or amount of calcium deposition is sufficiently radiodense. In many cases, therefore, they are not detected during life. But the better the radiographic technique and vigilance of the observer, the more likely they are to be seen. Hyaline plaques are demonstrated best by films taken at about 120 kV and calcified plaques, by films taken at about 80 kV. In addition right and left 45 degree anterior oblique views (as described on p. 96) are an essential complement to the PA film both for the detection and delineation of plaques whether these are on the chest wall or the diaphragm because they display many of them tangentially at maximum radiodensity which the PA film may fail to do (Anton, 1968). These views also possess the important advantage of providing different sight lines of the lungs thus helping to confirm or exclude the signs of intrapulmonary fibrosis.

On the standard PA film uncalcified plaques appear as ill-defined misty opacifications of the middle or lower zones of the lung fields when they lie at right angles, *en face*, to the X-ray beam; or as slightly to moderately protuberant linear or ovoid opacities along the costal or diaphragmatic margins when they are more or less parallel to the beam (Fletcher and Edge, 1970). As a rule these appearances are fairly obvious but slight *en face* haziness and small peripheral opacities (which have a tendency to be contiguous with and run along subcostal rims in the lower mid-zones) may easily be missed if the lung fields are not scrutinized systemically and oblique views omitted (*Figure 9.7*).

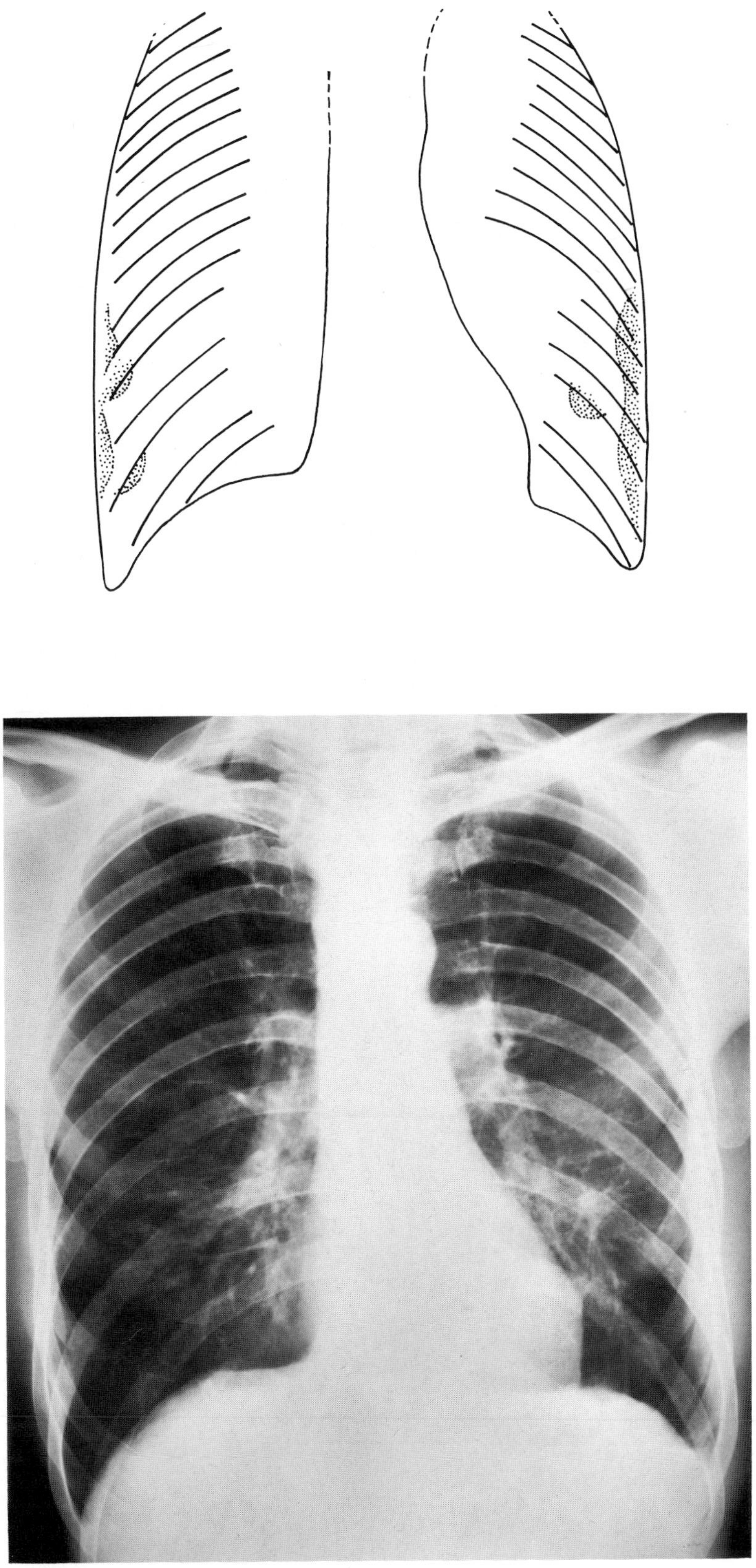

Figure 9.7(a)

(b)

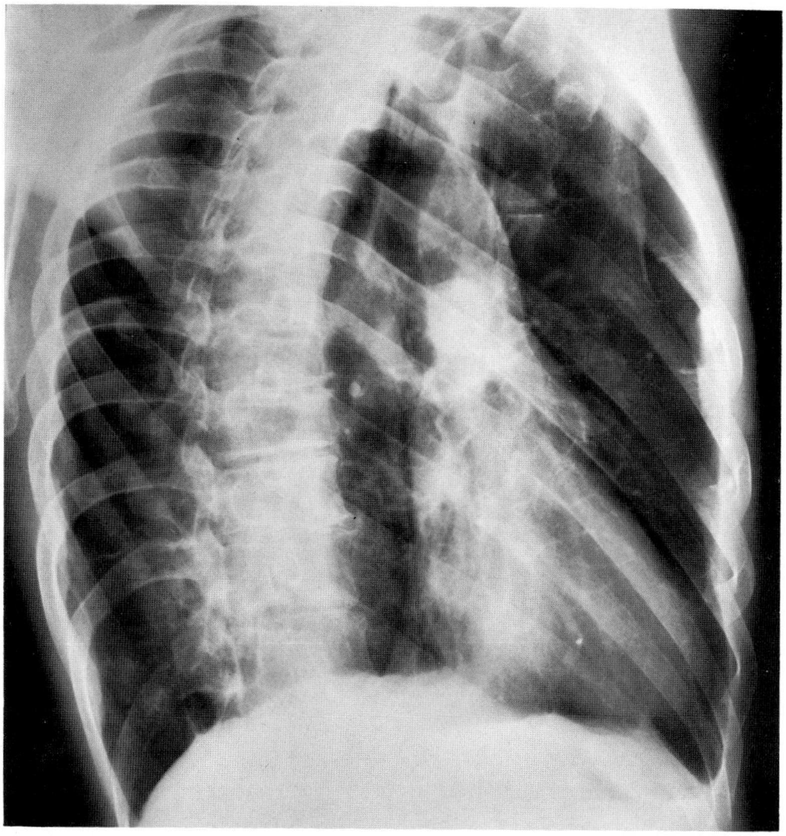

Figure 9.7 Mild hyaline plaque formation visible on both costal margins in the mid and lower zones. (a) The ill-defined haze in the left mid zone is due to a plaque seen en face *(see diagram). (b) Some of the plaques are shown in sharper relief when tangential to the X-ray beam in the right anterior oblique view. Calcification is not evident in any of the lesions. No evidence of DIPF in either film. Insulation worker for 18 years before and after the Second World War*

'Companion shadows' along the lateral chest walls caused by muscular interdigitations or folds of extrapleural costal fat, although uncommon, must be carefully distinguished from uncalcified plaques; they are usually bilateral, but not necessarily symmetrical, and their similarity on the two sides is evident (*see* Chapter 5, *Figures 5.4* and *5.5*). Oblique views are valuable in differentiation.

Calcified plaques *en face* have an irregular, unevenly dense, and sometimes dramatic pattern which has neither a segmental nor a lobar distribution thus indicating their extra-pulmonary site. Peripherally, they are seen as very opaque, usually discontinuous, thick lines along the chest wall, diaphragm or cardiac border (*Figure 9.8*). In many cases, however, the opacities are small and easily overlooked (especially in 'too-white' films) unless they are systemically sought (*Figure 9.15*); they are sometimes seen in the absence of any evidence of plaques on the chest wall. Care must be taken not to mistake calcified costal cartilages for plaques—in particular when these are seen through the shadow of the diaphragm. Radiographic development of calcified plaques is shown in *Figure 9.9*. There should be no confusion between opacities caused by intrapulmonary disease and pleural plaques if anterior oblique views are taken.

Bilateral calcified plaques may occasionally draw attention to unsuspected (if mild) past asbestos exposure. (*Figure 9.10*). However, it must also be emphasized that the appearances of both hyaline and calcified plaques can result from causes other than asbestos exposure (*Figure 9.11*).

Diagnosis

During life this rests entirely on radiographic evidence. Plaques are always bilateral but by no means of equal extent. Bilateral pleural calcification, of course, may also be the result of old tuberculous disease, empyema or haemothorax due to sharp or blunt trauma or other causes, but this is rare and such changes are generally unilateral. Whether calcified or not plaques are distinguished by their sharp outline when viewed tangentially and by their absence from the costophrenic angles and apices of the lung fields. By contrast, diffuse pleural thickening is often ill-defined and irregular irrespective of the angle from which it is viewed, and the costophrenic sulci or lung apices are commonly obliterated.

As stated earlier radiographic evidence of diffuse intrapulmonary fibrosis (asbestosis) is absent in more than half the cases although physical signs and defects of lung function alone may suggest its presence in some of them; so that thorough investigation along these lines is necessary in each subject (*see* next section). In a minority of cases, however, asbestosis may be of advanced degree. Hence, pleural plaques do not indicate the existence of asbestosis any more than do asbestos bodies in the sputum.

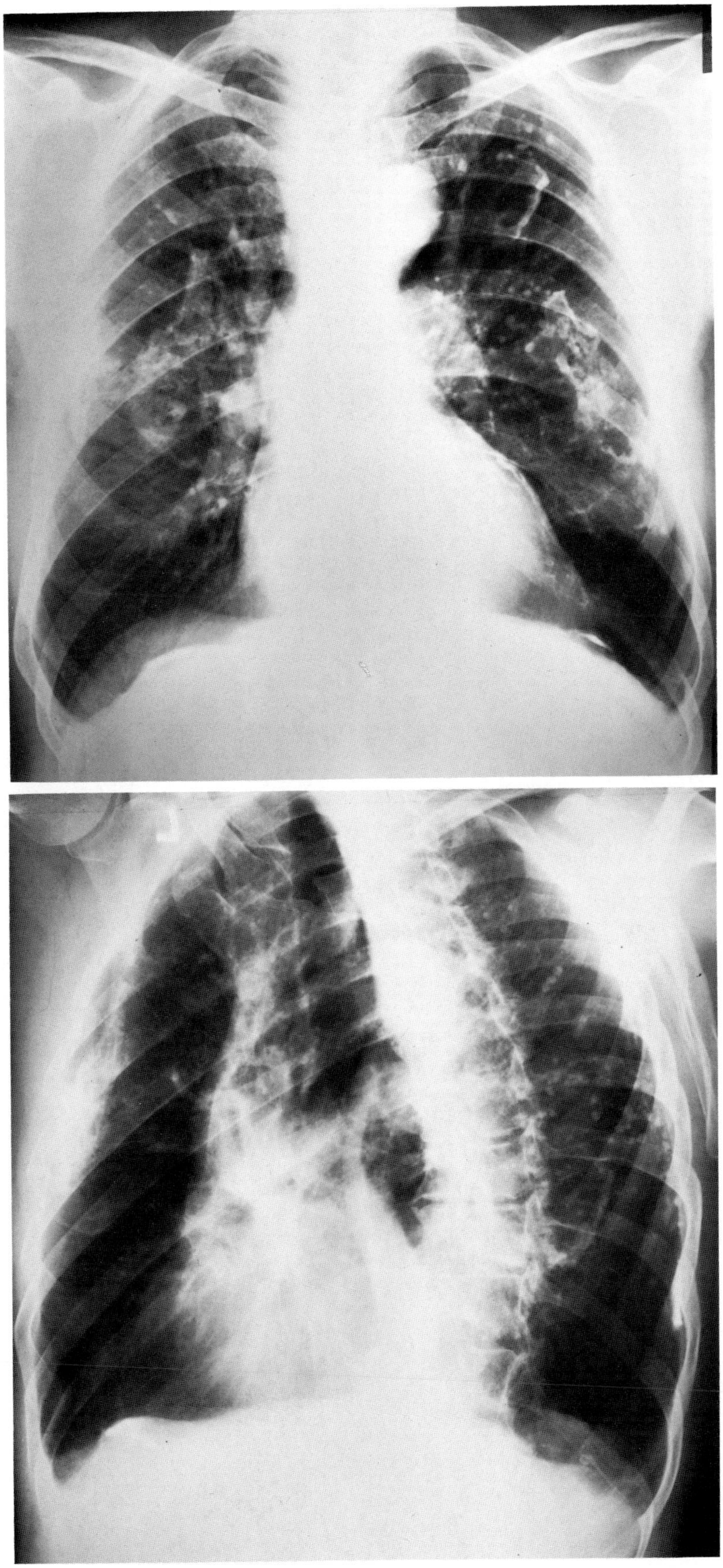

Figure 9.8 Bilateral calcified pleural plaques on chest walls and diaphragm. (a) Note irregular outline and variable density of the large lesion seen en face *and the rim, of calcification along the left cardiac border. The small rounded lesions also represent calcification in plaques and are not intrapulmonary. (b) The large plaque in the right lung field on the PA film is seen end-on against the chest wall (left field). No evidence of DIPF in either film. Ex-insulation worker (1925 to 1932) aged 65. No crepitations in lungs. Lung function: severe airflow obstruction and hyperinflation only*

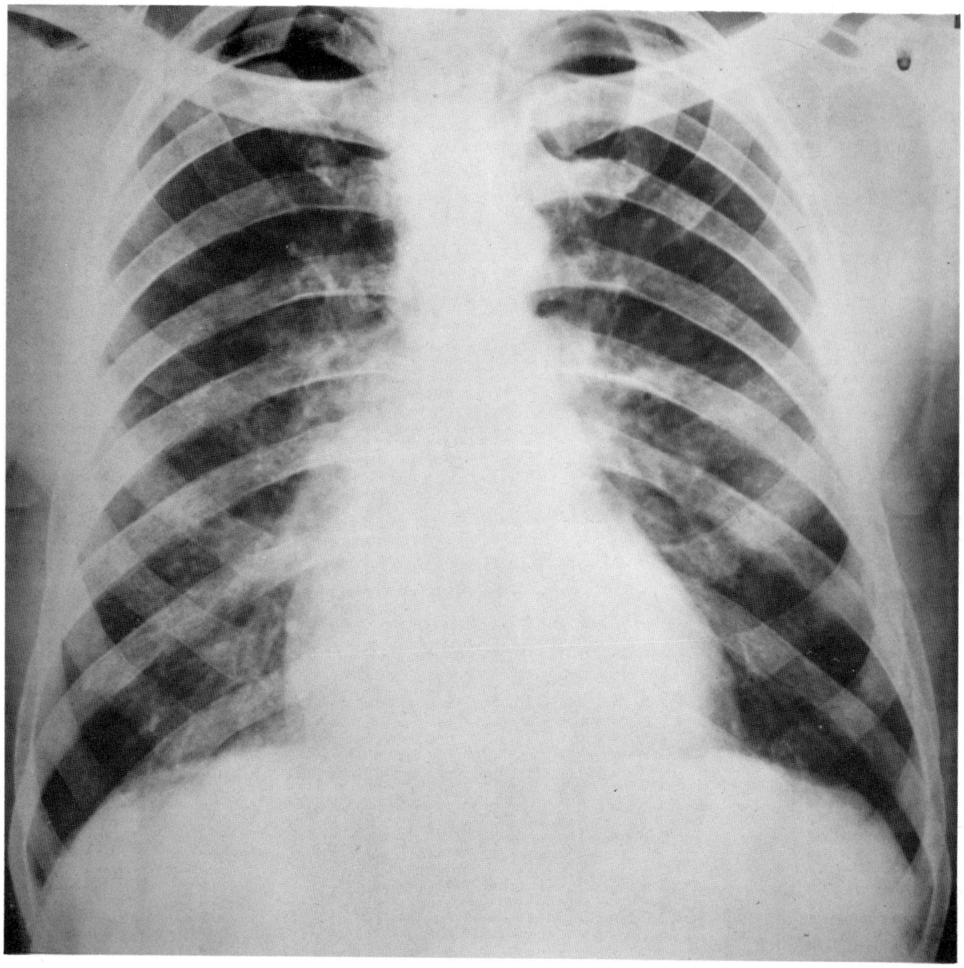

Figure 9.9(a) 1948

In general, dyspnoea in a patient with bilateral pleural plaques is more likely to be due to airflow obstruction with or without emphysema or to cardiovascular disease than to asbestosis: for example, the case illustrated in *Figure 9.8*.

It has also to be borne in mind that the appearances of widespread plaque formation may mask the early signs of tuberculosis and carcinoma of the lung.

Ultrasound techniques are capable of detecting plaques which are invisible on conventional radiographs but they are not practical for routine purposes.

Prognosis and complications

Plaques themselves have no effect on life expectancy and are not known to give rise to any complications.

It has been suggested that there may be an increased incidence of lung cancer in individuals with pleural plaques. However, a Finnish study of pleural plaques did not reveal any association between plaques and carcinoma of the lung, but in cases where these lesions coincided lung fibrosis was also present (Kiviluoto, Meurman and Hakama, 1979) (*see* next section). Although a malignant mesothelioma which apparently arose from the surface of a plaque has been reported there is no evidence to suggest that plaques are precursors of this tumour (Lewinsohn, 1974).

To summarize

The pathogenesis of pleural plaques in asbestos-exposed persons is a fascinating enigma but their bilateral presence at autopsy and in chest radiographs is, for practical purposes, like asbestos bodies, an index only of past asbestos exposure if other causes are excluded. They do not imply co-existent asbestosis as clinical and pathological evidence of this is present in less than 50 per cent of cases. On occasion, bilateral calcified plaques are seen in individuals with no known asbestos exposure (*Figure 9.11*).

ASBESTOSIS

Definition

Asbestosis or asbestos pneumoconiosis, first recognized by Murray in 1907, is a bilateral diffuse interstitial pulmonary fibrosis (DIPF) caused by fibrous asbestos mineral dusts.

Incidence and prevalence

Accurate statistics of the incidence and prevalence of asbestosis are few, and valid comparisons between similar

Figure 9.9(b) 1973

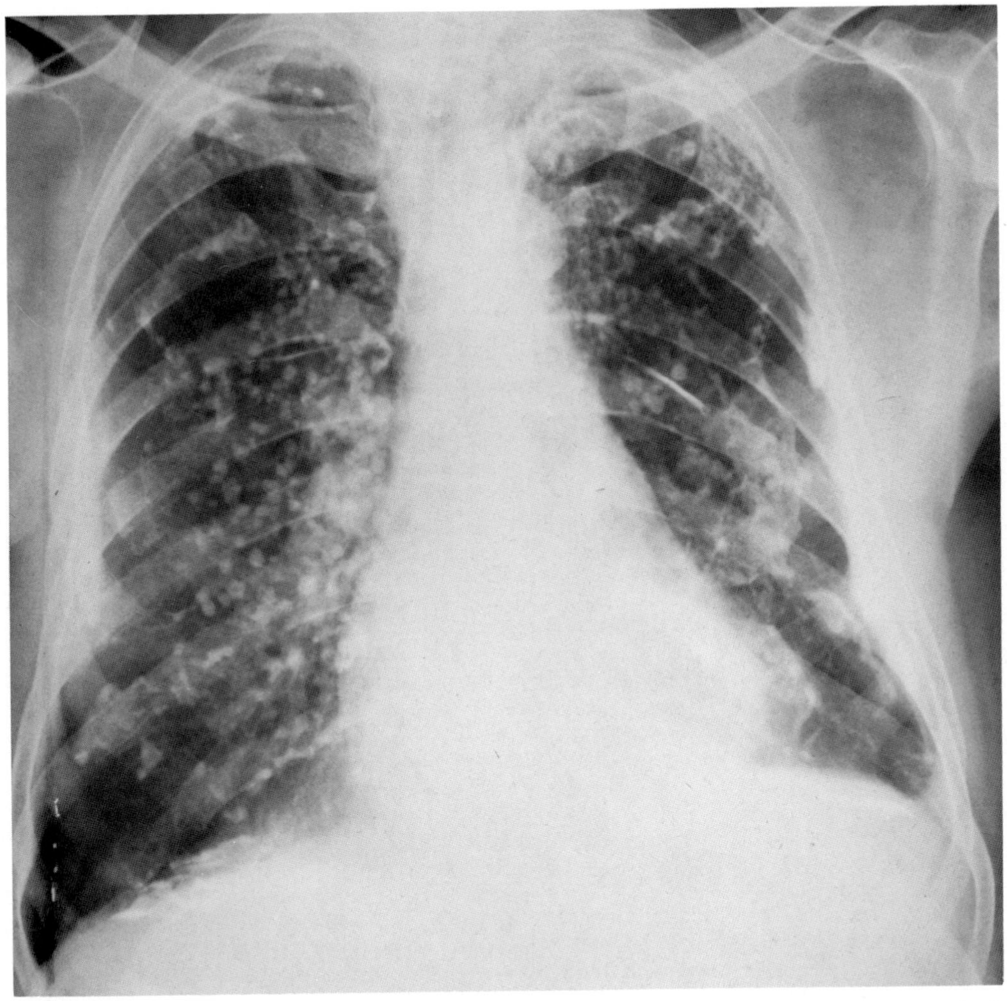

Figure 9.9 Development of widespread calcified plaques of different patterns in costal and diaphragmatic parietal pleura over 25 years (a) 1948, (b) 1973. Asbestos insulation worker 40 years. Died aged 70. Post mortem confirmed parietal pleural plaques. Gross evidence of intrapulmonary fibrosis absent but mild asbestosis demonstrated microscopically with numerous asbestos bodies

and dissimilar asbestos industries in one country or in different countries are not possible. In general, it is true to say that the disease has been most common in persons who worked in milling and disintegrating ore, in heat and sound insulation (lagging, stripping and spraying), and in shipyards. Figures are derived from surveys (usually radiographic) of specific industries, compensation records and death certificates. Cases first diagnosed for compensation purposes (the trend of which in the UK is shown in *Table 1.2*, p. 3) are of little value as they represent only those individuals who have been referred for examination and are not readily related to numbers 'at risk' in the industry in which they worked; and the accuracy of death certificates, in this respect, is severely limited.

Nevertheless, there is no doubt that an overall rise in the incidence of asbestosis occurred in most industrial countries since the 1930s. This was due to the cumulative effect of the years of exposure when there was little dust control; to a great increase in the use of asbestos during and after the Second World War; and to an increased awareness of the existence of the disease and accuracy of diagnosis in latter years. It has also to be remembered that there is a considerable time lag between exposure and development of evident disease. However, where the incidence of asbestosis in longitudinal clinical and radiographic surveys of a given industry is related to dust count records it has been shown to decline with the application of strict dust control measures. Following controls imposed in the UK by the Asbestos Industry Regulations (1931) since 1933 a striking decline in new cases of asbestosis occurred in the asbestos cement and textile industries (Knox, Doll and Hill, 1965; Smither, 1965; Smither and Lewinsohn, 1973); but similar control was not applied to some other industries (for example, insulation) until 1970 (Asbestos Regulations, 1969). In the chrysotile industry in Rhodesia during the period 1963 to 1967, 39 cases of asbestosis were diagnosed in 8336 workers (0.5 per cent) (Gelfand and Morton, 1970) and in South Africa for the period 1960 to 1971, 19 cases in 1350 workers (1.4 per cent) (Sluis-Cremer, 1973).

An 'attack rate' of asbestosis of approximately 0.6 per cent has been observed in a random sample of employees of a British naval dockyard, first examined in 1966, when re-examined in 1977 (McMillan, Sheers and Pethybridge, 1978). And an incidence 1.1 per cent per year over the 6½ years from 1965 to 1972 was found by Murphy *et al.* (1978) in shipyard pipe insulators in the USA. As there was an 80 per

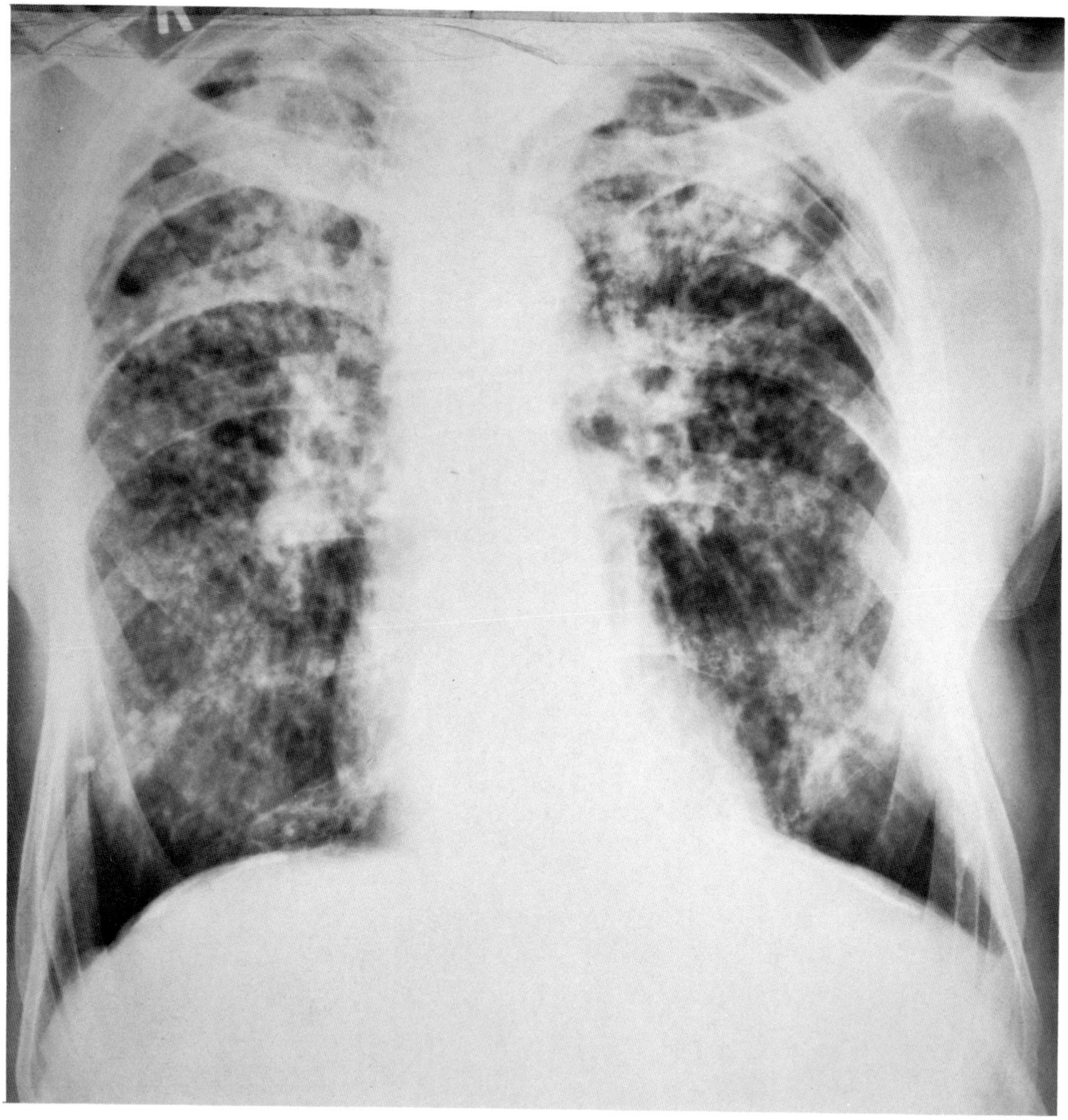

Figure 9.10 Category 3rA silicosis in a crusher and grinder of flint and ochre ore for eight years. This work was done on the same site as an asbestos processing factory. Subsequently odd jobs brought him into close proximity with various parts of this factory for 20 years. Note the dense linear opacities indicative of calcification in both leaves of the diaphragm. Biopsy of lung ten years before death showed numerous asbestos bodies and confirmed silicosis. Post mortem: calcified plaques present in both leaves of diaphragm and smaller plaques on the costal surfaces, but no asbestosis

cent reduction in the total amount of asbestos used in this period this rate is probably an expression of the time lag from the days of heavier exposure.

There is no epidemiological evidence as to whether asbestosis is more likely to develop as a result of exposure to one particular type of fibre rather than another because asbestos workers have, in general, been exposed to different types of fibre in one process or successively in a variety of processes over the years. And, although a survey of asbestos cement workers suggests that exposure to crocidolite may have a greater fibrogenic effect than a similar total exposure to chrysotile (Weill *et al.*, 1977), this is not supported by recent work with animals (Davis *et al.*, 1978).

For the acquisition of systematic prospective information it is necessary to keep accurate records of the types of asbestos used in an industrial process and during what periods, and a diary of fibre count levels obtained by accurate sampling instruments in workers' breathing zones and in the 'background' air so that these data can be correlated with the development or absence of asbestos-related disease.

The most valuable diagnostic criteria to be sought in periodic surveillance of asbestos exposed working populations are persistent, bilateral, late inspiratory basal crepitations (*see* p. 256), irregular opacities in the chest radiograph (*see* p. 257) and reduction in VC and Tl (*see* p. 257) (Murphy *et al.*, 1978). The order in which these abnormalities first present themselves may, however, differ in individual subjects.

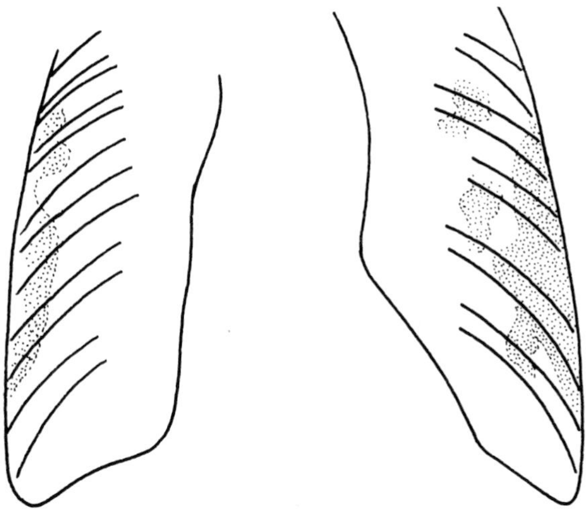

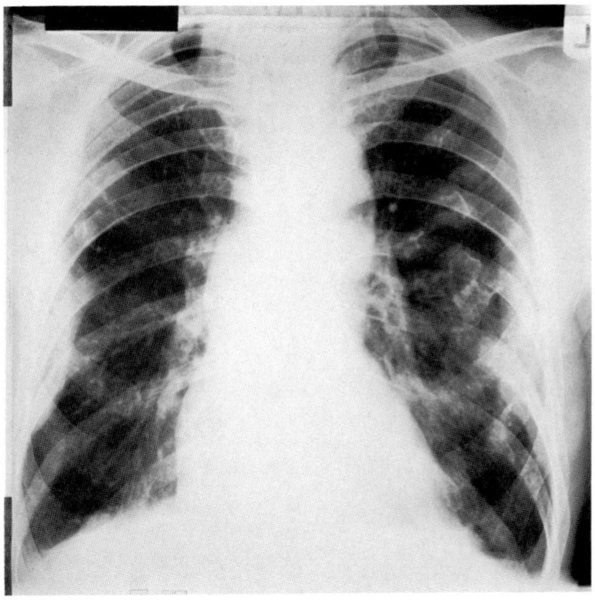

Figure 9.11 Bilateral hyaline and calcified plaques in a coal-miner. No occupational exposure to asbestos. Such appearances may follow the resolution of bilateral pneumothoraces

Pathology

Macroscopic appearances The external features of the lungs depend very much on the extent and severity of disease. The pulmonary pleura in most cases is thickened, varying from a slight, diffuse loss of translucency (due to a thin layer of fibrosis) to widespread fibrosis (with fusion of both pulmonary and parietal layers) which tends to be most evident over the lower half of the lungs. Multiple air cysts (or blebs) are absent. Circumscribed hyaline plaques of the parietal pleura, with or without calcification, may also be present in less than half the cases.

When the lungs are sliced sagittally the appearances vary according to the severity of the disease (*Figure 9.12*). In the early stages its presence may only be discernible to the touch: that is, the tissues feel firmer and more resilient than normal and the pleural margins and subpleural intralobular septa of the lower lobes stand out prominently. With disease of moderate severity these changes are more pronounced and a network of grey-coloured or more deeply pigmented irregular fibrosis is visible in the subpleural regions of the lower lobes and, to a lesser extent in the middle lobe and lingula to a depth of about 1 to 2 cm. When disease is advanced the lower parts of the lungs are pale and much indurated, and the interlobular septa are obviously thickened and fibrosed. At this stage irregular fibrosis is coarse and extends more deeply from the pleura and interlobular septa into the lung. Demarcation from adjacent normal lung tissue is often ill-defined in contrast to most instances of DIPF due to other causes which are usually sharply outlined. Whether slight or advanced the fibrosis is distributed mainly in proximity to the diaphragmatic and posterolateral pulmonary pleura of both lower lobes and, to a lesser degree of the middle lobe and lingula (*Figure 9.12*). In advanced disease the subpleural zones of the bases of the upper lobes may be involved in addition to the more extensive fibrosis of the lower lobes. *Reversal of this predominantly basal distribution points to some other lung pathology and not to asbestosis* (*see* Chapter 4, p. 78 *et seq.*). As a rule the extent of fibrosis is roughly equal in both lungs.

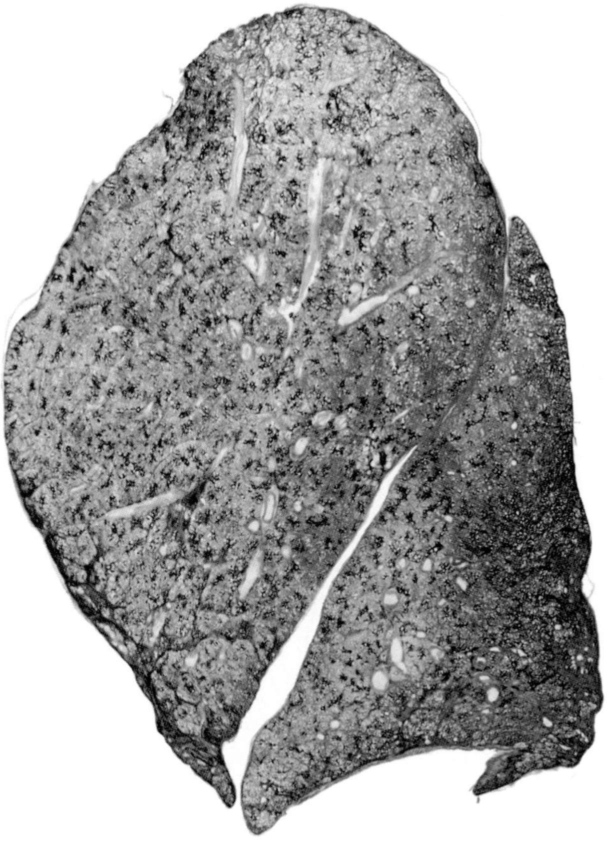

Figure 9.12 Asbestosis of moderate degree involving the posterior and basal zones of the lower lobe which is reduced in size, and the lingula and lower part of the upper lobe anteriorly. The fibrosis is limited to the lower half of the lung, does not involve the more central parts of the lobes and cyst formation is absent. The numerous macules are those of 'city dwellers' lung' due to the deceased having lived and worked in London from the 1920s to the early 1950s. (Compare with Figures 4.14 *and* 4.15*)*

In the early stages of asbestosis there is no evidence of fibrosis either to sight or touch and the lungs are of normal size whereas in advanced disease they are small, pale and rubbery.

The fibrotic areas occasionally contain small cysts within a subpleural zone approximately 1 cm in depth but these are few and rarely larger than 3 mm in diameter, so that a cystic appearance is never more than slight and limited (Hourihane and McCaughey, 1966). Illustrations of widespread irregular fibrosis with multiple large cysts seen in some publications as exemplifying asbestosis almost certainly represent some other pathological process (*see* Chapter 4). In some cases (usually those whose exposure occurred many years ago) there are minute discrete, grey-black macules, 1 to 2 mm diameter, throughout the lungs resembling those seen on 'town dwellers' lung'.

Small, partly pigmented crescents of subpleural fibrosis up to 1 cm thick are occasionally present at the apices of the upper lobes (*see* Microscopic appearances). Rarely, solid masses of grey fibrosis which, as a rule, are not more than about 5 cm in their greatest dimension and are often unilateral have been seen in an upper lobe of individuals whose early work in the asbestos industry occurred before the late 1940s, but not in those who entered later (*see* Pathogenesis, p. 255).

The hilar lymph nodes show no gross abnormality.

It is sometimes said that emphysema (of unspecified type) is a feature of asbestosis but this has not been my experience. Although, in advanced disease some degree of hyperinflation of the upper lobes may exist, irregular (scar) emphysema of the fibrotic lower lobes is not seen. Panlobular emphysema appears to be remarkably uncommon.

Bronchiectasis, recorded in earlier texts, is rarely seen but, if present, is not a consequence of asbestosis which is distributed distal to the bronchi.

Silicotic nodules may be found in the lungs of men who worked crushing and milling ore at asbestos mines and, in the USA in some asbestos cement workers. Rarely large fibrotic masses ('massive fibrosis'), which are also associated with additional exposure to free silica, may be seen. A very rare reported finding is that of necrobiotic nodules of varying size associated with rheumatoid arthritis or circulating rheumatoid factor but lacking the concentric dust pigmentation of typical Caplan nodules (*see* next section).

Microscopic appearances The initial stages of the disease in animals are described in the next section (Pathogenesis). Although some intra-alveolar desquamation of Type I cells seem to occur, there is no evidence that a desquamative fibrosing 'alveolitis' (DIPF) (*see* Chapter 4)—a semi-acute disorder—is a feature of the early stages of human asbestosis. Next, a thin reticulin network gradually evolves in relation to damaged alveolar epithelium and envelops cells and asbestos fibres. Collagenous fibrosis then replaces the reticulin fibres until these alveoli are more or less obliterated. Hence, the primary lesions—the earliest stage identifiable in man—is a plastering of the alveoli from within the lumen of the respiratory bronchioles and not a mural fibrosis (Wagner, 1965). Patchy bronchiolitis obliterans may develop. At this stage structures distal to the respiratory bronchioles are not involved, but later the fibrosis spreads peripherally into the alveolar ducts, atria and alveolar walls obliterating many alveoli especially in the subpleural regions (Gloyne, 1932–33; Caplan *et al.*, 1965; Hourihane and McCaughey, 1966). It is now a DIPF (*Figure 9.13*). In spite of this obliteration the elastic network of alveolar walls is often seen to be intact when elastic tissue stains are used indicating that much of the fibrosis is intra-alveolar (Webster, 1970). But in areas where the fibrosis is solid, alveolar architecture is completely replaced by a mass of collagen which has a peculiarly strong affinity for haematoxylin. Numerous macrophages—some of which contain short asbestos fibres—may be present in neighbouring patent alveoli the walls of which are thickened by fibrosis and cellular infiltration. Prominent hyperplasia of smooth muscle or lymph follicles or excess of elastin (elastosis) are not seen, but condensation of the elastic framework of alveolar walls may be present when fibrosis is advanced owing to collapse and obliteration of many alveolar spaces. Granulomas of foreign body or sarcoid type are absent. This is discussed in more detail in Chapter 4.

Cytoplasmic hyaline material may be present in Type II pneumocytes but appears to be a non-specific reaction to injury (Warnock, Press and Churg, 1980).

Asbestos bodies, intact or fragmented, are usually numerous, and often occur in clusters within and adjacent to areas of fibrosis, in macules of carbon pigmentation and elsewhere in the lungs (*Figure 9.13b*). Ashcroft and

(a)

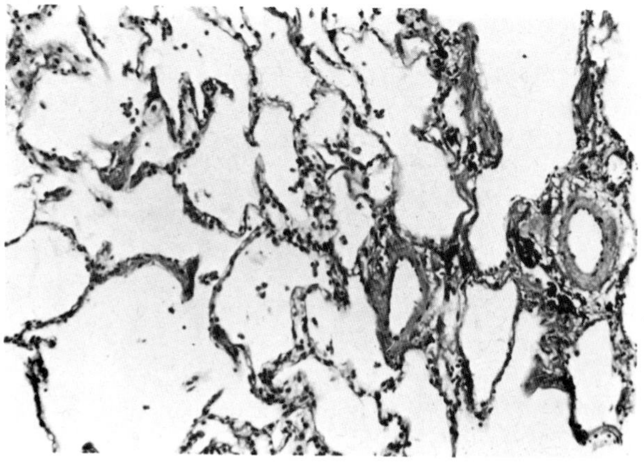

(b)

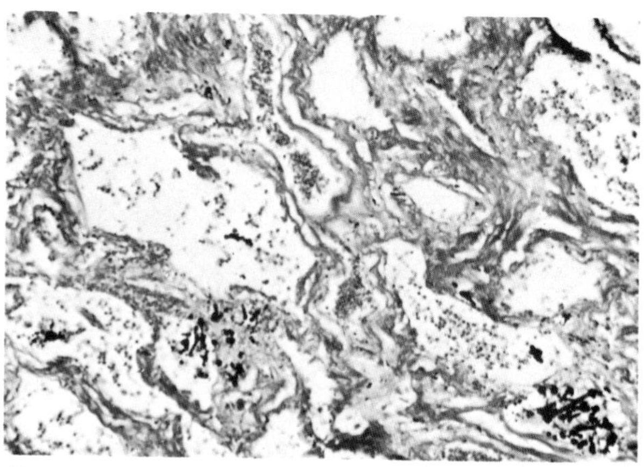

Figure 9.13 (a) Very early stage of asbestosis showing peribronchiolar fibrosis. The alveolar walls are little involved at this stage. (Biopsy: original magnification × 250, reproduced at × 60; van Giesen stain). (b) Asbestosis of moderate to severe degree. Collagenous fibrosis is widespread in the alveolar walls and alveolar spaces are partly obstructed. Clusters of whole and fragmented asbestos bodies which, in the right lower quadrant, are incarcerated by fibrosis. (Original magnification × 50, reproduced at × 100, van Giesen stain)

Heppleston (1973) showed that the concentration of asbestos fibres increases in proportion to the degree of pulmonary fibrosis up to asbestosis of moderate degree, but that no such correlation exists in disease which they interpreted as advanced asbestosis nor with its morphology (*see* Chapter 4).

Microscopically, fibrosis may be found when its presence is not suspected or is uncertain on gross examination. The early pathological changes precede clinical, physiological and radiographic evidence of the disease process. In order that the *extent of lung involvement* can be properly assessed the International Union against Cancer (1965) recommended that at least six blocks of tissue should be taken from specified sites as follows:

(1) Apex of right upper lobe, pleural surface.
(2) Right middle lobe, lateral pleural surface.
(3) Right lower lobe, middle of basal surface.
(4) Left upper lobe, central section.
(5) Lingula, central section.
(6) Left lower lobe, central basal section.

This can be combined with a system of grading *severity of fibrosis* to obtain a standard method of assessing the *degree of asbestosis* in the lungs as a whole (Hinson *et al.*, 1973). There are four grades of *extent of lung involvement:*

(1) none;
(2) less than 25 per cent;
(3) 25 to 50 per cent;
(4) over 50 per cent.

And there are five grades of *severity of fibrosis*:

(1) *None.*
(2) *Minimal.* Slight proliferation of reticulin fibres around respiratory bronchioles with asbestos bodies. Usually confined to lower lobes.
(3) *Slight.* Proliferation of reticulin fibres confined to the walls of respiratory bronchioles of scattered acini. Occasional asbestos bodies and fibre fragments in their walls and lumina either free or in macrophages. More acini and alveolar ducts are involved as disease advances. This grade is classed as an 'asbestos reaction' rather than asbestosis.
(4) *Moderate.* Increased peribronchiolar reticulin fibre proliferation some of which is replaced by collagen. Bronchiolar vessels are also involved. The lesions are fairly widespread (though individual) throughout the sections and there is septal thickening. Cuboidal metaplasia of the alveolar epithelium of respiratory bronchioles and alveolar ducts is present in some cases.
(5) *Severe.* Large areas of collagenous fibrosis distorting bronchioles which may be narrowed to clefts. Some alveoli around these survive and are lined by cuboidal epithelium. The walls of distal alveoli are thickened by fibrosis and usually contain many asbestos bodies and fibres.

However, it must be said that this grading method is not generally accepted although a better agreed system has not, to my knowledge, yet been proposed.

To this should be added a standardized simple method of quantifying the content of asbestos fibres.

A proportion of asbestos fibres is visible by light and more easily by phase contrast microscopy but the majority can only be detected by the electron microscope (Timbrell, Pooley and Wagner, 1970). The composition of fibres (serpentines and amphiboles) in industrial dusts and lung tissue can be positively identified by X-ray diffraction, thermal analysis and electron microprobe techniques. But these methods cannot distinguish between the fibrous and non-fibrous habits or varieties of asbestos minerals. To do this microscopy—in particular electron microscopy—is necessary (Campbell, 1978; Stanley, 1978) (*see* Appendix: Identification of Minerals).

The large fibrotic lesions consists of diffuse hyaline fibrosis. But in asbestos miners they include areas of concentric fibrosis which are sometimes necrotic or calcified and associated with endarteritis, and the quartz content of their lungs is greater than that in control lungs (Solomon *et al.*, 1971).

Subpleural crescents of apical fibrosis consist of dense collagen in which asbestos bodies may be found but evidence of tuberculosis is absent. Their significance is uncertain.

Necrobiotic nodules of rheumatoid disease are microscopically similar to subcutaneous rheumatoid nodules and lack the striking features of classic Caplan nodules (*see* Chapter 8). They have been found in areas of asbestosis—which may be of minimal amount—and when large may be more fibrotic although still exhibiting the characteristic cell reaction. Asbestos (or 'ferruginous') bodies have been observed in the lungs of all of the few reported cases (Mattson, 1971; Morgan, 1964; Rickards and Barrett, 1958; Tellesson, 1961). However, the nodules are not so clearly related to asbestos dust as they are to coal dust, and it is open to question whether the DIPF in these cases is an expression of 'rheumatoid lung' or of asbestosis (*see* Chapter 4).

There is little dust and negligible fibrosis in the hilar lymph nodes although asbestos fibres may be found when obscuring carbon is removed by incineration.

Pathogenesis (*see also* Chapter 4)

Chrysotile, crocidolite, amosite and anthophyllite are all capable of causing asbestosis; but it is possible that chrysotile is most active in this respect.

The most important factor determining its development is the product of the level and duration of asbestos exposure experienced by the worker; that is, a dose × time relationship. A linear relationship between the development of asbestosis and increasing dust exposure has been demonstrated in Canadian chrysotile workers by McDonald *et al.* (1980). In short, the incidence and the severity of asbestosis increases as exposure dose is augmented. The 'residence time' of fibres in the lungs may also be significant (Sluis-Cremer, 1970). The fibre content of the lungs increases with length of exposure but varies considerably in different individuals (Beattie and Knox, 1961); and, as stated already (p. 240), is greater with increasing severity of asbestosis up to disease of moderate degree (Ashcroft and Heppleston, 1973; Beattie and Knox, 1961). However, the relationship between radiographic appearances and dust exposure is weaker and that between impairment of lung function and mortality stronger in asbestosis than in coal pneumoconiosis (Rossiter, 1972).

The degree to which inhaled fibres penetrate to the periphery of the lungs is determined by their diameter and, to a lesser extent, their shape (*see* pp. 47 and 238) which, in turn depend upon the physical properties of airborne particles generated by different industrial processes. Other factors include the worker's physical activity and whether or not he is an habitual mouth breather.

In experimental animals the inhalation of all four asbestos types is followed by deposition of fibres in alveoli of, and beyond, some respiratory bronchioles, desquamation of some Type I alveolar cells, proliferation of Type II cells and an influx of alveolar macrophages. The macrophages, unlike those seen in animals exposed to quartz particles, are all mature cells (Miller *et al.*, 1978). A reticulin network forms and is subsequently converted to collagenous fibrosis which lines and later occupies alveolar walls. With increasing exposure more respiratory units are involved and the fibrosis spreads into alveolar ducts, atria and alveoli; and coalescence of the lesions results in diffuse interstitial fibrosis. Fibrosis continues to progress after animals are removed from exposure (Holt, Mills and Young, 1966; Hiett, 1978; Suzuki, 1974; Wagner *et al.*, 1974; Webster, 1970). Although there are certain species differences in response to different types of asbestos (Wagner, 1965) the crucial behaviour of alveolar macrophages appears to be common to all, and it is likely that the initial events seen in animals reflect the earliest stage of asbestosis in man.

As described already in Chapter 4 (pp. 73, 74) it is fibres which are too long to be completely engulfed and are poorly transported by macrophages and not short fibres which are apparently responsible for fibrogenesis (*see* Davis, 1979). This is exemplified by an experiment in rats in which the length distribution of inhaled anthophyllite fibres recovered from the lungs by bronchopulmonary lavage and those remaining in the lungs following lavage were measured sequentially over a period of 205 days. Fibres shorter than 5 μm were cleared from the lungs via the airways more efficiently than longer fibres but fibres in excess of 50 μm in length were not removed by this route. And although fibres about 200 μm long were present in all the lungs examined, the longest recovered by lavage, after fibres deposited in the airways had been cleared, was about 100 μm and this decreased to 60 to 70 μm after 205 days (Morgan, Talbot and Holmes, 1978). Apart from the fact that fibres of this size cannot be wholly engulfed by macrophages they will be more likely to bridge the alveolar ducts and alveoli than short fibres. These observations correspond to the lavage findings in human beings referred to on p. 240. It is of interest in this respect that of airborne fibres produced in various processes in the asbestos industry about 90 per cent on the whole are reported to be under 5 μm in length (Gibbs, 1978); that is, those most likely to reach the alveolar regions and subsequently to be cleared from them. If substantial numbers of short fibres are present in lungs with asbestosis (and, perhaps, with other types of diffuse fibrosis) this may be due to impairment of the clearance of fibres of any length from areas of fibrosis (Morgan and Holmes, 1980).

After ingesting crocidolite fibres alveolar and peritoneal macrophages of rats show an increase in surface membrane receptors for the C3 component of complement and for IgG (Miller and Kagan, 1976). And chrysotile ingested by macrophages induces a rapid, massive and selective release of lysosomal enzymes (Davies *et al.*, 1974). It has also been shown that chrysotile, crocidolite amosite and anthophyllite activate both classic and alternative (properdin) complement pathways and, in the presence of normal human serum, generate a chemotactic factor for peripheral blood leucocytes. Neither of these effects is produced by crystalline silica particles or glass wool fibres. These observations suggest the possibility that activation of the complement system and enzyme release may play an important role in the development of asbestosis in man (Wilson, Gaumer and Salvaggio, 1977; Hasselbacher, 1979). Miller and Kagan (1977) observed deposition of complement components on the surface of alveolar macrophages from rats which had inhaled UICC crocidolite over a period of six months but not when alveolar macrophages from 'non-dusted' rats were allowed to phagocytose crocidolite *in vitro*.

The increased prevalence of circulating antinuclear antibody (which is not sex-dependent) and rheumatoid factor in individuals with asbestosis but not in asbestos-exposed persons without evidence of asbestosis (*Table 4.3*) raises the possibility, discussed in Chapter 4, that immunological events may participate in pathogenesis especially as antinuclear antibody titres tend to rise slowly with the passage of time (Turner-Warwick and Parkes, 1970; Turner-Warwick, 1977; Lange, 1980a). The fact that the characteristics of antinuclear antibody associated with asbestosis are different from those of antinuclear antibody in so-called 'connective tissue' diseases of the lung (*see Table 4.2*) suggests that its origin and mode of action (if any) are different. The prevalence of non-organ-specific complement fixing antibodies is not increased above normal in asbestosis as it is in cryptogenic fibrosing 'alveolitis' (Turner-Warwick and Haslam, 1971).

Human antibodies against denatured collagen seem to be well authenticated and the possibility (for which there is some experimental evidence) that anticollagen antibodies might be capable of stimulating fibroblasts to an increased synthesis and secretion of collagen requires investigation, but at present there is no evidence of such antibody activity in asbestosis; if it exists it is conceivable that it would contribute to progression of the disease after asbestos exposure has ceased. Similarly, the possibility that sensitization of lymphocytes may play a role requires elucidation.

Reduction in the proportion and absolute numbers of circulating T lymphocytes, but not of B lymphocytes, and impairment of T cell function has been reported in patients with radiographic evidence of asbestosis (Kang *et al.*, 1974; Kagan *et al.*, 1977a and b; Lange and Skibinski, 1977; Haslam *et al.*, 1978). In a more recent study of a small number of patients with asbestosis Gaumer *et al.* (1979) were unable to confirm impaired function of T cells in the peripheral blood in response to mitogens (phytohaemagglutinin and concavalin A) but they did not record smoking habits. However, it appears probable that the number of T suppressor (rosette-forming) cells are diminished in asbestosis, but confirmation is awaited. These cytological changes, which seem to be related in some way to the fibrotic response, are associated with cutaneous anergy for 'recall' antigens such as tuberculin (PPD) and *Candida albicans* (Pierce and Turner-Warwick, 1980). This suggests the possibility of impaired function of one or more components of the cellular immune response. The possible significance of defective suppressor T lymphocyte function in the development of carcinoma of the lung in individuals with asbestosis is discussed later (p. 271). Lymphocyte sensitization to DNA has been shown to occur in some ANA-positive patients with asbestosis—and also cryptogenic fibrosing 'alveolitis'—which implies that delayed hypersensitivity may sometimes contribute to lung damage in both diseases (Haslam, Turner-Warwick and Lukoszek, 1975). Indeed, impairment of cell-mediated immunity, as indicated by lack of response to recall antigens, is most pronounced in asbestos workers with asbestosis and circulating ANAs, but is present to a lesser extent in those without asbestosis but with circulating ANAs (Lange *et al.*, 1978).

An apparent association between the HLA antigen B27 (*see* Chapter 4) and asbestosis poses the question that some individuals may be more susceptible than others to the damaging effect of asbestos on the lungs (Matej and Lange, 1976; Merchant *et al.*, 1975). A trend towards an increased frequency of HLA B27 which is not present in a large number of unaffected asbestos workers and control subjects, has been demonstrated among asbestos workers with radiographic evidence of DIPF. And, furthermore, the workers with pulmonary fibrosis and HLA B27 had a significantly shorter duration of exposure to asbestos than those without this antigen, although the mean profusion score of radiographic opacities was the same in both. Recently more detailed controlled studies, which were designed to compare HLA phenotypes in asbestos workers with asbestosis compared with those of compatible age and asbestos exposure but no evidence of lung disease, have not shown any statistical difference in the prevalence to B27 in those with asbestosis and the controls (Evans, Lewinsohn and Evans, 1977; Gregor *et al.*, 1979; Huuskonen, Tiilikainen and Alanko, 1979). Although Darke *et al.* (1979) found this phenotype twice as frequently in dockyard workers with asbestosis as in those without theirs was not a case control study. There is a suggestion that B5, apparently more common in individuals who do not develop asbestosis, may play a protective role (Evans, Lewinsohn and Evans, 1977), as may B18 (Huuskonen, Tiilikainen and Alanko, 1979).

However, the general conclusion from controlled studies is that there is no significant or consistent difference in the frequency of HLA phenotypes on the A, B and C loci in persons with asbestosis compared with control subjects. Hence, it is not possible, on present evidence to identify individuals who may have an undue susceptibility or resistance to developing asbestosis (Turner-Warwick, 1979).

The occurrence of massive fibrotic lesions has been virtually-confined to asbestos miners and it appears to be a 'mixed dust fibrosis' in which quartz plays a significant role (Solomon *et al.*, 1971). However, the solid, fibrotic upper lobe lesions referred to on p. 252 were probably associated with tuberculous infection for the cases in our experience were found to have had tuberculosis or tuberculous contacts in the past, or clusters of calcified hilar lymph nodes on the relevant side. Furthermore, we have not seen these lesions in individuals whose asbestos exposure commenced after the 1940s. A recent claim that bilateral massive, upper lobe fibrosis was solely or primarily caused by asbestos is not supported by convincing evidence (Green and Dimcheff, 1974).

Clinical features

Neither symptoms nor physical signs are pathognomonic as they are found in DIPF due to a variety of other causes. It is of interest that a recent survey of dockyard workers showed that clinical, physiological and radiographical abnormalities only occurred in older men who had been exposed to asbestos before the introduction of strict protective measures (Harries and Lumley, 1977).

Symptoms

These are of insidious onset and the time lag between their first being noticed by the patient and his earliest past exposure to asbestos varies considerably; in some cases (especially when exposure has been heavy) this period may only be a few years, but in others it may be so long that he has forgotten that he worked in contact with asbestos. This emphasizes the need for direct questioning when taking an occupational history.

As a rule the most important symptom is breathlessness on effort, slight at first, being experienced only on undue effort, and then increasing in severity until finally it may be present at rest. In most cases this increase occurs slowly over a period of many years, and in others there may be very little change over a decade. When breathlessness has become at least moderate in degree some patients complain of chest tightness and inability to breathe in deeply and, in some cases, to yawn due (as in any advanced DIPF) to substantially increased stiffness—or reduced compliance—of the lungs. A proportion of patients, however, never complain of breathlessness.

Cough is absent in early disease but is present in the later stages of most, though not all, cases. It is usually 'dry' or productive of only small quantities of viscid mucoid sputum. This may be difficult to raise and thus provoke paroxysms of coughing. Paroxysms may also be related to effort. But some patients with advanced asbestosis, however, have remarkably little cough.

Sputum, when present, is usually mucoid and tends to be raised in the first two hours after getting up in the morning. Cough and sputum throughout the day appear to be exceptional rather than the rule (Elmes, 1966), although in smokers bronchial catarrh is usual.

Haemoptysis is not caused by asbestosis. When it does occur complicating bronchial carcinoma may be responsible and must be sought.

Chest pain is not a feature of asbestosis. But poorly localized aching, chest tightness or transient, sharp pains are sometimes complained of by patients with severe dyspnoea and may arise from overtaxed intercostal and other chest wall muscles. Complaints of persistent and sometimes oddly distributed pain, apparently of psychoneurotic origin, are apt to be encountered in those who are anxious about asbestos-related disease and its much publicized consequences. However, it must be remembered that persistent pain may be the first evidence of carcinoma of the lung or malignant mesothelioma of the pleura (*see later*).

Lassitude is not uncommon in advanced disease.

Physical signs

Clubbing of fingers and toes is an inconstant sign. It is present in varying severity in approximately half the cases of more advanced asbestosis and less often in those with mild disease. It may or may not increase as fibrosis progresses.

Rapid onset or worsening of existing clubbing may signal the presence of complicating bronchial carcinoma. Hypertrophic pulmonary osteoarthropathy is rarely, if ever, seen in uncomplicated asbestosis. Methods of recording the hyponychial angles objectively have been devised to reduce observer variation and to note changes in severity of clubbing with the passage of time (Bentley and Cline, 1970; Regan *et al.*, 1967).

Clubbing is deemed to be present when the angle is 195 degrees or more. Using this technique Huuskonen (1978) recorded clubbing in 32.2 per cent of 133 cases of asbestosis of all grades of severity: in 22 per cent with ILO/UC category 1/0 to 1/1 irregular opacities and in 55 per cent with category 2/3 or higher. However, the test is not practical in routine clinical work and, in any case, this sign has no value in the diagnosis of asbestosis (*see* Diagnosis).

Equilateral impairment of expansion affecting the lower chest wall occurs with advancing disease. Measurement of expansion from full expiration to full inspiration round the maximum circumference of the chest each time the patient is examined is a helpful index of progression. When disease is of slight amount expansion is usually 'normal' (that is, about 2½ inches (6.3 cm) or more) but, when advanced, may be reduced to ½ inch (1.2 cm) or less. Some reduction occurs naturally with age. This sign is only of value in following individual patients and, due to its wide variability, has no relevance in epidemiological surveys.

Crepitations, the most important physical sign, are discussed in Chapter 1 (p. 23). Their presence is closely related to duration of asbestos exposure (Murphy *et al.*, 1978). They are heard bilaterally early in the development of the disease, patchily, in the basal regions of the lower lobes usually posteriorly but often first in the lower axillae, and sometimes in the middle lobe and ligular regions. At this stage they are of fine, crisp quality (that is, high pitched, about 700 Hz), are unaltered by cough and may only be heard at the end of *full* inspiration especially after a short period of breath-holding at low lung volume. They often precede respiratory symptoms and may antedate abnormality of routine lung function tests and chest radiographs. As fibrosis progresses fine to medium quality crepitations (about 400 Hz) are present throughout inspiration but *not* in expiration, and gradually become bilaterally widespread in the lower lobes, middle lobe and lingula; they are rarely heard anteriorly over the upper lobes. In the presence of bilateral diffuse thickening of the pleura they may be difficult to detect due to impairment of sound conduction and, possibly, to reduction in expansion of the lungs. A consistent feature of the crepitations of any DIPF is their persistent and repetitive pattern in each respiratory cycle. Crepitations in many other lung diseases may be provoked or discharged by coughing, are often present in expiration and are frequently coarser or lower pitched (about 250 Hz).

A recent study has shown that in patients with 'diffuse interstitial lung disease' diagnosed both clinically and by biopsy bilateral fine crepitations ('crackles') were present in about 60 per cent of cases of asbestosis and UIP, in about 50 per cent of cases of desquamative fibrosing 'alveolitis' (*see* Chapter 4), and in 40 per cent of cases of extrinsic allergic 'alveolitis'; but less often in patients with sarcoidosis, chronic bronchitis and emphysema. Coarse quality crepitations were predominant in chronic bronchitis and emphysema and were usually accompanied by rhonchi (Epler, Carrington and Gaensler, 1978). (*See also* Chapter 1, p. 23.)

Wheezes and rhonchi are not caused by asbestosis but are present concurrently in some cases, though infrequently. Pleural friction may sometimes be heard, especially at the lung bases, but is not related to parietal pleural plaques (if present) nor always to evidence of diffuse pleural fibrosis.

Loss of weight is not a feature and, although it may occur in advanced disease, it should prompt suspicion of carcinoma of the lung. Similarly, central cyanosis is rarely seen except in advanced disease, usually after effort, and is not severe in the absence of co-existent airflow obstruction. The signs of pulmonary heart disease may ultimately develop but are most uncommon.

Investigations

Sputum In general, examination of sputum for asbestos bodies is of no practical value as their presence merely confirms exposure to asbestos in persons with a known occupational history but does not prove the existence of asbestos-related disease; and, vice versa, their absence does not indicate freedom from such disease. However, the finding of these bodies may be of some help in cases where both the clinician and patient are in doubt as to whether a past occupation involved asbestos exposure.

Broncho-alveolar lavage fluid from patients with asbestosis and cryptogenic DIPF contains a higher percentage of polymorphonuclear leucocytes and higher average concentrations of IgG, IgA and α-antitrypsin than fluid from normal individuals and from workers with asbestos exposure but no lung fibrosis. Asbestos fibres which are of similar length to those found in the sputum but shorter than those present in the lung tissue may be recovered from individuals with asbestos exposure (*see* p. 240) (Bignon *et al.*, 1978b).

Erythrocyte sedimentation rate This is sometimes raised in individuals with moderate to advanced asbestosis in the absence of any other evident disease. The significance of this finding remains to be explained.

Serology The association of ANAs and RFs with asbestosis is discussed in Chapter 4 and on p. 254. Apart from the different characteristics of ANA in asbestosis compared with 'connective tissue' disease of the lungs it is of no diagnostic assistance.

Lung function Lung function tests have four applications:

(1) As an important aid in establishing diagnosis.
(2) To evaluate progress of established disease.
(3) For periodic observation of healthy asbestos workers.
(4) In epidemiological surveys.

(1) *Diagnostic* Physiological tests alone cannot prove the diagnosis of asbestosis; they reveal only the abnormal patterns of function which characterize diffuse interstitial fibrosis (fibrosing 'alveolitis') from any cause. But in combination with occupational history, abnormal physical signs and chest radiographs they give strong confirmatory evidence of the presence of the disease and indicate its severity. For this reason they are an essential part of the investigation of suspected cases of asbestosis.

The earliest detectable abnormality of lung function appears to be an increase in static elastic pressure (decreased compliance) which precedes symptoms and physical signs of lung disease, definitive changes in other parameters of lung function and radiographic abnormality (Jodoin *et al.*, 1971); but this test is not suitable for routine use as it is complex, causes some discomfort to the subject and demands a high degree of cooperation. However, consistent impairment of VC in the absence of significant airflow obstruction or other chronic chest disease reflects reduction of compliance and is the most sensitive routine test for the early detection of asbestosis (Becklake *et al.*, 1970; Gandevia, 1967; Thomson, Pelzer and Smither, 1965) and correlates better with dust exposure than Tl (Becklake *et al.*, 1972).

For practical purposes, the most important tests are those which determine the lung volumes (TLC, RV, FRC and VC), ventilatory capacity (FEV_1, FVC and FEV per cent) and Tl; assessment of arterial oxygen saturation if a useful additional, but not requisite, test. Determination of compliance is not essential in establishing the diagnosis.

In the early stages of the disease slight hyperventilation may occur on effort due to hypoxaemia resulting from reduction in gas transfer in the absence of any abnormality of lung function tests at rest or of radiographic changes. With increased fibrosis the changes in function are those of the 'restrictive syndrome' (*see* Chapter 1). TLC and FRC are diminished but RV is either little changed (so that RV/TLC is increased) or is decreased. VC, FVC and FEV_1 are reduced—and to a severe degree when disease is advanced—but the FEV_1/FVC percentage is usually normal or greater than normal. Airflow obstruction, therefore, is uncommon but when present is usually related to cigarette smoking and co-existent chronic obstructive bronchitis. However, it has been suggested that it may also be caused by asbestos fibrosis at respiratory bronchiolar level both in man (Fournier-Massey and Becklake, 1975; Muldoon and Turner-Warwick, 1972) and guinea pigs (Hiett, 1978), although epidemiological studies of function in asbestos workers have so far failed to substantiate this (*see* next section). Detailed correlation of physiological data with the pathology of the small airways in a sufficient number of cases is required to resolve the problem. In addition, Tl is impaired and Kco usually reduced (*see* Chapter 1). Carbon dioxide exchange is not affected.

Regional lung function studies using radioactive xenon-133 have shown, when compared with a normal group, that patients with asbestosis have impaired ventilation of the lower zones of their lungs whereas those with radiographic evidence of calcified plaques, but not of intrapulmonary fibrosis, do not have this abnormality (Seaton, 1977).

(2) *Progression of established disease* Once the diagnosis of asbestosis is established, progress of the disease can be adequately assessed at subsequent re-examination by VC, FVC and FEV_1. Decline in VC and FVC values greater than that due to the normal ageing effect over a period with a normal FEV_1/FVC percentage indicates progress of fibrosis in the absence of other causes of the 'restrictive syndrome'. The VC is the most sensitive index of progression of asbestosis (Becklake *et al.*, 1970). However, if there is a substantial increase of respiratory symptoms, abnormal physical signs or radiographic appearances it is desirable to repeat the more comprehensive tests.

(3) *Periodic observation of healthy asbestos workers* The suggestion made by Leathart (1960) that the VC of all asbestos workers 'should be measured at regular intervals and that a progressive decline should be taken as a warning of impending disease' is good practical advice. VC, FVC and FEV_1 should be recorded in each new entrant to an asbestos hazard to establish his normal values, and annually in all healthy asbestos workers (*see also* Preventive measures).

(4) *Epidemiological surveys* Lung function tests play an essential role and the simple ventilatory tests are the most practical for the purpose. Vital capacity and Tl do not, however, appear to be more sensitive than radiographic changes in detecting slight or early asbestosis (Becklake *et al.*, 1970; Weill, Waggenspack and Bailey, 1973; Weill *et al.*, 1975). But in individual cases periodic clinical examinations, ventilatory function tests and chest radiographs are essential. The possibility that crocidolite exposure alone causes significantly smaller lung volumes and lower forced expiratory flow rates and Tl values than 'pure' chrysotile exposure (Weill *et al.*, 1977) requires confirmation though the difficulty in evaluating the type and amount of past asbestos exposures is, in most instances, insuperable. No clear decrease in Tl was observed, however, with increasing exposure in Canadian chrysotile miners and millers (McDonald *et al.*, 1974). Although the reliability and consistency of reduced Tl as one of the criteria for the diagnosis of 'asbestosis' in insulation workers has been confirmed, the value of this test in epidemiological surveys appears to need further assessment (Murphy *et al.*, 1978).

The suggestion, already referred to, that asbestosis might cause airflow obstruction has not been supported to date by epidemiological studies in which no increase in the prevalence of obstruction in healthy asbestos workers and in individuals with asbestosis compared with non-exposed populations has been demonstrated (Murphy *et al.*, 1971b and 1972; Wallace and Langlands, 1971; Woitowitz, 1970). Although some reduction in closing volume has been reported in asbestos workers its significance is uncertain (Peress *et al.*, 1975) as neither closing volume nor closing capacity appear to correlate with duration of asbestos exposure or with asbestos dust indices (Konietzko *et al.*, 1974).

Radiographic appearances

As described in Chapter 5 (p. 96) PA and suitably angled right and left anterior oblique views should be taken in all new cases of suspected asbestosis and periodically in those with established disease. Good technique is of paramount importance.

Intrapulmonary By contrast with silicosis and coal pneumoconiosis the appearances of asbestosis are predominant in the lower halves of the lung fields. This, however, is also true in some cases of DIPF due to other causes (*see* Diagnosis).

The earliest abnormalities are usually found in *both lower zones* near the costophrenic angles and may be verified and, sometimes identified, more easily by anterior oblique views than the standard PA views. The first perceptible changes consist of more fine vessel opacities than are normal in these regions with thickening of the vascular markings where they branch and divide. Linear opacities which look like extensions of vascular markings may reach the periphery often crossing over each other to give a net-like appearance (*Figure 9.14*). Initially the opacities are tenuous and difficult

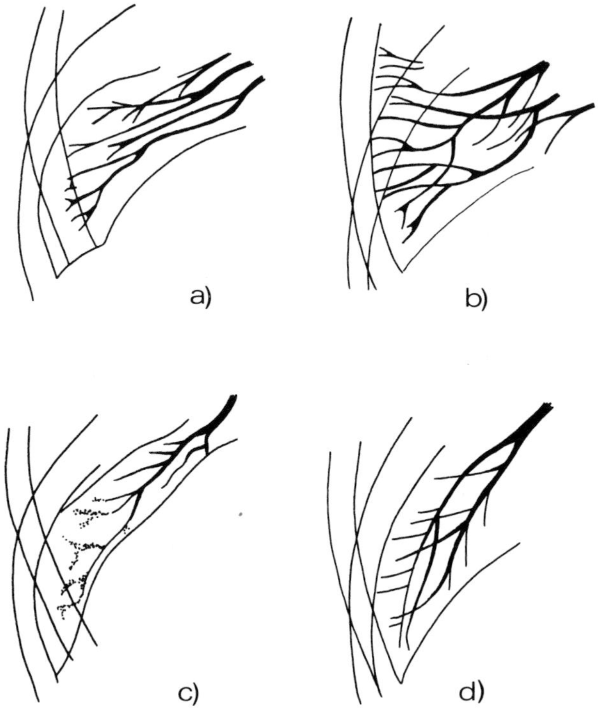

Figure 9.14 Diagram showing the various radiographic patterns of early asbestosis. (a) More small vessel markings than is normal; (b) vessel markings tend to be thickened where they branch and divide, an appearance occasionally seen in normal chests. Vessels may have the same calibre over the peripheral 2 or 3 cm and extend to the pleural margin. Branches cross giving a coarse net-like appearance; (c) fine, 'nodular' opacities 1 to 2 mm in diameter accompanying the smaller peripheral vessels; (d) horizontal linear pattern resembling Kerley's B lines. Some of these lines are continuous with vessel markings and do not reach the pleural margin. (Reproduced by courtesy of Drs D. E. Fletcher and J. R. Edge and the Honorary Editor of Clinical Radiology*)*

to define with confidence but they become progressively thicker and, when few, may resemble Kerley's B lines although often they do not reach the pleura (*Figure 5.13b*, p. 107). Another early abnormality consists of minute bead-like opacities, 1 to 2 mm in diameter, close to distal branches of the pulmonary arteries in the costophrenic angles (Fletcher and Edge, 1970) (*Figure 9.15*).

Identification of these early changes may be facilitated by the use of a good hand lens and a bright light source (*see* Chapter 5) but, as might be expected, disagreement between observers is apt to occur at this stage. Computerized tomography appears to be more sensitive than conventional radiographs in detecting early fibrosis (*see* Chapter 5, p. 111) but is not routinely practical.

There is some evidence that basal DIPF is significantly more common among asbestos workers who smoke than those who do not (Weiss, 1971; Harries, Rossiter and Coles, 1976; Weiss and Theodos, 1978). This may be due to synergism rather than to independent additive effects of the two exposures (Samet *et al.*, 1979).

As asbestosis progresses linear and irregular opacities become thicker and spread into the middle zones but rarely reach the upper zones (*Figures 9.16* and *9.17*). Appearances suggesting cystic spaces, which are not more than about 3 mm in diameter, sometimes develop in the lower zones but this is the exception rather than the rule and they appear to be caused, at least in some cases, by the effects of superimposition of different tissue radiodensities (*see* Chapter 5, p. 109). A coarse, 'honeycomb' pattern is not a feature of asbestosis.

In the majority of cases the appearances of basal intrapulmonary fibrosis sometimes are symmetrical or almost so, but are more prominent on one side. This may be due to the more extensive general opacity caused by diffuse pleural thickening on that side. They are never unilateral.

As indicated in *Table 5.3*, p. 99 the ILO U/C International Classification of Radiographs (1971) codifies irregular opacities as categories s, t and u according to a crude scale of thickness. But there is greater difficulty in assigning these categories than is the case with categories p, q and r and, hence, more observer disagreement. For routine clinical purposes, the 12 point scale of profusion is more of a hindrance than a help. The 'short classification', however, is useful.

Pleural The costophrenic and cardiophrenic angles are frequently obliterated—a sign which may develop at a fairly early stage (*Figure 9.16*). Evidence of a greater or lesser degree of diffuse pleural thickening which usually takes the form of an ill-defined haze in both middle and lower zones (sometimes more on the one side than the other) is commonly present. When diffuse thickening of the pleura is advanced and extensive evidence of basal intrapulmonary fibrosis may be obscured on standard radiographs but is usually demonstrable by using increased kV and anterior oblique views. However, it does not necessarily match the pleural changes in severity. In a small number of cases evidence of diffuse pleural thickening is not detectable. The heart outline may be blurred due to superimposition of the radiodensities of the heart and fibrosis of parietal pericardium, lungs and pleura (so-called 'shaggy heart') (*Figure 9.17c*); but this appearance, which is frequently described in textbooks, is exceptional and non-specific. In contrast to diffuse pleural thickening bilateral pleural plaques are observed in only a minority of cases of asbestosis—less than half (*see* p. 242). They may be few or multiple and extensive. Very occasionally crescentric, cap-like opacities are present at the apices of the lung fields; their significance is uncertain but they may represent old tuberculous disease.

In far advanced asbestosis enlargement of the heart and proximal pulmonary artery shadows due to pulmonary hypertension may be seen.

Development and progression The signs of fibrosis develop slowly but as they advance the area of the lung fields often diminishes due to fibrotic contraction. The line of the lesser fissure (which is often thickened) shifts downwards and there may be crowding of the vascular pattern in the lower zones. It is important to note that radiographic progression is slow and often shows little change over five,

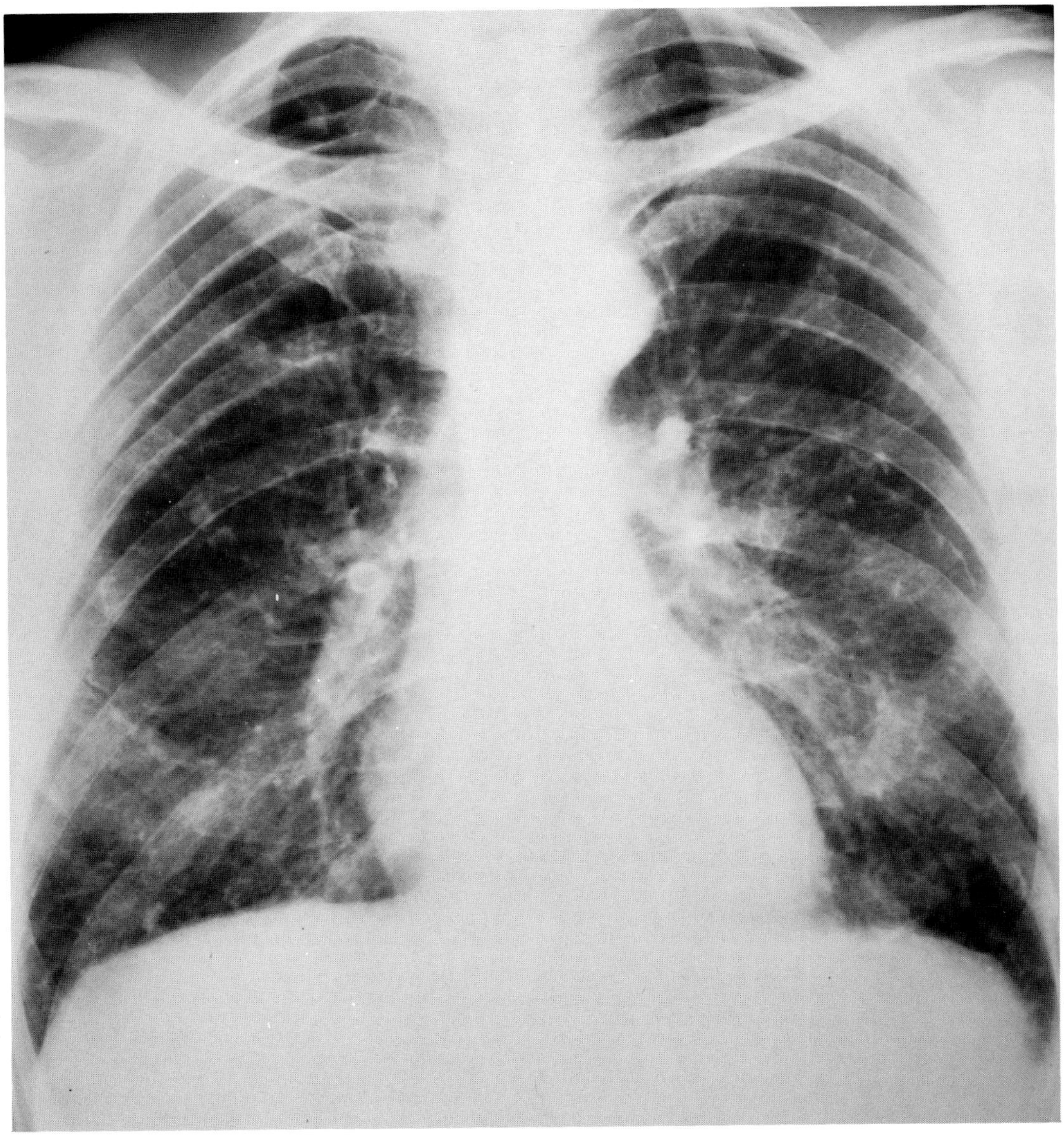

Figure 9.15(a)

ten or more years (*Figure 9.17*) sometimes ceasing altogether; indeed, many cases do not progress after diagnosis (Coutts *et al.*, 1980). It may, however, be quicker in some individuals than in others due to different conditions of past dust exposure and, possibly, to idiosyncracy; and may only be detected some years after exposure has ceased. Becklake *et al.* (1979) found radiographic changes of intrapulmonary fibrosis—mainly in the form of 'attacks' rather than 'progression'—in six (9.1 per cent) of 66 men some ten to 20 years after they had left the Quebec chrysotile production industry in which they had worked for two or more years. There was no apparent association with age or smoking habits. Current films were compared with films taken at the time of leaving the industry. Although error in evaluating radiographic appearances in films taken about 20 years apart may occur due to technical differences the authors were satisfied that their findings were not attributable to this. By contrast, in a follow-up study of 253 dockyard workers Rossiter, Heath and Harries (1980) observed that radiographic parenchymal abnormalities increased and occurred more frequently in those who had been more heavily exposed to asbestos, and in smokers compared with non-smokers.

Other features Discrete, rounded opacities, small or large, are not a feature of asbestosis. When present they may be related to other past occupational dust exposure: for example, coal mining or foundry fettling, or to another dust hazard in the same occupation (*Figure 9.18*). But in the asbestos industry minerals in the host rock are likely to be responsible. The banded ironstones in which crocidolite and amosite are found may contain considerable quantities of quartz: as much as 20 per cent has been recorded in the dust from ore-crushing mills (Solomon, 1969). Hence, large opacities due to massive silicosis or to 'mixed dust fibrosis' may occur in amphibole miners and millers (Solomon *et al.*, 1971) (*Figure 9.19*) (*see* p. 267), but not in those exposed to chrysotile or to amphiboles which have been thoroughly separated from the host rock. Similarly, because the host

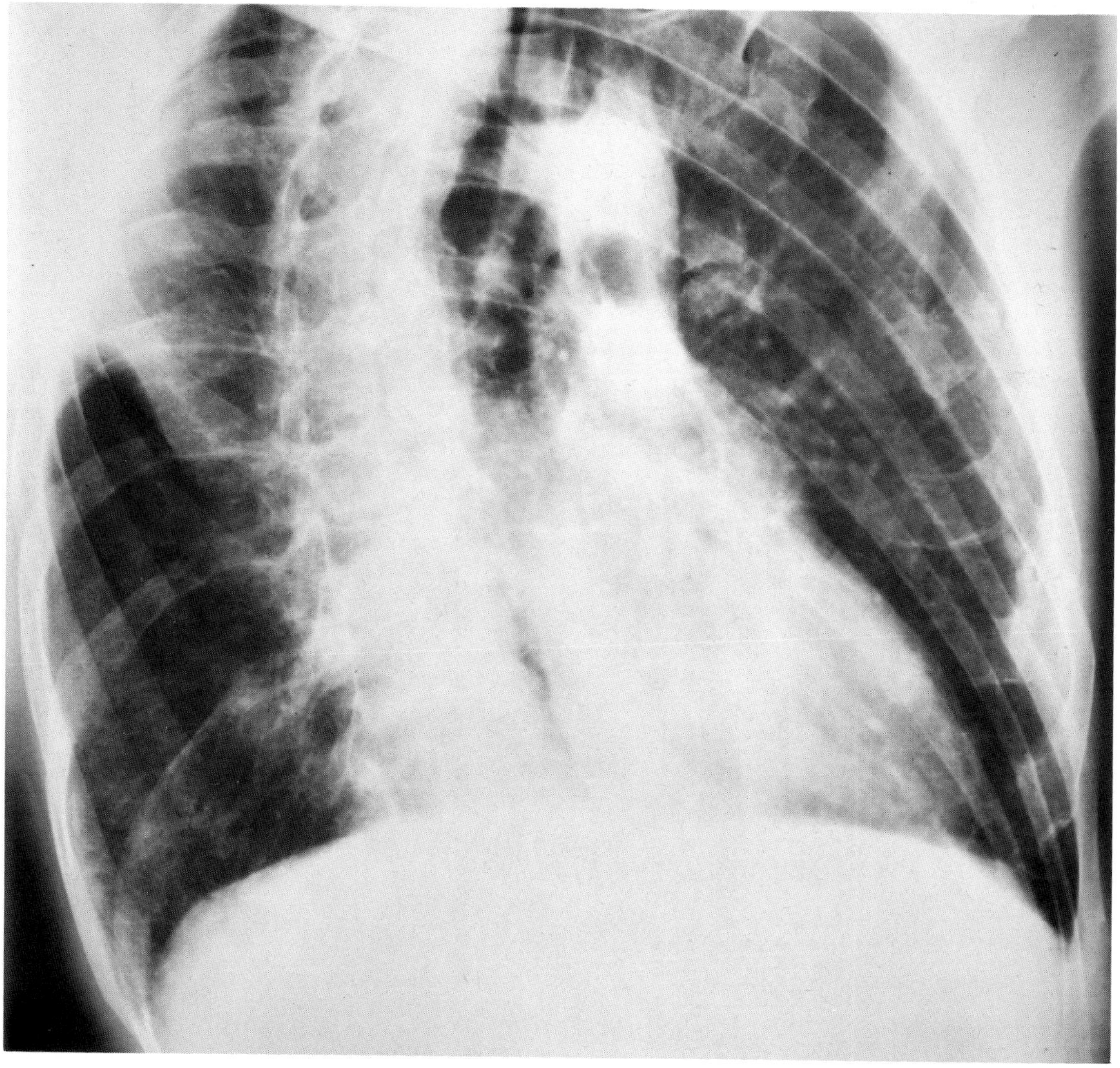

Figure 9.15(b)

rocks of crocidolite and amosite also contain the iron minerals magnetite and hematite siderosis (p. 113) may also be seen in some asbestos miners and millers. However, rounded opacities are occasionally observed in individuals who have worked in asbestos processing or manufacturing industries. In which case they are likely to be due to exposure to 'dirty' fibre which still contained host rock dust or to some other free silica contamination of the process.

Round opacities (up to about 2 cm diameter) indicative of 'rheumatoid' necrobiotic nodules have been described in asbestos workers with and without accompanying evidence of asbestosis. They may closely resemble typical Caplan lesions (*see Figure 8.30*) (Mattson, 1971; Morgan, 1964; Rickards and Barrett, 1958; Telleson, 1961). But these appearances are evidently rare and their significance in relation to asbestosis uncertain (*see* p. 253); they may be associated with a non-asbestos dust component or be 'spontaneous' rheumatoid nodules. Greaves (1979) has reported a case in which there was no gross or microscopical evidence of asbestosis.

Basal bronchiectasis, demonstrable by bronchography (Leathart, 1960), is rarely seen.

Diagnosis

This is not as straightforward as it might seem for three reasons.

(1) Asbestosis possesses no pathognomonic clinical, physiological or X-ray features.
(2) Not all individuals with similar exposures to asbestos develop asbestosis.
(3) DIPF due to a variety of other causes may resemble or be mistaken for asbestosis clinically (*see* Chapter 4).

If DIPF due to another cause occurs in an asbestos exposed individual it may not be recognized as such and is likely to be accepted as asbestosis—a not uncommon mistake. It is clear, therefore, that if the *post hoc propter hoc* fallacy is not avoided a disease which may be responsive to some form of treatment may remain undiagnosed (at least until too late for treatment to be effective) or the individual encumbered with the disadvantage of an incorrect diagnosis of asbestosis.

Hence, given evidence of past occupational asbestos

(c)

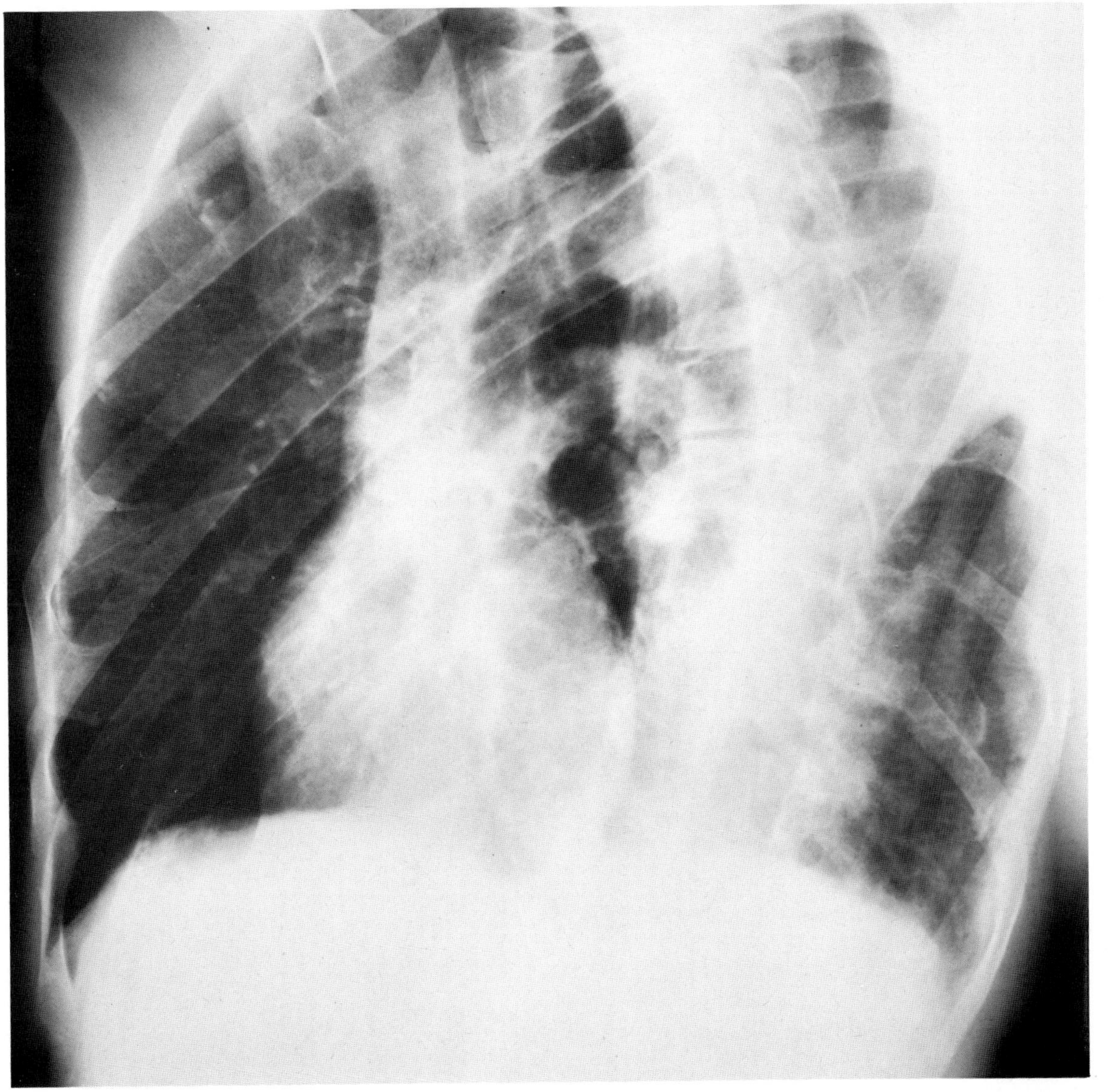

Figure 9.15 Appearances of clinically early asbestosis (DIPF). (a) Fine irregular opacities (Category s) in both lower zones especially the costophrenic angles (b) and (c). Small calcified pleural plaques are also present and are most clearly demonstrated in the 45 degree anterior oblique views. Note: hyaline plaques in left lower zone of the left anterior oblique view (that is, right lung field) No diffuse pleural thickening evident and costophrenic angles sharply defined. Insulation worker, aged 52 with 30 years intermittent exposure to asbestos. No respiratory symptoms; ballroom dancer. Fine persistent inspiratory crepitations both lower lobes. Lung function: slight reduction of TLC, Tl and Kco

exposure the diagnosis of asbestosis rests firstly upon establishing the clinical features of asbestosis described earlier (pp. 255–259); and secondly, upon excluding DIPF due to other causes or to disease which may simulate it.

To elicit an adequate history of occupational or para-occupational exposure an intimate knowledge of the asbestos industry and the use of its products is necessary and some attempt should be made to assess whether cumulative exposure (dose × time) has been light, moderate or heavy. By itself a history of exposure does not prove the presence of asbestosis. Asbestos bodies in the sputum or radiographic evidence of bilateral pleural plaques may confirm exposure but do not establish the existence of asbestosis; equally their absence does not exclude it.

Clinical criteria

Asbestosis

(1) *Abnormal physical signs* Persistent, bilateral, basal late-inspiratory crepitations of high to medium frequency which occur early in the evolution of the disease are the important sign which is only exceptionally absent (*see* p. 256). Coarse quality crepitations in inspiration *and* expiration suggest some other disease.

Finger clubbing has no discriminative value as it is observed in only some cases of asbestosis and occurs with a variety of diseases including DIPF due to other causes.

(2) *Abnormalities of lung function* Namely, reduction of TLC, VC and Tl with or without slightly increased RV.

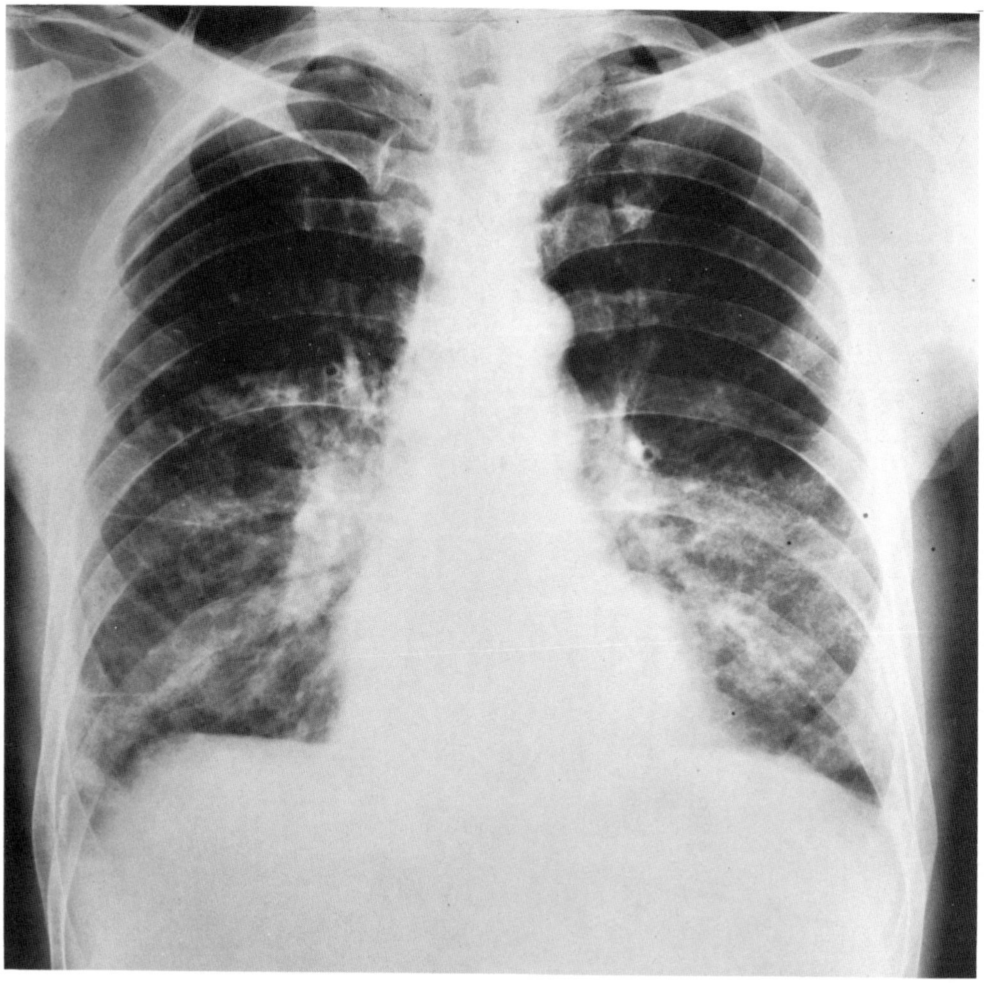

Figure 9.16(a)

Kco is usually, but not always, reduced. These parameters, however, are not necessarily impaired to an equal or comparable degree.

(3) *Radiographic abnormalities* (pp. 257–259, *Figures 9.15* to *9.17*) The important points are: (a) the appearances and distribution of the abnormalities; and (b) their mode of development and progression. Involvement of the upper zones is rarely seen and then only when the lower and mid-zone changes are far advanced. In most cases there is evidence of bilateral, *diffuse* thickening of the pleura which may range from very slight (obliteration of the costophrenic angles) to severe and widespread. Development occurs slowly over a number of years, and progression is also gradual and at some point may cease; but the rate of change varies from case to case.

In passing it should be noted that severe hyperinflation of the lungs may occasionally compress their lower parts sufficiently to give a superficial resemblance to diffuse intrapulmonary, bilateral, basal fibrosis (*Figure 9.20*).

Other types of DIPF (chronic fibrosing 'alveolitis') or disease which simulates DIPF

(1) Evidence of causes of DIPF other than the asbestos minerals (for example, extrinsic allergens, connective tissue diseases and certain drugs, *see Tables 4.4*, p. 77 and *5.2*, p. 97, must be sought.

In some instances, and unlike asbestosis, the development and progression of dyspnoea may occur over a short period of time and may be accompanied by constitutional symptoms.

(2) *Abnormal physical signs* Crepitations of similar quality, timing and distribution to those of asbestosis may be present or absent. In some cases medium to coarse quality crepitations are heard mainly in the upper lobe regions and are often predominant anteriorly—a sign not observed in asbestosis.

(3) *Changes in lung function* These are similar to those of asbestosis and thus have no discriminative value.

(4) *Radiographic appearances* These are the most important means of discrimination and can conveniently be considered as follows:

(a) *Distribution* Predominant involvement of the upper and mid-zones by irregular opacities which may be coarse and sometimes more prolific on one side than the other with the lower zones remaining partly or wholly free is fairly common and is not due to asbestosis (*Figures 9.21, 9.22,* and *9.23*). In some cases the abnormalities first appear in the upper zones even though the lower zones may be most affected at a later stage (*Figures 9.21* and

(b)

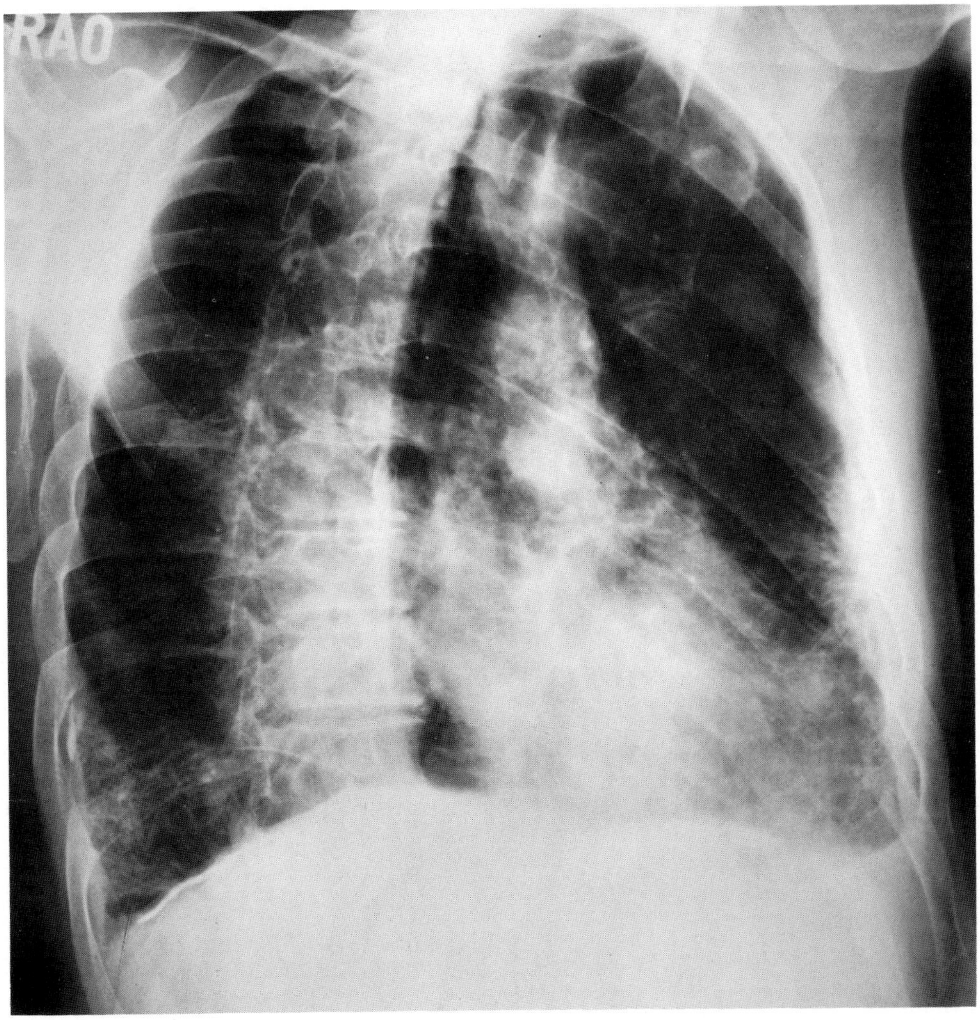

Figure 9.16 (a) Moderately advanced asbestosis: category 't' irregular opacities. Note: (1) freedom of the upper zones in both PA and 45 degree right anterior oblique view (b). (2) Presence of bilateral diffuse pleural thickening. (3) Calcified plaques in the oblique view which are not evident in (a). Insulation worker for 34 years, aged 59. Moderate dyspnoea after climbing 14 stairs. Persistent medium inspiratory crepitations in both lower lobes middle and lingula; none in the upper lobes. Lung function: moderately severe restriction and impairment of Tl with slight reduction of Kco

9.22). Equal involvement of all zones, is also against a diagnosis of asbestosis (*Figure 9.24*). However, a distribution identical to or closely resembling that of asbestosis can be caused by other pathology: for example, rheumatoid disease, chronic sarcoidosis, cryptogenic fibrosing 'alveolitis', multiple neurofibromatosis (*Figure 9.25*) and lymphangitis carcinomatosa (*Figure 9.26*) (*see Table 5.2*).

Such cases can usually be differentiated by noting the remaining radiographic features in this list and by evidence of the relevant underlying disease.

Although one or both costophrenic angles may be clear and of normal appearance in occasional cases of proven asbestosis this is uncommon. When seen it should at least raise the question of another disease.

(b) *Development and progression* These often occur with much greater rapidity than the rate of change seen in asbestosis: that is, in a period ranging from months to two or three years (*Figures 9.21, 9.22, 9.27* and *9.28*). If this situation is observed in disease with bilateral basal distribution the likelihood that it is asbestosis should be seriously questioned. Sometimes isolated changes of DIPF which have no continuity with basal abnormalities may appear in the upper or middle zones, unilaterally or bilaterally, in a short period of time. Occasionally, however, though the distribution and other features are not those of asbestosis, the rate of change may be slow (*Figures 9.24* and *8.29*).

(c) *'Honeycomb' pattern* The appearances of multiple cysts, often seemingly thick-walled, may be localized or widespread and in some cases may develop fairly quickly. Cystic translucencies range from about 5 to 10 mm in diameter, sometimes larger. This is not the behaviour of asbestosis (*Figures 9.21, 9.27* and *9.29*).

(d) *Diffuse bilateral pleural thickening* By contrast with asbestosis this is commonly absent in other types of DIPF though it may be present (sometimes unilaterally) in rheumatoid and other connective tissue diseases (*Figures 9.22, 9.23, 9.24* and *9.27*). It is rarely seen in cryptogenic fibrosing 'alveolitis' (Turner-Warwick, Burrows and

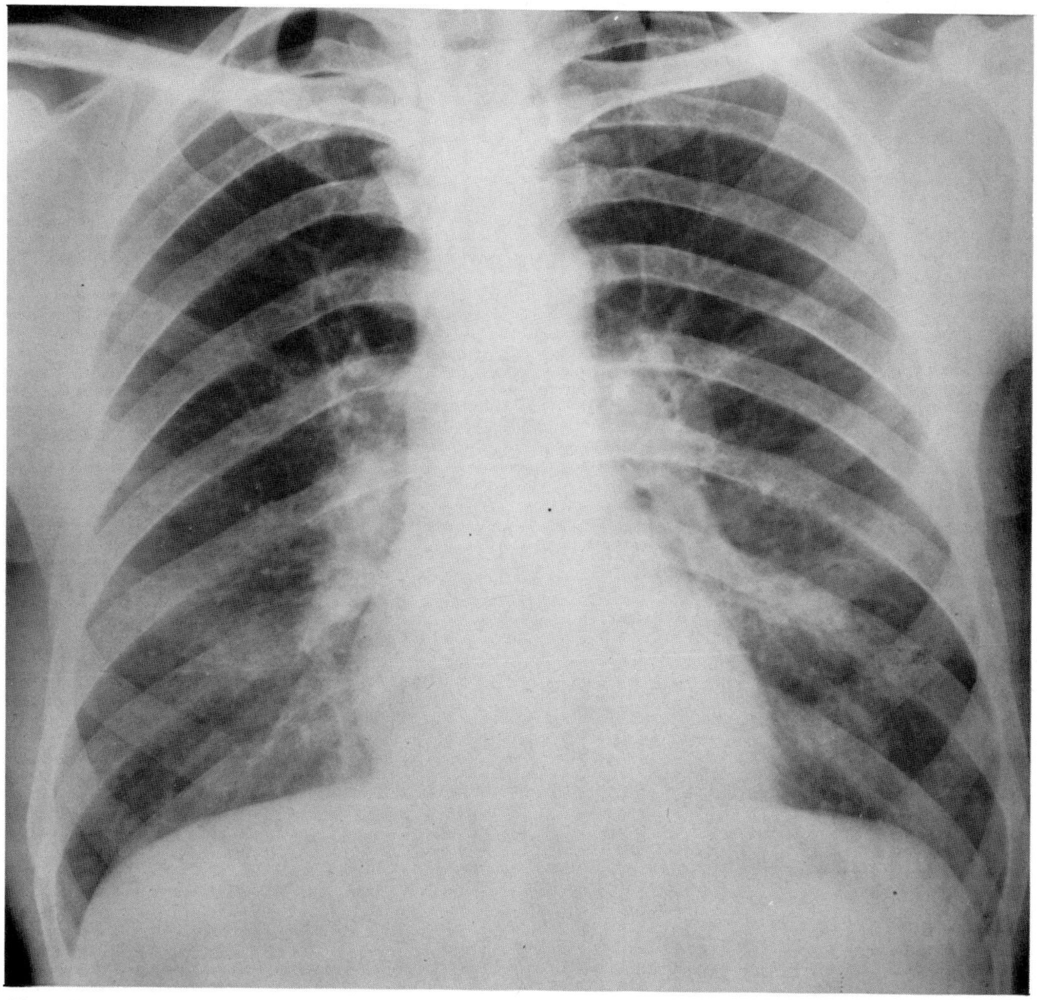

Figure 9.17(a) 1957

Johnson, 1980), chronic extrinsic allergic 'alveolitis' (*Figures 9.28* and *11.7*) and multiple neurofibromatosis (*Figure 9.25*).

(e) *Spontaneous pneumothorax* This may occur in cryptogenic fibrosing 'alveolitis', chronic extrinsic allergic 'alveolitis', chronic beryllium disease and other diseases with multiple cyst formation owing to rupture of an air bleb, but it is most exceptional in asbestosis.

Rarely a non-asbestos DIPF, or fibrosing 'alveolitis', may occur in an individual who already has asbestosis. This is likely to be expressed by an unexpected and atypical alteration in established radiographic appearances (*Figure 9.30*).

Hence, the diagnosis of asbestosis should be questioned if the overall radiographic features are unlike those generally associated with asbestosis, and if some other cause of DIPF is present. In this respect it is evident that comparison of current with earlier chest radiographs (if available) is absolutely essential.

Experience of many cases with occupational asbestos exposure suggests that the level of exposure (dose × time) has usually been moderate to heavy in most of those with asbestosis but light or sometimes moderate, in many of those with non-asbestotic DIPF.

The importance of taking PA and appropriately angled RAO and LAO films of good quality in individuals seen for the first time and in those who show unusual changes later cannot be too strongly emphasized (*see* Chapter 5, p. 96).

The clinical diagnosis of asbestosis, therefore, depends on the following criteria:

(1) Evidence of occupational exposure to asbestos minerals.
(2) Persistent bilateral basal, inspiratory crepitations.
(3) Relevant lung function abnormalities.
(4) Radiographic evidence of bilateral basal DIPF often with diffuse pleural thickening.
(5) Rigorous exclusion of simulative disease and its causes.

Of these (1) and (5) and at least two of the remaining criteria are necessary.

Circulating ANAs and RFs are, in general, of no value in differential diagnosis apart from the fact that high titres of RF may suggest rheumatoid lung disease rather than asbestosis. The presence or absence of avian precipitins in individuals with previous exposure to birds may be of limited help in differentiation.

In a small number of cases it may be very difficult to determine with reasonable confidence whether or not the disease with which one is confronted is asbestosis. In this situation, and to ensure that treatable disease is not missed, lung biopsy may be necessary. A good sample of lung tissue should then be taken at thoracotomy because needle and

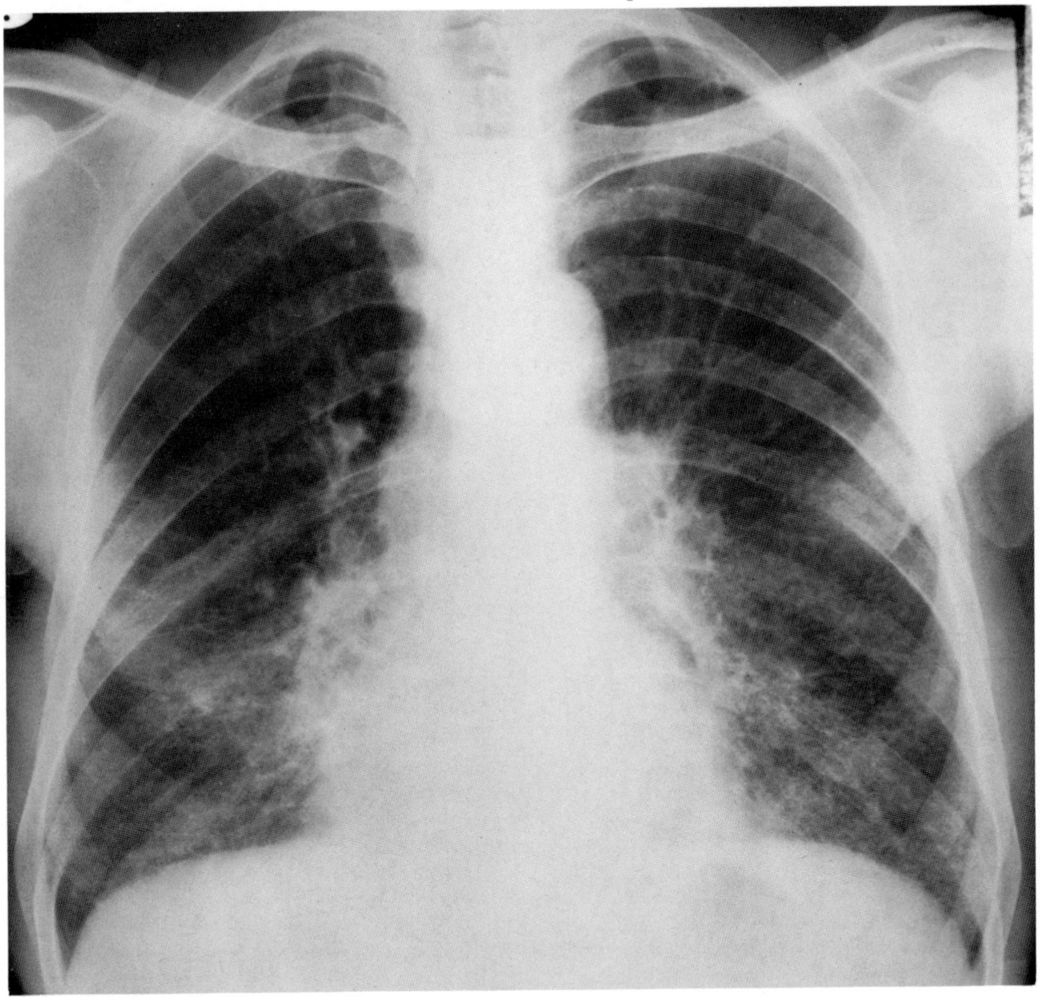

Figure 9.17(b) 1969

drill techniques often fail to obtain relevant samples or, owing to their small size, to resolve the diagnosis (Scott and Hunt, 1975). The chief considerations for or against this investigation in patients with past asbestos exposure can be tabulated as follows.

(1) *Lung biopsy is indicated if one or more of these conditions is present:*
(a) atypical development, distribution, progression and character of the radiographic appearances;
(b) constitutional symptoms;
(c) the presence of a disorder known to be associated with DIPF or one of the causes of simulative disease.
(2) *Lung biopsy is contra-indicated if:*
(a) the development, distribution, progression and radiographic appearances are consistent with asbestosis (*see* pp. 257 to 259);
(b) the conditions listed under the foregoing headings (1) (b) and (c) are excluded.

Post-mortem and microscopical criteria

These have been discussed on pp. 251 to 253. The problems involved in differentiating other forms of DIPF from asbestosis are examined in Chapter 4, pp. 75 to 82. It is pointed out there that microscopy in some of these cases reveals significant hyperplasia of elastin, smooth muscle or lymphoid tissue which is not seen in asbestosis. Examples of these from asbestos-exposed individuals with difffuse, mural fibrosis unlike asbestosis are shown in *Figures 4.16, 4.17,* and *4.18* which correspond respectively to *Figures 9.24, 9.27* and *9.23*.

In asbestosis of moderate to severe degree the electron microscopic asbestos fibre count is usually substantially in excess of about 60 million fibres/g of dried lung, sometimes as high as 300 to 400 million, and in slight disease it may be as low as 20 million fibres/g. But values of the latter order and below may sometimes be found in other forms of DIPF if there has been exposure to asbestos. Counts in the lungs of 'control' urban populations may be as much as 8 million/g. With a modified Ashcroft–Heppleston (1973) phase-contrast light microscopy technique *mean* fibre levels have been found to be about 28 million/g of dried lung in severe asbestosis and about 5 million/g in mild asbestosis; and are not often less than 3 million/g when asbestosis is present (Whitwell, Scott and Grimshaw, 1977).

In 'control' urban lungs counts are usually under 50000/g. It must be pointed out, however, that, due to the subjectivity of this method (which chiefly identifies amphiboles) there is considerable variation in the results of different observers which has to be taken into account.

The relationship of asbestos bodies to the fibre content of

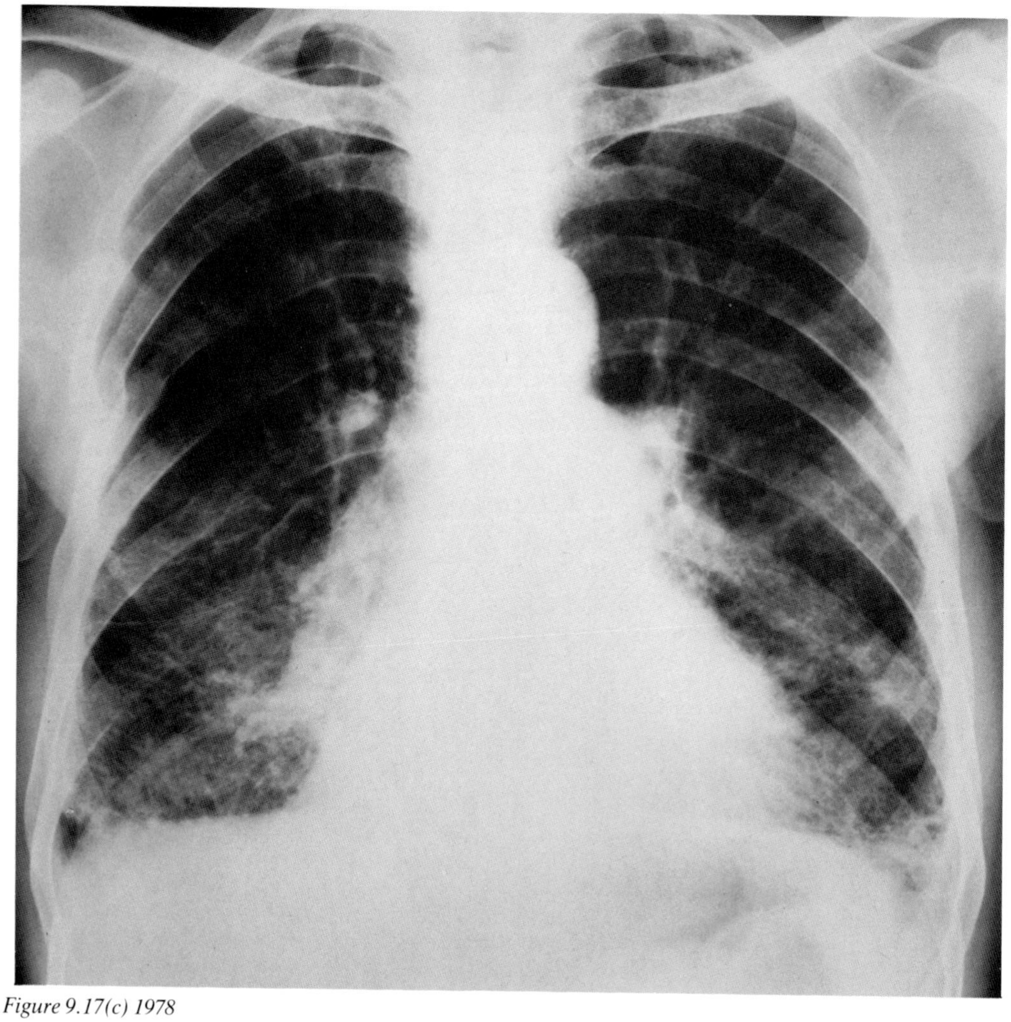

Figure 9.17(c) 1978

Figure 9.17 Progression of asbestosis over 20 years. Operator of disintegrator and crusher of crude asbestos fibre from 1956 to 1959. (a) 1957, no evident abnormality. (b) 1969, slight to moderate asbestosis: category 's'. Note: clear upper zones, and minimal evidence of diffuse pleural thickening. Asbestosis with many asbestos bodies confirmed by biopsy. Clinically: persistent fine paninspiratory crepitations in both lower lobes, middle lobe and lingula with moderate restrictive and gas transfer defects. (c) 1978, advanced disease (category t/u). Note downward displacement of lesser fissure; evidence of diffuse pleural thickening with obliteration of the costophrenic angles, indefinite ('shaggy') cardiac outline, and clear upper zones. Severe respiratory disability

the lungs has been referred to already on pp. 239 and 240. In asbestosis intact bodies or fragments are usually found fairly readily.

To summarize

Individuals with occupational exposure to asbestos appear to fall into four categories in regard to DIPF:

(1) Those who never develop asbestosis.
(2) Those who develop asbestosis which may or may not be progressive.
(3) Those who develop some causally unrelated form of DIPF or fibrosing 'alveolitis'.
(4) Rarely, those who already have asbestosis and subsequently develop some other form of chronic fibrosing 'alveolitis'.

From what has been said, therefore, it will be clear that the diagnosis of asbestosis during life may be less straightforward than is often thought. When confronted with this problem it is wise to have Lewinsohn's (1977) sound advise in mind:

> 'Asbestosis is not a clearcut entity. . . and very often a mistaken diagnosis can be made which, if communicated to the individual concerned before all diagnostic avenues have been explored and the disease confirmed, can lead to psychological stress and breed ill-will in a community.'

Prognosis

The development and severity of asbestosis is related more to prolonged than to intermittent asbestos exposure but individual susceptibility both to development and

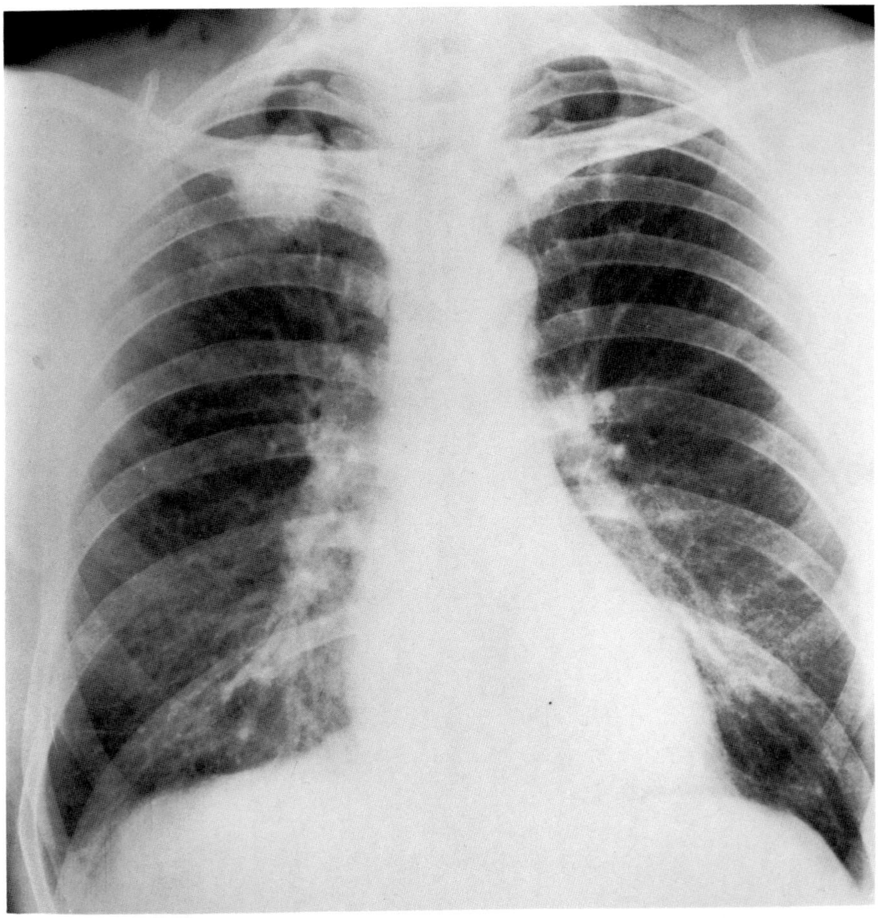

Figure 9.18 Coal pneumoconiosis with PMF in right upper zone and slight to moderate asbestosis (1980). Coal-miner at the 'dump end' of a coal conveyor underground for five and a half years (1936 to 1942). Very dusty conditions. 1961 to 1968: fitter assembling asbestos cement panels in a power station; but chief exposure occurred in the earlier years of this period when he was in proximity to asbestos insulation workers. Open lung biopsy revealed coal pneumoconiosis, mild asbestosis and moderate numbers of asbestos bodies in 30 μm sections

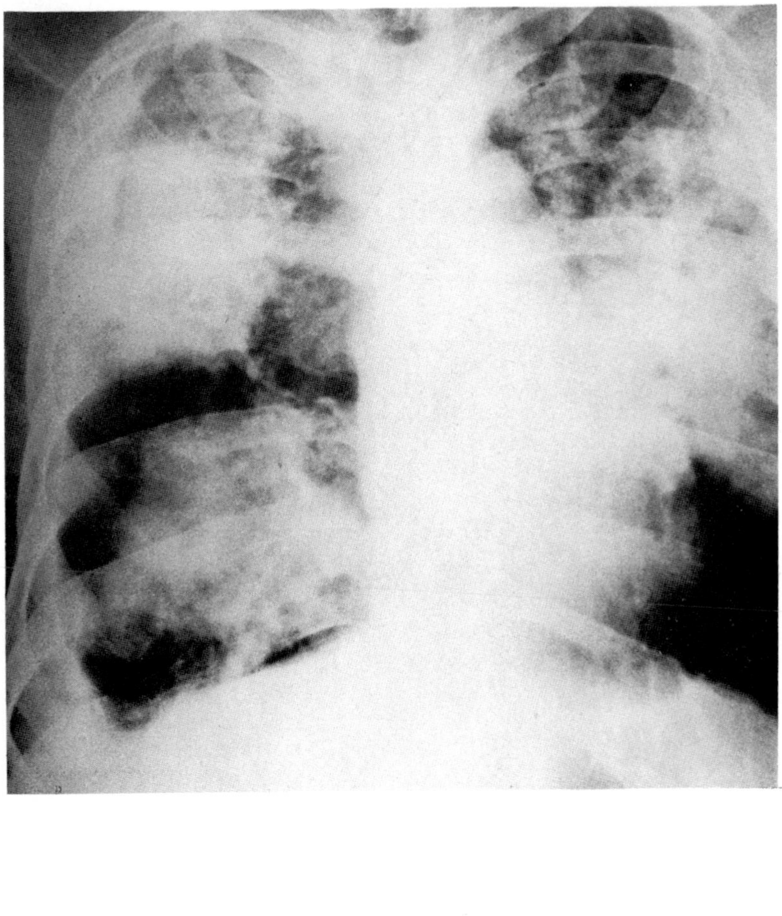

Figure 9.19 Radiograph of a young man with about 10 years' high dust exposure in a North Cape (S. Africa) crocidolite-mine. In addition to the large opacities, smaller round opacities are present as well as evidence of extensive pleural thickening over the right lung. (Reproduced by courtesy of Dr A. Solomon and colleagues and the Editor of Environmental Research*)*

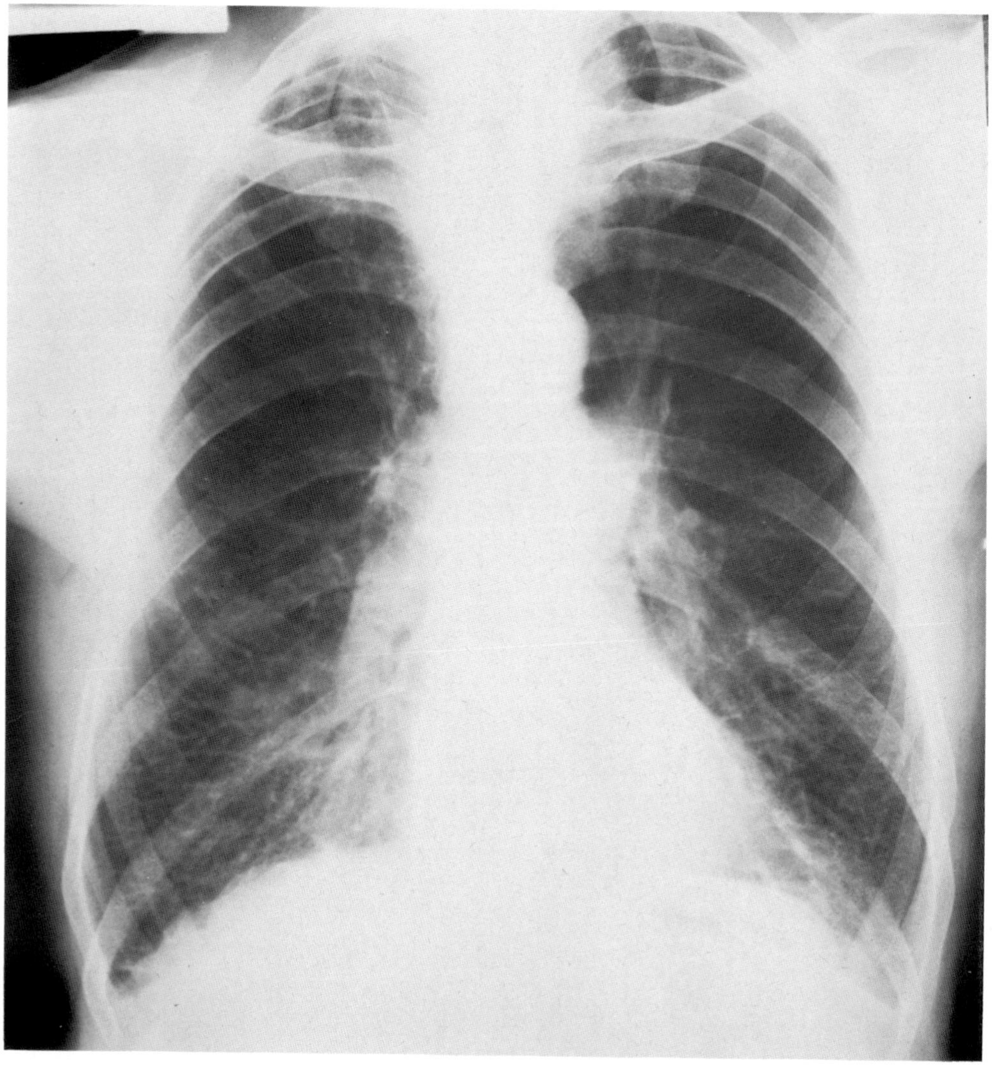

Figure 9.20 Severe hyperinflation of both upper lobes causing appearances simulating slight DIPF in both lower zones. No occupational hazard

progression of the disease appears to vary considerably; among men with an apparently similar history of exposure some ultimately have severe asbestosis, some mild and others no evident disease. As a general rule, however, once acquired asbestosis tends to progress slowly sometimes many years after exposure has ended but progression may cease at any stage. Slow progression is exemplified by those patients (who may be in their sixth or seventh decades) in whom the disease proclaims itself, or first comes under medical supervision, 20 or more years after they left the responsible industry.

Whether removing workers with minimal asbestosis from further exposure prevents progression is not known for certain although there is some experimental evidence to suggest that it continues after exposure ceases (Wagner *et al.*, 1974). At present there is no means of identifying those who are likely to develop advanced disease in the long run and those who are not. The presence of circulating ANAs or RFs does not appear to influence the rate of progression of disease.

The possibility that increased serum activity of angiotensin-converting enzyme in some cases of asbestosis might identify those with progressing disease is worth investigating (*see* Chapter 4).

In the UK severe respiratory disability occurs at a later age today than 30 or so years ago—usually after the fourth decade. This is due primarily to disease being, on the whole, less severe than previously as a result of the application of dust control measures in industries subject to the 1931 Asbestos Industries Regulations which came into force in 1932. The average age of death among men with asbestosis increased from about 49 years before 1940 to about 60 years in the early 1960s (Buchanan, 1965). In the asbestos textile and cement industries only men with long exposure to high dust concentrations in the past die of non-malignant respiratory disease at an earlier age than men in the general populations (Newhouse, 1969); and of 3270 chrysotile miners and millers born before 1921 only about 3 per cent (who had experienced the highest level of exposure) died of cardiorespiratory disease (McDonald, 1973a). Although more advanced disease may occur in insulation and other workers who were not subject to the Asbestos Industries Regulations in the past and who were often exposed to uncontrolled concentrations of asbestos before 1970 when

(a)

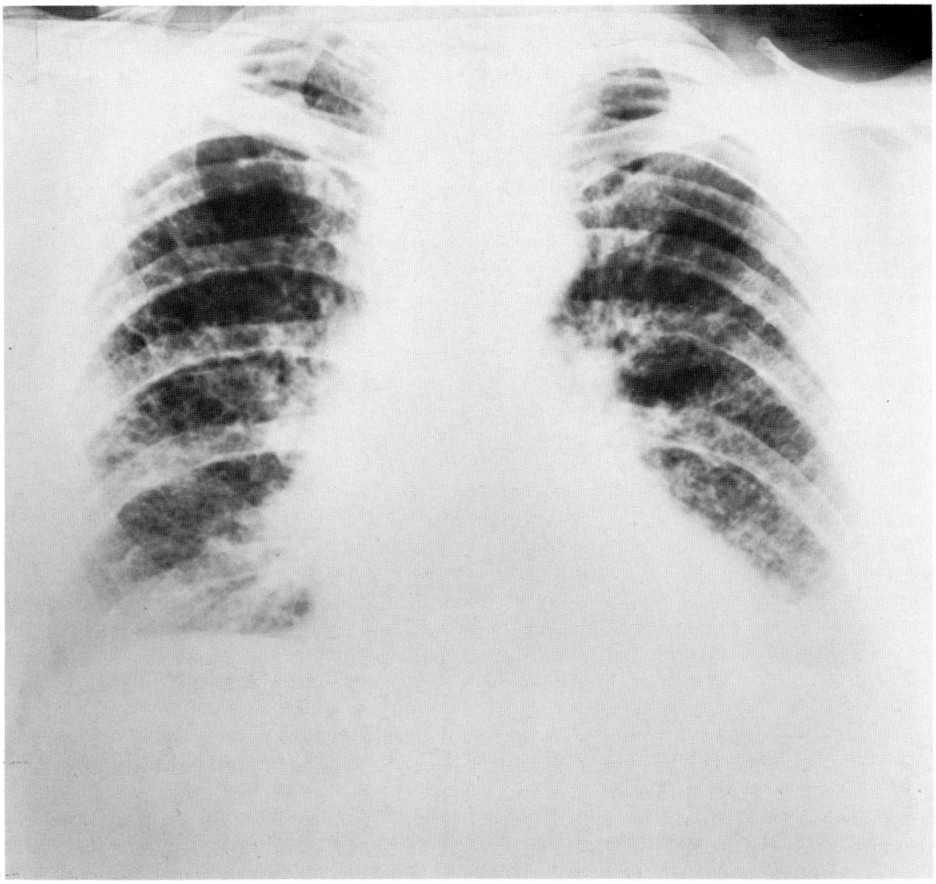

(b)

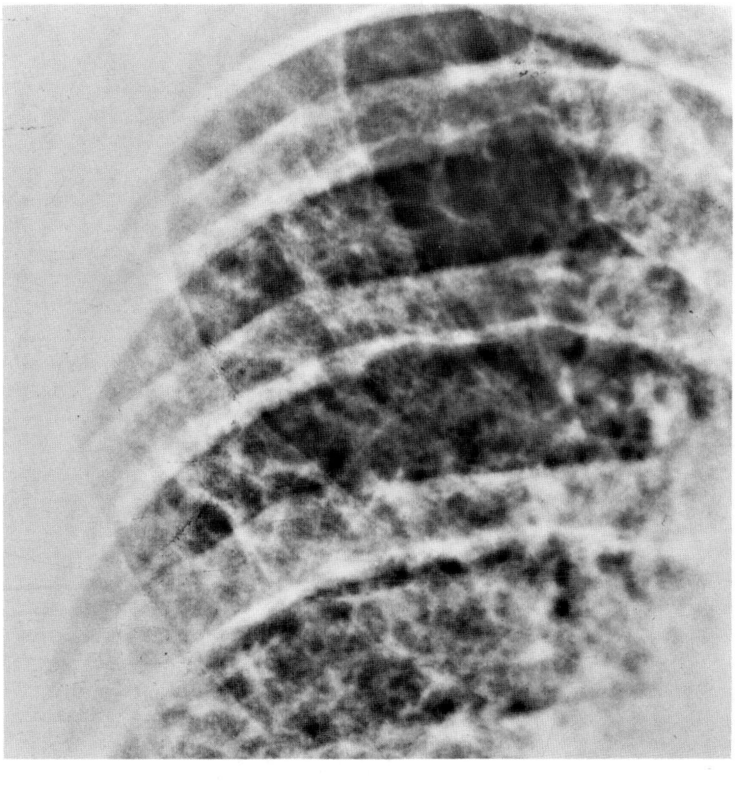

Figure 9.21 (a) Widespread irregular opacities in all zones with 'honeycomb' appearances showing progression over six years. The abnormal opacities in the upper zones (b) preceded those in the lower zones by two years. Maintenance man in an asbestos factory. Intermittent, slight exposure to asbestos. Clinically: *widespread medium, inspiratory crepitations in both upper and lower lobe areas partly altered by cough. Circulating ANA-positive. Asbestosis diagnosed.* Post mortem. *Naked eye: multiple air-blebs on the surface of the pulmonary pleura and coarse DIPF with multiple cysts up to 5 mm diameter in all lobes, the right upper lobe being extensively involved. Microscopically; DIPF with bronchiolectasis showing squamous metaplasia. No asbestos bodies found in multiple 30 μm sections.* Diagnosis: *cryptogenic fibrosing alveolitis. (Right upper zone, natural size)*

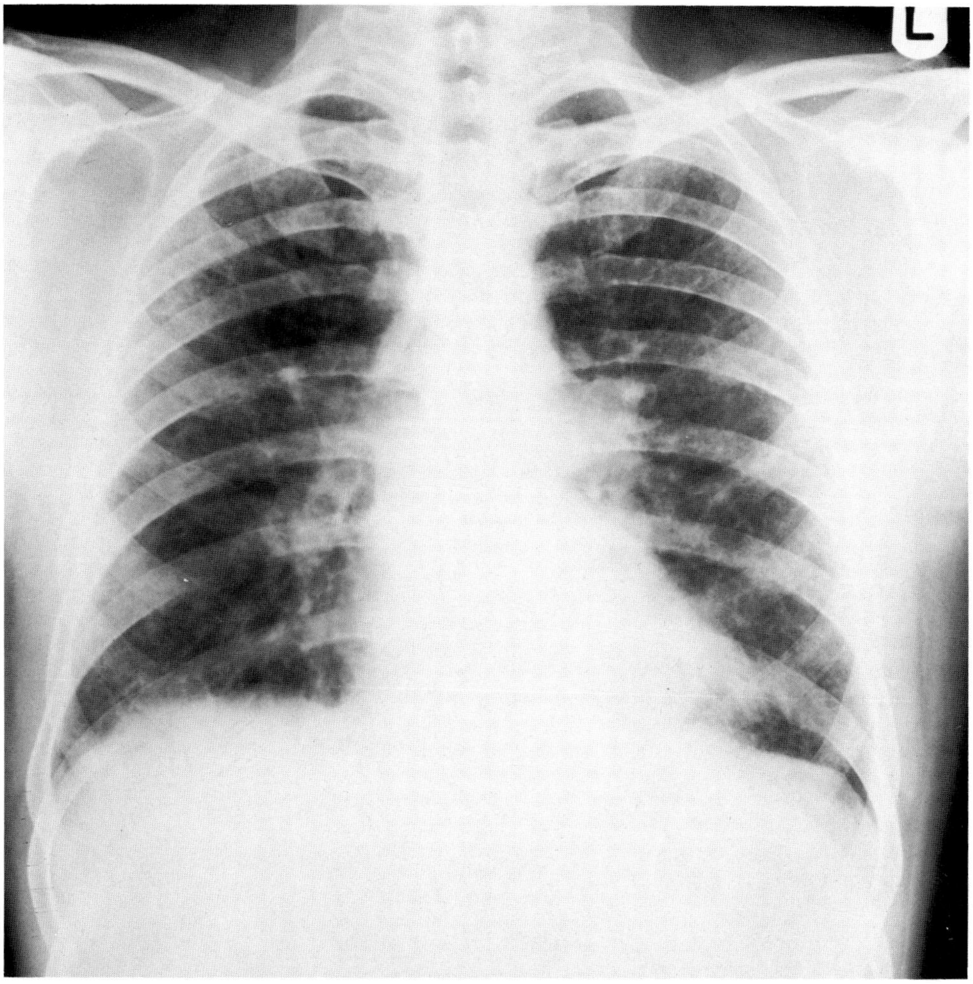

Figure 9.22(a) 1974

the Regulations came into force in Britain (*see* Preventive measures) the excess mortality due to asbestosis previously observed in insulation workers in Belfast ceased after 1965 (Elmes and Simpson, 1977). Hence, today many persons with asbestosis live a normal life span or die of unrelated causes but, because of longer survival, the risk of their developing the complication of bronchial carcinoma is correspondingly increased (*see* next section).

Complications

Carcinoma of the lung Wood and Gloyne (1934) first suggested that individuals with asbestosis might develop carcinoma of the lung and Merewether (1949), in the UK, reported that 14.7 per cent of men with asbestosis died of lung cancer between 1929 and 1947. The relationship was confirmed by Doll (1955) who showed that asbestos textile workers *with asbestosis* and ten or more years exposure had a ten-fold excess risk of acquiring the disease. By 1955 39.4 per cent of individuals with asbestosis died of carcinoma of the lung (21.6 per cent of males, 17.8 per cent of females) and at the end of 1963 just over 50 per cent died of an intrathoracic neoplasm (including four recorded 'mesothelioma of pleura') (Buchanan, 1965). A similar trend has been observed in the USA and elsewhere. This increase is attributable (at least in the UK) to a combination of improved life expectancy of individuals with asbestosis whose dust exposure during the 1930s to the 1950s was, in general, worse than it has been since and to the steady rise in cigarette consumption since the 1920s (*see Table 1.3,* p. 00). It appears that in individuals with asbestosis in Britain, who smoke, life expectancy is reduced by about ten years compared with non-smokers due, mainly, to bronchial carcinoma (Berry, 1981).

However, rigorous hygiene measures in a British asbestos textile factory over approximately 30 years following implementation of Asbestos Industry Regulations (1931) in 1932 resulted in there being little increase in mortality from bronchial carcinoma among workers who entered the industry after 1932 (Knox *et al.,* 1968), although a further eight and a half year follow-up of this group has shown a slight increase in mortality from the tumour (Peto *et al.,* 1977).

As a rule, the tumour arises in the vicinity of the fibrosis and, therefore, occurs chiefly in the lower parts of the lungs—usually the lower lobes (Hueper, 1966; Jacob and Anspach, 1965; Whitwell, Newhouse and Bennett, 1974). It may be of bronchial (central) or peripheral origin and its

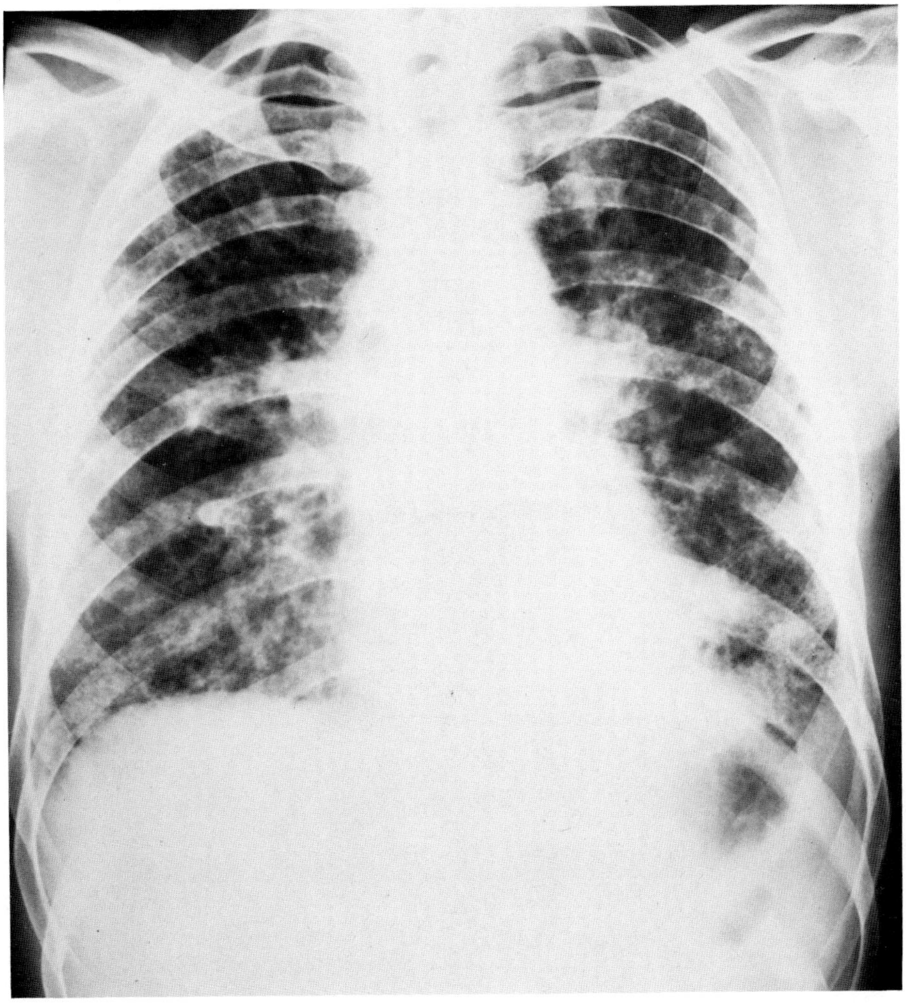

Figure 9.22(b) 1977

commonest histological type appears to be adenocarcinoma which is more frequently peripheral than are the other types (Hourihane and McCaughey, 1966; Hueper, 1966; Whitwell, Newhouse and Bennett, 1974). Animals exposed to asbestos have shown a greater frequency of adenocarcinoma than squamous carcinoma with Canadian and Rhodesian chrysotile and an equal frequency of both tumours with other types of fibre (Wagner *et al.*, 1974). Kannerstein and Churg (1972), however, did not find an overall excess of adenocarcinoma in a group of asbestos workers compared with a control series but, as Whitwell, Newhouse and Bennett (1974) point out, it is difficult to assess the significance of their findings which were based on disparate material derived from bronchial biopsy, secondary deposit biopsy, surgical specimens and post-mortem tissue.

Not unexpectedly the frequency of lung cancer is increased in the smokers compared with non-smokers (Whitwell, Newhouse and Bennett, 1974) but, as most of the information on this topic in asbestos workers has been derived in the main from epidemiological and not post-mortem studies, information concerning the presence or absence of asbestosis has been inadequate. The effects of smoking and asbestosis appear to be synergistic and multiplicative (Saracci, 1977). The question as to whether asbestos exposure alone (that is, without asbestosis) is related to lung cancer is discussed on p. 294.

Although a relationship between asbestosis and carcinoma of the lung is well established in man and supported by observations in animals (Wagner *et al.*, 1974) there is some difficulty in regarding the fibrosis as directly responsible for the tumour because an excess of lung cancer does not occur with other fibrotic pneumoconioses: for example, silicosis and coal pneumoconiosis (*see* Chapters 7 and 8). But on the other hand, there is an increased risk of bronchial carcinoma in cryptogenic fibrosing 'alveolitis', 'honeycomb lung' and DIPF associated with the 'collagen diseases' (Meyer and Liebow, 1965; Godeau *et al.*, 1974; Turner-Warwick, Burrows and Johnson, 1980). The apparent link (referred to earlier on p. 254) between impaired T lymphocyte function and clinical asbestosis (especially when advanced) in the absence of any evidence of lung cancer raises the possibility of reduced immune ('killer cell') surveillance and destruction of potentially neoplastic cells in asbestosis and a consequent increased propensity to develop malignancy. By contrast, patients with malignant pleural mesothelioma apparently have normal T lymphocyte responses and delayed hypersensitivity (Haslam *et al.*, 1978; Pierce and Turner-Warwick, 1980) (*see* p. 286).

(c)

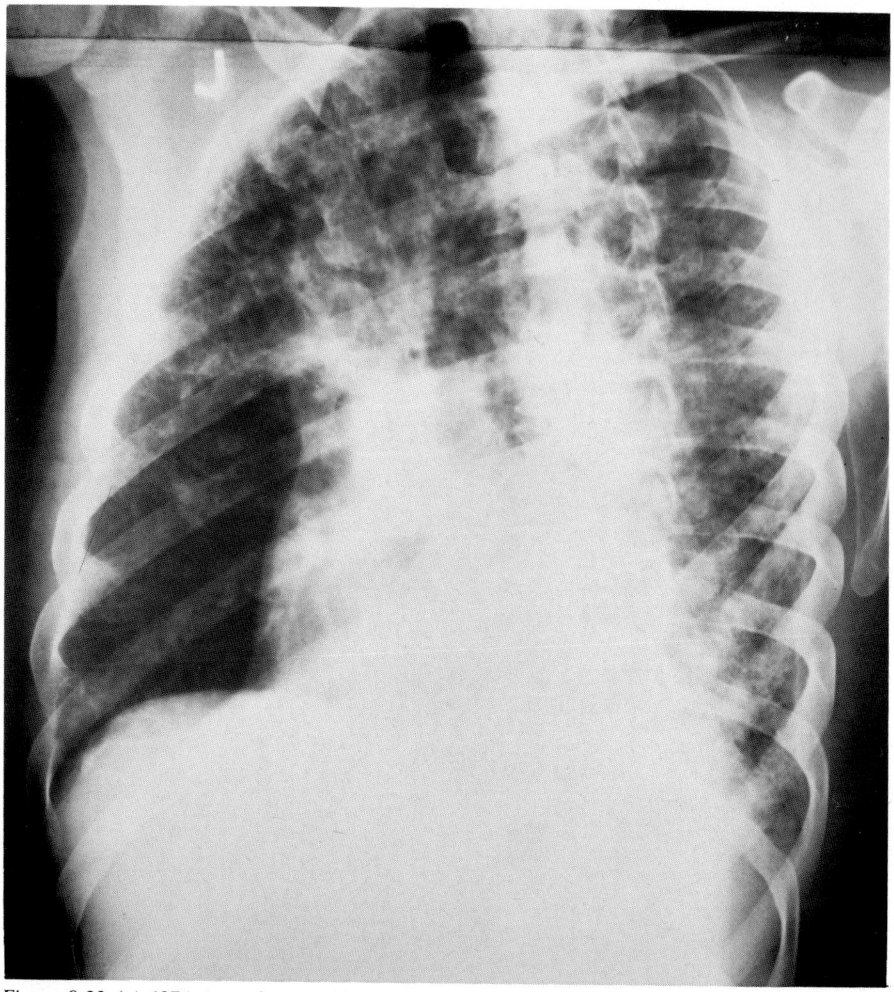

Figure 9.22 (a) 1974, irregular opacities in all zones (some breathlessness on exertion noted a year previously). Note involvement of right upper zone. (b) 1977, significant progression: coarse, irregular opacities in all zones with cystic appearances. (c) Left 45 degree anterior oblique view (same day) confirms widespread distribution and, in particular, the prominent involvement of the right upper lobe; but note that much of the right lower zone is free of opacities. Plumber and pipe fitter for 25 years; intermittent para-occupational proximity to insulation workers. Kept a budgerigar six years. Clinically: *coarse inspiratory and expiratory crepitations in all lobar areas. No arthropathy. Circulating RF and avian precipitins absent. Lung biopsy: DIPF with diffuse immunofluorescent staining by IgG; occasional asbestos bodies.* Post mortem: *Naked eye: Multiple small ('hobnail') airblebs on pulmonary pleura. Widespread patches of DIPF in all lobes especially in more central zones with numerous cysts from 2 to 7 mm diameter. Right upper lobe particularly affected. Microscopically: peribronchiolar and sub-pleural DIPF showing the features of mural type fibrosing 'alveolitis' in many areas with some muscular hyperplasia (*see Figures 4.16 *and* 9.24*). Very occasional asbestos bodies identified in multiple 30 μm sections.* Diagnosis: *cryptogenic fibrosing 'alveolitis'*

The possibility, therefore, that asbestosis is associated with a reduced ability for the lung to destroy potentially malignant cells requires to be explored by detailed longitudinal studies of individuals with asbestosis and matched controls from the point of view of the function of lymphocyte populations in bronchial washings and in the peripheral blood, especially as there is evidence that T lymphocyte function in the lungs of smokers without asbestosis is impaired by comparison with the function of these cells in the peripheral blood (Daniele *et al.*, 1977) (*see also* p. 56 and 254).

This risk of bronchial carcinoma complicating asbestosis must always be borne in mind especially in individuals who smoke and have had long exposure to asbestos. In order to identify the growth as early as possible it is advisable to examine workers with more than ten years exposure to asbestos routinely at yearly intervals.

Respiratory failure and pulmonary heart disease In advanced asbestosis respiratory failure, with or without congestive heart failure, may be precipitated by bacterial or viral pneumonia, but today pulmonary heart disease is seldom encountered in uncomplicated asbestosis and death from this cause is rare.

Tuberculosis A high rate of pulmonary tuberculosis was observed in the 1930s and 1940s in persons with asbestosis

(Middleton, 1936. Wood and Gloyne, 1934; Smither, 1965) but in recent years its frequency has been no higher than in the general population (Buchanan, 1965; Enterline, 1965; Smither, 1965). The earlier findings were merely a reflection of the greater prevalence of tuberculosis in the working urban population of that period. In fact, there is no evidence that asbestosis or asbestos exposure predispose to the development of tuberculosis.

Bronchiectasis In past years this sometimes developed in the lower lobes in association with extensive fibrosis of advanced asbestosis but is now rarely, if ever, seen.

Bronchitis and emphysema There is no evidence of a causal relationship between asbestosis and chronic obstructive bronchitis or emphysema although when fibrosis of the lower lobes is severe some hyperinflation of the upper lobes may occur.

Psychological disturbance Fear of life-threatening disease which, unfortunately, may be engendered by some types of publicity (*see* p. 238) is a cause of much anxiety in some patients. Although this is often successfully disguised, a multiplicity of symptoms resulting from physiological alterations caused by the 'hyperventilation syndrome' may be complained of (Pincus, 1978). This situation must be positively identified and thoroughly explained to the patient. Inconsistent and sometimes bizarre chest pains of psychophysiological origin may also occur. It should be borne in mind, too, that the patient's family may suffer distress on this account. The avoidance of uncritical or premature diagnosis of 'asbestosis' which is conveyed to the patient could spare unnecessary anxiety in many cases.

Treatment

There is no treatment at present known which will arrest or retard the progress of asbestosis and, although corticosteroids occasionally cause symptomatic improvement with some reduction of dyspnoea (possibly due to an effect on lung receptors), this appears to be short-lived. Today there should be no need to advise a worker with asbestosis to leave his job on account of dust exposure provided that it is known that the hygienic conditions are such that the level of airborne fibre accords with the currently recommended standards and that he is otherwise protected (*see* Preventive measures). A man with family commitments should not lightly be advised to change his job.

When the diagnosis is first made, reassurance which is realistic and seen by the patient to be founded on careful clinical and investigative examination must be given.

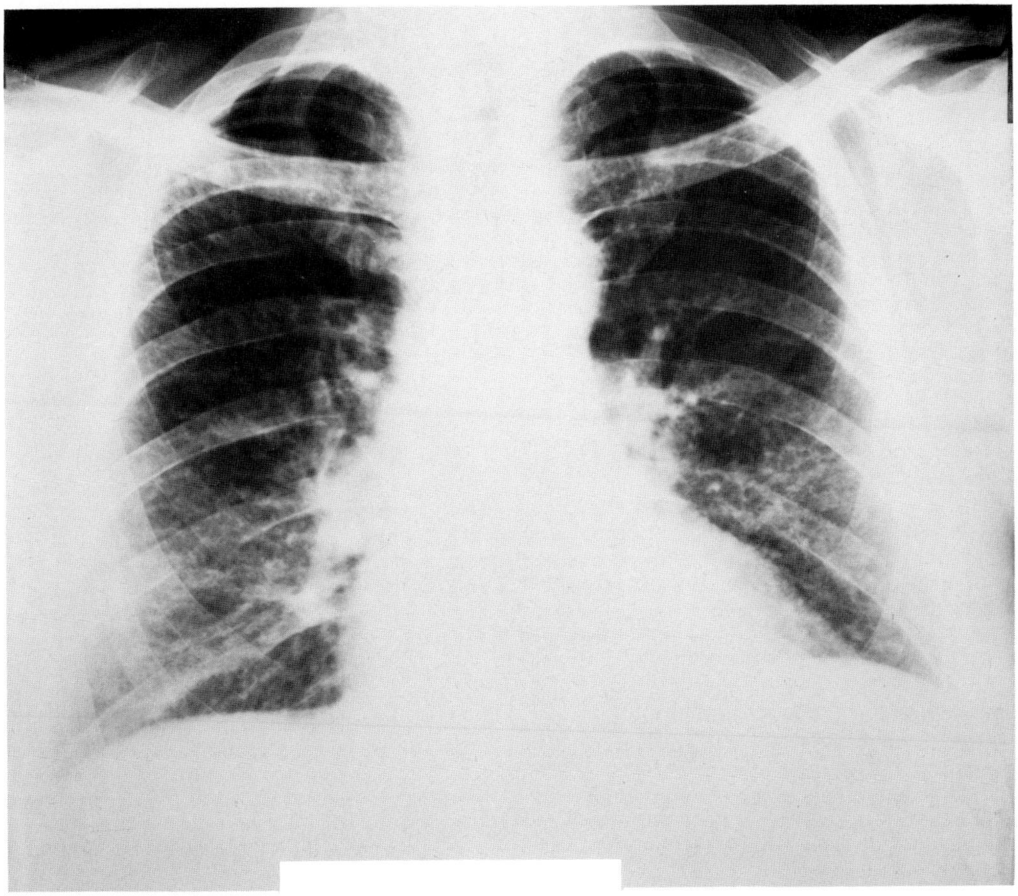

Figure 9.23(a)

(b)

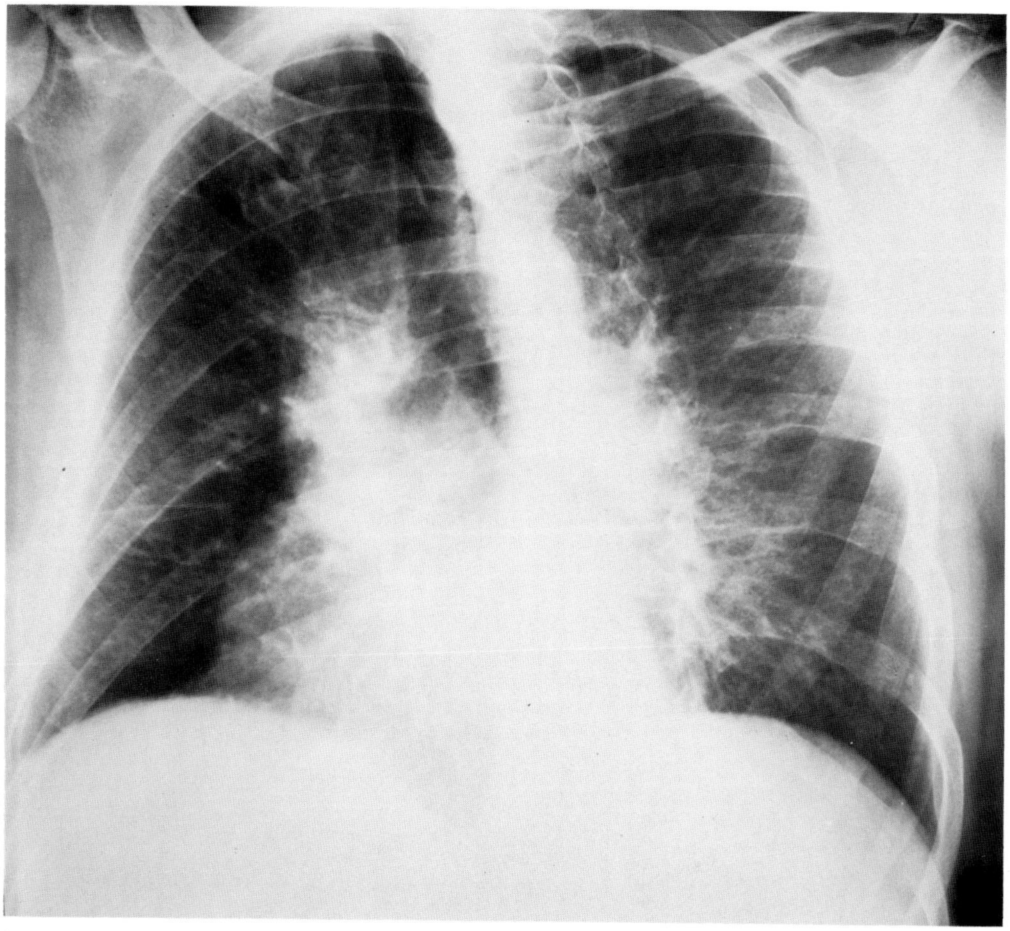

Figure 9.23 1975. (a) Fine irregular opacities in both lower zones and coarse irregular opacities in right upper zone. But note absence of opacities in the costophrenic angles in the left anterior oblique view (b). Appearances developed slowly over eight years following onset of rheumatoid arthritis two years earlier. Machinist milling and turning asbestos-containing brake linings from 1967 to 1977. Fibre count very low in work area in latter years. Clinically: transient inspiratory crepitations both lower lobes. Moderate restrictive and gas transfer defects with low Kco. Moderately severe rheumatoid arthritis with subcutaneous nodules. Lung biopsy: fibrosing 'alveolitis' of predominantly mural type with prominent lymphoid follicular hyperplasia; no asbestos bodies. Post mortem four years later. *Naked eye: widespread, fine, well-demarcated DIPF in all lobes with honeycomb cysts from 2 to 10 mm diameter. Microscopy verified biopsy findings* (see Figure 4.18). *No asbestos bodies found in multiple 30 μm sections.* Diagnosis: *'rheumatoid lung'*

Because the combination of asbestosis and smoking offers a high risk of developing bronchial carcinoma he should be strongly advised to stop smoking permanently. Patients with troublesome paroxysmal cough require an appropriate antitussive drug, and if sputum is viscid and difficult to raise, the simple remedies of an expectorant and inhalation of steam give considerable relief. Respiratory infections in patients with advanced asbestosis require prompt investigation and treatment.

Therapeutic measures for respiratory failure or bronchial carcinoma may ultimately be necessary; but, in the latter case, surgery may be impossible if fibrosis is advanced.

MALIGNANT MESOTHELIOMA OF PLEURA AND PERITONEUM

Until recent years this tumour, which arises from multipotential coelomic mesothelial cells of the pleura, pericardium and peritoneum was considered to be an exceptionally rare (Willis, 1967) but, nonetheless, real entity in that tissue cultures have shown that mesothelial cells can form fibroblastic tissue, and fibrous mesotheliomas can produce epithelial cells (Godwin, 1957; Sano, Weiss and Gault, 1950). In 1943 a link between asbestos exposure and pleural growths was suggested by Wedler. In 1946 Wyers noted the occurrence of 'endothelioma' (mesothelioma) of the pleura in an asbestos worker, and in 1960 the tumour was described in individuals with previous industrial or environmental contact with crocidolite more than 20 years earlier in the North West Cape Province of South Africa (Wagner, Slegg and Marchand, 1960). Since then the number of recorded cases of pleural and peritoneal tumours associated with past occupational or para-occupational exposure to asbestos has been increasing in the UK where the annual incidence is now computed to be at least 120 (Greenberg and Lloyd Davies, 1974) though 260 cases were recorded in death certificates in 1975 (Health and Safety Executive, 1979); in South Africa (Newhouse, 1977); in Australia (Milne, 1976); in the USA (Boron *et al.*, 1973; Selikoff, 1976); in Holland (Zielhuis, Versteeg and Planteijdt, 1975); in West Germany (Bohlig *et al.*, 1970) and in other countries (Newhouse, 1977). Between 1959 and 1976, 4539 cases were reported from 22 countries (McDonald and McDonald, 1977a). It is uncertain to what extent this is a real increase or the expression of a recently enhanced tendency to make this diagnosis rather than another; however, although the diagnosis is often erroneous (Greenberg and Lloyd Davies, 1974; McDonald, Magner and Eysson, 1973; Willis, 1973) the rise in incidence cannot be dismissed as a diagnostic artefact.

The 'attack rate' among occupationally exposed individuals is, in general, less than 7 per cent and the excess risk of malignant mesothelioma varies according to the type of industrial exposure (*Table 9.2*). It has been predicted that by AD 2000 the mortality from these tumours among men and women who worked at a London asbestos textile factory before 1964 will be between 7 and 11 per cent of the total mortality for men and somewhat higher for women (Newhouse and Berry, 1976).

In the USA crude incidence rates of the tumour are computed to range from 3.0 to 7.1 per million per year. Sex specific incidence rates adjusted by age to the 1970 population range from 4.4 to 11.1 per million per year in males and 1.2 to 3.8 per million per year for females (Hinds, 1978).

The tumour occurs in both sexes and, as a rule, the pleural origin is much more common than the peritoneal (Elmes and Simpson, 1976; Milne, 1976) though the latter site may be more frequent in women (Newhouse *et al.*, 1972) and, exceptionally, has been recorded as predominant in a series of male American insulation workers

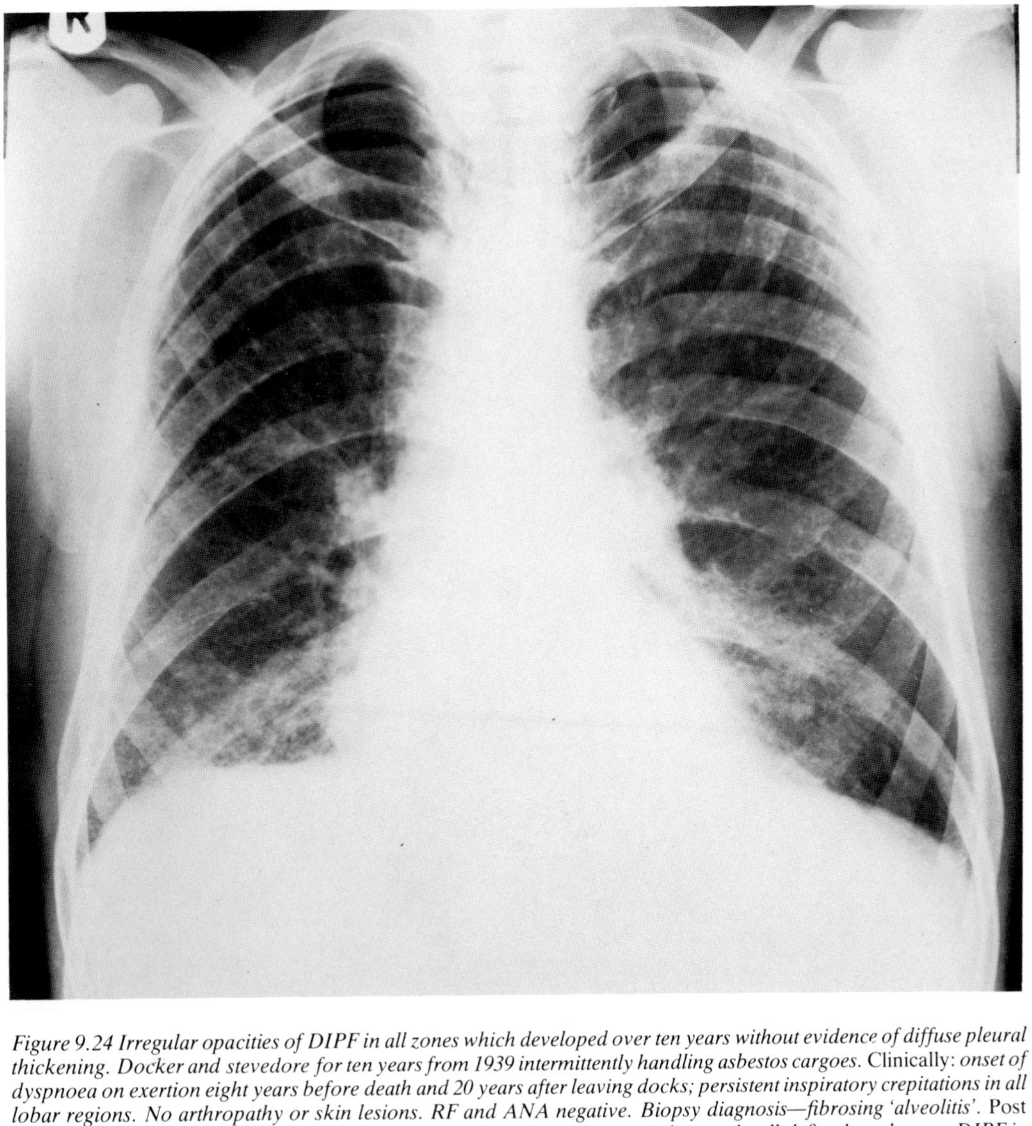

Figure 9.24 Irregular opacities of DIPF in all zones which developed over ten years without evidence of diffuse pleural thickening. Docker and stevedore for ten years from 1939 intermittently handling asbestos cargoes. Clinically: *onset of dyspnoea on exertion eight years before death and 20 years after leaving docks; persistent inspiratory crepitations in all lobar regions. No arthropathy or skin lesions. RF and ANA negative. Biopsy diagnosis—fibrosing 'alveolitis'.* Post mortem. *Naked eye: multiple 'hobnail' air blebs on pulmonary pleura. Widespread well-defined patchy grey DIPF in all lobes with numerous honeycomb cysts varying from 2 to 10 mm diameter. Appearances unlike those of asbestosis. Microscopically: DIPF of moderate severity with cystic dilatation of peripheral bronchioles and pronounced smooth muscle hyperplasia arranged in bizarre bundles. Occasional asbestos bodies in 30 μm sections.* (See Figure 4.16 *for histology of this case).* Diagnosis: *cryptogenic fibrosing 'alveolitis'*

Table 9.2 Percentage Proportion of all Deaths due to Malignant Mesothelioma in Cohorts Asbestos Workers and the General Population

	Mesothelioma	*Number of surveys*	*Total numbers*
Asbestos workers			
Insulation	5–9	6	26 500
Asbestos-using factories	1–7	5	10 000
Mining and milling of asbestos*	0–0.2	3	13 700
General population			
England and Wales } USA } Canada }	0.001		

*2 Chrysotile mines (Quebec and Italy)
1 Anthophyllite mine
Mixed fibre exposure in other two groups
(Adapted by courtesy of Dr J. C. Gilson and Editor of INSERM Symposium Series)

(Selikoff, 1976). Occasionally it occurs in more than one member of a family, but its site of origin or histological features are not necessarily similar. On present evidence its occurrence appears to be closely, but not uniquely, related to exposure to either crocidolite alone or a mixture of fibre types in the distant past—usually 20 or more years earlier and, in some instances, more than 40 years (*see* section on Pathogenesis).

In some cases exposure appears to have been solely non-occupational and environmental due, for example, to residence in close proximity to a dockyard or an asbestos-processing plant or factory (Wagner, Munday and Harington, 1962; Bohlig *et al.*, 1970; Newhouse and Thompson, 1965), and, apparently, to household contact with asbestos brought home by factory workers on their working clothes. By 1976 37 alleged mesothelial tumours

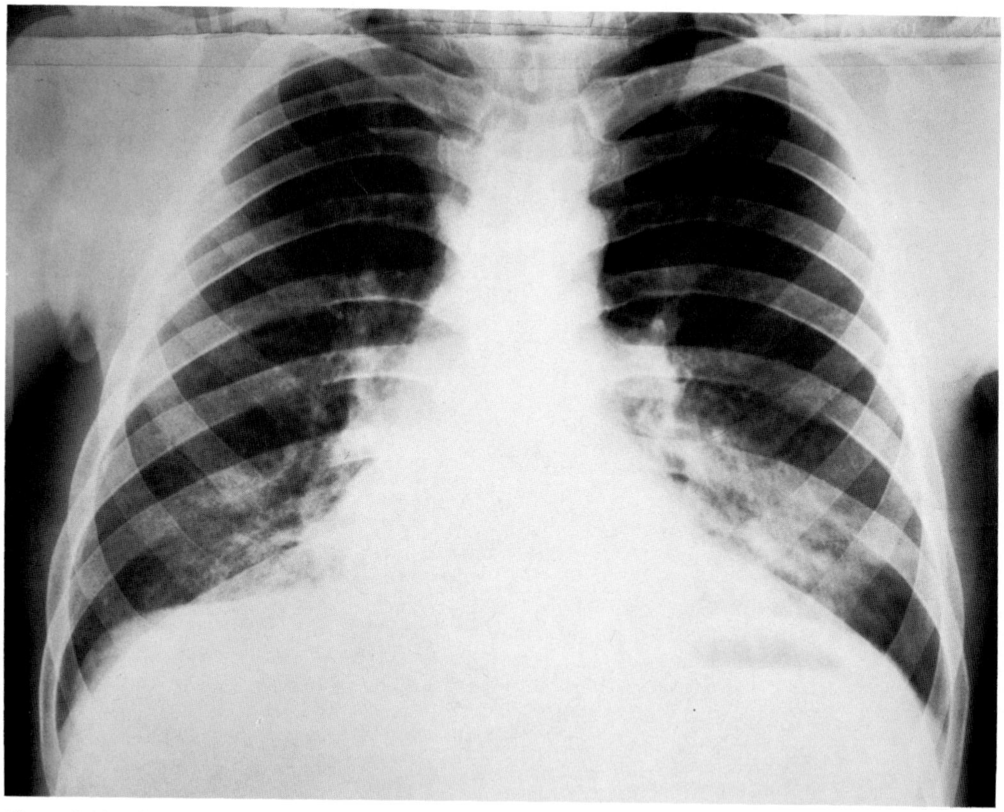

Figure 9.25 Bilateral basal irregular opacities associated with moderately advanced multiple neurofibromatosis (von Recklinghausen's disease). The appearances are not typical of those of DIPF, there is no diffuse pleural thickening and the costophrenic angles are clear. Machinist in an asbestos processing factory. Clinically: *no abnormal physical signs in the lungs.* Physiology: *lung volumes within normal limits but some reduction in Tl and Kco. The pathological features of the disease are those of cystic DIPF with some hyperplasia of smooth muscle adjacent to distal airways and of the neurilemmal (Schwann) cells of periarterial nerves. Glomus-like structures may be present in small pulmonary artery branches. These changes may also occur in patients with focal cutaneous hyperpigmentation ('cafe-au-lait' spots) only*

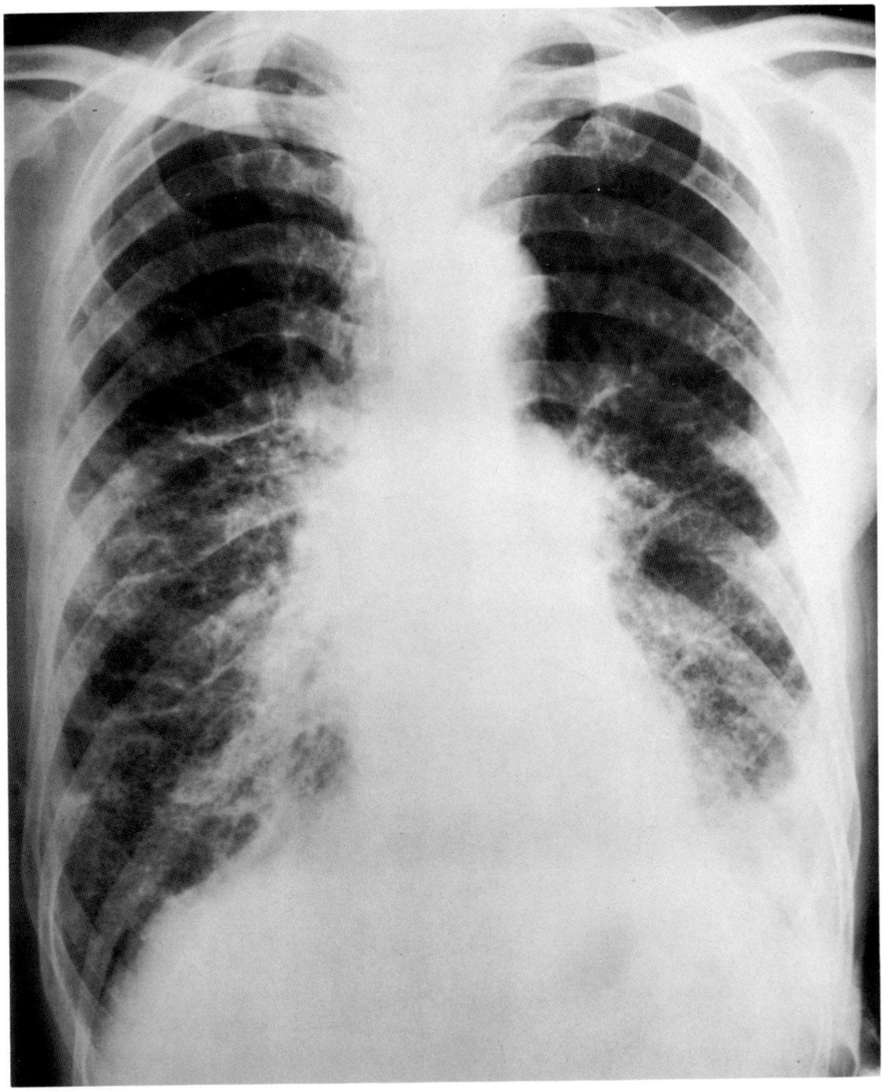

Figure 9.26 Widespread irregular opacities due to lymphangitis carcinomatosa. (Courtesy of Dr P. M. Bretland, London)

are said to have been related to such domestic exposure in nine different countries (Anderson *et al.*, 1976).

However, malignant mesothelioma may occur spontaneously, though very rarely, among the general public—including young children (Kauffman and Stout, 1964)—in the absence of any known exposure to asbestos (about 1 per million per year) (*Table 9.2*). And, according to various recent surveys, there is no evidence of exposure in about 15 per cent of these tumours in adults (Greenberg and Lloyd Davies, 1974; Milne, 1976; Wagner *et al.*, 1971; Webster, 1973; Whitwell, Scott and Grimshaw 1977); although in Holland occupational exposure has been reported in 100 per cent of cases (Zielhuis, Versteeg and Planteijdt, 1975).

Pathology

Macroscopic features

The tumour is ivory-white, grey or yellow, sometimes with reddish striae and it varies in extent from a hard sheet about 0.5 to 1.0 cm thick covering a limited part of the surface of the lung with some tendency to spread into interlobar fissures to a thick softer mass totally encasing one lung and invading it in lobulated fashion (*Figure 9.31*). All lobes of the lung are then much compressed and may be virtually obliterated. Both the pulmonary and the parietal pleura are involved and frequently there is massive direct invasion along interlobobar and interlobular fissures, into and around the pericardium (especially when the tumour is on the left side) and, sometimes, the contralateral pleura and the liver. Plaques may be present in the parietal pleura on both sides, but this is exceptional.

The cut surface of the tumour may be glutinous (due to the production of hyaluronic acid); in places there may be necrotic cavities which contain either viscid and sometimes haemorrhagic fluid or a fibrinous material, and are sometimes of considerable size.

It must be emphasized, however, that these gross appearances are *not* diagnostic. Tumours which may present identical features are adenocarcinoma originating peripherally in the lung or pseudomesotheliomatous

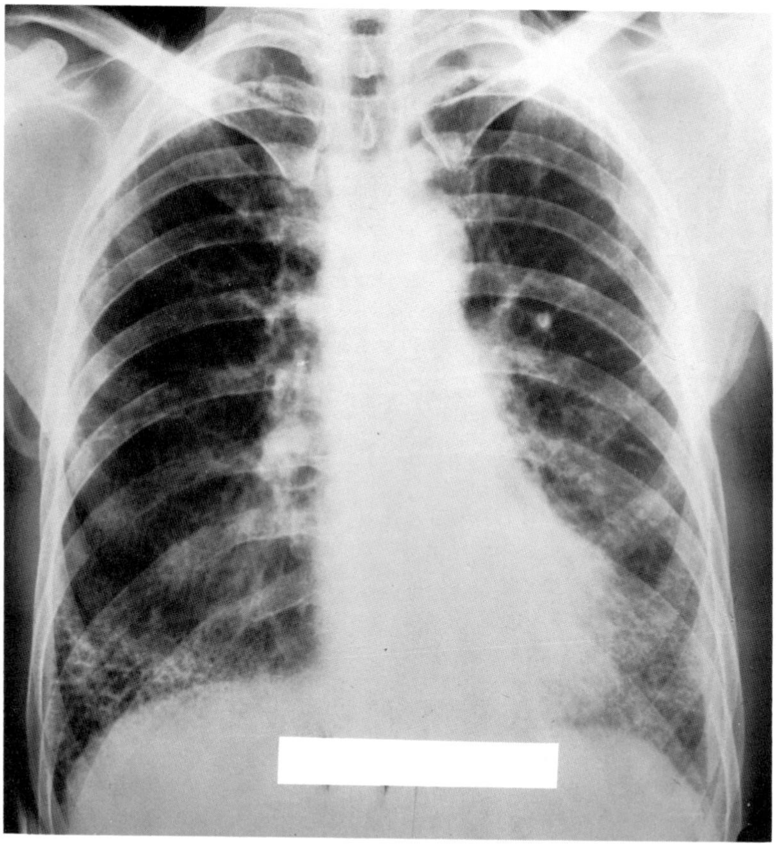

Figure 9.27 (a) 1972

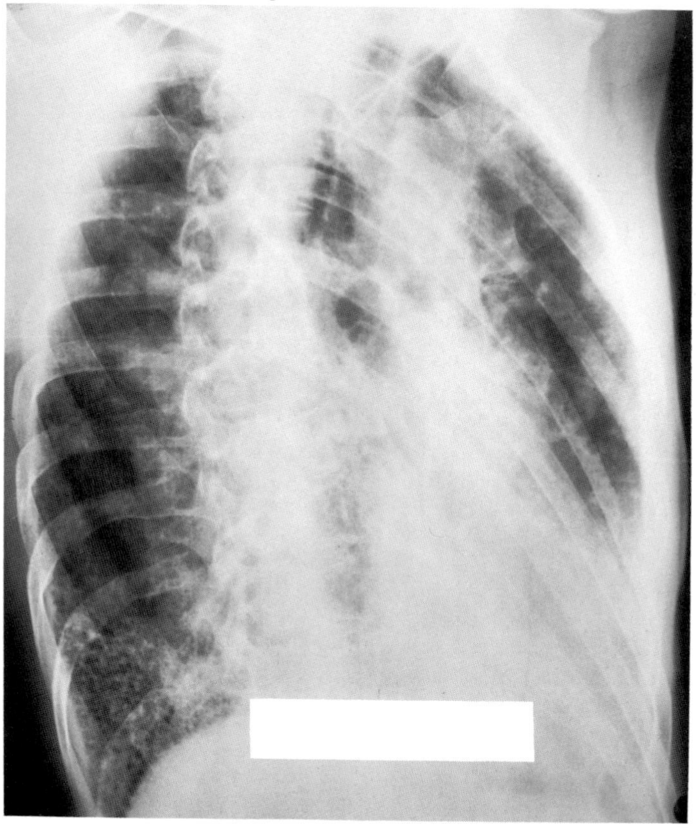

Figure 9.27 (b) 1972

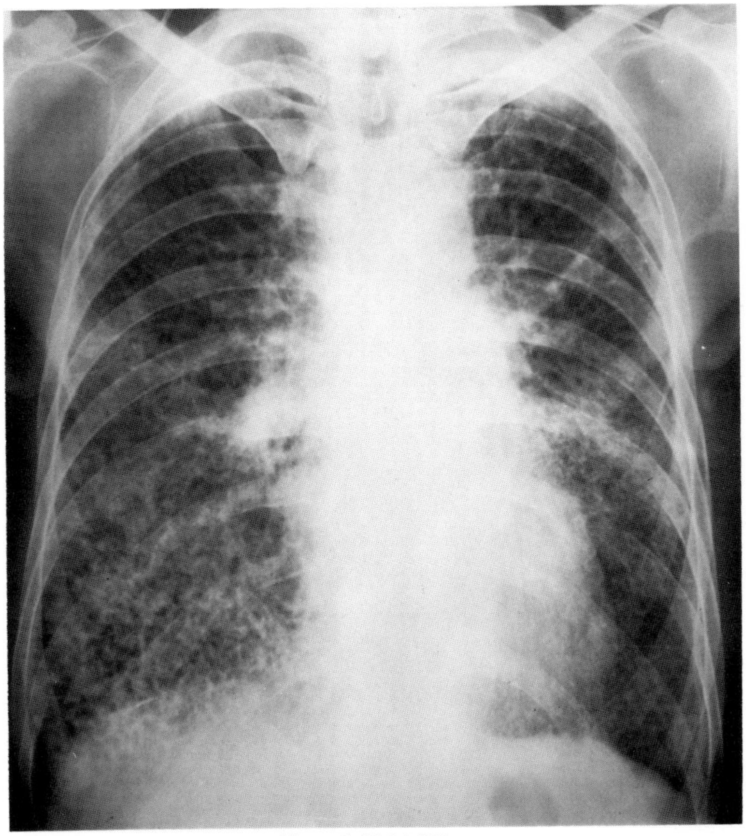

Figure 9.27 (c) 1974

Figure 9.27 (a) 1972, (b) 1972 and (c) 1974. Coarse DIPF pattern with multiple 'cystic' appearances involving all zones in (c). No evidence of diffuse pleural thickening in this film. Note small calcified plaque in right hemidiaphragm. The changes occurred in two years 30 years after the patient left the asbestos industry in which he worked as a disintegrator and mill operator of unprocessed fibre from 1938 to 1940. Clinically: *coarse, persistent, inspiratory and expiratory crepitations over all lobes. Lung function results typical of severe DIPF.* Post mortem. *Naked eye: severe, clear-cut DIPF with numerous thick-walled cysts 2 to 10 mm diameter involving right lung more than left. Appearances unlike asbestosis.* Microscopy: *severe DIPF with cystic bronchiolectasis heavily infiltrated by plasma cells particularly in right lung. Pronounced excess of elastin (elastosis) in these areas (*see Figure 4.17*). Some clusters of asbestos bodies away from the fibrotic areas. (Cryptogenic fibrosing 'alveolitis')*

carcinoma of lung (Harwood, Gracey and Yokoo, 1976); metastasis from carcinoma of pancreas, intestine and ovary; Hodgkin's lymphadenoma; fibrosarcoma and myosarcoma.

The peritoneal tumour presents similar gross post-mortem appearances which may vary from a confluent mass enclosing most of the abdominal organs to multiple nodules of the intestines, peritoneum and other organs (Entiknap and Smither, 1964), although matting of the visceral and parietal layers is unusual. A variable amount of glutinous ascitic fluid is often present. Invasion of the gut wall beyond the muscularis propria is rare (Hourihane, 1964). In some instances the liver and spleen may be encased by a thin layer of growth and in others the peritoneal cavity is obliterated and the viscera completely engulfed by the tumour. At laparotomy, however, it may be localized.

Spread of both pleural and peritoneal tumours to local lymph nodes (hilar, mediastinal or abdominal) is fairly common but is unusual in other organs. Nonetheless, contrary to opinion generally held until recently, distant metastatic deposits may occur in about half the cases of mesotheliomas in either site (Kannerstein and Churg, 1977; Edge and Choudhury, 1978; Roberts, 1976; Whitwell and Rawcliffe, 1971): in the contralateral lung, pericardium, heart, peritoneum, kidneys, suprarenals, liver, spleen, brain, pancreas and skeleton from pleural tumours; in liver, suprarenals, pleura, lung and pericardium from peritoneal tumours. Secondary invasion of pleura or peritoneum occurs by direct extension through the diaphragm (Thomson, 1970), and it is sometimes impossible to determine in which cavity the tumour originated. There is, apparently, no clear association between histological type and a propensity to blood-borne or lymph-borne metastasis (Roberts, 1976) although in one series a slight preponderance of tumours of 'mixed type' (*see* next section) was noted (Edge and Choudhury, 1978). Extension of the pleural tumour into the chest wall may cause rib erosion, and invasion of aspiration needle tracks and thoracotomy incisions is apt to occur.

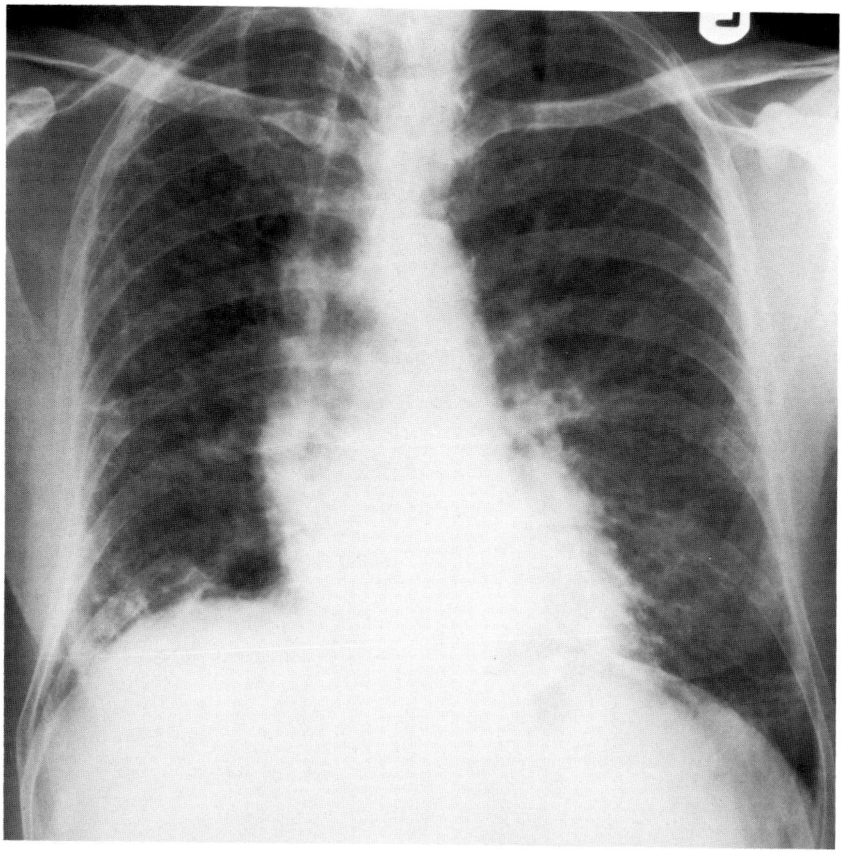

(a) 1973

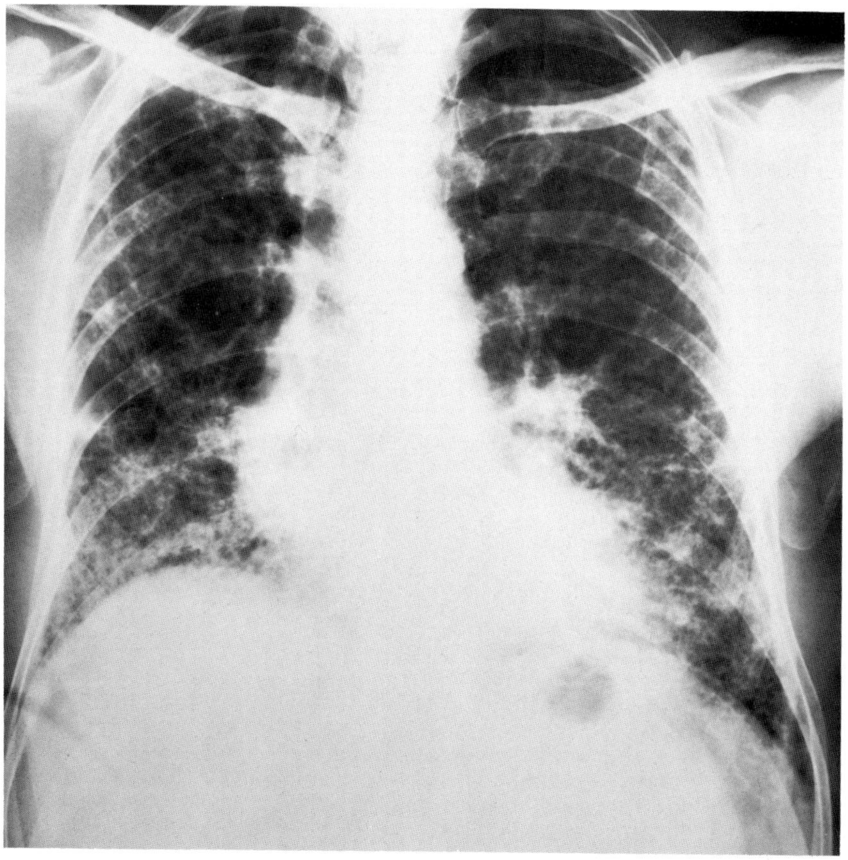

(b) 1974

Figure 9.28 (a) 1973 and ((b) 1974. Irregular opacities with cystic appearances in all zones, especially the lower, showing substantial progression in 18 months. Labourer in building (brick laying) and demolition industry from 1946 to 1974; para-occupational contact with asbestos insulation work for four years in 1950s. Bred budgerigars for 12 years until 12 months before film (a). Clinically: *coarse inspiratory and expiratory crepitations in all lobes. Lung function—severe restrictive and gas transfer defects. Avian precipitins present.* Post mortem. *Naked eye: multiple small air blebs on pulmonary pleura. Extensive well-defined DIPF both subpleurally and centrally with numerous cysts from 0.2 to 2 cm diameter. Changes more prominent in lower than upper halves of the lungs.* Microscopy: *highly vascularized DIPF with coarse honeycomb cysts and patches of desquamative alveolitis. Occasional asbestos bodies in 30 μm sections.* Diagnosis: *Avian extrinsic allergic, 'alveolitis' (bird fanciers' lung)*

(a) 1969

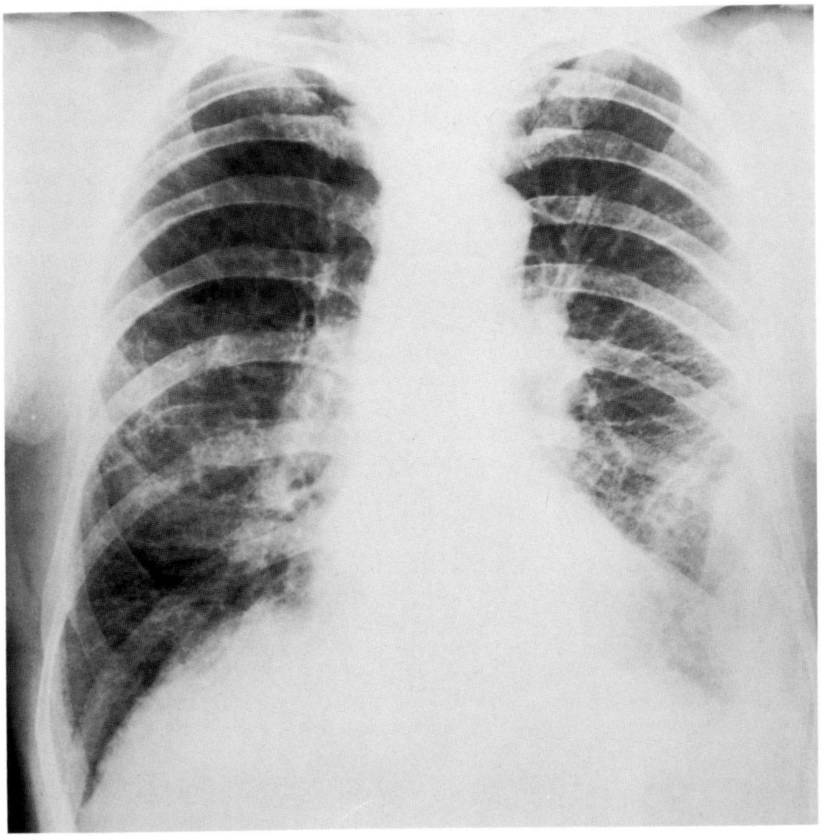

(b) 1976

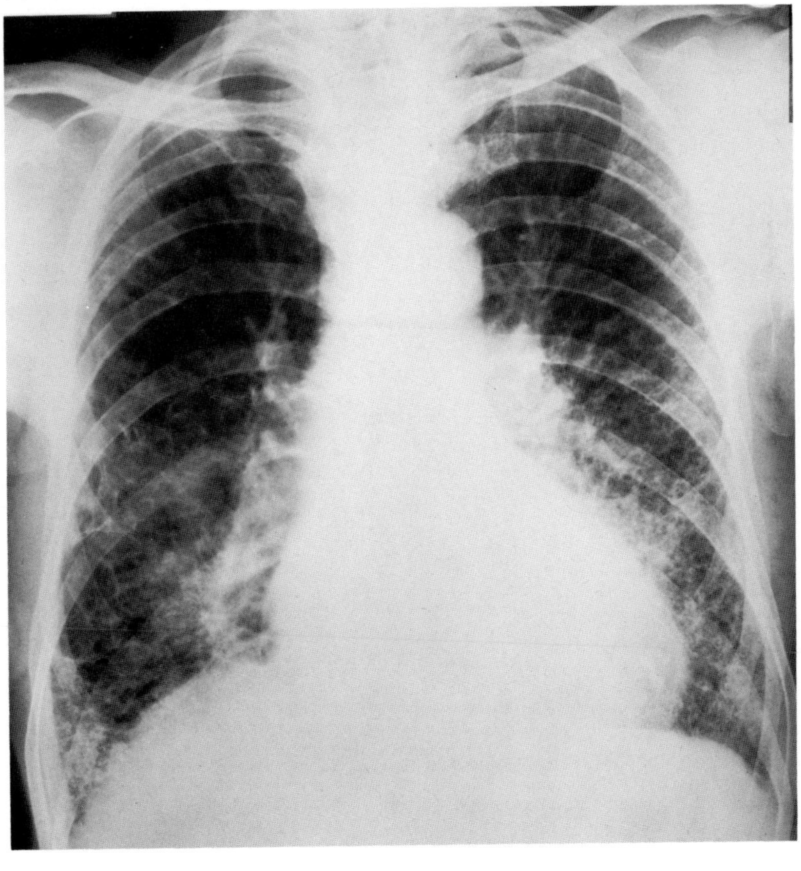

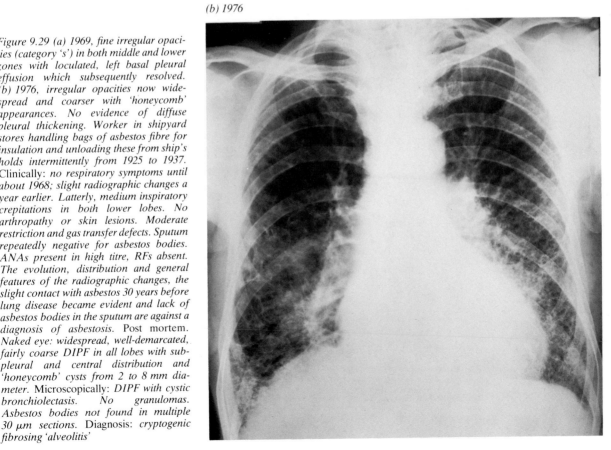

Figure 9.29 (a) 1969, fine irregular opacities (category 's') in both middle and lower zones with loculated, left basal pleural effusion which subsequently resolved. (b) 1976, irregular opacities now widespread and coarser with 'honeycomb' appearances. No evidence of diffuse pleural thickening. Worker in shipyard stores handling bags of asbestos fibre for insulation and unloading these from ship's holds intermittently from 1925 to 1937. Clinically: *no respiratory symptoms until about 1968; slight radiographic changes a year earlier. Latterly, medium inspiratory crepitations in both lower lobes. No arthropathy or skin lesions. Moderate restriction and gas transfer defects. Sputum repeatedly negative for asbestos bodies. ANAs present in high titre, RFs absent. The evolution, distribution and general features of the radiographic changes, the slight contact with asbestos 30 years before lung disease became evident and lack of asbestos bodies in the sputum are against a diagnosis of asbestosis.* Post mortem. *Naked eye: widespread, well-demarcated, fairly coarse DIPF in all lobes with subpleural and central distribution and 'honeycomb' cysts from 2 to 8 mm diameter.* Microscopically: *DIPF with cystic bronchiolectasis. No granulomas. Asbestos bodies not found in multiple 30 μm sections.* Diagnosis: *cryptogenic fibrosing 'alveolitis'*

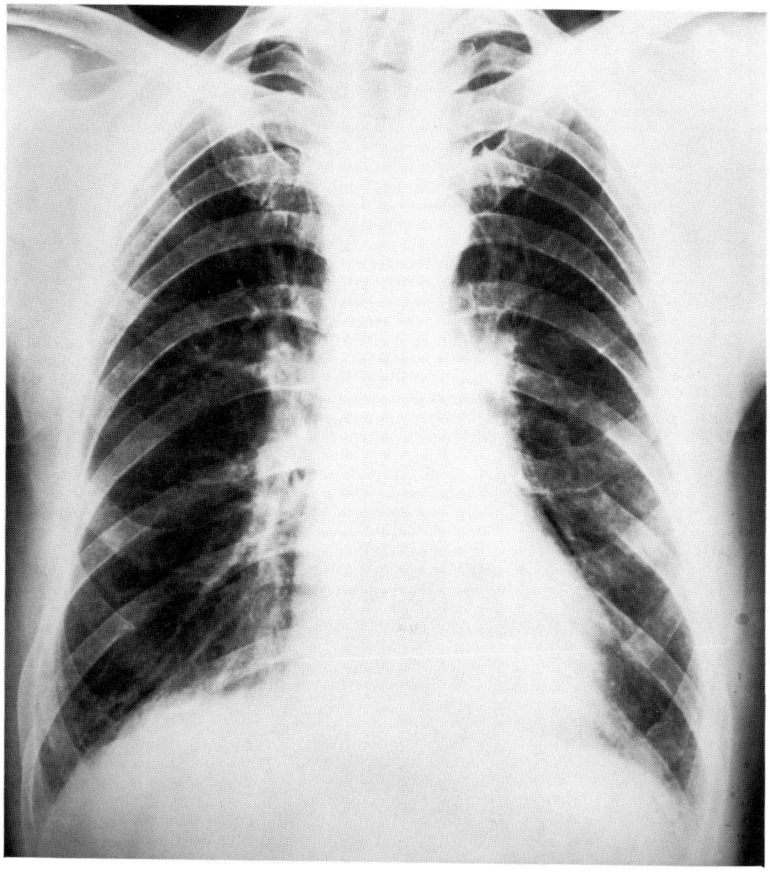

(a) 1965

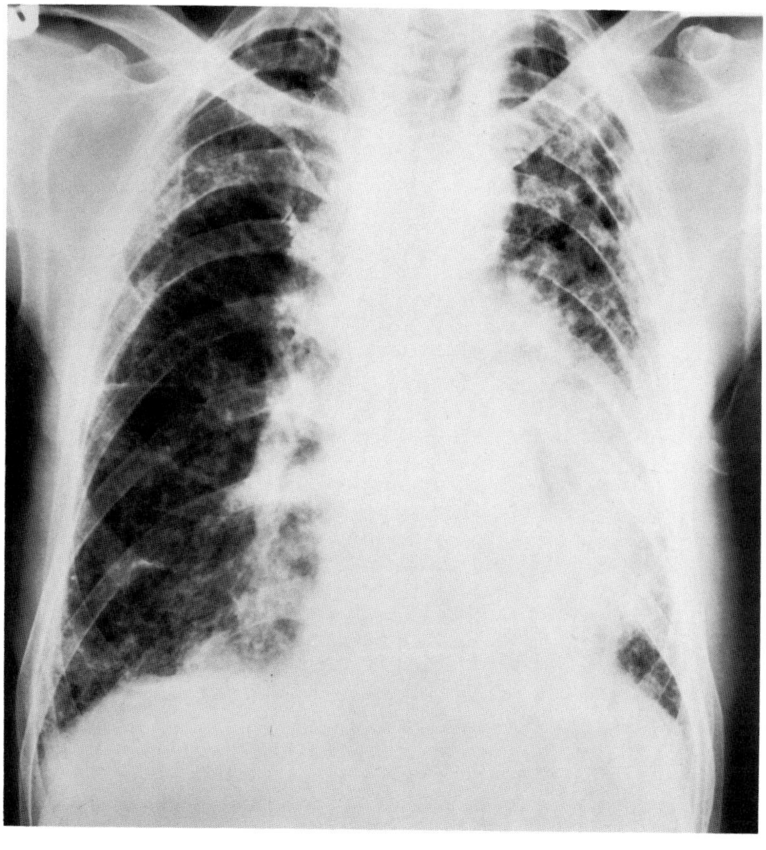

(b) 1975

Figure 9.30 Development of chronic fibrosing 'alveolitis' in a 65 year old man who had been an asbestos insulation worker for five years in the late 1930s. (a) 1965, appearances consistent with mild asbestosis in both lower zones. (b) 1975, coarser irregular opacities which developed quickly over four years are now widespread especially in the upper zones where there are cystic appearances. However, part of the abnormality on the left was due to bronchial carcinoma. Post mortem *naked eye. Ill-defined, irregular, grey fibrosis subpleurally in the bases of both lower lobes. Also separate, well-demarcated areas of coarser DIPF with multiple cysts varying from 3 to 8 mm diameter, mainly anterior in both upper lobes (left more than right), middle lobe and lingula, and more central lobar involvement. Scirrhous-type growth in left hilum spreading into lower lobe. Microscopy: fine subpleural DIPF in lower lobes associated with numerous asbestos bodies but no bronchiolectasis. Elsewhere coarse DIPF with cystic bronchiolectasis and occasional asbestos bodies. No granulomas. Squamous carcinoma of left lung.* Diagnosis. *Asbestosis, cryptogenic fibrosing 'alveolitis' and carcinoma of left lung. (Extrinsic allergic 'alveolitis' was not excluded)*

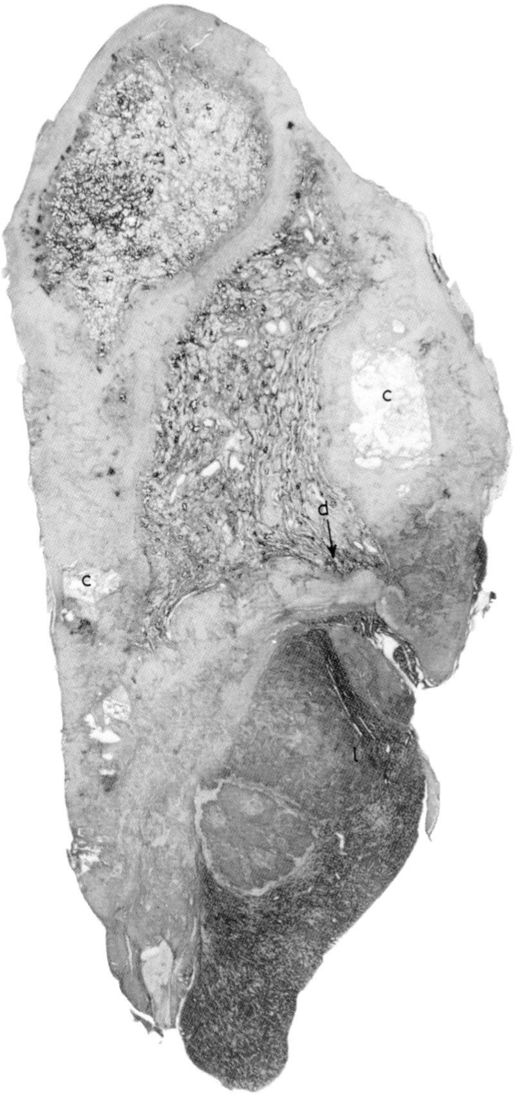

Figure 9.31 Malignant mesothelioma of the pleura of the right lung in a man exposed to an asbestos hazard for 18 months 25 years before his death. Note the encasement and compression of the lung by the tumour, its extension into the fissures with necrotic cavities (c) in the tumour mass. The tumour has spread through the diaphragm (d) into the liver (l)

Microscopic features

Characteristically mesothelial tumours are pleomorphic and there is much diversity from tumour to tumour, and in different areas of individual tumours and their metastatic forms because both epithelial and connective tissue (mesenchymal) elements are usually present. At one extreme the appearances closely resemble adenocarcinoma and, at the other, fibrosarcoma. Electron microscopy shows that typical and atypical epithelial cells and mesenchymal cells (which appear similar in ultrastructure to fibroblasts) are connected by a variety of transitional forms suggesting that malignant mesothelioma cells can differentiate into a number of different cell lines (Suzuki, Churg and Kannerstein, 1976).

Four distinct histological patterns are recognized (Whitwell and Rawcliffe, 1971):

(1) Tubulo-papillary type (predominantly epithelial).
(2) Sarcomatous type (predominantly mesenchymal).
(3) Undifferentiated cell type (predominantly epithelial).
(4) Mixed type.

Tubulo-papillary type (*Figure 9.33*)

This consists predominantly of serpiginous, glandular tubules lined by regularly ordered, low columnar or cuboidal cells with a few mitotic figures; in some places the cells are flat and in others appear as branching papillary projections covering a fine core of reticulin. The tumour cells in the lung and hilar lymph nodes may contain dust particles—a phenomenon rarely observed in carcinoma cells. A variable amount of more or less acellular collagen may be present. Cystic spaces are prominent in some tumours of this type.

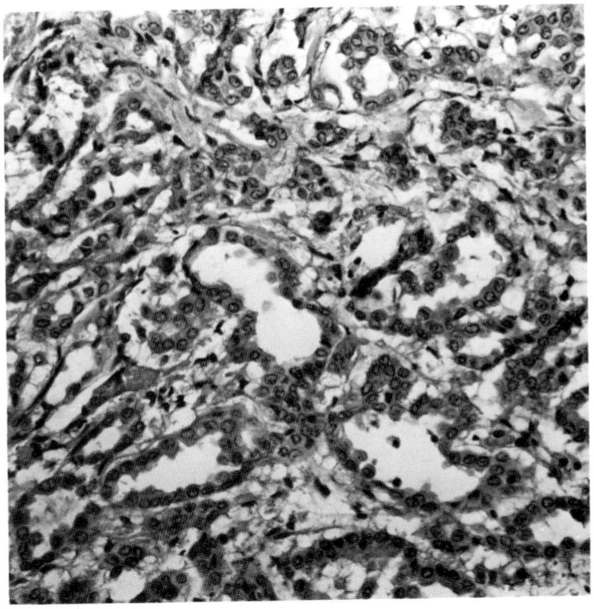

Figure 9.32 Malignant mesothelioma of tubulo-papillary type. (See text for description.) (Original magnification, × 380, reproduced at × 960; H and E stain; by courtesy of Dr J. C. Wagner)

In general, this is the commonest type of mesothelioma and, in many cases, is very difficult to distinguish from adenocarcinoma of lung, breast, stomach, pancreas, prostate or ovary if the primary tumour is not identified. Special staining techiques, however, are a valuable, if limited, aid in differentiation (*see* p. 284).

Sarcomatous type (*Figure 9.33*)

The pattern varies from that of a very cellular fascicular fibrosarcoma with uniform spindle cells, but sometimes with rounded cells of near-epithelial appearances, to virtually acellular masses of collagen fibres. Cell nuclei tend to be regular and mitotic figures, few. The acellular form may closely resemble a benign fibrous pleural plaque in places

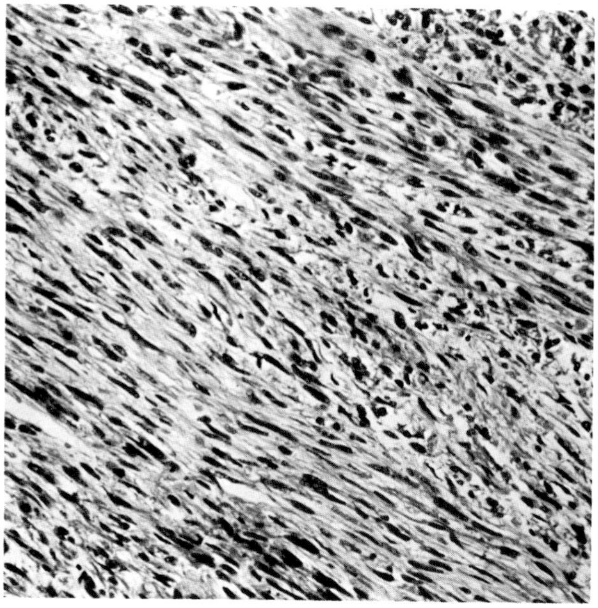

Figure 9.33 Malignant mesothelioma of sarcomatous type. Cellular fibrosarcomatous appearance. Note small spindle-shaped clefts. See text. (Original magnification × 380, H and E stain)

and extensive search of the tumour may be necessary before its sarcomatous character is identified.

This type of mesothelioma appears to be less common in the peritoneum than in the pleura (Kannerstein and Churg, 1977).

Secondary fibrosarcoma must be excluded and, on the whole, this is not difficult because the primary tumour is usually obvious both clinically and at post mortem. But this is not always the case and fibromyosarcoma of the uterus is an important exception.

Undifferentiated cell type

The cells are round or polygonal, occasionally fusiform, in shape; have a foamy cytoplasm and large frequently mitotic nuclei, and are similar to the cells which line tubulo-papillary structures. They may be found in clusters in other mesothelioma types (for example, in the cleft-like spaces which may be present in the collagen bundles of the sarcomatous type) but often they constitute a pure unmixed cellular sheet (supported by a more intricate framework of reticulin fibres (demonstrated by silver stains) than is usual in similar areas of a carcinoma (McCaughey, 1965). Furthermore, extensive search of the tumour often reveals tubular, papillary and sarcomatous elements. Sometimes the appearances are almost benign and this may be a source of misdiagnosis when the amount of tissue for examination is small.

Mixed type

This is a mixture of the other three types although one is usually predominant. Occasional clefts in a large collection of collagen fibres may be lined by tumour cells. Sarcomatous elements usually consist of fusiform cells with elongated, oval or, sometimes, large bizarre nuclei. Widespread examination of the tumour and metastatic deposits (for example, in local lymph nodes) may be necessary before its mixed nature is evident.

Staining reactions

Many malignant mesotheliomas produce a mucinous substance, hyaluronic acid, which it was hoped would help to identify them positively. It is chiefly *extracellular* and stains blue with Alcian Blue and Hale's colloidal iron (Pearce, 1968) but not with periodic acid Schiff (PAS) or mucicarmine. By contrast adenocarcinomas often produce an intracellular mucin which is usually PAS-positive but occasionally give the Alcian Blue reaction. The application of these stains before and after removing the mucoid substance with the enzyme hyaluronidase may cause reversion of previously positive Alcian Blue and colloidal iron reactions in mesotheliomas to negative (Wagner, Munday and Harrington, 1962). But, unfortunately, this is not consistent and is least helpful in those cases which are microscopically the most difficult. However, in many cases the PAS test is negative in mesothelioma sections which are pre-digested by the enzyme diastase (DPAS test) whereas a strongly positive reaction within cell cytoplasm and mucin in the lumina of neoplastic glands favours adenocarcinoma or pseudo-mesotheliomatous carcinoma of the lung (Harwood, Gracey and Yokoo, 1976). In spite of their limitations, therefore, the combination of these histochemical tests are valuable in the differentiation of a substantial number of difficult cases (Kannerstein, Churg and Magner, 1973). It has recently been suggested that specific glycosaminoglycan-degrading enzymes may be used to quantify hyaluronic acid in mesotheliomas (Arai *et al.*, 1979).

Asbestos bodies and fibres

These are present in the lungs of almost all cases whether the tumour is of pleural or peritoneal origin, and in 95 per

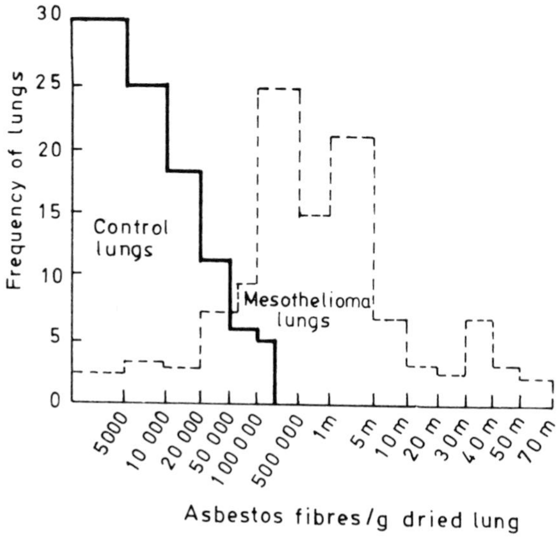

Figure 9.34 Comparison of asbestos fibre content of lungs from mesothelioma and normal control series. (From Whitwell et al.*, 1977. By permission of authors and editors of* Thorax*)*

cent of cases of asbestos-related pleural mesothelioma the fibre content of the lungs has been found to be greatly in excess of that in normal lungs (Whitwell, Scott and Grimshaw, 1977) (*see Figure 9.34*). The finding of bodies and fibres, however, does not help to identify a tumour as a malignant mesothelioma. Electron microscopy reveals that neither fibres nor bodies are present within the growth itself (Suzuki, Churg and Kannerstein, 1976).

Asbestosis

The association of asbestosis with pleural tumours is exceptional. It is present in, approximately, one-quarter of cases most of which have a higher fibre content than those with no asbestosis (Whitwell, Scott and Grimshaw, 1977), and is usually of mild degree. By contrast, it frequently accompanies the peritoneal tumours which are significantly associated with heavy asbestos exposure (Elmes and Simpson, 1976) and is often fairly advanced. This curious anomaly is discussed further in the section on pathogenesis.

Micro-diagnosis summarized

A definitive diagnosis of malignant mesothelioma cannot be made during life or at post mortem other than by microscopy.

Tissue for biopsy must be sufficiently large to permit, if possible, different features of the tumour to be identified. If it is too small or otherwise inadequate a large number of other primary or secondary tumours may be confused with mesothelioma as only epithelial or mesenchymal elements of the tumour, which are present in varying amounts, may be sampled. For example:

Primary tumours. Peripheral adenocarcinoma (pseudomesotheliomatous carcinoma) and scirrhous carcinoma of lung, fibroma, fibrosarcoma, leiomyoma, leiomyosarcoma, neurofibroma, neurofibrosarcoma.

Secondary tumours. Adenocarcinoma of undetermined origin or of stomach and pancreas, sarcomas (including fibromyosarcoma of uterus), reticulin-cell sarcoma, papillary carcinoma of ovary, seminoma, cystosarcoma of breast.

But even with adequate material in many cases—apart from those showing the characteristic diversity of cytohistological features—the diagnosis during life can only be putative as the histological features may be indeterminate and the existence of an occult primary growth, of which the tumour under investigation is a secondary manifestation, can rarely be excluded.

At post mortem a thorough search for a possible primary growth (which may be minute) is necessary, though occasionally it will be engulfed by an advanced secondary tumour and escape recognition. Indeed, Willis (1973) in emphasizing the difficulties involved, has asserted: 'No tumour, whatever its structure, can be regarded as a primary coelomic one until the most painstaking and exhaustive search of all viscera has failed to disclose a primary epithelial growth'. Although some pathologists may regard this as too sweeping a statement it is desirable to bear it in mind as a general rule in this particularly difficult field of oncological diagnosis both in practice and in the interpretation of reported cases. As Kannerstein and Churg (1977) pointed out, the diagnosis of malignant mesothelioma should not be 'a repository for tumours in which a primary site cannot be demonstrated'.

Peritoneal tumours are more likely to be wrongly diagnosed as malignant mesotheliomas in women than in men due to the range of potentialities of cells in the female pelvis (Kannerstein and Churg, 1977).

The use of exfoliative cytology of pleural fluid in diagnosis of the tumour during life is referred to on p. 290.

Pathogenesis

Experimental evidence in animals

All types of asbestos when inoculated intrapleurally in rats and other experimental animals cause malignant mesotheliomas which are histologically identical to the tumour in man (Reeves *et al.*, 1971; Smith *et al.*, 1965; Wagner, 1972). Wagner (1972a) showed that of the UICC reference asbestos samples (*see* p. 239) crocidolite produces the most tumours followed in order of potency by amosite, anthophyllite, chrysotile B (Canadian) and chrysotile A (Zimbabwean); but, using a higher dose of crocidolite, amosite and chrysotile A, Stanton and Wrench (1972) found that all three produced an equally high rate of tumours. The risk of animals developing the tumour at a given age was also shown to be proportional to the dose of crocidolite and chrysotile (Stanton and Wrench, 1972; Wagner, Berry and Timbrell, 1973).

The possibility that the mesothelioma-producing potential of asbestos might be due to natural oils and waxes in the fibres or to contaminating oils from the preparation of fibre or its storage in plastic and jute bags (Commins and Gibbs, 1969; Roe, Walters and Harington, 1966) have not been substantiated (Wagner and Berry, 1969; Wagner 1972); neither does it appear to be related to the metallic content of the fibres or to their contamination by trace metals (Harington, 1973), and the leaching out of magnesium from chrysotile apparently has no significant effect on the occurrence of mesotheliomas (Morgan *et al.*, 1977). Pathogenesis of the tumours seems rather to be related primarily to the length and diameter of asbestos fibres than to their physico-chemical properties. For the most part the responsible fibres are less than 3 μm in diameter but, by contrast, 'submicroscopic' fibres (that is, beyond the range of the light microscope) possess a much reduced tumour-producing potential (Stanton, 1973; Stanton and Wrench, 1972; Wagner and Berry, 1969). Indeed, fibres under 1 μm diameter and longer than 10 μm appear to be most oncogenic. The importance of fibre dimensions is emphasized by the fact that fibres of different internal structure and chemical composition to asbestos but of similar size (such as fibre glass and aluminium oxide) also induce mesotheliomas or sarcomas following *intrapleural* inoculation (Stanton, 1973; Pott, Huth and Friedrich, 1974). It has, therefore, been postulated that the genesis of these tumours may be due to a mechanical, solid-state surface, or Oppenheimer, effect (Bryson and Bischoff, 1967) though there appears to be no evidence that such a phenomenon occurs in man.

It should, however, be noted that implantation of asbestos in the pleural cavities of animals has no relevance to the mode of entry and distribution of asbestos fibres in human beings. But these experiments have demonstrated that the different types of asbestos applied directly to the pleural surfaces can all induce malignant pleural tumours in spite of their differing chemical compositions, and that trace metals and organic contaminants do not (*see also* section on man-made silicate fibres).

By contrast, the *inhalation* of asbestos fibre (UICC standard reference samples) by animals has produced only a very small number of mesotheliomas which were associated predominantly with crocidolite and Canadian chrysotile (Davis *et al.*, 1978; Wagner *et al.*, 1974). The aerodynamic properties of the fibres (*see* Chapter 3, p. 47) are decisive in determining their penetration to the subpleural regions of the lung.

Evidence in man

Malignant mesothelioma of the pleura was first related to exposure to crocidolite in the north-western Cape Province of South Africa and in Western Australia (Wagner, Sleggs and Marchand, 1960; McNulty, 1968) and this has been confirmed among women who worked filling gas mask filters with pure crocidolite during the Second World War (Jones, Pooley and Smith, 1976). Occupational exposure to pure chrysotile has been very uncommon but, when experienced, does not seem to have been associated with mesotheliomas (Elwood and Cochrane, 1964; McDonald, 1973b; Weiss, 1977). However, a very low incidence of the tumour has been reported in workers apparently exposed to pure chrysotile at the major mine in Quebec Province (McDonald and McDonald, 1977b), but when amphibole, as well as chrysotile, fibres were found in the lungs of some workers from this site (Pooley, 1976) it was discovered that crocidolite had in fact been processed there for gas mask manufacture during the Second World War. However, there is now convincing evidence that amosite may be responsible for some mesotheliomas in the USA (McDonald, 1980; McDonald and McDonald, 1980). Pure amosite exposure has been held responsible for the occurrence of mesotheliomas in a group of insulation workers in the USA (Selikoff *et al.*, 1972). But the only source of supply of this fibre during the relevant period was the Eastern Transvaal where crocidolite and amosite are intimately associated (*see* p. 234). The pleural tumour has also been reported in association with exposure to fibrous tremolite present in outcropping mineral deposits used in whitewash and stucco for the walls and roofs of houses in certain districts in Turkey (Yazicioglu *et al.*, 1980). No confirmed cases of mesothelioma appear to have resulted from pure anthophyllite exposure (Meurman, Kiviluoto and Hakama, 1974).

It is often claimed, as was originally thought, that malignant mesothelioma follows trivial exposure to asbestos in the remote past but both epidemiological and pathological evidence has clearly shown that it is, in fact, dose-related—though not so strongly as asbestosis. The tumour rate tends to increase with intensity and duration of asbestos exposure, and though duration may have been short in some cases, it has usually been intense (Newhouse, 1973; Newhouse and Berry, 1976; Peto, 1979) (note the analogy in experimental animals, p. 285). A dose relationship is substantiated by the fact that the content of asbestos fibres in the lungs of mesothelioma cases is significantly higher than in non-mesothelioma cases, and amphibole fibres are predominant (Pooley, 1973b; Whitwell, Scott and Grimshaw, 1977) (*see Figure 9.34*). In general, however, exposure levels tend to be less than those which produce asbestosis.

The paradoxical situation in which there is a clear association between mesothelioma and exposure to crocidolite dust in the Cape Province whereas the occurrence of tumours following exposure to the geologically intimately related crocidolite and amosite of the Transvaal is very rare has been explained by the fact that both the diameter and length of the Transvaal fibres are, on average, three times greater than the Cape fibres which imposes differences in aerodynamic behaviour (*see* Chapter 3). Fewer 'respirable' fibres of Transvaal asbestos are likely to be liberated and they have a higher settling rate and, hence, may be less likely to reach the periphery of the lung. The fibres of Australian crocidolite which is also associated with malignant mesothelioma (Jones, Pooley and Smith, 1976; Milne, 1976) are even smaller in diameter than those of Cape crocidolite (Timbrell, 1973).

There is no evidence that mesotheliomas of the pleura originate in parietal pleural plaques; and this is supported by radiographic evidence of bilateral calcified plaques or changes of asbestosis being found in only 12 per cent of one large series of mesothelioma cases (Elmes and Simpson, 1976).

Cigarette smoking is not related to the development of this tumour.

Preliminary studies of cellular immunity in mesothelioma of the pleura have produced somewhat contradictory results. Haslam *et al.* (1978) found no evidence of impaired T lymphocyte function either *in vitro* by PHA stimulation or *in vivo* by delayed hypersensitivity skin testing though Wagner (1978) has reported depressed lymphocyte transformation to PHA.

The possibility that the tumour might be caused in man by non-asbestos mineral fibres is being investigated and is discussed briefly on pp. 285 and 320.

Malignant mesotheliomas of the pleura have been found in agricultural communities in Turkey in regions where asbestos minerals are absent from the soil and rock formations though chrysotile fibres were identified in the lungs of one case and amphiboles in another; the origin of these fibres is obscure (Baris *et al.*, 1978a). A submicroscopic fibrous form of the mineral zeolite has, however, been identified in the soil and street dust and is under investigation (Baris *et al.*, 1978b) (*see* p. 318). Bilateral calcified pleural plaques are also common in these areas.

The pathogenesis of the peritoneal tumour is not understood. Although it can be induced in rats and mice by intraperitoneal injection of crocidolite (Davis, 1974) it does not follow feeding animals with asbestos, and there is no evidence at present that it is caused by asbestos fibres in food or drink penetrating the gut. Irradiated fibres injected into the right pleural cavity of rats have been shown to accumulate in peritoneal folds adjacent to the liver (Morgan, Holmes and Gold, 1971), but whether this observation has any relevance to human disease remains to be discovered. Although, in general, these tumours are much rarer than pleural mesotheliomas they have, in some series, been either of equal frequency (Newhouse and Berry, 1976) or more common (Selikoff, 1976). They appear to occur more often when asbestos exposure has been heavy (Elmes and Simpson, 1976); which might explain why asbestosis is more often associated with peritoneal than the pleural tumours, but not why it is so infrequently found with pleural mesotheliomas. In New York state an unusually high prevalence of cancer has been observed in the parents of women with peritoneal mesotheliomas but no occupational exposure to asbestos. It is not clear whether this suggests that the mesothelioma patients came from cancer-prone families (Vianna and Polan, 1978).

Evidently this is a complex problem which will probably require some years to resolve.

To summarize

(1) The production of mesothelial tumours by intrapleural and intraperitoneal injection of asbestos minerals in animals, though indicative of the actions they may have on these membranes, has little relevance to pathogenic events in man.
(2) Crocidolite is, apparently, the type of asbestos which is overwhelmingly, if not exclusively, causally related to mesotheliomas in man. At present the association of other fibres from past occupational exposure appears to be fortuitous but an open mind must be maintained until more information on the types of asbestos found in the lungs is available.
(3) The risk of developing asbestos-induced malignant mesothelioma is dose-related whether due to occupational or neighbourhood exposure and is not associated with trivial or casual contact with asbestos. The conditions which produced the tumours existed, in the main, many years ago. Hence, there is no evidence that the general public is at risk (Report of the Advisory Committee on Asbestos Cancers, 1973).
(4) There is no proof to date that ingested asbestos fibre is responsible for peritoneal mesothelioma and, in females, the tumour is easily confused with other pleomorphic tumours of pelvic origin.
(5) The possibility that other fibre types—including the man-made—might have oncogenic potential is, on present evidence, speculative.

Clinical features

Symptoms

The pleural tumour In the great majority of cases the presenting symptoms are pain in the chest and breathlessness on effort of gradual and insidious onset. The pain, which is the commonest early symptom (Elmes and Simpson, 1976) and is of heavy, nagging quality unrelated to movement or respiration, can often be ignored at first but later becomes severe and intractable due to involvement of intercostal nerves, and may be referred to the abdomen or the ipsilateral shoulder. Occasionally, local invasion of the brachial plexus may cause pain, paraesthesiae and muscular weakness (with wasting) on the ulnar side of the ipsilateral arm. Breathlessness gradually worsens due to expansion of the tumour until it is present at rest, but in some cases it increases quickly due to accumulation of fluid within the pleural space or in the tumour itself. In these circumstances it can usually be temporarily relieved by aspiration of the fluid. In a small number of cases the onset of pain or breathlessness may be acute and require emergency admission to hospital.

Lassitude, malaise and loss of weight are rarely early symptoms but are the rule later. In the absence of pre-existing chronic bronchitis or other lung disease cough is not a troublesome feature but, when the growth is advanced, it may be productive due to complicating respiratory infection. Haemoptysis does not occur. Some patients complain of distressing night sweats.

Because of the gradual onset of symptoms there is usually an interval of some three or four months between the patient first experiencing them and seeking medical advice (Elmes and Simpson, 1976). In the late stage of the disease dysphagia may be present due to oesophageal involvement.

The peritoneal tumour Again, the onset of symptoms, which are vague and variable, is insidious. At first there is a poorly defined or localized abdominal discomfort with loss of appetite and weight and, in some instances, constipation; but painless, diffuse swelling of the abdomen with increasing abdominal girth, which may be attributed to gaining weight, may be the first symptom. In about one-third of cases symptoms of intermittent upper or lower intestinal obstruction, which may or may not be associated with colicky pain, occur. Ultimately, however, the symptoms of complete obstruction are usual. Lethargy and weakness are common.

Physical signs

The pleural tumour When first seen the patient is usually in good general health but later when the disease is advanced he is ill, emaciated and dyspnoeic at rest.

Unilateral signs of pleural effusion or thickening are frequently present in greater or lesser degree and the chest wall may be tender or painful on palpation, and in advanced disease is flattened and immobile. Palpable or visible tumour masses may be present particularly after thoracotomy or needling of the chest. Persistent basal crepitations indicative of asbestosis are exceptional; they were detected in only six of 267 cases of pleural mesothelioma reported by Elmes and Simpson (1976). Signs of mediastinal shift to the opposite side are infrequent and are usually associated with rapidly developing effusion and dyspnoea. For reasons which are not clear the tumour occasionally presents with an ipsilateral spontaneous pneumothorax but this is not often detectable clinically. Pericardial friction is sometimes heard due to extension of the tumour into the sac.

Finger clubbing is seldom seen. It was observed in 9.5 per cent of cases by Elmes and Simpson (1976) who also noted an occasional case of hypertrophic pulmonary osteoarthropathy.

When invaded by tumour the liver may be palpable well below the costal margin but is not often tender. Rarely is there any clinical evidence of local lymph node metastasis and signs of superior mediastinal obstruction are most exceptional.

Occasionally, the features of Horner's syndrome on the side of the tumour are seen with impaired sweating of the face and, sometimes of the shoulder, arm and hand of that side due to invasion of the paravertebral sympathetic nerve chain (Stanford, 1976).

The peritoneal tumour Abnormal signs are often absent on initial examination but soon some diffuse abdominal fullness is evident and the signs of ascites may be present but difficult to elicit with certainty. Later the abdomen is much distended and its girth may increase rapidly; at this stage firm masses are usually palpable by direct or bimanual palpation, though it is not possible to relate these to any abdominal organ. The patient is now ill and emaciated. Jaundice is not seen.

The signs of asbestosis are also present in many cases.

Investigations

Radiographic appearances

Though yielding no pathognomonic signs the chest radiograph is the most informative of routine investigations.

The pleural tumour The appearances vary according to the stage at which the disease is first seen, its distribution and whether or not it is associated with effusion. The most important changes are as follows:

(1) Irregular, lobulated, well-demarcated protuberant opacities which line part of all of one inner chest wall and extend to a greater or lesser degree into the lung field, sometimes surrounding it completely (*Figures 9.35* and *9.46*). Dense elongated opacities due to the spread of tumour along the greater or lesser fissures may be seen (*Figure 9.31*). At an early stage the opacities may be indistinguishable from those of hyaline pleural plaques but they are unilateral. Occasionally, the appearances of a hilar mass are predominant and usually caused by the greater part of the tumour being in the mediastinum at this stage.

(2) A unilateral pleural effusion above with lobular opacities along the coastal margin or near the hilum may or may not be discernable (*Figure 9.36*). If fluid is aspirated the deliberate induction of a pneumothorax may demonstrate the outline of the tumour clearly in upright or decubitus positions. Some cases present the appearances of diffuse irregular pleural thickening (fibrosis) with crowding of ribs, scoliosis and mediastinal shift towards the affected side. Ultimately the hemithorax may be completely opaque. Tomography may help to define the distribution of the tumour.

(3) Evidence of bilateral calcified pleural plaques or of

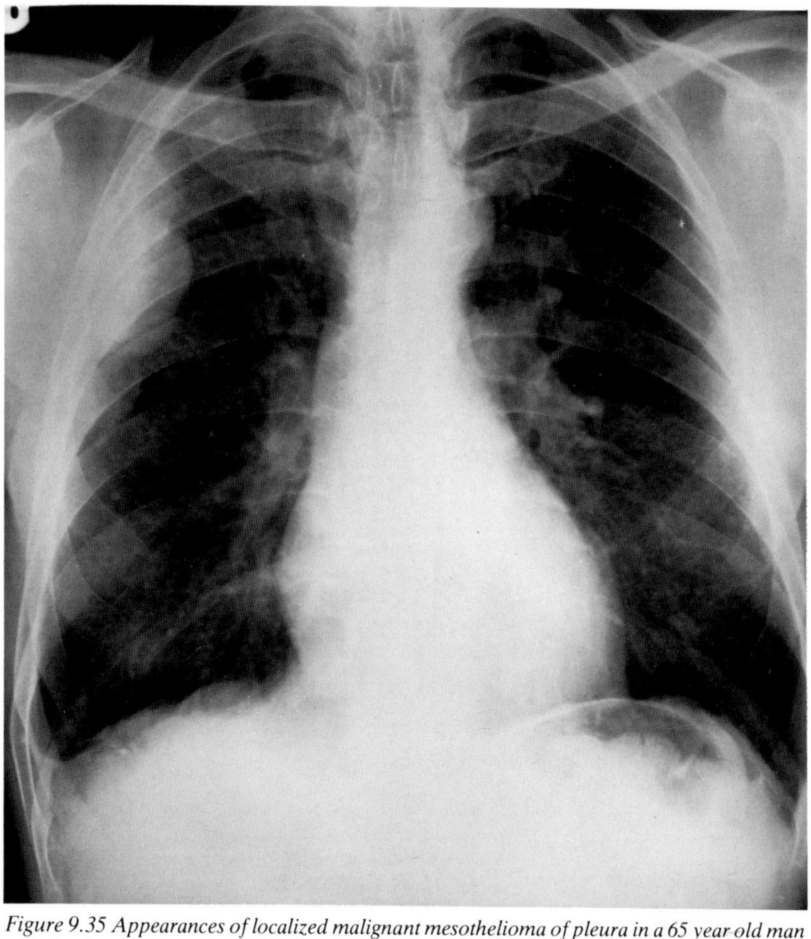

Figure 9.35 Appearances of localized malignant mesothelioma of pleura in a 65 year old man who had worked as a steam locomotive boiler maker for 45 years. Asbestos insulation, frequently carried out in his vicinity. Erosion of right 1st, 2nd, 3rd and 4th ribs evident four months later. Post mortem, *Naked eye: tumour mass enclosed most of right lung. Microscopy: mesothelioma confirmed; no evidence of asbestosis but moderate numbers of asbestos bodies present in 30 μm lung sections*

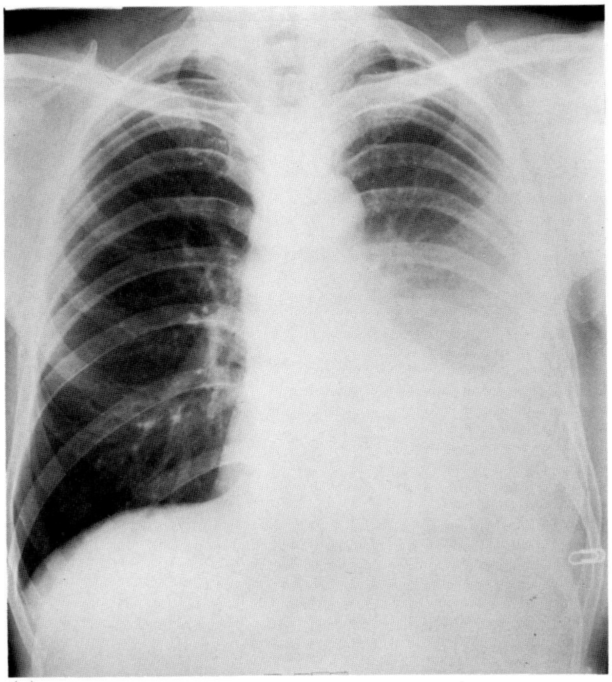

(a)

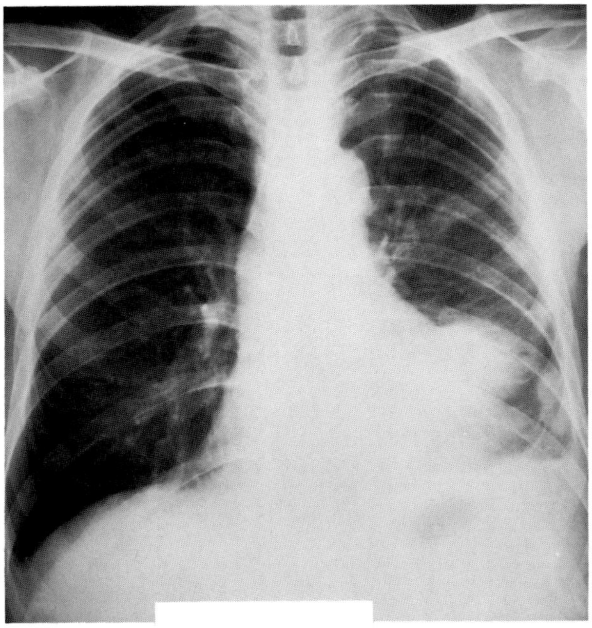

(b)

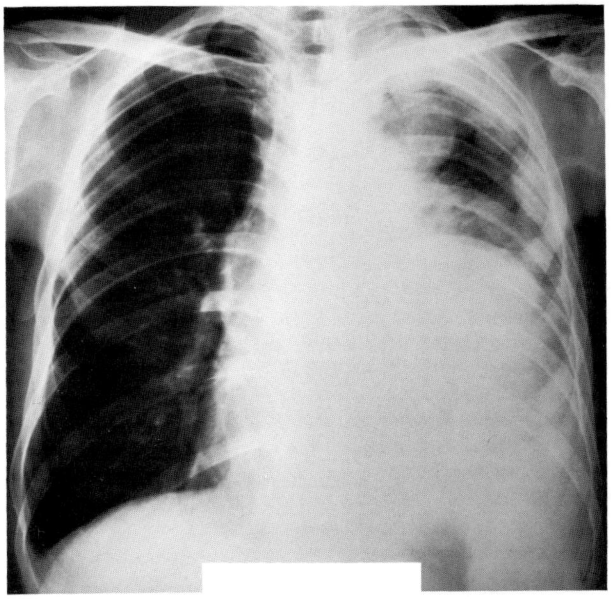

(c)

Figure 9.36 Stages in the development of a diffuse malignant pleural mesothelioma. Asbestos insulation worker 29 years. (a) March, 1972. Left pleural effusion. (b) July, 1972. Massive opacities localized to left lower zone. (c) December, 1972. Widespread, massive, lobulated opacities. Right lung field normal throughout. Post mortem, *naked eye: left lung surrounded by soft, lobulated, partly necrotic tumour mass. Deposits of tumour within the lung, hilar lymph nodes and liver.* Microscopy: *mesothelioma of mixed type. Minimal asbestosis and moderate numbers of asbestos bodies*

basal DIPF (asbestosis) may be present but is most uncommon; Elmes and Simpson (1976) observed one or the other or both in 34 per cent of their cases of pleural mesotheliomas.

(4) Exceptionally the signs of pleural infiltration or of discrete tumour deposits or the pattern of malignant lymphangitis in the lung on the opposite side may occur late in disease.

The peritoneal tumour The signs of bilateral calcified pleural plaques or of DIPF (asbestosis) are present in the chest film in many cases; they were seen in 13 of the 14 patients in the Elmes and Simpson (1976) series and precede the development of the tumour. Occasionally there is evidence of invasion of the pleura on one or both sides in advanced disease. In some cases, however, there is no abnormality. Radiography of the abdomen may be of little value due to generalized opacification but, when associated with a history of asbestos exposure and an abnormal chest film, the following radiographic features point to the possibility of mesothelioma (Young and Reddy, 1980):

(1) evidence of small or large bowel obstruction, with or without ascites;
(2) displacement of intra-abdominal structures by soft tissue masses;

(3) diffuse extrinsic indentation of the bowel with submucosal infiltration and encapsulation shown by barium meal or enema.

Examination of pleural fluid

The fluid is sterile and usually clear and yellow. Frequently it is glutinous and to such a degree as to make aspiration difficult.

Aspiration of pleural fluid is usually indicated to relieve discomfort and dyspnoea. Its examination may be of some value in excluding or establishing other pathology. Experienced cytologists may be able to diagnose the tumour by recognition of exfoliated cells which clearly show the cytoplasmic differentiation of mesothelial cells and possess nuclei showing the criteria of malignancy (Butler and Berry, 1973; Roberts and Campbell, 1972), though repeated fluid samples may be required to achieve this. But normal mesothelial cells found in a pleural effusion of any type assume bizarre appearances: giant and vacuolated forms and clumps of cells are common (Hinson, 1958) and special stains are of little help (Butler and Berry, 1973). In general, therefore, there is much difficulty in distinguishing malignant mesothelial cells with certainty from normal variants. Of the cases reported by Elmes and Simpson (1976) cytological examination provided the correct diagnosis in only 4 per cent. However, it has recently been claimed that the three different types of malignant mesothelioma cells can be identified in pleural fluid by electron microscopy and differentiated from cells of metastatic cancer, though with extreme difficulty in the case of adenocarcinoma (Legrand and Pariente, 1974; Suzuki, Churg and Kannerstein, 1976). If this technique proves to be accurate and practicable a considerable advance towards confident early diagnosis of the tumour will have been made.

Detection of hyaluronic acid in the fluid by electrophoretic and chromatographic techniques may provide *corroborative* evidence in favour of mesothelioma in spite of the fact that a small number of false negatives occur with authentic mesotheliomas and false positives with other tumours (Boersma, Degand and Havez, 1973).

Biopsy of tumour tissue

This may be necessary to attempt a more confident diagnosis but especially to exclude other types of growth which may be amenable to some form of treatment. The number of correct diagnoses increases with the amount of tissue obtained, but, for the reasons explained on p. 285, is still relatively small. Elmes and Simpson (1976) found that the diagnosis of mesothelioma was correct in 26 per cent of needle specimens, 38 per cent of thoracotomy specimens and 70 per cent of surgical excision specimens. In considering the use of these techniques the propensity for mesothelial tumours to advance along needle tracks and thoracotomy scars has to be borne in mind; in fact, 80 per cent of palpable masses of the tumour in the chest wall have been related to these sites (Elmes and Simpson, 1976). Hence, these methods of investigation should not be undertaken lightly or routinely.

In the case of the peritoneal tumour laparotomy is usually unavoidable as aspiration often fails but a definite diagnosis is apparently achieved in only a minority of cases (Elmes and Simpson, 1976; Kannerstein and Churg, 1977). Here also the tumour may infiltrate through incisions.

Erythrocyte sedimentation rate (ESR)

This is raised at an early stage in most cases and is higher in patients with blood stained effusions or no effusion than in those with serous effusions (Elmes and Simpson, 1976).

Examination of sputum

Asbestos bodies, if found, will alert the clinician to the possibility of malignant mesothelioma if a history of past exposure to the mineral has not been elicited. Mesothelial cells are not found.

Diagnosis

During life

In most cases this can be no more than a presumption. The important features are as follows:

(1) A history of past exposure to asbestos—especially to crocidolite—is usual.
(2) A latent period of 20 years or more between exposure to asbestos and development of the tumour.
(3) Insidious onset of symptoms and good general health in the early stage of the disease with raised ESR.
(4) Usually no clinical evidence of lymphadenopathy or other metastases.
(5) Asbestos bodies in sputum or lung tissue (biopsy), confirming exposure.
(6) The appearances of the chest radiograph bearing in mind, however, that these may be imitated by other tumours (*Figures 9.37, 9.38* and *9.39*).
(7) Demonstration of malignant mesothelial cells and hyaluronic acid in the fluid, and the biopsy appearances of the tumour with exclusion as far as possible of other tumour types.

Post mortem

(1) In most cases the tumour exhibits the gross features described previously and shown in *Figure 9.31* which, though suggesting its identity, can be caused by other neoplasms (*see* pp. 277 to 278).
(2) A searching necropsy fails to reveal a primary growth of which the suspected mesothelioma could be a metastatic deposit.
(3) The microscopical criteria described earlier must be satisfied.

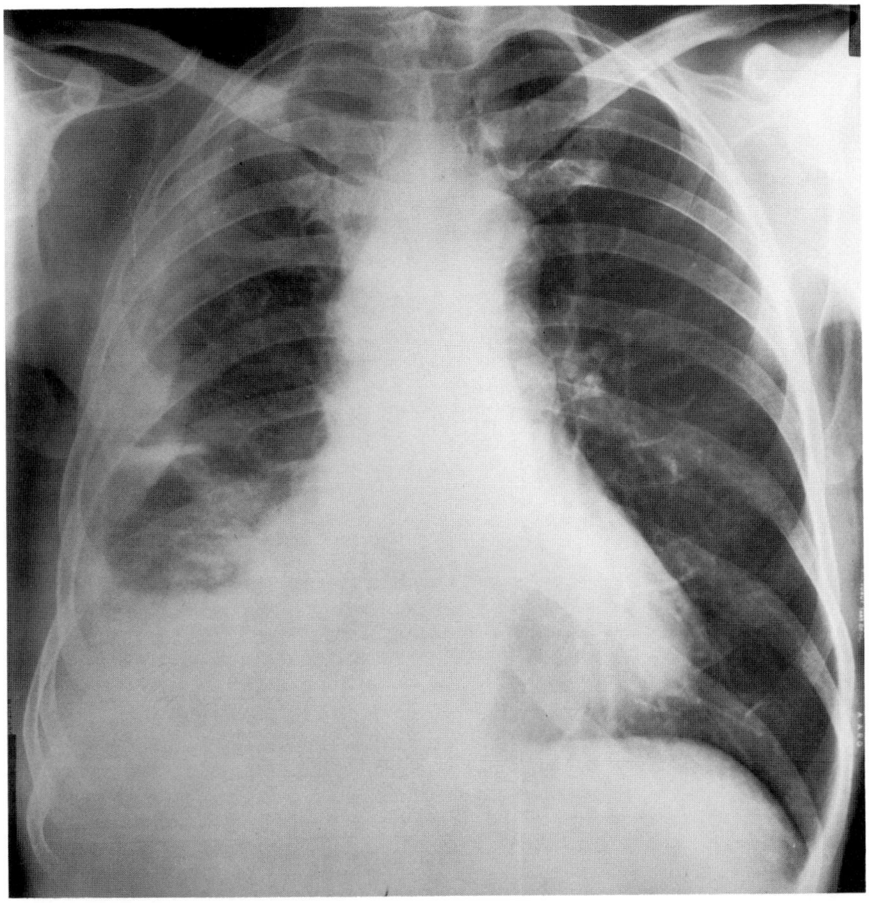

Figure 9.37 Appearances caused by carcinoma of the lung in a man who worked for one month in an asbestos processing factory 30 years before death. Post mortem, *naked eye: right lung was surrounded by a massive, partly necrotic nodular, tumour mass with invasion of the fissures. No evidence of metastasis outside the lung. Microscopy: large cell carcinoma. Only two asbestos bodies found on intensive search of 30 μm sections. No DIPF*

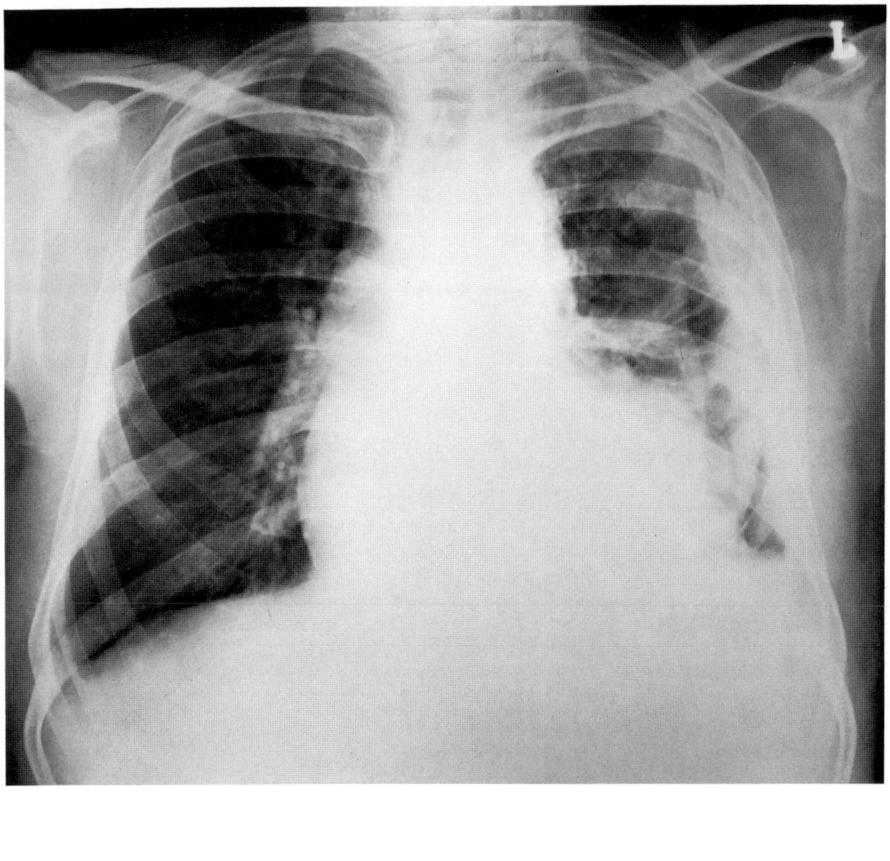

Figure 9.38 Appearances caused by secondary carcinoma in a shipyard plumber with intermittent exposure to asbestos insulation during Second World War. Right lung field clear. Post mortem, *naked eye: left lung surrounded by hard tumour mass with encysted fluid. A few small tumour deposits in right lung. Massive invasion of hilar and mediastinal lymph nodes by tumour. No gross evidence of tumour elsewhere. Microscopy: tumour—poorly differentiated adenocarcinoma. Lung—areas of lymphangitis carcinomatosa. No DIPF. Only two asbestos bodies found in 30 μm sections. Pancreas—transitional areas of gland acini and adenocarcinoma.* Diagnosis: *secondary tumour of lung from primary adenocarcinoma of pancreas. Initial post mortem diagnosis: tubulo-papillary mesothelioma*

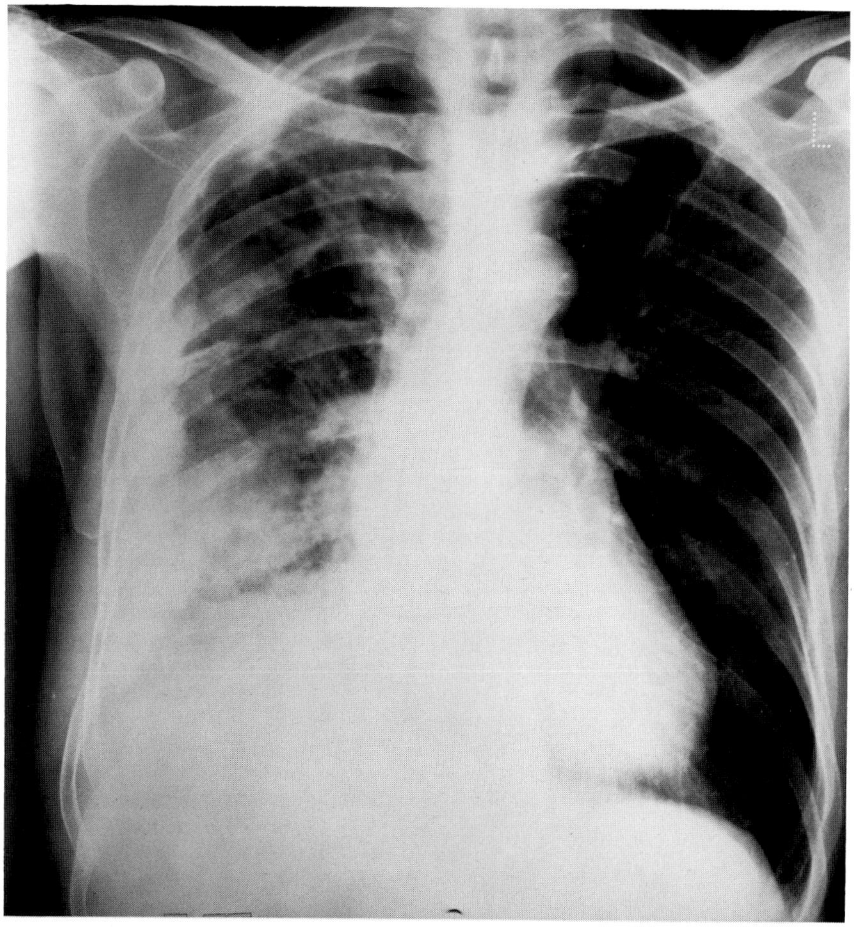

Figure 9.39 Leiomyosarcoma of lung. Builder's labourer for 45 years, occasional contact with asbestos materials. Tumour was regarded as mesothelioma during life. Post mortem, *naked eye: large lobulated fleshy tumour surrounding most of right lung; massive involvement of hilar lymph nodes. No evidence of tumour elsewhere in body. Microscopical features of leiomyosarcoma, not mesothelioma. Occasional asbestos bodies in 30 μm sections. No asbestosis*

Multiple haematogenous secondary deposits are the exception rather than the rule but they do not invalidate the diagnosis if the microscopical features are unambiguous.

Differential diagnosis

Clinically this includes all causes of subacute or 'chronic' unilateral pleural effusion, chronic pleural thickening and the exclusion of any suspicion of a primary growth elsewhere. Bronchial carcinoma may be most difficult to differentiate as it is common whereas mesothelioma is not, and, at times, may present unusual features. Biopsy is often unhelpful and sputum cytology, bronchoscopy and bronchography are uninformative in mesothelioma. In the future, electron microscopy of exfoliated cells or the identification of specific antibodies against tumour antigens may permit early diagnosis.

Today pleural disease of insidious onset in individuals over middle age should cause the diagnosis of malignant mesothelioma to be considered although a history of asbestos exposure must not be allowed to blind one to the more likely possibility of some other disease. The most important goal, however, is to distinguish between benign and treatable malignant disease otherwise the exercise is academic.

Mesothelioma should never be diagnosed at necropsy on gross appearances alone nor without thorough examination along the lines already outlined.

Prognosis

The outlook is uniformly fatal. Elmes and Simpson (1976) found that the average period between the onset of illness and death was 16 months in the case of pleural tumours and nine months with peritoneal tumours; though some patients with the pleural tumour may survive as long as four or five years (Whitwell and Rawcliffe, 1971). As the disease advances there is increasing weight loss and, in the case of pleural tumours, progressive dyspnoea and often severe and intractable chest pain. Death usually occurs from respiratory failure or bronchopneumonia, but occasionally as a result of invasion of the pericardium causing haemorrhage and tamponade. With peritoneal tumours there is malnutrition and electrolyte imbalance resulting from anorexia and frequent vomiting and, in some cases, progressive ascites. Complete intestinal obstruction is common terminally, but bronchopneumonia may intervene before this happens.

Treatment

Aspiration of intrathoracic fluid at regular intervals relieves breathlessness. Initially, this may be required daily but later, only occasionally, as less fluid accumulates. However, increasing thickness and hardness of the tumour mass ultimately makes this impossible. Diuretics are not effective in preventing accumulation of fluid (Elmes and Simpson, 1976), but installation of a cytotoxic agent into the cavity may have a limited success though without reducing pain.

Where feasible excision by pleuropneumonectomy has been advocated but it is a formidable procedure which only appears to be justifiable if the tumour is of pure epithelial type and confined to pleura and lung (Butchart *et al.*, 1976).

Radiotherapy and systemic cytotoxic drugs have not been shown to be effective either in causing shrinkage of the tumour or significant relief of pain; indeed there is some evidence to suggest that they may encourage the tumour to spread (Elmes and Simpson, 1976).

Attempts to halt the progress of the tumour by enhancing the patient's immune response have been made using three-weekly intradermal injections of viable BCG in a small number of cases following pleurectomy. Significantly longer survival and greater symptomatic relief than in patients treated by other means have been claimed (South African MRC, 1977). Further information is awaited. However, if specific antibodies could be raised against tumour antigens these might prove to be more effective.

In short, the treatment of malignant mesothelioma is essentially palliative and may tax the clinician's skill in terminal care. Pain should be relieved by analgesics in the early stages of the disease and by narcotics later when repeated nerve-root blockade or section may also be necessary. Bouts of excessive sweating may require the use of anhidrotic drugs.

SKIN CORNS

Asbestos corns (or warts) were a common feature in workers handling asbestos fibres and textiles until recent years. They are callosites on the dorsal and palmar surfaces of the hands (especially the knuckles and finger tips) and on the forearms. They consist of pronounced thickening and hyperkeratosis of the surface epithelium with some fibrosis of the dermis, round cell infiltration and occasional foreign body giant cells in the papillary layer (Alden and Howell, 1944; Schwartz, Tulipan and Birmingham, 1957). Asbestos fibres are invariably present, amphiboles apparently being more culpable than chrysotile. Interestingly, they do not ever appear to have been associated with local malignancy of the skin.

The corns, which may be tender on pressure, persist for years unless the spicules of fibre are removed. The worker usually learns to do this himself. Though uncommon today they are still seen occasionally but, apart from drawing attention to past asbestos exposure which may have been overlooked, they are of no importance.

DISORDERS PRESUMED TO BE RELATED TO ASBESTOS EXPOSURE

BENIGN PLEURAL EFFUSION AND LONE DIFFUSE PLEURAL THICKENING

Unilateral pleural effusion is occasionally encountered among asbestos workers with or without evidence of DIPF (asbestosis) when they are seen in hospital or during routine radiographic survey of an industrial population (Chahinian, *et al.*, 1973; Collins, 1968; Gaensler and Kaplan, 1971; Leménanger *et al.*, 1976; Mackenzie and Harries, 1970; Sheers and Templeton, 1968). The effusion may be recurrent either on the same side or on alternate sides and, in many cases, resolves spontaneously. In some instances the stage of effusion may not be observed but the radiographic appearances of residual diffuse pleural thickening or fibrosis are seen.

'Benign asbestos pleural effusion' is considered to be a specific asbestos-related entity by some authors (Becklake, 1976; Eisenstadt, 1964 and 1965; Gaensler and Kaplan, 1971; Sheers, 1979). The development of the effusion may be acute with fever, chest pain, leucocytosis and raised ESR; or chronic with few or no symptoms. No correlation appears to exist between its occurrence and the duration of exposure to asbestos which is reported to vary from ten months to 30 years, or the interval since last exposure which has varied from zero to 31 years (Chahinian *et al.*, 1973). Asbestos fibres may be found in the fluid—which is sometimes blood-stained—but rarely in the pleura, and asbestos bodies may be present in the sputum (Chahinian *et al.*, 1973). Biopsy shows some collagenous thickening of parietal and pulmonary pleura which may be infiltrated with lymphocytes (Chahinian *et al.*, 1973; Sluis-Cremer and Webster, 1972). Radiographic evidence of hyaline or calcified pleural plaques is recorded in a few cases.

However, pleural effusion, whether single or recurrent, and diffuse pleural thickening are common disorders the causes of which are very numerous (Crofton and Douglas, 1975). And although this is not the place to set these out in detail it is important not to overlook, among those usually listed, past chest trauma (remarkably often forgotten both by the patient and the clinician); uncommon infections some of which may be difficult to identify; rheumatoid disease in which effusions may last for months (Hunninghake and Fauci, 1979); drugs such as nitrofurantoin (which may cause acute effusion), methysergide (which may cause chronic effusion), oxprenolol (a possible cause of progressive diffuse pleural thickening: Page, 1979), and those (of which there are many) which induce systemic lupus erythematosus (Rosenow, 1972) including practolol (Erwteman, Braat and van Aken, 1977; Hall, Morrison and Edwards, 1978); thrombo-embolic disease; sarcoidosis (Nicholls, Friend and Legge, 1980); the post-myocardial infarction syndrome (Dressler, 1959); Waldenström's macroglobulinaemia (Teo and Lee, 1978), and lymphatic hypoplasia with or without primary lymphoedema—the so-called 'yellow nail syndrome' (Beer, Pereira and Snider, 1978). These few examples serve to emphasize the wide range of possible causes of pleural effusion. In five cases of so-called 'asbestos pleurisy' described by Leménanger *et al.* (1976) the differential cell count of the fluid revealed eosinophils in excess of 40 per cent in three and 70 per cent polymorphonuclear leucocytes in another; and, although asbestos fibres were demonstrated by electron microscopy in all, abnormalities which the authors admit could have accounted for the effusions were present in four; namely, rheumatoid arthritis, chronic bronchial infection, Rickettsia-positive serology, and empyema. Even in the presence of circulating RF the effusions have sometimes been attributed to asbestos rather than to rheumatoid disease in which effusions are known to occur without rheumatoid arthritis (Leading article, 1978b; Torrington, 1978). But in most of the cases reported as due to asbestos systematic and exhaustive exclusion of all known causes has rarely been carried out. Furthermore, thorough investigation of pleural effusions in general leaves a substantial number unexplained (Storey, Dines and Coles, 1976).

The identification of asbestos bodies or fibres in association with an apparently inexplicable pleural effusion is, of course, no guarantee of a causal relationship as these would be expected in any asbestos worker whether pleuropulmonary disease is present or not.

Clearly, it is essential to determine whether or not radiographic evidence of pleural effusion or diffuse pleural thickening in large numbers of patients seen randomly in chest clinic and similar practice is associated with past exposure to asbestos. Surprisingly there appears to be only one comprehensive survey of this type reported: namely, that of the British Thoracic and Tuberculosis Association and MRC Pneumoconiosis Unit (1972), referred to already on p. 241, which found 'no strong association between pleural shadowing and asbestos exposure' in 3868 patients of whom an appreciable number could have been exposed to asbestos. Until similar surveys are done in different geographical areas this problem will not be satisfactorily resolved (*see* Murphy, 1980).

It is suggested, therefore, that at present the case for asbestos minerals being a specific cause of isolated, benign pleural effusions or diffuse pleural fibrosis without accompanying intrapulmonary fibrosis is not proven, and that such current terms as 'asbestos pleural effusion' and 'asbestos pleurisy' are not justifiable; although further investigation may well vindicate them.

On the other hand, effusions detected on routine radiographs of a group of naval dockyard workers proved to be early evidence of malignancy (Harries, 1976). Hence, bronchial carcinoma and malignant mesothelioma of the pleura must always be kept in mind as possible causes of an effusion which develops in an asbestos worker of middle age or over, irrespective of whether he has overt evidence of asbestosis. Unfortunately, some cases diagnosed as diffuse, unilateral, pleural 'fibrosis' following a benign 'asbestos effusion' are ultimately found to have malignant mesotheliomas even after a span of two or three years.

CARCINOMA OF LUNG IN THE ABSENCE OF ASBESTOSIS

A link between asbestosis (DIPF) and carcinoma of the lung is proven and is discussed on pp. 270–272, but there is also a widespread belief that a causal relationship between asbestos exposure alone (that is, without asbestosis) and carcinoma of the lung is established. This rests on a number of epidemiological studies of respiratory cancer hazards in working populations exposed to asbestos. These have shown an excess of bronchial carcinoma by comparison with control groups which occurs almost exclusively in smokers (Berry, Newhouse and Turok, 1972; Enterline, 1976; Selikoff, Hammond and Churg, 1968; Selikoff, Hammond and Seidman, 1973; Selikoff, 1976; Selikoff, Seidman and Hammond, 1980). The majority of these studies appear to agree that an excess of lung cancer exists but there is pronounced disagreement as to the magnitude of the relative risk which ranges from 1.2 to 9.2. There are a number of reasons for this disparity: in the majority of studies the wrong population was used to estimate numbers of deaths; in some surveys death certificates for the 'at risk' populations were adjusted from data in other (for example, hospital) medical records though comparison was made with expected deaths derived from uncorrected death certificates (*see* Chapter 1, p. 25); in the majority of studies the level and duration of exposure is unknown; and standardization of smoking habits is rarely possible (Enterline, 1976). But the most important weakness in this thesis is that, in spite of the large numbers of subjects involved in these surveys, there have been very few necropsies to confirm the diagnosis of primary carcinoma of the lung and the *absence* of evidence of asbestosis, both macroscopical and microscopical.

It is of interest that, in a study of 264 men who started work between 1935 and 1945 in a factory using chrysotile only and who were followed up to 1974, the standardized mortality ratio for lung cancer was reported to be 0.93, and two men died of asbestosis (Weiss, 1977). Similarly, no excess of deaths from carcinoma of the lung and from all causes has been found in a mortality study dating from 1942 to 1979 of workers (male and female) who manufactured friction materials with chrysotile. But there were a few cases of malignant mesothelioma of the pleura associated with a short period prior to 1944 when crocidolite was used instead (Newhouse, Berry and Skidmore, 1980).

As stated earlier the development of asbestosis and lung cancer in asbestos workers and experimental animals is related to the duration of exposure to asbestos—the exposure-response relationship for lung cancer in man being essentially linear (Newhouse, 1973; Wagner *et al.*, 1974; McDonald, 1980), and smoking greatly increases the cancer risk. Indeed, it has been suggested that the carcinogenic agents in cigarette smoke may be adsorbed onto fibres which are deposited in the periphery of the lung provoking tumours of peripheral origin (Rossiter and Berry, 1978).

It is, of course, conceivable that the combination of lighter exposure to asbestos (dose × time) than that which usually causes asbestosis and a critical level of smoking (dose × time) might induce bronchial carcinoma in advance of, or in preference to, asbestosis. If asbestos exposure, which is too low to cause asbestosis, really does increase the incidence of tobacco-induced cancer, the lungs of lung cancer patients in cities might be expected to contain significantly more asbestos bodies than a series of control lungs without cancer or industrial disease from a population of similar age and sex distribution (*see* p. 240). Whitwell, Scott and Grimshaw (1977) have shown that this is not so and that there is a very similar fibre content in the lungs both of the cancer patients and of the controls; and more recently Churg and Warnock (1979) reported that the numbers of asbestos bodies in the lungs of an American urban population did not correlate with the presence of bronchial carcinoma.

It must be concluded, therefore, that the evidence available to date has not established that asbestos exposure causes carcinoma of the lung in the absence of antecedent asbestosis. But to answer this question with certainty extensive necropsy studies, carefully controlled and matched in all relevant respects and employing standardized methods of microscopical assessment and accurate fibre analysis of the lungs, are necessary. The need for such investigation has recently been stressed by Seal (1980).

The Report of the Advisory Committee on Asbestos Cancers (1973) indicated that there is no increased risk of developing lung cancer to the general public from the low levels of asbestos which may occur in general air pollution; and the observations of Whitwell, Scott and Grimshaw (1977) referred to already support this.

CARCINOMA OF LARYNX

Carcinoma of the larynx is known to be linked with cigarette smoking but an association between asbestos exposure and an increased incidence of this tumour which appears to develop ten years earlier than in patients with no known asbestos exposure was reported by Stell and McGill (1973 and 1975). Other studies have suggested that the association with asbestos, which is largely confined to smokers, is stronger than the association with smoking alone (Libshitz *et al.*, 1974; Morgan and Shettigara, 1976). However, in 4463 deaths among 11 379 chrysotile production workers followed from 1926 to 1975 there was no excess due to laryngeal carcinoma—21 cases in all (McDonald *et al.*, 1980). And no evidence of a relationship between the tumour and asbestos exposure was found in an unselected group of 305 male and 206 female patients attending a London Hospital (Newhouse, Gregory and Shannon, 1979); in 47 males with laryngeal cancers in Washington State (Hinds, Thomas and O'Reilly, 1979); and in 60 cases investigated in Italy (Bianchi *et al.*, 1978). The importance of the combination of alcohol with smoking and development of the tumour has been emphasized by McMichael (1978) who also noted ethnic associations.

At present, therefore, it is incorrect to regard asbestos exposure as a proven cause of this uncommon tumour.

OTHER FORMS OF NEOPLASIA

This topic is given only brief mention as it lies outside the scope and purpose of this book.

A relationship between asbestos exposure and neoplasia of the gastro-intestinal tract and reticulo-endothelial system has been reported in some surveys but not in all. Miller (1978) has calculated that there is an approximately three-fold increased risk of gastro-intestinal malignancy in asbestos workers 20 or more years after first exposure. However, the problem requires further investigation as no increase was observed in an earlier study of asbestos workers in the UK (Ministry of Labour, 1967), and no correlation was found between the numbers of asbestos bodies in the lungs and the presence of gastro-intestinal carcinoma in an American urban population (Churg and Warnock, 1979).

PREVENTIVE MEASURES

SUBSTITUTION

Alternative materials are used to replace asbestos in a variety of applications, the most notable being the wide range employed for thermal and acoustic insulation: these include glass, rock and slag wools, diatomite, vermiculite, perlite, cork, expanded polystyrene and polyvinyl chloride (PVC), and polyurethane foam. But for many, often life-saving purposes such as fire-resistant materials, there is no satisfactory substitute. In these circumstances crocidolite has been replaced in the UK by one of the other types of asbestos since the Asbestos Regulations 1969 were enacted.

CONTROL

To ensure conditions of safety codes of practice are essential. These can be briefly considered from four standpoints: conveyance and storage of asbestos fibre, factory conditions, other occupational conditions and waste disposal. In the UK all are controlled by the Asbestos Regulations 1969 which came into force in May, 1970 (Department of Employment and Productivity, 1970). Detailed instructions for all contingencies are provided by the Environmental Control Committee of the British Asbestos Research Council in 'Control and Safety Guide' booklets which are revised periodically. And the British Health and Safety Executive has now published its recommendations (1979).

(1) Conveyance and storage of fibre

Fibre is now kept in sealed polythene or impermeable paper bags which prevent exposure to spillage previously experienced by dockers, truck loaders and factory workers.

(2) Factory conditions

Where wet processes are used, as in the production of asbestos cement products, there is very little dust. But dusty, dry processes (such as milling) can be effectively controlled by total or partial enclosure with effective exhaust ventilation and, where enclosure is not possible (as in machining and sawing asbestos products), by hoods subjected to 'low-volume high velocity' exhaust ventilation.

Exhaust ventilation, both local and general, must carry the dust-laden air away and filter out the dust efficiently so that it does not return to the factory or escape to the outside air. Filtered dust is sealed in polythene bags.

Where a worker is likely to be exposed to an asbestos-dust risk, personal protective equipment must be worn. This consists of standard respirator masks, positive-pressure respirators powered by a portable mechanism, air-line breathing apparatus and also closely fitting overalls of synthetic fibre to which little dust adheres.

Dust on floors and other surfaces is removed at frequent intervals by portable industrial vacuum cleaners. If these are not available floors are wetted or spread with damp sawdust before sweeping.

(3) Other occupational conditions

Air-line respirators and impervious suits which are decontaminated in a shower before being removed are used in British naval dockyards for work in the heavy dust concentrations encountered during removal of old lagging, acoustic board and sprayed asbestos coatings in ships and submarines: for lower dust concentrations, nylon overalls and positive pressure power respirators are used. The area of operation is thoroughly vacuum cleaned after completion. Similar principles apply to demolition of old asbestos installations.

Where possible, old lagging is soaked with water before it is removed to suppress liberation of dust and, when removed placed in polythene bags which are then sealed for disposal. Under conditions where the wet method is not practicable air-line breathing apparatus must be employed in addition to protective equipment. Stripping should be done when other workers are not in the vicinity but, if this is impossible, they too should wear protective equipment. After completion of the operation, the area should be vacuum cleaned.

The dust produced by the spraying of asbestos for thermal and acoustic insulation and other purposes can be greatly reduced by wetting the fibre before it is fed into the spray-gun, and by confining the work area by plastic sheeting to prevent dissemination by wind and draughts. Approved respirators and protective clothing should be worn throughout the operation. In the UK recommendations on asbestos insulation practice have been made by the Health and Safety Commission (1978a).

Drilling, sawing and shaping of asbestos cement sheeting should be segregated and the workers should wear protective equipment.

(4) Disposal of waste

Fine dust and loose fibre should be placed in impermeable polythene sacks which can be tightly sealed, and insulation waste can be deposited on polythene sheeting which is folded to form a sealed envelope. All waste should be transported in closed containers which carry a warning as to their contents. Empty containers are cleared out by vacuum cleaning. The waste is deposited in a pit and covered by at least 230 mm of consolidated earth or other dry waste (Asbestos Research Council, 1973).

Levels of airborne dust

These are 'monitored' in two ways: by personal sampling instruments worn by the worker in his 'breathing zone', and by instruments designed to sample the general factory air. Sampling is carried out either for short specified periods or continuously over prolonged periods. Fibre counts on membrane filters by phase-contrast light microscopy and gravimetric methods used in conjunction have been recommended (Report of the Advisory Committee on Asbestos Cancers, 1973), and means of standardization suggested (Gibbs *et al.*, 1977). However, non-asbestos fibres can be confused with asbestos fibres on routine counting by phase contrast microscopy and lead to spuriously high asbestos counts (Middleton, 1978). For this reason and because asbestos fibres beyond the resolution of the light microscope cannot be identified by these methods the routine use of total counts by electron microscopy has been suggested, though the pathogenic significance of minute fibres is in doubt (*see* Chapter 4, p. 74).

The Health and Safety Commission (UK) (1978b) has proferred advice on methods by which technical inadequacies and observer error in identification and counting of fibres can be reduced and has established a Reference Laboratory at the Institute of Occupational Medicine, Edinburgh, to standardize counting techniques.

Environmental dust standards in industry (TLVs)

These vary from country to country and are constantly under review and are thus in a state of flux. In the UK the Hygiene Standards Committee of the British Occupational Hygiene Society made various recommendations in 1968 and 1973 but the newly formed Health and Safety Executive will concern itself with the matter in future. In the USA the responsible body is the National Institute for Occupational Safety and Health. In principle, standards are based on maximal average concentrations or numbers of fibres of specified diameter and length which should not be exceeded over an eight hour working day or a shorter defined period. The International Labour Office (1974) has also issued a guidance booklet.

It is worth noting, in this context, that Peto (1978) has pointed out that 'accurate dose-response data at levels below 2 fibres/ml are unlikely to be available for the forseeable future and the biologically plausible assumption that excess cancer (bronchial carcinoma and malignant mesothelioma) mortality is approximately proportional to dust level should be provisionally accepted.

Medical examination of workers

Medical examination of healthy asbestos workers should be done every one to two years (*see* p. 25) and include good quality, full-size chest radiographs and a record of VC, FVC and FEV_1. Ideally, details of current dust-count levels should be included in these records.

Employment of young persons

Special provisions applying to 'young persons' are laid down by the British Asbestos Regulations 1969.

'TALC' PNEUMOCONIOSIS

Talc pneumoconiosis was first described by Thorel (1896), since when it has not always been clear to what type of lung pathology this term has referred. Radiographic appearances may be those of a nodular disease (such as silicosis, coal pneumoconiosis or sarcoidosis) or of DIPF; and both are sometimes seen in the one individual. In fact, pathologically three different basic lesions occur—irregular quasi-nodular fibrosis, DIPF and foreign body granulomas. The reason for much of this diversity is that in industry and commerce the term 'talc' often embraces a variety of minerals other than talc itself. Hence, the commonly used term, 'talcosis', is inappropriate.

Table 9.3 Typical Mineralogical Composition of some Commercial Grades of Talc

	Weight per cent					
	1	*2*	*3*	*4*	*5*	*6*
Talc	95	90	89	50	49	45
Chlorite	3	4	8	49	15	12
Magnesite	—	0.6	—	—	31	37
Dolomite	1	0.8	—	trace	—	4
Tremolite	—	—	—	—	trace	—
Serpentine	—	—	—	—	*	—
Quartz	—	trace	trace	trace	—	—
Opaques	—	—	—	trace	trace	trace
Percentage reflectance	94	89	84	70	70	64

*Serpentine identified by X-ray diffraction but included by thermogravimetry in chlorite figure.
Mineralogical compositions obtained by X-ray diffractometry; weight percentages derived from thermogravimetric data. Percentage reflectance gives an indication of whiteness.
1 Chinese talc—cosmetic grade.
2 Italian (Pinerolo) talc—cosmetic grade.
3 French (Luzenac) talc—high quality.
4 French (Luzenac) talc—industrial grade.
5 Norwegian talc—industrial grade.
6 Unst talc (Shetland)—industrial grade.

Reproduced by courtesy of Dr H. E. Highley and HMSO

Definition and mode of occurrence of talc

Talc is a hydrated magnesium silicate with the formula $Mg_3Si_4O_{10}(OH)_2$ although calcium, aluminium and iron are always present in variable amounts. It occurs in sheets which readily cleave and break down to form flat, flaky plates and, to a lesser degree, short rolled sheets. It is usually formed in one of two ways: either by low-grade thermal metamorphism of siliceous dolomites or by hydrothermal alteration—frequently accompanied by dynamic metamorphism—of magnesium-rich ultrabasic rocks (*see* Chapter 2). In consequence, other minerals are almost invariably present in association with talc. These include serpentines (usually antigorite but, rarely, chrysotile), chlorites, quartz, magnesite, calcite and the amphiboles tremolite and anthophyllite. Magnesium silicate mineral remnants such as olivine, enstatite and diopside may also be present. According to the geographical area of origin, therefore, talc deposits exhibit a wide variety of mineral assemblages which differ in occurrence and proportion. This is exemplified in *Tables 9.3* and *9.4*. Intergrowths of tremolite and anthophyllite, usually in prismatic crystalline form, may be intimately associated with talc but in some geological regions (notably New York State) which appear to be uncommon, if not exceptional, they may occur in true fibrous (that is, asbestos) form and persist after beneficiation.

High purity (high grade) white talcs from the Italian Alps, Pyrenees, China and India were formed from siliceous dolomite and dolomite limestones and contain little or no quartz although this mineral may be encountered in small amounts in the mining of Italian talc. Domestically-produced Norwegian talc is, however, of fairly low grade and usually contains chlorite, magnesite and, possibly, non-fibrous tremolite and trace amounts of quartz. The 'talc' from the famous mines of St. Lawrence County in New York State frequently contains as much as 50 per cent or more of tremolite with less than 25 per cent talc, and significant amounts of anthophyllite and quartz occur in some samples (Weiss and Boettner, 1967). In these deposits a significant proportion of both tremolite and anthophyllite is of true fibrous habit. The variable composition of some New York State 'talc' samples is shown in *Table 9.4*. Californian (Death Valley) 'talc' is associated with non-fibrous tremolite, quartz, serpentine and calcite. Talc from the Vermont area, on the other hand, is associated with

Table 9.4 Varieties of Commercial 'Talc' from New York State (Gouverneur District)

	1	*2*	*3*	*4*	*5*	*6*	*7*	*8*	*9*	*10*
Tremolite	68	98	17	—	78	38	29	15	88	46
Anthophyllite	—	—	20	—	—	—	45	78	4	39
Talc	—	1	63	—	4	—	—	7	1	5
Serpentine*	—	1	—	80	18	54	26	—	4	4
Quartz	31	—	—	—	—	—	—	—	2	4
Others	1	—	—	20	—	8	—	—	1	2

Figures indicate percentage composition.
Dashes indicate no determination made.
*Either massive or fibrous.
By courtesy of Johns-Manville Research and Engineering Center, New Jersey

magnesite and dolomite, but there are no asbestos minerals and quartz is either absent or present in trace amounts (Boundy *et al.* 1979) and quartz is either absent or of negligible amount. Canadian 'talc', which comes mainly from the Madoc district of Ontario, has a similar geological origin to that of St. Lawrence County and contains considerable quantities of tremolite and dolomite, and some quartz which may remain in variable amount in the final product. In the UK only a small quantity of impure (low grade) talc is produced in the Shetlands and this has decreased in recent years due to its previous use in the roof felting industry being much restricted.

Low grade talcs, therefore, may contain in excess of 50 per cent impurities and significant amounts of quartz, tremolite and anthophyllite (of prismatic or fibrous habit according to origin) may be present in some. Where talc is associated with substantial quantities of tremolite and anthophyllite it is often known as *asbestine*. The presence of chrysotile is rare, though it occurs occasionally as a result of intrusion in some low grade talcs. But *sepiolite* fibres (also an hydrated magnesium silicate), which are occasionally found in talc samples may be mistaken for chrysotile as they have a very similar appearance and can only be differentiated by microprobe analysis and high magnification electron microscopy (Pooley and Rowlands, 1977).

Under the light microscope talc appears as flat, angular, polygonal plates (that is, platy, non-fibrous talc) and occasionally as short 'fibres' which are, in fact, rolled talc sheets; whereas tremolite and anthophyllite both consist of prismatic, acicular crystals and, occasionally, true fibres. The term 'fibrous' talc is only applicable to 'talc' in which these amphiboles occur in true fibrous habit and are predominant (*Figure 9.40*). Talc and tremolite are strongly birefringent, but anthophyllite is only weakly so. However, electron microscopy and diffraction and X-ray diffraction are needed for positive identification. The inability of light and phase contrast microscopy to distinguish rolled talc plates and talc shards from asbestos fibres must be borne in mind when considering the total fibre content of industrial talcs (Boundy *et al.* 1979).

Steatite is the term used to describe the massive, fine-grained (cryptocrystalline) variety of talc; *soapstone* is a term loosely applied to impure talcose rocks containing variable amounts of talc and other minerals.

Pyrophyllite (*see* Chapter 2) is sometimes wrongly referred to as 'talc' in industry. It is an hydrated alumino-silicate with very similar properties to talc but, except in its purest form, it contains quartz in abundance.

Hence, the term *talc* should be confined to the description of a mineral containing at least 95 per cent platy talc with no amphibole and negligible quartz content. And it is important to reiterate that, with the exception of such regions as New York State and Madoc, Ontario, tremolite and anthophyllite in talc occur mainly in prismatic crystalline form and not in fibrous form; and to emphasize that statements such as 'talc is closely related to asbestos', now often seen in medical and public health literature, are most misleading (*see* Chapter 2, p. 39).

Most of the talc used for industrial purposes in the UK before and since the Second World War has come from Norway, France, China and Italy. Total imports from all sources was 56300 tonnes in 1977 (Highley, 1978). However, during the War all these sources of supply were cut off and were apparently replaced mainly by Canadian and, possibly, some American 'talc'. The use of these talcs which contain substantial quantities of fibrous tremolite and anthophyllite may have had an influence on the type of pneumoconiosis which has been sporadically observed in some 'talc'-exposed workers in the UK since the War. After 1970 imports of 'tremolitic talc' into the UK have been recorded separately and are not much in excess of 1000 tonnes annually (Highley, 1974), being 1592 tonnes in 1977 (Highley, 1978).

Uses of talc

The valuable qualities of talc in industry are its extreme softness, whiteness (when pure), good hiding power, high surface area, high slip or lubricating power, chemical inertness, low electrical and heat conductivity, oil adsorption properties and high refractoriness. Because of this great versatility talc in a variety of grades is put to a large number of industrial uses, but only the most common are referred

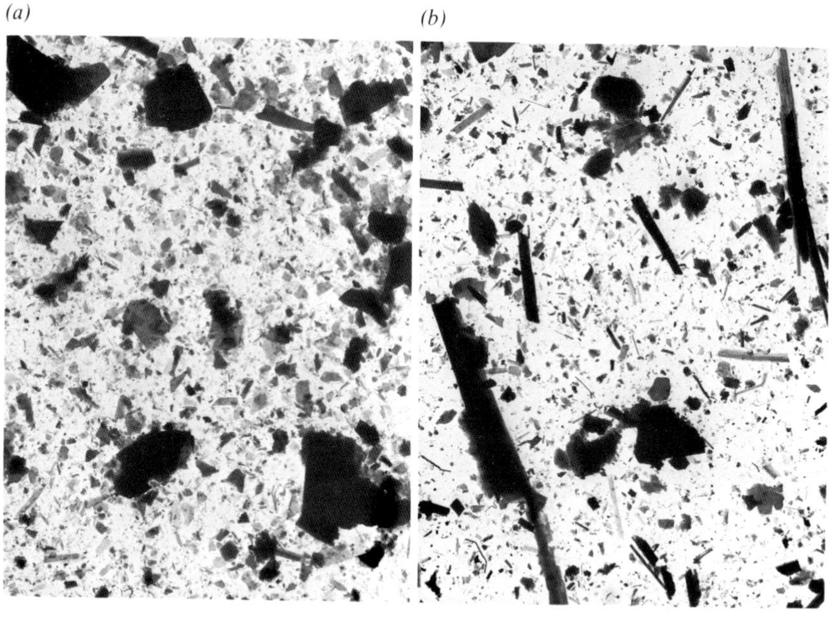

Figure 9.40 (a) Talc plates, good quality cosmetic talc. (b) Talc plates and tremolite, the acicular crystals and fibres of which are evident by their long axes. This is typical of industrial grade talc used in the USA. (Electron micrographs; original magnification × 5000, reproduced at × 4000; by courtesy of Johns-Manville Research and Engineering Center, New Jersey)

to. In the UK the greatest consumption of talc occurs in the paint, pharmaceutical and cosmetics industries.

Paints

High grade talc is used in the paint industry as a filler and inert extender because of its whiteness and laminar form. But 'fibrous talc' (asbestine) is also widely employed because its good suspending powers reduce settling in the can, and it also increases the mechanical strength of paint films. However, it appears that the term 'asbestine' is also being used in the paint industry in the UK for some grades of talc which do not contain fibrous minerals (Highley, 1974). The paint industry is the main consumer of tremolitic 'talc' in the UK.

Cosmetic and pharmaceutical industries

High grade talcs are used in large quantities in these industries: for example, face powders, talcum powders, other cosmetic preparations and dermopaediatric powders, and for polishing tablets. The particle size of good cosmetic grade talc lies between 0.3 to 50 μm (Hamer, Rolle and Schelz, 1976) but only a fraction of the particles are of 'respirable' size. Quartz and other harsh minerals should be absent or only trace amounts present, and, apart from chlorite which, as a holder of perfume, may be acceptable, the only impurities should be calcium sulphate. But, this level of purity may not always exist in poor quality preparations (*see* p. 300). The best cosmetic talcs come from Italy, China and Vermont (USA). Talc used in the British cosmetic industry is specifically controlled for asbestos minerals whether of fibrous habit or not (Phillipson, 1980).

Ceramics

Both talc and steatite are employed in small amounts in the ceramics industry for a variety of purposes. Talc mixed with clay and alumina and fired at 1250 to 1400 °C forms *cordierite* (a pseudo-hexagonal crystalline aluminium magnesium iron silicate) which is used for such things as coil formers, fuse cores, rheostat blocks, fire bars, electric insulators and the manufacture of saggers and other types of refractory kiln equipment. Steatite together with ball clay and a barium carbonate flux fired between 1200 and 1350 °C is widely employed in electronic ceramics; for example, in condenser end-plates, stand-off insulators, valve holder bases, valve electrode spacers and panel bushes. In the USA—but not in the UK—talc is used as a substitute for feldspar in the manufacture of earthenware bodies, especially for wall tiles and dinner ware.

Roof felting industry

Here the lubricating properties of talc are used for dusting roofing felts to prevent the layers sticking when rolled, and to increase, resistance to fire and weather. Low grade talcs are employed but, in the UK, they have recently been largely replaced by silica sand.

Rubber industry

Again the lubricating properties are exploited as a dusting agent to prevent adhesion of the rubber in the moulds and to provide smooth extrusion but, in recent years, this use has declined considerably. Talc is also used as a filler in hard rubber goods such as accumulator cases and valves (which may require grinding, hence the term 'rubber-grinder'), in cable manufacture and as an inert filler in some plastic polypropylene compounds. Small quantities of 'tremolitic talc' are employed for these purposes in the UK.

Fertilizer industry

Significant amounts of low grade talc are used as an anti-caking agent in the manufacture of fertilizers.

Refractory materials

Low grade talc is used as a refractory filler for moulds and cores in both ferrous and non-ferrous castings.

Paper industry

Because of its whiteness, good retention and ability to improve the gloss, opacity and brightness of paper talc may be substituted for china clay as a coating and filler of paper. Although this use is very small in the UK it is increasing rapidly in the USA due to the availability of a 'micronized' talc in which particle size ranges from 5 μm to less than 0.5 μm (Roe, 1975).

Textile industry

Finely ground French talc is used for 'loading' and bleaching cotton sacks, cordage, string and rope.

Miscellaneous

Talc is used as a dusting agent for glass moulds and as a polishing medium for chocolate, peanuts, rice and chewing gum; and until the 1950s, was employed to dust moulds for the manufacture of lead accumulator plates before coating. It is also used as a carrier for insecticides, in oil adsorption treatment of leather, for dusting of furs, and in shoe manufacture to prevent the adherence of layers of leather.

Sources of exposure

Mining is carried out by both open-pit and underground methods. The milling operations involve jaw and roll crushers, screens and pebble mills. Cases of DIPF have been recorded in miners and millers of New York State 'talc' (Siegel, Smith and Greenburg, 1943; Greenburg, 1947; Kleinfeld *et al.*, 1964a). Bagging of the milled material is also a potential risk.

Radiographic appearances consistent with silicosis have been reported in Italian talc-miners mainly in ILO Category 'q' (Pettinati *et al.*, 1964), but the quartz content falls progressively during milling and preparation for factory use in which there appears to be no risk of silicosis (Dettori, Scansetti and Gribaudo, 1964). Some working milling and bagging high-grade, allegedly quartz-free, talc in the Hamata area of Egypt have, however, been found to have either 'nodular' or conglomerate opacities (El-Ghawabi, El-Samra and Mehasseb, 1970).

Industrial applications

Exposure to fibrous tremolite and to quartz in industries normally using low-grade talc probably occurred to some extent in the UK during the Second World War due to substitution by Canadian and American 'talc' and pyrophillite, and stocks may have continued for some years after the war. Recent analysis of imported bulk talc samples in powder and rock form by means of X-ray diffraction, thermal gravimetric and differential thermal analysis, and electron microprobe analysis has shown that the major contaminating minerals were chlorite, carbonates and quartz with tremolite in only a minority; although in one sample tremolite was the major mineral phase, apparently in fibrous form (Pooley and Rowlands, 1977).

Exposure has occurred in the roof felting and shingle industry where talc is distributed liberally on the felt surfaces prior to rolling to prevent adhesion and may be used as a filler in asphalt coating; in the rubber industry where the powder is blown on to the tacky rubber surface (for example, during extrusion of tubes and sheets) or dusted onto rubber goods before storage; in the mouldings of accumulator plates; in leather finishing; and in preparing the mix for electrical ceramics, tiles and refractory kiln bodies. In all these processes only low grade talc is required and, therefore, accessory minerals may be present. It should be noted that before and during the Second World War women worked in the rubber trade, especially in tyre extruding, and were probably exposed to considerable quantities of mixed dust.

Talc heated above a temperature of 1000 °C (as is required in the manufacture of some ceramics) yields *clinoenstatite* (a prismatic magnesium silicate) and cristobalite which is strongly fibrogenic (*see* Chapters 2 and 7). However, in this form, it gives rise to little dust.

Exposure to tremolite and anthophyllite, probably mostly in non-fibrous form, may occur in the manufacture of some types of paints.

Talc employed in the manufacture of cosmetic, toilet and pharmaceutical talcum powder is normally of high purity. However, X-ray diffraction analysis of 21 powders obtained through retail channels in the USA showed that few consisted of pure talc. Quartz, ranging from 2 to 5 per cent, was found in eight, and in a single sample was 35 per cent. Detectable amounts of 'fibrous' tremolite and anthophyllite were reported to be present in ten, and chrysotile in two; other mineral phases identified were platy serpentine, chlorite, pyrophyllite, mica and carbonate minerals (Rohl *et al.*, 1976). It should, however, be pointed out that overlap of diffraction peaks of chlorite—commonly present in talc—and chrysotile make identification of the latter difficult or impossible unless other analytical methods are used (*see* Appendix: Identification of Minerals).

Strict specifications to ensure high purity of cosmetic talc have recently been laid down by the Toilet Preparations Federation in the UK and the Cosmetic Toiletry and Fragrance Association in the USA, and methods of characterizing talc for this purpose described (Hamer, Rolle and Schelz, 1976).

Millman (1947) recorded the case of a man with small discrete, radiographic opacities interpreted as indicative of pneumoconiosis (though this was not proven) who had spent years in a cosmetic factory weighing, mixing and sifting talc containing less than 0.5 per cent of free silica.

In the USA, apart from the cosmetic industry, much of the industrial 'talc' used has probably been fibrous.

Because talc is expensive substitutes for filler and low grade dusting applications are used in a variety of processes, and have been for some years. In the UK one of the most important of these has been powdered slate which contains significant quantities of quartz; and china clay by-product, which contains small amounts of quartz, and mica have been employed in the roof felt industry. But, apart from substitution, ground flint and silica sands have been used as surfacing materials for some roof felts, and asbestos has been exploited as an asphalt filler to produce a fire- and weather-resistant material. These points may need to be borne in mind when evaluating a past occupational risk.

Epidemiology

There have been very few controlled epidemiological studies of the incidence and prevalence of pneumoconiosis in workers exposed to industrial talc although, since 1896, many cases of disease resembling either silicosis or asbestosis have been reported (Hildick-Smith, 1976).

In 1970 a study of 39 men mining and milling talc containing fibrous tremolite and anthophyllite for a mean period of 16.2 years (ranging from 11 to 22 years) in New York State discovered only one man (2.6 per cent) with radiographic changes consistent with pneumoconiosis. Whereas among 35 men with a similar mean period of exposure at a neighbouring talc mining and milling plant (presumably similar mineralogically) examined in 1964, 12 (34 per cent) had radiographic evidence of pneumoconiosis. The average dust count in 1970 at the first plant (in which dust controls were installed at the start of operations in 1948) was 18 mppcf of talc with an average of 43 fibres longer than 5 μm; and in the second plant the average count done in 1969 was 23 mppcf with an average of 159 fibres longer than 5 μm. Hence, although dust control reduced the incidence of pneumoconiosis in the first plant, the fibre count was still excessively high. It was thus concluded that fibrous tremolite and anthophyllite are less fibrogenic than other asbestos types at comparable dust exposures (Kleinfeld, Messite and Langer, 1973).

In a group of 70 mine employees producing cosmetic grade talc (free of amphiboles and quartz) compared with a matched control group of agricultural workers there was no evidence of pneumoconiosis and ventilatory function tests in the two were similar, but an increase of phlegm production was noted in the talc miners who smoked (Hildick-Smith, 1977). However, a recent study of New York State talc miners and millers showed that respiratory symptoms were little more prevalent than in a control population of 'potash miners' though ventilatory function was significantly decreased and the presence of 'pleural thickening' and calcification was greater than in the controls (Gamble, Fellner and Dimeo, 1979).

Mortality statistics of talc miners and millers in New York State showed that pulmonary heart disease was a significant complication of pneumoconiosis in the early 1960s but this was reduced by half in the later period 1965–69 though the number of deaths was, in fact, very small—nine compared with four; but over the period 1940–69 it was recorded as responsible for 29 of a total of 108 deaths. The overall proportional mortality from carcinoma of the lung for this period (1940–69) was approximately four times that expected and was predominant in 60 to 79 age group rather than the 40 to 59 age group; but in the years 1965 to 1969 it was approximately the same as the generally expected rate. However, data of smoking habits were not available and expected mortality was calculated from all deaths among white males in the USA in 1955 (Kleinfeld, Messite and Zaki, 1974) (*see also* p. 310).

In Italy Rubino *et al.* (1976 and 1979) compared the causes of death among men who had worked for more than one year between 1920 and 1950 mining and milling Piedmont talc (which, in its natural state, is pure and is used in the cosmetic and pharmaceutical industries) with mortality among agricultural workers with similar social and economic conditions in an area some 38 miles distant, and also with expectation of death in the Italian male population. The miners were exposed to dust containing about 5 per cent free silica whereas the millers were exposed to a content of about 0.5 per cent and to a lower total dust concentration. An excess mortality due to silicosis and silico-tuberculosis occurred in the miners but there was no increase in mortality from lung cancer in either the miners or millers.

Hence, epidemiological studies, in general, indicate that prolonged industrial exposure to cosmetic grade talc is not associated with the development of pneumoconiosis or cancer of the lung though exposure to industrial grade talc (depending upon its composition) may result in silicosis, 'mixed dust fibrosis' (*see* Chapter 7) and DIPF (asbestosis). The question of lung cancer in talc workers exposed to fibrous tremolite and anthophyllite is incompletely resolved.

Pathology

Macroscopic appearances

Fibrous adhesions of the pleural surfaces are often present and in some cases may be dense, and hyaline and calcified plaques have been observed in the diaphragmatic, mediastinal and costal parietal pleura in cases in which there may have been a significant exposure to 'fibrous talc' (Kleinfeld *et al.*, 1963). The cut surfaces of the lungs reveal one or other of two different patterns of fibrosis. On the one hand, small ill-defined nodules somewhat larger than silicotic nodules (but lacking their compact concentric arrangement) or the appearances of 'mixed dust fibrosis' (*see* Chapter 7) may be scattered throughout the lungs, though with some partiality for their middle zones. Some confluence of these lesions which are grey, grey-white or sometimes greenish in colour may occur (McLaughlin, Rogers and Dunham, 1949); and, occasionally, there are large coalescent, fibrotic masses some of which may contain ischaemic cavities similar to those seen in the PMF of coal pneumoconiosis (Hunt, 1956) (*see* Chapter 8). Typical silicotic nodules are also sometimes seen when there has been exposure to industrial talc containing significant quantities of quartz. On the other hand, the appearances are identical to those of asbestosis: they are predominant in the lower halves of the lungs and are usually accompanied by some diffuse thickening of the pulmonary pleura. Both the nodular and diffuse patterns of fibrosis are sometimes present in the same lung.

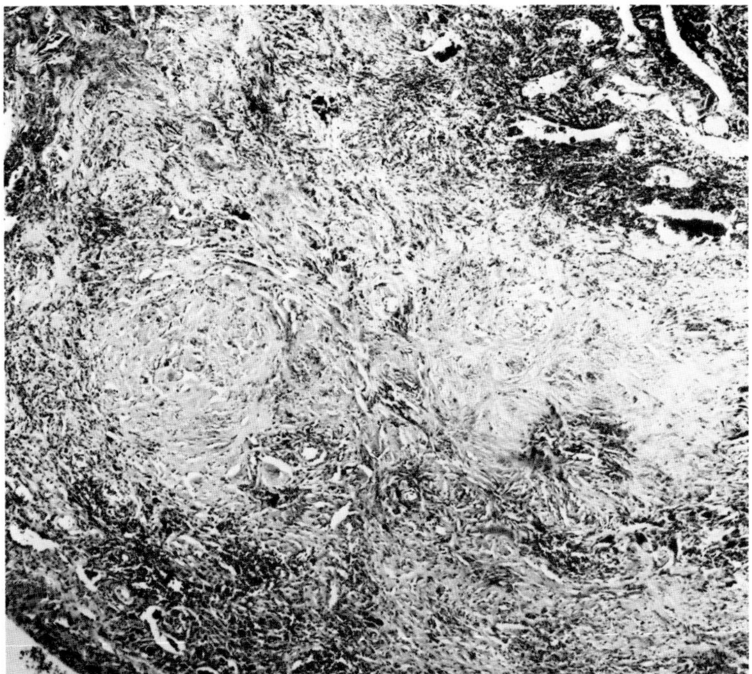

Figure 9.41 Ill-defined nodular lesions in a rubber worker exposed for many years to 'talc' dust. The fibrosis is relatively acellular and shows only a suggestion of the concentric pattern of typical silicotic nodules. (Original magnifications × 55, reproduced at × 36; H and E stain.)

Microscopic appearances

The primary reaction to talc mine dust in the human lung consists of an accumulation of macrophages around blood vessels in the vicinity of respiratory bronchioles with the formation of small, stellate lesions which contain some reticulin fibres but negligible collagen. Numerous acicular or platy particles which are strongly birefringent under crossed polaroid lenses are present in and adjacent to the lesions both within and outside macrophages (Schepers and Durkan, 1955a). Talc particles in the lungs indicate exposure to a talc-containing mineral but are not necessarily proof of talc-associated disease. If the majority of the particles are greater than 5 μm diameter the possibility of intravenous injection of talc-contaminated drugs should be considered (Abraham and Brambilla, 1979).

Three distinct types of lesion may subsequently occur:

(1) Ill-defined nodular lesions.
(2) Diffuse interstitial pulmonary fibrosis (DIPF).
(3) Foreign body granulomas.

Ill-defined nodular lesions consist of irregular, acellular collagenous tissue (*Figure 9.41*) which in places, may show incomplete whorling identical to the arrangements of immature silicotic nodules, and is associated with a relatively high quartz content in the lungs. Often the lesions have the irregular stellate form of a 'mixed dust fibrosis' and, similarly, they appear to represent a modification of the silicotic reaction by talc (*see* Chapter 7). Likewise, they vary considerably in size and may ultimately form large confluent masses. Numerous macrophages containing birefringent particles surround the lesions and these particles are readily identifiable within the lesions. Sometimes there are necrotic areas of amorphous, finely granular material which colours yellow with van Giesen's stain (Hunt, 1956). Adjacent endarteritis with intimal hyperplasia is common.

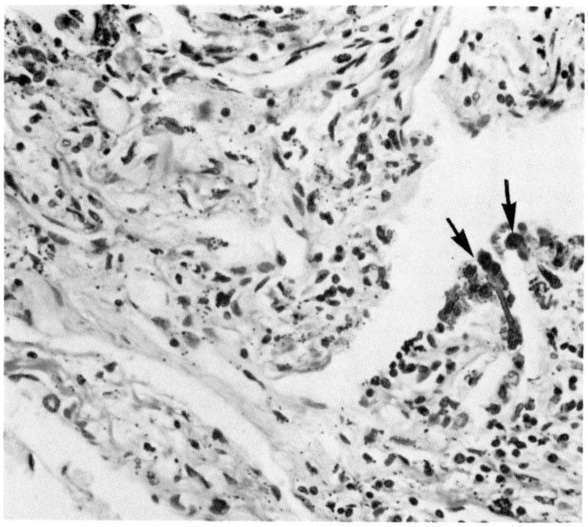

Figure 9.42 Slight DIPF with pronounced cellularity and ferruginous bodies due to tremolite or anthophyllite bodies (arrowed) in this section. Elsewhere acellular DIPF with occasional small 'honeycomb' cysts (not seen in this field). Polarized light also revealed numerous, highly birefringent, platy particles. Exposure to mixed 'talc' materials for 30 years. (Original magnification × 380, reproduced at × 285. H and E stain). (See Figure 9.48 *for radiographic appearances in this case)*

Diffuse interstitial pulmonary fibrosis (DIPF) originates around respiratory bronchioles and has the same appearances as asbestosis; many alveolar spaces are obliterated in advanced disease. But in some areas there may be pronounced infiltration of alveolar walls by macrophages containing birefringent talc particles and in others they lie free within the walls. Endarteritis may be present. 'Ferruginous bodies', which are identical with asbestos bodies (but have been misleadingly called 'talc bodies'), are readily found in and adjacent to the fibrosis and are demonstrated by the same techniques (*see* p. 240); they may contain tremolite or anthophyllite (*Figure 9.42*). The bodies are also sometimes seen in small numbers in some cases with ill-defined nodular lesions; this may imply past exposure to fibrous tremolite or to some other asbestos mineral. Schepers and Durkan (1955a) found that when the tremolite asbestos content of the lung ash from talc miners was low such bodies were sparse. (*See* Addendum 2, p. 332.)

Foreign body granulomas may also occur in variable degree in association with ill-defined nodular disease and DIPF; and, rarely, they are the only lesions (*Figure 9.43*). They consist of macrophages, epithelioid cells and foreign body giant cells all of which contain doubly refractile particles of talc; and asteroid bodies may be observed in some giant cells (Kleinfeld *et al.*, 1963). A reported case of multiple sarcoid-type granulomas in a man who cleaned factory ventilators in which 'talc' dust was deposited seems to have been one of coincidental sarcoidosis (Miller *et al.*, 1971).

Birefringent polygonal particles in and around all these lesions can be identified as platy talc crystals, and the fibrous particles as tremolite or anthophyllite by combining electron microscopy, differential thermal analysis, thermal gravimetric analysis and X-ray diffraction (Pooley and Rowlands, 1977). Many talc plates lie sideways to the line of vision and, by light microscopy, may give the impression of particles of fibrous habit. Talc crystals visible by the light microscope vary from 0.5 to 5 μm in size but many may be less than 0.5 μm and thus can only be identified by electron microscopy; however, it is improbable that 'submicron' particles occur in the lungs in the absence of larger particles.

Analysis of the lungs of talc miners and millers in New York State showed that those with the ill-defined nodular type of lesions contained considerable quantities of talc and small amounts of quartz but little tremolite or anthophyllite; whereas those with DIPF contained large quantities of fibrous tremolite and, occasionally, anthophyllite in addition to talc (Schepers and Durkan, 1955a).

The three distinctive lesions of 'talc' pneumoconiosis may occur alone or in various combinations in one individual according to the composition of the dusts to which he was exposed. But none of these lesions possesses any pathognomonic features.

Pathogenesis

Schepers and Durkan (1955a) postulated that talc modifies the reaction of the lungs to quartz. This is supported by their observation in experimental animals that the fibrogenic effect of quartz when combined with talc appears to be reduced although granulomatous lesions and fibrosis may

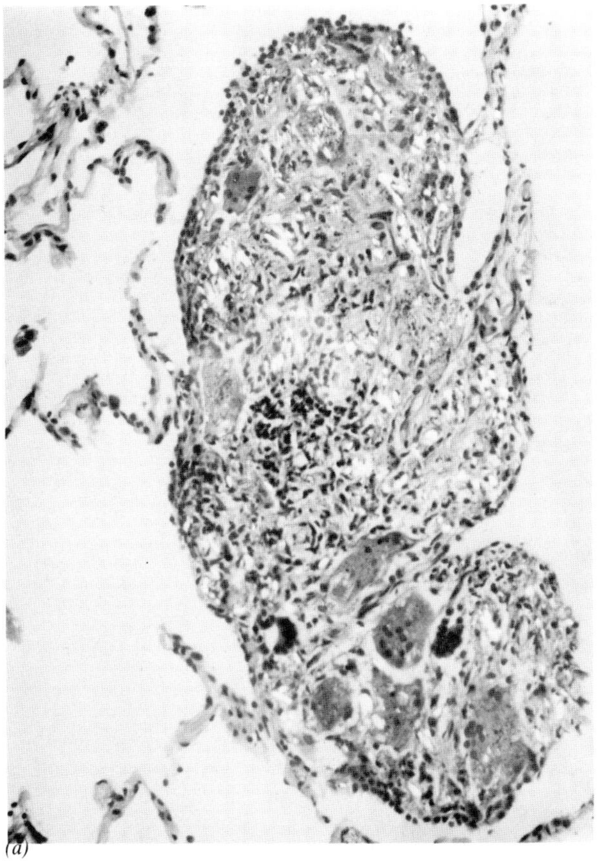
(a)

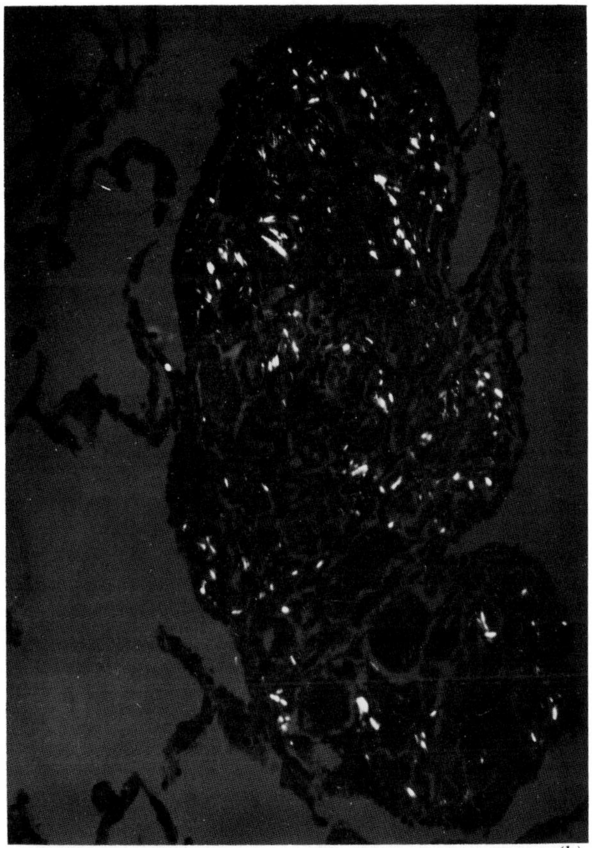
(b)

*Figure 9.43 (a) Foreign body granuloma in a worker exposed to talc dust in the rubber industry for ten years. Note the cellularity and giant cells, and the normality of the adjacent alveolar walls. No tremolite bodies found. (Biopsy. Original magnification × 240, reproduced at × 800. H and E stain). (b) Polarized light demonstrates the presence of birefringent talc plates. (c) Electron micrograph of the lesion: talc and mica-like plates (original magnification × 3000). (Courtesy of Drs S. Steel and F. D. Pooley). (*See Figure 9.47 *for radiographic appearances)*

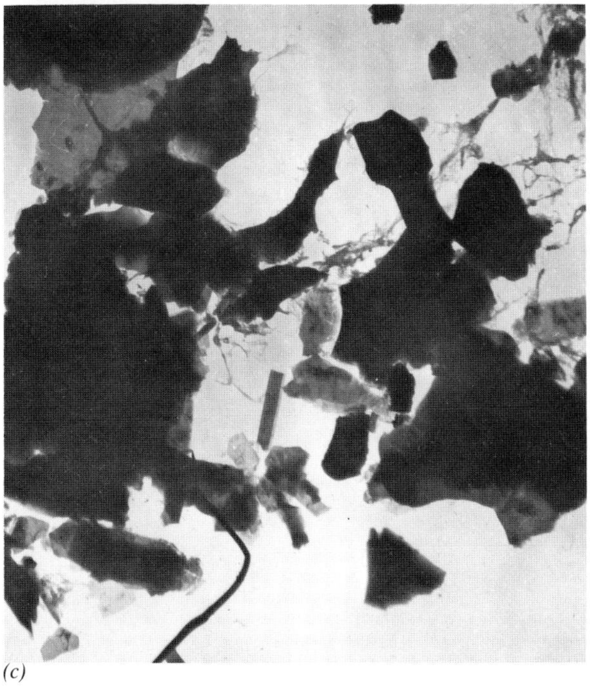
(c)

result—that is, a 'mixed dust fibrosis' (Schepers and Durkan, 1955b).

In general, among the many investigations of 'talc' which have been conducted in animals rarely has the precise nature of the mineral used been specified, its particle size indicated or the details of administered doses defined. However, two important recent studies have furnished this information precisely. Wehner *et al.* (1977) exposed hamsters to the inhalation of high grade cosmetic talc consisting of 95 per cent (w/w) platy talc and trace quantities of carbonates, chlorite and rutile but no quartz or amphiboles; and the mass mean aerodynamic diameter of the particles was 6 μm. Total doses up to nearly 2000 times those to which babies are exposed during toilet care had no effect on survival or the degree of histopathological change compared with control animals. In short, no fibrosis or increased incidence of neoplasia in the lungs was observed. Wagner *et al.* (1977) exposed rats to inhalation of high grade talc consisting of 92 per cent talc, 3 per cent chlorite, 1 per cent carbonate minerals and 0.5 to 1 per cent quartz (w/w) in doses which, at their highest level, exceeded those used by Wehner *et al.* (1977) about three-fold. A slight degree of respiratory bronchiolar fibrosis which was little more than that in the control animals was found and there was no excess of tumours. By contrast, talc calcined at 1200 °C produces intense collagen fibrosis in animals due, probably, to the presence of cristobalite (Lüchtrath and Schmidt, 1959) (*see* p. 300 and Chapter 2).

Pure talc particles 0.3 to 10 μm in size are apparently capable of penetrating the cell membranes but not the nuclear membranes of fibroblasts in culture (Henderson *et al.*, 1975). What significance this may have—if any—in human disease remains to be elucidated.

Tremolite particles 3 μm or less in size produce only small localized lesions of cellular perivascular infiltration, but fibres 20 to 50 μm in length cause a progressive DIPF in animals (Schepers and Durkan, 1955b). This, of course, is similar to the behaviour of other asbestos fibres referred to already in the section on Pathogenesis of Asbestosis. Schepers and Durkan (1955b) also demonstrated that tremolite fibres 20 to 50 μm in length provoke the formation in animal lungs of ferruginous bodies which are identical to those seen in asbestosis and some cases of 'talc' pneumoconiosis in man.

Foreign body granulomas are caused by talc itself. They have been observed in the peritoneum, fallopian tubes and ovaries contaminated by talc from surgical glove dusting powder (German 1943; Roberts, 1947), and following intraperitoneal injection in animals (Blümel, Piza and Zischka-Konorska, 1962). They may also occur—though rarely—in human lungs as a result of the inhalation of pure talc (Moskowitz, 1970) (*Figure 9.43*) and the intravenous introduction by drug addicts of dissolved talc-dusted tablets into the pulmonary circulation (Hopkins and Taylor, 1970; Smith, Graf and Silverman, 1978). Birefringent talc crystals may be seen in such lesions through crossed polarizers.

Calcified pleural plaques, which only appear to occur in 'talc' workers exposed to fibrous 'talc' and asbestine, are probably due to contaminating fibrous anthophyllite or some extraneous asbestos exposure.

To summarize

'Talc' pneumoconiosis is an enigma. Indeed, whether pneumoconiosis attributable to pure talc really occurs is uncertain. Explanations of the various types of lung disease associated with occupational exposure to the heterogenous dusts referred to as 'talc' (or French chalk) may be tabulated as follows.

(1) *Nodular silicosis or 'mixed dust fibrosis' may be due to:*
   (a) Quartz contamination of talc: for example, in talc mining and in low grade talcs used in industry.
   (b) Quartz or some other form of free silica in additional minerals used in the same industrial process (*see* p. 300).
   (c) Cristobalite in calcined talc in certain processes.

(2) *DIPF may be due to:*
   (a) Association of fibrous tremolite or anthophyllite with talc. Mainly encountered in mining and milling, and occasionally in the use of low grade industrial talcs but otherwise, rarely.
   (b) Use of an asbestos mineral in the same process for which talc is used: for example, as a filler for asphalt in some roofing felts (*see* p. 300).

(3) *Foreign body granulomas:*
   Appear to be caused by pure platy talc, but are rare. No convincing evidence that subsequent fibrosis occurs.

The finding of birefringent talc plates in the lungs does not establish a causal relationship with associated disease except, perhaps, in the case of foreign body granulomas.

Clinical features

Symptoms

There may be no symptoms for years but ultimately dyspnoea on effort, often with cough and sputum, are complained of in many cases and are more commonly associated with advancing DIPF-type disease than with the ill-defined nodular form. Dyspnoea in the latter is usually found in individuals with radiographic evidence of large confluent masses and related scar emphysema. Symptoms tend to develop after about 15 to 20 years of exposure to industrial talc dust. Occasionally, when dust concentrations have been very high, severe dyspnoea has developed within about two years with rapidly progressive 'nodular' type disease (Alvisatos, Pontikakis and Terzis, 1955).

The chief symptoms associated with foreign body granulomas alone are usually progressive dyspnoea and unproductive cough which may be of mild or severe degree.

Physical signs

There are no abnormal physical signs in the early stages nor in many cases of the later stages of predominantly 'nodular' disease. When large confluent masses are present chest expansion and breath sounds may be locally reduced.

In disease of the diffuse fibrotic type the range of abnormal physical signs is the same as that observed in asbestosis (*see* p. 256) or any other form of bilateral basal DIPF.

In the case of lone granulomatous disease abnormal signs may be absent or there may be widespread fine, late, inspiratory crepitations.

Investigations

Lung function

The 'nodular' form of the disease—as in the case of silicosis—causes little if any abnormality in its early stages, but later a restrictive defect develops with decreased compliance, ventilation–perfusion imbalance, impaired gas transfer and hypoxia on effort with oxygen desaturation. In advanced cases oxygen desaturation may be present at rest (Alvisatos, Pontikakis and Terkis, 1955). In the diffuse fibrotic form the functional abnormalities are similar to those seen in asbestosis. In general, abnormal values are appreciably greater in persons with diffuse fibrosis who have been exposed to 'tremolitic talc' than in those with 'nodular' disease (Kleinfeld *et al.*, 1964a, b), although the correlation between functional abnormalities and the radiographic appearances is poor and impairment of the same parameters of lung function which mark the earliest stages of asbestosis has been observed before radiographic evidence of this type of 'talc' pneumoconiosis is apparent (Kleinfeld *et al.*, 1965).

In foreign body granulomatous disease static lung volume and compliance may be reduced and Tl, diminished. This may only be evident after exercise or may be present at rest with significant reduction in systemic arterial oxygen (Pa_{O_2}).

Radiographic appearances

As might be anticipated from the different types of lesion associated with 'talc' minerals the appearances of 'talc' pneumoconiosis vary widely.

(1) Nodular This consists either of opacities some 3 to 5 mm in diameter identical to those of silicosis or of appearances similar to 'mixed dust fibrosis' (*see* Chapter 7). These changes sometimes favour the middle lung fields but may be distributed throughout all zones (*Figure 9.44*). There are large opacities like those of silicotic conglomerations or coal PMF which may show evidence of cavity formation (Hunt, 1956; Kipling and Bech, 1960) (*Figure 9.45*). One such case was associated with rheumatoid arthritis and the microscopical features of rheumatoid activity in the lung lesions (*Figure 9.46*).

Exceptionally, very small, widely disseminated opacities (about 2 to 3 mm in diameter) similar to the miliary lesions of sarcoidosis or tuberculosis and due to multiple foreign body granulomas may be seen (*Figure 9.47*).

(2) Diffuse interstitial pulmonary fibrosis (DIPF) The features are the same as those of asbestosis (*see* pp. 257–258) (*Figure 9.48*).

(3) Mixed Both types of appearance may occur in combination (*Figure 9.49*). This is probably uncommon and other causes of diffuse fibrosis should be considered before

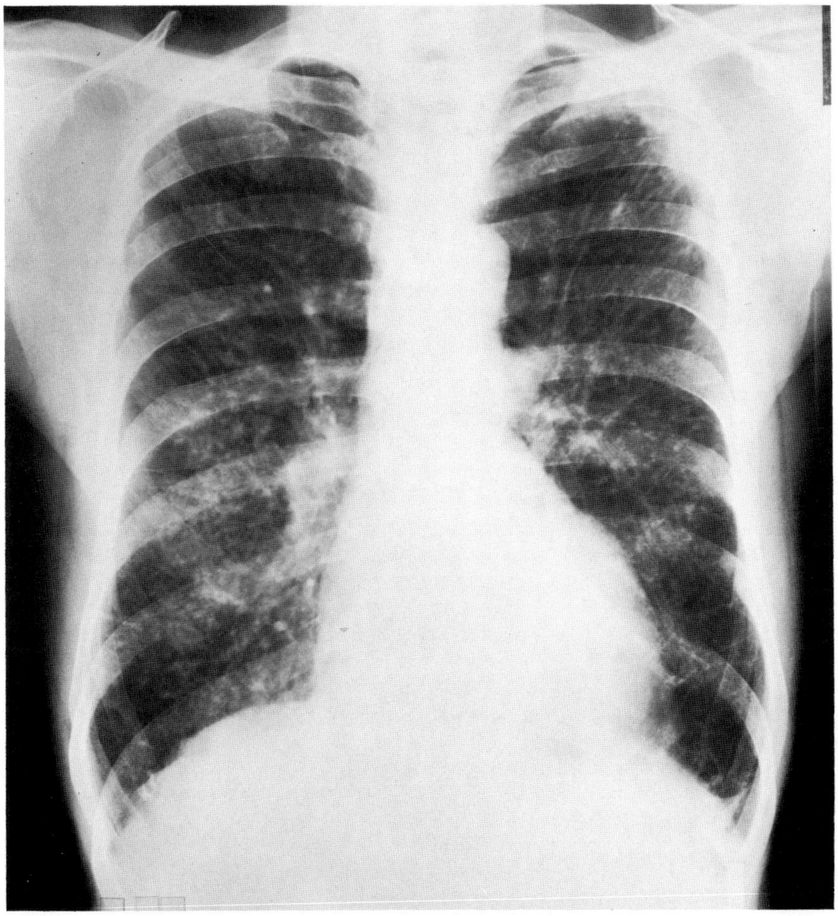

Figure 9.44 Discrete silicotic type opacities (category 'q') in a machine operator and cutter in the roof felting industry. Constant use of 'French chalk'. Microscopy, *nodules 'mixed dust fibrosis' (similar to* Figure 9.41*) and small areas of DIPF with occasional whole and fragmented tremolite bodies*

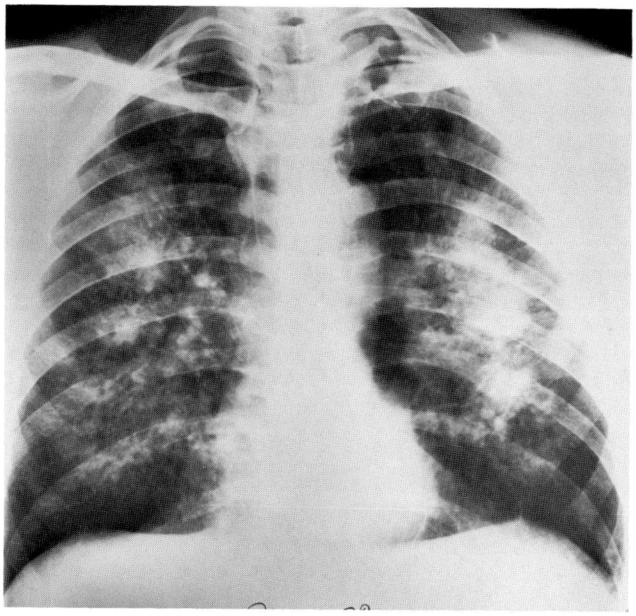

Figure 9.45 Bilateral conglomerate lesions in an operator of a rubber extruding machine for 18 years before and during the Second World War. No evidence of DIPF

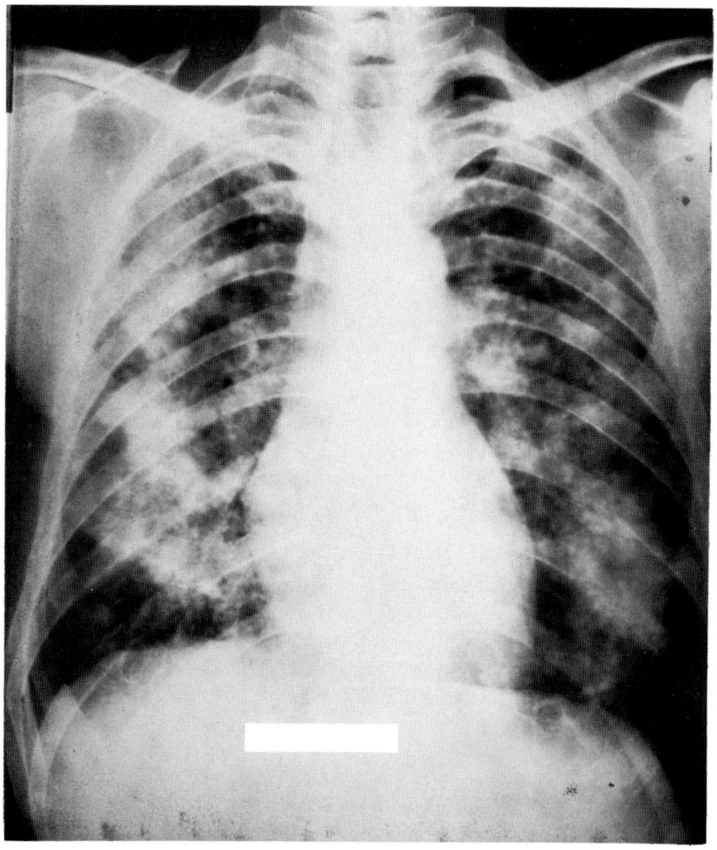

Figure 9.46(a) 1950

Figure 9.46(b) 1955

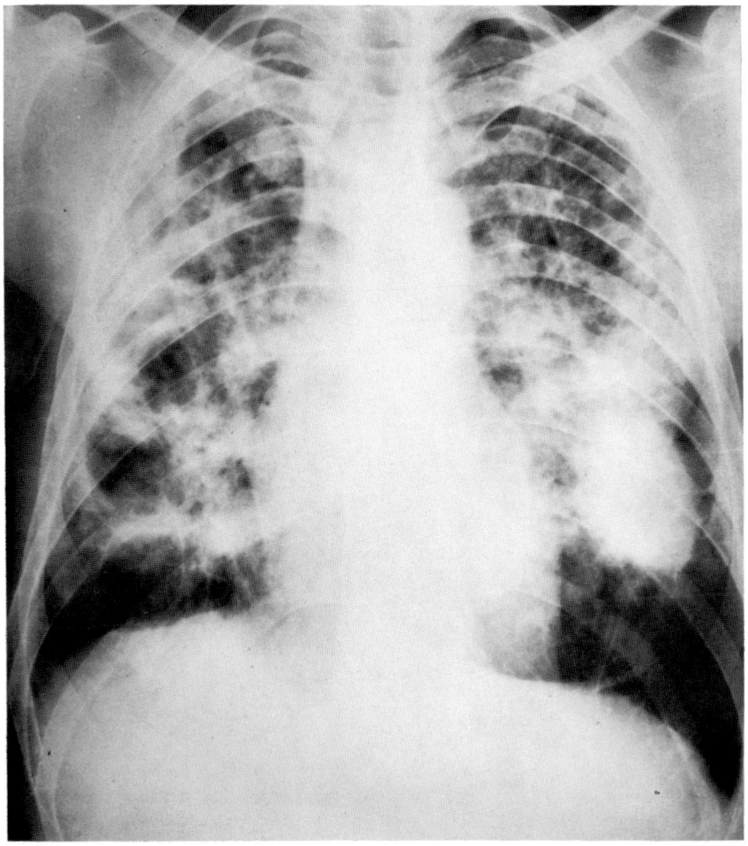

Figure 9.46 *Massive rheumatoid 'talc' pneumoconiosis in a caster of lead battery accumulator plates for 22 years until 1954. 'French chalk' from Canada, China and Egypt used liberally as a parting powder. Polyarthropathy developed in 1954. (a) 1950, appearances similar to conglomerate silicosis. No evidence of DIPF. (b) 1955, cavities now evident in masses in the right lung. The left upper zone lesion has disappeared but a faint cavity outline remains; the lower zone opacity has increased in size.* M. tuberculosis *never isolated. (c) Segments of two rheumatoid nodules set in randomly arranged cellular fibrosis are seen on both sides of the section. Note palisading of fibroblasts in the peripheral zones and the partly necrotic appearance of the nodules, but the absence of pigmented rings. Many lesions elsewhere consisted of hyalinized and necrotic collagen. No evidence of tuberculosis and no tremolite bodies found. Numerous talc plates revealed by polarized light. (Original magnification × 160. H and E stain). (Courtesy of Dr A. C. Hunt)*

Figure 9.46(c)

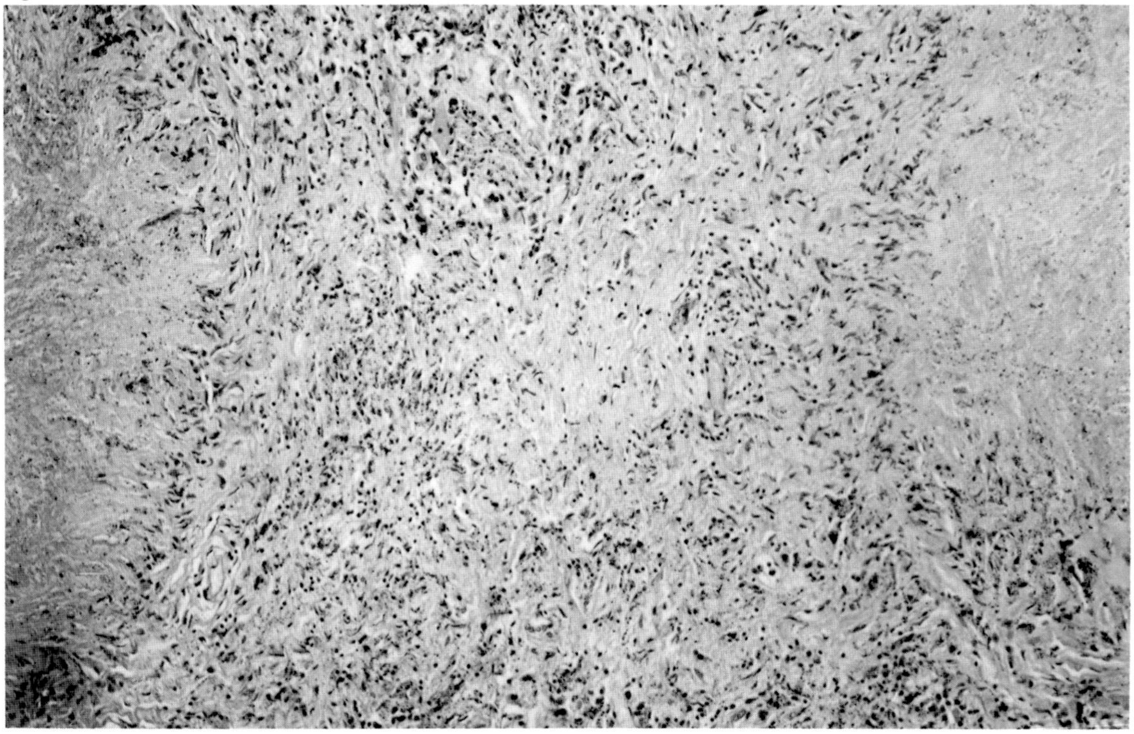

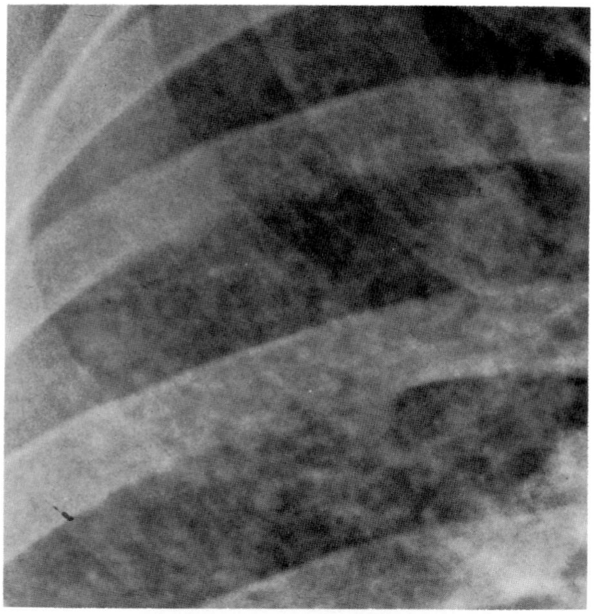

*Figure 9.47 Faint miliary opacities due to multiple foreign body granulomas in a rubber worker exposed to talc powder (*see Figure 9.43*). Similar appearances present throughout both lung fields. Unchanged during five years observation. No clinical stigmata of sarcoidosis. Kveim test negative. Serum calcium and proteins normal. Tuberculin test positive; cultures for* M. tuberculosis *negative. No evidence of drug addiction*

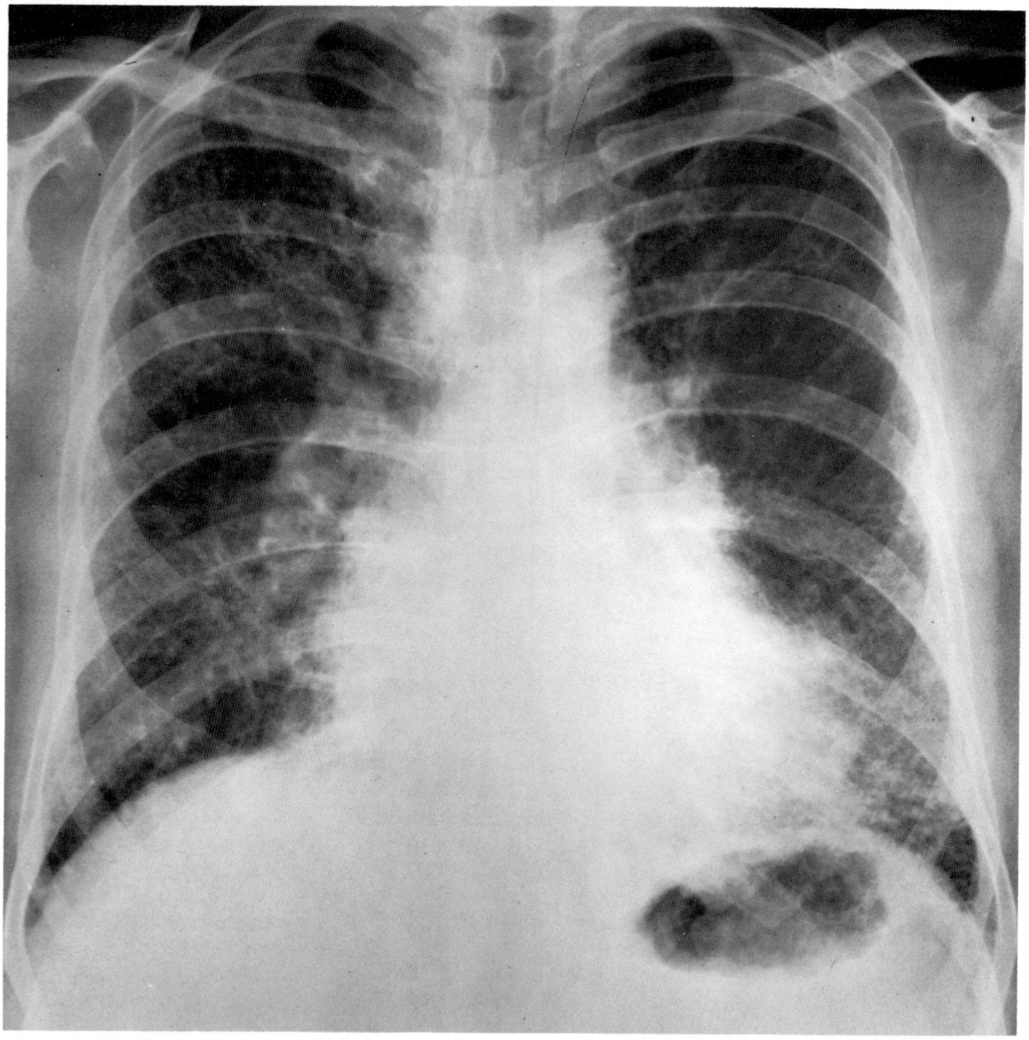

*Figure 9.48 Widespread DIPF in a man who weighed, mixed and bagged high grade talc powders from many sources for 30 years. Post mortem microscopy indicated the presence of tremolite (*see Figure 9.42*). No arthropathy or connective tissue disease. RF negative*

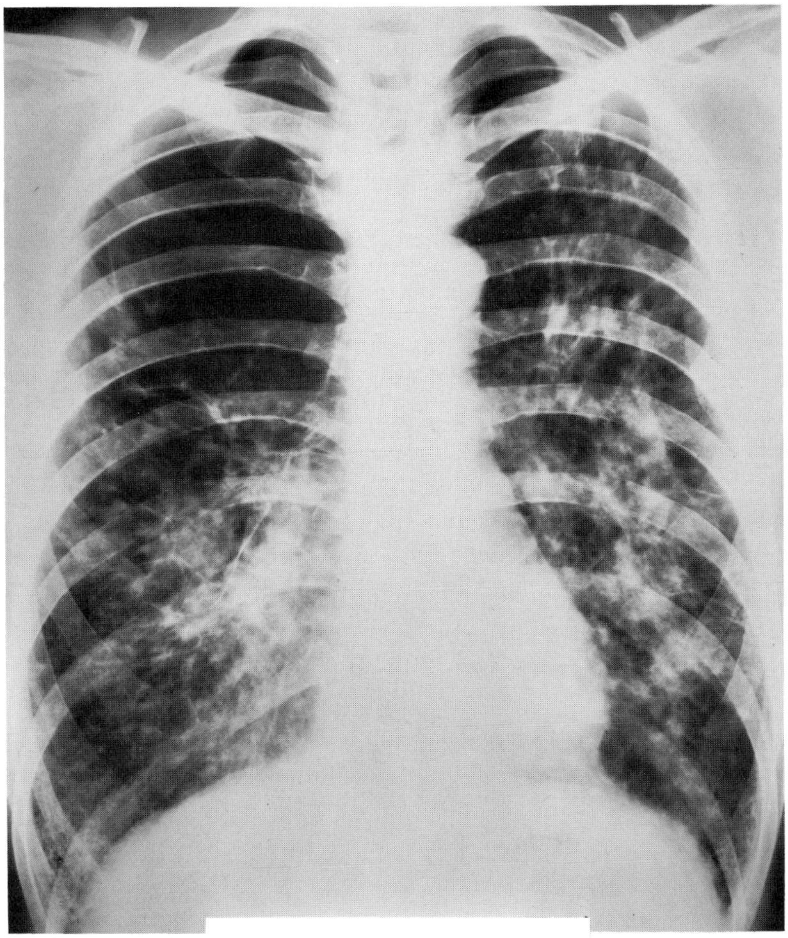

Figure 9.49 'Talc' pneumoconiosis with bilateral 'nodular' opacities (category 2rB) and appearances of DIPF in both lower zones and costophrenic angles. Large bullae in both upper zones. Persistent inspiratory crepitations present in the lower lobe, lingular and middle lobe areas. No arthropathy; RF negative. Rubber moulder from 1937 to 1939; extruding machine operator from 1939 to 1965. During the Second World War low grade Canadian and American 'tremolite talc' used, but before and after only French Lugansac talc was employed

attributing it to fibrous tremolite or anthophyllite—in particular, exposure to other asbestos minerals.

(4) Pleural There may be evidence of diffuse, bilateral pleural thickening with obliteration of the costophrenic angles. Bilateral calcified plaques are occasionally associated with exposure to talc containing fibrous tremolite or anthophyllite, or to some other unrelated asbestos mineral (Kleinfeld *et al.*, 1963; Yazicioglu *et al.*, 1980).

Diagnosis

This rests upon the past occupational history and a known exposure to 'talc', and on the appearances of the chest radiograph. However, it is often impossible to obtain precise details of the type (or types) of 'talc' used in an industry 20 or more years ago, although this is sometimes available from the manufacturer's or supplier's records. It should be borne in mind that a worker may speak of having handled 'french chalk' (talc) when in fact the material may have been powdered slate or china clay by-product, and that some industries which employed talc may also have used asbestos or quartz-containing minerals (as, for example, in roofing felt manufacture). It is also to be remembered that women have sometimes been exposed to industrial grade talc in various industries (chiefly rubber) in the past.

The diagnosis can be made in the majority of cases without lung biopsy but, if this proves necessary, sufficient tissue should be taken (preferably by thoracotomy) not only to enable adequate demonstration of the pathology but for positive mineral identification. The differential diagnosis lies chiefly between quiescent tuberculosis, silicosis or some unrelated type of DIPF and, in the case of the granulomatous type of disease, sarcoidosis.

After death, and in particular in cases encountered for the first time, the diagnosis is made virtually certain by the combination of an accurate history of industrial exposure, the presence of one or more of the pathological entities described, of numerous highly birefringent platy and acicular particles and, in some cases, of ferruginous bodies especially in those with DIPF. If the occupational history is uninformative positive identification of the minerals may be necessary. However, it should be recalled that the identification of talc proper serves only as a marker of occupational exposure.

Prognosis

As a rule, 'talc' pneumoconiosis tends to progress very slowly even after exposure to the dust has ceased and although a variable degree of respiratory disability may occur life expectancy appears rarely to be significantly shortened. But in those cases where there is massive confluent fibrosis or extensive DIPF pulmonary heart disease may ultimately cause death in congestive heart failure. However, as indicated in the Epidemiology section this is a rare event, though death may result from respiratory failure especially when there is concurrent lung disease.

Occasionally, when there has been exposure to very high concentrations of 'talc' dust progression to advanced massive fibrosis with severe respiratory disability occurs within a few years due, almost certainly, to a high quartz content (Alivisatos, Pontikakis and Terzis, 1955).

Complications

In general, there is no evidence that 'talc' pneumoconiosis predisposes to the development of tuberculosis although it may when there has been exposure to industrial 'talc' with a high quartz content. Colonization by 'opportunist' mycobacteria or aspergilli may occur in advanced disease.

Rheumatoid 'talc' pneumoconiosis does not seem to have been described but Hunt's (1956) case was an example as later re-examination of the microsections confirmed (*Figure 9.46c*).

Bronchial carcinoma is not associated with exposure to 'non-fibrous talc' but excess mortality from this tumour (possibly associated with DIPF) 20 or more years after commencement of employment has been reported in miners and millers in the Gouveneur mining area in New York State (Brown, Dement and Wagoner, 1979). This was not evident in earlier investigations (Van Ordstrand, 1970; Kleinfeld, Messite and Zaki, 1974) (*see* p. 301). Malignant mesothelioma does not seem to have been described among workers in asbestiform talc though it is apparently related to fibrous tremolite in certain country districts of Turkey (*see* p. 286). Continued study of this problem is obviously needed. It is interesting that follow-up of 136 patients who had undergone talc pleurodesis 14 to 40 years earlier revealed no increased incidence of cancer and no pleural mesothelioma (Research Committee of BTA and MRCPU, 1979).

An association between 'talc' pneumoconiosis and coronary artery disease in talc miners in the USA has been suggested (Nash and Nash, 1978) but requires epidemiological investigation. At present there is no evidence of a causal relationship.

Although talc crystals have been found in ovarian carcinomas there is nothing to indicate that they were the cause of the tumour (Henderson *et al.*, 1971; Henderson, Hamilton and Griffiths, 1979). But investigation of the problem continues.

Treatment

In general, no treatment is effective apart from that required for concurrent lung disease or, in the case of advanced pneumoconiosis, for congestive heart failure or respiratory failure. But when the pneumoconiosis consists of foreign body granulomas a substantial, if not complete, regression appears to be possible with large daily doses (40 to 60 mg) of prednisolone (Moskowitz, 1970; Smith, Graf and Silverman, 1978). Whether or not such improvement is permanent remains to be established, but it indicates that lung biopsy is justifiable in individuals whose chest radiographs suggest the granulomatous type of disease.

Prevention

Dust suppression measures have been applied to the mining, crushing and milling of 'talc' for some years past. Finely milled talc has a particle size which may range from 0.5 to 25 μm. Exhaust ventilation and enclosure of dusty processes have been introduced into most large industries but some small factories or work places may still be dusty. In circumstances where efficient dust suppression cannot be applied respirators are required. Good housekeeping is essential to prevent dust accumulation, and monitoring of airborne dust in the worker's breathing zone is desirable.

A detailed record of the type and source of 'talc' and of other relevant non-talc minerals used in an industrial should be kept.

Threshold Limit Values recommended by the American Conference of Governmental Industrial Hygienists (1979) take into account the different biological effects of the non-fibrous and fibrous forms of 'talc': that is, talc proper, tremolite asbestos and anthophyllite.

PNEUMOCONIOSIS ASSOCIATED WITH OTHER SILICATES

KAOLIN (CHINA CLAY)

Description of disease

Mainly nodular or massive fibrosis of the lungs associated with past exposure to kaolin dust which is apparently free of accessory quartz or contains small amounts.

Nature and origin of kaolin

The kaolin, or china clay, group of clay minerals consists predominantly of *kaolinite* which is a hydrous aluminium silicate (approximately composition $Al_2O_3.2SiO_2.2H_2O$) with a platy pseudohexagonal, non-fibrous morphology under the electron microscope (Beutelspacher and van der Marel, 1968).

Kaolinite is formed by the hydrothermal alteration of aluminosilicates such as feldspars in granites (as in Cornish china clay), by residual weathering of granites and by erosion of kaolinized granite and its subsequent deposition (as in the large sedimentary kaolin deposits in some of the eastern states of the USA). Hence, these clays contain a wide variety of mineral impurities in their natural state.

Cornish china clay consists of 10 to 40 per cent kaolinite, the residue being chiefly quartz, mica and feldspar; Georgia kaolin contains 85 to 95 per cent kaolinite, the remainder being largely quartz and a variety of other silicates; and North Carolina kaolin is 10 to 40 per cent kaolinite with quartz, muscovite and altered feldspars (Patterson and Murray, 1975).

Although commercial kaolins contain very little quartz the raw material from which they are produced (which is used for fillers and dusting powders in various industries) may contain appreciable amounts. For example, in Cornwall, 3.7 tonnes of coarse, mainly quartz, sand are produced for each tonne of china clay (Highley, 1980).

Cornish kaolin is obtained by means of directing a high pressure jet of water onto the walls of the open pit and subjecting it to differential sedimentation in water so that impurities such as grit, sand and mica are removed while the kaolin remains suspended. The water is largely removed either by the use of filter presses or by drawing off, and the plastic residue transferred to drying kilns. Moisture content is thus reduced to about 10 per cent and the clay residue is either shovelled or conveyed on a moving belt to storage hoppers. Spray drying of high-grade clays is increasingly being used. It is then either bagged mechanically (but, until recent years, this was done by hand shovel) or bulk-loaded into trucks for transportation. Some quartz may remain in the lower grade clays.

In the USA the clay is obtained in moist lumps by open-cast mining and then piped as a slurry through degritting and segregating units. Beneficiation is done by dry or wet methods. Lower quality kaolin is produced by the dry method which includes air flotation to remove grit. The wet method, which produces grades of kaolin with uniform properties, has been more extensively and highly developed in recent years. Here the clay is passed as a slurry through various refining processes to apron, drum or rotary driers and then, in the dried state, to pulverizers. To produce material with a high degree of whiteness and brightness and better abrasive powers for certain industrial uses it is calcined at about 1050 °C thus converting kaolinite largely into mullite (an aluminium silicate) and cristobalite (*see* Chapter 2 and 7).

Uses of kaolin

Kaolin has many industrial applications. It is used as a filler to give body to paper pulp, for coating paper to produce a smooth surface, for the manufacture of china (or white-ware) in which the quartz content must be less than 5 per cent, and for stoneware. Residual kaolin is used for these purposes in the UK, and secondary kaolin of high purity in the USA. Kaolin also has important uses as a filler and extending agent in rubber, paints, inks, plastics and insecticides; in the manufacture of refractory bricks, crucibles, saggars and glass; and a refractory grog is produced by calcining it at high temperatures. It is employed as a mild abrasive in soaps and toothpastes and as a stiffener of textiles. Kaolin of high purity and small particle size is used for medicinal and cosmetic purposes.

Sources of exposure

Exposure has occurred mainly in the china-clay industry. After the clay left the driers all parts of the process some years ago were dusty; and, although ventilation and enclosure methods now do much to reduce the dust, brushing clay spilt from conveyors, cleaning driers, bagging and bulk loading may still be dusty activities (Sheers, 1964).

Other sources of significant exposure have been, and may still be, found in the manufacture of paper, rubber and plastics. In the pottery and refractory industries exposure may also occur to dusts of other minerals—such as flint, feldspar, graphite and quartzite sand.

It is of interest that silicosis due to quartz and cristobalite associated with kaolin has been reported in the Missouri firebrick industry. The cristobalite probably originated from pulverization for re-use of previously fired bricks (Lesser, Zia and Kilburn, 1978).

Prevalence

In a radiographic survey of 553 Cornish kaolin-processing workers evidence of pneumoconiosis was found in 9 per cent (Sheers, 1964) and among 1130 similar workers in Georgia, in 3.7 per cent (Edenfield, 1960). Of 914 processing workers in Ayyat, United Arab Republic, six had pneumoconiosis—two with confluent masses (Warraki and Herant, 1963).

Duration of exposure to the dust was apparently significant in the Cornish workers in that 23 per cent of those exposed to high dust concentrations in milling, bagging and loading for more than 15 years had pneumoconiosis by contrast with 6 per cent of men similarly exposed for five to 15 years. Among all 553 cases there were 12 (2.2 per cent) with confluent masses and 30 (5.4 per cent) with ILO Category 2 or 3 opacities (Sheers, 1964).

Hence, only a small number of similarly exposed workers developed radiographic evidence of pneumoconiosis and then only after a prolonged period.

Pathology

Macroscopic appearances

The pulmonary pleura of lungs which contain massive lesions is usually thickened.

Lesions which simulate immature silicotic nodules have been found in some cases (Lynch and McIver, 1954; Hale *et al.*, 1956), but as a rule there are dust macules like those of coal pneumoconiosis, although of a greyish hue.

Massive confluent lesions, which favour the upper parts of lungs, are well circumscribed, grey to blue-grey in colour, and although firm to the touch, are not as hard as conglomerate silicotic masses.

Microscopic appearances

Numerous dust-laden macrophages and extracellular dust particles are present around bronchiolar arteries and fill adjacent alveolar spaces. Proliferation of reticulin fibres support both cells and dust particles.

Nodules and massive confluent lesions consist of randomly distributed collagenous fibres, some of which are hyalinized, and large quantities of dust in similar fashion to the PMF of coal and carbon pneumoconiosis; they are infiltrated and surrounded by innumerable dust-laden macrophages. Evidence of tuberculosis does not seem to have been found (Hale *et al.*, 1956; Edenfield, 1960), but obliterative endarteritis is prominent in the vicinity of the lesions and is responsible for the necrosis which is sometimes observed in them.

Lynch and McIver (1954) noted 'conspicuous fibrosis of alveolar walls' in one of their cases a photomicrograph of which is consistent with DIPF. A slight degree of DIPF with much cellular infiltration including dust-containing macrophages has also been observed in a few cases of Cornish china clay workers both in the presence and absence of nodular or massive fibrotic lesions (Hinson, 1972; Wagner, 1972b) (*Figure 9.50*). However, it remains to be proved that this is, in fact, caused by the kaolin dust.

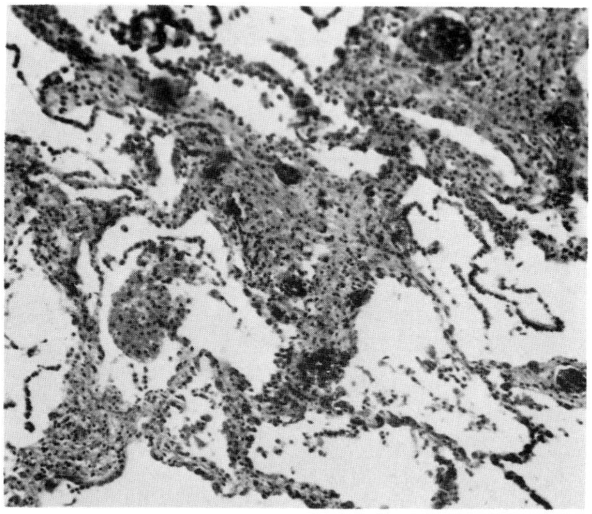

Figure 9.50 Section of lung from a china clay worker showing nodular lesions consisting of many macrophages and other cells and some collagenous fibrosis. There is limited extension of fibrosis into some alveolar walls. (Original magnification ×40. H and E stain). (Courtesy of Dr J. C. Wagner)

Analysis of lung-dust in a Cornish case revealed a large amount of kaolin and about 1 per cent of quartz; and in a case from Georgia with confluent masses the lungs contained some 98 per cent kaolin and no trace of quartz. The size of kaolin particles in the Cornish case ranged from 1.0 to 2.0 μm and in the case from Georgia, from 0.5 to 1 μm (Hale *et al.*, 1956).

Kaolinite is weakly birefringent.

Pathogenesis

The question is whether kaolin is wholly or partly responsible for these lesions or whether other causative factors are involved.

Although it has been claimed that some quartz always accompanies particles of kaolin (Policard and Collet, 1954) only trace amounts, as just noted, have been reported in lungs containing large quantities of kaolin; but there appear to be very few reports of sensitive lung analysis. This is analogous to the situation in carbon and coal pneumoconiosis. The high concentrations of dust experienced by some workers and the predominantly small size and low density of kaolin particles favours the deposition of dust in the lungs. Incidentally, it should be remembered that some cristobalite and also β-quartz is formed when kaolinite is heated to temperatures in excess of 950 °C (Mányai *et al.*, 1970) (*see* p. 311).

Tuberculous infection has been suggested as the factor which, in combination with kaolin dust, determines the development of these lesions (Edenfield, 1960). And, although this has not been evident in human disease, fibrotic lesions have been produced in the lungs of experimental animals by a combination of kaolin and chromogenic opportunist mycobacteria (Byers and King, 1959) or *M. tuberculosis* (var. *muris*) (Byers, King and Harrison, 1960).

Most experimental observations have shown that kaolinite alone does not cause collagenous fibrosis in the lungs of rats or guinea pigs (Kettle, 1934; King, Harrison and Nagelschmidt, 1948; Attygalle *et al.*, 1954; Schmidt and Lüchtrath, 1958; Goldstein and Rendall, 1970), although a mild degree was reported in rats by Martin, Daniel and Le Bouffant (1977). But it does provoke a diffuse accumulation of cells—including giant cells—in the alveolar walls and spaces; and there is some aggregation of cells with slight proliferation of supporting reticulin fibres, but no nodulation. By contrast, combinations of kaolinite and quartz give rise to pronounced collagen fibrosis (Schmidt and Lüchtrath, 1958).

Kaolin particles actively adsorb antigens and are known to be a good adjuvant to immune reactions. Thus, it has been proposed that antigen attached to retained dust particles might localize an antigen–antibody reaction (Vigliani and Pernis, 1958). There is, however, no evidence that this occurs in man, although analysis of the protein composition of the hyaline tissue of massive fibrosis in a Cornish china clay worker showed it to be rich in globulins (73 per cent) and relatively low in collagen content (27 per cent) (Vigliani and Pernis, 1958).

After phagocytosis by human and guinea-pig alveolar macrophages *in vitro* kaolinite particles are apparently capable of causing the release of lysosomal and cytoplasmic marker enzymes (Davis, Mortara and Green, 1975) but are only significantly cytotoxic when not coated with serum protein as they are *in vivo* (Low, 1978).

To summarize

The pathogenesis of kaolin pneumoconiosis is far from clear. It may be due—if kaolinite alone is responsible—to the effect of a large dust load in the lungs as is believed to be the case in pure carbon pneumoconiosis (*see* Chapter 8), but it is likely that quartz, tuberculous infection, or occasionally cristobalite play a significant role (at least in some cases); and immunological factors may be involved though this remains speculative. The cytotoxic and fibrogenic potential of kaolinite alone, however, appears to be extremely low.

Clinical features

Symptoms

There are no symptoms associated with discrete lesions but breathlessness on effort, cough and sputum may be present when there are confluent masses, and in some of these cases disability is severe (Edenfield, 1960). There is no conclusive evidence that disability was caused by pneumoconiosis attributed to kaolin in the English cases reported by Sheers (1964).

Physical signs

The same conditions apply as in the case of coal and carbon pneumoconiosis (*see* Chapter 8).

Investigations

Lung function

No comprehensive studies of kaolin workers have been reported; but in the majority of cases without confluent massing, normal values are to be expected unless coincidental lung disease is present. In the case of confluent masses the situation is the same as that encountered with the similar lesions of coal pneumoconiosis.

Radiographic appearances

These are similar to the range of abnormal opacities seen in coal pneumoconiosis. Some cases with confluent massing have signs of bullous emphysema (Hale *et al.*, 1956). Signs consistent with DIPF do not seem to have been recorded.

Prognosis

In the absence of masses, the prognosis for health and life-span appears to be normal but, when these are present, slowly increasing respiratory disability occurs; pulmonary heart disease may develop and ultimately cause death.

Treatment

No treatment, other than for concurrent lung disease, is effective.

Prevention

In the kaolin industry, wet methods, exhaust ventilation, enclosure of some sections, vacuum cleaning of the factory floor and other surfaces where dust accumulates have been introduced in the UK and similar measures have been applied in the USA. Control of dust in the bagging areas, however, is difficult.

BALL CLAYS AND STONEWARE CLAYS

Ball clays consist essentially of kaolinite and, like china clay, they originated by natural decomposition of feldspathic rocks but were subsequently transported from their site of origin by rivers. During this journey the ratio of quartz to kaolin increased on account of loss of clay so that a larger quantity of quartz is present than in primary china clay.

These clays are mined by opencast and underground methods in Dorset and Devon in the UK, and in Tennessee and Kentucky in the USA. The 'free silica' content of Devon and Dorset ball clays has been reported to range from 5 to 30 per cent (Patterson and Murray, 1975; Thomas, 1952). Their main use is for china or whiteware, sanitary pottery ware and electrical porcelain, refractory products and porcelain enamel slips.

Pneumoconiosis has occurred among workers milling and preparing these clays (Thomas, 1952) and because of their fairly high quartz content it is of silicotic type although poorly formed immature silicotic nodules may be present. The clinical features and radiographic appearances are similar to those of silicosis.

FULLER'S EARTH

Very few cases of pneumoconiosis supposedly caused by these clays have been reported and most of these were incompletely studied.

The geological identities of 'fulling' clays and important differences in their terminology are referred to in Chapter 2 (p. 35). 'Fuller's earth' may refer to fine-grained *calcium montmorillonite* clays or *bentonite* (*see* next section), and to *attapulgite* (palygorskite) clays which are mineralogically unrelated to the montmorillonites but possess similar adsorptive properties.

Large deposite of calcium montmorillonite occur in the UK at Redhill, Surrey, Woburn in Bedfordshire and near Bath, Somerset (production has increased steadily since 1948); and in the USA, in Arkansas, Mississippi and Illinois. In Georgia and Florida deposits of attapulgite are extensively worked.

Fuller's earth is mined by open-cast (tractor-scrapers and dragline excavators) and underground mining methods. It is dried in rotary driers and graded into a granular or fine powder by air flotation or elutriation. Until recent times the vicinity of driers, mills and bagging areas was very dusty.

The quartz content of Redhill fuller's earth is extremely low, except in intercalated sand layers, and is about 0.8 per cent of the milled product with only a trace amount in elutriated fractions which have a particle size of less than 5 μm (Bramwell, Leech and Dunstall, 1940). By contrast, quartz is more abundant in the Illinois montmorillonite deposits (Grim, 1933) and, although it may be present in mill dust it is largely removed by the subsequent air flotation processes. However, appreciable amounts of quartz—up to about 20 per cent—may be found in some deposits.

The word 'fuller' derives from the verb 'to full' which means the cleaning and thickening of cloth or wool. The highly adsorbent property of fuller's earth enables it to remove grease and oily material with great efficiency. It has a wide variety of uses: to clarify mineral, vegetable and animal oils; in refining mineral oils; as a carrier for herbicides and insecticides; as an adsorbent of alkaloids and vitamins; as a binder in foundry sands; as a filtering agent; as a stabilizing agent in emulsion paints; and as a filler in cosmetics, mud packs, toilet and baby powders.

Only three post-mortem studies appear to have been recorded and these were upon men who had been exposed to Nutfield fuller's earth. The fundamental lesions are round, firm—but not hard—black 'nodules' varying from 2 to 7.5 mm diameter and more in the upper than the lower parts of the lungs (Campbell and Gloyne, 1942; Tonning,

1949; Sakula, 1961); in one case they tended to run into small confluent masses in the upper lobes. Hilar lymph nodes are black.

The lesions are situated mainly around bronchiolo-vascular bundles and consist of aggregations of macrophages containing brownish particles some of which are extracellular; they are enmeshed by a network of reticulin fibres. Foreign body giant cells are absent. There is, therefore, a close resemblance to the lesions of kaolin pneumoconiosis and the non-collagen macules of coal pneumoconiosis. Reticulin proliferation but little collagenous fibrosis is present in the nodules and some extension into contiguous alveolar walls as been described (Tonning, 1949). Numerous birefringent particles may be seen in the nodules (Sakula, 1961) and are probably montmorillonite which is moderately birefringent. X-ray and electron diffraction studies in Sakula's (1961) case showed the patterns of montmorillonite but no evidence of quartz.

In a radiological survey of 49 fuller's earth workers in Illinois there were two (apparently occupied mainly in milling and bagging) whose films showed large confluent shadows indistinguishable from those which occur in coal miners and some cases of silicosis. No post-mortem examinations were done (McNally and Trostler, 1941). Discrete opacities were also observed in a small group of fuller's earth workers in Germany but various proportions of quartzose sand had been added to the clay in the past and there was also a significant content of naturally occurring quartz (Gärtner, 1955).

It is possible that montmorillonite may cause pneumoconiosis in some cases but quartz was probably the decisive factor in the Illionois and German cases. Tuberculous infection has not been observed. The problem of pathogenicity remains unsolved as post-mortem studies have been so few, and recorded animal experiments have been inconclusive and not related to the lungs (McNally and Trostler, 1941; Campbell and Gloyne, 1942). If fuller's earth (calcium montmorillonite) does possess fibrogenic potential it would seem to be of very low order.

In general, this pneumoconiosis, which is evidently rare, appears to occur only after long exposure to high concentrations of 'fuller's earth' dust; it is represented by small, discrete low-density opacities (which occasionally show some tendency to confluence) mainly in the upper halves of the lungs. It runs a benign course, and does not shorten life expectancy. Respiratory disability without radiographic evidence of pneumoconiosis has been reported in some fuller's earth workers and was apparently due to non-specific chronic airways obstruction.

Exposure to fuller's earth in industrial processes and from cosmetic preparations is most probably harmless.

BENTONITE

Bentonite consists of fine-grained clays containing not less than 85 per cent montmorrillonite. The name originates from the occurrence of such clays at Fort Benton in Wyoming in the USA. It is sodium montmorillonite with high swelling properties which has a greater capacity for water adsorption and cation exchange than other plastic clays. Similar clays are found in Italy, Greece, Spain and elsewhere.

The bentonite clays were deposited as airborne volcanic ash and later subjected to alteration by sea and ground water. All bentonites contain mineral impurities of varying type and quantity which include kaolinite, cristobalite and other forms of free silica. The Wyoming clay is associated with sandstone and siliceous shale and is reported to have a 'free silica' content varying from less than 1 per cent to about 24 per cent (Phibbs, Sundin and Mitchell, 1971).

Mining is carried out by the open-cast method, which is not a source of dust hazard, and the clay is then crushed and milled. Crushing and milling is done indoors and is a very dusty process. After crushing the clay is dried in oil-fired cylindrical driers. The 'free silica' in airborne and settled mill-dust has been found to consist of 'appreciable amounts of cristobalite' (Phibbs, Sundin and Mitchell, 1971) which was almost certainly formed by high-temperature conversion of quartz during the volcanic period and not by the heat of the driers which does not exceed about 800 °C. Bentonite from Wyoming (the world's largest producer) is imported into the UK in the crude form and milled and processed here.

The chief uses of bentonite are in oil-well drilling muds and oil refining, as a bonding material for foundry sands, in various adsorbents, in insecticides and fungicides, in ceramics and as a fire retardant. And also as a filtering agent (especially in clarifying wine), cosmetics and animal feeds, as a slurry to make tunnel and dam foundations impermeable to water, as a suspension agent for drilling fresh water muds and as a lubricant in sinking piles and caissons.

Bentonite itself is not fibrogenic in the lungs of experimental animals but causes local accumulations of large cells with foamy cytoplasm which stains strongly positive with periodic acid Schiff, and a mild proliferation of reticulin. When mixed with quartz, however, collagen fibrosis occurs but is not as severe as that produced by quartz alone (Timar, Kendrey and Juhasz, 1966).

Pneumoconiosis reported in bentonite millers developed fairly rapidly, was disabling and, in some cases, fatal (Phibbs, Sundin and Mitchell, 1971). It is undoubtedly due to the free silica content—chiefly cristobalite—of the clay. In short, it is silicosis. However, pneumoconiosis does not seem to have been reported in relation to other types of exposure to bentonite but vigilance would seem to be advisable in some of its uses.

SEPIOLITE AND MEERSCHAUM

These are two varieties of an amphibole hydrous magnesium silicate with the same formula which are related to attapulgite. Sepiolite has an earthy, clay-like form and meerschaum ('sea foam'), a compact nodular form. Both consist of microscopic lath-like fibres without associated free silica. The fibres of sepiolite are elongated and axially parallel whereas those of meerschaum are much shorter (Beutelspacher and van der Marel, 1968).

Sepiolite is used for many of the same purposes as bentonite but also as a suspending agent for cosmetics and paints, as a colour holder in copying papers and for toughening epoxy resins. Meerschaum has a limited use in the manufacture of decorative pipes, cigar and cigarette holders and ornamental objects.

Neither form of this mineral appears to be associated with the development of a pneumoconiosis. However, it has been suggested that sepiolite which is the predominant amphibole in the soil of a tobacco-growing region of south eastern Bulgaria may be responsible for calcified pleural plaques encountered there (Burilkov and Michailova, 1972) (*see also* p. 243). The problem is under investigation.

THE MICA GROUP

This group is referred to in Chapter 2 (p. 33). Its most important members in industry are *muscovite, phlogopite* and *vermiculite.*

Unmanufactured mica is classed either as *sheet mica* or *scrap and flake mica.*

Muscovite is the best sheet mica. It occurs as large laminated crystals or 'books or leaves' in granitic pegmatite which is rich in quartz. Its chief sources are the Bihar and Madras areas of India, Brazil and West Africa.

Phlogopite, a lesser source of sheet mica, is found in pegmatite-rich sedimentary rocks which also contain quartz. Its largest resources are in Canada and the Malagasy Republic.

Scrap and flake mica were originally the poor quality remainders from the milling and processing of sheet mica. But due to increased industrial demand, smaller size mica crystals and flake mica have been mined for this purpose from pegmatite, schist and clay deposits since early in this century. Hence, they are likely to contain variable amounts of quartz.

After mica from the mines has been crushed, washed and screened it has, since the mid-1960s, been reduced to a high degree of purity by the use of acid cationic or alkaline anionic–cationic flotation methods. Previously small amounts of contaminating minerals were likely to have been present.

Uses

Sheet mica is used for electrical insulators; for vacuum tubes and capacitators in the electronics industry; in the windows of furnaces and as a liner for the gauge glass of high pressure steam boilers; and as splittings cemented by an organic or inorganic binder into sheets which are hot-pressed and cut, milled or stamped into a variety of shapes for many purposes.

Scrap and flake mica is employed in oil well drilling; in the manufacture of roofing felt to prevent adhesion and improve weather-proofing; in the protective coatings of cables and welding rods; as a filler in asphalt products, cements and acoustic plastics; and, in very fine mesh, for paints and other decorative materials. Biotite, which was previously employed to a minor degree in the crushed state as a filler and coating in the rubber and roof felt industries, is now rarely, if ever, used.

Clinical and pathological considerations

It is very doubtful that a pneumoconiosis is caused by exposure to dust of the mica group of minerals *alone.* Certainly silicosis has occurred in Indian muscovite-miners in Bihar owing to the high quartz content of associated pegmatite rocks (Government of India Ministry of Labour, 1953 and 1956), and this remains a potential risk. When crude mica is crushed and milled, quartz is usually present in the dust and is not separated out until the later stages of refinement. However, remarkably little radiographic evidence of silicosis was found in one survey of muscovite and pegmatite miners in North Carolina (Dressen *et al.,* 1940) although in another survey of 79 men in the same region who milled mica which was not thought to contain 'free silica', seven were reported to have evidence of pneumoconiosis (Vestal, Winstead and Joliot, 1943).

Very few workers exposed to mica dust have been reported to have radiographic appearances consistent with a pneumoconiosis and of these the abnormalities have usually been of a minor order and other causes not excluded. A radiographic survey of 61 workers processing muscovite with less than 1 per cent of free silica showed no clear evidence of pneumoconiosis (Heimann *et al.,* 1953). Radiographic appearances consistent with DIPF were observed in one muscovite-grinder in North Carolina (Dressen *et al.,* 1940) and evidence of pleural calcification on chest films has been regarded in some cases as being due to mica (Smith, 1952; Kleinfeld, 1966), but in these the possibility of additional exposure to asbestos minerals (including fibrous tremolite) was not excluded.

Diffuse pigmented fibrosis was found at autopsy in the lungs of a man who had prolonged exposure to dusting powders in the rubber industry; the fibrotic areas contained numerous birefringent crystals (the mica minerals, incidently, are all strongly birefringent) which on X-ray diffraction proved to be biotite, and 'free silica' was absent (Vorwald, 1960). Because of the variety of mineral dusts to which this man could have been exposed Vorwald concluded that there was considerable 'uncertainty' that biotite was responsible and he was unable to eliminate other possible causes.

Pimental and Menezes (1978) reported a case of a woman exposed to muscovite dust for seven years during grinding and packing operations who suddenly developed respiratory symptoms for the first time after a 'common cold'. Two years later fine crepitations were present in both lungs and the chest radiograph showed 'bilateral reticulo-micronodular shadows and some nodular densities in the left lower lobe. After three years she died in respiratory failure. Post-mortem examination revealed extensive areas of 'diffuse fibrosis' with honeycombing. Microscopically alveolar walls were thickened and contained collagen fibres and muscovite particles, and sarcoid-type granulomas were present in the liver. However, the features of this case suggest sarcoidosis rather than a pneumoconiosis.

Because the micas are strongly birefringent and, therefore, readily visible by polarized light they may be wrongly regarded as the cause of co-existent lung disease in individuals with occupational exposures.

The majority of observers have shown that muscovite, biotite and sericite in the lungs of experimental animals produce only local macrophage accumulations with mild reticulin proliferation (King, Gilchrist and Rae, 1947; Tripsa and Rotura, 1966; Goldstein and Rendall, 1970), and the changes are those of a foreign body response to an inert dust which resolves in about 12 months (Vorwald, 1960). Intratracheal injection of 50 mg of muscovite in rats results in alveolar lipoproteinosis after 84 days and very slight collagen formation after 290 days, but not in acellular collagenized lesions (Kaw and Zaidi, 1973; Martin, Daniel and Le Bouffant, 1977). Hence, the micas evidently do not cause a fibrotic pneumoconiosis in animals. Neither is there any evidence of macrophage cytotoxicity or collagenous fibrosis in the tracheobronchial lymph nodes of guinea pigs followed at intervals for one year after intratracheal injection of muscovite, though there is some reticulin accumulation (Shanker *et al.*, 1975).

The available evidence (which has rarely included satisfactory details of past occupational dust exposures and differential diagnosis), therefore, gives little support to the belief that the mica minerals themselves cause a fibrotic pneumoconiosis in man. The demonstration and doubtful significance of biotite in Vorwald's (1960) case can hardly be regarded as proof of a causal relationship.

Vermiculite is the name given to a family of micaceous magnesium-aluminium silicates derived from hydrothermally altered biotite. The group is often classed with the clay minerals. Vermiculite is flaky, of light weight and has the property of expanding—or 'exfoliating'—to some 12 times its original size when heated. It is obtained in various parts of the world (especially in the USA) by open-cast mining, after which the ore is crushed and transported generally in the unheated—that is, unexpanded—form which is less bulky than the expanded form. When received by the expanding plant, prepared vermiculite is subjected to a furnace temperature of about 1100 °C, cooled, passed over separators to remove any impurities and packed in paper bags.

Expanded vermiculite is a good lightweight thermal insulator, is fireproof and resists decomposition, and has the properties of a mineral sponge. Its uses in industry include insulation granules for industrial and domestic buildings, as an aggregate for fireproof concrete, refractory bricks and pipe-lagging and, combined with gypsum, for fireproof building plasters; it is also used in soil conditioners, fertilizers and pesticides. Hence, expanded vermiculite is a valuable substitute for the asbestos minerals.

It is important, therefore, that there appears to be no evidence of any harmful effect to the lungs resulting from mining and crushing vermiculite or from the preparation and use of the expanded vermiculite. Furthermore, vermiculite does not cause fibrosis of the lungs in animals (Goldstein and Rendall, 1970), nor malignant mesothelioma after intrapleural injection in rats (Hunter and Thompson, 1973).

SOME OTHER NATURAL SILICATES

OLIVINE

'Olivine' is a generic term for a group of orthosilicate minerals which consist essentially of magnesium-rich *forsterite* ($Mg_2.SiO_4$) and iron-rich *fayalite* ($Fe_2.SiO_4$). They are mined by open-cast and underground methods and then dry-crushed. Crushed olivine has been widely used as a substitute for quartz since the 1930s. It is employed for a variety of refractory materials such as firebricks, heat resistant concrete, ceramic bodies for saggars, insulators and sparking plugs; in foundry moulds, paints and parting powders (to replace quartzite sands); and in the production of magnesia (MgO). The refractory properties are due mainly to forsterite.

There is, apparently, no record of olivine causing pneumoconiosis in man; and, in the rat lung, forsterite causes only a minimal foreign body reaction and no fibrosis (King *et al.*, 1945; Governa, Durio and Comai, 1979). Indeed, it was introduced as a substitute for flint and silica sands to eliminate silicosis in foundries.

Forsterite is the chief breakdown product of asbestos when subjected to high temperatures such as are generated in brake shoes during braking (*see* p. 236).

VOLCANIC SILICATE GLASSES

Pumice and pumicite

These volcanic silicate glasses (*see* Chapter 2, p. 40), as might be expected from their formation by violent expansion of dissolved gases in viscous silicic lavas such as rhyolite, may be associated with a variable amount of free silica in the form of microscrystals of quartz, tridymite and cristobalite, and as amorphous silica. This has been variously estimated as between 1 to 5 per cent by Faraone and Majon (1958) and 20 to 25 per cent—about one quarter of which is crystalline and the rest amorphous—by Pancheri and Zanetti (1963) in pumice on the Island of Lapari. Thus, the amount of free silica present varies from deposit to deposit but is generally low.

They are usually obtained by open-cast mining in the USA, Italy and Greece. Extraneous material is removed by screening through meshes of different sizes and, in general, pumice and pumicite used in industrial processes will contain little, if any, free silica; and high quality powders, none. The presence of a significant amount of crystalline material, in fact, would adversely affect the products.

Both have been employed increasingly in recent years as aggregate for building block lightweight concrete, and in pozzolan-portland cement. Pumice concrete is more resistant to heat than ordinary concrete. Because of its low bulk density pumice has valuable heat and sound insulating properties and is used for loose-fill insulation and in acoustic plasters. High quality pumice and pumicite are also used as abrasives especially for fine polishing operations, and in some scouring powders and soaps.

Pneumoconiosis has been described, usually without associated tuberculosis, in men who worked on crushers, pulverisers, drying kilns and screens—the last two processes carrying the greatest risk—at the Lipari Island quarries in the Mediterranean. It is, therefore, sometimes referred to as '*liparosis*' although it has the histological features of silicosis or 'mixed dust fibrosis' (Holt, 1957). Radiographically it may progress to large, multiple conglomerate opacities (ILO Category C) which in some cases have a curious propensity for the lower halves of the lung fields (Pancheri and Zanetti, 1963). However, pneumoconiosis does not seem to have been described in similar workers in the USA nor, apparently, among men exposed to pumice or pumicite in any of their industrial applications. Undoubtedly, therefore, pumice and pumicite themselves are inert, and the presence of free silica is required to cause fibrosis.

Perlite

This is a metastable volcanic silicate glass some ores of which occasionally contain small amounts of quartz ranging, for example, from 1 to 3 per cent (Anderson *et al.*, 1956) though high grade perlite does not contain any crystalline material (Cooper, 1975). It has found increasing use in industry since the Second World War in competition with pumice owing to its ability to be expanded ('popped') by heating between 760 to 1200 °C to a very light material possessing the valuable properties of low density, low thermal conductivity and high sound adsorption. It is mined by open pit methods chiefly in western USA and, on a smaller scale, in Greece, Hungary, Italy, Sardinia, Turkey and the USSR. The ore is passed through crushers, grinders and screens until appropriate particle size for introduction into the furnace is achieved. Quartz is usually absent or substantially less than 1 per cent in perlite intended for 'expansion' as its presence in any significant amount impairs the quality of the product.

Expanded perlite is used mainly in plasters and wall boards in combination with gypsum but also as an aggregate in lightweight concretes, and as a filtration medium and paint filler. Because it possesses excellent insulating and fire resistant capacities it is employed for sound adsorbing materials and loose-fill insulations. Like pumice, therefore, it is a good substitute for asbestos in certain insulation products. It is also used in foundry sand mixtures, as an extender and filler in paints, enamels, plastics and rubber, and as a soil conditioner.

Perlite is non-fibrogenic in the lungs of experimental animals (Vorwald, 1953) and a preliminary survey of 240 perlite workers with up to 23 years exposure in different parts of the industry did not reveal radiographic evidence of an associated pneumoconiosis (Cooper, 1975) nor any significant reduction of FEV_1 or FEV_1/FVC (Cooper, 1976). But as only 28 of the men X-rayed, all of whom represented only 13 of 62 existing perlite producing plants, had more than 15 years exposure, continued surveillance—preferably of the whole industry—is desirable.

It may be concluded that perlite itself is unlikely to cause pulmonary fibrosis but the possibility that occasionally some ores may contain quartz in excess of 2 to 3 per cent has to be borne in mind.

THE KYANITE GROUP

These consist of *andalusite, kyanite* and *sillimanite* which are anhydrous aluminium silicates with the same formula ($Al_2O_3.SiO_2$) but different crystal structures. They occur in different metamorphic rocks such as gneisses and schists. Sillimanite has an acicular, whiskery form with interlaced and interlocked quartz and other minerals which are not removed by benificiation (Bennet and Castle, 1975).

They are invaluable for the manufacture of high-grade refractories which are chemically inert under acidic or basic conditions, and capable of withstanding higher temperatures than fireclay bodies. Hence, they are used in the manufacture of porcelains for laboratory ware, sparking plugs and thermocouple tubing, and in special alumina-silica refractory bricks and mortars when high resistance to ware and temperature is required.

The raw ores are calcined at about 1550 °C for 24 hours, dry crushed and then milled with water in cylindrical mills. The resulting slip is mixed with varying amounts of clay for processing whatever type of ware is required. Formed brick and tiles are dried and again fired at different temperatures. The calcination and crushing processes are potentially dusty. Calcination at this temperature converts these minerals to mullite ($3Al_2O_3.2SiO_2$) which may occur in lath and needle form, cristobalite and glass. But the quantity of cristobalite formed depends upon the amount of alkaline or other fluxes (naturally associated with the minerals or added) present because these favour its conversion to the glassy phase. If there is much glass formation little or no cristobalite may be produced. Thus, according to the circumstances there may be variable amounts of cristobalite in 'respirable' dust. Some corundum may also be formed (*see* Chapter 13).

There appear to be no authentic cases of pneumoconiosis caused by these silicates on record. The minimal abnormality of chest radiographs reported by Middleton (1936) in four out of 15 sillimanite workers he examined is of doubtful significance. But small, irregular fibrotic nodules were described by Gärtner and van Marwyck (1947) in the lungs of a sillimanite furnace worker and attributed to mullite but it seems more probable that cristobalite was responsible.

Goldstein and Rendall (1970) showed that, in animals, uncalcined sillimanite causes localized accumulations of cells with some loose reticulin formation but no collagen; though slight fibrosis was described by Jötten and Eickhoff (1944). There were no lesions of silicotic type.

In summary

Exposure to the dust of these clay minerals when calcined may, under certain conditions, give rise to a silicosis hazard from cristobalite so that regular medical surveillance and analysis of airborne dust in the manufacture of alumina refractories is desirable. In their uncalcined form, however, there is no convincing evidence that andalusite, kyanite or sillimanite cause pneumoconiosis.

WOLLASTONITE

This is a monocalcium silicate ($Ca.SiO_3$) which is found in contact–metamorphic deposits of limestones and in igneous rocks. Hence, it is sometimes associated with quartz. It occurs in acicular and fibrous forms, the aspect ratio of the 'fibres' being usually about 7 or 8:1 (Elevatorski, 1975). It is moderately birefringent. Its chief source is the USA, but it is also mined in Mexico, Finland and elsewhere.

Wollastonite has only been exploited for industrial use since 1952. It is most extensively employed in the ceramic industry to improve the mechanical properties of the ware and as an important substitute for sand and flint in the prevention of silicosis (*see* p. 139). It is also widely used in paints to increase weather resistance and reduce oil absorption. And, as it possesses a high resistance to heat, it is assuming importance as a substitute for asbestos minerals in insulation mainly as mineral wool made into tiles, boards and blankets.

Because of the fibrous or semi-fibrous habit of this mineral it is important to know if it is likely to offer any hazard to health even though its molecular structure is different from the asbestos minerals. Shasby *et al.*, (1979) examined 104 mine and mill workers in the USA by respiratory questionnaire, physical examination, lung function tests and chest radiographs. They found no association between respiratory symptoms and increasing exposure; no significant abnormalities of ventilatory capacity, TLC or Tl; and no radiographic evidence of pleural plaques or of irregular opacities suggestive of DIPF. But as only about one-third of the men studied had more than 15 years exposure prolonged follow-up of this population is advisable.

As far as is known at present wollastonite is not harmful to the lungs.

ZEOLITES

These are a family of hydrous aluminium silicates with sodium and calcium as their principal bases. They occur in vesicular cavities and fissures in basic lavas (or tuffs) and may be associated with small quantities of other silicates and quartz. However, for commercial purposes they are obtained by quarrying sedimentary volcanic deposits originally formed in fresh water and marine environments. Of the many different species (more than 35) the most important commercially are *chabazite, erionite* (which has a needle-like form), *faujasite* and *mordenite* which consists of ultrathin, submicroscopic fibres (Mumpton, 1975).

They possess remarkable adsorptive properties so that they have been used increasingly during the past decade as ion exchange systems, gas purifiers, in adsorption and other molecular sieves for the separation and collection of radioactive wastes, in petroleum refining, animal feeds and agricultural products. They are also employed in pozzolanic cements and concrete, as dimension stone, as fillers for paper and, after calcination at about 1300 °C, for light weight aggregates.

There appears to be no record of pneumoconiosis associated with these minerals. However, interest has recently been focused on them following the observation of calcified pleural plaques and malignant pleural mesothelioma in agricultural populations with no evident contact with asbestos minerals in the central uplands of Turkey. Although the plaques do not shorten life expectancy malignant mesothelioma is said to account for about 50 per cent of deaths in two villages. Diffuse pleural fibrosis has also been observed. Both villages stand on volcanic rock which is used for building. This rock contains a submicroscopic, fibrillar zeolite which is also found in the soil and street dust (Baris *et al.*, 1978b; Baris, Artvinli and Sahin, 1979). A preliminary study has demonstrated the presence of a fairly large number of long fibres (probably erionite) 75 per cent of which are less than 0.25 μm in diameter (Pooley, 1979), although, at present, a relationship between zeolites and these chest disorders is speculative. However, in view of the period during which these minerals have been exploited industrially and of an expected boom in their use in the next decade it is obviously important to determine whether their fibrous forms possess any oncogenic or other pathogenic potential. But, as pointed out in the next section, relevant animal experiment should be by inhalation.

It is of interest that many buildings of the Mayan regions in southern Mexico have recently been found to be constructed of zeolite blocks with a high mordenite content and that the same tuff is still being quarried today in Oaxaca for use in local buildings. Early ranch houses in the American West were built of locally quarried erionite (Mumpton, 1975).

MAN-MADE SILICATE FIBRES

Since the later 1890s a variety of man-made silicate fibres have been increasingly used for thermal and acoustic insulation, in textiles and for plastic re-inforcement; and, latterly, their use has expanded further in the substitution of asbestos minerals. This has raised the question as to whether synthetic fibres cause pneumoconiosis or malignancy in man in view of the fact that fibrous particles of less than 2.5 μm in diameter—irrespective of their chemical composition—have been shown to cause malignant tumours in animals when introduced directly into their pleural or peritoneal cavities.

Man-made fibres fall into three main groups:
slag wools,
rock wools,
glass wools and filaments.

The mineral wools are made from melts of specific argillaceous limestones and smelter slags sometimes with the addition of wollastonite or kaolinite; glass wool (or fibre glass) is made from borosilicate or calcio-alumina silicate glass (Hill, 1977). All are glassy minerals which, unlike the asbestos minerals, are amorphous silicates. 'Melts' at a temperature of 1000 to 1500 °C are 'fiberized' by drawing, blowing or centrifugal methods (Klingholz, 1977). The diameters and lengths of fibres differ according to the use for which they are required and are manufactured to a controlled 'nominal' (specified) diameter. Filaments for textiles and reinforcements of plastics and similar materials have a large diameter ranging from 12 to 20 μm and only a very small number of 'respirable' fibres occur in the process. For insulation (which forms the major part of commercial production) fibres are usually about 6 μm in diameter but a proportion (8 per cent or less) may be smaller than 3 μm in diameter. Filaments less than 1 μm in diameter may be produced for acoustic insulation and for certain limited specialized purposes (such as laboratory filter papers). But they represent only about 1 per cent of world production (Hill, 1978).

The fibres are commonly coated with a binder which is usually a biologically inert, fully polymerized, thermosetting resin but may be mineral oil. Unlike asbestos fibres which split longitudinally into numerous fibrils of much smaller diameter mineral fibres break transversely into shorter fragments with the same diameter (Assuncao and Corn, 1975) (*Figure 9.51*).

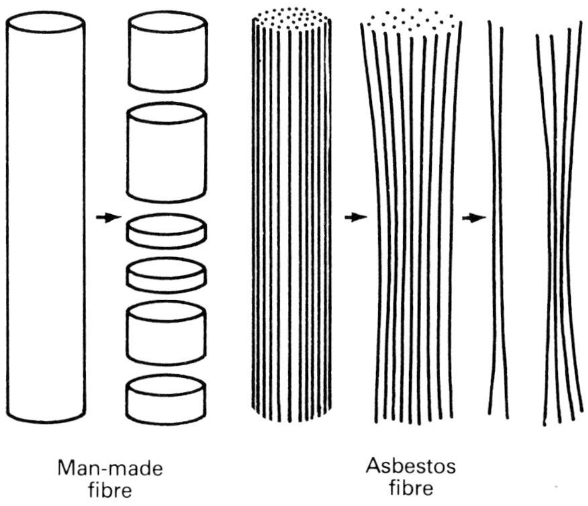

Figure 9.51 Mode of fracture of man-made and asbestos fibres compared. (Adapted from Klingholz, 1977. By kind permission of the Editor of Annals of Occupational Hygiene*)*

Sources of exposure

Dust is generated during handling the various wools, in insulation operations and in sawing, grinding and cutting board containing these fibres. Such operations cause fibre breakage which may give rise to some particles small enough to remain airborne for a short time. However, it has been shown that chamfering, cutting and machining of glass fibre re-inforced calcium silicate insulating board with the exhaust ventilation switched off produces airborne fibres with an average length of 100 μm and an almost uniform diameter of 12 μm. Fibres of these dimensions have a high settling velocity, are quickly removed from the airborne dust and are unlikely to reach the lower respiratory tract (Hounam, 1973). If inhaled they will be deposited in the upper respiratory tract (*see* Chapter 3).

The average range of concentration of 'respirable' fibres evolved during the manufacture of continuous filament and insulation wools is, in general, reported to be about 0.03 to 0.2 fibres/ml (Hill, 1977). In a study of the exposure of employees to mineral wool fibres in five different plants producing man-made fibres the size and length distribution of the fibres were found to be remarkably consistent in spite of differences in the manufacturing and handling processes. About 80 per cent of the fibres were less than 50 μm in length and about 10 per cent, less than 10 μm in length. Approximately 50 per cent were less than 3 μm in diameter but very few less than 1 μm in diameter. Compared with a similar study of fibrous glass manufacture the overall airborne concentrations of both types of fibre were of the order of 0.1 fibres/ml of which the 'respiratory' fraction (fibres less than 3 μm in diameter) accounted for about 50 per cent (Esmeu *et al.* 1978).

Respiratory effects in man

Slag and rock wools have been produced since the late 1840s and glass wool since about 1930 yet no clearly authenticated cases of causally related lung disease have been reported even though fibres of 'respirable' dimensions have been present in most products since manufacture began (Klingholz, 1977).

Two cases of acute respiratory infections and a third with bronchiectasis were attributed to fibre glass exposure but without satisfactory proof (Hill, 1977). The presence of glass fibres in the lungs in such cases does not, of course, establish a pathogenic relationship.

Epidemiological studies have provided additional information. Radiographic surveys of workers with long periods of exposure in the rock and slag wool industry (Carpenter and Spolyar, 1945), the fibre glass industry (Wright, 1968; Nasr, Ditcheck and Scholtens, 1971), the glass and rock wool industry and in insulation work (Keane and Zavon, 1966; Hill *et al.,* 1973) have not revealed any evidence of pneumoconiosis. Similarly, investigation of respiratory symptoms and lung function in workers exposed to fibre glass and glass and rock wools have not identified any abnormality attributable to them (Bjure, Soderholm and Widimsky, 1964; Utidjian and de Treville, 1970; Hill *et al.,* 1973).

A review of 416 men retiring from plants manufacturing fibre glass insulation materials from 1945 to 1972 revealed no excess of respiratory cancers and no mesotheliomas (Enterline and Henderson, 1975). An investigation in 1972 of the causes of mortality among 1448 glass wool production workers initially employed between 1940 and 1949 and exposed for five years or more to airborne fibres of 1.8 μm mass median diameter likewise disclosed no excess of respiratory malignancy (Bayliss *et al.,* 1976). Another recent survey of workers in five fibre glass plants did not discover any excess of malignant or non-malignant respiratory disease among them (Enterline and Marsh, 1979). These studies incidently appear to have covered time-lag for the development of putative malignancy adequately.

Post-mortem examination of the lungs of individuals exposed to fibre glass for 16 to 32 years compared with the lungs of unexposed control urban subjects showed no evidence of fibrosis or tissue response which could be attributed to the glass dust. Furthermore, the quantity and dimension of fibres present in the fibre glass workers lungs were similar to those in the 'control' lungs suggesting that any glass fibres deposited in the workers' lungs over the years were largely removed by the normal clearance mechanisms (Gross, 1976).

Fibres from the 'wools' may cause some irritation of the nose and throat with sneezing, but itching of the skin of the hands, wrists, neck, waist and ankles is the most irksome complaint among workers unaccustomed to handling these materials. This is due to the mechanical effects of superficially embedded fibres, and not to skin sensitization. The unpolymerized resins, amines and hardners in the coating of finished fibres are not reactive (Hill, 1977).

Experimental observations

As already indicated elsewhere the dimensions of fibres rather than their chemical composition appear to be the important factors in their ability to induce lung disease (pp. 73 and 254). It was early reported that neither uncoated nor plastic coated glass fibres inhaled or injected via the intratracheal route into rats, guinea pigs, rabbits and monkeys caused pulmonary fibrosis (Schepers and Delehant, 1955; Schepers, 1959). Later observations have shown that the inhalation by rats and hamsters of glass fibres with an approximate diameter of 0.5 μm and approximate length range of 5 to 20 μm cause neither fibrosis nor malignancy in their lungs, nor pleural tumours, irrespective of whether the fibres are coated (with resin or starch-like binders) or uncoated; and that in spite of heavy exposure little glass dust is found in the lungs as a result, apparently, of its rapid clearance (Gross, 1976).

In a more recent experiment with rats lasting 17 to 19 days in which glass fibres of 1.5 μm mean diameter and either 5 μm or 60 μm in length were instilled *via* the trachea little difference was found in the clearance rates of the long versus the short fibres, although short fibres were successfully engulfed by macrophages and transported to the lymph nodes whereas long fibres were not. Long fibres caused well-demarcated, foreign body granulomas containing numerous giant cells and glass fibres. But neither long nor short fibres provoked any fibrosis. A few short fibres were seen in the lymph nodes of animals exposed only to long fibres (Bernstein, Drew and Kuschner, 1980). But earlier, Wright and Kuschner (1977) found mild local DIPF 2 years after intratracheal injection of short fibres—about 5 μm. However, intratracheal instillation is unphysiological and, compared with inhalation, causes excessively high local concentrations of fibres. (*See* Addendum, page 332).

The situation is very different when fibres are introduced directly into the coelomic 'cavities' of animals. Experiments in which glass fibres ranging from less than 5 μm to more than 10 μm in length and less than 2.5 μm in diameter were implanted in the pleural or peritoneal 'spaces' of rats have resulted in sarcomatous tumours classed as mesotheliomas—though the criteria for this diagnosis are not always given (Stanton and Wrench, 1972; Wagner, Berry and Timbrell, 1973; Pott, Huth and Friedrich, 1974). Stanton *et al.* (1977) have since investigated 17 fibrous glasses of diverse type and dimensions by introducing them into the pleural 'spaces' of rats and shown that, as the diameter of the fibres is reduced below 1.5 μm and their length increased above 8 μm, the yield of 'pleural sarcoma' increases; when all the fibres are shorter than 8 μm they are inactivated by phagocytosis and no statistically significant excess of tumour occurs. But under similar circumstances, fibres of asbestos and synthetic aluminium silicate, as well as glass fibres, also possess tumour-producing potential if they are thinner than 0.5 μm and longer than 10 μm or 20 μm (Wagner, Berry and Timbrell, 1973; Maroudas, O'Neill and Stanton, 1973). However, the induction of small numbers of malignant tumours (classed as mesotheliomas) in rats by intrapleural inoculation of such diverse *non-fibrous* substances as ultrafine non-crystalline silicon dioxide, barium sulphate, aluminium oxide and powdered glass (Stanton and Wrench, 1972; Wagner, Berry and Timbrell, 1973) suggests that neither the fibrous form nor a particular chemical composition is essential for the production of malignancy in this animal species.

Such implantation experiments are not likely to have any relevance to human pathology for these reasons:

(1) The direct introduction of glass fibres (or other substances) into the pleural or peritoneal cavities of animals as in no way analogous to their normal mode of entry into the human body; and the numbers of fibres implanted is almost certainly greatly in excess of any accumulation—assuming that this occurs—which might conceivably result from inhalation.
(2) The animal used almost exclusively in these experiments has been the rat in which it is known that sarcomatous tumours can be readily induced in different anatomical sites by the surgical implantation of a variety of chemically dissimilar solids due, it is postulated, to so-called 'solid-state surface' oncogenesis (Bischoff and Bryson, 1964; Brand, 1975) (*see also* p. 285); but this phenomenon shows striking species differences and there is no evidence to suggest that it occurs in man.

To summarize

(1) The results of epidemiological surveys, human post-mortem studies and inhalation experiments in animals to date have provided no evidence that man-made fibres are responsible for disease of the lungs or pleura in man, and are, therefore, reassuring.
(2) Animal experiments and observations of human lungs suggest that glass fibres are efficiently cleared from the lungs.
(3) The production of malignant tumours in animals by direct implantation experiments is unlikely to have any relevance to human exposure.
(4) Nonetheless, continued careful monitoring of the occupational environment and medical surveillance of those involved in the manufacture and use of man-made fibres is desirable for three main reasons. *First,* a great increase in the production and use of existing and new types of fibres of very small diameter can be expected. *Second,* epidemiological—especially mortality—studies may not yet have been done in large enough numbers and over a sufficiently long period. *Third,* the possibility of related malignancy even though this would not seem to apply to human exposure.

Hence, a collaborative investigation is under way in many European countries which includes methods of collating epidemiological data on a large scale, techniques for identifying, collecting and counting fibres, and further study of possible biological effects (Rossiter, 1977). Results will be awaited with interest.

The American College of Chest Physicians (1976) has stressed that, in order to obtain evidence from animals which might have relevance to man, inhalation experiments are essential.

Threshold limit values

Although fibrous glass is classed as a 'Nuisance Particulate' by the ACGIH the US Department of Health, Education and Welfare (1977) has recommended strict limitations to the concentration of fibres having specific diameters and lengths over an average working week on the grounds that fibrous glass causes pulmonary fibrosis and is carcinogenic. This recommendation, however, has been critized on the grounds that it is 'not founded on any scientific or medical basis' (Gross, 1978).

CARBON FIBRE

It is convenient to make brief mention of this topic here for want of a more appropriate place.

A family of carbon fibres prepared by oxidizing polyacrylonitrile fibre under tension at 220 °C and then heating the product to between 1100 and 2500 °C in an inert atmosphere was introduced by Phillips in 1968 and has since been extensively used in the aircraft industry for the reinforcement of plastics instead of asbestos and glass fibre because of its superior flexural properties.

There appears to be no evidence that carbon fibre has caused pneumoconiosis in man but the possibility that it might is sometimes raised. Holt and Horns (1978) have shown experimentally that it is difficult to produce a cloud of dust particles in the 'respirable' range from carbon fibre. Many of the fibres being longer than 100 μm and more than 10 μm in diameter. Furthermore, inhalation of carbon fibre dust by guinea pigs has not been followed by detectable pathological effects in their lungs. Thus, although these authors suggest that long-term exposure experiments are required to establish that carbon fibres are completely innocuous there is, currently, no reason to suspect that they are harmful to man.

CODA

The British Health and Safety Commission has recently stated that it 'regards mineral fibres with suspicion' because it considers that current data 'neither assert safety nor establish health risk' (Lancet, 1979). The need for critical appraisal of animal and epidemiological studies in this respect, however, is clearly essential.

REFERENCES

Abraham, J. L. and Brambilla, C. (1979). Particle size for differentiation between inhalation and injection pulmonary talcosis. *Am. Rev. resp. Dis.* **119** (Supplement), 196

Alden, H. S. and Howell, W. M. (1944). The asbestos corn. *Archs Derm. Syph.* **49,** 312–314

Alivisatos, G. P., Pontikakis, A. E. and Terzis, B. (1955). Talcosis of unusually rapid development. *Br. J. ind. Med.* **12,** 43–49

Amandus, H. E., Lapp, N. L., Jacobson, G. and Reger, R. B. (1976). Significance of irregular small opacities in radiographs of coal miners in the USA. *Br. J. ind. Med.* **33,** 13–17

American College of Chest Physicians (1976). The pulmonary response to fibreglass dust. Report of the Committee on Environmental Health. *Chest* **69,** 216–219

Anderson, A. E., Gealor, R. L., McCune, R. C. and Sprys, J. W. (1973). Asbestos emissions from brake dynamometer tests. Paper 730549 Automobile Engineering Meeting, Detroit 1973. New York; Society of Automobile Engineers, Inc.

Anderson, H. A., Lilis, R., Daum, S. M., Fischbein, A. S. and Selikoff, I. J. (1976). Household-contact asbestos neoplastic risk. *Ann. N.Y. Acad. Sci.* **271,** 311–323

Anderson, F. G., Selvig, W. A., Baur, G. S., Colbassani, P. J. and Bank, W. (1956). Composition of perlite. Report of Investigations 5199. Washington DC; US Bureau of Mines

Anjilvel, L. and Thurlbeck, W. M. (1966). The incidence of asbestos bodies in the lungs of random necropsies in Montreal. *Can. med. Ass. J.* **95,** 1179–1182

Anton, H. C. (1968). Multiple pleural plaques. Part 1. *Br. J. Radiol.* **41,** 341–348

Arai, H., Kang, K-Y., Sato, H., Satoh, K., Nagai, H., Motomiya, M. and Kono, K. (1979). Significance of the quantification and demonstration of hyaluronic acid in tissue specimens for the diagnosis of pleural mesothelioma. *Am. Rev. resp. Dis.* **120,** 529–532

Asbestos International Association (1979). Asbestos cement products. Health and Safety Publication. Recommended Control Procedure No 2 (RCP 2)

Asbestos Research Council (1973). Recommended Code of Practice for Handling and Disposal of Asbestos Waste Materials

Asbestos Research Council (1976). Obtained from PO Box 40. Rochdale, Lancs., UK

Ashcroft, T. and Heppleston, A. G. (1973). The optical and electron microscopic determination of pulmonary asbestos fibre concentration and its relation to the human pathological reaction. *J. clin. Path.* **26,** 224–234

Assuncao, J. and Corn, M. (1975). The effects of milling on diameters and lengths of fibrous glass and chrysotile asbestos fibres. *Am. ind. Hyg. Ass. J.* **36,** 811–819

Attygalle, D., Harrison, C. V., King, E. H. and Mohanty, G. P. (1954). Infective pneumoconiosis 1. The influence of dead tubercle bacilli (BCG) on the dust lesions produced by anthracite, coal mine dust, and kaolin in the lungs of rats and guinea pigs. *Br. J. ind. Med.* **11,** 245–259

Bader, M. E., Bader, R. A. and Selikoff, I. J. (1961). Pulmonary function in asbestosis of the lung; an alveolar-capillary block syndrome. *Am. J. Med.* **30,** 235–242

Bader, M. E., Bader, R. A., Tierstein, A. S. and Selikoff, I. J. (1965). Pulmonary function in asbestosis: serial tests in a long term prospective study. *N.Y. Acad. Sci.* **132,** 391–405

Bader, M. E., Bader, R. A., Tierstein, A. S., Miller, A. and Selikoff, I. J. (1970). Pulmonary function and radiographic changes in 598 workers with varying duration of exposure to asbestos. *J. Mt Sinai Hosp.* **37,** 492–499

Bamber, H. A. and Butterworth, R. (1970). Asbestos hazard from protective clothing. *Ann. occup. Hlth* **13,** 77–79

Baris, Y. I., Artvinli, M. and Sahin, A. A. (1979). Environmental mesothelioma in Turkey. *Ann. N. Y. Acad. Sci.* **330,** 423–432

Baris, I., Elmes, P. C., Pooley, F. D. and Sahin, A. (1978). Mesotheliomas in Turkey. *Thorax* **33,** 538

Baris, Y. I., Sahin, A. A., Ozesmi, M., Kerse, I., Ozen, E., Kolacan, B., Altinors, M. and Goktepeli, A. (1978). An outbreak of pleural mesothelioma and chronic fibrosing pleurisy in the village of Karain Urgup in Anatolia. *Thorax* **33,** 181–192

Bayliss, D. L., Dement, J. M., Wagoner, J. K. and Blejer, H. P. (1976). Mortality patterns among fibrous glass production workers. *Ann. N.Y. Acad. Sci.* **271,** 324–335

Beattie, J. and Knox, J. F. (1961). Studies in mineral content and particle size distribution in the lungs of asbestos textile workers. In *Inhaled Particles and Vapours, I,* edited by C. N. Davies, pp. 419–433. Oxford and New York; Pergamon

Becklake, M. R. (1976). Asbestos-related diseases of the lung and other organs: their epidemiology and implications for clinical practice. *Am. Rev. resp. Dis.* **114,** 187–227

Becklake, M. R., Fournier-Massey, G., McDonald, J. C., Siemiatycki, J. and Rossiter, C. E. (1970). Lung function in relation to chest radiographic changes in Quebec asbestos workers. In *Pneumoconiosis. Proceedings of the International Conference, Johannesburg, 1969,* edited by H. A. Shapiro, pp. 233–236. Cape Town; Oxford University Press

Becklake, M. R., Liddell, F. D. K., Manfreda, J. and McDonald, J. C. (1979). Radiological changes after withdrawal from asbestos exposure. *Br. J. ind. Med.* **36,** 23–28

Becklake, M. R., Rossiter, C. E. and McDonald, J. C. (1972). Lung function in chrysotile asbestos mine and mill workers of Quebec. *Archs Envir. Hlth* **24,** 401–409

Beer, D. J., Pereira, W. and Snider, G. L. (1978). Pleural effusion associated with primary lymphedema: a perspective on the yellow nail syndrome. *Am. Rev. resp. Dis.* **117,** 595–599

Bennett, P. J. and Castle, J. E. (1975). Kyanite and related minerals. In *Industrial Minerals and Rocks,* 4th edition, edited by Stanley F. Lebond, pp. 729–736. New York; American Institute of Mining, Metallurgical and Petroleum Engineers, Inc.

Beutelspacher, H. and van der Marel, H. W. (1968). Atlas of electron microscopy of clay minerals and their admixtures. Amsterdam, London, New York; Elsevier Publishing Company

Bentley, D. and Cline, J. (1970). Estimation of clubbing by analysis of shadowgraph. *Br. med. J.* **3,** 43

Bernstein, D. M., Drew, R. T. and Kuschner, M. (1980). Experimental approaches to exposure to sized glass fibres. *Environ. Hlth Perspec.* **34,** 47–57

Berry, G. (1981). The mortality of workers certified by pneumoconiosis medical panels as having asbestosis disease. *Br. J. ind. Med.* **38,** 130–137

Berry, G., Newhouse, M. L. and Turok, M. (1972). Combined effect of asbestos exposure and smoking on mortality from lung cancer in factory workers. *Lancet* **2,** 476–479

Bhagavan, B. S. and Koss, L. G. (1976). Secular trends in prevalence and concentration of pulmonary asbestos bodies—1940–1972. *Archs path-lab. Med.* **100,** 539–541

Bianchi, C., Di Bonito, L., Castelli, M. and Brollo, A. (1978). Exposition à l'amiante dans le cancer du larynx. *Pathologica* **70,** 403–408

Bignon, J., Atassi, K., Jaurand, M. C., Yamine, J., Kapleau, H., Geslin, P., Solle, E. and Bientz, M. (1978b). Etude cytologique et biochimique du liquide du lavage broncho-alveolaire (LBA) dans la fibrose pulmonaire idiopathique et l'asbestose. *Rev. fr. Mal-Resp.* **6,** 353–358

Bignon, J., Depierre, A., Bonnard, G., Gani, J. and Brouet, G. (1973). Mise en evidence des corps ferrugineux par micro-filtration de l'expectoration. *Nouv. Presse med.* **2,** 1697–1700

Bignon, J., Sebastien, P., Gaudichet, A. and Bientz, M. (1978a). Analysis of mineral particles recovered by broncho-alveolar lavage for diagnosis of dust related lung diseases. *Am. Rev. resp. Dis.* **117** (suppl), 218

Bischoff, F. and Bryson, G. (1964). Carcinogenesis through solid state surfaces. *Prog. exp. Tumour res.* **5,** 85–133. Basel/New York; Karger

Bjure, J., Soderholm, B. and Widimisky, J. (1964). Cardio-pulmonary function studies in workers dealing with asbestos and glass wool. *Thorax* **19,** 22–27

Blümel, G., Piza, F. and Zischka-Konorsa, W. (1962). Tierexperimentelle Untersuchungen der Gerwerbereaktion auf Starke-und Talkumpuder nach intraperitonealer Anwendung. *Wiener Klinische Wochenschrift* **74,** 12–13

Boersma, A., Degand, P. and Havez, R. (1973). Diffuse mesothelioma: biochemical stages in the diagnosis, detection and measurement of hyaluronic acid in the pleural fluid. In *Biological Effects of Asbestos,* edited by P. Bogovski *et al.* pp. 65–67. Lyon; International Agency for Research on Cancer

Bohlig, H., Dabbert, A. F., Dalquen, P., Hain, E. and Hinz, I. (1970). Epidemiology of malignant mesothelioma in Hamburg. *Envir. res.* **3,** 365–372

Boron, M., Couston, A., Livornese, L. and Schalet, N. (1973). Mesothelioma following exposure to asbestos: a review of 72 cases. *Chest* **64,** 641–646

Boundy, M. G., Gold, K., Martin, Jr., K. P., Burgess, W. A. (1979). Occupational to non-asbestiform talc in Vermont, In *Dusts and Disease.* Edited by R. Lemen and J. M. Dement, pp. 365–378. Illinois; Pathotox Publishers, Inc.

Bramwell, A., Leech, J. G. C. and Dunstall, W. S. (1940). Montmorillonite in fuller's earth. *Geol. Mag.* **77,** 102–112

Brand, K. G. (1975). Foreign body induced sarcomas. In *Cancer I,* edited by F. F. Becker, pp. 485–511. New York and London; Plenum Press

British Occupational Hygiene Society (1973). Hygiene standards for airborne amosite asbestos dust. *Ann. occup. Hyg.* **16,** 1–5. Review of the hygiene standard for chrysotile asbestos dust. *Ann. occup. Hyg.* **16,** 7

British Thoracic and Tuberculosis Association and the Medical Research Council Pneumoconiosis Unit (1972). A survey of pleural thickening: its relation to asbestos exposure and previous pleural disease. *Envir. Res.* **5,** 142–151

Brown, D., Dement, J. M. and Wagoner, J. K. (1979). Mortality patterns among miners and millers occupationally exposed to asbestiform talc. In *Dusts and Disease.* Edited by R. Lemen and J. M. Dement, pp. 317–324. Illinois; Pathotox Publishers Inc.

Bryks, S. and Bertalanffy, F. D. (1971). Cytodynamic reactivity of the mesothelium. Pleural reaction to chrysotile asbestos. *Archs envir. Hlth* **23,** 469–472

Bryson, G. and Bischoff, F. (1967). Silicate-induced neoplasms. *Prog. exp. Tumour resp.* **9,** 77–164. Basel/New York; Karger

Buchanan, W. D. (1965). Asbestosis and primary intrathoracic neoplasms. *Ann. N.Y. Acad. Sci.* **132,** 507–518

Burilkov, T. and Michailova, L. (1970). Asbestos content of soil and endemic pleural asbestosis. *Envir. Res.* **3,** 443–451

Burilkov, T. and Michailova, L. (1972). Uber den sepiolitgehalt des bodens in gebieten mit endomischen pleuraverkalkungen. *Int. Arch. Arbeitsmed.* **29,** 95–101

Butchart, E. G., Ashcroft, T., Barnsley, W. C. and Holden, M. P. (1976). Pleuropneumonectomy in the managements of diffuse malignant mesothelioma of the pleura. *Thorax* **31,** 15–24

Butler, E. B. and Berry, A. N. (1973). Diffuse mesotheliomas: diagnostic criteria using exfoliative cytology. In *Biological Effects of Asbestos,* edited by P. Bogovski *et al.,* pp. 68–73. Lyon; International Agency for Research on Cancer

Byers, P. D. and King, E. J. (1959). Experimental and infective pneumoconiosis with coal, kaolin and mycobacteria. *Lab. Invest.* **8,** 647–664

Byers, P. D., King, E. J. and Harrison, C. V. (1960). The effect of triton, a surface active polyoxethylene ether, on experimental infective pneumoconiosis. *Br. J. exp. Path.* **41,** 472–477

Campbell, A. H. and Gloyne, S. R. (1942). A case of pneumonokoniosis due to the inhalation of fuller's earth. *J. Path. Bact.* **54,** 75–79

Campbell, W. J. (1978). Identification of selected silicate minerals and their asbestiform varieties. In *Proceedings of the Workshop on Asbestos: Definitions and Measurement Methods,* Gaithersburg, Maryland, 1977. pp 201–220. National Bureau of Standards Special Publication 506

Caplan, A., Gilson, J. C., Hinson, K. F. W., McVittie, J. C. and Wagner, J. C. (1965). II a preliminary study of observer radiation in the classification of radiographs of asbestos-exposed workers and the relation of pathology and X-ray appearances. *Ann. N.Y. Acad. Sc.* **132,** 379–386

Carpenter, J. L. and Spolyar, L. W. (1945). Negative chest findings in a mineral wool industry. *J. Indiana med. Ass.* **38,** 389–390

Carroll, W. G. (1962). The manufacture of brake linings. *Br. Plastics* **35,** 414–417

Cartier, P. (1949). Contribution à l'étude de l'amiantose. *Archs Mal. Prof. Med.* **10,** 589–595

Cartier, P. (1965). Discussion on pleural plaques. *Ann. N.Y. Acad. Sci.* **132,** 387–388

Cate, C. C. and Burrell, R. (1974). Lung antigen induced cell-mediated immune injury in chronic respiratory disease. *Am. Rev. resp. Dis.* **109,** 114–123

Cauna, D., Totten, R. S. and Gross, P. (1965). Asbestos bodies in human lungs at autopsy. *J. Am. med. Ass.* **192,** 371–373

Chahinian, Ph., Hirsch, A., Bignon, J., Choffel, C., Pariente, R., Brouet, G. and Chrétien, J. (1973). Les pleurésies asbestosiques non tumorales. *Rev. Fr. Mal. resp.* **1,** 5–38

Chahinian, P., Ramachandar, K., Schechter, R., Holland, J. F. and Becesi, J. G. (1976). Immunocompetence in patients with diffuse malignant mesothelioma. Proc. of 3rd Inter. Symposium on Detection and Prevention of Cancer. NY. No. 406

Churg, A. M. and Warnock, M. L. (1979). Number of asbestos bodies in urban patients with lung cancer and gastrointestinal cancer and in matched controls. *Chest* **76,** 143–149

Churg, A. M., Warnock, M. L. and Green, N. (1979). Analysis of the cores of ferruginous (asbestos) bodies from the general population. 11 True asbestos bodies and pseudoasbestos bodies. *Lab. Invest.* **40,** 31–38

Codling, B. W. and Chakera, T. M. H. (1972). Pulmonary fibrosis following therapy with melphalan for multiple myeloma. *J. Clin. Path.* **25,** 668–673

Collins, T. F. B. (1968). Pleural reaction associated with asbestos exposure. *Br. J. Radiol.* **41,** 655–661

Commins, B. T. and Gibbs, G. N. (1969). Contaminating organic material in asbestos. *Br. J. Cancer* **23,** 358–362

Cooke, W. E. (1924). Fibrosis of the lungs due to the inhalation of asbestos dust. *Br. med. J.* **2,** 147

Cooke, W. E., McDonald, S. and Oliver, T. (1927). Pulmonary asbestosis. *Br. med. J.* **2,** 1024–1027

Cooper, W. C. (1975). Radiographic survey of perlite workers. *J. occup. Med.* **17,** 304–307

Cooper, W. C. (1976). Pulmonary function in perlite workers. *J. occup. Med.* **18,** 723–729

Coutts, I. I., Gilson, J. C., Kerr, I. H., Parkes, W. R. and Turner-Warwick, M. (1980). Progression of intrapulmonary fibrosis due asbestos exposure. (To be published)

Cralley, L. J., Keenan, R. G., Lynch, J. R. and Lainhart, W. S. (1968). Source and identification of respirable fibres. *Am. ind. Hyg. Ass. J.* **29,** 129–135

Crofton, J. and Douglas, A. (1975). *Respiratory diseases.* 2nd edition. Oxford and Edinburgh; Blackwell Scientific Publications

Daniele, R. P., Dauber, J. H., Altose, M. D., Rowlands, D. T. and Gorenberg, D. J. (1977). Lymphocyte studies in asymptomatic cigarette smokers. *Am. Rev. resp. Dis.* **116,** 997–1005

Darke, C., Wagner, M. M. F. and Grant McMillan, G. H. (1979).

HLA-A and B antigen frequencies in an asbestos exposed population with normal and abnormal radiographs. *Tissue Antigens* **13,** 228–232
Davies, P., Allison, A. C., Ackerman, J., Butterfield, A. and Williams, S. (1974). Asbestos induces selective release of lysosomal enzymes from mononuclear phagocytes. *Nature* **251,** 423–425
Davis, G. S., Mortara, M. and Green, G. M. (1975). Lysosomal enzyme release from human and guinea alveolar macrophages during phagocytosis. *Clin. Res.* **23,** 346A (abstract)
Davis, J. M. G. (1965). Electron microscope studies of asbestosis in man and animals. *Am. N.Y. Acad. Sci.* **132,** 98–111
Davis, J. M. G. (1972). The effects of polyvinyl pyridine-N-oxide (P204) on the cytopathogenic action of chrysotile asbestos *in vivo* and *in vitro*. *Br. J. exp. Path.* **53,** 652–658
Davis, J. M. G. (1974). Histogenesis and fine structure of peritoneal tumours produced in animals by injections of asbestos. *J. Nat. Cancer Inst.* **52,** 1823–1828
Davis, J. M. G. (1979). Current concepts of asbestos fiber pathogenicity. In *Dusts and Disease (occupational and environmental exposures to selected fibrous and particulate dusts)*. Edited by R. Lemen and J. M. Dement, pp 45–49. Illinois; Pathotox Publishers Inc
Davis, J. M. G., Beckett, S. T., Bolton, R. E., Collings, P. and Middleton, A. P. (1978). Mass and number of fibres in the pathogenesis of asbestos-related lung disease in rats. *Br. J. Cancer* **37,** 673–688
Davis, J. M. G. and Gross, P. (1973). Are ferruginous bodies an indication of atmospheric pollution by asbestos? In *Biological effects of asbestos,* edited by P. Bogorski *et al.* pp. 238–242. Lyon; International Agency for Research on Cancer
Davis, J. M. G., Gross, P. and de Treville, R. T. P. (1970). 'Ferruginous bodies' in guinea pigs. *Archs Path.* **89,** 364–373
Department of Employment and Productivity (1970). *Asbestos: Health Precautions in Industry.* Health and Safety at work, 44. London; HMSO
Dettori, G., Scansetti, G. and Gribaudo, C. (1964). 'Relievi sull' uiquinamento ambientale nell' industria del talco. *Medna Lav.* **55,** 453–455
Doll, R. (1955). Mortality from lung cancer in asbestos workers. *Br. J. ind. Med.* **12,** 81–86
Doll, R. (1971). The age distribution of cancer. Implications for models of carcinogenesis. *J. R. statist. Soc.* **134,** 133–155
Donna, A. and Cappa, A. P. M. (1967). Contributo sperimentale allo studio della pneumoconiosi da asbesto altivata pneumoconiotica dell'asbesto di chrisolito nel ratto. *Medna Lav.* **58,** 1–12
Doniach, I., Swettenham, K. V. and Hathorn, M. K. S. (1975). Prevalance of asbestos bodies in a necropsy series in East London: association with disease occupation and domiciliary address. *Br. J. ind. Med.* **32,** 16–30
Dressen, W. C., Dallavalle, J. M., Edwards, T. I. and Sayers, R. C. (1940). *Pneumoconiosis among Mica and Pegmatitie Workers.* US Pub. Hlth Serv. Publ. Hlth Bull. No. 250, Washington
Dressler, W. (1959). The post-myocardial infarction syndrome. *Archs intern. Med.* **103,** 28–42
Edenfield, R. W. (1960). A clinical and roentgenological study of kaolin workers. *Archs envir. Hlth* **1,** 392–406
Edge, J. R. (1976). Asbestos related disease in Barrow-in-Furness. *Envir. Res.* **11,** 244–247
Edge, J. R. and Choudhary, S. L. (1978). Malignant mesothelioma of the pleural in Barrow-in-Furness. *Thorax* **33,** 26–30
Eisenstadt, H. B. (1964). Asbestos pleurisy. *Dis. Chest* **46,** 78–81
Eisenstadt, H. B. (1965). Benign asbestos pleurisy. *J. Am. med. Ass.* **192,** 419–421
El-Ghawabi, S. H., El-Samra, G. H. and Mehasseb, H. (1970). Talc pneumoconiosis. *J. Egypt. med. Ass.* **53,** 330–340
Elevatorski, E. A. (1975). Wollastonite. In *Industrial minerals and rocks,* 4th edition, edited by Stanley F. Lebond, pp. 1227–1233. New York; American Institute of Mining, Metallurgical and Petroleum Engineers Inc.
Elmes, P. C. (1966). The epidemiology and clinical features of asbestosis and related diseases. *Postgrad. med. J.* **42,** 623–635
Elmes, P. C. (1974). Incorrect diagnosis of asbestosis. *Postgrad. med. J.* **50,** 250–251
Elmes, P. C. and Simpson, M. J. C. (1976). The clinical aspects of mesothelioma. *Q. J. Med.* **45,** 427–449
Elmes, P. C. and Simpson, M. J. C. (1977). Insulation workers in Belfast. A further study of mortality due to asbestos exposure (1940–75). *Br. J. ind. Med.* **34,** 174–180
Elwood, P. C. and Cochrane, A. L. (1964). A follow-up study of workers from an asbestos factory. *Br. J. ind. Med.* **21,** 304–307
Enterline, P. E. (1965). Mortality among asbestos products workers in the United States. *Ann. N.Y. Acad. Sci.* **132,** 156–165
Enterline, P. E. (1976). Estimating health risks in studies of the health risks of asbestos. *Austr. Rev. resp. Dis.* **113,** 175–180
Enterline, P. E. (1979). Mortality of workers in the man-made mineral fibre industry. Conference on Biological Effects of Minerals, Sept. 25–27, 1979. IARC, Lyon
Enterline, P. A. and Henderson, V. (1975). The health of retired fibrous glass workers. *Archs envir. Hlth* **30,** 113–116
Enterline, P. E. and Marsh, G. M. (1979). Environment and mortality of workers from a fibrous glass plant. In *Dusts and Disease.* Edited by R. Lemen and J. M. Dement. pp. 221–231. Illinois; Pathotox Publishers Inc.
Enticknap, J. B. and Smither, W. J. (1964). Peritoneal tumours in asbestosis. *Br. J. ind. Med.* **21,** 20–31
Epler, G. R., Carrington, C. B. and Gaensler, E. A. (1978). Crackles (rales) on the interstial pulmonary diseases. *Chest* **73,** 333–339
Erwteman, T. M., Braat, M. C. P. and van Aken, W. G. (1977). Interstitial pulmonary fibrosis: a new side effect of practolol. *Br. med. J.* **2,** 297–298
Esmeu, N. A., Hammad, Y. Y., Corn, M., Whittier, D., Kotsko, N., Haller, M. and Kahn, R. A. (1978). Exposure of employees to man-made mineral fibres; mineral wool production. *Envir. resp.* **15,** 262–277
Evans, C. C., Lewiasohn, H. C. and Evans, J. M. (1977). Frequency of HL-A antigens in asbestos workers with and without pulmonary fibrosis. *Br. med. J.* **1,** 603–605
Fahr, T. and Feigel, F. (1914). Kristallbildung in der Lunge. *Dt. med. Wschr.* **40,** 1548–1549
Faraone, G. and Majon, L. (1958). Determiazioni conimetriche e granulometriche nelle varie fasi lavorative della industria della pomice in Canneto-Lapari (Messina). *Acta Med. Leg. et Soc.* **11,** 83–94
Ferris, B. G., Ranadive, M. V., Peters, J. M., Murphy, L. H., Burgess, W. A. and Pendergrass, H. P. (1971). Asbestosis in ship repair workers. *Archs envir. Hlth* **23,** 220–225
Fletcher, D. E. and Edge, J. R. (1970). The early radiological changes in pulmonary and pleural asbestosis. *Clin. Radiol.* **21,** 355–365
Fondmiare, A. and Desbordes, J. (1974). Asbestos bodies and fibres in lung tissues. *Envir. Hlth Perspect.* **9,** 147–148
Fortschungbericht Asbest (1978). Untersuchungen über die Gesundheitsgefahren durch Stäube asbesthatiger Bremsbeläge. Hauptverbandes der gewerblichen Berufsgenossenschaften e.V., pp. 100–102. Bonn
Fournier-Massey, G. and Becklake, M. R. (1975). Pulmonary function profiles in Quebec asbestos workers. *Bull physio-path. resp.* **11,** 429–445
Francis, D. Jussuf, A., Mortensen, T., Sikjaer, B. and Viskum, K. (1977). Hyaline pleural plaques and asbestos bodies in 198 randomized autopsies. *Scand. J. resp. Dis.* **58,** 193–196
Gaensler, E. A. and Kaplan, A. I. (1971). Asbestos pleural effusion. *Ann. intern. Med.* **74,** 178–191
Gamble, J. F., Fellner, W. and Dimeo, M. J. (1979). An epidemiological study of a group of talc workers. *Am. Rev. resp. Dis.* **119,** 741–753
Gandevia, B. (1967). Pulmonary function in asbestos workers: a three year follow-up study. *Am. Rev. resp. Dis.* **96,** 420–427
Gärtner, H. (1947). Über Lungenbefunde bei einem Korundschmelzer. *Z. ges. Inn. Med.* **2,** 761–764

Gärtner, H. (1955). Die Bleicherde-Lunge. *Arch. Gewerbepath. Gewerbehyg.* **13,** 508–516

Gärtner, H. and von Marwyck, C. (1947). Lugenfibrose durch Sillimanit. *D. med. Wschr.* **72,** 708–710

Gaumer, H. R., Kaimal, J., Schuyler, M. and Salvaggio, J. (1979). Suppressor cell function in patients with asbestosis. *Am. Rev. resp. Dis.* **119** (Supplement), 216

Gaumer, H. R., Wilson, M. R. and Salvaggio, J. E. (1977). Activation of the alternative complement pathway by asbestos fiber. *Am. Rev. resp. Dis.* **115,** (2), 56

Gelfand, M. and Morton, S. A. (1970). Asbestosis in Rhodesia. In *Pneumoconiosis. Proceedings of the International Conference, Johannesburg, 1969,* edited by H. A. Shapiro, pp. 204–208. Cape Town; Oxford University Press

German, W. M. (1943). Dusting powder granulomas following surgery. *Surgery Gynec. Obstet.* **76,** 501–507

Gibbs, G. W. (1978). Discussion. In *Proceedings of Asbestos Symposium, Johannesburg 1977.* Edited by H. W. Glen, pp. 28–30. Department of Mines. National Institute of Metallurgy. S. Africa; Randburg

Gibbs, G. W. (1979). Etiology of pleural calcification: a study of Quebec chrysotile asbestos miners and minerals. *Archs envir. Hlth* **34,** 76–83

Gibbs, G. W., Baron, P., Beckett, S. T., Dillen, R., du Toit, R. S. J., Kuponen, M. and Robock, K. (1977). A summary of asbestos fibre counting experience in seven countries. *Ann. occup. Hyg.* **20,** 321–332

Gilson, J. C. (1966). Health hazards of asbestos. Recent studies on its biological effects. *Trans. Soc. occup. Med.* **16,** 62–74

Gilson, J. C. (1976). Asbestos cancers as an example of the problem of comparative risks. In *Environmental Pollution and Carcinogenic Risks,* p. 111. INSERM Symposia. Series Vol. 52. IARC Scientific Publications. No. 13

Gloyne, S. R. (1931). Presence of asbestosis bodies in faeces in case of pulmonary asbestosis. *Tubercle* **12,** 158–159

Gloyne, S. R. (1932–33). The morbid anatomy and histology of asbestos. *Tubercle* **14,** 445–451; 493–497; 550–558

Godeau, P., de Saint-Maur, P., Herreman, G., Rault, P., Cenac, A. and Rosenthal, P. (1974). Carcinoma bronchiolo-alvéolaire et scléroderma. *Sem. Hôp. Paris* **50,** 1161–1168

Godwin, M. C. (1957). Diffuse mesotheliomas. *Cancer* **10,** 298–319

Gold, C. (1967). A simple method of detecting asbestos in tissues. *J. clin. Path.* **20,** 674

Goldstein, B. and Rendall, R. E. G. (1970). The relative toxicities of the main classes of minerals. In *Pneumoconiosis. Proceedings of the International Conference, Johannesburg, 1969,* edited by H. A. Shapiro, pp. 429–434. Cape Town; Oxford University Press

Governa, M., Durio, G. and Comai, M. (1979). Changes in rat lung produced by olivine dust inhalation. *Pathologica* **71,** 745–753

Governa, M. and Rosanda, C. (1972). A histochemical study of the asbestos body coating. *Br. J. ind. Med.* **29,** 154–159

Government of India Ministry of Labour (1953). *Silicosis in Mica Mining in Bihar.* Report No. 3. Office of the Chief Adviser Factories

Government of India Ministry of Labour (1956). Silicosis among hand drillers in mica mining in Bihar. Report No. 12. Office of the Chief Adviser Factories

Graham, J. and Graham, R. (1967). Ovarian cancer and asbestos. *Envir. Res.* **1,** 115–128

Greaves, I. A. (1979). Rheumatoid 'pneumoconiosis' (Caplan's syndrome) in an asbestos worker: a 17 years' follow-up. *Thorax* **34,** 404–405

Green, R. A. and Dimcheff, D. G. (1974). Massive bilateral upper lobe, fibrosis secondary to asbestos exposure. *Chest* **65,** 52–55

Greenburg, L. (1947). The dust exposure in tremolite talc mining. *Yale J. biol. Med.* **19,** 481–501

Greenberg, M. and Lloyd Davies, T. A. (1974). Mesothelioma Register, 1967–1968. *Br. J. ind. Med.* **31,** 91–104

Gregor, A., Singh, S., Turner-Warwick, M., Lawler, S. and Parkes, W. R. (1979). The role of histocompatability (HLA) antigens in asbestosis. *Br. J. Dis. Chest* **73,** 245–252

Grim, R. E. (1933). Petrography of fuller's earth deposits, Olmstead, Illinois, with a brief study of some non-Illinois earths. *Econ. Geol.* **28,** 344–363

Gross, P. (1976). The biological categorization of inhaled fibre glass dust. *Archs envir. Hlth* **31,** 101–107

Gross, P. (1978). Critique of NIOSH Criteria Document on fibrous glass. *J. occup. Med.* **20,** 519–520

Gross, P., Cralley, L. J. and de Treville, R. T. P. (1967). 'Asbestos' bodies: their non-specificity. *Am. ind. Hyg. Ass. J.* **28,** 541–542

Gross, P., de Treville, R. T. P. and Haller, M. N. (1969). Pulmonary ferruginous bodies in city dwellers. *Archs envir. Hlth* **19,** 186–188

Hale, L. W., Gough, J., King, E. J. and Nagelschmidt, G. (1956). Pneumoconiosis of kaolin workers. *Br. J. ind. Med.* **13,** 251–259

Hall, D. R., Morrison, J. B. and Edwards, F. R. (1978). Pleural fibrosis after practolol therapy. *Thorax* **33,** 822–824

Hamer, D. H., Rolle, F. R. and Schelz, J. P. (1976). Characterization of talc and associated minerals. *Am. ind. Hyg. Ass. J.* **37,** 296–304

Harington, J. S. (1973). Chemical factors (including trace elements) in etiological mechanisms. In *Biological Effects of Asbestos,* edited by P. Bogovski, *et al.,* pp. 304–311. Lyon; International Agency for Research on Cancer

Harington, J. S., Gilson, J. C. and Wagner, J. C. (1971). Asbestos and mesothelioma in man. *Nature, Lond.* **232,** 54–55

Harries, P. G. (1971). *The Effects and Control of Diseases Associated with Exposure to Asbestos in Devonport Dockyard.* Gosport; Institute of Naval Medicine

Harries, P. G. (1976). Experience with asbestos disease and its control in Great Britain's naval dockyards. *Envir. res.* **11,** 261–267

Harries, P. G. and Lumley, K. P. S. (1977). Royal Naval Dockyard Asbestosis Research Project—Survey of registered asbestos workers. *J. Roy. naval Med. Serv.* **43,** 133–148

Harries, P. G., Mackenzie, F. A. F., Sheers, G., Kemp, J. H., Oliver, T. P. and Wright, D. S. (1972). Radiological survey of men exposed in naval dockyards. *Br. J. ind. Med.* **29,** 274–279

Harries, P. G., Rossiter, C. E. and Coles, R. M. (1976). Royal Naval Dockyards Asbestosis Research Project. Main morbidity study of the total population at Devonport, Chatham, Portsmouth and Rosyth dockyards. *RN Clinical Research Working Party No. 1.* Institute of Naval Med., Alverstoke, Gosport

Harwood, T. R., Gracey, D. R. and Yokoo, H. (1976). Pseudomesotheliomatous carcinoma of the lung. *Am. J. clin. Path.* **65,** 159–167

Haslam, P., Lukoszek, A., Merchant, J. A. and Turner-Warwick, M. (1978). Lymphocyte responses to phytohaemagglutinin in patients with asbestosis and pleural mesothelioma. *Clin. Exp. immun.* **31,** 178–188

Haslam, P., Turner-Warwick, M. and Lukoszek, A. (1975). Antinuclear antibody and lymphocyte responses to nuclear antigens in patients with lung disease. *Clin. Exp. Immun.* **20,** 379–395

Hasselbacher, P. (1979). Binding of immunoglobulin and activation of complement by asbestos fibres. *J. Allergy Clin. Immunol.* **64,** 294–298

Hatch, D. (1970). Possible alternative to asbestos as a friction material. *Ann. occ. Hyg.* **13,** 25–29

Health and Safety Commission. (1978a). Asbestos work on thermal and acoustic insulation and sprayed coatings. London; HMSO

Health and Safety Commission. (1978b). Asbestos. Measurement and monitoring of asbestos in air. London; HMSO

Health and Safety Executive (1979). Asbestos Vols. 1 and 2. Advisory Committee on Asbestos, Final Report. London; HMSO

Heard, B. E. and Williams, R. (1961). The pathology of asbestosis with reference to lung function. *Thorax* **16,** 264–281

Heimann, H., Moskowitz, S., Iyer, C. R. H., Gupta, M. N. and Mankiker, N. S. (1953). Note on mica dust inhalation. *Arch ind. Hyg. occ. Med.* **8,** 531–532

Henderson, W. J., Blundell, G., Richards, R., Hext, P. M., Volcani, B. E. and Griffiths, K. (1975). Ingestion of talc particles by cultured lung fibroblasts. *Envir. res.* **9**, 173–178

Henderson, W. J., Hamilton, T. C. and Griffiths, K. (1979). Talc in normal and malignant ovarian tissue. *Lancet* **1**, 499

Henderson, W. J., Joslin, C. A. F., Turnbull, A. C. and Griffiths, K. (1971). Talc and carcinoma of the ovary and cervix. *J. Obstet. Gyn. Br. Comwlth,* **78,** 266–272

Hendry, N. W. (1965). The geology, occurrences and major uses of asbestos. *Ann. N.Y. Acad. Sci.* **132,** 12–21

Hickish, D. E. and Knight, K. L. (1970). Exposure to asbestos during brake maintenance. *Ann. occup. Hyg.* **13,** 17–21

Hiett, D. M. (1978). Experimental asbestosis: an investigation of functional and pathological disturbances II. Results for chrysotile and amosite exposures. *Br. J. ind. Med.* **35,** 135–145

Highley, D. E. (1974). *Talc.* Mineral Dossier No. 10. Mineral Resources Consultative Committee. London; HMSO

Highley, D. E. (1978). Personal communication

Hildick-Smith, G. Y. (1976). The biology of talc. *Br. J. ind. Med.* **33,** 217–229

Hildick-Smith, G. Y. (1977). Talc—recent epidemiological studies. In *Inhaled Particles IV,* edited by W. H. Walton and B. McGovern, pp. 655–664. Oxford; Pergamon Press

Hill, J. W. (1977). Health aspects of man-made mineral fibres. A review. *Ann. occup. Hyg.* **20,** 161–173

Hill, J. W. (1978). Man-made mineral fibres. *J. Soc. occup. Med.* **28,** 134–141

Hill, J. W., Whitehead, W. S., Cameron, J. D. and Hedgecock, G. A. (1973). Glass fibres: absence of pulmonary hazard in production workers. *Br. J. ind. Med.* **30,** 174–179

Hinds, M. W. (1978). Mesothelioma in the United States. Incidence in the 1970s. *J. occup. Med.* **20,** 469–471

Hinds, M. W., Thomas, D. B. and O'Reilly, H. P. (1979). Asbestos, dental X-rays, tobacco and alcohol in the epidemiology of laryngeal cancer. *Cancer* **44,** 1114–1120

Hinson, K. F. W. (1958). Laboratory diagnosis. In *Carcinoma of the Lung. Neoplastic Disease at Various Sites Vol. 1,* edited by J. R. Bignall, pp. 143–150. Edinburgh and London; E. and S. Livingstone Ltd

Hinson, K. F. W. (1971). Personal communication

Hinson, K. F. W. (1972). Personal communication

Hinson, K. F. W. (1973). Personal communication

Hinson, K. F. W., Otto, H., Webster, I. and Rossiter, C. E. (1973). Criteria for the diagnosis of grading asbestosis. In *Biological Effects of Asbestos,* edited by P. Bogovski *et al.,* pp. 54–57. Oxford; Pergamon Press

Hodgson, A. A. (1966). Fibrous Silicates. Lecture Series, 1965, No. 4. London; The Royal Institute of Chemistry

Hodgson, A. A. (1977). Nature and paragenesis of asbestos minerals. *Phil. Trans. R. Soc. London* **286,** 611–624

Holt, P. F. (1957). *Pneumoconiosis,* p. 174. London; Edward Arnold

Holt, P. F. and Horns, M. (1978). Dust from carbon-fibre. *Envir. Resp.* **17,** 276–283

Holt, P. F., Mills, J. and Young, D. K. (1966). Experimental asbestosis in the guinea pig. *J. Path. Bact.* **92,** 185–195

Hopkins, G. B. and Taylor, D. G. (1970). Pulmonary talc granulomatosis. *Am. Rev. resp. Dis.* **101,** 101–104

Hounam, R. F. (1973). Investigations of airborne dust produced during the machining of glass fibre reinforced calcium silicati, insulating board and 'Marinite' asbestos reinforced board. Report by Health Physics and Medical Division. Harwell, UK; Atomic Energy Research Establishment

Hourihane, D. O'B. (1964). The pathology of mesotheliomata and an analysis of their association with asbestos exposure. *Thorax* **19,** 268–278

Hourihane, D. O'B. and McCaughey, W. T. E. (1966). Pathological aspects of asbestosis. *Postgrad. med. J.* **42,** 613–622

Hourihane, D. O'B., Lessof, L. and Richardson, P. C. (1966). Hyaline and calcified pleural plaques as an index of exposure to asbestos. A study of radiological and pathological features of 100 cases with a consideration of epidemiology. *Br. med. J.* **1,** 1069–1074

Hromek, J. (1962). Large scale incidence of characteristic pleural changes in the inhabitants of the western section of the former Jihlava region. *Rozhledy v. Tuberkulose* **22,** 405–414

Hueper, W. C. (1966). Occupational and environmental cancer of respiratory tract. *Recent Results in Cancer Research* **3,** 43–44. Berlin; Springer

Hunninghake, G. W. and Fauci, A. S. (1979). Pulmonary involvement in the collagen vascular diseases. *Am. Rev. resp. Dis.* **119,** 471–503

Hunt, A. C. (1956). Massive pulmonary fibrosis from inhalation of talc. *Thorax* **11,** 287–294

Hunter, B. and Thomson, C. (1973). Evaluation of the tumorigenic potential of vermiculite by intrapleural injection in rats. *Br. J. ind. Med.* **30,** 167–173

Huuskonen, M. S. (1978). Clinical features mortality and survival of patients with asbestosis. *Scand. J. work Env. and Hlth* **4,** 265–274

Huuskonen, M. S., Tiilikainen, A. and Alanko, K. (1979). HLA-B18 antigens and protection from pulmonary fibrosis in asbestos workers. *Br. J. Dis. Chest* **73,** 253–259

International Labour Office (1974). Asbestos: health risks and their prevention. *Occup. Safety and Health Services No. 30,* Geneva; ILO

International Union Against Cancer (1965). Working group on asbestos and cancer. *Archs envir. Hlth* **11,** 221–229

Jacko, M. G., Du Charme, R. T. and Somers, J. H. (1973). Brake and clutch emissions generated during vehicle operation. Paper 730548 Automobile Engineering Meeting, Detroit 1973. New York; Society of Automotive Engineers, Inc.

Jacob, G. and Anspach, M. (1965). Pulmonary neoplasia among Dresden asbestos workers. *Ann. N.Y. Acad. Sci.* **132,** 536–548

Jaurand, M-C., Kaplan, H., Thiollet, J., Pinchon, M-C., Bernadin, J-F and Bignon, J. (1979). Phagocytosis of chrysotile fibres by pleural mesothelial cells in culture. *Am. J. Path.* **94,** 529–532

Jodoin, G., Gibbs, G. W., Macklem, P. T., McDonald, J. C. and Becklake, M. R. (1971). Early effects of asbestos exposure on lung function. *Am. Rev. resp. Dis.* **104,** 525–535

Jones, B. M., Edwards, J. H. and Wagner, J. C. (1972). Absorption of serum proteins by inorganic dusts. *Br. J. ind. Med.* **29,** 287–292

Jones, J. S. P., Pooley, F. D. and Smith, P. G. (1976). Factory populations exposed to crocidolite asbestos: a continuing enquiry. In *Environmental Pollution and Carcinogenic Risks,* edited by C. Rosenfeld and W. Davis, pp. 117–120. Lyon; International Agency for Research on Cancer

Jones, J. S. P. and Sheers, G. (1973). Pleural plaques. In *Biological Effects of Asbestos,* edited by P. Bogovski *et al.,* pp. 243–248. Lyon; International Agency for Research on Cancer

Jötten, K. W. and Eickhoff, W. (1944). Lungenveränderungen durch Sillimanistaub. *Arch. Gewerbepath. Gewerbehyg.* **12,** 223–232

Kagan, E., Solomon, A., Cochrane, J. C., Kuba, P., Rocks, P. H. and Webster, I. (1977a). Immunological studies of patients with asbestosis. II studies in circulating lymphoid cell numbers and humoral immunity. *Clin. exp. Immun.* **28,** 268–275

Kagan, E., Solomon, A., Cochrane, J. C., Beissner, E. I., Gluckman, J., Rocks, P. H. and Webster, I. (1977b). Immunological studies of patients with asbestosis. I studies of cell-mediated immunity. *Clin. exp. Immun.* **28,** 261–267

Kang, K. Y., Sera, Y., Okochi, T. and Yamamura, Y. (1974). T lymphocytes in asbestosis. *New Engl. J. Med.* **291,** 735–736

Kang, K. Y., Yagura, T., Sera, Y., Yokoyama, K. and Yamamura, Y. (1973). Antinuclear factor in pneumoconioses and idiopathic pulmonary fibrosis. *Med. J. Osaka Univ.* **23,** 249–256

Kannerstein, M. and Churg, J. (1972). Pathology of carcinoma of the lung associated with asbestos exposure. *Cancer* **30,** 14–21

Kannerstein, M. and Churg, J. (1977). Peritoneal mesothelioma *Human Path.* **8,** 83–94

Kannerstein, M., Churg, J. and Magner, D. (1973). Histochemistry in the diagnosis of malignant mesothelioma. *Ann. Clin. Lab. Sci.* **3,** 207–211

Kannerstein, M., Churg, J., McCaughey, W. T. E. and Selikoff, I. J. (1977). Pathogenic effects of asbestos. *Arch. Path. Lab. Med.* **101,** 623–628

Kauffman, S. L. and Stout, A. P. (1964). Mesothelioma in children. *Cancer* **17,** 539–544

Kaw, J. L. and Zaidi, S. H. (1973). Effect of mica dust on the lungs of rats. *Exp. Path.* **8,** 224–231

Kay, S. and Silverberg, S. G. (1971). Ultrastructural studies of a malignant fibrous mesothelioma of the pleura. *Arch. Path.* **92,** 449–455

Keal, E. E. (1960). Asbestosis and abdominal neoplasms. *Lancet* **2,** 1211–1216

Keane, W. T. and Zavon, M. R. (1966). Occupational hazards of pipe insulators. *Archs envir. Hlth* **13,** 171–184

Kettle, E. H. (1934). Infective pneumoconiosis: infective silicatosis. *J. Path. Bact.* **38,** 201–208

King, E. J., Gilchrist, M. and Rae, M. V. (1947). Tissue reaction to sericite and shale dusts treated with hydrochloric acid: an experimental investigation. *J. Path. Bact.* **59,** 324–327

King, E. J., Harrison, C. V. and Nagelschmidt, G. (1948). Effect of kaolin on the lungs of rats. *J. Path. Bact.* **60,** 435–440

King, E. J., Rogers, N., Gilchrist, M., Goldschmidt, V. W. and Nagelschmidt, G. (1945). The effect of olivine on the lungs of rats. *J. Path. Bact.* **57,** 488–491

Kipling, M. D. and Bech, A. D. (1960). Talc pneumoconiosis. *Trans. Ass. ind. med. Offrs* **10,** 85–93

Kilviluoto, R. (1960). Pleural calcification as a roentgenologic sign of non-occupational anthophyllite-asbestosis. *Acta radiol.,* Suppl. 494

Kiviluoto, R. and Meurman, L. (1969). Results of asbestos exposure in Finland. In *Pneumoconiosis. Proceedings of the International Conference, Johannesburg 1969,* edited by H. A. Shapiro, pp. 190–191. Cape Town; Oxford University Press

Kiviluoto, R., Meurman, L. O. and Hakama, M. (1979). Pleural plaques and neoplasia in Finalnd. *Ann. N.Y. Acad. Sci.* **330,** 31–33

Kleinfield, M. (1966). Pleural calcifications as a sign of silicatosis. *Am. J. med. Sci.* **251,** 215–224

Kleinfeld, M., Giel, C. P., Majeranowski, J. F. and Messite, J. (1963). Talc pneumoconiosis. *Archs envir. Hlth* **7,** 101–115

Kleinfeld, M., Giel, C. P., Majeranowski, J. F. and Shapiro, J. (1964a). Pulmonary ventilatory function in talcosis of the lung. *Dis. Chest* **46,** 592–598

Kleinfeld, M., Giel, C. P., Majeranowski, J. F. and Zaki, M. H. (1967). Mortality among talc miners and millers in New York State. *Archs envir. Hlth* **14,** 663–667

Kleinfeld, M., Giel, C. P., Shapiro, J. and Swencicki, R. (1965). Effect of talc duct inhalation on lung function. *Archs envir. Hlth* **10,** 431–437

Kleinfeld, M., Giel, C. P., Shapiro, J., Kooyman, O. and Swencicki, R. (1964b). Lung function in talc workers. *Archs envir. Hlth* **9,** 559–566

Kleinfeld, M., Messite, J. and Langer, A. M. (1973). A study of workers exposed to asbestiform minerals in commercial talc manufacture. *Envir. res.* **6,** 132–143

Kleinfeld, M., Messite, J. and Zaki, M. H. (1974). Mortality experiences among talc workers: a follow-up study. *J. occup. Med.* **16,** 345–349

Klingholz, R. (1977). Technology and production of man-made mineral fibres. *Ann. occup. Hyg.* **20,** 153–159

Knight, K. L. and Hickish, D. E. (1970). Investigation into alternative forms of control of dust generated during the cleaning of brake drum assemblies and drums. *Ann. occup. Hyg.* **13,** 37–39

Knox, J. F., Doll, R. S. and Hill, I. D. (1965). Cohort analysis of changes in incidence of bronchial carcinoma in a textile asbestos factory. *Ann. N.Y. Acad. Sci.* **132,** 526–535

Knox, J. F., Holmes, S., Doll, R. and Hill, I. D. (1968). Mortality from lung cancer and other causes among workers in an asbestos textile factory. *Br. J. ind. Med.* **25,** 293–303

Konietzko, N., Gerke, E. and Schlehe, H. (1974). Verschlussvolumen bei asbestaubexponierten. *Prax Pneumol.* **28,** 829–831

Lancet (1979). Health risks of man-made mineral fibres. Health and Safety Commission. **2,** 162

Lange, A. (1980a). An epidemiological survey of immunological abnormalities in asbestos workers. I. Nonorgan and organ-specific autoantibodies. *Environ. Res.* **22,** 162–175

Lange, A. (1980b). An epidemiological survey of immunological abnormalities in asbestos workers. Serum immunoglobulin levels. *Environ. Res.* **22,** 176–183

Lange, A. and Skibinski, G. (1977). T and B cells and delayed-type skin reactions in asbestos workers. *Scand. J. Immunol.* **6,** 720

Lange, A., Smolik, R., Chmielarczyk, W., Garncarek, D. and Gielgier, Z. (1978). Cellular immunity in asbestosis. *Arch. immunol. Therap. Exp.* **26,** 899–903

Langer, A. M., Rubin, I. and Selikoff, I. J. (1970). Electron microprobe analysis of asbestos bodies. In *Pneumoconiosis. Proceedings of the International Conference, Johannesburg, 1969,* edited by H. A. Shapiro, pp. 57–69. Cape Town; Oxford University Press

Langer, A. M., Baden, V., Hammond, E. C. and Selikoff, I. J. (1971). Inorganic fibres, including chrysotile in lungs at autopsy; preliminary report. In *Inhaled Particles, III,* edited by W. H. Walton, pp. 683–692. Woking; Unwin

Langlands, J. H. M., Wallace, W. F. M. and Simpson, M. J. C. (1971). Insulation workers in Belfast. 2. Morbidity in men still at work. *Br. J. ind. Med.* **28,** 217–225

Leading article (1978a). Television Medicine. *Br. med. J.* **1,** 323–324

Leading article (1978b). Respiratory complications of rheumatoid disease. *Br. med. J.* **1,** 1437–1438

Leathart, G. L. (1960). Clinical, bronchographic, radiological and physiological observations in ten cases of asbestosis. *Br. J. ind. Med.* **17,** 213–225

Leathart, G. L. (1968). Pulmonary function tests in asbestos workers. *Trans. Soc. occup. Med.* **18,** 49–55

Le Bouffant, L., Bruyere, S., Martin, J. C., Tichonx, G. and Normand, C. (1976). Quelques observations sur les fibres d'amiante et les formations minerals diverses rencontrees dans les poumons asbestosiques. *Rev. Fr. Mal. Resp.* **4** (Suppl. 2), 121–140

Le Bouffant, L., Martin, J. C., Durif, S. and Daniel, H. (1973). Structure and composition of pleural plaques. In *Biological Effects of Asbestos,* edited by P. Bogovski *et al.,* pp. 249–257. Lyon; Intern. Agency for Res. on Cancer

Legrand, M. and Pariente, R. (1974). Ultrastructural study of pleural fluid in mesothelioma. *Thorax* **29,** 164–171

Leménanger, J., Rousselot, P., Mandard, J. C., Le Bouffant, L. and Borel, B. (1976). Les pleurésies bénignes de l'asbeste. *Rev. Fr. Mal. Resp.* **4** (Suppl. 2), 75–86

Lesser, M., Zia, M. and Kilburn, K. H. (1978). Silicosis in kaolin workers and firebrick makers. *S. med. J.* **71,** 1242–1246

Lewinsohn, H. C. (1974). Early malignant changes in pleural plaques due to asbestos exposure: a case report. *Br. J. Dis. Chest* **68,** 121–127

Lewinsohn, H. C. (1977). Asbestosis—a diagnostic enigma. *J. occup. Med.* **19,** 607–610

Libshitz, H. I., Wershba, M. S., Atkinson, G. and Southard, M. E. (1974). Asbestos and carcinoma of the larynx. *J. Am. med. Ass.* **228,** 1571–1572

Low, R. B. (1978). Effects of kaolinite on amino acid transport in incorporation into protein by rabbit pulmonary alveolar macrophages. *Am. Rev. resp. Dis.* **117**Suppl. (abstract), 243

Lüchtrath, H. and Schmidt, K. G. (1959). Uber Talkum und Steatit, ihre Beziehungen zum Asbest Sowie ihre Wirhung beim intrachealer Tierrersuch an Ratten. *Beitr Silikosforsch.* **61,** 1–60

Lumley, K. P. S. (1971). Asbestos dust levels inside firefighting helmets with chrysotile asbestos covers. *Ann. occup. Hyg.* **14,** 285–286

Lumley, K. P. S. (1977). Physiological changes in asbestos pleural disease. In *Inhaled Particles IV,* edited by W. H. Walton and B. McGovern, pp. 781–787. Oxford; Pergamon Press

Lumley, K. P. S., Harries, P. G. and O'Kelley, F. J. (1971). Buildings insulated with sprayed asbestos: a potential hazard. *Ann. occup. Hyg.* **14,** 255–257

Lynch, J. R. (1968). Brake lining decomposition products. *J. Air Pollut. Control Ass.* **18,** 824–826

Lynch, K. M. and Cannon, W. M. (1948). Asbestosis: VI Analysis of forty necropsied cases. *Dis. Chest* **14,** 874–885

Lynch, K. M. and McIver, F. A. (1954). Pneumoconiosis from exposure to kaolin dust. *Am. J. Path.* **30,** 1117–1127

Lynch, K. M. and Smith, W. A. (1935). Pulmonary asbestosis: carcinoma of the lung in asbesto-silicosis. *Am. J. Cancer* **24,** 56–64

Mackenzie, F. A. F. and Harries, P. G. (1970). Changing attitudes to the diagnosis of asbestos disease. *J. R. nav. med. Serv.* **56,** 116–123

McCaughey, W. T. E. (1965). Criteria for diagnosis of diffuse mesothelial tumours. *Ann. N.Y. Acad. Sci.* **132,** 603–613

McDonald, A. D. (1980). Mineral fibre content of the lung in mesothelial tumours. In *Biological Effects of Mineral Fibres.* WHO/International Agency for Research on Cancer, Lyon (In press)

McDonald, A. D. and McDonald, J. C. (1980). Malignant mesothelioma in North America. *Cancer* **46,** 1650–1656

McDonald, A. D. and McDonald, J. C. (1977b). Mesothelioma and asbestos-fibre type. *Am. Rev. resp. Dis.* **115** (Suppl.) 229

McDonald, A. D., Magner, D. and Eyssen, G. (1973). Primary malignant mesothelial tumours in Canada, 1960–1968. *Cancer* **31,** 869–876

McDonald, J. C. (1973a). Asbestosis in chrysotile mines and mills. In *Biological Effects of Asbestos,* edited by Bogovski *et al.,* pp. 155–159. Lyon; Intern. Agency for Res. on Cancer

McDonald, J. C. (1973b). Cancer in chrysotile mines and mills. In *Biological Effects of Asbestos,* edited by P. Bogovski *et al.,* pp. 189–194. Lyon; Intern. Agency for Res. on Cancer

McDonald, J. C. (1980). Asbestos and lung cancer: has the case been proven? *Chest* **78,** 374–376

McDonald, J. C., Liddell, F. D. K., Gibbs, G. W., Eyssen, G. E. and McDonald, A. D. (1980). Dust exposure and mortality in chrysotile mining, 1910–1975. *Br. J. ind. Med.* **37,** 11–24

McDonald, J. C. and McDonald, A. D. (1977a). Epidemiology of mesothelioma from estimated incidence. *Prev. Med.* **6,** 426–446

McDonald, J. C., Backlake, M. R., Gibbs, G. W., McDonald, A. D. and Rossiter, C. E. (1974). The health of chrysotile asbestos mine and mill workers of Quebec. *Archs envir. Hlth* **28,** 61–68

McLaughlin, A. I. G., Rogers, E. and Dunham, K. C. (1949). Talc pneumoconiosis. *Br. J. ind. Med.* **6,** 184–194

McMichael, A. J. (1978). Increases in laryngeal cancer in Britain and Australia in relation to alcohol and tobacco consumption trends. *Lancet* **1,** 1244–1246

McMillan, G. H. G., Sheers, G. and Pethybridge, R. (1978). A radiological follow-up study of the effect of asbestos in dockyard workers in Devonport. *J. Roy. naval Med. Serv.* **64,** 88–104

McNally, W. D. and Trostler, I. S. (1941). Severe pneumoconiosis caused by inhalation of fuller's earth. *J. ind. Hyg. Toxicol.* **23,** 118–126

McNulty, J. C. (1968). Asbestos mining Wittenoom, Western Australia. In *First Australian Pneumoconiosis Conference, 1968,* pp. 447–474. Sydney; Joint Coal Board

Mányai, S., Kabai, J., Kis, J., Süveges, E. and Timàr, M. (1970). The effect of heat treatment on the structure of kaolin and its *in vitro* haemolytic activity. *Envir. Res.* **3,** 187–198

Marchand, F. (1907). Uber eigentümliche Pigmentkristalle in den: lungen. *Ver. Deutsch Path. Gesell* **10,** 223–228

Maroudas, N. G., O'Neill, C. H. and Stanton, M. F. (1973). Fibroblast anchorage in carcinogenesis by fibres. *Lancet* **1,** 807–809

Martin, J. C., Daniel, H. and Le Bouffant, L. (1977). Short and long term experimental study of the toxicity of coal-mine dust and some of its constituents. In *Inhaled Particles IV,* edited by W. H. Walton and B. McGovern, pp. 361–370. Oxford; Pergamon Press

Matej, H. and Lange, A. (1976). HLA and diseases. First International Symposium on HLA and Diseases. 256 Paris; INSERM

Mattson, S. B. (1971). Caplan's syndrome in association with asbestosis. *Scand. J. resp. Dis.* **52,** 153–161

Merchant, J. A., Klouda, P. T., Soutar, C. A., Parkes, W. R., Lawler, S. D. and Turner-Warwick, M. (1975). The HL-A system in asbestos workers. *Br. med. J.* **1,** 189–191

Merewether, E. R. A. (1949). *Annual Report Chief Inspector of Factories, 1947.* London; HMSO

Merewether, E. R. A. and Price, C. W. (1930). *Report on Effects of Asbestos on the Lungs and Dust Suppression in the Asbestos Industry.* London; HMSO

Meurman, L. (1966). Asbestos bodies and pleural plaques in a Finnish series of autopsy cases. *Acta path. microbiol. scand.* Suppl. 181

Meurman, L. O. (1968). Pleural fibrocalcific plaques and asbestos exposure. *Envir. Res.* **2,** 30–46

Meurman, L. O., Kivilnoto, R. and Hakama, M. (1974). Mortality and morbidity among the working population of anthophyllite miners in Finland. *Br. J. ind. Med.* **31,** 105–112

Meyer, E. C. and Liebow, A. A. (1965). Relationship of interstitial pneumonia honey-combing and atypical epithelial proliferation to cancer of the lung. *Cancer* **18,** 323–350

Middleton, E. L. (1936). Industrial pulmonary disease due to the inhalation of dust. *Lancet* **2,** 59–64

Middleton, A. P. (1978). On the occurrence of fibres of calcium sulphate resembling amphibole asbestos in samples taken for the evaluation of airborne asbestos. *Ann. occup. Hyg.* **21,** 91–93

Miller, A., Teirstein, A. S., Bader, M. E., Bader, R. A. and Selikoff, I. J. (1971). Talc pneumoconiosis. Significance of sublight microscopic mineral particles. *Am. J. Med.* **50,** 395–402

Miller, A. B. (1978). Asbestos fibre dust and gastro-intestinal malignancies review of literature with regard to a cause/effect relationship. *J. chron. Dis.* **31,** 23–33

Miller, K. (1979). Alterations in the suface-related phenomena of alveolar macrophages following inhalation of crocidolite asbestos and quartz dusts: an overview. *Envir. Res.* **20,** 162–182

Miller, K. and Kagan, E. (1976). The *in vivo* effects of asbestos on macrophage membrane structure and population characteristics of macrophages: a scanning electron microscope study. *J. retic. Soc.* **20,** 159–171

Miller, K. and Kagan, E. (1977). Immune adherence reactivity of rat alveolar macrophages following inhalation of crocidolite asbestos. *Clin. exp. Immun.* **29,** 152–158

Miller, K., Webster, I., Handfield, R. I. M. and Skikne, M. I. (1978). Ultrastructure of the lung in the rat following exposure to crocidolite asbestos and quartz. *J. Path.* **124,** 39–44

Millman, N. (1947). Pneumoconiosis due to talc in the cosmetic industry. *Occup. Med.* **4,** 391–394

Milne, J. E. H. (1976). Thirty two cases of mesothelioma in Victoria, Australia: a retrospective survey related to occupational asbestos exposure. *Br. J. ind. Med.* **33,** 115–122

Ministry of Labour (1967). *Problems Arising from the Use of Asbestos.* HM Factory Inspectorate. London; HMSO

Morgan, A., Davies, P., Wagner, J. C., Berry, G. and Holmes, A. (1977). The biological effects of magnesium-leached chrysotile asbestos. *Br. J. exp. Path.* **58,** 465–473

Morgan, A. and Holmes, A. (1980). Concentrations and dimensions of coated and uncoated asbestos fibres in human lungs. *Br. J. ind. Med.* **37,** 25–32

Morgan, A., Holmes, A. and Gold, C. (1971). Studies of the solubility of constituents of chrysotile asbestos *in vivo* using radioactive tracer techniques. *Envir. Res.* **4,** 558–570

Morgan, A., Talbot, R. J. and Holmes, A. (1978). Significance of fibre length in the clearance of asbestos fibres from the lung. *Br. J. ind. Med.* **35,** 146–153

Morgan, R. W. and Shettigara, P. T. (1976). Occupational asbestos exposure, smoking and laryngeal carcinoma. *Ann. N.Y. Acad. Sci.* **271,** 308–310

Morgan, W. K. C. (1964). Rheumatoid pneumoconiosis in association with asbestosis. *Thorax,* **19,** 433–435

Moskowitz, R. (1970). Talc pneumoconiosis: a treated case. *Chest* **58,** 37–41

Muldoon, B. C. and Turner-Warwick, M. W. (1972). Lung function studies in asbestos workers. *Br. J. Dis. Chest* **66,** 121–132

Mumpton, F. A. (1975). Commercial utilization of natural zeolites. In *Industrial Minerals and Rocks,* 4th edition, edited by Stanley J. Lebond, pp. 1262–1274. New York; American Institute of Mining, Metallurgical and Petroleum Engineers, Inc.

Murphy, R. (1980). Asbestos related disease: difficulties in diagnosing occupationally related illness. Frontiers in medicine 9. *Comprehensive Therapy* **6,** 6–13

Murphy, R. L. H., Ferris, B. G., Burgess, W. A., Worcester, J. and Gaensler, E. A. (1971b). Effects of low concentration of asbestos: clinical environmental, radiological and epidemiological observations in shipyard covered and pipe controls. *New Engl. J. Med.* **285,** 1271–1278

Murphy, R. L. H., Gaensler, E. A., Ferris, B. G., Fitzgerald, M., Solliday, N. and Morrisey, W. (1978). Diagnosis of Asbestosis. Observations from a longitudinal survey of shipyard pipe coverers. *Am. J. Med.* **65,** 488–498

Murphy, R. L., Levine, B. W., Faio, J. A. B., Lynch, J. and Burgess, W. A. (1971a). Floor tile installation as a source of asbestos exposure. *Am. Rev. resp. Dis.* **104,** 576–580

Murphy, R. L. H., Jr., Gaensler, E. A., Redding, R. A., Keelan, P. J., Smith, A. A., Goff, A. M. and Ferris, B. G. (1972). Low exposure to asbestos. Gas exchange in ship pipe coverers and controls. *Archs envir. Hlth* **25,** 253–264

Murray, M. (1907). Report, Department, Commission on Compensation of Industrial Disease. Cd. 3496, pp. 127–128. London; HMSO

Nash, D. T. and Nash, S. D. (1978). Talcosis and coronary artery disease. *Mt. Sinai J. Med. (NY)* **45,** 265–270

Nasr, A. N. M., Ditchek, T. and Scholtens, P. A. (1971). The prevalence of radiographic abnormalities in the chest of fibre glass workers. *J. occup. Med.* **13,** 371–376

National Cancer Institute. (1975). Third National Cancer Survey: Incidence Data. Ed. by S. J. Cutler and J. L. Young Jr. *Nat. Cancer Inst. Monogr.* **41,** 1–454

Navrátil, M. and Dobiáš, J. (1973). Development of pleural hyalinosis in lung from studies of persons exposed to asbestos dust. *Envir. Res.* **6,** 455–472

Navrátil, M., Moravkova, K. and Trippe, F. (1978). Follow-up study of pleural hyalinosis in individuals not exposed to asbestos dust. *Envir. Res.* **15,** 108–118

Newhouse, M. L. (1969). A study of the mortality of workers in an asbestos factory. *Br. J. ind. Med.* **26,** 294–301

Newhouse, M. L. (1973). Asbestos in the work place and the community. *Ann. occup. Hyg.* **16,** 97–107

Newhouse, M. L. (1977). The grographical pathology of mesothelial tumours. *J. occup. Med.* **19,** 480–482

Newhouse, M. L. and Berry, G. (1976). Predictions of mortality from mesothelial tumours in asbestos factory workers. *Br. J. ind. Med.* **33,** 147–151

Newhouse, M. L., Berry, G. and Skidmore, J. W. (1980). A mortality study of workers manufacturing friction materials with chrysotile asbestos. *Inhaled Particles and Vapours V.* Pergamon, Oxford. (In press)

Newhouse, M. L., Gregory, M. M. and Shannon, H. (1979). Aetiology of carcinoma of the larynx. Conference on Biological Effects of Mineral Fibres, September 25–27, 1979. Lyon; IARC

Newhouse, M. L. and Thompson, H. (1965). Mesothelioma of pleura and peritoneum following exposure to asbestos in the London area. *Br. J. ind. Med.* **22,** 261–269

Newhouse, M. L., Berry, G., Wagner, J. C. and Turok, M. E. (1972). A study of the mortality of female asbestos workers. *Br. J. ind. Med.* **29,** 134–141

New York City Department of Air Resources (1971). Spraying of asbestos prohibited, local law 49. In *Air Pollution Control Code of the City of New York,* sect. 1403, 2–9. 11(B)

Nicholls, A. J., Friend, J. A. R. and Legge, J. S. (1980). Sarcoid pleural effusion: three cases and review of the literature. *Thorax* **35,** 277–281

Nicholson, W. J. (1976). Case study 1: asbestos—the TLV approach. *Ann. N.Y. Acad. Soc.* **271,** 152–169

Noro, L. (1968). Occupational and 'non-occupational' asbestosis in Finland. *Am. Ind. Hyg. Ass. J.* **29,** 195–201

Pancheri, G. and Zanetti, E. (1963). L'aspetto radiologico della silicosi da pomice (liparosi). *Rass. med. ind.* **32,** 432–445

Patterson, S. H. and Murray, H. H. (1975). Clays. In *Industrial Minerals and Rocks,* 4th edition, edited by Stanley J. Lefond, pp. 519–595. New York; American Institute of Mining, Metallurgical and Petroleum Engineers, Inc.

Pearce, A. G. E. (1968). *Histochemistry. Theoretical and Applied.* London; Churchill

Peress, L., Hoag, H., White, F. and Becklake, M. R. (1975). The relationship between closing volume, smoking and asbestos dust exposure. *Clin. Res.* **23,** (Abstract), 647A

Peto, J. (1978). The hygiene standard for chrysotile asbestos. *Lancet* **1,** 484–489

Peto, J. (1979). Dose-response relationship for asbestos-related disease: implications for hygiene standards. Part II. Mortality. *Ann. N.Y. Acad. Sci.* **330,** 195–203

Peto, J., Doll, R., Howard, S. V., Kinlen, L. J. and Lewinsohn, H. C. (1977). A mortality study among workers in an English asbestos factory. *Br. J. ind. Med.* **34,** 169–173

Pettinati, L., Coscia, G. C., Francia, A. and Ghemi, F. (1964). Aspetti radiologie clinici della pneumoconiosi nell' industria estrattiva del talco. *Medna Lav.* **55,** 58–63

Phibbs, B. P., Sundin, R. E. and Mitchell, R. S. (1971). Silicosis in Wyoming betonite workers. *Am. Rev. resp. Dis.* **103,** 1–17

Phillips, L. N. (1968). Carbon fibre reinforced plastics. *Chem. ind.* 526–528

Phillipson, I. M. (1980). Talc quality. *Lancet* **1,** 48

Pierce, R. and Turner-Warwick, M. (1980). Skin tests with tuberculin (PPD), *Candida albicans* and Trichophyton spp. in cryptogenic fibrosing alveolitis and asbestos related lung disease. *Clin. Allergy* **10,** 229–237

Pimentel, J. C. and Menezes, A. P. (1978). Pulmonary and hepatic granulomatous disorders due to the inhalation of current and mica dusts. *Thorax* **33,** 219–227

Pincus, J. H. (1978). Hyperventilation syndrome. *Br. J. hosp. Med.* **19,** 312–313

Policard, A. and Collet, A. (1954). Étude experimentale des effets pathologique du kaolin. *Schweiz. Zr. allg. Path. Bakt.* **17,** 320–325

Pooley, F. D. (1972). Electron microscope characteristics of inhaled chrysotile asbestos fibre. *Br. J. ind. Med.* **29,** 146–153

Pooley, F. D. (1973a). Methods for assessing asbestos fibres and asbestos bodies in tissue by electron microscopy. In *Biological Effects of Asbestos,* edited by P. Bogovski *et al.,* pp. 50–53. Lyon; International Agency for Research on Cancer

Pooley, F. D. (1973b). Mesothelioma in relation to exposure. In *Biological Effects of Asbestos,* edited by P. Bogovski *et al.,* pp. 222–225. Lyon; International Agency for Research on Cancer

Pooley, F. D. (1975). The identification of asbestos dust with an electron microscope microprobe analyses. *Ann. occup. Hyg.* **18,** 181–186

Pooley, F. D. (1976). An examination of the fibrous mineral content of asbestos lung tissue from the Canadian chrysotile mining industry. *Envir. Res.* **12,** 281–298

Pooley, F. D. (1979). Evaluation of fiber samples taken from the vicinity of two villages in Turkey. In *Dusts and Disease.* Edited by R. Lemen and J. M. Dement. pp. 41–44. Illinois; Pathotox Inc.

Pooley, F. D., Oldham, P. D., Chang-Hyun Um and Wagner, J. C. (1970). The detection of asbestos in tissues. In *Pneumoconiosis. Proceedings of the International Conference, Johannesburg, 1969,* edited by H. A. Shapiro, pp. 108–116. Cape Town; Oxford University Press

Pooley, F. D. and Rowlands, N. (1977). Chemical and physical properties of British talc powders. In *Inhaled Particles IV,* edited by W. H. Walton and B. McGovern, pp. 639–646. Oxford; Pergamon Press

Pott, F., Huth, F. and Friedrich, K. H. (1974). Tumorigenic effect of fibrous dusts in experimental animals. *Envir. Hlth Perspect.* **9,** 313–315

Raunio, V. (1966). Occurrence of unusual pleural calcification in Finland. *Ann. Med. Inter. Fenn* **55** (Suppl), 47

Reeves, A. L., Puro, H. E., Smith, R. G. and Vorwald, A. J.

(1971). Experimental asbestos carcinogenesis. *Envir. Res.* **4**, 496–511

Regan, G. M., Tagg, B. and Thomson, M. L. (1967). Subjective assessment and objective measurement of finger clubbing. *Lancet* **1**, 530–800

Report of the Advisory Committee on Asbestos Cancers to the Director of the International Agency for Research on Cancer. (1973). In *Biological Effects of Asbestos*, edited by P. Bogovski *et al.*, pp. 341–346. Lyon; International Agency for Research on Cancer

Research Committee of the British Thoracic Association and the Medical Research Council Pneumoconiosis Unit (1979). A survey of the long-term effects of talc and kaolin pleurodesis. *Br. J. Dis. Chest* **73**, 285–288

Rickards, A. G. and Barrett, G. M. (1958). Rheumatoid lung changes associated with asbestosis. *Thorax* **13**, 185–193

Rickards, A. L. and Badami, D. V. (1971). Chrysotile asbestos in urban air. *Nature, Lond.* **234**, 93–94

Roberts, G. A. (1976). Distant visceral metastasis in pleural mesothelioma. *Br. J. Dis. Chest* **70**, 246–250

Roberts, G. B. S. (1947). Granuloma of the fallopian tube due to surgical glove talc. Siliceous granuloma. *Br. J. Surg.* **34**, 417–423

Roberts, G. H. (1971). The pathology of parietal pleural plaques. *J. clin. Path.* **24**, 348–353

Roberts, G. H. and Campbell, G. M. (1972). Exfoliative cytology of diffuse mesothelioma. *J. clin. Path.* **25**, 577–582

Roe, F. J. C., Walters, M. A. and Harington, J. S. (1966). Tumour initiation by natural and contaminating asbestos oils. *Int. J. Cancer.* **1**, 491–495

Roe, L. A. (1975). Talc and pyrophyllite. In *Industrial Minerals and Rocks*, 4th edition, edited by Stanley J. Lefond *et al.*, pp. 1127–1147. New York; American Institute of Mining, Metallurgical and Petroleum Engineers, Inc.

Rohl, A. N., Langer, A. M., Klimentidis, R., Wolff, M. S. and Selikoff, I. J. (1977). Asbestos content of dust encountered in brake maintenance and repair. *Proc. R. Soc. Med.* **70**, 32–37

Rohl, A. N., Langer, A. M., Selikoff, I. J., Tordini, A., Klimentidis, R., Bowes, D. R. and Skinner, D. L. (1976). Consumer talcums and powders: mineral and chemical characterization. *J. Toxicol. envir. Hlth* **2**, 255–284

Rosenow, E. C. (1972). The spectrum of drug-induced pulmonary disease. *Ann. intern. Med.* 977–991

Ross, J. G. (1931). *Chrysotile Asbestos in Canada*, pp. 128–130. Ottawa; Canada Dept of Mines

Rossiter, C. E. (1972). Evidence of dose-response relation in pneumoconiosis. *Trans. Soc. occup. Med.* **22**, 83–87

Rossiter, C. E. (1977). Workshop on the biological effects of man-made mineral fibres (MMMF). Current and future research. Round table discussions. *Ann. occup. Hyg.* **20**, 179–187

Rossiter, C. E. and Berry, G. (1978). The interaction of asbestos exposure and smoking on respiratory health. *Bull. europ. physiopath. resp.* **14**, 197–204

Rossiter, C. E., Bristol, L. J., Cartier, P. H., Gilson, J. C., Grainger, T. R., Sluis-Cremer, G. K. and McDonald, J. C. (1972). Radiographic changes in chrysotile asbestos mine and mill workers in Quebec. *Archs envir. Hlth* **24**, 388–400

Rossiter, C. E., Heath, J. R. and Harries, P. G. (1980). Royal naval dockyards asbestosis research project. Nine-year follow-up study of men exposed to asbestos in Devonport dockyard. *J. R. Soc. Med.* **73**, 337–344

Rous, V. and Studený, J. (1970). Aetiology of pleural plaques. *Thorax* **25**, 270–284

Rubino, G. F., and Scansetti, G., Piolatto, G. and Romano, C. A. (1976). Mortality study of talc miners and millers. *J. occup. Med.* **18**, 186–193

Rubino, G. F., Scansetti, G., Piolatto, G. and Gay, G. (1979). Mortality and morbidity among talc miners and millers in Italy. In *Dusts and Disease*. Edited by R. Lemen and J. M. Dement, pp. 357–363. Illinois; Pathotox Publishers Inc.

Sakula, A. (1961). Pneumoconiosis due to fuller's earth. *Thorax* **16**, 176–179

Samet, J. M., Epler, G. R., Gaensler, E. A. and Rosner, B. (1979). Absence of synergism between exposure to asbestos and cigarette smoking in asbestosis. *Am. Rev. resp. Dis.* **120**, 75–82

Sano, M. E., Weiss, E. and Gault, E. S. (1950). Pleural mesothelioma. *J. thorac. Surg.* **19**, 783–788

Saracci, R. (1977). Asbestos and lung cancer: an analysis of the epidemiological evidence on the asbestos-smoking interaction. *Int. J. Cancer* **20**, 323–331

Sayers, R. R. and Dreesen, W. C. (1939). Asbestosis. *Am. J. publ. Hlth* **29**, 205–214

Schepers, G. W. H. (1959). Pulmonary histologic reactions to inhaled fiberglass-plastic dust. *Ann. J. Path.* **35**, 1169–1183

Schepers, G. W. H. and Delahant, A. B. (1955). An experimental study of the effects of glass wool on animal lungs. *Arch. Ind. Hlth* **12**, 276–279

Schepers, G. W. H. and Durkan, T. M. (1955a). The effects of inhaled talc-mining dust on the human lung. *Archs ind. Hlth* **12**, 182–197

Schepers, G. W. H. and Durkan, T. M. (1955b). An experimental study of the effects of talc dust on animal tissue. *Archs ind. Hlth* **12**, 317–328

Schmidt, K. G. and Lüchtrath, H. (1958). Die Wirkung von frischen und gebranntem Kaolin auf die Lunge und das Bauchfell von Ratten. *Beitr. Silikosforsch.* **58**, 1–37

Schwartz, L., Tulipan, L. and Birmingham, D. J. (1957). *Occupational Diseases of the Skin*, 3rd edition, p. 846. London; Kimpton

Scott, J. K. and Hunt, R. (1975). The diagnosis of asbestosis. *Br. J. Dis. Chest* **69**, 51–56

Seal, R. M. E. (1980). Current views on pathological aspects of asbestosis. The unresolved questions and problems. In *Biological Effects of Mineral Fibres*. WHO/International Agency for Research on Cancer, Lyon (In press)

Seaton, D. (1977). Regional lung function in asbestos workers. *Thorax* **32**, 40–44

Sébastien, P., Bignon, J., Gaudichet, A., Dufour, G. and Bonnand, G. (1976). Les pollutions atmorphériques urbaines par l'asbeste. *Rev. Fr. Mal. resp.* **4**, (Suppl. 2) 51–62

Sébastien, P., Fondimare, A., Bignon, J., Mouchaux, G., Desbordes, J. and Bonnand, G. (1977). Topographic distribution of asbestos fibres in human lung in relation to occupational and non-occupational exposure. In *Inhaled Particles IV*, edited by W. H. Walton and B. McGovern, pp. 435–444. Oxford; Pergamon Press

Selikoff, I. J. (1965). The occurrence of pleural calcification among asbestos insulation workers. *Ann. N.Y. Acad. Sci.* **132**, 351–367

Selikoff, I. J. (1976). Asbestos disease in the United States 1918–1975. *Rev. Fr. Mal. resp.* **4**, (Suppl. 2), 7–24

Selikoff, I. J. and Hammond, E. C. (1970). Asbestos bodies in the New York City population in two periods of time. In *Pneumoconiosis. Proceedings of the International Conference, Johannesburg, 1969*, edited by H. A. Shapiro. Cape Town; Oxford University Press

Selikoff, I. J., Churg, J. and Hammond, E. C. (1964). Asbestos exposure and neoplasia. *J. Am. med. Ass.* **188**, 22–26

Selikoff, I. J., Hammond, E. C. and Churg, J. (1968). Asbestos exposure, smoking and neoplasia. *J. Am. med. Ass.* **204**, 106–112

Selikoff, I. J., Hammond, E. C. and Churg, J. (1972). Carcinogenicity of amosite asbestos. *Archs envir. Hlth* **25**, 183–186

Selikoff, I. J., Hammond, E. C. and Seidman, H. (1973). Cancer risk of insulation workers in the United States. In *Biological Effects of Asbestos*, edited by P. Bogovski *et al.*, pp. 209–216. Lyon; Int. Agency for Res. on Cancer

Selikoff, I. J., Seidman, H. and Hammond, E. C. (1980). Mortality effects of cigarette smoking among amosite asbestos factory workers. *J. Nat. Cancer. Inst.* **65**, 507–513

Shanker, R., Sahu, A. P., Dogra, R. K. S. and Zaidi, S. H. (1975). Effect of intratracheal injection of mica dust on the lymph nodes of guinea pigs. *Toxicology* **5**, 193–199

Shasby, D. M., Petersen, M., Hodous, T., Boehlecke, B. and Merchant, J. (1979). Respiratory morbidity of workers exposed to wollastonite through mining and milling. In *Dusts and*

Disease. Edited by R. Lemen and J. M. Dement, pp. 251–256. Illinois; Pathotox Publishers Inc.
Sheers, G. (1964). Prevalence of pneumoconiosis in Cornish kaolin workers. *Br. J. ind. Med.* **21**, 218–225
Sheers, G. (1979). Asbestos-associated disease in employees of Devonport dockyard. *Ann. N.Y. Acad. Sci.* **330**, 281–287
Sheers, G. and Templeton, A. R. (1968). Effects of asbestos in dockyard workers. *Br. med. J.* **3**, 574–579
Siegal, W., Smith, R. A. and Greenburg, L. (1943). The dust hazard in tremolite talc mining including roentgenological findings in talc workers. *Am. J. Roentg.* **49**, 11–29
Simson, F. W. (1930). Annual Report, 1929, p. 64. Johannesburg; South African Institute for Medical Research
Simson, F. W. and Strachan, A. S. (1931). Asbestos bodies in the sputum: a study of specimens from fifty workers in an asbestos mill. *J. Path. Bact.* **34**, 1–4
Sluis-Cremer, G. K. (1970). Asbestosis in South African asbestos miners. *Envir. Res.* **3**, 310–319
Sluis-Cremer, G. K. (1973). Quoted by McDonald, J. C. In *Biological Effects of Asbestos,* edited by P. Bogovski *et al.*, pp. 155–159. Lyon; Int. Agency for Res. on Cancer
Sluis-Cremer, G. K. and Webster, I. (1972). Acute pleurisy in asbestos exposed persons. *Envir. Res.* **5**, 380–392
Smith, A. R. (1952). Pleural calcification resulting from exposure to certain dusts. *Am. J. Roentgen.* **67**, 375–382
Smith, R. H., Graf, M. S. and Silverman, J. F. (1978). Successful management of drug-induced talc granulomatosis with corticosteroids. *Chest* **73**, 552–554
Smith, W. E., Miller, L., Elsasser, R. E. and Hubert, D. D. (1965). Tests for carcinogenicity of asbestos. *Ann. N.Y. Acad. Soc.* **132**, 456–488
Smither, W. J. (1965). Secular changes in asbestosis in an asbestos factory. *Ann. N.Y. Acad. Sci.* **132**, 166–181
Smither, W. J. and Cross, A. A. (1972). Health hazards (asbestos—its effects and safety precautions). *Trans. Inst. Marine Eng.* **84**, 35–41
Smither, W. J. and Lewinsohn, H. C. (1973). Asbestos in textile manufacturing. In *Biological Effects of Asbestos,* edited by P. Bogovski *et al.*, pp. 169–174. Lyon; Int. Agency for Res. on Cancer
Solomon, A. (1969). The radiology of asbestosis. *S. Afr. med. J.* **43**, 847–851
Solomon, A., Goldstein, B., Webster, I. and Sluis-Cremer, G. K. (1971). Massive fibrosis in asbestosis. *Envir. Res.* **4**, 430–439
South African Medical Research Council (1977). Fifth Annual Report 1975–1976. National Research Institute for Occupational Diseases, Johannesburg, 35–36
Speil, S. and Leineweber, J. P. (1969). Asbestos minerals in modern technology. *Envir. Res.* **2**, 166–208
Stanford, F. (1976). Sympathetic nerve involvement with mesothelioma of the pleura. *Br. J. Dis. Chest* **70**, 134–137
Stanley, H. D. (1978). The detection and identification of asbestos and asbestiform minerals in talc. In *Proceedings of the Workshop on Asbestos: Definitions and Measurement Methods,* Gaithersburg, Maryland, 1977. pp. 325–338. National Bureau of Standards Special Publication 506
Stansfield, D. and Edge, J. R. (1974). Circulating rheumatoid factor and antinuclear antibodies in shipyard workers with pleural plaques. *Br. J. Dis. Chest* **68**, 166–170
Stanton, M. F. (1973). Some etiological considerations of fibre carcinogenesis. In *Biological Effects of Asbestos,* edited by P. Bogovski *et al.*, pp. 289–294. Lyon; Int. Agency for Res. on Cancer
Stanton, M. F., Layard, M., Tegeris, A., Miller, E., May, M. and Kent, E. (1977). Carcinogenicity of fibrous glass: pleural response in the rat in relation to fiber dimension. *J. Nat. Cancer Inst.* **58**, 587–597
Stanton, M. F. and Wrench, C. (1972). Mechanisms of mesothelioma induction with asbestos and fibrous glass. *J. Nat. Cancer Inst.* **48**, 797–821
Steel, S. J. and Winstanley, D. P. (1968). Trephine biopsy of the lung and pleura. *Thorax* **24**, 576–584
Stell, P. M. and McGill, T. (1973). Asbestos and laryngeal carcinoma. *Lancet* **2**, 416–417
Stell, P. M. and McGill, P. M. (1975). Exposure to asbestos and laryngeal carcinoma. *J. Laryng. Otol.* **89**, 513–517
Storey, D. D., Dines, D. E. and Coles, D. T. (1976). Pleural effusion. A diagnostic dilemma. *J. Am. med. Ass.* **236**, 2183–2186
Susuki, Y. (1974). Interaction of asbestos with alveolar cells. *Envir. Hlth Perspect.* **9**, 241–252
Suzuki, Y. and Churg, J. (1969). Formation of the asbestos body. A comparative study with three types of asbestos. *Envir. Res.* **3**, 107–118
Susuki, Y., Churg, J. and Kannerstein, M. (1976). Ultrastructure of human malignant diffuse mesothelioma. *Am. J. Path.* **85**, 241–251
Taskinen, E., Ahlman, K. and Wiikeri, M. (1973). A current hypothesis of the lymphatic transport of inspired dust to the parietal pleura. *Chest* **64**, 193–196
Tellesson, W. G. (1961). Rheumatoid pneumoconiosis (Caplan's syndrome) in an asbestos worker. *Thorax* **16**, 372–377
Teo, S. K. and Lee, S. K. (1978). Recurrent pleural effusion in Waldenström's macroglobulinaemia. *Br. med. J.* **2**, 607–608
Thomas, R. W. (1952). Silicosis in the ball-clay and china-clay industries. *Lancet* **1**, 133–135
Thompson, V. C. (1965). Clinical aspects of diffuse mesothelial tumours. *Thorax* **20**, 248–251
Thomson, J. G. (1970). The pathogenesis of pleural plaques. In *Pneumoconiosis. Proceedings of the International Conference, Johannesburg, 1969,* edited by H. A. Shapiro, pp. 138–141. Cape Town; Oxford University Press
Thomson, J. G., Kaschula, R. O. C. and Macdonald, R. R. (1963). Asbestos as a modern urban hazard. *S. Afr. med. J.* **37**, 77–82
Thomson, M. L., Pelzer, A. M. and Smither, W. J. (1965). The discriminant value of pulmonary function tests in asbestosis. *Ann. N.Y. Acad. Sci.* **132**, 421–436
Thorel, C. (1896). Die Specksteinlunge. *Beitr. path. Anat.* **20**, 85–101
Timár, M., Kendrey, G. and Juhasz, Z. (1966). Experimental observations concerning the effects of mineral dust on pulmonary tissue. *Medna Lav.* **57**, 1–9
Timbrell, V. (1965). The inhalation of fibrous dusts. *Ann. N.Y. Acad. Sci.* **132**, 255–273
Timbrell, V. (1970). The inhalation of fibres. In *Pneumoconiosis. Proceedings of the International Conference, Johannesburg, 1969,* edited by H. A. Shapiro, pp. 3–9. Cape Town; Oxford University Press
Timbrell, V. (1973). Physical factors as etiological mechanisms. In *Biological Effects of Asbestos,* edited by P. Bogovski *et al.*, pp. 295–303. Lyon; Int. Agency for Res. on Cancer
Timbrell, V. (1975). Alignment of respirable asbestos fibres by magnetic fields. *Ann. occup. Hyg.* **18**, 299–311
Timbrell, V., Pooley, F. and Wagner, J. C. (1970). Characteristics of respirable asbestos fibres. In *Pneumoconiosis. Proceedings of the International Conference, Johannesburg, 1969,* edited by H. A. Shapiro, pp. 120–125. Cape Town; Oxford University Press
Timbrell, V. and Rendall, R. E. G. (1971/72). Preparation of UICC standard reference samples of asbestos. *Powder Tech.* **5**, 279–287
Tobacco Research Council (1970). Personal communication
Tonning, H. O. (1949). Pneumoconiosis from fuller's earth. *J. ind. Hyg. Toxicol.* **31**, 41–45
Torrington, K. G. (1978). Rapid appearance of rheumatoid pleural effusion. *Chest* **73**, 409–411
Tripsa, R. and Rotura, G. (1966). Recherches experimentales sur la pneumoconiose provoquée par la poussierre de mica. *Medna Lav.* **57**, 493–500
Turner-Warwick, M. (1977). Immune reactions in pulmonary fibrosis. *Schweiz. med. Wschr.* **107**, 171–175
Turner-Warwick, M. (1979). HLA phenotypes in asbestos workers. *Br. J. Dis. Chest* **73**, 243–244
Turner-Warwick, M., Burrows, B. and Johnson, A. (1980). Cryptogenic fibrosing alveolitis: clinical features and their influences on survival. *Thorax* **35**, 171–180

Turner-Warwick, M. and Haslam, P. (1971). Antibodies in some chronic fibrosing lung diseases 1. Non-organ-specific antibodies. *Clin. Allergy* **1,** 83–95

Turner-Warwick, M. and Parkes, W. R. (1970). Circulating rheumatoid and anti-nuclear factors in asbestos workers. *Br. med. J.* **3,** 492–495

Um, Chang-Hyun (1970). Study of the secular trend in asbestos bodies in lungs in London. 1936–1966. *Br. med. J.* **2,** 248–251

US Department of Health, Education and Welfare (1977). Criteria for a recommended standard, occupational exposure to fibrous glass. National Institute for Occupational Safety and Health. Washington, DC; US Government Printing Office

Utidjian, H. M. D. (1973). Criteria documents. *J. occup. Med.* **15,** 374–379

Utidjian, H. M. D. and de Treville, R. T. P. (1970). Fibrous glass manufacturing and health reports of an epidemiological study. In *Proceedings of the 35th Annual Meeting of the Industrial Health Foundation, Pittsburgh.* Industrial Health foundation, 10–18

Utidjian, H. M. D., Gross, P. and de Treville, R. T. P. (1968). Ferruginous bodies in human lungs. *Archs envir. Hlth* **17,** 327–333

Van Ordstrand, H. S. (1970). Talc Penumoconiosis (Editorial). *Chest* **58,** 2

Vestal, T. F., Winstead, J. A. and Joliot, P. V. (1943). Pneumoconiosis among mica and pegmatite workers. *Ind. Med. Surg.* **12,** 11–14

Vianna, N. J. and Polan, A. K. (1978). Non-occupational exposure to asbestos and malignant mesothelioma in females. *Lancet* **1,** 1061–1063

Vigliani, E. C. and Pernis, B. (1958). Immunological factors in the pathogenesis of the hyaline tissue of silicosis. *Br. J. ind. Med.* **15,** 8–14

von Hayek, H. (1960). *The Human Lung.* Trans. V. E. Krahl. New York; Hafner

Vorwald, A. J. (1953). Quoted by Cooper, W. C. (1975)

Vorwald, A. J. (1960). Diffuse fibrogenic pneumoconiosis. *Ind. Med. Surg.* **29,** 353–358

Vorwald, A. J., Durkan, T. M. and Pratt, P. C. (1951). Experimental studies of asbestosis. *Archs ind. Hyg. occup. Med.* **3,** 1–43

Wagner, J. C. (1963). Asbestosis in experimental animals. *Br. J. ind. Med.* **20,** 1–12

Wagner, J. C. (1965). The sequelae of exposure to asbestos dust. *Ann. N.Y. Acad. Sci.* **132,** 691–695

Wagner, J. C. (1972a). The significance of asbestos in tissue. In *Recent Results in Cancer Research.* 39. Edited by E. Grundmann and H. Tulinius, pp. 37–46. London; Heinemann; Berlin, Heidelberg, New York; Springer

Wagner, J. C. (1972b). Personal communication

Wagner, J. C. (1977). General epidemiology of pleural and lung cancers. In *Colloque amainte et canceragenese humaine,* pp. 65–68. Chambre syndicate de l'Amiante et le Syndicat de l'Amiante-Ciment, 10 Rue de la Pepiniere 75008, Paris

Wagner, J. C. (1978). Susceptibility to asbestos-related diseases. In *Proceedings of Asbestos Symposium, J'burg, South Africa, 1977,* edited by H. W. Glen, pp. 109–113. Randburg; Department of Mines, Nat. Inst. Metallurgy

Wagner, J. C. and Berry, G. (1969). Mesotheliomas in rats following inoculation with asbestos. *Br. J. Cancer* **23,** 567–581

Wagner, J. C., Berry, G., Cooke, T. J., Hill, R. J., Pooley, F. D. and Skidmore, J. W. (1977). Animal experiments with talc. In *Inhaled Particles IV,* edited by W. H. Walton and B. McGovern, pp. 647–652. Oxford; Pergamon Press

Wagner, J. C., Berry, G., Skidmore, J. W. and Timbrell, V. (1974). The effects of inhalation of asbestos in rats. *Br. J. Cancer* **29,** 252–269

Wagner, J. C., Berry, G. and Timbrell, V. (1970). Mesothelioma in rats. In *Pnneumoconiosis. Proceedings of the International Conference, Johannesburg, 1969,* edited by H. A. Shapiro, pp. 216–219. Cape Town; Oxford University Press

Wagner, J. C., Berry, G. and Timbrell, V. (1973). Mesotheliomata in rats after inoculation with asbestos and other materials. *Br. J. Cancer* **28,** 173–185

Wagner, J. C., Sleggs, C. A. and Marchand, P. (1960). Diffuse pleural mesothelioma. *Br. J. ind. Med.* **17,** 260–271

Wagner, J. C., Munday, D. E. and Harington, J. S. (1962). Histochemical demonstration of hyaluronic acid in pleural mesotheliomas. *J. Path. Bact.* **84,** 73–78

Wagner, J. C., Gilson, J. C., Berry, G. and Timbrell, V. (1971). Epidemiology of asbestos cancers. *Br. med. Bull.* **27,** 71–86

Wagner, M. M. F. (1979). *Immunology and asbestos.* Symposium on Biological Effects of Mineral Fibres, Lyons. September, 1979

Wallace, W. F. M. and Langlands, J. H. M. (1971). Insulation workers in Belfast. Comparison of a random sample with a controlled population. *Br. J. ind. Med.* **28,** 211–216

Walther, E. (1970). Dust problems in the use of asbestos products. In *Pneumoconiosis. Proceedings of the International Conference, Johannesburg, 1969,* edited by H. A. Shapiro, pp. 37–41. Cape Town; Oxford University Press

Warnock, M. L. and Churg, A. M. (1980). Asbestos bodies. *Chest* **77,** 129

Warnock, M. L., Press, M. and Churg, A. (1980). Further observations on cytoplasmic hyaline in the lung. *Human Path.* **11,** 59–65

Warraki, S. and Herant, Y. (1963). Pneumoconiosis in china clay workers. *Br. J. ind. Med.* **20,** 226–230

Webster, I. (1970a). The pathogenesis of asbestosis. In *Pneumoconiosis. Proceedings of the International Conference, Johannesburg, 1969,* edited by H. A. Shapiro, pp. 117–119. Cape Town; Oxford University Press

Webster, I. (1973). Asbestos and malignancy. *S. Afr. med. J.* **47,** 165–171

Wedler, H. W. (1943). Asbestos und lungenkrebs. *Dtsch. med. Wschr.* **69,** 575–576

Wehner, A. P., Zwicker, G. M., Cannon, W. C., Watson, C. R. and Carlton, W. W. (1977). Inhalation of talc baby powders by hamsters. *Fd. Cosmet. Toxicol.* **15,** 121–129

Weill, H., Rossiter, C. E., Waggenspack, C., Jones, R. N. and Ziskind, M. M. (1977). Differences in lung effects resulting from chrysotile and crocidolite exposure. In *Inhaled Particles IV,* edited by W. H. Walton and B. McGovern, pp. 789–796. Oxford; Pergamon Press

Weill, H., Waggenspack, C. and Bailey, W. (1973). Radiographic and physiologic patterns amongst workers engaged in manufacture of asbestos cement products. *J. occup. Med.* **15,** 248–252

Weill, H., Ziskind, M. M., Waggenspack, C. and Rossiter, C. E. (1975). Lung function consequences of dust exposure in asbestos cement manufacturing plants. *Archs envir. Hlth* **30,** 88–97

Weiss, W. (1969). Cigarette smoking and diffuse pulmonary fibrosis. *Am. Rev. resp. Dis.* **99,** 67–72

Weiss, W. (1971). Cigarette smoking, asbestos and pulmonary fibrosis. *Am. Rev. resp. Dis.* **104,** 223–227

Weiss, W. (1977). Mortality of a cohort exposed to chrysotile asbestos. *J. occup. Med.* **19,** 737–740

Weiss, B. and Boettner, E. A. (1967). Commercial talc and talcosis. *Archs envir. Hlth* **14,** 304–308

Weiss, W. and Theodos, P. A. (1978). Pleuropulmonary disease among asbestos workers in relation to smoking and type of exposure. *J. occup. Med.* **20,** 341–345

Whitwell, F., Newhouse, M. L. and Bennett, D. R. (1974). A study of the histological cell types of lung cancer in workers suffering from asbestosis in the United Kingdom. *Br. J. ind. Med.* **31,** 298–303

Whitwell, F. and Rawcliffe, R. M. (1971). Diffuse malignant pleural mesothelioma and asbestos exposure. *Thorax* **26,** 6–22

Whitwell, F., Scott, J. and Grimshaw, M. (1977). Relationship between occupations and asbestos-fibre content of the lungs in patients with pleural mesothelioma, lung cancer and other diseases. *Thorax* **32,** 377–386

Willis, R. A. (1967). *Pathology of Tumours,* pp. 181–183. London; Butterworths

Willis, R. A. (1973). *The Spread of Tumours in the Human Body.* 3rd edition, pp. 56–60. London; Butterworths

Wilson, M. R., Gaumer, H. R. and Salvaggio, J. E. (1977). Activation of the alternative complement pathway and generation of chemostatic factors by asbestos. *J. Allergy Clin. Immun.* **60,** 218–222

Woitowitz, H. J. (1970). Berufliche Asbeststaubexposition und obstruktive Ventilationsstrorungen. *Int. Arch. Arbeitsmed.* **27,** 244–256

Wood, W. B. and Gloyne, S. R. (1934). Pulmonary asbestosis. *Lancet* **2,** 1383–1385

Wright, G. W. (1968). Airborne fibrous glass particles. Chest roentgenograms of persons with prolonged exposure. *Archs envir. Hlth* **16,** 175–181

Wright, G. W. (1969). Asbestos and health. *Am. Rev. resp. Dis.* **100,** 467–479

Wright, G. W. and Kuschner, M. (1977). The influence of varying lengths of glass and asbestos fibres on tissue response in guinea pigs. In *Inhaled Particles IV,* edited by W. H. Walton and B. McGovern, pp. 455–472. Oxford; Pergamon Press

Wyers, H. (1946). Thesis presented to the University of Glasgow for the Degree of Doctor of Medicine

Wyers, H. (1949). Asbestosis. *Postgrad. med. J.* **25**, 631–638

Yazicioglu, S., Ilçayto, R., Balci, K., Şayli, B. S. and Yorulmaz, B. (1980). Pleural calcification, pleural mesotheliomas and bronchial cancers caused by tremolite dust. *Thorax* 564–569

Young, J. R. and Reddy, E. R. (1980). Peritoneal mesothelioma. *Clin. Rad.* **31,** 243–247

Zielhuis, R. L., Versteeg, L. P. J. and Planteijdt, H. J. (1975). Pleural mesothelioma and exposure to asbestos: a retrospective case-control study in the Netherlands. *Int. Arch. occup. envir. Hlth* **36,** 1–18

Zolov, C., Burilkov, T. and Babadjov, L. (1967). Pleural asbestosis in agricultural workers. *Envir. Res.* **1,** 287–292

Zoltai, T. (1978). History of asbestos-related mineralogical terminology. In *Proceedings of Workshop on Asbestos: Definitions and Measurement Methods,* edited by C. C. Gravatt *et al.* Washington DC; NBS – SP – 506

Zoltai, T. (1979). Asbestiform and acicular mineral fragments. *Ann. N.Y. Acad. Sci.* **330,** 621–643

Zussman, J. (1979). The minerology of asbestos. In *Asbestos,* **1,** *Properties, Applications and Hazards,* edited by L. Michaels and S. S. Chissick, pp. 45–65. Chichester, New York, Brisbane and Toronto; John Wiley

Addendum

1 Ratio of asbestos bodies to fibres in lungs

This appears to be inconstant in persons with a low level of exposure. An average of 1:10000 has been reported in the general population (Churg and Warnock, 1980) and from 1:20 to 1:100 in individuals with moderate to heavy exposure (Sébastian *et al.*, 1977). There appears to be no precise value above which asbestosis is always found (Churg and Warnock, 1981).

2 'Talc bodies'

It is important to note that bodies sometimes form on rolled talc sheets (or plates) and may closely resemble tremolite (asbestos) bodies.

Churg, A. and Warnock, M. L. (1980). Asbestos fibres in the general population. *Am. Rev. resp. Dis.* **122**, 669–678

Churg, A. and Warnock, M. L. (1981). Asbestos and other ferruginous bodies. Their formation and clinical significance. *Am. J. Path.* **102**, 447–456

3 Man-made silicate fibres

The animal experiments with glass fibres referred to on page 319 are not comparable in respect of duration nor in the mode, dosage and dimensions of the fibres administered. Gross (1982) has summarized the current situation thus: 'The development of slight peribronchiolar fibrosis when thin, long fibres were injected intratracheally requires confirmation by inhalation studies which are not yet completed. The authors of the intratracheal injection study (Wright and Kuschner, 1977) suggested that the peribronchiolar fibrosis may be caused by the unnatural technique employed'. This caveat, applies equally to experiments with all mineral and synthetic fibres. Gross (1982) also stresses that epidemiological studies which 'involved many thousands of men who had been exposed to man-made vitreous fibres for as long as 40 years' have not revealed an increased risk of 'lung cancer or non-malignant respiratory disease'.

Further light on the effect of length and diameter of glass fibres administered by intratracheal instillation in rats—but in much smaller doses than those used by Wright and Kuschner (1977)—on fibre clearance and solubility in the lung has recently been shed by Morgan, Holmes and Davison (1982). Fibres less than 3 μm diameter and about 10 μm long are cleared efficiently—most probably by macrophages; whereas those about 30 μm long are not cleared to any significant degree over at least 1 year. Furthermore, fibres dissolve in the lung at a rate which is dependent on their length: those too long (30–60 μm) to be contained within a single macrophage dissolve relatively rapidly, often undergoing fragmentation; but short fibres (5–10 μm) dissolve more slowly and uniformly. The authors conclude that this leaching out of long fibres suggests that in man they are unlikely to cause the pathological effects which are associated with virtually insoluble amphibole fibres. The apparent clearance of longer fibres reported by Bernstein, Drew and Kuschner (1980) (*see* page 319), they believe, may be accounted for by their dissolution.

Gross, P. (1982). Review Article. Man-made vitreous fibers: present status of research on health effects. *Int. Arch. Occup. Environ. Hlth.* **50**, 103–112

Morgan, A., Holmes, A. and Davison, W. (1982). Clearance of sized fibres from the rat lung and their solubility *in vivo. Ann. occup. Hyg.* **25**, 317–331

10 Beryllium Disease

Beryllium disease is a multisystem disorder caused by dusts, fumes or mists of beryllium metal or its salts but, because their most common and important mode of entry into the body is the respiratory tract, their effects are predominantly pulmonary. It has two forms: an *acute,* non-specific, chemical tracheo-bronchopneumonia; and a *chronic* epithelioid granulomatous disorder which ends in diffuse fibrosis capable of causing severe respiratory disability.

It is now uncommon owing to the operation of stringent hygiene measures since the 1950s in industries processing and using beryllium materials. Nonetheless it has a disproportionate medical importance for these reasons:

(1) The application of beryllium metal and its compounds has greatly increased in recent years and will continue to expand. Hence, an awareness of the possible modes of exposure is important.
(2) The possibility of accidental or unrecognized exposure to high concentrations of beryllium dusts or fumes.
(3) If not diagnosed and treated acute disease may be fatal and chronic disease, disabling and sometimes fatal.
(4) The chronic form of the disease may develop many years after exposure, and is largely determined by individual susceptibility or hypersensitivity. Furthermore, its histological appearances are those of a sarcoid-type granuloma and, when disseminated, it may resemble sarcoidosis clinically in many respects.
(5) Progression from acute to chronic disease may occur without further contact with beryllium compounds.
(6) Because new cases are now likely to be seen singly and infrequently their prompt treatment will depend upon beryllium exposure being considered in diagnosis.
(7) The possibility that chronic disease might predispose to the development of carcinoma of the lung.

BERYLLIUM AND ITS COMPOUNDS

Metallic beryllium and its compounds are extracted from beryl ore, beryllium aluminium silicate ($3BeO.\ Al_2O_3\ 6SiO_2$), found in granite pegmatites. Beryl is obtained as a by-product or co-product of mining mica, feldspar and other pegmatite minerals in Brazil, Argentina, Zimbabwe, South Africa and the USA. Compounds used in industrial processes are the oxides, hydroxides, sulphates, fluorides, nitrates and synthetic silicates.

Extraction is carried out by the *sulphate* or *fluoride processes* in which ore is melted and treated either with concentrated sulphuric acid or sodium silicofluoride. Both methods produce beryllium hydroxide from which the oxide, *beryllia,* is derived by calcination at 1000 °C. Chloride, fluoride and oxyfluoride salts are produced by electrolytic reduction. In Britain beryllium extraction was not established on a large scale until the end of the 1950s before which the metal was imported in the form of beryllium–copper master alloy.

Properties

Beryllium has the important properties of being the only stable light-weight metal possessing a high strength-to-density ratio, extreme hardness, good electric and thermal conductivity and high resistance to corrosion and temperature fluctuations. It has a low neutron absorbing capacity (and is thus an excellent moderator and reflector of neutrons), it yields a profusion of neutrons when bombarded by α particles, and its low atomic number, 4, renders it translucent to X-rays. When alloyed with other metals it lends its properties to them even in concentrations as low as 2 per cent; the commonest alloy, beryllium–copper, has non-magnetic and non-sparking qualities.

Beryllium oxide is most stable and is endowed with very high thermal conductivity (being superior to alumina in refractory properties especially at temperatures higher than 1900 °C), low thermal expansion, dielectric properties and low neutron absorption. It is prepared by calcination at about 1600 °C ('high-fired') or between 500 and 1100 °C ('low-fired'). The 'high-fired' variety is believed to be biologically less active than the 'low-fired', possibly because of differences in crystal structure (Crossman and Vandemark, 1954), but because of the likelihood of cross contamination it is difficult to be certain of this (Tepper, 1972). Low-fired beryllium oxide is more soluble *in vivo* than high-fired oxide and, on the whole, the halides are more soluble than either. This may have some bearing on clearance of beryllium from the lungs.

The vapour pressures of the halides are such that hazardous concentrations of all except the fluoride can be generated when they are subjected to temperatures as low as 158 °C, and the volatilization of beryllium oxide is greatly increased in the presence of water vapour (Tepper, Hardy, and Chamberlin, 1961). Vapour evolved condenses as fume.

All the compounds and the metal itself are potentially hazardous to health. But beryl ore is not believed to be harmful to man, although prolonged exposure to its dust has apparently caused lesions consistent with beryllium disease in rats and monkeys (Stokinger, 1966).

BERYLLIUM ALLOYS

A 'master alloy' of beryllium and copper is produced by the reaction of beryllium oxide, carbon and copper in a carbon arc furnace and usually contains 4 per cent beryllium. 'Industrial alloys' of copper, nickel, aluminium, manganese and zinc are prepared from the master alloy and usually contain 2 per cent or less beryllium.

BERYLLIUM PHOSPHORS

A *phosphor* is a substance which phosphoresces when stimulated by external radiation. Beryllium phosphors containing beryllium oxide were used in the manufacture of fluorescent lighting tubes until about 1949 in the USA and the early 1950s in Britain when, owing to outbreaks of beryllium disease, they were discontinued and replaced by halophosphates. However, stores of unused tubes occasionally survived for some years after.

APPLICATIONS AND SOURCES OF EXPOSURE

Occupational

During extraction of ore and the manufacture of master and industrial alloys fume or dust are evolved by annealing furnaces and forging, knocking-out and fettling castings; by hot-rolling industrial alloy in strip mills; and by heating, milling and hot and cold processing blocks of metal. Metallurgical grade beryllium is usually produced by isostatic pressing of beryllium metal rather than by casting. By this means the density of the metal ingot can be varied according to the pressure applied. Depending upon the purpose for which it is required the metal may be cut into small sections, machined or milled to fine particle size. Low density metal gives rise to considerably more dust when machined than high density metal. Any operation involving heat treatment of 2 per cent alloy is potentially dangerous, and chronic disease due to 1.8 per cent alloy has been recorded (Israel and Cooper, 1964).

Blocks of pure metal undergo corrosion in a humid atmosphere (which may be present under some storage conditions) forming white beryllium oxide powder on their surfaces. This powder is easily disturbed and becomes airborne.

Beryllium has important uses in the construction of space vehicles, space mirrors and satellite antennae; in glass windows of X-ray tubes; as a reflector to increase neutron flux in atomic reactors; and as a filler in moulded plastics. It is employed as a rocket fuel because it contains more energy per unit volume than any other solid and chemically stable material. Analysis of rocket exhaust products has indicated the presence of about 50 per cent beryllium oxide, 40 per cent fluoride and a remainder mainly chloride (Robinson, Schaffner and Trachtenberg, 1968). However, apparently this fuel is not activated until the rocket is outside the earth's atmosphere. Static firing of rocket motors for research purposes is done either in enclosures in which the exhaust is scrubbed and filtered or in desert areas under favourable meteorological conditions with the operators sealed off from the atmosphere and subsequent decontamination of affected areas (Maxwell, 1971).

The beryllium alloys have a very wide application in modern technology: beryllium–copper is used extensively in the electrical and electronics industries, in computers and the couplings of underwater cables, in strong non-sparking tools for use under conditions where there is risk of explosion, and in the moving parts of engines. Beryllium–nickel is employed for dies and drill bits, and many components requiring high resistance to wear and extreme heat. Beryllium–aluminium possesses greater toughness and resilience than aluminium.

Machining and drilling operations of the metal and its alloys throw off metallic particles of mostly 'non-respirable' size, but a proportion may be less than 10 μm. When the amount of waste is substantial dry machining is used to facilitate its recovery and much dust is generated. When cutting oils are employed the operation causes little waste as these capture most of the particles but, should the oils be re-used for other operations not involving beryllium alloys, they may present an unsuspected source of exposure. Wet grinding, honing and polishing may give rise to mists carrying beryllium particles. Deburring metallic compounds with high-speed burrs generates dust in close proximity to the operator's face (Benoit, 1967).

Welding of beryllium alloys and the reclamation of scrap metals containing beryllium alloys by melting down in a furnace produces beryllium oxide fume. These are important causes of unsuspected exposure if the nature of the metal alloys is not known: for example, if wrongly labelled.

Beryllium oxide is used in refractory ceramics such as crucibles, and a wide variety of technical ceramics for the electronics industry; in microwave windows and, with metallic beryllium in metal ceramics—or *cermets* (that is, materials consisting of a ceramic heat-bonded to a metal)—in rocket motor parts, nose-cones and in the manufacture of the blading of jet engines. Technical ceramic shapes are slip-cast and pressed by cold and hot methods. These and refractory shapes are fettled and finished by wet grinding. In the absence of efficient hygiene control these processes can cause accumulation of beryllium-containing dust on floors, benches and ledges.

The beryllium halides have some use in the manufacture of lantern mantles and as catalysts in certain organic chemical reactions.

The manufacture and use of beryllium phosphors in fluorescent and neon lighting tubes were responsible for many cases of disease in the past. Established about 1940 and active until 1950 or thereabouts this industry caused about half the recorded cases of chronic beryllium disease up to 1966 (Hardy, Rabe and Lorch, 1967), many cases not being manifest until some ten years after exposure ceased. All stages of manufacture were potentially dangerous as phosphor dust containing beryllium oxide was released from natural and accidental spillage. Breakage of fluorescent tubes by accident or deliberately during disposal also gave rise to dust. Limited use of beryllium oxide in phosphor powder mixtures apparently still continues, however, for certain types of specialized electronic equipment. Beryllium silicate, which may contain about 0.5 per cent beryllium oxide as an impurity, is employed to coat high-energy cathode ray tubes for radar and similar installations and appears to have been used in Italy for fluorescent lamps until 1967 (Ambrosi *et al.*, 1968).

The use of beryllium compounds by laboratory workers—chemists and physicists—has occasionally caused disease (Agate, 1948; McCallum, Rannie and Verity, 1961); and cleaning exhaust ventilation ducts, dust collectors, cyclones and high-efficiency filters for air-scrubbing in dry beryllium processes and the replacing of filters are potential sources of significant exposure.

Although most of these processes and operations have been subjected to rigorous industrial hygiene controls for years past the possibility of hazardous contamination exists wherever beryllium and its compounds are used. Hence, because disease may result from very limited exposure, the efficiency of these controls is of paramount importance (*see* p. 354). Breakdown of dust and fume control systems or rupture of storage containers can cause sudden, high-level contamination of factory atmosphere. Today plant maintenance personnel and workers in specialized ceramic and engineering industries are those most likely to develop disease.

As a general principle it should be noted that because particles of beryllium metal or its compounds are so very light they may remain airborne for prolonged periods.

Para-occupational

Men not actually working in beryllium processes may, for example, be exposed to risk when in the vicinity of ill-protected furnaces melting down non-ferrous metal scrap. Spillage of powdered beryllium metal or beryllium compounds from containers and subsequent brushing up are potential sources of concentrated exposure to dockers, transport workers and store keepers. Office staff in beryllium plants have been known to develop disease (Sander, 1950).

Neighbourhood

Occasional cases of disease have occurred in the past in the general population living in the vicinity of beryllium plants. These were mostly women who cleaned or laundered the working clothes of their husbands who were beryllium workers. Contamination of the atmosphere by emissions from factory smoke stacks or exhaust systems was probably less important (Sussman, Lieben and Cleland, 1959), although a tendency for cases to occur in the direction of the prevailing wind has been observed (Lieben and Metzner, 1959). However, the significance of these cases is that, though exposed to such low concentrations of beryllium, many developed more severe disease than the beryllium workers themselves; thus pointing to the likelihood of individual susceptibility and an immunological pathogenesis (Sterner and Eisenbud, 1951).

Other

Mantles of gas camping lanterns may consist of nitrates of thorium, cerium and beryllium on rayon fabric. During the first few minutes after lighting a new mantle significant amounts of beryllium oxide (about 200 μg) are emitted into the air and may also be deposited on the inner surface of the lantern cap (Griggs, 1973).

THE NATURAL HISTORY OF BERYLLIUM DISEASE

Beryllium compounds cause ocular and skin lesions by direct contact, and respiratory and systemic lesions almost exclusively by entry into and absorption from, the upper respiratory tract and lungs (but *see* case referred to on p. 340).

ACUTE DISEASE

This was originally described in Germany by Weber and Englehardt (1933) and later in the USA by Van Ordstrand, Hughes and Carmody (1943). It is caused very largely by the soluble salts and its severity is determined by intensity of exposure. Hence, it is rarely seen today because, apart from occasional accidental massive contamination, strict hygienic control of processes effectively prevent the accumulation of high beryllium concentrations in the factory atmosphere.

Non-respiratory disease includes conjunctivitis, corneal ulceration, allergic blepharitis and allergic contact dermatitis. Entry of salts into skin abrasions cause chemical ulcers and, if embedded subdermally, chronic granulomas. Beryllium fluoride is chiefly responsible, beryllium sulphate and ammonium beryllium fluoride being less active.

Respiratory disease follows excessive, usually accidental exposure, to dusts, fumes or mists. Transient rhinitis, tracheitis and bronchitis of varying severity, according to the degree of exposure, occur and are due almost entirely to the soluble salts. Chemical pneumonia results from inhalation of the less soluble salts and of beryllium oxide fume which consist of particles capable of reaching the alveoli. After massive exposure it occurs within 72 hours and follows a fulminant course; with lower concentrations it may be of insidious and slow development but is classified as 'acute' if it occurs within 12 months (Tepper, Hardy and Chamberlin, 1961). Illness similar to metal fume fever (*see* Chapter 13) has also been described (Gelman, 1936) but not generally reported. It seems probable that it was caused by fume of associated metals and not beryllium.

Skin disease may occur independently of respiratory disease but, after resolution, tends to recur earlier and more severely on second exposure when it may be associated with lung disease; a phenomenon consistent with acquired hypersensitivity.

Acute chemical pneumonia occurred chiefly in the beryllium extraction industry but is now unlikely to be encountered apart from the rare accidental and unexpected conditions referred to earlier.

It is important to note that although acute disease usually resolves completely, either spontaneously or as a result of corticosteroid treatment, it occasionally progresses to chronic disease—sometimes rapidly (Freiman and Hardy, 1970; Jones Williams, 1977).

CHRONIC DISEASE

This is a completely different syndrome—first described by Hardy and Tabershaw in 1946—from that of acute disease although, as just stated, it may follow it after a variable period in a small number of cases—about 6 per cent (Hardy, Rabe and Lorch, 1967). It is usually associated with exposure to low-fired beryllium oxide or with work with beryllium metal and alloys. As a rule symptoms develop insidiously and the delay in their onset since last exposure may range from a period of months to more than ten years—exceptionally up to 20 years (Hardy and Chamberlin, 1972). But sudden exacerbation may follow surgery, pregnancy and respiratory infection (*see* p. 343). The disease may exhibit most, but not all, of the clinical, pathological, lung function and radiographical abnormalities of sarcoidosis chiefly involving the lungs. However, a restricted dissemination of granulomas may also occur in the skin and other viscera, and this is sometimes found in the absence of overt lung disease. These features are discussed in detail under the relevant headings.

EPIDEMIOLOGY

Both forms of the disease may occur at any age but the incidence according to sex has changed over the years. 'Neighbourhood cases' of chronic disease were more commonly observed in women than in men in the 1950s due, probably, to their laundering contaminated clothing; indeed, most of these cases are most likely to have been caused in this way. The 'attack rate' of chronic disease is low. Even with exposure to the high concentrations of beryllium oxide or beryllium salts which often existed before hygiene controls were introduced it was approximately 1 per cent in extraction plants and 4 per cent in the fluorescent lamp industry (Preuss, 1975).

The most valuable source of information is the US Beryllium Case Registry in which all known cases in that country have been recorded since 1952 (Tepper, Hardy and Chamberlin, 1961). By the end of 1978, 892 cases were on file. Of these 408 (46 per cent) were known to have died and the status of the living was known in 361 (40 per cent) (Sprince *et al.*, 1978). Before 1949–50, when hygiene control of beryllium industries was introduced, most of the cases occurred in the fluorescent lamp industry—almost in epidemic proportions. Since the 1960s the majority of new cases have arisen in workers in beryllium extraction and ceramic industries, in atomic research and in machining beryllium alloys especially in the aviation and space exploration industries. In Britain a comparable registry is being compiled and since 1948 35 cases have been recorded (Jones Williams, Nosworthy and Williams, 1980); though at the end of 1980 the number had risen to 42 (Jones Williams, 1980). However, it is virtually certain that an unknown number, either not reported or undiagnosed, have occurred.

Of 76 new cases added to the US Beryllium Case Register since 1966, 53 were men and 23 women which contrasts with the preponderance of women in the late 1940s following employment during the Second World War; and the average age of onset in both sexes tended to be younger—the mean age for both being 46 years whereas prior to 1949 the mean age for men was 53 years and for women, 52 years. Delay in onset of disease was much shorter in cases developing after 1949 than in those which occurred before. In the majority of those reported before 1949 the period was over ten years whereas in most of those reported after this date it was under a year, in spite of the fact that the beryllium levels to which they had been exposed were considerably lower than in the pre-1949 group. This paradox is explained by an increased awareness of the disease and effectiveness of diagnosis by physicians, and the limitation of exposure to defined industries in latter years. After 1966 there were no cases of acute disease although two were classed as 'subacute'. The majority of patients in this series, who had been exposed after 1949 (29 of 36), gave a history of handling or machining beryllium metal and alloys in the aircraft industry, electronics, and the manufacture of nuclear reactors (Hasan and Kazemi, 1974).

Mortality figures are unreliable and comparisons not possible due to different methods of reporting and the fact that the usually given overall mortality does not specify causes of death. However, of 60 patients with chronic beryllium disease seen between 1940 and 1966 17 (28 per cent) were dead by 1966; 13 from 'cor pulmonale' and two from respiratory diseases (Stoeckle, Hardy and Weber, 1969).

ABSORPTION AND EXCRETION OF BERYLLIUM COMPOUNDS

Information in man is incomplete but it appears that after inhalation the soluble compounds are cleared fairly readily from the lungs although a variable quantity may remain; whereas the relatively insoluble beryllium oxide is very slowly eliminated and is retained for long periods due, it is suggested, to its being bound to tissue proteins and only gradually released (Reeves, 1968). Excretion occurs mainly via the kidneys and the amount depends upon the solubility of the compounds inhaled (Klemperer, Martin and Van Riper, 1951). A proportion which is not excreted, and is greater in acute than chronic disease, is stored in the liver, spleen, lymph nodes and skeleton (Tepper, Hardy and Chamberlin, 1961). Mobilization and excretion of beryllium in the urine may continue for years so that urinary concentrations at any given time reflect only the amount released and not the total body burden (Preuss, 1975). There is no evident correlation between the presence or severity of disease and the quantity of beryllium excreted (Klemperer, Martin and Van Riper, 1951; Lieben, Dattoli and Vought, 1966).

Beryllium and its compounds are not absorbed through unbroken skin but readily enter cracks and abrasions; they are poorly absorbed from the gastro-intestinal tract and no toxic effects from this route are on record (Preuss, 1975). Beryllium apparently crosses the placental 'barrier' but no disease in infants has been attributed to this (Tepper, Hardy and Chamberlin, 1961).

PATHOLOGY

As this book is concerned with lung disorders the pathology and pathogenesis of beryllium disease of other organs is given only brief mention.

ACUTE DISEASE

Upper respiratory tract

The mucosa is oedematous and hyperaemic.

Lungs

Macroscopic appearances

In fatal cases, the lungs are heavy and have a firm, liver-like consistency. The pleura is not thickened although there may be some recent deposition of fibrin. Their cut surfaces have a pink to blue-grey colour, and a frothy, often blood stained fluid can be expressed from them. The trachea, bronchi and bronchioles are oedematous and red, and may contain haemorrhagic exudates. The hilar and bronchopulmonary lymph nodes are enlarged (Hazard, 1959; Sprince, Kazemi and Hardy, 1976).

Microscopic appearances

Alveolar spaces and walls are engorged with a proteinaceous fluid exudate which contains lymphocytes, large monocytes, plasma cells and cellular debris but few neutrophil leucocytes (Vorwald, 1966); and foamy desquamated Type II pneumocytes may be present in the spaces. Organization of this exudate frequently occurs and is continuous with similar early organization within the walls.

Although occasional giant cells may be observed, granulomas (*see* next section) are uniformly *absent* (Freiman and Hardy, 1970).

The only abnormality to be found in the lungs of persons who have recovered from the illness may be a very slight excess of connective tissue elements (Vorwald, 1966).

There is nothing characteristic in any of these appearances which are also seen in other chemical pneumonias.

Outside the lungs, centrilobular necrosis of the liver and coagulation necrosis of bone marrow have also been reported (Tepper, Hardy and Chamberlin, 1961).

CHRONIC DISEASE

Lungs

Macroscopic appearances

The visceral pleura is thickened and there may be extensive adhesion with the parietal pleura. In some cases multiple, thick-walled blebs, similar to those seen in 'honeycomb lung', are present on the lung surfaces. The lungs are heavy and their cut surfaces reveal areas of grey-white, diffuse fibrosis which is usually present in all lobes though, in some cases, only parts of the lungs are affected. Thick walled cysts—up to 1 cm or more in diameter—are often associated with the fibrotic areas, and scattered fibrotic nodules which may reach 3 cm in diameter are occasionally found (*Figure 10.1*). No particular distribution appears to be favoured. The hilar lymph nodes are usually only slightly enlarged but exceptions to this are seen.

None of these features is pathognomonic.

Microscopic appearances

In the majority of cases the appearances are those of diffuse cellular infiltration of alveolar walls and sarcoid-type granulomas, though the latter may be inconspicuous. The degree of cellular infiltration differs greatly in different cases; histiocytes predominate but there are also numerous lymphocytes and a variable number of plasma cells. The histiocytes tend to form into groups ranging from a few cells to large well-demarcated granulomas but in some cases they are disseminated widely in alveolar walls and are difficult to differentiate from lymphocytes.

The granulomas, which are also diffusely, though sometimes scantily, scattered in sub-pleural, septal, peribronchial, and perivascular sites and, occasionally, in the walls of blood vessels, consist of epithelioid and Langhan's-type giant cells. Lymphocytes are prominent and are important in the immunopathology of the disease. Central eosinophilic necrosis is usually absent or only slight but may sometimes be pronounced due, possibly, to high beryllium content (Jones Williams, 1977). It is also seen in florid sarcoidosis especially in the mediastinal lymph nodes (Carlens, Hanngren and Ivemark, 1974). Pleural involvement too, though uncommon, occurs in sarcoidosis (Beekman *et al.*, 1976); hence, this is not a differentiating feature of beryllium disease.

The epithelioid cells which characterize the granulomas are indistinguishable from similar cells in sarcoidosis, Kveim test granulomas, extrinsic allergic 'alveolitis' (farmers' lung), and non-caseating tuberculosis (Jones Williams, 1977). Inclusion bodies of crystalline or Schaumann type are often present in epithelioid and giant cells especially in the fibrotic stage of the disease. Jones Williams (1960) found one or both of these types of body in 62 per cent of 52 cases of chronic beryllium disease and also in 88 per cent of 17 cases of sarcoidosis, but only in 6 per cent of 100 cases of caseating tuberculosis. Schaumann bodies are calcium and iron impregnated conchoidal bodies often containing central, birefringent crystals which may consist of calcite (Jones Williams, 1960). The presence of inclusion bodies has no diagnostic significance. Light microscopy, histochemistry, enzyme content and electron microscopy indicate that the morphology of granulomas in all these

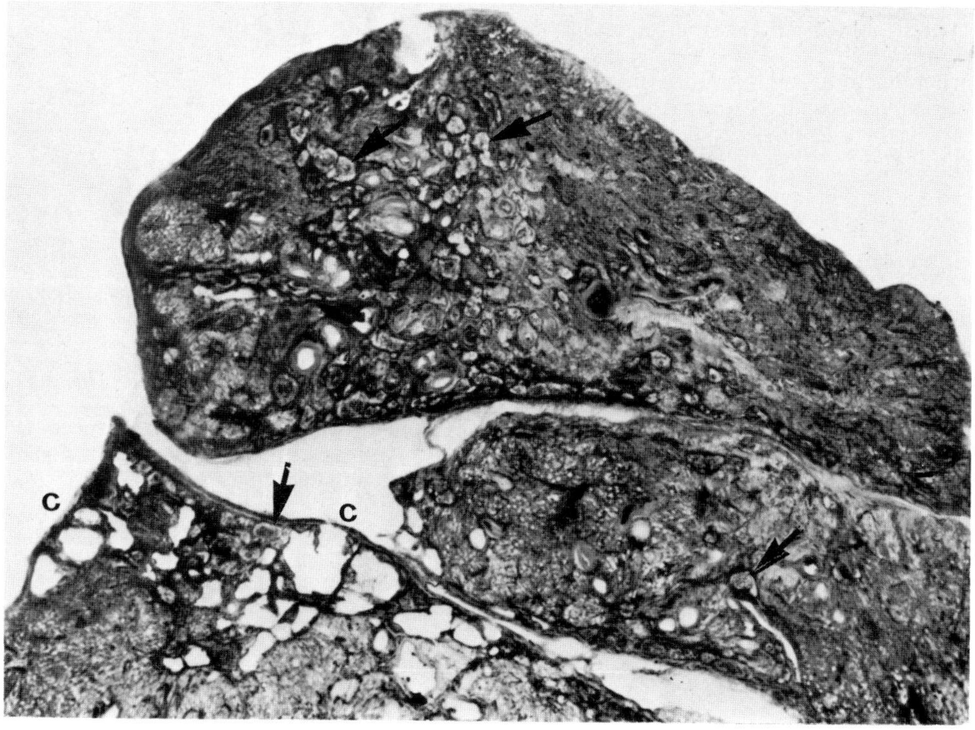

Figure 10.1 Chronic beryllium disease showing small fibrotic nodules resembling silicotic nodules (arrowed) and cystic areas (c). The upper and middle lobes are much contracted due to fibrosis and the pulmonary pleura is moderately thickened; this is particularly evident round the middle lobe and apex of lower lobe. Patches of irregular, diffuse fibrosis are also present in each lobe. (Paper-mounted lung section)

disorders is identical (Jones Williams, 1958; Jones Williams and Williams, 1967; Williams, Jones Williams and Williams, 1969; James and Jones Williams, 1974). The distinction can only be made by the detection of beryllium in the tissues and, during life, by evidence of beryllium hypersensitivity (*see* Immunological features).

Freiman and Hardy (1970) have shown that the histology of chronic beryllium disease tends to fall into one of three categories which they designate as Group I (subdivided into sub-groups A and B) and Group II according to the relative degrees of cellular infiltration of alveolar walls, granuloma formation and the number of conchoidal and Schaumann bodies present (*see Table 10.1* and *Figures 10.2* to *10.5*). Cases which are difficult to classify usually fall into sub-group IB.

Conchoidal bodies are found in about two-thirds of Group I cases and less often in Group II cases (Jones Williams, 1967a; Freiman and Hardy, 1970). The presence of widespread cellular infiltration of alveolar walls and poorly circumscribed granulomas may favour beryllium disease rather than sarcoidosis. Cellular infiltration, when extensive, is associated with a poor prognosis (Freiman and Hardy, 1970).

Ultimately the granulomas are interlaced with reticulin fibres and then obliterated by collagenous fibrosis, which becomes densely eosinophilic and converted to hyaline material. The demonstration of intact reticulin in this material by silver staining may help to distinguish it from caseation (Jones Williams, 1977) though the differentiation is difficult and does not provide an unequivocal criterion (Mitchell *et al.*, 1977).

Well-demarcated, dense, 'hyalinized' nodules (which also sometimes occur in sarcoidosis) are present in about 40 per cent of cases. They vary from very few to large numbers

Table 10.1 Histological Classification of Chronic Beryllium Disease

Histological characteristics	*Group I*		*Group II*
	Sub-group IA	*Sub-group IB*	
Interstitial (alveolar wall) cellular infiltration	Moderate to marked		Slight or absent
Granuloma formation	Poorly formed or absent	Well formed	Numerous and well formed
Conchoidal bodies	Variable; frequently present and numerous		Few or absent

By courtesy of Freiman and Hardy, 1970, and the Editor of *Human Pathology*

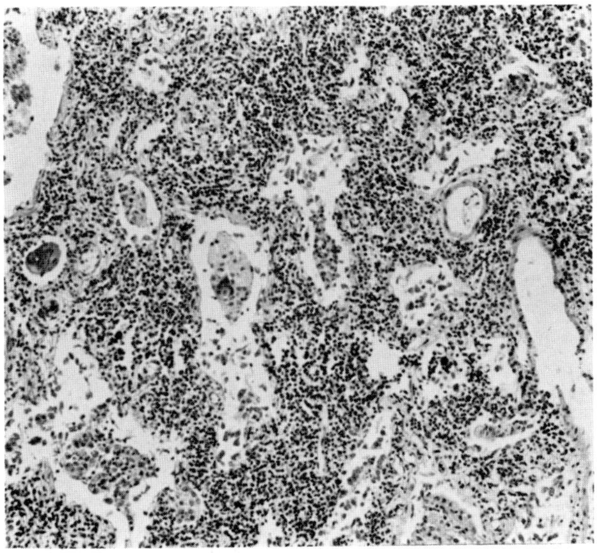

Figure 10.2 Chronic beryllium disease, Group IA. Extensive interstitial cellular infiltration without granuloma formation. (Magnification × 25)

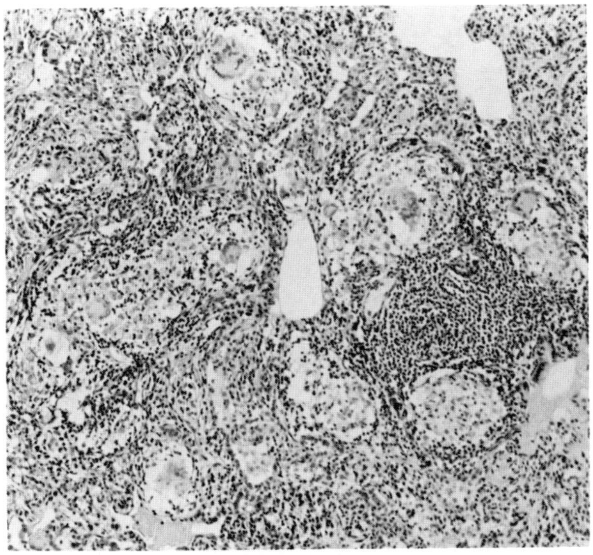

Figure 10.3 Chronic beryllium disease, Group IB. Pronounced interstitial cellular infiltration and well-formed sarcoid-type granulomas with Langhan's giant cells. (Magnification × 25)

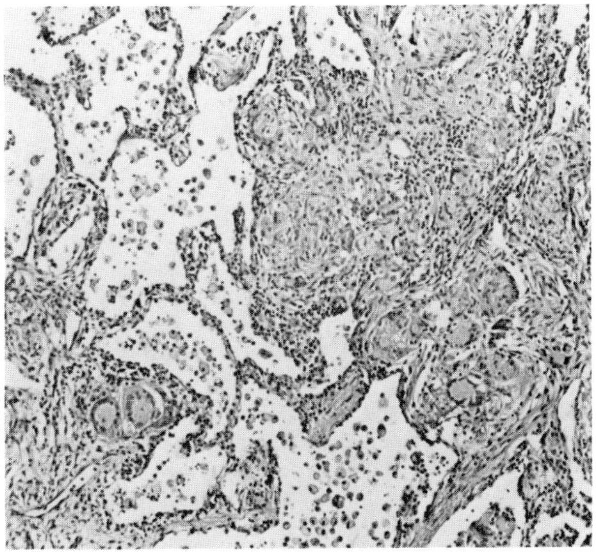

Figure 10.4 Chronic beryllium disease, Group II. Minimal interstitial cellular infiltration and well-formed sarcoid-type granulomas. (Magnification × 25)

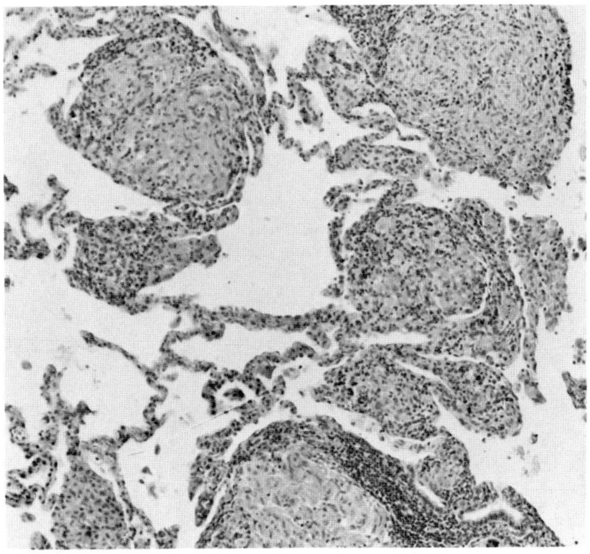

Figure 10.5 Chronic beryllium disease, Group II. Appearances identical with idiopathic sarcoidosis. Prominent granuloma formation and negligible interstitial cellular infiltration. (Magnification × 25)

Figures 10.2 to 10.5 are reproduced by courtesy of Drs Freiman and Hardy and the Editor of Human Pathology

in which case they may be the predominant lesions; and, they are also found in the hilar lymph nodes. Their peripheral zone consists of a narrow ring of fibrosis and their central area, of hyalinized collagen which may contain some black pigment. The nodules closely resemble silicotic lesions although some are distinguished by remnants of granulomas at their periphery (*Figures 10.1* and *10.6*). The presence of these nodules in association with Group II lesions may be helpful in differentiating chronic beryllium disease from sarcoidosis (Freiman and Hardy, 1970).

Diffuse interstitial pulmonary fibrosis of moderate to advanced degree adjacent to granulomas, some of which may be partly or wholly fibrotic, is also evident in about half the cases, and may be associated with honeycombing.

Endarteritis is sometimes present in areas of fibrosis. Emphysema of scar—or 'irregular'—type may occur in relation to fibrosis but is not a characteristic feature.

Extra-pulmonary

Granulomas may also be found in the skin, cervical, intrathoracic and abdominal lymph nodes, the liver, spleen, pancreas, kidneys, suprarenal glands, bone marrow,

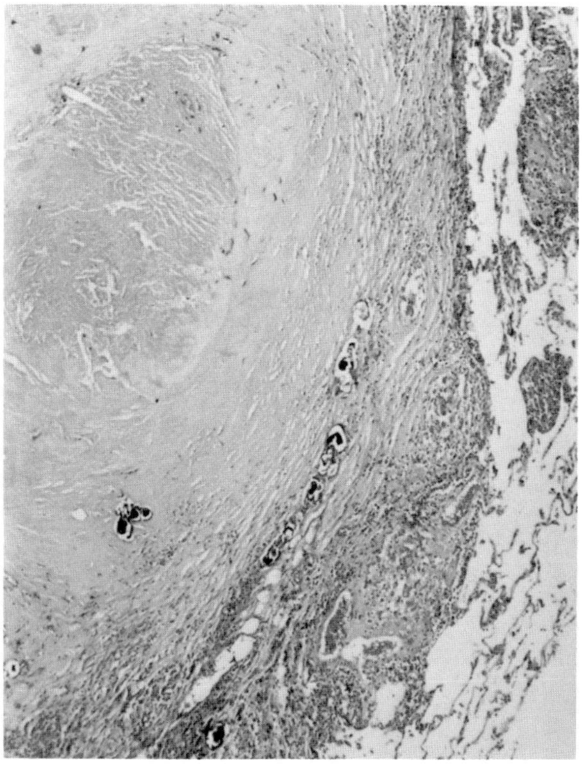

*Figure 10.6 Chronic beryllium disease. Fibrotic nodular lesion with necrotic hyalinized central zone. Calcified inclusions (small densely black areas) are present in the fibrotic zone and granulomatous infiltration can be seen at the periphery. Granulomas are also present in close proximity to the nodule, the appearances of which are similar to a typical silicotic lesion (*Figure 7.4*); the distinguishing features are the inclusions and adjacent granulomas. Magnification × 10; reproduced by courtesy of Drs Freiman and Hardy and the Editor of* Human Pathology*)*

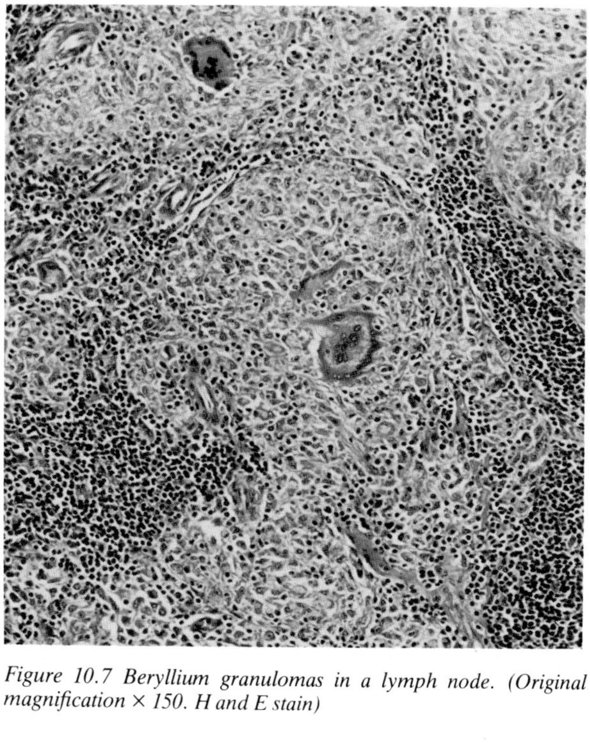

Figure 10.7 Beryllium granulomas in a lymph node. (Original magnification × 150. H and E stain)

skeletal muscle, and central nervous system; and there is some evidence that the myocardium may occasionally be involved (Sprince, Kazemi and Hardy, 1976) (*Figure 10.7*). Skin granulomas may precede lung disease and, unlike those seen in sarcoidosis, may ulcerate (Jones Williams, 1967 a and b and 1971). An apparently unique case of chronic beryllium ulceration of a finger followed by extensive local lymphatic spread and later by granulomas of the lungs has been reported; the beryllium content at all the sites involved was high (Jones Williams and Kilpatrick, 1974). Although skin granulomas are usually due to intradermal implantation of beryllium salts they may occasionally follow respiratory exposure. Stoeckle, Hardy and Weber (1969) found four examples among 60 cases of respiratory exposure only.

BERYLLIUM CONTENT OF THE LUNGS

This bears little or no relationship to the type and severity of disease nor, indeed, to its presence; and it may be distributed unevenly in the lungs. Analysis of other organs—liver, kidney, spleen, bone—has also revealed wide variations in content (Tepper, Hardy and Chamberlin, 1961). Small amounts of beryllium are sometimes found in the lungs of persons with no known industrial exposure to beryllium compounds. This is usually attributed to the fact that urban air may contain small amounts of beryllium from the ash of some fossil fuels. For example, from 0.0001 to 0.003 $\mu g/m^3$ was detected in air samples from some 30 metropolitan areas in the USA (Chambers, Foster and Cholak, 1955).

However, beryllium disease is rarely seen without there being some beryllium in the lungs and mediastinal lymph nodes. Its detection depends upon sensitive techniques and an adequate amount of tissue for analysis. A recent analytical study of lung tissue and mediastinal nodes from known cases of beryllium disease, sarcoidosis and normal controls revealed some practical information (Sprince, Kazemi and Hardy, 1976):

(1) In the control and sarcoid cases the lungs and lymph nodes contained only minute amounts of beryllium which were uniformly less than 0.02 $\mu g/g$ of dried tissue.
(2) In 66 cases of beryllium disease the beryllium content of the lungs was in excess of 0.02 $\mu g/g$ of dried tissue in 82 per cent and the overall mean value was 1.19 $\mu g/g$ (range = 0.004 to 45.7 $\mu g/g$). In mediastinal nodes the average level was 3.41 $\mu g/g$ (range = 0.056 to 8.50 $\mu g/g$). Levels in peripheral lymph nodes, however, were lower than those in the lungs and mediastinal nodes.

Hence, although overlap of beryllium content evidently occurs the level in the lungs and mediastinal nodes in beryllium disease is, in general, considerably higher than it is in sarcoidosis or control cases. Thus, analysis of these tissues may be of diagnostic value if the concentration found is relatively high but, if low, should be treated with some reserve.

BIOCHEMICAL ABNORMALITIES

There is often an increase in urinary calcium in patients with chronic beryllium disease and, if renal function is impaired, hypercalcaemia results. The underlying reason for the high urinary calcium is obscure but, as beryllium is known to be excreted by the tubules (Underwood, 1951), cellular intoxication at this level is a possible explanation. It is not attributed to immobilization of the patient but to the activity of the disease (Tepper, Hardy and Chamberlin, 1961; Stoeckle, Hardy and Weber, 1969). Renal failure, however, is rare unless calculi develop (*see* Complications). Steroid therapy results in return to normal of the urinary calcium levels. Both hypercalcaemia and renal calculi, of course, may also occur in sarcoidosis.

Hyperuricaemia develops in some cases of chronic beryllium disease and also in a proportion of patients with sarcoidosis. This appears to be due to impaired renal clearance rather than to an increased production of uric acid, but its cause is not understood. There is no correlation between hyperuricaemia and the nature and duration of exposure to beryllium, severity of disease, or the presence of beryllium in the urine (Kelley, Goldfinger and Hardy, 1969) (*see* Complications).

Serum alkaline phosphatase activity has usually been reported to be normal (Tepper, Hardy and Chamberlin, 1961) but, *in vitro,* is inhibited in varying degree according to the experimental conditions used (Tepper, 1972). Though serum angiotensin-converting enzyme (ACE) and serum lysozyme levels are significantly raised in sarcoidosis compared with healthy controls (Studdy *et al.,* 1978; Rohrbach and Deremee, 1979; Selroos and Grönhagen-Riska, 1979). Sprince, Kazemi and Fanburg (1980) found no increase in serum ACE in chronic beryllium disease and suggested that the test may be useful in differentiating this disorder from sarcoidosis. But Torii *et al.* (1980) have reported that serum ACE and lysozyme activity is similarly increased in both sarcoidosis and chronic beryllium disease. These discrepitant findings may, perhaps, be due to differences in disease activity in cases selected for study. However, if normal serum ACE levels in chronic beryllium disease can be verified this would certainly provide a valuable additional diagnostic index.

IMMUNOLOGICAL FEATURES

CIRCULATING IMMUNOGLOBULINS

An increase in circulating immunoglobulins has been repeatedly observed during exacerbations of chronic disease and this has prompted speculation that humoral antibodies may be involved. The concentrations of immunoglobulins are often raised but the Ig types affected have varied in different reports: in one the predominant increase was in IgA in 17 of 35 patients with chronic disease (Deodhar, Barna and van Ordstrand, 1973); in another it was IgG in five or six patients with disease and 13 of 22 individuals with beryllium exposure but no evidence of disease (Resnick, Roche and Morgan, 1970). The significance of these findings is uncertain but, as IgG and IgA are often elevated in sarcoidosis especially in female and black patients (Buckley and Dorsey, 1970; Goldstein, Israel and Rawnsley, 1969), Ig levels are of little practical value in diagnosis.

The status of ANA and RF in chronic beryllium disease does not seem to be known but a significant increase in both, which is not correlated with the activity or extent of the disease, may be present in sarcoidosis (Oreskes and Siltzbach, 1968, Veien *et al.,* 1976).

SKIN REACTIVITY

Beryllium patch test

Hypersensitivity to beryllium may be detected by the development of an erythematous reaction in 48 to 72 hours after patch testing with a solution of beryllium sulphate or nitrate (Curtis, 1959). Skin granulomas may develop in three to four weeks. However, a positive response may occur in beryllium exposed individuals with acute dermatitis or granulomatous lesions but no systemic involvement in the lungs or elsewhere; and a small proportion of patients with chronic disease does not react at all (Stoeckle, Hardy and Weber, 1969). Furthermore, as Curtis showed, the test itself can induce hypersensitivity because control individuals with no beryllium exposure who are negative on initial testing react positively when the test is repeated. For these reasons and the further possibility that exacerbation of existing beryllium disease might be provoked (Sneddon, 1955) it is generally regarded as unsuitable in clinical and industrial medical practice. But Jones Williams, Nosworthy and Williams (1980) found that there were no complications in 20 patch-tested cases of beryllium disease 16 of which were positive. A positive reaction is reversed by corticosteroids (Norris and Peard, 1963; Ambrosi *et al.,* 1968).

Kveim test

The Kveim test is usually negative (Stoeckle, Hardy and Weber, 1969; Jones Williams, Nosworthy and Williams, 1978), and, provided that the Kveim suspension exhibits little cross-reactivity (Siltzbach, 1976), it is a valuable adjunct to differential diagnosis. However, this test is negative in 10 to 15 per cent of cases of subacute sarcoidosis and 30 to 35 per cent of cases of chronic sarcoidosis (Mitchell *et al.,* 1977). Prospective study of the Kveim test in a large number of cases of beryllium disease does not appear to have been carried out.

Tuberculin test

Although the response to the tuberculin test has not been studied with the same epidemiological vigour in beryllium disease as in sarcoidosis the available evidence indicates that it is generally negative in chronic disease (Stoeckle, Hardy and Weber, 1969; Izumi *et al.,* 1976; Price *et al.,* 1977; Jones Williams, Nosworthy and Williams, 1978). In a factory survey in Japan there appeared to be a tendency for more healthy beryllium workers to be non-reactors than comparable groups of non-exposed workers. This was thought to imply beryllium sensitization and, possibly, an increased risk of developing beryllium disease (Izumi *et al.,* 1976). However, continuing study of these workers over another three years has not supported this. Three new cases of beryllium disease were tuberculin positive before its onset and negative at the time of diagnosis (Nishikawa and Izumi, 1978).

The behaviour of the lepromin reaction in chronic disease is not known.

Lymphocyte transformation and macrophage migration inhibition (see p. 59)

T lymphocytes from individuals with beryllium hypersensitivity are highly reactive *in vitro* when incubated with beryllium compounds or the insoluble oxide and undergo blastogenic transformation; whereas, under similar conditions, lymphocytes from non-sensitive donors do not exhibit blastogenesis. Moreover, there is a good correlation between the clinical severity of chronic disease and the degree of transformation (Hanifin, Epstein and Cline, 1970; Deodhar, Barna and van Ordstrand, 1973; Preuss, 1975). Similarly, lymphocytes from patients with chronic beryllium disease or hypersensitivity to beryllium are readily stimulated to transformation by the mitogen phytohaemagglutinin (PHA) whereas lymphocytes from patients with active sarcoidosis have a depressed response (Jett, 1971; Morison, 1976). Although, at present, there is some inconsistency in results from different laboratories due to lack of standardization, the beryllium lymphocyte transformation test appears to be a valuable and accurate index of beryllium hypersensitivity (*see* pp. 348 to 349).

Cell-free supernatant fluid from positive beryllium lymphocyte transformation preparations contain a macrophage migration inhibition factor (MIF) which is immunologically specific. Beryllium added to lymphocytes from non-sensitized donors does not stimulate either blast transformation or MIF production (Henderson *et al.*, 1972). But the beryllium MIF test (Be MIF test) is positive in some patients with chronic disease—provided that they are not receiving steroid treatment—and in a small number (14 per cent) of healthy beryllium workers, though not in sarcoidosis patients (Marx and Burrell, 1973; Price *et al.*, 1977). The suppression of positivity of the test by steroids is reversed if they are discontinued for two to three weeks. A positive response probably weakens with time but, at present, little is known about this. There is some indication that a positive Be MIF test correlates with tuberculin negativity (Price *et al.*, 1977).

Cellular and immunological components of bronchoalveolar lavage fluid

It is not yet known whether the significant increase in lymphocyte content and reduction in IgG/albumin ratio which has been found in the fluid of patients with sarcoidosis (Weinberger *et al.*, 1978) occurs in chronic beryllium disease but information on this topic will be of great interest and might be of help in indicating activity of the disease.

The relevance of some of these tests to diagnosis is referred to later in the appropriate section.

PATHOGENESIS

As stated earlier acute and chronic beryllium disease are two distinct syndromes and their pathogenesis is completely different.

ACUTE DISEASE

This is always associated with an excessive exposure to beryllium dusts, fumes or mists. The soluble salts are largely responsible for upper respiratory symptoms and less soluble compounds of small particle size, for bronchopneumonic disease. It is clearly dose-related and the result of an acute toxic effect.

Acute, non-specific, chemical pneumonia identical to that seen in man has been produced in various species of animals by beryllium oxide and the soluble salts of which beryllium fluoride is the most toxic (Hall *et al.*, 1950; Stokinger *et al.*, 1953).

The fact that acute disease may exceptionally progress to chronic disease suggests development of hypersensitivity to beryllium remaining in the lungs.

CHRONIC DISEASE

Immunological aspects

The fact that the development of chronic disease is often separated from beryllium exposure by latent periods of variable, sometimes prolonged, duration; and that the attack-rate among workers is low and not evidently dose-related (*see* p. 336) points, as Sterner and Eisenbud (1951) originally suggested, to involvement of immunological factors. The immunological features of human disease—delayed response to the beryllium patch test, depressed tuberculin reactivity, lymphocyte blast transformation and the presence of Be MIF—strongly support this and indicate a cell-mediated Type IV reaction. The underlying reason as to why such a reaction should occur is not understood. Although the existence of a 'beryllium antigen' seems now to be accepted its identity is not known. As the beryllium ion is too small to act as a complete antigen it is possible that it achieves antigenicity by attaching itself to a protein or other macromolecule and, thus functions as a hapten. Animals inoculated with Freund's adjuvant in which mycobacteria are replaced by beryllium develop antibodies to the antigen and granulomas which, however, are not as widely dispersed nor as rich in epithelioid cells as those caused by the complete (mycobacterial) adjuvant (Salvaggio, Flax and Leskowitz, 1965). Unanue, Askonas and Allison, (1969) made the interesting observation that beryllium sulphate is a potent adjuvant in increasing antibody response to antigen (*Maia squinada haemocyanin*) after its uptake by mouse macrophages and that this effect does not depend upon beryllium and the antigen being present in the same cell.

Skin hypersensitivity to beryllium can be passively transferred to normal guinea pigs by the injection of lymphocytes, but not serum, from beryllium-sensitized guinea pigs (Cirla, Barbiano di Belgiojoso and Chiappino, 1968). It also appears that transient contact sensitivity to beryllium can be transmitted by transfer factor (TF) from lymphocytes of human donors with strong cellular immunity to beryllium to human recipients 'primed' with subsensitizing doses of beryllium fluoride. Fourteen of 38 recipients (37 per cent) developed a positive patch test to beryllium fluoride 24 hours or more after receiving the TF but this reactivity lasted more than a week in only four cases (Epstein and Byers, 1979). Further investigation is needed to confirm these findings and their significance: whether, for example, nonspecific transfer factor might not work equally well.

Inhalation of beryllium sulphate by guinea pigs in which cutaneous hypersensitivity to beryllium has previously been established and reinforced by repeated injections has been shown to result in a much diminished response in their lungs compared with those of non-sensitized animals (Reeves, 1980). It is not known whether this apparent immunization to beryllium disease of the lungs occurs in man.

Rabbits in which delayed hypersensitivity to beryllium sulphate has been induced develop antigen-specific alveolar macrophage migration inhibition. Beryllium sulphate is highly toxic to isolated alveolar macrophages *in vitro* causing swelling of mitochondia and disruption of the cell membrane and cellular sap, but, in striking contrast to the situation so far observed in man and guinea pigs, it *depresses* lymphocyte transformation in sensitized rabbits which show delayed skin reactivity and macrophage inhibition (Kang *et al.*, 1977). Species difference might explain the depressed lymphocyte response but this requires clarification.

Unlike beryllium salts zirconium compounds, which may cause non-caseating granulomas of the skin in man, have not been found to induce delayed hypersensitivity in experimental animals (*see* Chapter 6, p. 124). This may be due to the relatively soluble beryllium salts being rapidly and widely dispersed after injection whereas insoluble zirconium compounds are poorly dispersed, so that access to immunologically competent cells will be facilitated in the case of beryllium salts but severely limited in that of insoluble zirconium compounds (Kang *et al.*, 1977).

The significance of an increase in circulating Igs in human disease has not been explained but there is no evidence to suggest that humoral factors are involved in pathogenesis.

To summarize: Although the mechanisms are by no means clear there is now little doubt that immunological activity plays a key role in the pathogenesis of beryllium disease.

Other aspects

The phagocytosis of beryllium by alveolar macrophages of rats and guinea pigs *in vitro* appears to depend on the solubility of beryllium compounds: the soluble are not taken up whereas insoluble particles are, and are probably localized in phagolysosomes (Hart and Pittman, 1980). The fact that 'low-fired' beryllium oxide is much more toxic—and more soluble—than 'high-fired' oxide (*see* p. 334) in the lungs of a variety of animals does not, however, appear to have any proven relevance to the development of human disease (Tepper, 1972).

Although beryllium has been shown experimentally to cause disturbances in the activity of various enzymes *in vitro* and *in vivo* and abnormalities of protein and nucleic acid metabolism in animals, apart from serum ACE, these observations do not appear to have any application to man (Reeves, 1977). Imbalance of suprarenal gland activity, observed in beryllium-treated guinea pigs, has been postulated as the basic 'triggering' factor in exacerbation of chronic beryllium disease (Clary and Stokinger, 1973) (*see* p. 336). However, there is no evidence that this occurs in man and, though reduction in suprarenal reserve has been reported in patients with chronic beryllium disease (Orlova and Ozerova, 1966), this may be an effect of the disease rather than a factor in its cause.

Why chronic beryllium disease resembles sarcoidosis so closely in some respects while exhibiting a few striking exceptions in others remains to be explained. Important exceptions are these:

(1) Uveitis and erythema nodosum have not been encountered and isolated bilateral hilar lymphadenopathy occurs only rarely in beryllium disease.
(2) Unlike beryllium disease a large majority of patients with sarcoidosis recover spontaneously and only a few with chronic—so-called stages II and III—disease progress to fibrosis.

CARCINOGENESIS

Beryllium, in the form of the oxide or certain compounds has been shown to cause malignancy in animals which, however, is specific to certain species. Rats and monkeys develop lung cancer and rabbits, osteosarcoma after inhalation; whereas guinea pigs show no evidence of malignancy at any site following either inhalation or injection (Reeves, 1977).

Analysis of the total population of two major beryllium-extraction companies in the USA did not show any excess of lung cancer in beryllium exposed individuals but did reveal a slight increase in those with lung disease including beryllium disease (Mancuso, 1970). An interesting point to emerge from this study was that the incidence of lung cancer in beryllium workers showed an inverse relationship to the length of their exposure in the industry, and it has been suggested that human beings may resemble guinea pigs in being susceptible to beryllium disease but resistant to the development of lung cancer (Reeves, 1977). In a study of 4000 beryllium workers referred to by Utidjian (1973) there was no significant excess of respiratory tract cancers.

However, more recent studies of workers in the US beryllium industry suggest that they have an excess risk of lung cancer which is not apparently explained by smoking or personal characteristics alone (Infante, Wagoner and Sprince, 1980; Mancuso, 1980; Wagoner, Infante and Bayliss, 1980). No particular cell type of tumour has been identified (Smith and Suzuki, 1980). Confirmation of these findings is clearly necessary. In Hardy's opinion (1980) 'more knowledge is needed to clarify what part beryllium plays, at what dose, in the production of lung cancer with or without what factors'.

CLINICAL FEATURES

SYMPTOMS

The beryllium US Case Registry figures have shown that respiratory disease is the commonest mode of presentation (Hardy, Rabe and Lorch, 1967).

In *acute disease,* depending upon the magnitude of exposure, there is irritation of the nose and pharynx with copious mucoid nasal discharge and mild epistaxis; paroxysmal cough which raises bloodstained sputum when pneumonitis is present, but is non-productive in its absence; a burning, tight sensation in the centre of the chest, and moderate breathlessness on effort. These symptoms commence within about 72 hours of heavy exposure. In persons who have worked with soluble acid salts there may also be irritation of the eyes, and, in some cases, an itching, burning skin rash of exposed parts of the body, without respiratory symptoms. When the onset is slower, or sub-acute (usually within a few weeks of first exposure), there is cough of gradually increasing severity which is frequently paroxysmal and small quantities of sputum which may be bloodstained, progressively increasing breathlessness on exertion, and pronounced lassitude with anorexia and loss of weight. If these symptoms persist for more than 12 months the disease is said to be chronic.

In *chronic disease* symptoms develop insidiously, commonly within a month to some five years—rarely as much as 25 years (*see* p. 336)—after last exposure, but, as previously stated they may become established after the patient has partly recovered from acute disease. The most common is dyspnoea on exertion which is, in some cases, the only symptom. The next most common is an irritating, usually unproductive, cough which is worse in the mornings and after exertion and may be paroxysmal, ending in retching and vomiting; it is possible that this may be due to granulomas in bronchial walls (Tepper, Hardy and Chamberlin, 1961). Occasionally there is mucoid, or less often, purulent sputum, and, though haemoptysis has been recorded, it is rare. Breathlessness on effort may gradually increase and, in cases of advanced disease, become severe when it may be accompanied by anorexia, malaise, lassitude and loss of weight. But progression of the symptoms of early disease is prevented and those of advanced disease alleviated by steroid treatment (*see* Treatment). Sudden worsening of dyspnoea, sometimes with chest pain, may be caused by spontaneous pneumothorax (*see* Complications).

Chronic disease, however, may be symptomless or associated with only slight cough and mild breathlessness on effort but, as noted earlier, sudden exacerbation can occur in relation to respiratory infection, surgery, pregnancy or re-exposure to beryllium compounds.

PHYSICAL SIGNS

In *acute disease* there is low-grade fever, central cyanosis, rapid heart and respiratory rates, and widespread crepitations over the lungs. Contact dermatitis which may result from exposure to the acid salts is of papulovesicular type, sometimes weeping and oedematous, on the hands, arms, trunk, head and neck. Conjunctivitis is often associated with pronounced conjunctival oedema.

In cases of mild *chronic disease* there may be no abnormal signs but in more advanced disease, finger clubbing is present in about 20 per cent of cases (Stoeckle, Hardy and Weber, 1969), there may be central cyanosis, and pleural friction with persistent crepitations (which predominate in the upper or lower parts of the lungs according to the distribution of the disease) are usual. In uncomplicated disease the liver is sometimes slightly enlarged, but not tender (Hall *et al.*, 1959).

During exacerbation or rapid progression of chronic disease there may be fever up to about 38.9°C (102°F) with rigors, and in advanced disease there may be signs of congestive heart failure but this is uncommon today. Pronounced cachexia was also a feature of the disease in the past but is now rarely seen.

Skin granulomas, indistinguishable from those of 'idiopathic' sarcoidosis, may develop at some stage of the illness but, unlike the persistent lesions caused by local traumatic implantation of particles of beryllium compounds, they resolve with steroid therapy or remission of the disease. Lupus pernio and erythema nodosum do not occur.

INVESTIGATIONS

LUNG FUNCTION

The functional abnormalities of *acute disease* are the same as those found in pneumonia or pulmonary oedema and consist of hypoxaemia and hypercapnoea resulting from uneven distribution of ventilation and perfusion (*see* Chapter 1), and airways obstruction. The severity of these changes depends upon the extent of the disease. Unless resolution is incomplete and the disease becomes chronic function subsequently returns to normal.

The abnormalities seen in *chronic disease* are in no way specific; they may occur equally in sarcoidosis, extrinsic allergic 'alveolitis' and DIPF from any cause. In the early stages reduction in gas transfer, arterial hypoxaemia—especially on effort—and increase in alveolar–arterial oxygen tension difference are present. These changes are probably due mainly to multiple granulomas and cellular infiltration of alveolar walls as they can be reversed significantly by steroid treatment. With more advanced disease, when a varying amount of nodular or diffuse fibrosis can be expected, combined 'restrictive' and gas transfer defects, the degree of which reflect the severity of the disease, are present. They are unaffected by steroids. Gas transfer tends to deteriorate less over the years than other functional parameters (Andrews, Kazemi and Hardy, 1969).

Obstruction or reduction of air flow, apparently unrelated to smoking, has been noted in a minority of patients with chronic beryllium disease or sarcoidosis (Andrews, Kazemi and Hardy, 1969; McCarthy and Sigurdson, 1978). This may be due to granulomatous infiltration or fibrosis in terminal and respiratory bronchioles or to reduced elastic recoil. It is possible, too, that some larger airways may be involved.

Patients with both restrictive and obstructive defects have more hypoxaemia and greater respiratory disability over a five-year period than those with a predominantly gas transfer defect (Andrews, Kazemi and Hardy, 1969).

Spontaneous improvement in hypoxaemia and the alveolar–arterial oxygen tension difference has been reported over a three-year period in 13 of 20 workers (who had not changed their smoking habits) following a substantial reduction in peak air concentrations of beryllium in their factory environment during that time (Sprince *et al.*, 1978). Whether this was due to resolution of granulomas as a result of reduced exposure is uncertain, but is possible.

RADIOGRAPHIC APPEARANCES

Acute disease

Abnormal changes in the lung fields lag behind the symptoms and clinical signs by one to three weeks. Serial films show the development, first of a diffuse haziness and then of widespread, large, 'woolly' opacities similar to those of pulmonary oedema which correlate with areas of consolidation. As the patient recovers the opacities clear and, in most cases, appearances return to normal in a few months (*Figure 10.8*).

In subacute disease very small, discrete opacities appear throughout both lung fields (*Figure 10.9*) but with

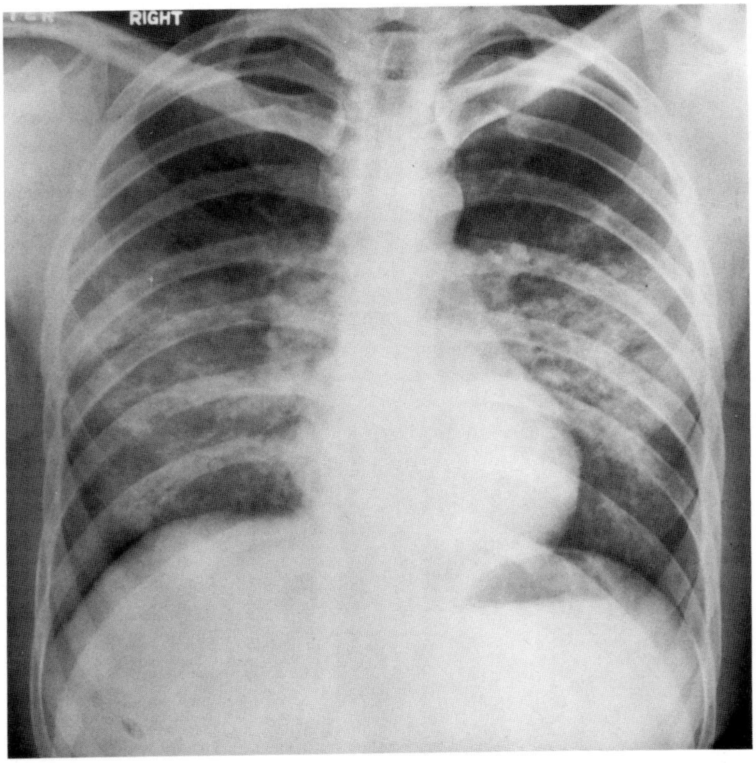

Figure 10.8 Acute beryllium disease in a male metallurgist. Complete recovery and clearing of the radiograph followed. (By courtesy of Dr Harriet Hardy)

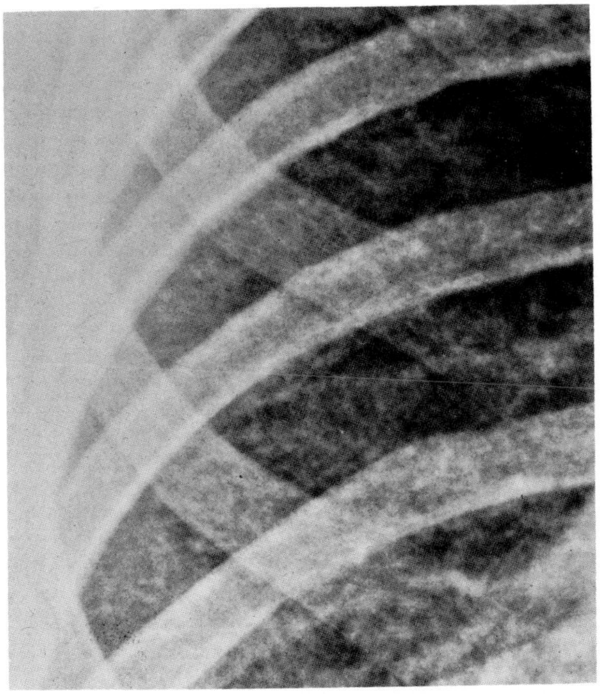

Figure 10.9 Small, discrete opacities, similar in both lung fields, which developed without further exposure following an episode of acute disease six years earlier and appeared to resolve completely. Subsequently chronic disease, including recurrent renal calculi, became established. Case of an atomic research worker subjected to accidental beryllium contamination in the 1940s. (Courtesy of Dr Harriet Hardy)

corticosteroid treatment may disappear within a few weeks. In some cases the opacities may be slightly larger.

Chronic disease

There is a variety of abnormal appearances which may occur within weeks of the onset of symptoms, but which are in no way pathognomonic. Abnormal opacities which are bilateral, but not necessarily equally so, have been classified as 'granular' (discrete opacities up to 1 mm in diameter), 'nodular' (discrete opacities 1 to 5 mm in diameter) and 'linear' (Stoeckle, Hardy and Weber, 1969), and the following variations are seen (Weber, Stoeckle and Hardy, 1965).

(1) Fine, discrete ('granular'), widespread opacities which remain unchanged for years (*Figure 10.10*) and in some cases become unusually dense due to microscopic calcification in granulomatous lesions. Rarely, small opacities may first appear some years after acute disease without further exposure to beryllium.
(2) Similar type opacities confined mainly to the lower zones of the lung fields with subsequent development of condensed irregular opacities in these zones sometimes with increased translucency in the upper zones. This indication of lung contraction takes a few years to appear.
(3) Small, discrete round opacities in the upper and mid-zones which may progress to linear shadows indicative of fibrosis with contraction of the upper zones and translucent areas of cyst formation (*Figure 10.11*).
(4) Widespread, discrete, larger ('nodular') shadows which increase progressively in size, and the subsequent development of numerous, translucent areas due to cysts and emphysematous bullae. Confluent opacities may

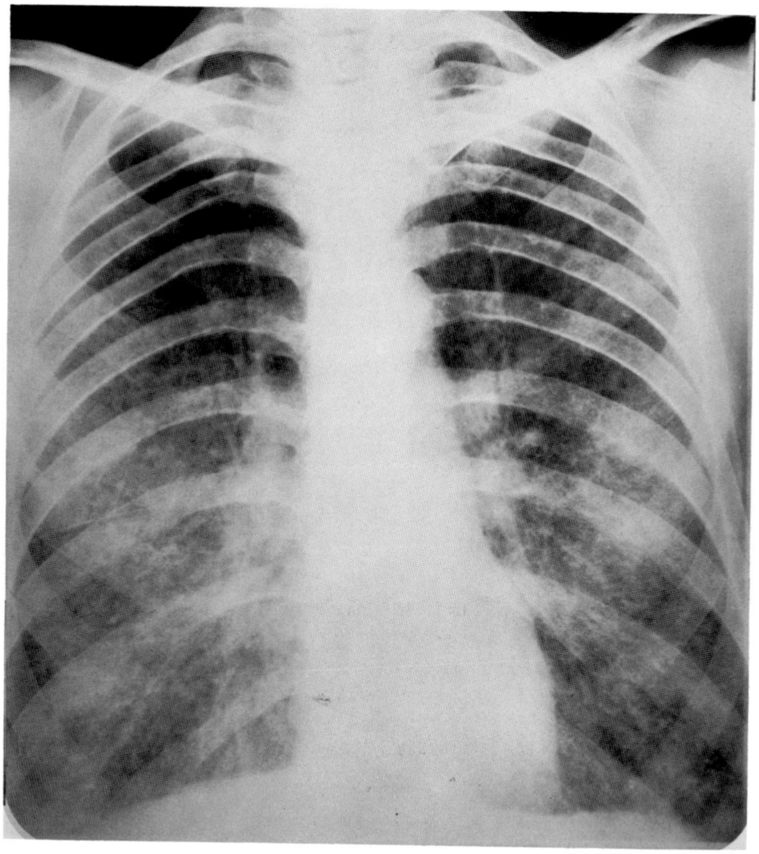

Figure 10.10 Widespread minute opacities and larger ill-defined opacities in both middle and lower zones in chronic beryllium disease. Chemical process worker exposed to beryllium intermittently for three years during the late 1940s in a laboratory manufacturing phosphors for fluorescent lamps and screens. Weight loss, central cyanosis, moderate finger clubbing, persistent crepitations in lower lobes of the lungs, and severe respiratory disability. Poor response to corticosteroids. Death from cardiorespiratory failure four years after initial symptoms. Microscopical confirmation of diagnosis post mortem

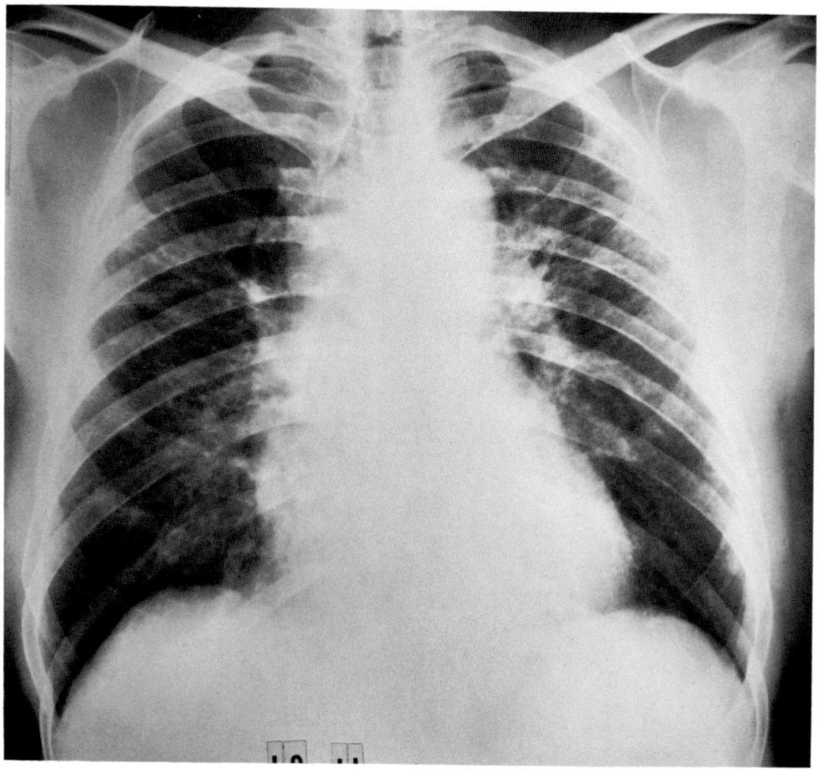

Figure 10.11 Appearances of irregular fibrosis in both upper zones with some contraction of right upper lobe (lesser fissure elevated) which evolved from a few small indefinite rounded opacities six years earlier. Mild respiratory disability. Intermittent renal colic. No abnormal physical signs in lungs apart from localized wheezing. Lung function: mild restrictive and gas transfer defects. Kveim and tuberculin tests negative. Bronchial biopsy: sarcoid-type granulomas. Beryllium present in urine; approximately 0.3 mg/day. Be MIF test positive before steroid treatment; Be lymphocyte transformation positive while receiving prednisolone. Press operator producing ingots of different densities from powdered beryllium metal—1955 to 1975

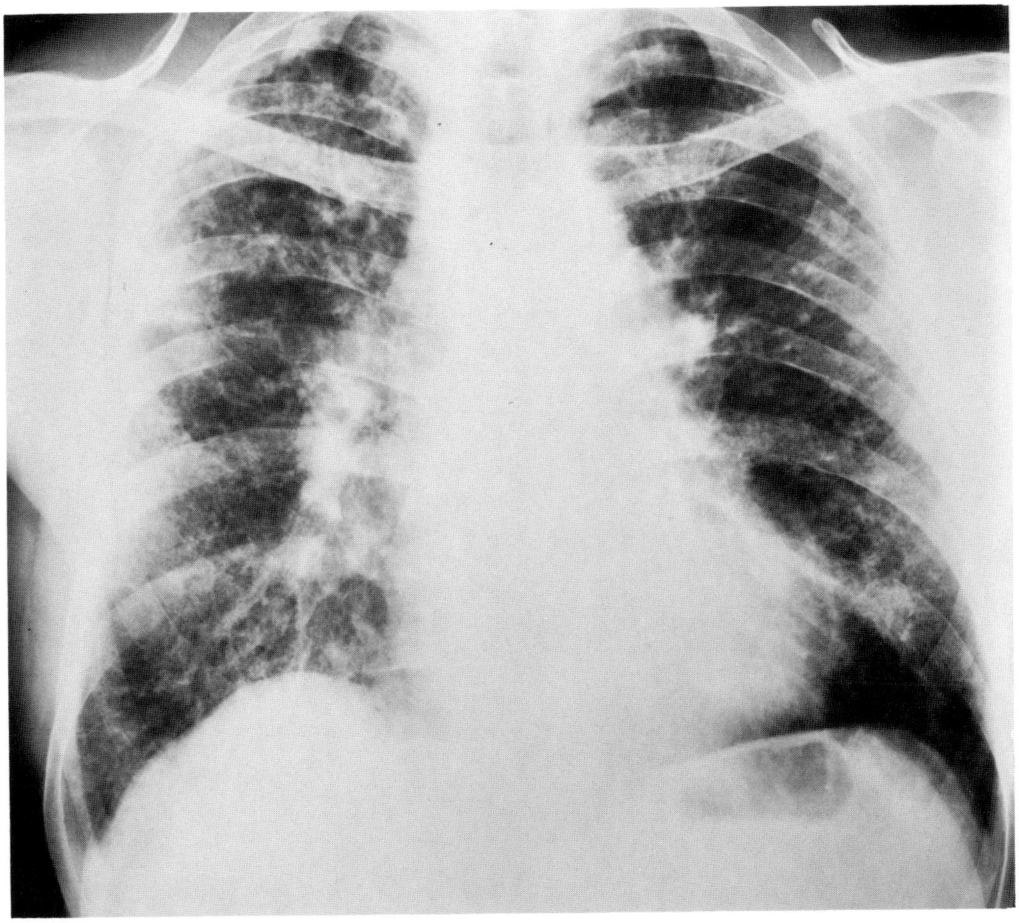

Figure 10.12 Multiple, dense, rounded opacities and evidence of diffuse pleural thickening. Irregular opacities of DIPF in right costophrenic angle. Foundry man pouring ladles of molten beryllium into moulds for four years during the late 1950s. No 'silica' exposure. Dyspnoea on effort noted ten years later. Investigations 14 years after leaving foundry. Sputum consistently culture negative for M. tuberculosis. *Tuberculin and Kveim tests negative. Beryllium patch test positive. Lung biopsy: sarcoid-type granulomas with moderate numbers of lymphocytes and occasional hyalinized nodules. Lung function: moderate restrictive and gas transfer defects*

appear later giving an appearance identical with nodular silicosis or irregular PMF (*Figure 10.12*). In other cases, as the signs of irregular fibrosis progress, 'nodular' opacities tend to regress. Contraction and distortion of the upper halves of the lungs due to fibrosis may be severe and the trachea much displaced and deformed.

(5) 'Nodular' opacities may become strikingly dense and contrasted due to the presence of calcification (*Figure 10.13*). They are then similar to calcified silicotic lesions or the small, calcified lesions of the 'rheumatoid' variant of coal pneumoconiosis. These probably represent calcified hyaline nodules.

(6) 'Nodular' opacities with bilateral enlargement of hilar lymph node shadows. Hilar node enlargement is uncommon and very rarely more than moderate in degree and, exceptionally, may be seen in the absence of any abnormality in the lung fields (Sprince, Kazemi and Hardy, 1976). This contrasts with the situation in sarcoidosis. In some cases the nodes become calcified.

(7) The changes may be entirely those of bilateral DIPF (*Figure 10.14*).

Occasionally discrete opacities regress, decreasing both in number and density, but never disappear completely. In most cases, however, the abnormalities increase progressively, though usually very slowly. A rapid increase is usually associated with exacerbation of disease. It is rare for no radiographic change to take place over a decade.

The commonest abnormality consists of a mixture of 'granular' (very small), 'nodular' and 'linear' (irregular) opacities and the least common is that of 'granular' opacities alone (*Figure 10.10*).

Evidence of pleural thickening involving mainly the upper zones (*Figure 10.12*) or of pneumothorax (*Figure 10.13*) is seen in a small proportion of cases (*see* Complications).

The effect of corticosteroid treatment on radiographic appearance is referred to in the section on Treatment.

SKIN TESTS

Kveim test

As this is usually negative in chronic beryllium disease it is most valuable in differentiating it from sarcoidosis, and is

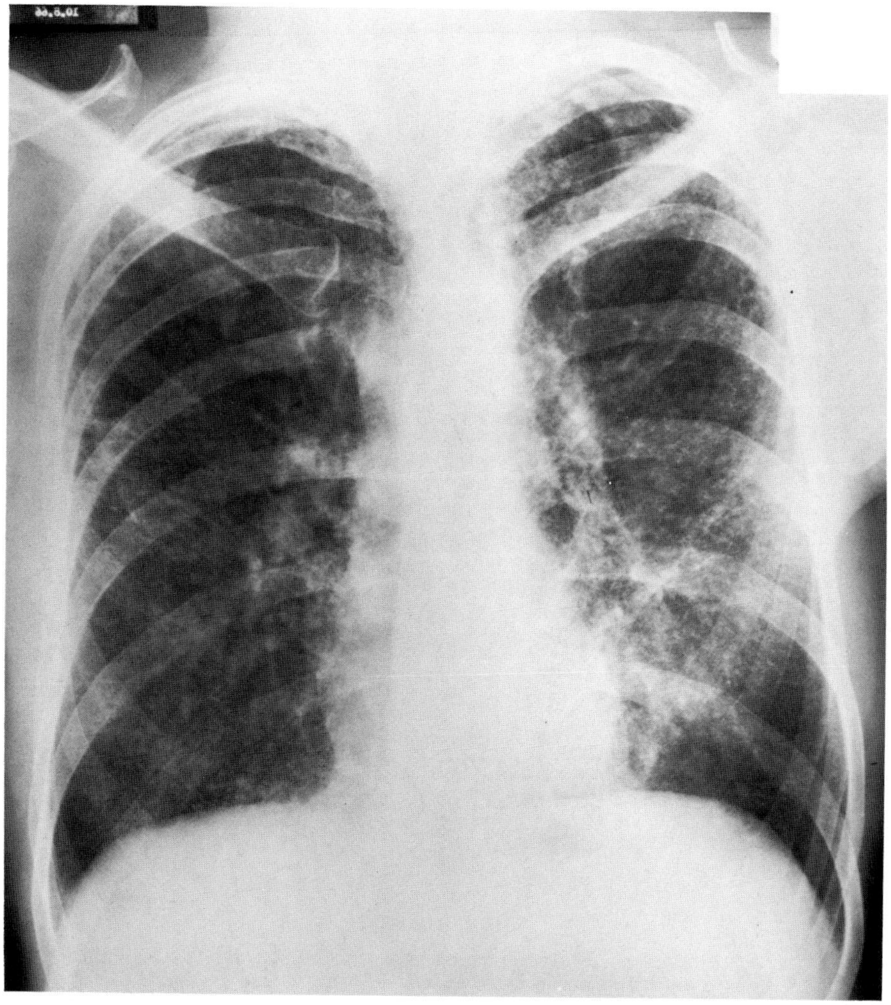

Figure 10.13(a) 1966

thus helpful in diagnosis. The necessity for minimal cross-reactivity of the suspension used has already been referred to on p. 341.

Tuberculin test

This is almost always negative in chronic disease.

Beryllium patch test (*see* p. 341)

This consists of applying gauze soaked with 2 per cent beryllium sulphate or nitrate or 1 per cent fluoride to the skin of the forearm for 48 hours. A positive reaction is indicated by a local erythematous rash with some induration which occurs in about 72 hours and persists for at least a week; or by the development of nodules which consist of sarcoid-type granulomas within 30 days. The former reaction points only to hypersensitivity but the latter suggests the likelihood of disease (James, 1976). However, as already explained, the test is not regarded as suitable in clinical practice. Furthermore, its use in a worker in conditions of potential beryllium exposure is clearly undesirable as it may induce sensitization and, thereby, increase the possibility of his developing disease if he returns to the same work.

If this test is employed it is essential to observe and record both its early and late results.

IN VITRO HYPERSENSITIVITY TESTS (*see* p. 342)

The experimental basis for the lymphocyte blast transformation and Be MIF tests has been established by Jones and Amos (1974, 1975).

Lymphocyte blast transformation

This involves exposing the patient's lymphocytes to a beryllium salt (usually beryllium sulphate) under special conditions and determining the percentage of blast formation by morphological cell counts or by the uptake of tritiated thymidine. Blast transformation of cells from patients with hypersensitivity to beryllium or chronic disease is also provoked by PHA in place of beryllium salts. The beryllium lymphocyte transformation test is strongly

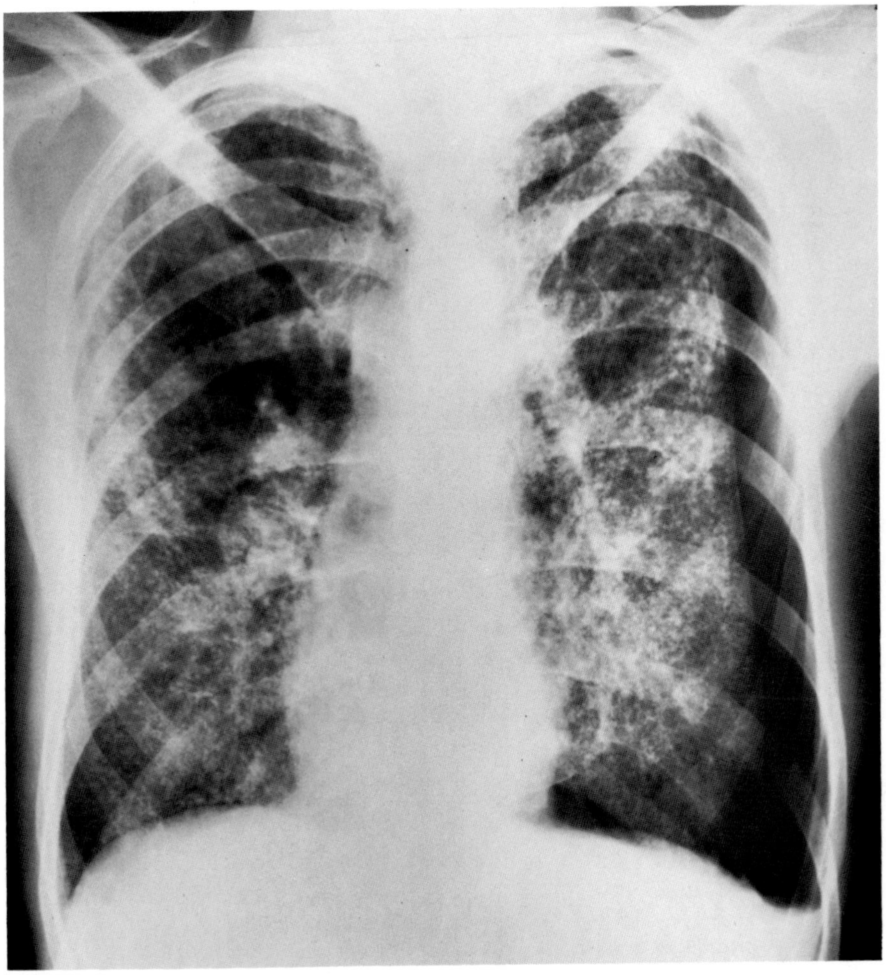

(b) 1977

Figure 10.13 Widespread, small, apparently calcified lesions in an operative who milled and machined beryllium-copper alloys for three years in the mid-1950s. (a) 1966, appearances on diagnosis; (b) 1977, increase in discrete opacities and development of left spontaneous hydro-pneumothorax which re-expanded without incident. Beryllium and Kveim patch tests negative. Be lymphocyte transformation test positive and Be MIF negative while receiving prednisolone. Lung biopsy: sarcoid-type granulomas with numerous conchoidal bodies; some nodular fibrosis. Lung function: moderately severe restrictive and gas transfer defects

and persistently positive in the majority of cases of chronic disease (Preuss, Deodhar and van Ordstrand, 1980); indeed, Jones Williams has found positive results in 100 per cent of 15 cases tested. Unlike the Be MIF test it is *not* suppressed by corticosteroids. The response to intradermal PHA in patients with chronic disease does not appear to have been tested.

Be MIF

The patient's white cells are separated from 20 ml of whole blood and incubated with three different concentrations of beryllium sulphate. The supernatant fluid is then added to guinea-pig macrophages in migration chambers and the extent of migration of the cells measured (Price *et al.*, 1977). The test is positive in many cases of chronic disease but not as consistently as the lymphocyte transformation test, and it has the disadvantage of being suppressed by corticosteroids. A test—at present experimental—which claims greater sensitivity and reproducibility is described by Price *et al.* (1980).

Positive results of either of these tests indicate beryllium-induced Type IV hypersensitivity but do *not* necessarily imply the presence of disease. On present evidence the lymphocyte transformation test appears to be much superior to the Be MIF test.

BIOPSY AND BERYLLIUM ASSAY

Removal of an adequate amount of pulmonary or other tissue is often needed to establish the diagnosis in spite of the development of the *in vitro* hypersensitivity tests. Biopsy may also be helpful in prognosis.

For the purpose of assay 1 g of tissue (but not less than 0.02 g) is sufficient, and this must be sent to the laboratory in a chemical clean borosilicate glass container. Because the

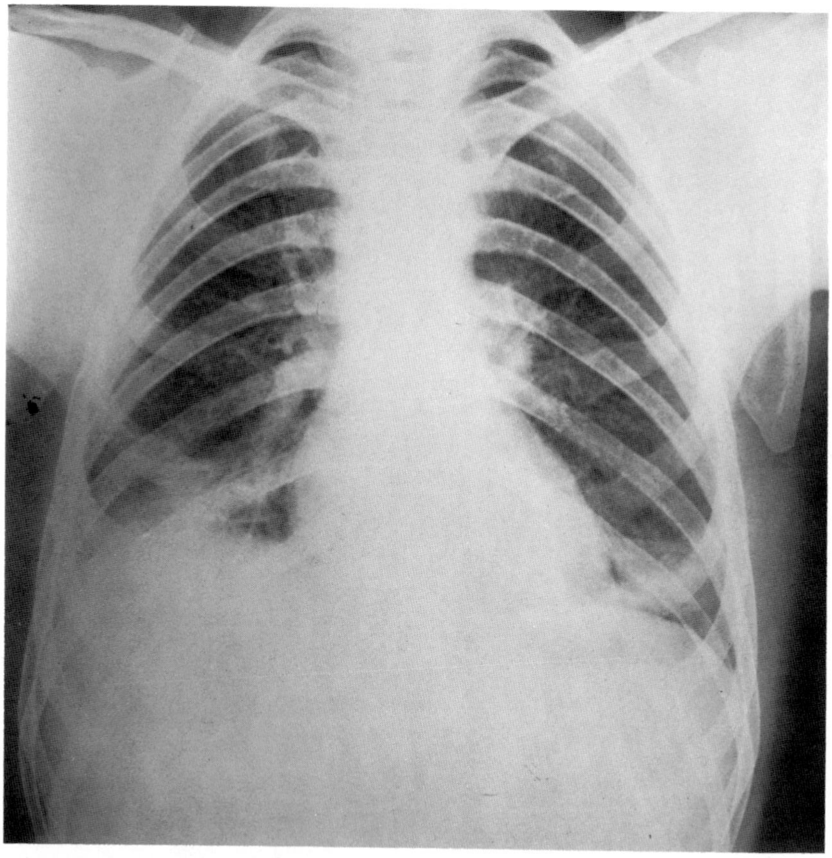

(a) 1949

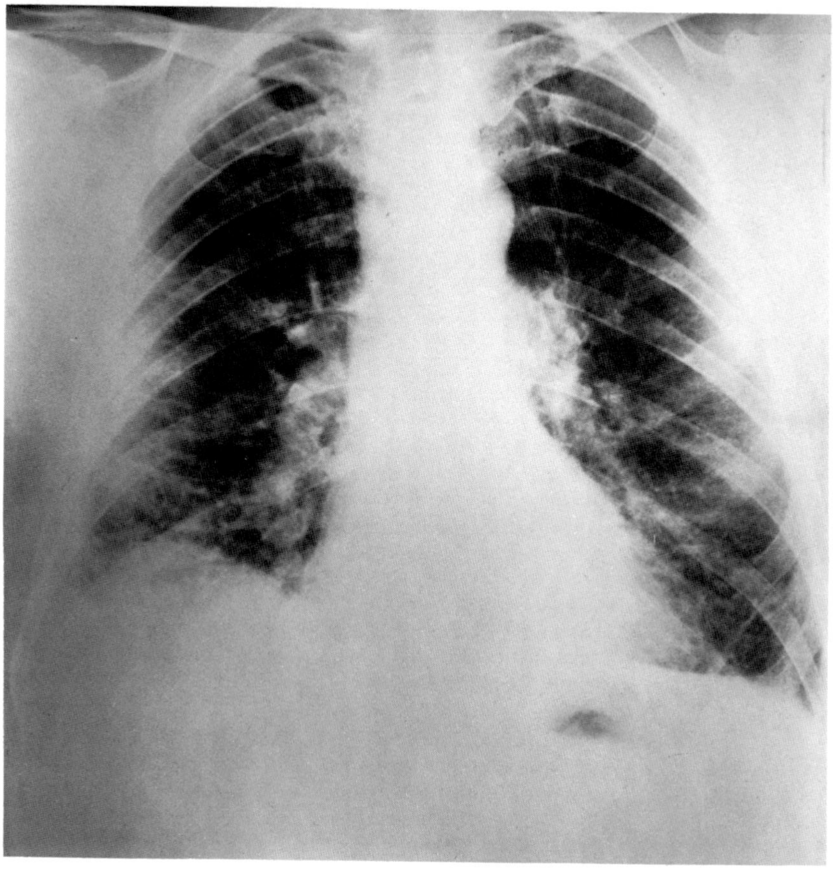

(b) 1974

Figure 10.14 Case of an industrial research laboratory worker from 1940 to 1948 who experimented with mixtures containing beryllium oxide and fired and crushed the end-products which contained beryllium silicates. (a) 1949, small low density, discrete opacities in both lung fields and changes consistent with bilateral, basal pneumonic consolidation. (b) 1974, appearances of bilateral DIPF predominant in the middle and lower zones with diffuse pleural thickening especially on the right. Lung function: severe restrictive and gas transfer defects, and increased inequality of ventilation-perfusion ratios. Post mortem, *naked eye: extensive pleural thickening and widespread grey-coloured DIPF with small cysts in the lower parts of the lungs. Microscopy: DIPF with occasional sarcoid-type granulomas containing numerous conchoidal bodies as deeply stained by haematoxylin* beryllium content of the hilar lymph nodes is likely to be higher than that of the lungs mediastinoscopy may sometimes be justifiable.

The presence of widespread cellular infiltration of alveolar walls (Group I disease—*see* p. 338) is a better guide to prognosis than the number of granulomas and may be helpful in distinguishing chronic beryllium disease from sarcoidosis.

Beryllium can be identified by conventional and micro-emission spectrography in minute portions of tissue in paraffin or frozen sections by volatilization with a laser beam and examination of the vapour in the spectrographic arc (Robinson *et al.*, 1968). The drawbacks of spectrographic methods, however, are interference by other elements, especially iron, and the fact that they are very time consuming. Beryllium oxide can be identified within the epithelioid cells of granulomas by the combination of ion microprobe mass analysis (IMMA) with electron beam micro-analysis and scanning electron microscopy (Abraham, 1978). A modified atomic absorption technique which is both simple and sufficiently sensitive for most analytical purposes is applicable in a variety of ways to the analysis of air and biological materials (Bogowski, 1968). A quantitative IMMA technique, which is capable of analysing small amounts of needle and transbronchial biopsy material, appears to be the most sensitive of these tests and it correlates well with bulk chemical analysis of larger samples of the same tissues (Abraham, 1980). Failure to detect beryllium in individuals who have been exposed to it is usually due to inadequate techniques.

URINE

As pointed out earlier, the presence of beryllium is only an indication that at some time it has been assimilated into the body. Gas chromatographic analysis—which is sensitive, reliable, rapid and reproducible—is capable of detecting beryllium in a sample as small as 1 ml (Foreman, Gough and Walker, 1970).

Measurement of excretion of urinary calcium may be a help in observing the course of chronic disease because transient hypercalcuria appears to be correlated with activity of the disease (Stoeckle, Hardy and Weber, 1969).

DIAGNOSIS

ACUTE DISEASE

The diagnosis of acute nasopharyngitis, tracheobronchitis or pneumonitis depends mainly upon the recognition that a toxic beryllium compound has been inhaled—usually one to two days before the onset of the symptoms. Other features supporting the diagnosis are *low* fever and rapid loss of weight. As already described, the appearances of the chest radiograph are in no way characteristic and laboratory tests cannot distinguish this disease from pneumonic disease due to other causes except in the negative sense that evidence of bacterial or viral infection is lacking. Blood counts, ESR, serum protein levels and urinalysis do not help as they show no significant abnormality (Tepper, Hardy and Chamberlin, 1961).

CHRONIC DISEASE

Diagnosis is often difficult in view of the protean manifestations of the disease and its resemblance to other granulomatous disorders—especially sarcoidosis; and, at times, may be impossible. Prolonged observation of the patient is sometimes needed before the diagnosis can be made with any certainty.

The criteria upon which diagnosis is based are as follows:

(1) *A history of exposure to beryllium.* This is an essential requirement. It may demand a most comprehensive enquiry into occupational details over at least 20 years. And the possibility of unsuspected exposure in such work as scrap metal reclamation and welding operations which may involve beryllium alloys has to be borne in mind. Furthermore, the possibility of para-occupational exposure (such as work near an annealing furnace) must be borne in mind. In some instances the manufacturer may be able to supply a detailed analysis of processes involved and the concentrations of beryllium in the work place air over a period of some years.
(2) *Lung function tests.* The physiological defects which may occur (referred to on p. 344) are helpful in confirming the presence of disease of the gas-exchanging region of the lungs consistent with beryllium disease, but have no specific diagnostic value.
(3) *Radiographic appearances.* These include any of the abnormalities in the chest radiograph just described. In some cases serial films may be required to detect the changes. Evidence of bilateral hilar node enlargement is uncommon, not prominent and generally associated with signs of intrapulmonary disease (usually, miliary to nodular size opacities), though very occasionally these are absent (Sprince, Kazemi and Hardy, 1976). It is noteworthy that, in contrast to sarcoidosis, complete or permanent resolution of abnormalities in the chest film rarely occurs even under the influence of steroid treatment, and progression is common.
(4) Negative Kveim test.
(5) Beryllium and PHA lymphocyte blast transformation tests positive even during steroid treatment.
(6) Be MIF test may be positive but not during steroid treatment.
(7) The presence of beryllium in the tissues in an amount greater than 0.02 μg/g dried tissue or in the urine.
(8) Histological features. The importance of cellular infiltration of alveolar walls in Group I disease and of conchoidal bodies and hyalinized nodules in Group II disease in differential diagnosis is referred to on p. 338.

DIFFERENTIAL DIAGNOSIS

With the accumulation of cases in the US and UK Beryllium Case Registries the merging of the clinical manifestations of chronic beryllium disease with those of sarcoidosis has become increasingly evident. The few remaining differences are the extent of cellular infiltration of alveolar walls, a negative Kveim test, the comparative rarity of bilateral hilar node enlargement, and a tendency for the lung disease (unlike that in most cases of sarcoidosis) to progress. This raises two important points. *First,* that sarcoidosis may be wrongly diagnosed as beryllium disease. However, epidemiological studies have shown that the chance occurrence of sarcoidosis in an individual exposed to beryllium in industry is improbable (Hardy, 1956). This fact and the deployment of the diagnostic procedures just described should enable positive differentiation to be made in most cases (*Table 10.2* contrasts the main features of both disorders). *Second,* that the possibility of beryllium disease should always be kept in mind in cases presenting as sarcoidosis.

Normal or low levels of serum ACE and lysozyme may favour chronic beryllium disease and high levels, sarcoidosis. But this has still to be confirmed (*see* p. 341).

Other diseases which may have to be eliminated are:

(1) Tuberculosis of miliary, bronchopneumonic or fibro-cavernous type.
(2) Histoplasmosis in endemic areas. This is excluded by the histoplasmin skin test, complement fixation test, cultures of *H. capsulatum* and biopsy of lung tissue.
(3) Other forms of pneumoconiosis. These include siderosis, stannosis, silicosis, 'mixed dust fibrosis' and coal pneumoconiosis and, in most cases, the occupational history serves to make the distinction. Neither symptoms nor abnormality of lung function are associated with siderosis or stannosis (*see* Chapter 6).
(4) Chronic extrinsic allergic 'alveolitis' (farmers' lung and similar disorders). Although this produces clinical, physiological and radiographical features which are identical to chronic beryllium disease the occupational history, identification of beryllium in lung tissue and lack of precipitating antibodies (in recent cases) establish the difference. Furthermore, cellular, sarcoid-type granulomas which are a feature of chronic beryllium

Table 10.2 Comparative Features of Chronic Beryllium Disease and Sarcoidosis*

		Chronic beryllium disease	*Sarcoidosis*
Clinical features	Anorexia and weight loss	common	rare
	Granulomas of skin	implantation only	not common (approx 7%)
	Splenomegaly	rare	occasional
	Parotitis	rare	uncommon (about 4%)
	Ocular lesions	never	occasional (15%)
	Nervous system involvement	never	uncommon (4%)
	Peripheral lymphadenopathy	none	occasional (15%)
	Lupus pernio	never	uncommon
	Erythema nodosum	never	fairly common in Britain (about 32%)
Radiographic features	Bilateral hilar node enlargement	very rare	common
	Spontaneous regression of lung disease	occasional but never complete	common, often complete
Skin tests	Beryllium patch test	often positive (erythema with induration in 48–72 hours; granulomas in three to four weeks)	negative
	Kveim test	negative	positive in most cases
	Tuberculin test	negative or low reactivity in a few cases	negative in chronic disease, positive in a minority of cases of early disease
Immunological features	Circulating IgA and G	often increased	often increased
	Be lymphocyte transformation test	positive	negative
	Be MIF test	positive in absence of steroid treatment	negative
Biochemical features	Hypercalcaemia	occasional (about 10%)	occasional, usually transient (11%)
	Hypercalcuria	occasional	occasional (about 15%)
	Serum angiotensin converting enzyme	not increased?	increased in active disease
Beryllium content	Tissue	fairly high in mediastinal lymph nodes	absent
		moderate in lungs	absent
	Urine	often, but not always present	absent
Histology	Granulomas	indistinguishable	indistinguishable
	Inclusion bodies	indistinguishable	indistinguishable
	Cellular infiltration of alveolar walls	prominent	inconspicuous

*Prevalence of the various features of sarcoidosis derived mainly from the worldwide review by James *et al.* (1976)

disease are absent in chronic extrinsic allergic 'alveolitis' (*see* Chapter 11).

The occurrence of granulomas in beryllium disease compared with extrinsic allergic 'alveolitis' can be summarized as follows:

	Acute	*Chronic*
Beryllium disease	Absent	Moderate to numerous
Extrinsic allergic 'alveolitis'	Numerous	Absent

(5) Lymphangitis carcinomatosa. This may cause dyspnoea and radiographic changes similar to those of chronic beryllium disease but lack of exposure to beryllium, rapid deterioration in health and, probably, identification of a primary growth should point to the diagnosis.

PROGNOSIS

ACUTE DISEASE

Recovery within one to six months is the rule in the majority of cases but fulminant disease (usually associated with accidental exposure) carries a risk of death in some 7 per cent of cases (Tepper, Hardy and Chamberlin, 1961). Episodes of pneumonitis may recur, however, following recovery if the subject is re-exposed to beryllium and, as has been described, a proportion of individuals may later develop chronic disease without further exposure to beryllium.

Occasionally, evidence of acute disease in the chest radiograph may persist for almost a year before finally disappearing.

CHRONIC DISEASE

Prognosis in the individual cannot be predicted with certainty and different patterns of evolution of the disease occur, any one or all of which may be observed in the same patient.

The minority of individuals who experience no symptoms and in whom the only evidence of the disease, apart from beryllium assay and biopsy, is the chest radiograph may remain asymptomatic for a decade or more (Tepper, Hardy and Chamberlin, 1961), but at any time, symptoms and impairment of lung function may develop without evident change in the radiographic appearances.

The majority of persons have symptoms and the impaired pattern of lung function, described already, to the point of being slightly or moderately disabled though able to lead a fairly normal life for years. But should exacerbation of disease occur it is usually followed by increase of disability. When exacerbations are accompanied by fever and rigors the prognosis tends to be poor (Tepper, Hardy and Chamberlin, 1961). Severely disabling disease is of very variable duration—from about one to 20 years in corticosteroid-treated patients (Hardy, Rabe and Lorch, 1967). It may end in death from respiratory failure and pulmonary heart disease which, in some cases, may be precipitated by repeated episodes of spontaneous pneumothorax (*see* next section).

Although corticosteroids have a substantial ameliorating effect upon the course of chronic disease, complete resolution, either spontaneous or as a result of treatment, has not been reliably reported. But if it is not understood that long periods of remission occur in some cases these may be interpreted as a 'cure', and although some reduction of discrete radiographic opacities may occur during corticosteroid treatment this is never complete and they tend to reappear when it is stopped.

It has already been pointed out that there is a distinct relationship between the histological features and the degree of morbidity and life expectancy. Prognosis is significantly worse in patients with Group I (*see Figures 10.2* and *10.3*) lesions than in those with Group II lesions.

COMPLICATIONS OF CHRONIC DISEASE

PULMONARY HEART DISEASE

This has been the commonest, but not necessarily inevitable, complication of chronic disease and more often the cause of death than respiratory failure (Tepper, Hardy, Chamberlin, 1961).

MYOCARDITIS

Very rarely granulomatous myocarditis may occur (Sprince, Kazemi and Hardy, 1976).

SPONTANEOUS PNEUMOTHORAX

A fairly common complication, it has been observed in about 15 per cent of cases, may be recurrent and bilateral, and, in some cases, the immediate cause of death (*Figure 10.13*).

CARCINOMA OF THE LUNG

As already noted on p. 343 there is some evidence which suggests an excess risk of cancer of the lung, apparently unrelated to smoking, in beryllium workers. But this needs confirmation.

PULMONARY TUBERCULOSIS

There is no increased tendency for persons with chronic disease to develop tuberculosis; on the contrary, it has been remarkably uncommon (Tepper, Hardy and Chamberlin, 1961).

RENAL CALCULI

In a small proportion of cases these lead to renal failure.

GOUT

Gout has been recorded as a rare complication of the hyperuricaemia of chronic disease (Kelley, Goldfinger and Hardy, 1969).

RHEUMATOID ARTHRITIS

An alleged association of rheumatoid arthritis with chronic disease has not been supported by the available evidence (Tepper, Hardy and Chamberlin, 1961).

EFFECTS OF TREATMENT

The complications of corticosteroid therapy have been recorded, but only in very few cases (Hardy, Rabe and Lorch, 1967).

TREATMENT

Administration of corticosteroids is associated with a significant reduction in mortality and increased survival (Hardy, Rabe and Lorch, 1967), although it is difficult to be certain whether this is wholly due to their influence or partly to other causes (Freiman and Hardy, 1970).

Acute disease must be treated immediately with rest and prednisone 60 to 80 mg daily. If it is of fulminant type oxygen—preferably under positive pressure—will be necessary. Antibiotic agents are not indicated except in the event of secondary infection.

When chronic disease is first diagnosed predisolone should be commenced at an initial dose of 15 to 30 mg daily or 30 to 60 mg on alternate days and later adjusted according to progress (Stoeckle, Hardy and Weber, 1969). This usually causes a reduction of symptoms and serum globulins, improvement in general health, gas transfer and, in some cases, radiographic appearances. Patients with sub-group IA and sub-groups IB lesions respond equally well (Freiman and Hardy, 1970), but when fibrosis is established, no improvement can be expected. If treatment is started early progression of fibrosis may seem to be arrested but deterioration of lung function is not always prevented. However, no controlled trials of corticosteroid treatment appear to have been done due, no doubt, to the comparative rarity of the disease and ethical principles involved, but in sarcoidosis such trials indicate that steroids have no significant effect on long-term results (Mitchell and Scadding, 1974).

When corticosteroids are discontinued there may, in some patients, be prolonged remission. In others, symptoms and abnormalities of lung function and chest radiographs reassert themselves; in which case life-long maintenance of these drugs may be advisable, though the rationale of such treatment is questionable.

The effect of chloroquine and immunosuppressant drugs which appear to cause temporary improvement in some sarcoidosis cases (Mitchell and Scadding, 1974) does not seem to have been reported in beryllium disease.

Chelating agents—such as aurintricarboxylic acid (ATA) and edathamil (EDTA)—are ineffective.

Supportive treatment of pulmonary heart disease, congestive heart failure and respiratory failure may ultimately be required.

When acute or chronic disease has been diagnosed the worker should not return to any job which may incur the risk of exposure to beryllium in any form.

Skin ulcers must be curetted to remove the toxic particles, otherwise permanent healing will not occur; skin granulomas require early and wide excision.

PREVENTION

Preventive measure cannot be considered in detail—they are fully described by Breslin (1966) and Utidjian (1973)—but are briefly summarized.

CONTROL OF WORK ENVIRONMENT

The objective is to prevent contamination of the factory air and of the worker's skin and clothing. Routine beryllium processes should be segregated from the rest of the factory, preferably in a room subjected to a negative atmosphere.

Beryllium extraction, reduction furnaces and alloy production should be completely enclosed and exhaust ventilated, and beryllium liquids and slurries contained in closed vessels. Partial enclosure (for example, hoods) combined with low-volume high-velocity exhaust ventilation to exert a strong negative air pressure is required for grinding, deburring, drilling, machining and ceramic operations. High velocity exhaust systems are attached to tools such as drills and grinding wheels. General exhaust ventilation is also applied to the factory or workroom atmosphere and the extracted air scrubbed and filtered by different methods according to whether the processes are dry or wet, so that no beryllium is discharged into the environmental air.

Rigid work practices are necessary to maintain a high standard of cleanliness and housekeeping. Any spillage must be dealt with promptly by wet mopping or a special vacuum cleaning system. Surfaces which are normally inaccessible (such as ventilation ducts, beams and lighting fixtures) should be vacuum cleaned at regular intervals. A specified code of practice is required for the maintenance of machinery (for example, lathes and grinders) and for entering enclosures.

In the USA there are special provisions to control the levels of beryllium emmitted by industrial plants and rocket motor firing.

PROTECTION OF PERSONNEL

All employees must be regularly informed of the dangers of beryllium and of any existing potential hazard, and frequently briefed about necessary preventive measures.

Special protective clothing (overalls, head gear, underwear and socks) must be worn and laundered on the factory site, and not taken home. An ideal arrangement consists of a locker room divided in the middle by showers and other washing facilities with the workers work clothes housed on one side and his normal street clothes on the other. In this way, 'clean' and 'contaminated' areas are clearly demarcated. Protective footwear must be provided and, for some processes (for example, handling soluble compounds and bulk materials or cleaning contaminated machines) impervious gloves must be worn.

Respirators of approved design must be used whenever the actual or projected level of beryllium is likely to exceed the recommended eight hour time-weighted average, and also during the maintenance and cleaning of machinery and exhaust ventilation ducts and changing of dust-collector bags. They may also be required for furnace operations, and must be easily accessible in areas where massive accidental contamination could occur. Continuous flow air-line respirators or self-contained breathing units which maintain positive pressure during inhalation are required in any atmosphere likely to exceed 1000 μg Be/m³. Frequent inspection and maintenance of all respiratory devices is essential.

An established emergency procedure must be in force for any process which carries a potential risk of massive contamination and should include special visual and auditory alarm signals, prompt evacuation of the area and by the donning of respirators by personnel who remain to deal with the emergency and by workers leaving the area if they have to walk any distance.

AIR SAMPLING

Both the general factory air and the worker's breathing zone should be sampled. To sample the general air a static instrument is placed in a position which is representative of the conditions over the working area, usually at a height of 4 to 6 feet from the floor, and operates over a period of a day or more. And to sample the breathing zone the instrument is placed in a fixed position near the worker's nose or mouth, either worn on his clothing or held in the zone by a technician for the required sampling time. Samples are collected and analysed both as time-weighted and peak concentration values *at least* quarterly or, in work areas where values are in excess of the standards, every 30 days. Sampling of peak concentrations must continue for a minimum of 30 min.

Records of all sampling schedules and the types of personal protection used must be maintained and preserved for at least 20 years.

DISPOSAL OF SOLID WASTE MATERIAL

Any metal, wood, rags or paper which become contaminated should be removed in sealed containers and buried in ground approved for the purpose.

MEDICAL SURVEILLANCE

(1) *Pre-employment examination* A careful clinical examination, with a good quality full-sized, standard chest film (14 × 17 in or 35.6 × 43.2 cm) and ventilatory function tests must be done. Individuals with respiratory tract disease should not be accepted for work in any process using beryllium for, although there is no evidence that they are more liable to develop beryllium disease than healthy persons, it could make later differential diagnosis extremely difficult. Hence, any chronic lung disease (including other occupational disorders) and evidence of atopy, such as hay fever, asthma or eczema should exclude the applicant; as should any evidence of past or present skin sensitization. And, because of the effect which pregnancy is reported to have, women of child-bearing age should also be excluded.

(2) *Routine examination of employees* Completion of a medical history questionnaire, clinical examination, ventilation function tests (FEV_1 and FVC) and a full-sized, standard chest film should be done annually in all workers. It is recommended that employees in refinery, alloy or ceramic processes should have ventilatory function tests performed monthly. Any undue decline in weight or ventilatory capacity indicates the necessity for further investigation. The skin should be examined at regular intervals for evidence of contact dermatitis, granulomas and ulcers.

As indicated on pp. 341 and 348, the beryllium patch test is contra-indicated for any person likely to be accepted into the industry. But the use of the lymphocyte transformation test is recommended as a valuable indication of the development of beryllium hypersensitivity and the possibility of disease. Indeed, it could provide an early warning of the development of beryllium hypersensitivity if done at pre-employment examination and subsequently at intervals during work in the industry.

A detailed record of his work, air-sampling results and medical examinations must be kept for each employee.

(3) *Medical examination after leaving employment* Yearly supervision of ex-workers with no evident disease should be continued for at least 15 years after their last potential contact with beryllium.

(4) *Notification* In the UK beryllium disease, in any of its forms, is notifiable under the terms of the Factories Act, 1961 (Section 83).

REFERENCES

Abraham, J. L. (1978). Recent advances in pneumoconiosis: the pathologist's role in etiologic diagnosis. In *The Lung: Structure, Function and Disease,* edited by W. M. Thurlbeck and M. R. Abell, p. 128. Int. Acad. of Path. Mono. Baltimore; Williams and Wilkins

Abraham, J. L. (1980). Microanalysis of human granulomatous lesions. *8th Int. Conf. on Sarcoidosis and other Granulomatous Diseases.* Edited by W. Jones Williams and B. H. Davies, pp. 767–768. Cardiff; Alpha Omega Publishing Ltd

Agate, J. N. (1948). Delayed pneumonitis in a beryllium worker. *Lancet* **2,** 530–533

Ambrosi, L., Sartorelli, E., Sbertoli, C. and Secchi, G. C. (1968). Two cases of chronic pulmonary granulomatosis caused by beryllium. *Med. Lav.* **59,** 321–333

Andrews, J. L., Kazemi, H. and Hardy, H. L. (1969). Patterns of lung dysfunction in chronic beryllium disease. *Am. Rev. resp. Dis.* **100,** 791–800

Beekman, J. F., Zimmet, S. M., Chun, B. K., Miranda, A. and Katz, S. (1976). Spectrum of pleural involvement in sarcoidosis. *Archs intern. Med.* **136,** 323–330

Benoit, M. P. (1967). Open bench top deburring of metallic beryllium. *J. occup. Med.* **9,** 170–174

Bogowski, D. L. (1968). Rapid determination of beryllium by a direct-reading atomic absorption spectrophotometer. *Am. ind. Hyg. Assoc. J.* **29,** 474–481

Breslin, A. J. (1966). *Occupational Health Aspects,* edited by H. E. Stokinger, pp. 245–321. New York and London; Academic Press

Buckley, C. E. and Dorsey, F. C. (1970). A comparison of serum immunoglobulin concentrations in sarcoidosis and tuberculosis. *Ann. intern. Med.* **72,** 37–42

Carlens, E., Hanngren, A. and Ivemark, B. (1974). The concomitance of feverish onset of sarcoidosis and necrosis formation in the lymph nodes. In *Proceedings of the VI International Conference on Sarcoidosis,* edited by K. Iwai and Y. Hosada, p. 409. Tokyo; University of Tokyo Press

Chambers, L. A., Foster, M. S. and Cholak, J. (1955). A comparison of particulate loadings in the atmosphere of certain American cities. In *Proceedings of 3rd National Air Pollution Symposium, Standard Research Institute, Pasadena, California,* p. 24

Cirla, A. M., Barbiano di Belgiojoso, G. and Chiappino, G. (1968). La ipersensibilità ai composti di berillio; trasferimento passivo nella cavia mediante cellule linfoidi. *Boll. Ist. sieroter. milan* **47,** 663–668

Clary, J. J. and Stokinger, H. E. (1973). The mechanism of delayed biological response following beryllium exposure. *J. occup. Med.* **15,** 255–259

Crossman, G. C. and Vandemark, W. C. (1954). Microscopic observations correlating toxicity of beryllium oxide with crystal structure. *Arch. ind. Hyg. occup. Med.* **9,** 481–487

Curtis, G. H. (1959). The diagnosis of beryllium disease, with special reference to the patch test. *Arch. ind. Hlth* **19,** 150–153

Deodhar, S. D., Barna, B. and Van Ordstrand, H. S. (1973). A study of the immunological aspects of chronic berylliosis. *Chest* **63,** 309–313

Epstein, W. L. and Byers, V. (1979). Transfer of contact sensitivity to beryllium using dialyzable leukocyte extracts (transfer factor). *J. Allergy clin. Immun.* **63,** 11–115

Foreman, J. K., Gough, T. A. and Walker, E. A. (1970). The determination of traces of beryllium in human and rat urine samples by gas chromatography. *Analyst* **95,** 797–804

Freiman, D. G. and Hardy, H. L. (1970). Beryllium disease. *Hum. Path.* **1,** 25–44

Gelman, I. (1936). Poisoning by vapours of beryllium oxyfluoride. *J. ind. Hyg. Toxicol.* **18,** 371–379

Goldstein, R. A., Israel, H. L. and Rawnsley, H. M. (1969). Effect of race and stage of disease on the serum immunoglobulins in sarcoidosis. *J. Am. med. Ass.* **208,** 1153–1155

Griggs, K. (1973). Toxic metal fumes from mantle-type camp lanterns. *Science* **181,** 842–843

Hall, R. H., Scott, J. K., Laskin, S., Stroud, C. A. and Stokinger, H. E. (1950). Acute toxicity of inhaled beryllium III. Observations correlating toxicity with physico-chemical properties of beryllium oxide dust. *Archs ind. Hyg. occup. Med.* **2,** 25–48

Hanifin, J. M., Epstein, W. L. and Cline, M. J. (1970). *In vitro* studies of granulomatous hypersensitivity to beryllium. *J. invest. Derm.* **55,** 284–288

Hardy, H. L. (1956). Differential diagnosis between beryllium poisoning and sarcoidosis. *Am. Rev. Tuberc. pulm. Dis.* **74,** 885–896

Hardy, H. L. (1972). *Beryllium Disease.* US Public Health Service Bulletin No. 2173. The Toxicology of Beryllium. pp. 9–10

Hardy, H. L. (1980). Beryllium disease: a clinical perspective. *Environ. Res.* **21,** 1–9

Hardy, H. L. and Chamberlin, R. I. (1972). Beryllium Disease. In *Toxicology of Beryllium,* edited by Irving R. Tabershaw, pp. 9–16. U.S. Dept. Health, Education and Welfare. Public Health Service Publication No. 2173

Hardy, H. L. and Tabershaw, J. R. (1946). Delayed chemical pneumonitis occurring in workers to beryllium compounds. *J. ind. Hyg. Toxicol.* **28,** 197–211

Hardy, H. L., Rabe, E. W. and Lorch, S. (1967). United States Beryllium Case Registry (1952–1966). *J. occup. Med.* **9,** 271–276

Hart, B. A. and Pittman, D. G. (1980). The uptake of beryllium by the alveolar macrophage. *J. Reticuloendothelial Soc.* **27,** 49–58

Hasan, F. M. and Kazemi, H. (1974). Chronic beryllium disease: a continuing epidemiological hazard. *Chest* **65,** 289–293

Hazard, J. B. (1959). Pathologic changes of beryllium disease. *Archs ind. Hlth* **19,** 179–183

Henderson, W. R., Fukuyama, K., Epstein, W. L. and Spitler, L. E. (1972). *In vitro* demonstration of delayed hypersensitivity in patients with berylliosis. *J. invest. Derm.* **58,** 5–8

Infante, P. F., Wagoner, J. K. and Sprince, N. L. (1980). Mortality patterns from lung cancer and non-neoplastic respiratory disease among white males in the Beryllium Case Registry. *Environ. Res.* **21,** 35–43

Israel, H. L. and Cooper, D. A. (1964). Chronic beryllium disease due to low beryllium content alloys. *Am. Rev. resp. Dis.* **89,** 100–102

Izumi, T., Kobara, Y., Inui, S., Tokunaga, R., Orita, Y., Kitano, M. and Jones Williams, W. (1976). The first seven cases of chronic beryllium disease in ceramic factory workers in Japan. *Ann. N.Y. Acad. Sci.* **278,** 636–652

James, D. G. (1976). Discussion of current (1975) problem of differentiating between beryllium disease and sarcoidosis. *Ann. N.Y. Acad. Sci.* **278,** 664

James, D. G., Neville, E., Siltzbach, L. E., Turiaf, J., Battesti, J. P., Sharma, O. P., Hosoda, Y., Mikami, R., Odaka, M., Villar, T. G., Djurič, B., Douglas, A. C., Middleton, W., Karlish, A., Blasti, A., Olivieri, D., and Preuss, P. (1976). A worldwide review of sarcoidosis. *Ann. N.Y. Acad. Sci.* **278,** 321–333

James, E. M. V. and Jones Williams, W. (1974). Fine structure and histochemistry of epithelioid cells in sarcoidosis. *Thorax* **29,** 115–120

Jett, R. (1971). Immunological aspects of beryllium disease. Quoted by Tepper, L. B. (1972)

Jones, J. M. and Amos, H. E. (1974). Contact sensitivity *in vitro:* activation of actively allergized lymphocytes by a beryllium complex. *Int. Archs Allergy* **46,** 161–171

Jones, J. M. and Amos, H. E. (1975). Contact sensitivity *in vitro* II: The effect of beryllium preparations on the proliferative responses of specifically allergized lymphocytes and normal lymphocytes stimulated with PHA. *Int. Archs Allergy* **48,** 22–29

Jones Williams, W. (1958). A histological study of lungs in 52 cases of chronic beryllium disease. *Br. J. ind. Med.* **15,** 84–91

Jones Williams, W. (1960). The nature and origin of Schaumann Bodies. *J. Path. Bact.* **79,** 1, 193–201

Jones Williams, W. (1967a). The pathology of pulmonary sarcoidosis. *Proc. R. Soc. Med.* **60,** 986–988

Jones Williams, W. (1967b). The pathology of sarcoidosis. *Hosp. Med.* **2,** 21–27

Jones Williams, W. (1971). The beryllium granuloma. *Proc. R. Soc. Med.* **64,** 946–948

Jones Williams, W. (1977). Beryllium disease—pathology and diagnosis. *J. Soc. occup. Med.* **27,** 93–96

Jones Williams, W. (1980). Personal communication

Jones Williams, W. and Kilpatrick, G. S. (1974). Cutaneous and pulmonary manifestations of chronic beryllium disease. In *Proceedings of the VI International Conference on Sarcoidosis, 1972,* edited by K. Iwai and Y. Hosoda, p. 141–145. University of Tokyo

Jones Williams, W., Nosworthy, S. E. and Williams, W. R. (1980). UK Beryllium Case Registry. *8th International Conference on Sarcoidosis and other Granulomatous Diseases.* Edited by W. Jones Williams and B. H. Davies, p. 771. Cardiff; Alpha Omega Publishing Ltd

Jones Williams, W. and Williams, D. (1967). 'Residual bodies' in sarcoid and sarcoid-like granulomas. *J. clin. Path.* **20,** 574–577

Kang, K., Bice, D., Hoffman, E., D'Amato, R. and Salvaggio, J. (1977). Experimental studies in sensitization to beryllium, zirconium and aluminium compounds in the rabbit. *J. Allergy Clin. Immun.* **59,** 425–436

Kelley, W. N., Goldfinger, S. E. and Hardy, H. L. (1969). Hyperuricaemia in chronic beryllium disease. *Ann. intern. Med.* **70,** 977–983

Klemperer, F. W., Martin, A. P. and Van Riper, J. (1951). Beryllium excretion in humans. *Archs ind. Hyg.* **4,** 251–256

Lieben, J. and Metzner, F. (1959). Epidemiological findings associated with beryllium excretion. *Am. ind. Hyg. Ass. J.* **20,** 494–499

Lieben, J., Dattoli, J. A. and Vought, V. M. (1966). The significance of beryllium concentrations in urine. *Archs envir. Med.* **12,** 331–334

McCallum, R. I., Rannie, I. and Verity, C. (1961). Chronic pulmonary berylliosis in a female chemist. *Br. J. ind. Med.* **18,** 133–142

McCarthy, D. S., and Sigurdson, M. (1978). Lung function in pulmonary sarcoidosis. *Irish J. med. Sci.* **147,** 413–419

Mancuso, T. F. (1970). Relation of duration of employment and prior respiratory illness to respiratory cancer among beryllium workers. *Envir. Res.* **3,** 251–275

Mancuso, T. F. (1980). Mortality study of beryllium industry workers' occupational lung cancer. *Environ. Res.* **21,** 48–55

Marx, J. J. and Burrell, R. (1973). Delayed hypersensitivity to beryllium compounds. *J. Immun.* **111,** 590–598

Maxwell, W. R. (1971). (Rocket Propulsion Establishment, Ministry of Defence.) Personal communication

Mitchell, D. N. and Scadding, J. G. (1974). Sarcoidosis. *Am. Rev. resp. Dis.* **110**, 774–802

Mitchell, D. N., Scadding, J. G., Heard, B. E. and Hinson, K. F. W. (1977). Sarcoidosis: histopathological definition and clinical diagnosis. *J. clin. Path.* **30**, 395–408

Morison, W. L. (1976). Phytohaemagglutinin and transfer factor in the leucocyte migration inhibition test in patients with sarcoidosis. *Thorax* **31**, 87–90

Nishikawa, S. and Izumi, T. (1980). A three year prospective study on Mantoux reaction of factory workers exposed to beryllium oxide. *8th International Conf. on Sarcoidosis and Granulomatous Diseases.* Edited by W. Jones Williams and B. H. Davies, pp. 722–727. Cardiff; Alpha Omega Publishing, Ltd

Norris, G. F. and Peard, M. C. (1963). Berylliosis. Report of two cases with special reference to the patch test. *Br. med. J.* **1**, 378–382

Oreskes, I. and Siltzbach, L. E. (1968). Changes in rheumatoid factor activity during the course of sarcoidosis. *Am. J. Med.* **44**, 60–67

Orlova, A. A. and Ozerova, V. V. (1966). Functional state of the adrenal cortex in patients with chronic berylliosis treated with glucocorticoid preparation. *Gig. Truda Prof. Zabol.* **10**, 17–21

Preuss, O. P. (1975). Beryllium and its compounds. In *Occupational Medicine: Principles and Practical Applications,* edited by C. Zenz, pp. 619–636. Year Book Med.

Preuss, O. P., Deodhar, S. D. and van Ordstrand, H. S. (1980). Lymphoblast transformation in beryllium workers. *8th International Conf. on Sarcoidosis and Granulomatous Disease.* Edited by W. Jones Williams and B. H. Davies, pp. 711–714. Cardiff; Alpha Omega Publishing Ltd

Price, C. D., Eliott, J. A., Gladish, M. E., Major, P. C., Mentnech, M. S., Mull, J. C., Olenchock, S. A., Pearson, D. J., Spurgeon, D. E. and Taylor, G. (1980). Microdrop beryllium migration inhibition test. (Be MIF). *Proc. 8th Int. Conf. on Sarcoidosis and other Granulomatous Diseases.* Edited by W. Jones Williams and B. H. Davies, pp. 767–768. Cardiff; Alpha Omega Publishing Ltd

Price, C. D., Jones Williams, W., Pugh, A. and Joynson, D. H. (1977). Role of *in vitro* and *in vivo* tests of hypersensitivity in beryllium workers. *J. clin. Path.* **30**, 24–28

Reeves, A. L. (1968). Über die Retention von eingeatmetein Beryllium sulfat—Aerosol in Rattenlungen. *Arch. Gewerbepath. Gewerbehyg.* **24**, 226–237

Reeves, A. L. (1977). Beryllium in the environment. *Clin. Toxicol.* **10**, 37–48

Reeves, A. L. (1980). Delayed hypersensitivity in experimental pulmonary berylliosis. *8th International Conf. on Sarcoidosis and Granulomatous Diseases.* Edited by W. Jones Williams and B. H. Davies, pp. 715–721. Cardiff; Alpha Omega Publishing Ltd

Resnick, H., Roche, M. and Morgan, W. K. C. (1970). Immunoglobulin concentration in berylliosis. *Am. Rev. resp. Dis.* **101**, 504–510

Robinson, F. R., Brokeshoulder, S. F., Thomas, A. A. and Cholak, J. (1968). Microemission spectrochemical analysis of human lungs for beryllium. *Am. J. clin. Path.* **49**, 821–825

Robinson, F. R., Schaffner, F. and Trachtenberg, E. (1968). Ultrastructure of the lungs of dogs exposed to beryllium-containing dusts. *Archs envir. Hlth* **17**, 193–203

Rohrbach, M. S. and Demeree, R. A. (1979). Serum angiotensin converting enzyme activity in sarcoidosis as measured by a simple radiochemical assay. *Am. Rev. resp. Dis.* **119**, 761–767

Salvaggio, J. E., Flax, M. H. and Leskowitz, S. (1965). Studies in immunization. III The use of beryllium as a granuloma-producing agent in Freund's adjuvant. *J. Immun.* **95**, 845–854

Sander, O. A. (1950). Clinical report of illness in the neon sign industry. In *Symposium, Current Knowledge of Disease Encountered in the Handling of Beryllium and its Compounds: Clinical, Pathological and Engineering Data; USAEC. Report AECU—1921.* Massachusetts; Instit. Technol.

Selroos, O. and Grönhagen-Riska, C. (1979). Angiotensin converting enzyme. III Changes in serum level as an indicator of disease activity in untreated sarcoidosis. *Scand. J. resp. Dis.* **60**, 328–336

Siltzbach, L. E. (1976). Qualities and behaviour of satisfactory Kveim suspensions. *Ann. N.Y. Acad. Sci.* **278**, 665–668

Smith, A. B. and Suzuki, Y. (1980). Histopathologic classification of bronchogenic carcinomas among a cohort of workers occupationally exposed to beryllium. *Environ. Res.* **21**, 10–14

Sneddon, I. B. (1955). Berylliosis; a case report. *Br. med. J.* **1**, 1448–1449

Sprince, N. L., Kanarek, D. J., Weber, A. L., Chamberlin, R. I. and Kazemi, H. (1978). Reversible respiratory disease in beryllium workers. *Am. Rev. resp. Dis.* **117**, 1011–1017

Sprince, N. L., Kazemi, H. and Fanburg, B. L. (1980). Serum angiotensin I converting enzyme in chronic beryllium disease. *8th Internat. Conf. on Sarcoidosis and other Granulomatous Diseases.* Edited by W. Jones Williams and B. H. Davies, pp. 287–290. Cardiff; Alpha Omega Press

Sprince, N. L., Kazemi, H. and Hardy, H. L. (1976). Current (1975) problem of differentiating between beryllium disease and sarcoidosis. *Ann. N.Y. Acad. Sci.* **278**, 654–664

Sterner, J. H. and Eisenbud, M. (1951). Epidemiology of beryllium intoxication. *Archs ind. Hyg.* **4**, 123–151

Stoeckle, J. D., Hardy, H. L. and Weber, A. L. (1969). Chronic beryllium disease. *Am. J. Med.* **46**, 545–561

Stokinger, H. E. (1966). In *Beryllium. Its Industrial Hygiene Aspects,* edited by H. E. Stokinger, p. 168. New York and London: Academic Press

Stokinger, H.E., Spiegl, C.J., Root, R.E., Hall, R.H., Steadman, L.T., Stroud, C.A., Scott, J.K., Smith, F.A. and Gardner, D.E. (1953). Acute inhalation toxicity of beryllium IV, Beryllium fluids at exposure concentrations of one and ten milligrams per cubic metre. *Archs ind. Hyg. occup. Med.* **8**, 493–506

Studdy, P., Bird, R., James, D. G. and Sherlock, S. (1978). Serum angiotensin-converting enzyme (SACE) in sarcoidosis and other granulomatous disorders. *Lancet* **2**, 1331–1334

Sussman, V. H., Lieben, J. and Cleland, J. G. (1959). An air-pollution study of a community surrounding a beryllium plant. *Am. ind. Hyg. Assoc. J.* **20**, 504–508

Tepper, L. B. (1972). Beryllium. *C.R.C. Critical Review on Toxicology* **1**, 235–258

Tepper, L. B., Hardy, H. L. and Chamberlin, R. I. (1961). *The Toxicity of Beryllium Compounds.* Amsterdam; Elsevier

Torii, Y., Yamamoto, M., Morishita, M., Sugiura, T. and Suzuki, T. (1980). Serum angiotensin converting enzyme and serum lysozyme in sarcoidosis and other granulomatous diseases. *Proc. Nara. Symp. Sarcoidosis and other Granulomatous Dis.* To be published

Unanue, E. R., Askonas, B. A. and Allison, A. C. (1969). A role of macrophages in the stimulation of airborne responses by adjuvants. *J. Immun.* **103**, 71–78

Underwood, A. L. (1951). *Studies on the Renal Excretion of Beryllium.* (USAEC Report UR-171.) University of Rochester

Utidjian, H. M. D. (1973). Criteria for recommended standards: occupational exposure to beryllium and its compounds. *J. occup. Med.* **15**, 659–665

Van Ordstrand, H. S., Hughes, R. and Carmody, M. G. (1943). Chemical pneumonia in workers extracting beryllium oxide. *Cleveland Clin. Q.* **10**, 10–18

Veien, N. K., Hardt, F., Bendixen, G., Ringsted, J., Brodthagen, H., Faber, V., Geuner, J., Heckscher, T., Svejgaard, A., Sørensen, S. F., Wanstrup, J. and Wilk, A. (1976). Immunological studies in sarcoidosis: a companion of disease activity and various immunological parameters. *Ann. N.Y. Acad. Sci.* **278**, 47–51

Vorwald, A. J. (1966). Medical aspects of beryllium disease. In *Beryllium. Its Industrial Hygiene Aspects,* edited by H. E. Stokinger, pp. 167–200. New York and London; Academic Press

Wagner, J. K., Infante, P. F. and Bayliss, D. L. (1980). Beryllium and etiological agent in the induction of lung cancer, non-neoplastic respiratory disease and heart disease among industrially exposed workers. *Environ. Res.* **21**, 15–34

Weber, A. L., Stoeckle, J. D. and Hardy, H. L. (1965). Roentgenologic patterns in long-standing beryllium disease. *Am. J. Roentg.* **93**, 879–890

Weber, H. H. and Engelhardt, W. E. (1933). Über eine Apparatur zur Erzeugung niedriger Staubkonzentrationen von grosser Konstanz und eine Methode zur mikrogravinctrischen Staubbestimmung. Anwendung bei der Untersuchang con Stauben aus der Beryllium gewinnung. *Zentbl. GewHyg. Unfallerhüt.* **10**, 41–47

Weinberger, S. E., Kelman, J. A., Elsen, N. A., Young, R. C., Reynolds, H. Y., Fulmer, J. D. and Crystal, R. G. (1978). Bronchoalveolar lavage in interstial lung disease. *Ann. intern. Med.* **89**, 459–466

Williams, D., Jones Williams, W. and Williams, J. E. (1969). Enzyme histochemistry of epithelioid cells in sarcoidosis and sarcoid-like granulomas. *J. Pathol.* **97**, 705–709

11 Disorders Caused by Organic Agents (excluding Occupational Asthma)

INTRODUCTION

The range of extrinsic organic agents which can be inhaled as fine particulate matter or aerosols in occupational or other circumstances and give rise to lung disease is large. It includes vegetable dusts (notably fungal spores), proteins of animal and piscine origin, various pathognomonic micro-organisms (such as bacteria, Rickettsia and Chlamydia), vegetable and mineral oils, and certain organic chemicals.

This chapter is concerned with:

(1) hypersensitivity lung disease due to antigenic proteins or other matter;
(2) certain infectious diseases;
(3) pneumonic or granulomatous disease caused by oils;
(4) non-asthmatic disease caused by some organic chemicals.

Hypersensitivity lung disease is the result of different types of allergic reaction and takes two distinct forms — *asthma* and *extrinsic allergic bronchiolo-alveolitis* (hypersensitivity pneumonia in the USA). Occasionally both types of disorder occur in the same individual. The question of occupational asthma is dealt with in Chapter 12.

EXTRINSIC ALLERGIC BRONCHIOLO-ALVEOLITIS (HYPERSENSITIVITY PNEUMONIA)

This is a generic term for a common manifestation of a variety of causes. It can be defined as a clinical disorder due to the inhalation of particulate antigenic, organic material and is characterized in its *acute phase* by constitutional symptoms, the presence of specific precipitating antibodies (precipitins) in many cases, and by lymphocytic infiltration and sarcoid-type granulomas in the walls of alveoli and small airways; and, in its *chronic phase,* by an irreversible and often progressive diffuse intrapulmonary fibrosis. But it must be emphasized that the 'acute' phase is often clinically subacute and not an illness of abrupt onset. The majority of affected individuals are non-atopic.

Because, as explained in Chapter 4, the disease process involves respiratory bronchioles as well as alveoli the term 'alveolitis' falls short and bronchiolo-alveolitis is preferable (Seal, 1975). However, this being understood, allergic 'alveolitis' will be used throughout for convenience.

A large group of allergens is now known or believed to cause extrinsic allergic 'alveolitis' (*see Table 11.1*) and there appears to be no limit to the potential sources of such agents. The disease is usually associated with occupation or hobbies rather than with some random exposure because intensive or repeated low grade exposure to the responsible allergen is necessary to provoke sensitization. In Britain its commonest cause appears to be exposure to budgerigar (parakeet) proteins (Hendrick, Faux and Marshall, 1978a).

It must, however, be appreciated that the specific causal agent has only been identified in a small number of the disease types listed and evidence of an immunological mechanism (if, in fact, one is involved) is not always complete. The presence of precipitins in some cases is, of course, evidence of an immunological reaction but not necessarily of its involvement in pathogenesis. Furthermore, they are often present in the absence of disease. But the development of the clinical features of disease in association with repeated exposure to a particular material is a reasonably good indication of a causal relationship.

The pathology, pathogenesis and clinical characteristics will be considered first in general terms followed by an outline of features peculiar to each type of the disease.

PATHOLOGY

Acute disease

Details of the pathology of acute disease have been

Table 11.1 Types of Extrinsic Allergic 'Alveolitis'

Type	*Nature of responsible aerosol*	*Nature of antigen*
Farmers' lung	Mouldy hay, straw and grain	*M. faeni, T. vulgaris, T. thalpophilus*
Bird fanciers' lung	Droppings and feathers	Avian proteins
Bagassosis	Mouldy sugar cane	*T. sacchari*
Mushroom workers' lung	Compost dust	Thermoactinomycetes such as *Actinobifida dichotomica*. Mushroom spores
Malt workers' lung	Mouldy barley	*Aspergillus clavatus*
Suberosis	Mouldy cork bark dust	*Penicillium frequentans*
Maple bark strippers' lung	Mouldy bark dust	*Cryptostroma (Coniosporum) corticale*
Wood pulp workers' disease	Mouldy bark dust	*Alternaria*
Air-conditioner disease ('humidifier disease')	Dust or mist	(1) *T. vulgaris, T. thalpophilus* (2) Amoebae: *N. gruberi* and *Acanthamoeba* (see text)
Sewage sludge disease	Dust of heat-treated sludge	Gram-negative bacteria
Sauna-takers' disease	Contaminated steam	*Aureobasidium pullulans*
Sequoiosis	Mouldy sawdust of giant redwood	*Aureobasidium pullulans*. Graphium?
Cheese washers' lung	Mould dust	*Penicillium casei*. Acarids?
Dry rot lung	Mould dust	*Merulius lacrymans*
Wheat weevil lung	Mouldy grain and flour dust	*Sitophilus granarius*
Animal handlers' lung	Dust of dander, hair particles and dried urine of rats and gerbils	Serum and urine proteins
Fish meal workers' lung	Fish meal dust	Fish proteins
Diisocyanate 'alveolitis'	Dust and gas in manufacture of some adhesives, paints, etc.	TDI and HDI
Pyrethrum 'alveolitis'	Insecticide aerosol	Pyrethrum
Pituitary snuff takers' lung	Therapeutic snuff	Pig or ox protein

obtained almost entirely from biopsy material taken at varying intervals from the onset of symptoms. Bronchoscopically the large bronchi are usually intensely congested (Fuller, 1953).

Microscopic appearances

Initially there is oedema of the lungs with a predominantly lymphocytic infiltration and thickening of alveolar walls, and plasma cells are usually — but not always — prominent. Within the first two weeks, as oedema subsides, numerous non-caseating, sarcoid-type epithelioid granulomas with Langhan's giant cells develop (*Figure 11.1*). These changes were referred to as 'acute granulomatous pneumonitis' by Dickie and Rankin (1958).

The granulomas, many of which are surrounded by a narrow band of collagen fibres, are similar in appearance to

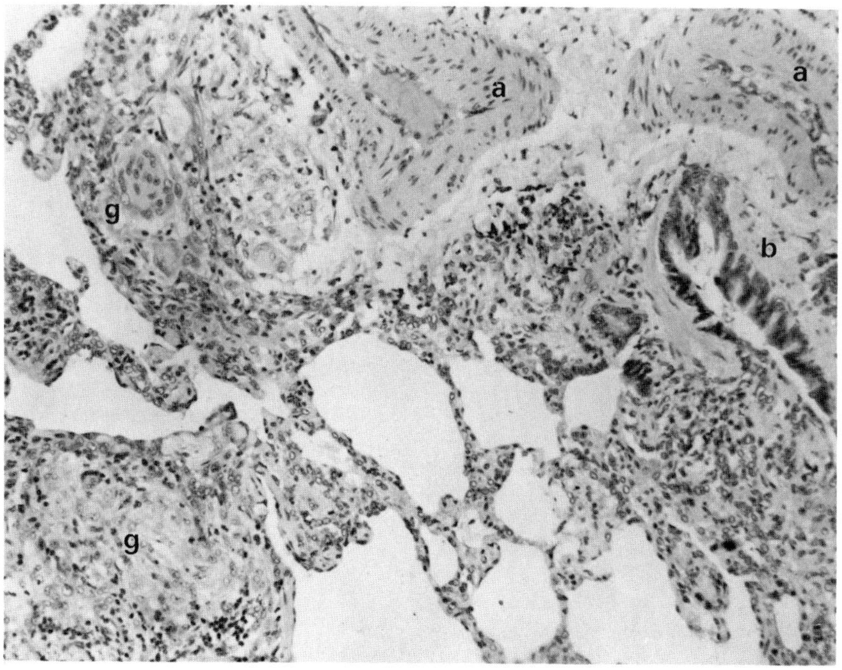

Figure 11.1 Acute extrinsic allergic 'alveolitis' in a farmer. Sarcoid-type granulomas (g) and infiltration of alveolar walls by lymphocytes and plasma cells; arteritis (a) and involvement of the wall of a bronchiole (b) with narrowing of its lumen. (Original magnification × 150, reproduced at ×120, H and E stain. Courtesy of Dr R. M. E. Seal)

those seen in sarcoidosis, chronic beryllium disease, tuberculosis without caseation, brucellosis and various fungal and protozoal infections (Jones Williams, 1967). But they sometimes contain birefringent bodies which are thought to be of vegetable origin (Molina, 1976). They occur in alveolar walls and in the walls of terminal and respiratory bronchioles which they may almost obliterate (*Figures 11.1* and *11.2*); and they tend to favour the centre of the lobule. Bronchiolitis is fairly common and the walls of related pulmonary arteries and arterioles are occasionally thickened by swelling of their muscle fibres and endothelial cells (Seal, 1975). Necrosing vasculitis, however, is not seen.

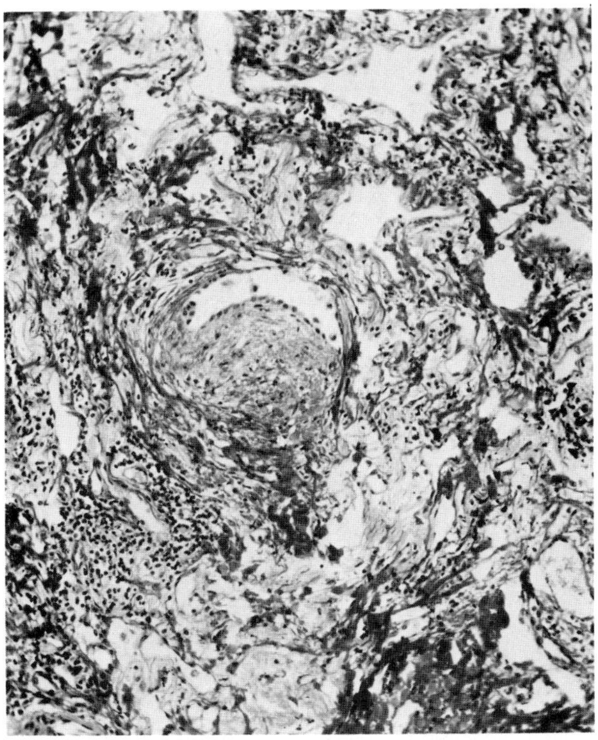

Figure 11.2 Subacute extrinsic allergic 'alveolitis' in a bird fancier showing a large granulomatous lesion in the wall of a bronchiole almost obstructing its lumen, round cell infiltration and early changes of DIPF. (Original magnification × 160, reproduced at × 120. van Giesen stain. Courtesy of Dr K. F. W. Hinson and the Editor of Human Pathology*)*

In contrast to sarcoidosis granulomas are not found in the hilar lymph nodes (Seal *et al.*, 1968).

An exceptional case of extremely acute disease in a young farmer showed numerous discrete, grey-coloured, miliary nodules throughout the lungs to the naked eye. The nodules consisted of large numbers of lymphocytes, epithelial cells and early reticulin formation, but relatively few plasma cells and neutrophils, and no granulomas. Acute necrosing 'alveolitis' was also present (Barrowcliff and Arblaster, 1968). It is possible, however, that this may have been a case of acute mycoplasma pneumonia which can produce *M.faeni*-like precipitins.

The granulomas resolve in about three or four months and are replaced by a substantial lymphocytic infiltration of alveolar walls and scattered lymphoid follicles with germinal centres. The inflammatory thickening of the walls is more pronounced than that seen in sarcoidosis. Some reticulin or fine collagen fibrosis may also be present. Hyalinized granulomas, like those seen in some cases of sarcoidosis and chronic beryllium disease, do not occur. This may reflect different rates of 'turn-over' of macrophages and their derivative epithelial cells (Spector, 1971).

Thermophilic actinomycetes have been isolated from lung biopsy specimens (Wenzel *et al.*, 1964) and fungal spores can sometimes be identified with special stains.

Little is known of the pathology during the transition period from acute to chronic disease.

Chronic disease

Macroscopic appearances

There may be some thickening of the pulmonary pleura though this is not often prominent. But in advanced disease multiple, thick-walled 'hob-nail' cysts ('air blebs') are common.

The cut surface of the lungs display the appearances of a fine DIPF which is confluent in places forming large, irregular, solid masses. Smooth-walled 'honeycomb' cysts up to 2 or 3 cm in diameter are often associated with the fibrosis. Characteristically these changes are distributed predominantly in the upper halves of the lungs but occasionally this is reversed, and advanced diseases may be generalized (*Figure 11.3*). In some cases the fibrosis is so delicate and the cysts so small that they are not readily identified if the lungs are not prepared by formalin perfusion or barium sulphate impregnation (*see* Appendix). Such fine fibrosis and dilated air-spaces may be mistaken for emphysema.

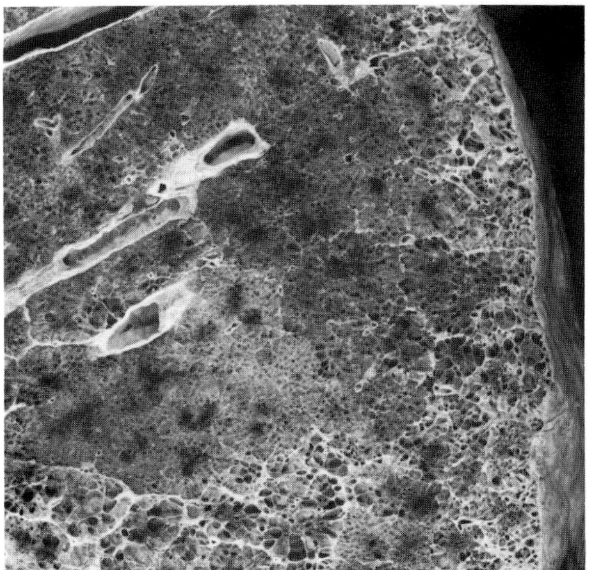

Figure 11.3 Naked eye appearances of chronic extrinsic allergic 'alveolitis' in a farm worker. Widespread, sharply demarcated DIPF with numerous small honeycomb cysts. Note diffuse thickening of pulmonary pleura. (Courtesy of Dr R. M. E. Seal)

Microscopic appearances

There is diffuse collagenous fibrosis of alveolar walls, around terminal and respiratory bronchioles and perivascular zones. Large tracts of collagen are often a feature of the fibrotic areas which may extend to the periphery of the lobule. Scattered bronchiolitis, which is said to occur in about one-third of cases, may be seen and is sometimes associated with centrilobular emphysema (Seal, 1975). Granulomas are absent but a few may still be found if the latent period since the episode of acute disease is not longer than about 12 months. Foreign-body giant cells containing birefringent material of uncertain identity may be present but plasma cells are usually absent, though substantial numbers may be found in the medulla of hilar lymph nodes (Seal *et al.*, 1968). Medial thickening of pulmonary arteries indicative of pulmonary hypertension will usually be seen in the more advanced cases.

PATHOGENESIS

The pathogenesis of extrinsic allergic 'alveolitis' involves immunological mechanisms and in all probability, other non-immunological factors. Its understanding is not helped by conflicting experimental results and controversy over the significance of the serological findings.

The features of farmers' lung and bird fanciers' lung which are the most common types of extrinsic allergic 'alveolitis' and, thus, the most extensively studied probably apply to all the other types (*see Table 11.1*).

The subject can be conveniently considered under three headings (Pepys, 1977):

(1) The nature of the inhaled material.
(2) The immunological reactivity of the subject.
(3) The circumstances of exposure.

The nature of the inhaled material

The most important characteristic is that the particles are small enough for a high proportion of them to reach and be deposited in the gas exchanging region of the lungs (*see* Chapter 3). The spores of thermophilic actinomycetes associated with farmers' lung, for example, range from 0.7 to1.5 μm in diameter and avian protein aggregates are considerably smaller. But, in addition, the chemical and biological properties have a significant effect in eliciting sensitization or other reactions.

Fractionation of responsible antigens shows that they, and hence their antigenic potential, are bewilderingly complex. For example, using immuno-electrophoretics four major and a number of minor antigens have been found in *M.faeni* associated with the mycelial cell wall and the spore coat, and some possess enzymatic activity. If, therefore, only spores are inhaled it appears likely that antibodies against the enzymes can only be produced if there is a limited degree of development and generation of the organism in the lungs (Edwards, 1978). Similarly, there is a variety of different antigens in pigeon dropping extracts and in pigeon serum (Fredericks, 1978), and it is probable that antigenic heterogeneity exists in the other disease types.

Purified fractions of antigenic mixtures are used for the evaluation of immunological responses and their possible contribution to pathogenesis. Standardization of antigens is necessary both for diagnostic and research purposes but the difficulties involved in achieving this are immense.

It is also possible that the material which harbours fungal spores may itself have a direct inflammatory effect in the lungs (*see* p. 364).

Immunological reactivity of the subject

Humoral immunity

Most affected individuals are non-atopic. Evidence which suggests that immune complexes are involved in pathogenesis is as follows:

(1) Large quantities of precipitating, complement-fixing, circulating antibodies are present in most patients with acute disease.
(2) The symptoms of acute disease (fever, rigors, myalgia, breathlessness) which are associated with intermittent high level exposure to the causal agent occur in four to eight hours after exposure.
(3) Bronchial provocation tests with inhaled extracts of the responsible agent reproduces all the features of acute disease in patients in four to eight hours, but not in controls (*see* Chapter 4). This is compatible with Type III allergy.
(4) Intradermal tests, with the relevant antigen results in an Arthus-type reaction in four to eight hours in symptomatic individuals.

This does not explain the characteristic feature of acute extrinsic allergic 'alveolitis'—sarcoid-type granulomas—which are not associated with Type III Arthus reactions. However, granulomas have been induced experimentally by injection of antigen–antibody complexes which are not complement fixing (Spector and Heesom, 1969). But the pathological features of the case of Barrowcliff and Arblaster referred to earlier are consistent with an Arthus reaction.

Precipitins against particular antigenic components may mediate reactions in one individual but not in another. Thus, they are often found in healthy (asymptomatic) persons who have had similar exposure as well as in those with disease. Precipitins to thermophilic actinomycetes are present in a proportion (about 18 per cent) of healthy farmers (Pepys, 1969). Avian precipitins in healthy persons appear to be found most commonly in poultry farmers, less often in pigeon fanciers and rarely in budgerigar and parrot fanciers (Pepys, 1977). This may reflect heavier exposure to dry droppings in the first two groups compared with the third.

There is some evidence that Type I allergy, which is mediated by reaginic IgE or by short-term sensitizing IgG antibodies (*see* Chapter 4), may be required for the development of the Type III reaction (Cochrane, 1971; Pepys, 1969). This may explain why precipitins are more often present in affected than in non-affected individuals (Pepys, 1978). However, specific precipitins are uniformly absent in some persons with proven extrinsic allergic 'alveolitis'. Nonetheless, in spite of the uncertainty about the part played by precipitins and their relevance in diagnosis they provide evidence of exposure and are the chief means by which most types of extrinsic allergic 'alveolitis' have been, and are, first identified.

In the chronic stage of farmers' lung disease the presence of circulating precipitins becomes progressively less common with the passage of time since the last acute episode. The period of transition from positive to negative appears to vary considerably (*see* section on farmers' lung). By contrast, in chronic budgerigar breeders lung precipitins are apparently permanent in most cases.

Although the complexity of antigens in farmers' lung makes quantification of the related antibodies difficult IgG, IgM and IgA antibodies are demonstrable by immunofluorescent and radio-immunoassay techniques (Parratt *et al.*, 1975; Patterson *et al.*, 1976). Similarly, IgG antibodies capable of fixing complement and smaller quantities of IgM and IgA antibodies have been demonstrated in pigeon fanciers' diseases and also in healthy individuals with similar exposure to birds (Fink, Tebo and Barboriak, 1969; Moore and Fink, 1975; Boren *et al.*, 1977). Deposits of IgG and complement have occasionally been found in lesions of pulmonary vasculitis (Ghose *et al.*, 1974), and IgM appears to be consistently present in the broncho-alveolar fluid in extrinsic allergic 'alveolitis' but not in sarcoidosis; and the IgG/albumin ratio is greater than 1 in the former but less than 1 in the latter (Weinberger *et al.*, 1978). Indeed, IgG and IgA levels in bronchial lavage fluid of individuals with bird (pigeon) fanciers' lung are significantly higher than in exposed, but healthy, persons (Calvanico *et al.*, 1980). The IgG subclass IgG_3 is increased in farmers' lung patients compared with 'control' farmers suggesting that they have a tendency to produce this antibody type (Stokes, Turton and Turner-Warwick, 1981).

Precipitin tests in routine use (usually agar gel diffusion techniques) are relatively insensitive and may fail to demonstrate antibodies in all cases whereas radio-immunoassay will detect them in most (Parratt and Boyd, 1976). This probably explains some — but not all — cases of precipitin-negative disease and may make the interpretation of some earlier investigations difficult to interpret.

Hay dust, *M. faeni* and pigeon serum antigens are capable of activating the C3 component of complement *in vitro* directly without the intervention of antibody — that is, by the alternative pathway (Berrens, Guikers and van Dijk, 1974; Edwards, Baker and Davies, 1974; Edwards, 1976; Marx and Flaherty, 1976; Bice *et al.*, 1977) (*see* Chaper 4, p. 58). It is suggested that after inhalation the antigens are rapidly ingested by macrophages causing them to secrete C3-cleaving enzymes. The resultant activated C3 (C3b) then stimulates macrophages to release other factors including fibrogenic factor, and leucocytes to produce tissue-damaging enzymes (Schorlemmer *et al.*, 1977) (*Figure 11.4*). But it is not clear whether the same antigens can activate both classic and alternative pathways nor whether the activation of one or other pathway is determined by the *nature* of the antigen, or by the *amount* of it inhaled. While this hypothesis explains some cases of precipitin-negative acute extrinsic allergic 'alveolitis' it does not readily account for the genesis of granulomas. However, transient granulomas with Langhans giant cells have been shown to develop eight days following intratracheal deposition of mouldy hay dust in unsensitized rats and rabbits, apparently without the intervention of a Type IV reaction (Edwards, Wagner and Seal, 1976, 1980). (*See also* Direct toxicity of organic dusts.) Other antigens which cause extrinsic allergic 'alveolitis' have not yet been shown to activate complement by the alternative pathway.

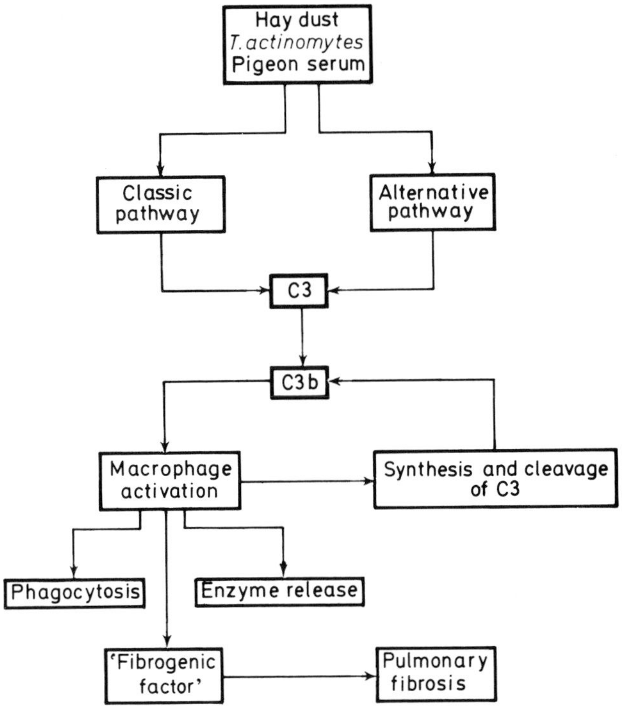

Figure 11.4 Schema of suggested interaction between the complement system and macrophages in extrinsic allergic 'alveolitis'

In a recent study of patients with farmers' lung a correlation was observed between complement fixation (consumption) and precipitins to *M. faeni* and, although precipitin levels fell over a 16-month period during which clinical recovery occurred, complement fixing antibody remained unchanged. Moreover, the complement fixation test successfully distinguished farmers' lung from unrelated respiratory disease in a control population exposed to a comparable antigen load (Berrens, de Ridder and de Boer, 1977). If this observation can be confirmed a valuable tool for diagnosis and epidemiological screening will be available.

Massive exposure of farm workers to a variety of saprophytic fungi when unsealing silos has been reported to cause disease which, though clinically identical to acute extrinsic allergic 'alveolitis', appears to be different in other respects. There was no past history of acute disease and no precipitins and the pathology (biopsy in one case) consisted of an acute, multifocal, inflammatory reaction without granulomas but with large numbers of fungi in the lungs. It has been suggested that this is a separate disorder caused by fungal toxins and not by immunological reactivity, and that the term 'pulmonary mycotoxicosis' might be used to refer to it although the nature of the toxins remains to be defined (Emanuel, Wenzel and Lawton, 1975). However, all these features could equally well be explained by activation of complement via the alternative pathway due to the heavy dust exposure (Edwards, Wagner and Seal, 1976). The new term is, perhaps, better avoided until the pathogenesis of this type of disease has been satisfactorily clarified.

Cell mediated immunity

In view of the granulomatous nature of extrinsic allergic

'alveolitis' it might be expected that Type IV allergy is involved but indisputable evidence of this has not been established in human disease. There is experimental evidence that particles coated with antigen can stimulate granuloma formation mediated by lymphoid cells in sensitized animals (Boros and Warren, 1973) and, in fact, many of the antigens which cause extrinsic allergic 'alveolitis' are particles with diffusible antigens on their surfaces. Hence, it is possible that these could induce Type IV as well as Type III allergy (Pepys, 1978). Indeed, Seal, Edwards and Hayes (1975) concluded from animal experiments that both Type IV hypersensitivity and a non-specific inflammatory response to many constituents of inhaled dust play a role in the total tissue response.

Due, possibly, to technical difficulties there are very few reports of lymphocyte sensitization tests with *M.faeni* or other farmers' lung antigens. But Marx *et al.* (1973) found macrophage inhibition factor (MIF) in some cases and studies of peripheral lymphocytes in patients with pigeon fanciers' lung have demonstrated positive specific lymphocyte transformation and MIF on exposure to antigen in many cases (Caldwell *et al.*, 1973; Hansen and Penny, 1974; Moore *et al.*, 1974; Fink, Moore and Barboriak, 1975; Sennekamp *et al.*, 1978). In one instance both bronchoalveolar and peripheral lymphocytes produced MIF after inhalation challenge with pigeon serum (Schuyler, Thigpen and Salvaggio, 1978). Specific lymphocyte transformation tests may remain positive for months, even years, in bird breeders' lung; whereas specific precipitins and MIF rapidly become negative after cessation of exposure (Allen, Basten and Woolcock, 1977). A small proportion of asymptomatic individuals also have T lymphocytes sensitized to pigeon antigens (Hansen and Penny, 1974; Moore *et al.*, 1974; Allen *et al.*, 1975; Fink, Moore and Barboriak, 1975; Sennekamp *et al.*, 1978), but whether or not this is a precursor of symptomatic disease remains to be discovered.

These findings, however, are confusing in that there are inconsistencies in the MIF and lymphocyte transformation tests. Some observers have found positive results with pigeon droppings but negative with serum, whereas others have found the reverse. But the recent observation that cells in bronchoalveolar fluid from patients with extrinsic allergic 'alveolitis' contain a high proportion of T lymphocytes is consistent with involvement of cell mediated immunity (Reynolds *et al.*, 1977; Weinberger *et al.*, 1978; Voisin *et al.*, 1979), though whether these cells possess specificity for the associated antigen has still to be established. The possibility that Type IV allergy plays a role in pathogenesis is supported by the production of identical disease in animals both with thermophilic actinomycete and pigeon antigens (Moore, 1978). Nevertheless, the full picture of Type IV allergy, as displayed by delayed skin test reactions has not been produced with antigens which are suitable for skin testing (Pepys, 1977).

In contrast to the high levels of T lymphocytes found in the lungs Turner-Warwick (1980) reported that, in a small number of cases of extrinsic allergic 'alveolitis' (farmers' and bird fanciers' lung), the response of blood T cells to PHA is significantly depressed in the majority and skin test responses to *C. albicans* and PPD antigens are reduced by comparison with matched control individuals. Thus, it is possible that a numerical and functional response of T cells in the lungs, with their depletion in the peripheral blood, rather than a particular type of immune reaction is the important factor in the genesis of the granulomas of extrinsic allergic 'aveolitis'. And the fact that these granulomas, unlike those of sarcoidosis and chronic beryllium disease, are evanescent might suggest that the causal agent does not persist whereas, in the other two, it does (Edwards, Wagner and Seal, 1980).

Circumstances of exposure

The mode of contact with the causal agent is relevant both to sensitization and elicitation of the reactions. Whereas ordinary low level, environmental exposure to an antigen is sufficient to give rise to specific IgE Type I allergy (asthma) in atopic subjects a much more intense exposure is needed to cause the production of precipitins in both non-atopic and atopic subjects. Heavy exposure may also induce IgE production in a proportion of non-atopic subjects: asthma probably occurs in about 10 per cent of patients with acute extrinsic allergic 'alveolitis' (Pepys and Jenkins, 1965). The amounts and duration of exposure to the various allergens believed to cause extrinsic allergic 'alveolitis' which are necessary for sensitization are, at present, unknown.

Intermittent heavy exposure to antigens causes acute disease which, if repeated, may become chronic and progressive. Continuous low level exposure — especially to avian antigens — is most likely to give rise to chronic progressive disease without any preceding 'acute' stage.

Direct toxicity of organic dusts

There is some experimental evidence to suggest that, due to a direct toxic effect on macrophages, the dust itself (for example, hay or bagasse) may contribute to the genesis of chronic disease in concert with the relevant micro-organism (Seal, Edwards and Hayes, 1975; Zaidi *et al.*, 1971; Bhattacharjee, Saxena and Zaidi, 1980). If relevant to man this possibility is obviously important.

Susceptibility to disease Only a very small proportion of people exposed regularly to the unknown causes of extrinsic allergic 'alveolitis' ever develop disease. This suggests that individual susceptibility is important in its development. Preliminary reports — the implications of which require further study—suggest that there may be an association between certain HLA antigens (notably B8) and the occurrence of farmers' lung and pigeon fanciers' lung (Allen *et al.*, 1975; Flaherty *et al.*, 1975; Berrill and Van Rood, 1977; Sennekamp, Rittner and Vogel, 1977); and also an indication that individuals with P_2 positive blood group may be less likely than other groups to develop pigeon fanciers' lung (Effler, Roland and Redding, 1976). However, Rodey *et al.*, (1979) found no significant association between any HLA specifications they tested and pigeon fanciers' lung.

The influence of smoking A survey of Devon farmers revealed that precipitins to *M.faeni* were significantly more common among non-smokers and ex-smokers than among smokers (Morgan *et al.*, 1973). This has subsequently been confirmed in respect of both avian and farmers' lung antigens in non-smokers with or without disease; although when sensitization has occurred the intensity of the antibody response appears to be unaffected by smoking habits

(Morgan *et al.*, 1975; Boyd *et al.*, 1977; Warren, 1977). The explanation may lie in the fact that particle deposition is greater in proximal than in distal airways in smokers compared with non-smokers so that relatively few particles penetrate to the periphery in smokers (*see* Chapter 3, p. 48).

To summarize

(1) Acute and subacute disease is caused by heavy, often intermittent, exposure to the extrinsic antigen. Repeated episodes may lead to irreversible, widespread fibrosis.
(2) Chronic, fibrotic disease, however, more commonly follows frequent and continued low-grade exposure because of the absence of acute illness.
(3) It seems likely that some or all of the pathogenic mechanisms just described may figure in the development of extrinsic allergic 'alveolitis' in varying degree at different stages, but that T lymphocyte activity in the lungs is particularly important.

CLINICAL FEATURES

Acute and subacute disease

Symptoms

Characteristically these occur about four to eight hours following heavy exposure to the offending antigen, though they may take several days to develop fully. They include headache (often severe), rigors, sweating, fever, anorexia, nausea and vomiting. 'Tightness' of the chest is a common complaint and breathlessness on effort is invariable and sometimes severe, cough which varies from occasional to frequent and harassing is usual, but sputum is absent or of small volume and mucoid in type. Haemoptysis is rare. Chest pain does not occur other than from cough fracture of ribs.

The pattern of symptoms, however, varies from patient to patient: in some they are chiefly constitutional; in others, respiratory. They may be mild or very severe. Because of the similarity of the symptoms to those of a variety of bacterial and viral diseases it is essential to obtain a detailed history of relevant exposure. This is especially true of subacute disease in which increasing breathlessness, fever and ill health may take some days to develop making its origin difficult to recognize.

Providing that there is no further exposure to the offending agent the symptoms usually subside after about 48 hours but they may not cease completely for seven to ten days. Some loss of weight may follow the episode and in some cases dyspnoea an effort may persist for a few months.

Repeated exposure may result in many episodes of acute symptoms and, in a small proportion of patients, a point may be reached when a reaginic (IgE) asthmatic response occurs immediately after exposure to be followed, several hours later, by the symptoms of acute extrinsic allergic 'alveolitis' (Pepys and Jenkins, 1965).

Physical signs

There is tachycardia and fever which may be as high as 46 °C (106°F) and, in patients whose symptoms are predominantly respiratory, dyspnoea at rest. Occasionally dyspnoea is sufficiently severe to demand hospital treatment. Central cyanosis is sometimes present and restlessness and apprehension may be prominent. These signs, which may take several days to become established, are often accompanied by considerable loss of weight.

Fine to medium pitched, often patchy, crepitations may be heard towards the end of full inspiration over the lower halves of the lung fields. They disappear completely with recovery. Wheeze is not a feature of the disease but may be present in a small number of patients (Pepys, 1969). Rhonchi are absent and there are no signs of consolidation or pleural effusion.

Chronic disease

Symptoms

After repeated acute episodes and a variable amount of sputum and dyspnoea on effort become permanent having increased progressively after each separate attack. Occasionally this occurs following a single episode of acute disease and where there has been recurrent exposure to low concentrations of mould dust, symptoms develop insidiously without an antecedent acute episode. In most cases of chronic disease dyspnoea gradually worsens without further exposure to antigen. There are no constitutional symptoms.

Physical signs

There are no characteristic signs. The patient is dyspnoeic on effort but not at first, at least until the disease reaches an advanced stage when central cyanosis may be present. Finger clubbing is rarely seen. Signs of widespread fibrosis with deviation of the trachea and impairment of chest expansion on the more affected side may be present. Crepitations (unlike acute disease) are not often heard and, in most cases, wheeze is absent. The rarity of finger clubbing and persistent crepitations contrasts with the findings in cryptogenic fibrosing 'alveolitis' in which clubbing is common and crepitations usually widespread.

The signs of pulmonary heart disease and congestive heart failure may be present in advanced disease.

INVESTIGATIONS

Acute and subacute disease

Lung function

The first changes to occur are arterial oxygen desaturation and reduction in arterial carbon dioxide tension due to hyperventilation. These are soon followed by a fall in VC, TLC and compliance, and the decrease in gas transfer tends to be proportional to the reduction in VC. In some cases the decrement in gas transfer is due to inequality of ventilation—perfusion ratios as is shown by a normal Kco and a significant increase in arterial oxygen tension on breathing pure oxygen. But in others there is an alveolar membrane component indicated by a low Kco. Evidence of airflow obstruction, as determined by FEV_1 and FVC, is absent but flow-volume curves reveal increased up-stream airflow resistance which is probably situated in the small airways due to their involvement by the disease process (Warren, Tse and Cherniack, 1978). The degree of impairment of these functional parameters varies from mild to severe according to the severity of the disease.

The abnormalities resolve within six weeks in most patients treated with corticosteroids (Hapke *et al.*, 1968) and in 12 months in the majority not treated, but impairment of gas transfer and compliance may still be present after the chest radiograph has returned to normal (Williams, 1963). Although lung function is normal between attacks in most cases, in a minority VC, compliance and gas transfer do not return fully to expected normal values. Lung function tests, therefore, are valuable in assessing response to treatment and prognosis, but not in diagnosis.

Radiographic appearances

In mild attacks the chest film may remain normal. Otherwise abnormalities vary from barely detectable changes to widespread coarse opacities similar to the appearances of acute beryllium disease (*see Figure 10.8*, p. 345) or acute pulmonary oedema.

The earliest changes consist of very fine, pin-point opacities (a 'ground glass' or miliary appearance) in the central two-thirds or lower zones of the lung fields, and may be so subtle as to be overlooked (*Figure 11.5*). They are often only detected in retrospect by comparison with films taken after the patient has recovered. The use of an AP in addition to a standard PA film viewed with a hand lens increases the likelihood of their detection.

More definite abnormalities consist of discrete, well-defined opacities ranging from pin-point size to about 3 mm in diameter in the middle and lower zones of the lung fields but frequently sparing the costophrenic angles (*Figure 11a*). In severe attacks larger, blotchy opacities are seen. However, the degree of radiographic abnormality correlates poorly with the severity of symptoms.

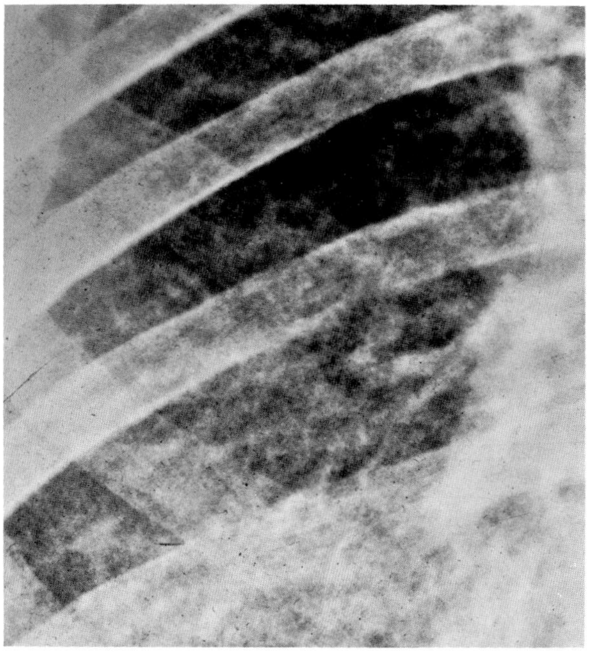

Figure 11.5 Small opacities due to acute extrinsic allergic 'alveolitis' in a farmer's wife. The appearances were uniformly distributed throughout both lung fields. Complete resolution occurred

Larger opacities usually disappear within two or three weeks after the onset of disease, but the fine type may last up to six months before clearing. If fine opacities fail to resolve in six to 12 months they are unlikely to do so, and will ultimately be replaced by the changes of chronic fibrotic disease (Hapke *et al.*, 1968).

Evidence of bilateral hilar node enlargement or of pleural effusion is not seen.

Serology

Precipitins specific to the antigen responsible for the disease are present in the majority of cases — about 90 per cent — if sufficiently sensitive tests are used.

Bronchial (inhalation) provocation tests

Some years ago it was shown that controlled inhalation of the relevant antigen is followed by a systemic reaction in four to eight hours after challenge accompanied by a transient rise in temperature, mild leucocytosis, restriction of ventilation and fall in FEV_1 and, in some instances, gas transfer (*Figure 11.6*). In a small proportion of cases this is preceded by an immediate asthmatic reaction with airflow obstruction (Pepys, 1969). More recently it has been confirmed that there are six practical measurements which indicate a positive late response to challenge: increase of body temperature (> 37.2 °C), circulating neutrophils (≥ + 2500/mm³), exercise minute ventilation (≥ + 15 per cent) and exercise respiratory frequency (≥ + 25 per cent); and decrease of circulating lymphocytes (≥ – 500/mm³ with lymphopenia) and FVC (≥ – 15 per cent). These confirmatory tests have specificities of approximately 95 per cent and sensitivities of 85 to 48 per cent. Auscultation and chest radiography and measurement of Tl and lung volume subdivisions are too insensitive to be useful. However, challenge doses sufficient to provoke significant changes in these tests may be potentially dangerous and are, if possible, better avoided (Hendrick *et al.*, 1980). But, in general, provocation tests are only indicated in suspect cases of extrinsic allergic 'alveolitis' in which precipitin tests are negative and chest radiographs, normal (Harries, Burge and O'Brien, 1980) (*see also* Chapter 12, p. 427).

Skin reactions

In general these are of little value due mainly to the fact that there are few suitable extracts available which do not cause non-specific reactions. An exception to this is an intracutaneous test with avian extract but it is unlikely to provide more information than specific precipitins (*see* Bird fanciers' lung). The Kveim test appears to be negative in many cases (Molina, 1976).

Haematology

There are no specific abnormalities. The sedimentation rate

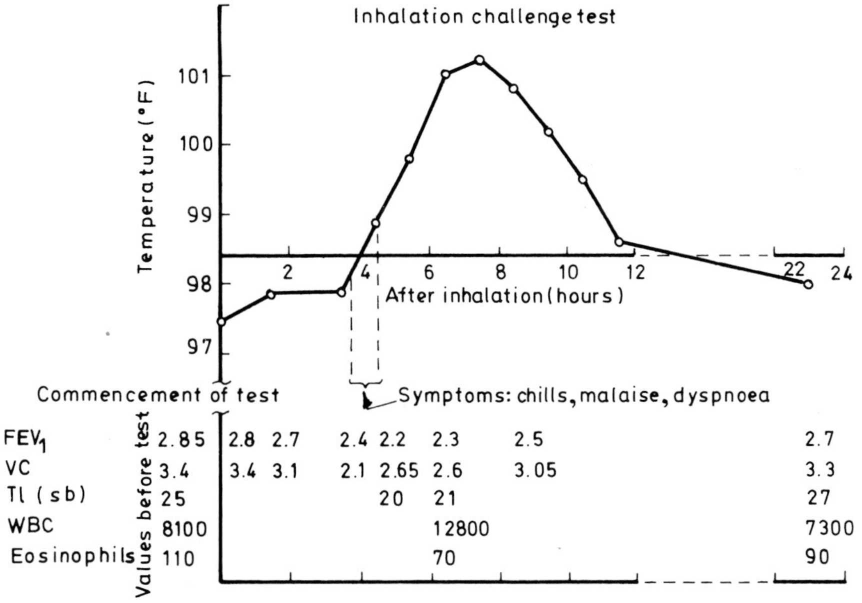

Figure 11.6 Systemic and pulmonary reactions to inhalation challenge with avian antigens in a patient with 'bird breeders' lung'. (Courtesy of Professor J. Pepys)

is raised and there is a mild polymorphonuclear leucocytosis but no eosinophilia. These changes are short-lived.

Sputum

There are no unusual features on naked eye or microscopical examination. But different strains of the *Thermoactinomyces* sp. can be cultured from specimens expectorated by patients who have been exposed to mouldy hay (*see* Farmers' lung), and the percentage of T lymphocytes among the total number of cells in broncho-alveolar lavage fluid is significantly increased (*see* Pathogenesis).

Lung biopsy

This is rarely necessary or justifiable. It is discussed briefly under Diagnosis.

Chronic disease

Lung function

Patterns of impaired function are variable. The most common pattern is a restrictive ventilatory defect, increased RV/TLC ratio and impaired gas transfer. However, in some patients there is reduction of gas transfer and compliance with or without decrease in lung volume, but no evidence of airflow obstruction. In others—about a third—there is slight to moderate, irreversible airflow obstruction (reduced FEV_1/FVC per cent and increase RV) which may be due to bronchiolitis obliterans of terminal and respiratory bronchioles as a sequela of gramulomatous infiltration (*see* Pathology). In yet other patients both types of functional impairment are combined (Dickie and Rankin, 1958; Hapke *et al.*, 1968). Compliance is usually reduced (increased elastic recoil), often considerably, but in some cases it is increased together with reduction of air flow indicating associated emphysematous changes (Warren, Tse and Cherniack, 1978).

There is sometimes a discrepancy between the symptoms complained of and the values of lung function tests at rest which may be near normal. This is analogous to the situation in early asbestosis and chronic beryllium disease.

Cardiac catheterization reveals the presence of pulmonary hypertension in some cases which appears to be caused by obliterative reduction of the vascular bed as pulmonary scintigraphy with I^{131} has shown (Bishop, Melnick and Raine, 1963; Molina, 1976).

Radiographic appearances

These vary according to the severity of the disease. They range from fine, linear or rounded, ill-defined opacities to coarse linear opacities which tend to radiate from the hilar regions and, in advanced disease, are accompanied by tracheal deviation and distortion, lobar contraction, and by small translucent areas caused by cyst formation (*Figures 11.7* and *11.8*). By contrast with acute disease these appearances predominate in the upper and middle zones, and are often more pronounced on one side. They are indistinguishable from fibrocavernous tuberculosis, chronic sarcoidosis, and, in some cases, allergic bronchopulmonary aspergillosis. Undue translucency of the lower zones may be present. Occasionally fibrotic appearances are more predominant in the middle or lower zones than in the upper zones.

Chronic disease may also be represented by small discrete opacities when these remain unchanged for about a year.

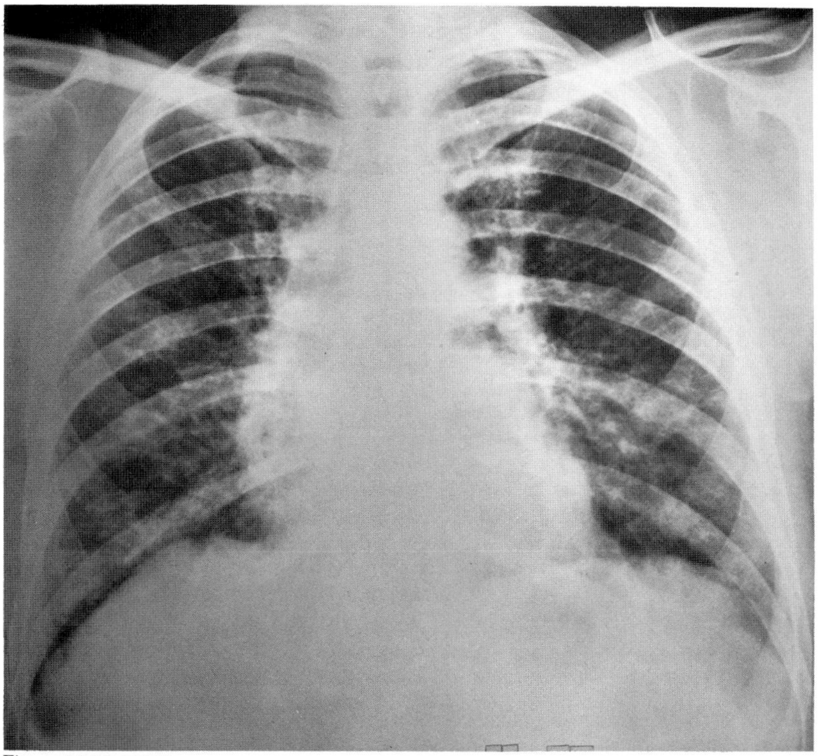

Figure 11.7(a) 1975

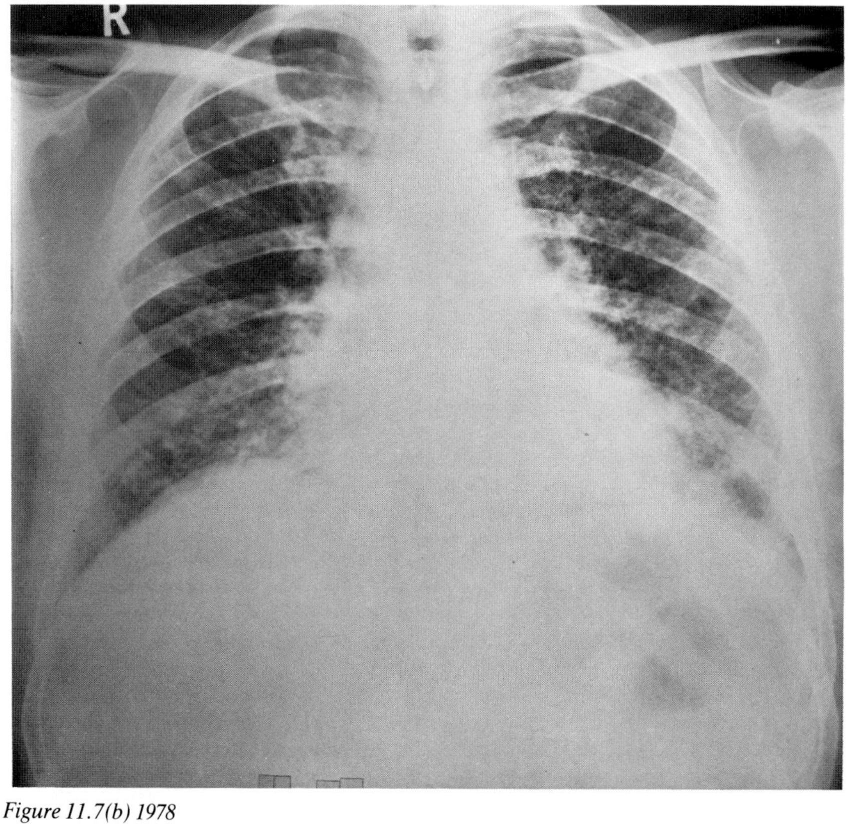

Figure 11.7(b) 1978

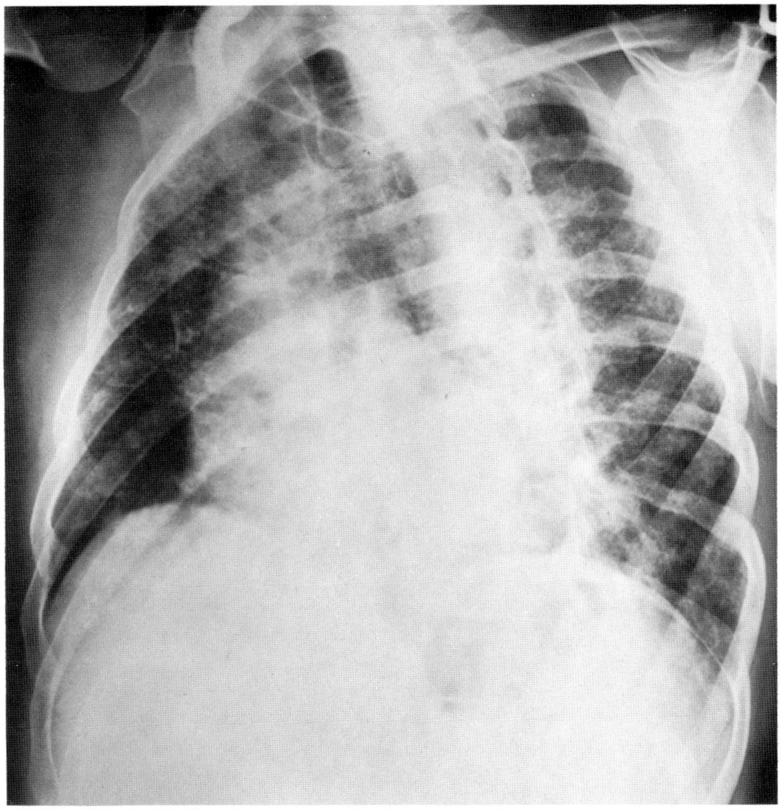

Figure 11.7(c)

Figure 11.7 Chronic extrinsic allergic 'alveolitis' in a cattleman handling straw, hay, grain and cattle bedding for 16 years. No definite episodes of acute disease but a heavy 'cold' and lassitude reported in the autumn of 1972. Productive cough, dyspnoea on effort and loss of weight three years later. (a) 1975. Widespread irregular opacities with no evident cystic appearances; disease of moderate severity. Clinically: pronounced finger clubbing and localized inspiratory crepitations. Precipitins M. faeni *positive in moderately high titre;* A. fumigatus *weakly positive;* T. vulgaris *negative. (b) 1978. Progression of small round and irregular opacities and increase in heart size due to pulmonary heart disease. Coarse inspiratory and expiratory crepitations in all lobar regions. (c) Left 45 degree anterior oblique view on same day shows particular involvement of the upper zone of the right lung.* Post mortem. *Naked eye: multiple 'hobnail' air blebs of the pulmonary pleura; widespread, fairly coarse DIPF with 'honeycomb' cysts up to 1.5 cm in diameter involving all lobes and sharply demarcated from adjacent normal lung. Microscopically: features of chronic extrinsic allergic 'alveolitis'; no granulomas. Death from cardiorespiratory failure*

They do not necessarily progress to the 'fibrotic' appearances just described. If serial chest films are not available these opacities could, in the presence of an acute respiratory illness be interpreted as evidence of acute extrinsic allergic 'alveolitis' or of some unrelated disease.

Serology

In the case of chronic disease the chance of demonstrating precipitins becomes less as the time since the last acute episode increases. Precipitins are still present in about 80 per cent of cases up to three years after an attack of acute farmers' lung disease, but in only about 20 per cent when the interval is longer than three years (Hapke *et al.*, 1968).

Lung biopsy

This is discussed in the next section.

DIAGNOSIS

Extrinsic allergic 'alveolitis' in its acute form must be distinguished at times from a variety of other respiratory diseases which occur fortuitously or originate from the same occupational environment. The chronic form may need to be differentiated from widespread fibrosis due to other causes.

The history is extremely important. It should include precise details of the occupational exposure. Careful

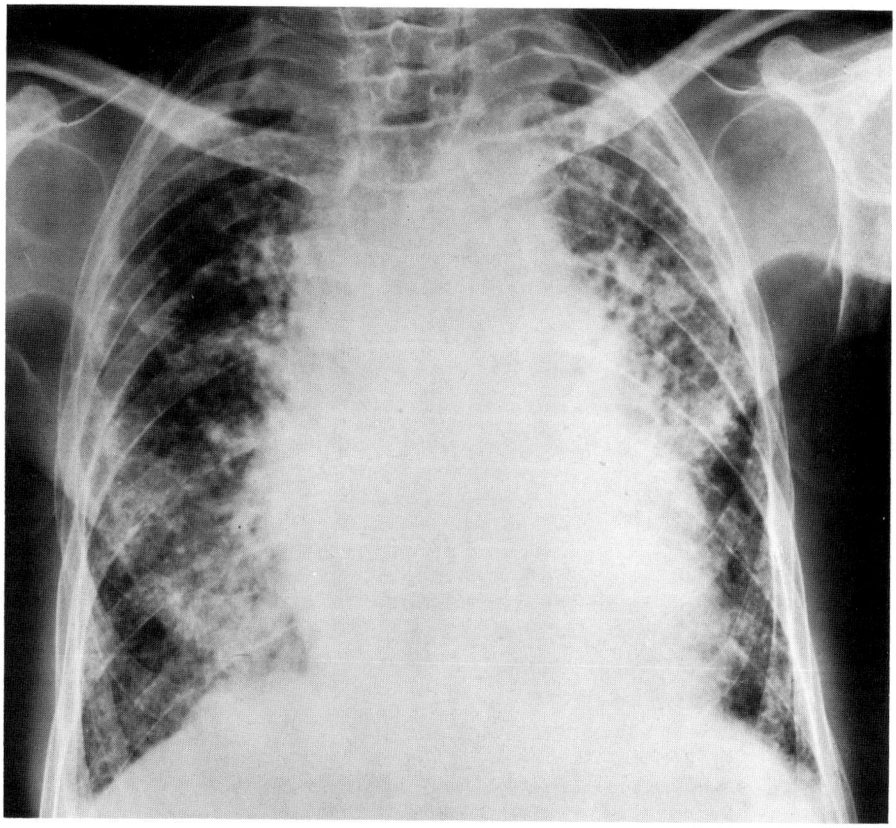

Figure 11.8 Advanced chronic extrinsic allergic 'alveolitis' in a farm worker with no history of initial episodes of acute disease. Coarse rounded and irregular opacities in all zones which tend to be predominant in the upper and middle zones. Large heart shadow due to severe pulmonary heart disease

enquiry into hobbies (such as pigeon racing and budgerigar breeding) and the keeping of domestic pets (for example, budgerigar or parrot) is also necessary in many cases of acute or chronic lung disease presenting for diagnosis. Of equal importance is the history of the development and nature of the symptoms. The historical details together with the associated clinical and radiographic features (and, in acute disease and a proportion of cases of chronic disease, the presence of specific precipitins) establish the diagnosis in the majority of cases.

The possibility that complement fixation, specific lymphocyte transformation and MIF tests may be value in diagnosis appears promising but remains to be verified (*see* Pathogenesis).

Bronchial provocation tests are rarely necessary except in cases in which proof of one of the rarer causes of extrinsic allergic 'alveolitis' is required.

Lung biopsy, as a rule, is not indicated but may be needed to exclude other causes of fibrosing 'alveolitis' in some cases of precipitin-negative acute disease and other causes of DIPF in chronic disease. Granulomas are readily found in most cases of acute and subacute disease (Reyes *et al.*, 1976).

Acute and subacute disease

The difference between the sudden onset of fever, rigors and dyspnoea of acute disease and the gradual development of ill health, fever, loss of weight, increasing breathlessness and widespread shadowing in the chest radiograph of subacute disease must be borne in mind. Of the two modes of presentation the subacute is probably more common and is more difficult to recognize promptly.

Diagnosis rests on a detailed history of occupation and the mode of onset of disease, characteristic constitutional and respiratory symptoms and signs, the presence of relevant precipitating antibodies and consistent radiographic appearances. Lung function tests are of no diagnostic help. It must be remembered that, in taking the history, the patient may not be aware that he has been in contact with the relevant antigenic source (for example, mouldy hay). In mild cases there are no dramatic symptoms.

The following diseases may need to be distinguished:

(1) *Influenza* Acute extrinsic allergic 'alveolitis' is most frequently confused with an influenzal illness, but the history of exposure and delayed onset of symptoms should lead to the correct diagnosis.

(2) *Acute bronchitis* Extrinsic allergic 'alveolitis' is differentiated by unproductive, or slightly productive cough; by rapidly developing breathlessness; by the presence of crepitations in the lower halves of the lung fields in the absence of rhonchi; and by a lack of response to treatment with antibiotics and bronchodilators.

(3) *Late asthma* (*see* Chapter 12) The time of onset may be identical. Differentiation may be difficult initially if, as is often the case, wheeze is absent and if mouldy hay or avian precipitins are present which is likely in farm workers and bird fanciers respectively. This applies especially to asthma due to storage mites ('barn allergy') which is referred to on p. 375 and in Chapter 12.

(4) *Atypical viral or mycoplasmal pneumonia* These are similar but the physical signs and radiographic signs of consolidation are distinct from extrinsic allergic 'alveolitis'. Serological tests may be required.

(5) *Miliary tuberculosis* Differentiation here rests mainly upon the occupational and clinical history, and upon the presence of precipitins. Resolution of radiographic abnormalities after treatment with antituberculosis drugs is of no diagnostic assistance as most cases of acute extrinsic allergic 'alveolitis' recover spontaneously. In both diseases the tuberculin test is often negative.

(6) *Allergic bronchopulmonary aspergillosis* May occur in atopic farm workers (who usually have a history of extrinsic asthma) after exposure to mouldy hay with a high content of aspergillus spores but the features of the disease are entirely different from those of farmers' lung. They consist of a more rapid onset after exposure, an asthmatic attack with evident wheeze, expectoration of solid brown plugs of sputum which contain fungal mycelia, eosinophilia of sputum and peripheral blood, immediate (Type I) and late (Type III) skin responses to extracts of *A. fumigatus* which do not occur in farmers' lung, and radiographic evidence of lung consolidation or collapse.

(7) *Psittacosis–ornithosis* (*see* p. 389) This disease, which affects birds of the parrot family, pigeons, and turkeys, may be acquired by farmers and people keeping or handling birds, or coming into contact with their droppings. It is distinguished by high titres of antibodies to Chlamydia group B and the fact that the radiographic appearances are usually those of patchy consolidation or collapse which is often unilateral. The presence of precipitins to thermoactinomycetes or avian proteins does not help differentiation.

(8) *Silo-fillers' disease* (*see* Chapter 13) Although the onset of symptoms may resemble that of acute extrinsic allergic 'alveolitis' it is usually more rapid, but in some cases it may be delayed for two or three weeks. As a rule the clinical and radiographic features are those of pulmonary oedema but occasionally they may be identical to those of acute extrinsic allergic 'alveolitis'. However, the nature of the exposure should point to the diagnosis. But it should be remembered that moulding of silo contents may ultimately occur and cause acute extrinsic allergic 'alveolitis' when they are disturbed after the silo is re-opened.

(9) *Sarcoidosis* In extrinsic allergic 'alveolitis' the work history, mode of onset of the illness, basal crepitations, absence of radiographic evidence of hilar lymphadenopathy and rapid recovery with resolution of radiographic abnormalities make confusion with sarcoidosis unlikely. Furthermore, the Kveim test is usually negative.

(10) *Acute fibrosing 'alveolitis'* The progressive nature of most cases of cryptogenic disease, rapid deterioration of the patient's condition especially in Hamman–Rich-type disease, and the absence of precipitins to a specific antigen distinguish this from extrinsic allergic 'alveolitis'. However, in some cases the possibility of previous administration of drugs capable of causing allergic 'alveolitis' may need to be excluded: for example, hydrochlorothiazide, nitrofurantoin and sodium cromoglycate (Beaudry and Laplante, 1973; Goldstein and Janicki, 1974; Sheffer, Rocklin and Goetzl, 1975).

Chronic disease

If chronic disease does not follow single or repeated episodes of acute disease, or if these have passed unrecognized, diagnosis can be very difficult. The difficulty is emphasized by the fact that there are no characteristic physiological or radiographic features, and that relevant precipitins are unlikely to be present more than three years after the last exposure, furthermore, precipitins may be found in farmers who have remained in intermittent contact with mouldy hay but have lung fibrosis due to another cause. And, unlike acute and subacute disease, there are no constitutional symptoms.

Diagnosis depends upon a careful and detailed history of work, hobbies, domestic pets, and past respiratory illnesses; and upon exclusion of other causes of lung fibrosis. Biopsy may be necessary in disease of insidious onset but can be indecisive when it has been present for more than 12 months as by then epithelioid granulomas have disappeared.

As stated previously the radiographic changes may take two forms:

(1) A widespread fibrotic pattern usually in the upper halves of the lung fields but sometimes in the lower halves.

(2) Widespread round opacities.

Differentiation may have to be made from the following diseases:

(1) *Fibro-cavernous tuberculosis* Past clinical, bacteriological and therapeutic history indicate the diagnosis in most cases, and in some *M. tuberculosus* can be cultured from the sputum. Occasionally, the organism isolated is *M.avium* which may originate from exposure to birds.

(2) *Chronic fungal disease* Certain pathogenic fungi are occasionally encountered in the same environmental conditions as some of the causal agents of extrinsic allergic 'alveolitis' and may cause disease with similar clinical and radiographic features. These include (but not in the UK) histoplasmosis, coccidioidomycosis and sporotrichosis. Differentiation in some cases might be difficult as only limited help can be expected from skin and serological tests in these diseases, although the relevant organisms may be recovered from the sputum (*see* later in this chapter).

(3) *Chronic sarcoidosis* Though this is irreversible, the absence of hilar lymphadenopathy and extrathoracic

stigmata of sarcoidosis together with a negative Kveim test in chronic extrinsic allergic 'alveolitis' should distinguish the two disorders. However, the reactivity of the tuberculin test may also be reduced in extrinsic allergic 'alveolitis' (Scadding, 1967). The clinical history is crucial.

Pathologically, the presence of plasma cells and the absence of sarcoid-type granulomas in hilar lymph nodes and other organs exclude sarcoidosis; and Schaumann bodies, common in sarcoidosis, are rare in extrinsic allergic 'alveolitis' (Seal *et al.*, 1968).

(4) *Other forms of DIPF* The lack of relevant occupational history and the fact that, in most cases, they favour the lower parts of the lungs differentiate them from chronic extrinsic 'alveolitis'. The histological features of both disease groups are sufficiently similar in most cases to make microscopical differentiation difficult or impossible. The possibility of fibrosis due to certain drugs has to be borne in mind (*see* Chapter 4).

(5) *Asbestosis* Difficulty may sometimes arise when exposure to asbestos and a known cause of extrinsic allergic 'alveolitis' have both occurred, although the two diseases should rarely be confused. However, both may occasionally be seen in the same patient. This question is discussed in more detail in Chapters 4 and 9.

(6) *Chronic beryllium disease* The occupational history is usually sufficient for differentiation. Otherwise beryllium and epithelioid granulomas are not found in chronic extrinsic allergic 'alveolitis' (*see* Chapter 10).

(7) *'Mixed dust fibrosis'* (*see* Chapter 7) The occupational history is usually sufficient. However, coincident chronic bird fanciers' lung may also be present on occasion.

PROGNOSIS AND COMPLICATIONS

Acute disease

After a single attack, complete recovery is the rule in two to 12 weeks if the patient ceases to be exposed to the offending antigen, but there are exceptions to this. After repeated attacks it becomes increasingly less likely, and the possibility of chronic disease is greater. Corticosteroids hasten the rate of recovery.

In a series of 44 patients who had acute disease about 70 per cent were asymptomatic three or more years later and about 30 per cent were mildly or moderately dyspnoeic on effort (Barbee *et al.*, 1968). Symptomatic recurrences are probably the most important factor in determining progressive disease (Braun *et al.*, 1979).

Spontaneous pneumothorax is a rare complication.

Chronic disease

Dyspnoea on exertion may steadily increase and, according to the severity of the disease, pulmonary hypertension with secondary polycythaemia may develop and eventually lead to fatal congestive heart failure. In the later stages emaciation may be a prominent feature. However, many patients are affected to only a minor degree and show little progression over years (Braun *et al.*, 1979).

It is probable that some cases of widespread pulmonary fibrosis which may be encountered in farm, mushroom and bagasse workers and people with relevant exposure to birds represent the end-point of unrecognized episodes of extrinsic allergic 'alveolitis' in the past.

TREATMENT

Acute disease

As soon as the diagnosis is made, the patient must be removed from exposure. This alone results in improvement. If the attack is severe he should be reassured and corticosteroids — the only treatment of any value — administered in the form of prednisolone in adequate dosage (about 40 mg/day) for two weeks followed by 20 mg daily until resolution of clinical and radiographic signs is complete.

It is possible that serial examination of broncho-alveolar lavage fluid for lymphocyte and Ig content may prove to be helpful in assessing response to treatment in some cases (Weinberger *et al.*, 1978).

Chronic disease

There is, of course, no treatment for fibrotic disease, but in some cases of moderately advanced disease acute lesions may also be present as a result of the most recent exposure to mouldy material and, in these, trial of corticosteroids is worthwhile.

FARMERS' LUNG

There is an old country tradition that mouldy hay has a baneful effect on the lungs. Over 100 years ago Icelandic farmers already referred to this by name as Heymaedi ('hay-shortness-of-breath') (Björnsson, 1960). But it was not until 1932 that it was first recorded in the medical literature by Campbell at Carlisle in the UK. He accurately described the characteristic features of acute disease in a group of farm workers exposed to mouldy hay but Pickles (1944) appears to have coined the term 'farmers' lung'. Other descriptions followed in England from Lancashire (Fawcitt, 1938), Yorkshire (Pickles, 1944), Devon (Fuller, 1953), in Wales (Staines and Forman, 1961), in Scotland and in Eire (Joyce and Kneafsey, 1955). Detailed study has also been done in the USA (for example, Dickie and Rankin, 1958;Emanuel *et al.*, 1964; Rankin *et al.*, 1967), Scandinavia (Törnell, 1946), Switzerland (Hoffman, 1946) and Australia (Cooper and Greenaway, 1961). The literature on the subject is now extensive. Extrinsic allergic 'alveolitis' due to exposure to mouldy hay and straw also occurs in cattle and horses (Pirie *et al.*, 1971; Pauli, Gerber and Schatzmann, 1972).

ORGANISMS ASSOCIATED WITH FARMERS' LUNG

Farmers' lung is characteristically associated with inhalation of the spores of thermophilic actinomycetes, a group of Gram-positive filamentous bacteria growing at temperatures between 30 and 65 °C. The species implicated include *Micropolyspora faeni* (previously identified erroneously with *Thermopolyspora polyspora*), *Thermoactinomyces* (*Micromonospora*) *vulgaris*, and *Saccharomonospora*

(*Thermomonospora*) *viridis*. They occur in hay and other substrates that have heated spontaneously and may be accompanied by such mesophilic actinomycetes as *Streptomyces griseus* and *S. albus*. *Thermoactinomyces vulgaris* was previously regarded as a very variable species (Kuster and Locci, 1964) but it now seems probable that it should be divided into at least two species, *T. vulgaris* and *T. thalpophilus* (Cross and Unsworth, 1977). Confusion has been caused by the proposal of the name *T. candidus* for strains corresponding most closely to the original description of *T. vulgaris* while retaining the latter name of strains corresponding to *T. thalpophilus* (Kurup, Barboriak and Fink, 1975). Thus, *T. candidus* should be considered a synonym of *T. vulgaris* while another species, *T. antibioticus*, probably synonymous with *T. thalpophilus*. *T. vulgaris* colonies appear to be more numerous in hay than *T. thalpophilus*, but *T. thalpophilus* colonies are stronger growing and produce an antibiotic inhibitory to *T. vulgaris*.

Antigenic preparations of isolates identified as *M. faeni* and *T. vulgaris* have been widely used to determine the presence of antibodies in exposed farm workers and in the diagnosis and epidemiological study of farmers' lung. However, most of the antigens '*T. vulgaris*' have originated from isolates of *T. thalpophilus* as a consequence of the stronger growth of this species. *T. vulgaris* differs antigenically from *T. thalpophilus* and may induce precipitins in exposed subjects more readily (Greatorex and Pether, 1975; Terho and Lacey, 1979). This may explain many precipitin-negative cases of farmers' lung and suggests that earlier work was probably incomplete (Cross and Unsworth, 1976, 1977). Recently, three specific *M. faeni* antigens have been identified which correspond to precipitins that occur only in individuals with disease, but not in those exposed but lacking disease symptoms (Treuhaft *et al.*, 1979).

The relative abundance of micro-organisms colonizing hay may vary between countries and with the method of hay-making used. Thus, hays associated with farmers' lung in Finland show less evidence of spontaneous heating and contain fewer actinomycete spores than British hays. Only *T. vulgaris* is sometimes abundant while precipitins to *T. vulgaris* are more frequent than those to *T. thalpophilus*. Precipitins to fungi of the *Aspergillus glaucus* group are also found (Terho and Lacy, 1979).

Aspergillus fumigatus antibodies sometimes occur but their significance in pathogenesis is uncertain (Pepys and Jenkins, 1965; Roberts, Wenzel and Emanuel, 1976; Katila and Mäntyjärvi, 1978).

Conditions for growth

Water is essential for the growth of fungi. Few can grow if the equilibrium relative humidity is less than 65 per cent (equivalent to 11 to 13 per cent water content in hay) and many require more water. If hay, straw or cereal grains are stored damp because of poor harvesting conditions and insufficient drying mould growth will occur, often accompanied by heating. The initial heating of damp plant material may be caused by respiration of plant cells, but subsequent respiration by micro-organisms plays an increasingly important part, until the plant cells are killed and heating is entirely microbial. The maximum temperature attained is related to water content, as shown for hay in

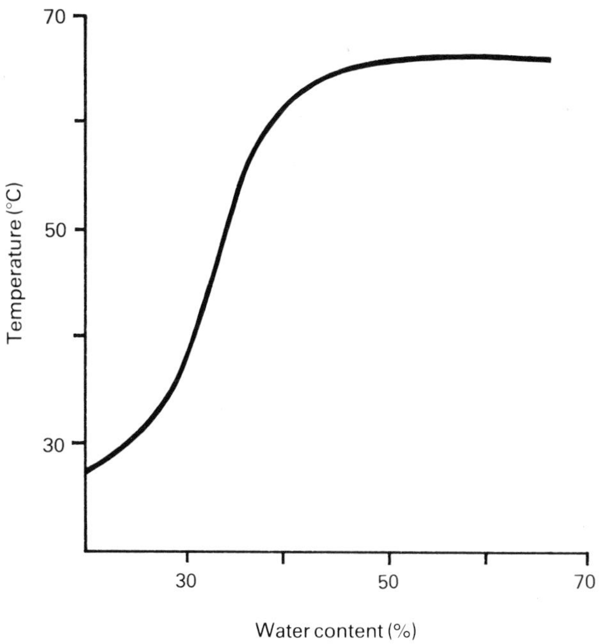

Figure 11.9 The relationship of the temperature generated in stored hay to its water content. (Courtesy of Dr J. Lacey and the Editor of World Crops*)*

Figure 11.9. Microbial heating is limited to a maximum of 65 to 70 °C, but chemical processes may sometimes be initiated leading to further heating, and eventually to spontaneous ignition. Heating is ultimately limited by loss of water from the material, so that it cools to ambient temperature.

Successive stages in the heating process are caused by a sequence of different micro-organisms, of which fungi and actinomycetes are probably the most important. When water content is low, the *Aspergillus glaucus* group of fungi predominates and, due to respiration, increases the water content of the fodder. This permits other fungi to become established leading, in turn, to the proliferation of a succession of fungus and actinomycete species which favour

Table 11.2 Characteristics of Different Hay Types

Hay type	*Water content at baling (%)*	*Maximum temperature reached (°C)*	*Spore content (millions/g)*	
			Fungi	*Actinomycetes and bacteria*
Very mouldy	35–50	50–65	10–100	350–1200
Mouldy	20–30	35–45	2–60	3–250
Good	15–20	22–26	0.1–7	0.5–8

By courtesy of Dr J. Lacey and the Editor of *World Crops*

increasing water content and temperature. Self-heating of fodder in this fashion encourages exuberant growth of such thermotolerant and thermophilic species as *T. thalpophilus, T. vulgaris, M. faeni* and *A. fumigatus* when the water content exceeds 35 per cent and the temperature rises to 50 °C or more (Festenstein *et al.*, 1965) (*Figure 11.10*). The characteristics of hay types are exemplified in *Table 11.2*.

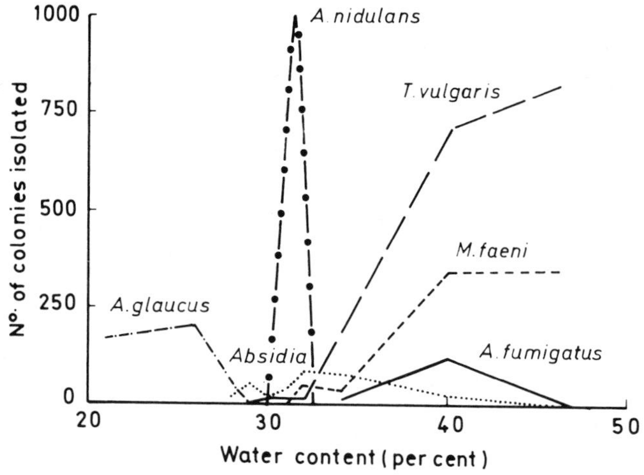

Figure 11.10 The effect of water content on the growth trends of some relevant fungi and actinomycetes in stored hay. (Courtesy of Dr J. Lacey and the Editor of World Crops*)*

For storage with little or no moulding, the water content of hay must be less than 20 per cent, and of grain about 14 per cent. The spore content of good hay will usually be less than 5 million spores/g dry weight, compared with over 100 million spores/g in mouldy hay, and sometimes in excess of 1000 million spores/g in a farmers' lung type hay (Gregory *et al.*, 1963).

When rainfall is high it is more difficult to make good hay without artificial drying, and the chances of moulding are therefore greater. This results in geographical and seasonal variations in the incidence of farmers' lung and other diseases related to hay moulding, e.g. mycotic abortion in cattle due to aspergillus or mucor infections (Hugh-Jones and Austwick, 1967).

The same principles relating water content and heating to fungal growth apply, in general, to grain, bagasse, mushroom compost and other substrates (*see* appropriate sections in this chapter).

Thus, farmers' lung is a disorder associated with cold and humid weather conditions often in mountainous and semi-mountainous regions.

SOURCES OF EXPOSURE

Turning and stacking hay in the field and removing it to storage present little hazard. Exposure most often occurs when stored mouldy hay crops are handled during such operations as opening bales of hay and straw for animal feeding and bedding and poultry bedding, and when moving and threshing mouldy grain. Many of these activities may be carried out in poorly ventilated barns, sheds, shippens or partly open buildings so that the spore cloud — which may consist of up to 1600 million spores/m^3 air (most of which are actinomycetes) (Lacey and Lacey, 1964) — is not diluted by clean air, and exposure is intense. The risk of exposure to mouldy material in these enclosed surroundings may occur at any time of the year, but is likely to be highest in the late winter and early spring months (Terho, Lammi and Heinonen, 1980).

However, in addition to farm workers, others who may be exposed to mouldy straw, hay, and grain include stable hands (including, until recent years, pit pony ostlers underground in coal-mines), poultry workers, attendants of zoo and circus animals, petshop workers and packers of glass and crockery who use straw.

INCIDENCE AND PREVALENCE

In the British Isles, and also elsewhere in Europe, acute disease may occur sporadically throughout the year but the incidence increases from September, reaches a peak from February to April and declines rapidly. Sporadic cases may occur at any time. For obvious reasons more cases have been reported in men than in women, although in Britain because farmers' wives are recorded as farm workers their sex is not identified. Children may also acquire the disease (Staines and Forman, 1961; Bureau *et al.*, 1979). The highest 'attack rate' is between the ages of 41 and 60 years. Staines and Forman (1961) found a varying regional prevalence of 11.5/100 000 of the farming population in East Anglia, 73.1 in South-West England and 193.1/100 000 in Wales; and they computed that a conservative estimate of the annual incidence might be about 1000. In Caithness (Scotland) the incidence of acute and chronic farmers' lung grouped together is 110/100 000 of the farming population (Boyd, 1971). In Orkney, Ayrshire and East Lothian the prevalence of precipitin-positive cases has been reported as 43, 36 and 0/1000 respectively (Grant *et al.*, 1972).

More recently, on the basis of disease associated with moderate to strong serological results, the prevalence rate for men ranged from 87/1000 in Devon to 302/1000 in mid-Wales (Morgan *et al.*, 1975); and in the farming population of Somerset the prevalence of both serologically positive and negative cases has been reported to be 23/1000 (Pether and Greatorex, 1976). Among 343 farm workers in North-West Ireland (Counties Sligo, Leitrim and Donegal) nine, of whom two had precipitins to *M.faeni*, were considered to have farmers' lung — a prevalence of 2.6 per cent (Shelley *et al.*, 1979). In Winconsin (USA) a prevalence of 9 to 12 per cent has been recorded in adult males exposed to mouldy hay (Madsen *et al.*, 1976).

Obviously prevalence rates are influenced by farming standards and vary according to whether diagnosis rests solely on symptomatology or on the acceptance of only precipitin positive cases and also upon the precipitin tests employed.

OTHER CONSIDERATIONS

Sputum

Thermophilic actinomycetes have apparently been isolated from the sputum of patients who have not been in contact with mouldy hay for three years but not from other individuals without such exposure (Greatorex and Pether, 1976). This suggests that spores may, perhaps, germinate and form vegetative cells in the lungs.

Persistence of precipitins

When there is no further exposure precipitins may disappear in three to five years after an acute episode (Rankin *et al.*, 1967; Hapke *et al.*, 1968) although, in about a third of cases, they are still present some ten years later (Braun *et al.*, 1979).

Additional factors in causation

There is some evidence that farmers' lung may not be due solely to thermoactinomycetes (*see* p. 364). When *M. faeni* alone is administered by intratracheal injection to guinea pigs they do not develop any lesions of allergic 'alveolitis' whereas with mouldy hay dust they do, and the reaction is still more severe with a mixture of both (Zaidi *et al.*, 1971). Furthermore, it appears that farmers with extrinsic allergic 'alveolitis' have also had significant exposure to many other respiratory pathogens (Marx *et al.*, 1977).

'Barn allergy'

This consists of rhinitis and allergic asthma in farm workers caused by hypersensitivity to storage mites resident in hay, straw and grain (*see* next Section and Chapter 12). Before a firm diagnosis of acute or subacute 'farmers' lung' is made, whether or not specific 'farmers' lung' precipitins are present, storage mite allergy should always be considered and trial treatment with sodium cromoglycate may help to prove it. In some cases, however, the diagnosis may only be reached by bronchial provocation tests and assessment of gas transfer (Cuthbert *et al.*, 1979).

PREVENTION

The chief aim is to dry hay or grain sufficiently by natural or artificial means (such as barn drying) and to prevent re-wetting during storage so that no moulding or heating can take place. Good ventilation of barns and storage buildings is required. Dust respirators of special design effectively prevent the inhalation of spores (Gourley and Braidwood, 1971), and should be worn by farm workers known to have had a previous attack of farmers' lung and who are likely to be exposed to mouldy material. However, many find masks difficult to tolerate and refuse to wear them during heavy work (Smyth *et al.*, 1975).

One per cent of concentrated propionic acid, well mixed with grain before it is loaded into the silo for storage, prevents the growth of fungi and bacteria and, thus, a rise in temperature favouring the growth of thermophilic organisms. A practical method of treating hay in this manner, however, has not yet been developed.

Substitution of silage for hay has been advocated as a preventive measure and is employed by some farmers.

Ideally, a farm worker who has had more than one acute attack should change his occupation, but usually he has no inclination or little aptitude for other work; and, if self-employed, change may be impossible.

GRAIN DUSTS

This is an appropriate point for brief general discussion of the composition and possible harmful effects of grain dusts, although they are also considered in Chapter 12.

Grain dust is a heterogeneous material consisting of particles from various cereals such as wheat, barley, oats, rye and maize. It may contain a large number of contaminants including seeds, pollens, bacteria and their endotoxins, fungi and their metabolites, insects such as the grain weevil, mites, mammalian debris, quartz, and chemical pesticides and herbicides. However, composition varies according to the geographic areas and climatic conditions in which the grain is grown, transported and stored.

On the whole little is known about the effects of pure grain dusts or their various contaminants on health. Certainly some of them are of 'respirable' size and they may constitute about 40 per cent of the total suspended dust though qualitative and quantitative details are lacking (Yoshida and Maybank, 1978). In regard to allergic lung disease — extrinsic allergic 'alveolitis' and asthma — the debris and excreta of mites and insects and the microflora are important. 'Barn allergy' has just been referred to, but *see also* Chapter 12, p. 430.

The presence of free silica due to contamination by soil containing quartz and from opaline 'silica cells' in wheat and other cereals is unlikely to present a silicosis risk because, in general, its amount is very small, although in one analysis it was reported to range from 1.2 to 6.5 per cent (Blackman, 1969; Farant and Moore, 1978). No radiographic evidence of silicosis was found in a survey of 3000 grain workers (Cotton and Dosman, 1978).

MICROFLORA OF GRAIN DUSTS (Lacey, 1980)

Grain dusts can be broadly grouped into two types according to whether they are produced during harvesting or storage. The microflora evolve continuously from harvest, through the early stage of storage of dry grain to the later stages of storage of moist grain and in accumulated grain deposits in silos and grain elevators. As cereal plants grow they may be infected by phytopathogenic fungi with airborne spores, and, as they ripen, both grain and straw are colonized by a variety of saprophytic fungi. Hence, combine harvester dust contains enormous numbers of spores and fungal hyphae as well as bacteria. Spores of *Cladosporium* spp. appear to be most abundant but those of *Verticillium paecilomyces*, *Alternaria*, *Epicoccum*, *Ustilago* and *Puccinia* are common.

Although *Cladosporium* and *Alternaria* spores are known to be allergenic (Hyde, 1972) a survey of British farm workers showed that 35 per cent had positive skin prick tests to *Aphanocladium album. Verticillium lecanii* and *Paecilomyces farinosus* extracts and that over 50 per cent had precipitins to these species; whereas only 18 per cent were skin-test positive to *Cladosporium* and *Alternaria* spp. (Darke *et al.*, 1976).

The composition of airborne dust from stored grain varies greatly according to the conditions of storage because the microflora change in relation to the aeration of the grain bulk, its water content and degree of spontaneous heating. As in the case of hay (*see* p. 373 and *Figures 11.9* and *11.10*), the more rising water content and heating increase the microflora the more prolific thermophilic and thermotolerant organisms—which are potential pathogens—become. The nature of airborne spores, therefore, is determined by the storage conditions and varies accordingly. As the water content and temperature increase respectively to about 30 per cent and 50 to 65 °C the greater the number of organisms such as *Absydia corymbifera, Mucor pusillus, T. vulgaris, M. faeni, A. fumigatus* and possibly others which may present a risk of extrinsic allergic 'alveolitis' or lung infection becomes. Near-anaerobic conditions, such as may occur in sealed silos, limit heating and microbial growth whereas aerated maltings favour the growth of *A. clavatus* and *A. fumigatus* (*see* maltworkers' lung). A recent study in grain elevators in Canada (Manitoba) has shown that the microflora was similar in all and consisted almost entirely of bacteria, *Penicillium*, yeasts, *Aspergillus flavus*, *A. fumigatus*, *T. vulgaris* and *Streptomyces albus*.

Barley grain for cattle fodder stored in concrete silos in different parts of Britain has also been studied. The grain, which contained 23 to 40 per cent water, was covered by straw or chopped wilted grass with or without a polyethylene or butyl rubber sheeting. Heating and moulding of the uppermost layer of grain was found to depend on the rate at which the grain was removed from the silo and on the efficiency of the top seal. Thus, the nature and number of organisms and airborne spores associated with grain stored by this method show very considerable variation. Species known to be potentially pathogenic for man and animals were most abundant in and immediately below the top seal, unless this formed silage, and when the temperature during unloading was in excess of 35 °C. Removing the top seal or unloading grain causes a rapid and large increase in the spore content of the air in silos.

It is not known if fungal enzymes and metabolites are potentially harmful to the lungs but, as has been noted on p. 363, it is suggested that they may cause 'pulmonary mycotoxicosis'.

Bacteria are universely present in grain and this raises the possibility that endotoxins of some species may be responsible for lung disease. Endotoxin of *Erwinia herbicola* is reported to be common in grain in Poland and has been suggested to be a cause of respiratory disease in farm workers (Dutkiewicz, 1978). But this organism is uncommon in Canadian grain elevators and British grain silos although it frequently colonizes plant surfaces before harvest.

The development of new techniques in harvesting and storing grain has to some extent increased the risks of microbial growth and the quantities of airborne dust produced. Preventive measures include: air-filtered driving cabs on combine harvesters; drying grain to a safe water content and maintaining this during storage until used; good ventilation of grain handling areas; treatment of grain for cattle fodder with propionic acid to prevent moulding; and ensuring rapid emptying of moist grain silos to prevent the production of large concentrations of spores of potentially pathogenic fungi. The recognition and prevention of respiratory disease from grain dust requires the cooperation of doctors, microbiologists and engineers.

BIRD FANCIERS' (BREEDERS') LUNG

This was first recorded in workers handling goose and duck feathers (Plessner, 1960) and in a budgerigar breeder (Pearsall *et al.*, 1960), but 'pneumonitis' of unknown cause in people exposed to pigeon excreta had, in fact, been reported by Feldman and Sabin in 1948. The disease is now known to be related to exposure to avian proteins in dry dust of the droppings, and sometimes of the feathers, of a variety of birds: pigeons, budgerigars (parakeets), parrots, turtle doves, turkeys and chickens (Reed, Sosman and Barbee, 1965; Hargreave *et al.*, 1966; Elman *et al.*, 1968; Hinson, 1970; Boyer *et al.*, 1974; Warren and Tse, 1974; Molina, 1976; Schatz *et al.*, 1976).

The *prevalence* of bird fanciers' lung is difficult to determine. It probably depends upon types of birds and modes of exposure to them. Among pigeon fanciers it is variously reported as 1/1000 (Molina, 1976), 1.4/1000 (Maesen, 1972), 6 per cent (Moore *et al.*, 1974) and 21 per cent (Christensen, Schmidt and Robbins, 1975); and among budgerigar fanciers in Britain it is calculated to lie between 0.5 and 7.5 per cent (Hendrick *et al.*, 1978a).

Atopic bird fanciers are apt to develop asthma with high levels of specific IgE antibodies, and it seems likely that this may protect them from acquiring allergic 'alveolitis' owing to partial airways obstruction reducing access of dust particles to the periphery of the lungs.

FEATURES OF EXPOSURE

Exposure occurs during cleaning out pigeon lofts, bird cages and hen houses. People likely to be exposed, therefore, include those who breed budgerigars or pigeons professionally or as a hobby, pet shop workers, aviary attendants, and budgerigar and parrot fanciers who may only keep one bird. Those who look after many birds (such as pigeon fanciers) experience intermittent exposure to high concentrations of dust at one- to two-weekly intervals during cage cleaning of lofts or cages and typical acute disease develops; whereas those who keep one or two pet birds at home are exposed more or less continuously to low concentrations of dropping dust, and in them the development of disease is gradual and insidious. These two modes of onset are, in fact, more clearly exemplified in this form of extrinsic allergic 'alveolitis' than in farmers' lung. However, typical acute disease appears to be rare among poultry farmers though it has been reported: tightness in the chest and cough are complained of by a minority after prolonged exposure (Elman *et al.*, 1968). Horses in contact with chickens have developed similar disease (Mansmann and Osborn, 1971).

Many persons with bird fanciers' lung give a history of repeated acute, febrile respiratory illnesses from which they recover rapidly when they cease contact with the birds, but recur — sometimes after slight exposure — when they return to their bird houses. When all contact with the birds is stopped complete clinical recovery is the rule although in some patients — especially those who have had a number of previous acute attacks — irreversible chronic disease may develop. When the onset is insidious and marked only by progressively increasing dyspnoea on effort, severe fibrosis is likely to be established by the time the patient is first seen. Occasionally it is fatal within two to three years of the first complaint of symptoms (Edwards and Luntz, 1974). But, as in the case of farmers' lung, not all persons exposed to avian antigens develop evidence of disease. The disease may occur in the children of pigeon and budgerigar enthusiasts and appears to be of more insidious onset than in adults (Stiehm, Reed and Tooley, 1967; Chandra and Jones, 1972).

PATHOLOGY AND IMMUNOLOGY

The pathology has already been described. Lung biopsy in

acute disease reveals infiltration of lymphocytes and plasma cells, reticulin proliferation and sarcoid-type granulomas in alveolar walls and spaces (Nash, Vogelpoel and Becker, 1967; Hensley *et al.*, 1969). Unlike allergic 'alveolitis' due to other causes large macrophages with pale vacuolated cytoplasm ('foam cells') are often seen in the granulomas. 'Honeycomb' cysts are common in chronic disease.

That avian antigens are casually responsible is demonstrated by the fact that acute respiratory and constitutional symptoms, basal crepitations and impaired gas transfer result about six hours after inhalation of a dilute aerosol of pigeon or budgerigar serum by patients who have previously had acute disease (Reed, Sosman and Barbee, 1965; Hargreave *et al.*, 1966). Precipitins and typical lesions of allergic 'alveolitis' with foam cells and granuloma formation occur in rats after prolonged inhalation of pigeon dropping dust (Fink, Hensley and Barboriak, 1969). If inhalation tests are used in diagnosis the initial extracts must be weak in order to avoid prolonged respiratory symptoms which may require treatment with corticosteroids.

Precipitins against avian antigens are found in the serum of the majority of patients with acute pigeon breeders' disease and in some 16 per cent of pigeon fanciers with no evidence of disease (Barboriak, Sosman and Reed, 1965), but they are absent in unexposed persons. Important factors in the antibody response are the total duration of exposure and the number of birds kept (Banham, Lynch and Boyd, 1978). They are also present in a majority of unaffected poultry farmers (Elman *et al.*, 1968); and there is a significantly higher prevalence of precipitins among symptomatic workers in the turkey raising and processing industry than among asymptomatic workers (Boyer *et al.*, 1974). In budgerigar fanciers the situation is remarkably different as precipitins are not found in exposed healthy subjects, although they are present in almost all those with allergic 'alveolitis' confirmed by inhalation tests (Faux *et al.*, 1971). These differences in correlation with disease are poorly understood but may be due to differing potency of the various antigens, as well as to a variable intensity of individual exposures.

The precipitating antibodies in pigeon breeders' disease are directed against pigeon IgG and IgM (Diment and Pepys, 1977) and an antigen (not present in the serum) which cross-reacts with pigeon γ-globulin and appears to be IgA derived from the intestinal tract (Tebo, Fredericks and Roberts, 1977). All are voided in the droppings but, due to subsequent enzyme activity, do not survive for more than a month (Edwards, Fink and Barboriak, 1969). All these antigens are apparently required to produce the disease and they exist together in the droppings, but not in the serum or feathers (Edwards, Barboriak and Fink, 1970). To detect specific antibodies to pigeon antigens a purified fraction of pigeon dropping extract is required as the whole extract causes a variety of non-specific reactions (Tebo, Moore and Fink, 1977).

Cross reaction between different antigens is sometimes observed. Precipitins against *M.faeni* and *Aspergillus fumigatus* have been found in some cases of bird fanciers' lung and precipitins against pigeon excreta are occasionally present in patients with farmers' lung. Furthermore, there appears to be a correlation between severity of disease and the variety of antibodies found. When antibodies against excreta extracts only are present the symptoms are mild, but when there are antibodies to the excreta, feathers, white of egg and the serum of pigeons the illness is more severe. Actinomycetes of *T.vulgaris* type have been identified in pigeon droppings due to ingestion of mouldy grain (Molina, 1976).

Intradermal tests with avian serum or extracts of droppings usually cause an immediate, Type 1, weal reaction followed later by an Arthus type reaction (Pepys, 1969). By contrast with farmers' lung the Arthus-type skin reaction to avian antigens is closely associated with the presence of precipitins and may, therefore, be a useful pointer to diagnosis.

CLINICAL FEATURES

Lung function returns to normal in most patients when they cease contact with the birds, but may continue to deteriorate if they remain exposed. As in farmers' lung, irreversible airways obstruction is sometimes present but can later recover completely (Nash, Vogelpoel and Becker, 1967; Dinda, Chatterjee and Riding, 1969). It is particularly important to identify the disorder in a child because permanent lung damage may develop unless contact with the birds is stopped.

Acute disease should not be confused with psittacosis for, although the symptoms may be somewhat similar, in psittacosis they develop after an incubation period of seven to 14, occasionally up to 30, days, and lung consolidation may occur (*see* p. 389). However, the possibility that both diseases can occur in the same patient must be borne in mind (Molina, 1976).

Chronic disease of insidious development due to continuous contact with birds in the home (chiefly budgerigars) is probably sufficiently prevalent, although uncommon, to cause possible diagnostic confusion in individuals who have worked in a known occupational dust hazard—for example, the asbestos industry, coal-mining, foundry—particularly as the keeping of budgerigars by the families of workers in these and other industries is fairly common.

In Britain about 0.3 per cent of the population keep pigeons whereas budgerigars are apparently kept in five to six million homes. On these estimates, if 12 per cent of the general population is exposed to budgerigars, then between 65 and 90/100 000 are likely to have bird fanciers' lung, though mildly in most cases. Hence, bird fanciers' lung is believed to be about ten times more common than farmers' lung because of the much larger population at risk — only about 1.1 per cent of the general population work in farming (Hendrick *et al.*, 1978a). Therefore, *when taking the occupational history of a patient with suspected lung disease the question of birds in the home or in hobby activity should never be omitted.*

False positive complement fixation titres to egg-grown respiratory virus preparations have been found in some patients with pigeon fanciers' lung and regarded as antibodies directed against antigens from hen's egg in which the test viruses were grown. Such antigens were, in fact, demonstrated in the virus preparations. Therefore, because of the clinical similarities between influenza and acute bird fanciers' lung, it is essential that a diagnosis of influenza should not be made in bird fanciers on the grounds of a single raised titre or a four-fold fall of complement fixation titre without appropriate control tests with avian antigens being made (Newman Taylor *et al.*, 1977).

PREVENTION

The most important precept in the management of patients with acute (or subacute) disease is permanent avoidance of contact with the offending birds; and it has to be remembered that antigen may persist in the birds' environment after they have been removed.

BIRD FANCIERS' LUNG, COELIAC DISEASE AND 'EGG EATERS' LUNG'.

An association between adult coeliac disease (gluten sensitive enteropathy) and diffuse interstitial pulmonary disease was reported by Hood and Mason (1970) and Lancaster-Smith, Benson and Strickland (1971) and later by Berrill *et al.* (1975), and it was thought likely that the lung disease might be an autoimmune fibrosing 'alveolitis'. But it was soon observed that avian precipitins were present in many of these patients (Lancaster-Smith *et al.*, 1974), and all of those studied by Berrill *et al.* (1975) proved to have had contact with birds. Thus, it was suggested that the lung pathology was bird fanciers' lung and that intestinal absorption of avian antigens might be a factor in its pathogenesis or persistence.

However, precipitins against avian antigens common to the pigeon, budgerigar and hen, but distinct from the antigens usually associated with bird fanciers' lung, have been found in patients with coeliac disease who were *not* exposed to birds (Morris *et al.*, 1971; Faux, Hendrick and Anand, 1978). This antigen is a component of hen egg yolk but not of bird droppings and is present in the birds' serum. It has been referred to as 'coeliac-associated' antigen to distinguish it from 'bird fanciers' lung-associated' antigen (Faux, Hendrick and Anand, 1978). Hence, the precipitins are unlikely to result from bird dust inhalation. There is, in addition, an association between the degree of intestinal mucosal damage and the presence of precipitins to 'coeliac-associated' antigen in coeliac patients (Hendrick *et al.*, 1978b). The source of the antigen is probably partly cooked or uncooked eggs in various foods.

It is not known whether the precipitins in the cases with lung disease reported by Berrill *et al.* (1975) were directed against 'bird fanciers' lung-associated or 'coeliac-associated' antigen but, as villous atrophy was present in all, it seems likely that they were of the latter category. But important evidence that the lung disease is not bird fanciers' lung is provided by two facts: that bronchial challenge tests with avian serum had no ill effects on lung function of affected patients (Benson *et al.*, 1972); and that no association has been found between villous atrophy and bird fanciers' lung (Hendrick *et al.*, 1978b).

It is possible, as Faux, Hendrick and Anand (1978) suggest, that because 'bird fanciers' lung-associated' antigens were found in eggs in addition to 'coeliac-associated' antigens some patients with bird fanciers' lung may respond unfavourably to eating eggs. Indeed, some of the patients studied by Hendrick *et al.* (1978b) disliked or avoided eggs which they thought caused gastro-intestinal discomfort, malaise and even dyspnoea on effort. Established bird fanciers' lung could be followed by 'egg eaters' lung' which might become particularly severe if the patient had coincident coeliac disease owing to defective mucosal processing of ingested avian antigens, even if there is no causal association between the two diseases. This might apply equally to farmers' lung as cases with coeliac disease have been reported (Robinson, 1976). Similarly, diffuse lung disease in patients with coeliac disease who do not keep birds might arise primarily as a result of ingested egg or other food antigens.

Another hypothesis, which needs investigation, has been suggested: namely, that antibodies to bird gut mucosa cross-react with the patients' gut mucosa and, thus, provoke simultaneous coeliac disease (Purtilo, Bonica and Yang, 1978).

Both coeliac disease and some types of fibrosing 'alveolitis' are more common in individuals with the HLA-8 antigen (Stokes *et al.*, 1972; Turton *et al.*, 1978) and it may be that the concurrence of the two disorders is the result of a common immunological dysfunction.

To summarize

When considering diagnosis it is important to bear in mind that patients with active coeliac disease are likely to have precipitins to bird serum even in the absence of exposure to birds or of lung disease so that, in patients with suspected bird fanciers' lung, the presence of antibodies requires careful interpretation. However, although the two precipitin groups are distinguishable, 'bird fanciers' lung-associated' precipitins are not pathognomonic of bird fanciers' lung nor does their absence exclude it (Hendrick *et al.*, 1978b). For this reason it may be necessary to perform bronchial challenge tests to establish the diagnosis of bird fanciers' lung; and, certainly, contact with the birds under suspicion should be discontinued. In view of the apparent lack of a strong association between bird fanciers' lung and coeliac disease routine jejunal biopsy is probably not desirable (Hendrick *et al.*, 1978b).

BAGASSOSIS

Bagasse is the fibrous cellulose residue of sugar-cane stalk after it has been crushed and the juice extracted. It consists of tough 'true fibre' and soft 'pith' tissue from the inner stalk. Pith absorbs water readily and, if present in any quantity, hinders drying. It is fibrous, tough and has good insulating qualities for heat and sound.

Sugar-cane is grown in the West Indies, India, Pakistan, Brazil, Cuba, Argentina, the southern USA, South Africa, Australia and Mexico. After the extraction of sugar, bagasse may be baled for storage.

Baling is done in a press similar to a hay baler. The bales are bound by steel wire and stacked in the open in such fashion as to allow ventilation. Stacks may be protected against rain by a covering of asbestos or plastic sheeting. The bagasse is stored for about 12 months, when it may be transferred to another plant for compression into smaller compact bales for transportation. The baling plant operates during the few months in the year when the crop is gathered.

Fresh bagasse stored in bales heats spontaneously to 54 °C in five days then cools to 40 °C before rising again after about 33 days to 49 °C. However, bagasse with a water content of 27 per cent heats to 49 °C in three days (Lacey, 1969). Hence, the growth of many different species of fungi and thermophilic and mesophilic actinomycetes is favoured in bagasse with this degree of moisture.

Fermentation of residual sugar by yeasts probably assists the initial heating.

Since the late 1950s the Ritter system of bulk storing unpithed or partly depithed bagasse has been used in some industrial plants. It consists of keeping large mounds of loose, unbaled bagasse wet with a 'biological' liquor containing molasses and lactic acid-producing bacteria until required for use. Continuous moistening with automatic sprinklers keeps the water content to a minimum of 50 to 60 per cent. The importance of this system is that it effectively eliminates the production of actmomycete-bearing dust during the mechanical processing of bagasse (Paturau, 1969; Lehrer *et al.*, 1978). Mouldy bagasse contains enormous numbers of fungal spores—probably as many as 500 000 000/g dry weight (Buechner, 1978)—and, although these were earlier identified as *T. vulgaris* (Seabury *et al.*, 1968), it is now known that they consist in fact chiefly of a much more abundant, but closely related, species of thermoactinomytes, *T. sacchari.*

Bagassosis has the same acute and chronic forms as farmers' lung, but is more often found in the acute form. It follows exposure to the dust of dry, mouldy bagasse but not of fresh or autoclaved bagasse. It was described in New Orleans (Jamison and Hopkins, 1941) and, although most of the reported cases have occurred in the southern states of the USA (Sodeman and Pullen, 1944; Buechner *et al.*, 1958, 1964), there have been many others in Britain (Castleden and Hamilton-Paterson, 1942; Hunter and Perry, 1946; Hargreave, Pepys and Holford-Strevens, 1968), Italy (Cangini, 1951), India (Ganguly and Pal, 1955; Viswanathan *et al.*, 1963), the Philippines (Dizon, Almonte and Anselmo, 1962), Spain (González de Vega *et al.*, 1966) and the West Indies (Hearn, 1968). It is apt to occur in sporadic outbreaks when workers are exposed to mouldy material.

USES OF BAGASSE

Bagasse has many possible uses and these are summarized in *Table 11.3*. Bagasse in briquettes is employed as a fuel to generate electricity in cane-producing areas, although it is now largely replaced by oil. Charcoal is produced by carbonization, and methane by anaerobic fermentation of the cellulose fraction. Manufacture of different types of paper and board has become increasingly important in recent years. Particle board can be moulded to any shape for the furniture container, motor car and ship-building industries and fibre board is used for acoustic and thermal insulation. Furfural, which is also known as furfuraldehyde and is produced by acid hydrolysis of the xylan in bagasse, is employed in the refining of lubricating oils and the manufacture of resins. Bagasse is also used in the production of viscose rayon and as a filler and extender in reinforced thermosetting plastics. For details of the many uses of bagasse *see* Paturau (1969).

SOURCES OF EXPOSURE

A potential risk of bagassosis exists in the following processes if bagasse is dry and mouldy: removing bales from stacks to the compressing plant, the compressing operation, opening or shredding of bales in the factory, hammer-milling bagasse to desired particle size, during various manufacturing operations (including the grinding of hard-board), and moving and turning bagasse for cattle and poultry bedding. In a British factory before the Second World War, bales were opened using a wet process, but when, in the altered circumstances of the war, they were opened dry, cases of bagossis occurred (Hunter and Perry, 1946).

The growth of bacteria and fungi in bagasse can now be prevented, however, by treating it when fresh with 1 per cent of propionic acid before or after milling. This has greatly increased the potential of bagasse in manufacture.

PATHOLOGY AND IMMUNOLOGY

The pathology of acute disease has the same features as acute farmers' lung, including granulomas (Sodeman and Pullen, 1943; Bradford, Blalock and Wascom, 1961; Buechner, 1962); but some cases are remarkable for the presence of large numbers of plasma cells both in the alveolar walls and spaces. Chronic disease consists of diffuse interstitial fibrosis with bronchiolectasis — mainly in the upper parts of the lungs—and pleural thickening (Buechner, 1962).

Table 11.3 Uses of Bagasse

SUGAR CANE →	Bagasse →	Utilization as fuel	Electricity
			Charcoal briquettes
			Methane and producer gas
		Fibrous products	Pulp and paper
			Paper board
			Fibre board
			Particle board
		Miscellaneous	Furfural
			Alpha cellulose
			Plastics
			Poultry litter and mulch
			Animal feed
			Bagasse concrete
			Soil amendment

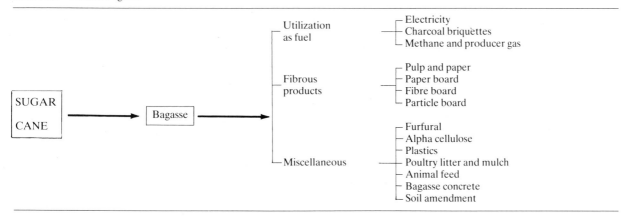

Adapted from *By-products in the Cane Sugar Industry* with permission of Dr J. M. Paturau and Elsevier Publishing Company.

Precipitins are present in some two-thirds of patients during or shortly after an acute attack of bagassosis, but disappear within one to three years (Salvaggio *et al.*, 1969). *Thermoactinomyces vulgaris* was thought to be the chief, if not only, antigenic source (Seabury *et al.*, 1968), and inhalation of extract of *T. vulgaris*, but not of *M.faeni*, by men suffering from bagassosis appeared to reproduce the symptoms of the disease. However, Lacey (1971a) subsequently identified the organism as *T. sacchari.* This explains why precipitins to genuine *T. vulgaris* extracts have not been demonstrated (Hargreave, Pepys and Holford-Strevens, 1968; Holford-Strevens, 1971). But when extracts of *T. sacchari* were tested by immuno-electrophoresis and agar-gel double diffusion against sera from patients with bagassosis in the USA and from exposed workers in Trinidad, characteristic precipitin reactions occurred (Lacey, 1971b). These reactions could not be altered by absorption of the sera with *T. vulgaris* extracts (Holford-Strevens, 1971). However, one of the subjects who reacted to extracts of *T. vulgaris* reacted similarly to extracts of *T. sacchari* (Lacey, 1971a) and immuno-electrophoresis suggests that the two species may contain some antigens in common.

Thus, *T. sacchari* appears to be the major source of antigen in mouldy bagasse which is responsible for bagassosis. However, it is possible, as may be the case in farmers' lung, that other components (in particular, bagasse dust itself) may be involved in pathogenesis. Experimental work lends some support to this possibility (Kawai *et al.*, 1972; Bhattacharjee *et al.*, 1980).

Allergic bronchopulmonary aspergillosis may occasionally occur in bagasse-exposed workers (*see* p. 393).

Serum IgG and IgA, but not IgM, levels are raised in acute bagassosis (Salvaggio *et al.*, 1969).

Bagasse contains a small amount of quartz (about 0–1 to 0–2 per cent) derived from the soil and, because of this, some authorities have suggested that bagassosis is a form of silicosis. There is no foundation for this belief and it is evident that the pathogenesis and pathology of the disease do not resemble silicosis in any way.

CLINICAL FEATURES

The symptoms, physical signs and radiographic appearances of both acute and chronic disease are similar to those of farmers' lung (*Figure 11.11*), but in a number of acute cases there is no evident abnormality of the chest film.

Lung function tests during acute disease reveal some reduction of TLC, VC and gas transfer which subsequently return to normal in most cases (Weill *et al.*, 1966). Vital capacity in exposed workers without disease may be significantly lower than in unexposed workers, but the reason for this has not been ascertained (Hearn 1968). However, a single episode of bagassosis can produce dyspnoea on effort, permanent reduction of lung volume and gas transfer, and hyperventiltion on exercise (Miller, Hearn and Edwards, 1971).

TREATMENT

As in the case of farmers' lung, the majority of patients with acute disease recover spontaneously in four to 12 weeks after being removed from exposure. Corticosteroids in adequate dose may hasten clinical recovery, but do not appear to influence the rate at which lung function returns to normal (Pierce *et al.*, 1968).

PREVENTION

The application of 1 per cent propionic acid to milled fresh bagasse before baling effectively prevents moulding even after bales are stored in the open for more than 12 months. However, the Ritter system and continuous moistening of large, loose mounds of bagasse have been used increasingly. This and carrying out grinding and shredding operations in the open, the use of exhaust ventiltion and enclosure of machinery (where possible) have greatly reduced both the incidence of the disease and the prevalence of *T. sacchari* precipitins in the workers (Lehrer *et al.*, 1978). High-efficiency respirators may be worn under some circumstances but are intolerable in hot and humid climates.

If more than one acute attack has occurred, the worker should be removed from further exposure to bagasse and should not transfer to agricultural work in which there could be contact with mouldy hay or fodder.

MUSHROOM WORKERS' LUNG

Mushroom workers' lung was first reported in the USA among Puerto Rican mushroom farm workers in 1959 (Bringhurst, Byrne and Gershon-Cohen, 1959) and is characterized by the same acute constitutional and respiratory symptoms and signs as farmers' lung, but only two cases of doubtful chronic disease appear to have been observed (Sakula, 1967; Jackson and Welch, 1970; Chan-Yeung, Grzybowski and Schonell, 1972). It appears to be remarkably uncommon considering that mushroom cultivation is carried out on a large scale in Britain, the USA and European countries, but it is probable that the illness is more common than reports suggest and often goes unrecognized.

Intensive methods of cultivation of various mushroom species have been used for some years. They involve the preparation of a compost consisting of wheat straw and fresh horse manure which is allowed to decompose in the open air for about three weeks and is then subjected to a temperature of 55 to 60 °C at 100 per cent humidity for five days in boxes indoors, allowing exuberant growth of thermophilic and thermotolerant actinomycetes, including *M. faeni* and *T. vulgaris*, and various fungi (Fergus, 1964; Craveri, Guicciardi and Pacini, 1966). The compost is then tipped from the boxes, the spawn added and mixed mechanically with the production of much dust which consists mainly of actinomycete spores. Random sampling of the air in a spawning shed has yielded counts of the order of 700×10^6 spores/m^3 (Stewart, 1974). During growth of the mushrooms the temperature is kept at about 20 °C and the humidity about 90 per cent. When the mushroom crop has been picked the growing sheds are heated to 60 °C after which the compost is taken out and deposited on a dumping ground. The spawning operation and the removal of compost are, therefore, the chief sources of exposure to spores and of outbreaks of disease. However, other species of thermoactinomycetes such as *Actinobifida dichotomica* may be present in the dust (Lacey, 1971a) which may also contain

(a)

(b)

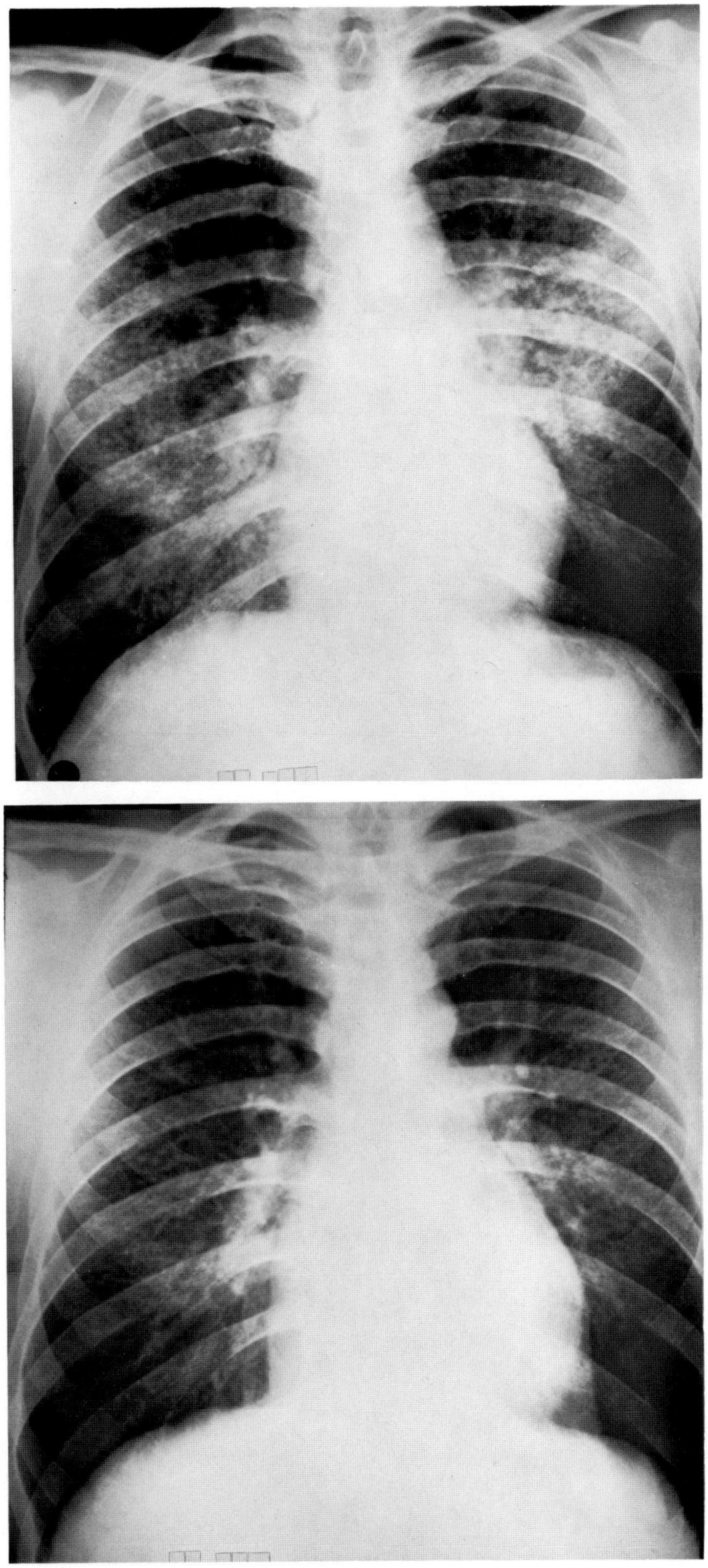

Figure 11.11 Subacute bagassosis in a worker in the UK handling mouldy bagasse for manufacture of laminated boards. Precipitins to the relevant organism present. (a) Multiple round mid-zone opacities preceded by a few months of lassitude, breathlessness and loss of weight. Note clear lower zones. (b) Resolution almost complete six weeks later. Ultimately complete recovery

large amounts of vegetable and animal particles derived from the compost (Sakula, 1967; Craig and Donevan, 1970).

CLINICAL AND IMMUNOLOGICAL FEATURES

In most instances affected workers attribute their symptoms to exposure to pasteurized compost in the spawning sheds. But there appears to be a remarkable variation of duration of exposure in relation to the development of symptoms. These usually first occur after some days or months of symptom-free work in the industry though occasionally they develop within a few hours of first exposure. In general the time between exposure and awareness of symptoms is from four to six hours (Chan-Yeung, Grzybowski and Schonell, 1972; Stewart, 1974).

The symptoms are those of acute extrinsic allergic 'alveolitis' described already. Cough and sputum are not troublesome but sputum may be bloodstained. Radiographic changes which range from bilateral miliary opacities in the middle and lower zones to confluent, ill-defined opacities in the same regions are usually present (Stewart, 1974).

Precipitins against *M. faeni* and *T. vulgaris* are found in very few cases even after concentration of the serum but precipitins to a variety of other thermophilic actinomycetes may be present, though none are common to all workers (Stewart and Pickering, 1974). Hence, with so rich a microflora as provided by mushroom compost it is probable that other organisms are involved. It is Lacey's (1971b) experience that thermomonospora-like organisms are more abundant than *M. faeni* and *T. vulgaris*.

However, the spores of mushrooms themselves may be a source of antigen. Acute symptoms of extrinsic allergic 'alveolitis' may be associated with inhalation of the spores of *Pleurotus florida*, a dual skin reaction to prick tests with the spore extract and serum precipitins against the organism (Schulz, Felton and Hausen, 1974). Of 17 mushroom farm workers who gave no precipitin reactions to *M. faeni* or *T. vulgaris* seven had precipitins to extracts of spores of the mushroom *Agaricus hortensis* but bronchial challenge with spore extract evoked no reaction in these patients. This may have been due to the dose being too low (Stewart and Pickering, 1974).

Whatever the identity of the causal allergens may be mushroom workers' lung is undoubtedly an allergic 'alveolitis'. It may be that, under different conditions, the disease is provoked by a variety of antigens from the compost itself, thermophilic actinomycetes, which are present in high concentrations in the compost, or the spores of different strains of mushrooms or permutations of all three (Stewart and Pickering, 1974).

It remains to be established why so few exposed indivuals are affected; why some workers react with severe constitutional symptoms after brief exposure whereas others take much longer to be sensitized; why, in some cases, the disease occurs shortly after a worker enters the industry but in others is delayed; and whether DIPF ever occurs (Stewart, 1974)

It has been suggested that nitrogen dioxide might be evolved by the compost (*see* Silo-fillers' disease, Chapter 13) and cause the disease (Bringhurst, Byrne and Gershon-Cohen, 1959), but there is no evidence that significant concentrations of the gas occur and no reason whatsoever to believe that it plays any part in the pathogenesis of mushroom workers' lung.

DIAGNOSIS AND PREVENTION

It is important to bear this form of extrinsic allergic 'alveolitis' in mind when a mushroom farm worker has an acute respiratory disease, especially as the illness is not necessarily severe. All the acutely ill patients in Stewart's (1974) group were first considered to have bronchopneumonia and were treated as such but without effect. A worker who has more than one acute attack should be advised to leave the industry and, probably, avoid any other work carrying a known risk of extrinsic allergic 'alveolitis'.

The most important preventive measure is good exhaust ventilation of the spawning houses and although rapid cooling of compost after initial heating has been recommended, it is probably ineffective. Respirators are not well tolerated and do not filter out airborne spores completely.

MALT WORKERS' LUNG

Although the features of acute extrinsic allergic 'alveolitis' in malt workers were first recorded in 1928 (Vallery-Radot and Giroud) the significance of this observation has only recently been recognized (Riddle *et al.*, 1968; Channel *et al.*, 1969). The disease occurs in distillery maltsmen and brewery workers. The prevalence of symptomatic disease with lung function changes in a few but without abnormal physical signs of radiographic changes is reported to be 5.2 per cent among workers in the Scottish malting industry (Grant *et al.,* 1976), but in the industry as a whole some cases may have been unrecognized. A chronic form of the disease does not seem to have been described, although chronic respiratory symptoms appear to be more common among malt workers than controls (Riddle, 1974).

In the malting process barley from the farms is dried in hot-air kilns, stored in silos for at least eight weeks, and dehydrated in steeping tanks with hypochlorite as a mild fungicide. It is then treated by traditional or mechanized processes. In the traditional process the barley is spread out on open concrete floors (open-floor malting) and allowed to germinate. The temperature of the grain is maintained at 18 °C by turning and raking the grain periodically (which also releases carbon dioxide and water) or by varying the thickness of the layer. The heat is produced by the respiration of the barley during germination. When the process has reached the desired stage of germination, it is stopped by drying the malt at 82 °C in a hot air kiln in which it is turned periodically to facilitate drying. It is then ready for the distillery. In modern maltings the process is partly or wholly mechanized (drum-method) so that dust exposure is either much reduced or eliminated and, correspondingly, so is the prevalence of disease. However, open-floor malting is believed to be essential for the characteristic flavour of high quality Highland malt whisky but, in this case, due, probably, to the fact that only high quality local, and not imported, barley is used the prevalence of extrinsic allergic 'alveolitis' is low (Grant *et al.*, 1976).

The disease is apparently caused by *Aspergillus clavatus* (Riddle *et al.,* 1968; Channel *et al.,* 1969). *A. clavatus* is a recognized contaminant of grain (Panasenko, 1967). Small amounts of inoculum may be present on grain or barley in the field, but there are also many opportunities of infection in the malting process and the suitable conditions on the malt floor lead to rapid proliferation. The spores are present in husks and malt grist, which implies that they can withstand the temperatures reached in the kilns (Channel *et al.*, 1969). Riddle *et al.* (1968) have suggested that the growth of fungi is encouraged by the presence of a large percentage of split corns, by maintenance of a higher floor temperature (24 °C) assisted by spraying the grain with water to shorten the germination time; and that the hypochlorite treatment encourages the growth of *A. clavatus* by suppression of other organisms. Malt workers may be exposed to spore dust, therefore, when turning barley on the malt floor and malt in the malt kilns, and also when cleaning the kilns (Channel *et al.*, 1969).

The sputum of all exposed workers, irrespective of whether or not they have evidence of disease, contains spores of *A. clavatus*. Precipitins against *A. clavatus* are present in the serum of men with symptoms in increasing prevalence according to their severity and also in a proportion of healthy employees, but not in normal unexposed employees nor in patients with suspected farmers' lung (Channel *et al.*, 1969). Skin prick tests suggest that symptoms are usually associated with a Type III reaction to *A. clavatus* (Grant *et al.*, 1976), and bronchial challenge tests with *A. clavatus* spores reproduce the disease in men who have previously suffered from it.

Some workers also have precipitins to *Aspergillus fumigatus, Penicillium granulatum, Penicillium citrinium* and *Rhizopus stolonifer*, which are common contaminants of malt floors, but without evidence of respiratory disease (Riddle, 1974).

When contamination of the malting process with *A. clavatus* is discovered clinical, radiographical and serological tests should be carried out on all exposed employees and the possibility of allergic 'alveolitis' considered in the event of acute respiratory disease.

The application of mechanical methods in some distilleries and breweries has greatly decreased or eliminated the chance of workers inhaling spores and of developing allergic 'alveolitis'.

SUBEROSIS

Cork workers in Portugal — who number more than 20 000 — are prone to lung disease which has been attributed to work dust (Cancella, 1959). In atopic workers it has the features of bronchial asthma with transient opacities in the chest radiograph, but in non-atopic workers it is an extrinsic allergic 'alveolitis' with the same clinical, physiological and radiographic features as farmers' lung (Ávila and Villar, 1968; Pimentel and Ávila, 1973). Persons with acute or subacute 'alveolitis' appear to recover completely when removed from the working environment.

Cork is the bark of *Quercus suber* L, a species of oak growing in Spain and Portugal. A wide variety of jobs are involved in its processing: sorting, grading and boiling cork bark in the open air; work in cork storage warehouses; cutting and preparing discs, stoppers ('corks') and other materials; and finishing, for example standing, grading and packing the products. Machine and other maintenance workers not directly involved with the process also work in the factory (Ávila and Lacey, 1974). Cork bark is burnt to produce a black pigment, Spanish black.

Cork bark may become mouldy after being boiled and stacked wet for straightening purposes in hot, damp warehouses. Dust which consists of cork and the spores of numerous different fungi, including *Penicillium frequentans* (Westling), is encountered in high concentrations during destacking and the preparatory manufacturing stages of discs and stoppers ('corks') (Ávila and Lacey, 1974).

The pathology of acute disease consists of infiltration of alveolar walls with lymphocytes, histocytes and, later, fibroblasts, and by the appearance of sarcoid-type granulomas with peripheral lymphocytic infiltration. In chronic disease there is dust pigmentation and DIPF with honeycombing and obliterative changes in small vessels (Ávila and Villar, 1968). The size of the spores of *P. frequentans* and some of the other airborne fungi will allow them to penetrate to alveolar level whereas cork particles tend to be larger (Ávila and Lacey, 1974), although they are consistently present in lung lesions (Pimentel and Ávila, 1973).

That *P. frequentans* is probably the chief cause of this form of extrinsic allergic 'alveolitis' is indicated by the facts that: (1) precipitins against *P. frequentans* are present in the sera of almost all (98 per cent) of affected workers but in only very few (7 per cent) unaffected workers; (2) extracts of the fungus give a Type III skin reaction in patients with disease; (3) bronchial challenge tests with the extract reproduce the symptoms; and (4) radiographic changes are significantly correlated with the concentration of airborne fungus spores (Ávila and Lacey, 1974). Although airborne cork particles are fewer and larger than the fungus spores it has been suggested that they may play some part in pathogenesis on the grounds that the incidence of precipitins correlates with the numbers of airborne cork particles and that cork particles are commonly present in the granulomatous lesions (Ávila and Lacey, 1974). However, the presence of cork particles in the lesions is not necessarily proof of cause. It is possible, nonetheless, that particulate cork might facilitate the production of disease by the fungus (*see* Bagassosis, p. 364).

There is no evidence that the dust of clean, non-mouldy cork causes lung disease. This point is important because exposure to cork dust in such activities as the cutting and buffing corn-containing products (for example, floor tiles) is fairly common.

MAPLE BARK STRIPPERS' DISEASE (CONIOSPOROSIS)

Acute respiratory disease in men who stripped the bark off maple trees was first reported by Towey, Sweany and Huron in 1932 since when a number of cases of allergic granulomatous 'alveolitis' have been reported (Emanuel, Lawton and Wenzel, 1962; Emanuel, Wenzel and Lawton, 1966; Wenzel and Emanuel, 1967). Although Towey, Sweany and Huron referred to the disorder as 'bronchial asthma' the clinical and radiographical features they described were typical of acute extrinsic allergic 'alveolitis'. The cause of the disease is inhalation of spores of *Cryptostroma (Coniosporum) corticale* which are ovoid and measure 4 to 5 μm in their greater axis. This fungus causes disease under the bark of maples, hickories, bass woods and sycamores (Gregory and Waller, 1951). Wenzel and Emanuel (1967) found that *C. corticale* was not present in maples before they were felled but developed during prolonged storage afterwards. Exposure to the spores occurred mainly in paper mills during stripping of logs by hand or mechanical means, sawing, and shaking small long chippings through screens to remove bark fragments. A chronic form of the disease does not seem to have been observed.

Precipitins specific for the spore extract are present in affected workers and also in exposed, but seemingly unaffected workers some of whom, however, have had subclinical disease (Emanuel, Wenzel and Lawton, 1966). Experimental work with *C. corticale* in rats supports the conclusion that delayed hypersensitivity plays an important role in maple bark disease (Tewksbury, Wenzel, and Emanuel, 1968).

Biopsy of lung tissue during the illness reveals sarcoid-type granulomas and some degree of diffuse interstitial fibrosis, and the presence of spores. The fungus can be grown from the tissue on Sabouraud's agar supplemented with an aqueous extract of maple wood (Emanuel, Wenzel and Lawton, 1966). The spores in the lungs closely resemble *Histoplasma capsulatum* but are distinguished by being stained black with Gomori's methenamine silver nitrate technique (Emanuel, Wenzel, and Lawton, 1966). Histoplasmin skin and complement fixation tests are negative.

Preventive measures consist of spraying logs during debarking with water containing detergent, remote control of some operations, the wearing of special respirators, monitoring of spore concentrations in the mill, and regular clinical, serological and X-ray examinations. The disease can be controlled by these means, but continual vigilance is necessary.

Similar type, prolonged exposure to the fungus *Alternaria* in logs during the preparation of wood pulp for the manufacture of paper may also cause allergic 'alveolitis' (*wood-pulp workers' disease*). Characteristic symptoms and radiographic changes occur and lung biopsy has shown features consistent with allergic 'alveolitis'. Bronchial challenge with *Alternaria* extract has reproduced symptoms of the disease (Schlueter, Fink and Henley, 1972).

AIR CONDITIONER DISEASE ('HUMIDIFIER FEVER')

'Humidifier fever' was described by Pestalozzi in 1959 and by HM Chief Inspector of Factories (1969) among printers who had been exposed to water mist sprayed into the workroom from humidifiers contaminated with algae and bacteria. Respiratory and constitutional symptoms consistent with extrinsic allergic 'alveolitis' have also been reported in relation to air conditioning systems contaminated with micro-organisms. The disorder was originally attributed to *M. faeni* spores released into the atmosphere of an office from a contaminated air conditioning system in the USA (Banaszak, Thiede and Fink, 1970). Subsequently episodes of disease have been associated with air conditioning systems in homes, offices, operating theatres and factories — especially in industries requiring carefully controlled humidity, such as printing, stationery and the manufacture of textiles (Fink *et al.*, 1971; Sweet *et al.*, 1971; Weiss and Soleymani, 1971; Hodges, Fink and Schlueter, 1974; Friend *et al.*, 1977; Medical Research Council Symposium, 1977; Campbell *et al.*, 1979). However, although in some respects the disorder may be similar to extrinsic allergic 'alveolitis' there are significant differences which suggest the existence of two distinct syndromes:

(1) extrinsic allergic 'alveolitis' which is predominant in the descriptions of disease in the USA and Switzerland (Scherrer *et al.*, 1978).
(2) 'humidifier fever' proper.

EXTRINSIC ALLERGIC 'ALVEOLITIS'

Symptoms, physical signs and lung function and radiographic changes are identical to those of acute, subacute or chronic extrinsic allergic 'alveolitis' due to other causes. Chronic disease appears to consist of the gradual onset of dyspnoea or exertion without previous acute disease. It does not appear to have been seen in Britain; the reason for this is not clear.

The illness has been attributed to thermophilic actinomycetes (*T. vulgaris* and *T. thalpophilus* — *see* p. 372) growing in water of air conditioning systems; and to spores of *Aureobasidium pullulans* (Pullularia) — the organism associated with *Sequoiosis* (*see* p. 385) — in steam from stagnant water poured over a heating element in a home sauna bath (*sauna-takers' disease*) (Metzger *et al.*, 1976). Serum precipitins to actinomycetes are present in some cases and, in a few, the antigen has been demonstrated in lung tissued by immunofluorescence. Inhalation challenge with cultured organisms has reproduced the illness (Fink *et al.*, 1976).

Because some outbreaks of legionnaires' disease have also been associated with contaminated water in air-conditioning or cooling tower systems the possibility that antibody to *Legionella pneumophilia* may be present in cases of extrinsic allergic 'alveolitis' related to such systems has been considered. But preliminary investigation suggests that there is probably no association between the organisms which cause the two diseases (Basich, Resnick and Fink, 1980).

'HUMIDIFIER FEVER'

This is an acute illness consisting of malaise, fever, myalgia, cough, tightness in the chest and breathlessness on exertion which usually resolves in 24 hours.

A feature of cases seen in Britain is that symptoms are worse at the beginning of a working week and improve during the rest of the week, but recur on re-exposure after an absence from work. This symptom pattern — apart from its clear asthmatic features (*Figure 11.12*) and recurrence on delayed re-exposure — is similar to that of 'mill fever' (*see* Chapter 12, p. 435). Investigation of four factories (printing, stationery and textiles) in Britain showed that only a minority of workers were affected but their symptoms were worse on Mondays ('Monday morning fever'). No radiographic changes were observed. Although airborne dust was not evident in any of the factories, the illness in all was associated with heavy contamination by a mixed growth of bacteria and fungi of water recirculated through humidifiers. In one factory Protozoa — mainly amoebae (*Naegleria gruberi*) and ciliates — were also present in abundance (Edwards, Griffiths and Mullins, 1976; Pickering *et al.*, 1976; Friend *et al.*, 1977; Medical Research Council Symposium, 1977). The incidence of the illness is highest in the winter months due, possibly, to greater recirculation of heated air during this period.

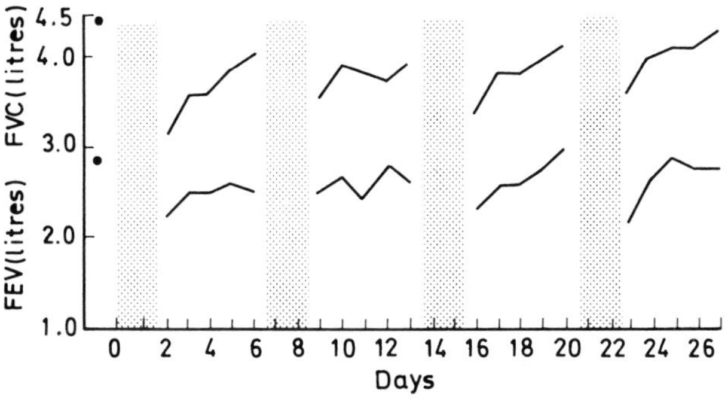

Figure 11.12 Spirometry during one month in a worker with intermittent malaise, cough and fever in a factory where air-conditioning units were contaminated with a variety of organisms. The stippled columns indicate weekends. Measurements taken at 16.00 hours each day. Indicates daily FVC and FEV_1 *measured at 16.00 hours when he was asymptomatic and working in an uncontaminated part of the factory. (Courtesy of Dr C. A. C. Pickering and the Editors of* Clinical Allergy*)*

Symptoms and reduction in ventilatory capacity may be most pronounced on return to work on a Monday and cease during the rest of the week like grades C1 and 2 byssinosis (*Figure 11.12*). (*See* Chapter 12.)

Specific responsible organisms have not been identified but serum precipitins against crude extracts of contaminated water are present both in affected and some healthy, similarly exposed, workers. In general no consistent relationships between precipitins and individual fungi or bacteria have been evident. However, antibodies against *Naegleria gruberi* and *Acanthamoeba* are found in affected workers when these amoebae are present in the humidifier systems (Edwards, Griffiths and Mullins, 1976; Medical Research Council Symposium, 1977); and precipitins to extracts of *B. subtilis* were constantly present in a group of badly affected workers exposed to a contaminated air-conditioning system in a printing factory (Parrot and Blyth, 1980). Bronchial challenge with extracts of contaminated water reproduces the illness in affected workers but not in normal unexposed control individuals (Friend *et al.*, 1977), though challenge with extracts of individual organisms caused no response (Pickering *et al.*, 1976). However, extracts of amoeba were not used. The pattern of the challenge reaction is similar in nature, rate of onset and duration to the 'late alveolar reaction' provoked by appropriate antigens in extrinsic allergic 'alveolitis' (Newman Taylor *et al.*, 1978).

A similar illness has been described in workers in sewage disposal plants in which sludge is reduced to powder by heat treatment. This so-called *'sewage sludge disease'* is associated with high concentrations of Gram-negative bacteria (Medical Research Council Symposium, 1977).

CONCLUSIONS

Evidently, the clinical features of 'humidifier fever' are very variable and the causal agents are yet to be clearly defined. Unlike typical acute (or subacute) extrinsic allergic 'alveolitis' where the source of exposure is usually well defined and dust concentrations high, the level of airborne material sufficient to cause an episode of 'humidifier fever' in susceptible individuals appears to be extremely low. It has been suggested that the febrile illness might be caused by bacterial endotoxins (especially when there is no evidence of lung involvement) or that soluble antigens might produce soluble aggregates and resultant complement consumption; whereas relatively insoluble antigens would remain in the gas-exchanging region of the lungs and could cause a granulomatous reaction. The pyrexial episodes of 'humidifier fever' might represent the first stage in a sequence of events which ends in a 'full' attack of extrinsic allergic 'alveolitis'. On the other hand, a mechanism other than immune-complex complement activation may be involved—possibly via the alternative pathway (Medical Research Council Symposium, 1977).

Whatever the solution of the problem proves to be two points are clear:

(1) The clinician must be aware of the existence of this 'disorder' and of the different forms it may take. A history of recurrent febrile illness, often with respiratory symptoms but normal chest radiograph, may call for investigation of the conditions in which the patient works including systematic observations at work. Inhalation challenge testing may be necessary for definitive diagnosis.

(2) Prevention of growth of organisms in humidifier systems. A rich flora grows readily in recirculated water resevoirs and some systems may release very small droplets into the air. The possibility of contamination is important, therefore, in air conditioned offices, factories, hospitals and laboratories. The growth of the organisms can be suppressed or prevented by input water filters or by steam injection of water which avoids recirculation and pooling. Heating of storage tanks to 60 or 70 °C and frequent cleaning (though difficult) may reduce, but not eliminate, the growth of organisms. Disinfectants are contra-indicated as they encourage the growth of some species of bacteria and are themselves likely to be inhaled (Medical Research Council Symposium, 1977).

Increased information about the prevalence of disease (which, on present evidence, appears to be low) is required because specially modified systems may be necessary only in situations where humidity control is particularly critical.

RARE CAUSES OF EXTRINSIC ALLERGIC 'ALVEOLITIS'

SEQUOIOSIS

A granulomatous 'alveolitis' has been reported in a man exposed to mouldy sawdust of the giant redwood (*Sequoia sempervirens*) in whose serum precipitins against extracts of saw-mill dust were found (Cohen *et al.*, 1967). The responsible organisms have not be positively identified, but may be *Graphium* or *Aureobasidium pullulans.*

CHEESE WASHERS' LUNG

The clinical features of extrinsic allergic 'alveolitis' have been observed in Swiss cheese makers engaged in washing moulds off the surface of cheeses. Symptoms tend to disappear when they are away from work. Apparently, some

10 to 15 per cent of workers are affected. Precipitins of IgG class against *Penicillium casei* were present in their sera (De Weck, Gutersohn and Bütikofer, 1969; Molina, 1976). But asthmatic symptoms also occur in cheese washers and may be difficult to differentiate from acute extrinsic allergic 'alveolitis'; indeed, both may occur together (Wuthrich and Keiser, 1970). Recently Molina (1976) has found Acarids of the Dermatophagoides type on the surface of cheese and preliminary investigation of Cantal cheese workers has shown specific serum precipitins against Acarid extracts. The cheese mites *Aleurobius farinae* and *Tyrolichus casei* may be implicated (Renaud *et al.*, 1979).

DRY ROT LUNG

Acute allergic 'alveolitis' with typical radiographic changes has been observed in association with asthma and shown to be due to the fungus *Merulius lacrymans* from extensive dry rot in the patient's home. Skin testing showed a dual reaction to the fungus extract and specific IgE and IgG precipitins were present. Complete recovery followed removal from exposure (O'Brien *et al.*, 1978). Asthma caused by the spores of this fungus is well known to occur (*see* Chapter 12).

WHEAT WEEVIL LUNG

For many years it has been known that asthma may occur in sensitive granary or farm workers exposed to grain and flour dust (Frankland and Lunn, 1965; Lunn, 1966). This may be caused by a variety of mites and fungi, but the wheat weevil (*Sitophilus granarius*) can give rise, not only to a pronounced immediate (Type I) allergy, but also to precipitating antibodies (Jimenez-Diaz, Lahoz and Canto, 1947). Delayed (Type III) sensitivity with constitutional symptoms, basal crepitations and impairment of gas transfer have been produced in an atopic worker by inhalation challenge three hours after an immediate asthmatic reaction. Precipitins against weevil extract were found in his serum after concentration, and intradermal injection of weevil extract caused a delayed, Arthus-type reaction (Lunn and Hughes, 1967). The source of the antigen is weevil protein.

ANIMAL HANDLERS' LUNG

Recurrent episodes of acute extrinsic allergic 'alveolitis' have been described in a research assistant handling rats for experimental purposes. Skin prick tests to rat serum were positive and precipitins against rat serum, urine and pelt, but not fur, were present. Rat urine contains large amounts of serum protein and was probably the chief source of antigen. The patient's symptoms recurred with radiographic changes on deliberate or inadvertent re-exposure to rats or mice. Thus, airborne proteins of the urine, dander and hair particles of rats and, possibly, other experimental animals are a source of antigen capable of provoking extrinsic allergic 'alveolitis' in laboratory workers (Carroll *et al.*, 1975).

Close contact with gerbils (small rodents also known as jerboas) is also reported to cause acute disease, presumably for similar reasons (Korenblat *et al.*, 1977).

FISH MEAL WORKERS' LUNG

Features of acute disease have been reported in an employee of a factory manufacturing animal foods in which fish meal was incorporated. Intracutaneous tests gave a dual response to fish meal extracts, and bronchial challenge was followed by basal crepitations and fall in Tl after five hours. Multiple serum precipitins against fish meal antigens were present (Ávila, 1971).

DIISOCYANATE 'ALVEOLITIS'

Organic isocyanates where are extensively used in the manufacture of synthetic rubbers, adhesives and paints, and as a catalyst in porcelain finishing are known to be a potent cause of asthma and are discussed in Chapter 12. But occasionally acute extrinsic allergic 'alveolitis', rather than asthma, may occur in individuals exposed to toluene diisocyanate (TDI) and, possibly, hexamethylene diisocyanate and can be reproduced by bronchial challenge (Charles *et al.*, 1976; Butcher *et al.*, 1977; Fink and Schlueter, 1978). Rabbits sensitized by intramuscular injection of a TDI-albumin conjugate have been shown to develop an Arthus-type reaction in the lungs on subsequent endotracheal challenge with antigen (Charles *et al.*, 1976).

PYRETHRUM 'ALVEOLITIS'

Repeated heavy exposure to a pyrethrum-based insecticide in the home is reported to have caused subacute extrinsic allergic 'alveolitis' with radiographic changes and granuloma-like lesions and DIPF on lung biopsy. Skin tests with pyrethrum produced a dual response (Carlson and Villaveces, 1977).

BACILLUS SUBTILIS 'ALVEOLITIS'

A minor epidemic of 'hypersensitivity pneumonitis' in six members of a family apparently caused by *B. subtilis* released from wood dust in the flooring of an old bathroom during its restoration has been described by Johnson *et al.* (1980). They suggest that this organism should be considered as a potential cause of irreversible lung damage in susceptible persons.

PAULI'S REAGENT 'ALVEOLITIS'

Acute extrinsic allergic 'alveolitis' caused by sodium diazobenzenesulphate (Pauli's reagent) used in chromatography has been reported in a atopic medical laboratory technicians by Evans and Seaton (1979). Bronchial challenge resulted in immediate and late airflow obstruction, and clinical, physiological, radiographic and histological evidence of allergic 'alveolitis'. Complete recovery followed withdrawal from exposure. The fact that other workers in the laboratory were unaffected and that this appears to be the first case on record suggests that the reaction was related to increased susceptibility due to the atopic status of the subject.

PITUITARY SNUFF TAKERS' LUNG

Cases of extrinsic allergic 'alveolitis' apparently caused by therapeutic snuffs containing powdered extracts of pig or ox pituitary glands in patients with diabetes insipidus were reported in the past (Mahon *et al.*, 1967; Harper *et al.*, 1970). But, as this method of treatment has now ceased, they no longer occur.

UNCERTAIN CAUSES OF EXTRINSIC ALLERGIC 'ALVEOLITIS'

CRYPTOCOCCUS NEOFORMANS

Miyagawa, Ochi and Takahashi (1978) have described 'hypersensitivity pneumonitis' which may have been provoked by this organism, the source of which is not obvious, in 42 Japanese individuals—mostly housewives.

FURRIERS' LUNG

Granulomatous lung disease has been described in an individual who had worked for years with animal furs (Pimentel, 1970).

COFFEE WORKERS' LUNG

An acute illness resembling extrinsic allergic 'alveolitis' has been recorded in a worker in a coffee roasting factory. Basal crepitations, 'mottling' of both lung fields and serum precipitins to coffee bean dust were present. Biopsy revealed infiltration of alveolar walls with lymphocytes, plasma cells and fibroblasts and, though giant cells were seen, there were no granulomas (van Toorn, 1970).

BAKELITE LUNG

Bakelite is a phenolic plastic produced by polymerization of phenol and formaldehyde. Pimentel (1973) described disease 'similar to extrinsic allergic alveolitis' in two workers exposed to bakelite dust. However, the mode of development of the illness in both cases was not like that of allergic 'alveolitis' and biopsy appearances were consistent with sarcoidosis, which was not excluded. Much reliance was placed on the presence of 'inclusions' of phenol compounds in some granulomas, but this is not necessarily proof of causation.

INFECTIOUS DISEASES AND ZOONOSES

These are discussed only briefly with the intention of concentrating on their occupational significance, diagnostic difficulties and prevention. Hence, the clinical, pathological, bacteriological and mycological details are brief and methods of treatment omitted as this information is fully presented in specialized standard works.

BACTERIAL INFECTIONS

Tuberculosis

The unusual susceptibility of patients with silicosis to develop tuberculosis is referred to in Chapter 7.

Although the prevalence of pulmonary tuberculosis in general has fallen dramatically since the 1950s it is an occasional occupational hazard in doctors, nurses and laboratory and pathology technicians, and is fairly common among seafarers (Oliver, 1979). But it is difficult to make an accurate assessment of the population at risk. All tuberculin negative staff in these categories should be inoculated with BCG and an annual chest radiograph is desirable. Seafarers under treatment are not normally permitted to serve at sea.

'Opportunist' mycobacteria

These organisms do not appear to cause occupationally related disease in the absence of pre-existing silicosis, coal pneumoconiosis or other forms of fibrotic pneumoconiosis (*see* Chapters 4, 7 and 8).

Brucellosis ('Undulant fever')

This is primarily a disease of farm animals and is uncommon in human beings not in contact with them. The responsible organisms are coccobacilli of the *Brucella* genus. In Britain cattle harbouring *B. abortus* are the chief cause of human disease; in the USA, where infection from this source has been virtually eliminated by controlled slaughter, the pig infected by *B. suis* is the culprit (Buchanan, Faber and Feldman, 1974); and in Mediterranean countries (but not in the UK), goats and sheep infected by *B. mellitensis*. Of the three species of the organism *B. mellitensis* is the most invasive.

A cow with brucellosis is most infectious during the month following calving, and the placenta, membranes and discharges are heavily contaminated with the organism which is also present in an aborted calf and in the cow's urine and faeces. Thus, the opportunity for widespread contamination of farm buildings, abattoirs and knacker's yards is evident, and infected dust or aerosol is readily produced. In Britain, therefore, people most likely to be at risk occupationally are dairy farmers, cattle breeders and dealers and their families, abattoir workers, knackers and veterinary surgeons. In the USA infection is chiefly associated with the slaughter of pigs and with the processing of pig meat. Disease due to *B. suis* does not apparently occur in Britain. Medical laboratory workers may also be infected and brucellosis has been placed first in the 'Top Ten' of laboratory acquired infections (Harrington, 1975)

Although human infection may occur via skin abrasions, the conjunctiva, mucous membranes and the gastro-intestinal tract (infected milk) the respiratory tract is the relevant route in the present context. The incidence of disease in Britain is probably about 300 cases a year (Leading article, 1975).

Clinically, the disease may be acute, subacute or chronic. There is also a subclinical or latent form which is not relevant here.

In *acute disease* with lung involvement — which occurs in only a small proportion of cases — there is cough, sputum, (acute bronchitis) haemoptysis, pleuritic pain, fever (which, characteristically, is undulant), headache, severe sweats, arthralgia and lymphadenopathy. The chest radiograph shows signs of bronchopneumonic consolidation often with hilar node enlargement. In *subacute disease* the symptoms are similar but less pronounced and, though severe fatigue is a feature, there are periods of spontaneous remission. Radiographically there is evidence of pulmonary infiltration or consolidation.

In *chronic disease* intermittent exacerbations of illness which resemble influenza, but without fever, occur over a number of years. Granulomas of sarcoid type are present in the lungs, liver, spleen and bone marrow (Ganado, 1975). The chest film may show scattered irregular opacities.

Diagnosis depends very much on the vital clues of the patient's occupation, local epidemiology and the clinical pattern of the illness. In acute disease high titres of agglutinating antibodies are usually present but in a few cases they are absent. Because brucella antibodies may be due to drinking infected milk in the past and can persist for several years, and because blood cultures for *B. abortus* are rarely positive, laboratory tests are of limited help (Henderson *et al.*, 1975). However, there is hope that a leucocyte migration inhibition test may prove to be of value in the diagnosis of chronic disease (Mann and Richens, 1973). In some circumstances lung biopsy appearances could be misinterpreted as farmers' lung.

Prevention rests on vaccination of female calves, slaughter of infected animals and pasteurization of milk. Heavy contamination of the air of abattoirs can be significantly reduced by slaughtering as few infected animals as possible at any one time (Buchanan, Faber and Feldman, 1974).

Tularaemia

Necrotic pneumonia with abscess formation and, in most cases, septicaemia caused by *Francisella tularensis (Pasteurella tularensis)* may occur among people handling carcasses and skins of infected wild rabbits, hares, squirrels and foxes, and as a laboratory acquired infection mainly in North America, though cases have been reported in Norway, Sweden and Japan. Sugar refinery workers in Czechoslovakia have apparently been affected by handling sugar beet imported from endemic areas (Černý, 1976). It appears to be unknown in Britain.

Diagnosis depends on the isolation of the organism or the presence of an increased or rising antibody titre in the blood.

Anthrax

When ingested by cattle, pigs, sheep or goats the spores of *Bacillus anthracis* germinate and cause disease. The hides, hair and wool of sick animals and the straw, hay and sacking associated with them are heavily contaminated by the organism and are thus a source of infection to man in a variety of ways. In Britain today anthrax is uncommon in farm animals but occasional cases are a source of infection to those who handle them. Anthrax is endemic in India, Pakistan, North and East Africa and the Near and Far East. Materials from these areas are potential sources of infection.

Imported materials which may be infected include: (1) hides and skins from endemic areas; those from the Argentine and Australasia are less likely to be affected; (2) wool, goat hair (cashmere and mohair), alpaca and camel hair from China, India and the Near East; and horse hair from China, Siberia and Russia; (3) crushed and dried bone from Pakistan and India and (4) hooves and horn from endemic areas.

Occupations in which there is a potential risk from these and other sources are: (1) tanning of skins and hides; (2) manufacture of glue and gelatin from imported bone and hooves; (3) production of fertilizers and charcoal for sugar refining from crushed bone; (4) sorting of goat, camel and alpaca hair; (5) mechanical opening and cleaning of imported wools; (6) processing of horse hair for the manufacture of brushes; (7) agricultural workers, knackers and veterinary surgeons in contact with sick animals; (8) dockers and transport workers handling infected material (such as hides) and medical and veterinary bacteriology laboratory staff may occasionally be at risk; (9) direct infection of medical and nursing staff by a patient with pulmonary anthrax and of the pathologist and his attendants who perform the autopsy may occur because, owing to its rarity, the disease is not often diagnosed during life, and thus is frequently fatal. Contaminated bone meal, is believed to be the most common source of potential infection in Britain today. A fatal case of pulmonary anthrax in London attributed to this source was reported by Enticknap *et al.* in 1968.

Pulmonary anthrax must be considered in any patient with pneumonia who works in a potential anthrax hazard. Its incidence is related to the number and size of anthrax-containing particles inhaled.

Though cutaneous anthrax is still seen occasionally in Britain pulmonary disease, which consists of haemorrhagic pneumonia with septicaemia, pleural effusions and recurrent haemoptysis is now rare but may be encountered in those areas of the world where anthrax is endemic (Plotkin *et al.*, 1960). This is due largely to effective preventive measures but also, to some extent, to the low infectivity of *B. anthracis* for man. For, in spite of the fact that enormous numbers of anthrax-contaminated particles — many less than 5 μm in diameter — may be present in the work-place air, only very few cases of inhalation anthrax occur (Brachman *et al.*, 1960).

Preventive measures consist of the following: (1) vaccination of susceptible animals; (2) cremation or deep burying in quicklime (anhydrous calcium oxide) of a diseased animal, preferably at the site of death, and burning of all contaminated materials; (3) restriction of movement of other animals in or out of the area inhabited by the affected animal; (4) in the UK disinfection of imported skins, hides, hair and wool by factories approved under the Anthrax Prevention Act, 1971 before use; (5) immunization of workers at substantial risk with alum precipitated vaccine by three intramuscular injections of 0.5 ml at three-weekly intervals and a fourth 0.5 ml injection six months later; (6) obligatory exhaust ventilation, protective clothing and proper washing facilities in all factories processing potentially contaminated material. Education of workers in the mode of transmission of spores, and the control of effluents and trade wastes are also necessary measures.

Anthrax is a notifiable industrial disease in Britain.

Psittacosis–ornithosis (Chlamydiosis)

Psittacosis refers to disease of psittacine birds (the parrot family) caused by the bacterium *Chlamydia psittaci*, formerly referred to as Bedsonia. *Ornithosis* refers to disease caused by the same organism in birds of other Orders. Hence, the terms indicate different hosts of a common agent and not different 'diseases', although the strains responsible for ornithosis appear to be less virulent for man than those from psittacine birds (Cullen, 1974). The continued use of the two terms, however, is unnecessarily confusing.

Of the 27 Orders of birds at least 17 are susceptible to infection. All the psittacines — for example, parrots, parakeets, macaws, cockatoos, budgerigars — appear to be susceptible and *Chlamydia* strains in Amazon parrots are especially virulent to man. the Passiformes or 'perching birds', which include canaries, are particularly susceptible and many species are sold in pet shops where they may be infected by diseased psittacines. Domestic and wild pigeons are commonly infected. Domestic waterfowl may acquire disease from infected gulls, waders and aquatic birds: duck pluckers are thus reported to be vulnerable to infection. Among the gallinaceous birds (domestic poultry and game birds) infection in turkeys is the most important to man, though disease has occurred in pheasant rearers. Fulmars, in common with other sea birds, are susceptible and were responsible for an outbreak of ornithosis among women plucking them for the table in the Faroe Islands. Other birds which may be infected and are found in aviaries and zoological gardens include toucans, humming birds and penguins (Keymer, 1974).

In Britain the birds most likely to cause human disease are parrots, racing pigeons and budgerigars, but turkeys and finches may occasionally be responsible (Anderson and Bridgewater, 1968; Anderson, 1973). There is an increasing demand for exotic birds as pets in the home and, following the Parrots and Miscellaneous Birds (Prohibition of Importation) Revocation Order 1966, they were freely imported in increasing numbers and sold in pet shops and markets. Many were sick or dead on arrival (Parry and Mason, 1972). In Britain the number of homes in which pet budgerigars are kept is referred to on p.377. Psittacosis is the commonest infectious disease in pet parrots and other psittacines (Keymer, 1972). Sea birds are a possible source of infection of harbour fish workers and oil rig personnel (Bourne, 1975). In the USA turkeys have been the cause of many outbreaks of ornithosis and occasional deaths (Leachman and Yow, 1958).

Human beings are infected by direct contact with sick birds, their excretions and carcasses. Many symptomless birds, however, excrete the organism. Infection can be endemic in aviaries. About 1 per cent of the general population in England have antibodies to *Chlamydia psittaci* and among people dealing with birds, about 5 per cent (Ramsay and Emond, 1978).

The symptoms of avian disease include lack of condition, listlessness, dirty plumage, distended abdomen and watery, green diarrhoea. The organism is present in urine, faeces and discharge from the nostrils and eyes. As the feathers are heavily contaminated the organism is disseminated in the surrounding air. At post mortem the air sacs are cloudy, the liver and spleen enlarged with small haemorrhages and necrotic foci, and there is a fibropurulent exudate on serosal surfaces. An impression smear made by touching a microscope slide on the surface of liver or spleen, heat fixing and staining with a modified Ziehl–Neelson stain reveals purple/red cytoplasmic inclusions (Levinthal–Coles–Lillie bodies) against a green counterstain. With dark-ground optics the inclusions appear green and the cells are outlined in red. Culture of the agent may be necessary to establish a definite diagnosis in some cases (Cullen, 1974).

People with occupations in which there may be a risk of psittacosis include: (1) pet shop owners and staff (Parry and Mason, 1972; Jernelius *et al.*, 1975); (2) attendants in aviaries, zoological gardens and bird sanctuaries; (3) employees in turkey farms and processing plants especially in the USA. The highest attack rate of disease is in killing, plucking, eviscerating and packing operations (Dickerson, Bilderback and Pessarra, 1976; Anderson, Stoesz and Kaufmann, 1978); (4) railway guards handling crates of pigeons carried in guards' vans and carriers delivering sick birds to dealers (Dew *et al.*, 1960); (5) workers repairing buildings and roofing heavily contaminated with pigeon excreta; (6) veterinary surgeons and pathologists (McKendrick, Davies and Dutta, 1973); (7) laboratory workers handling infected material from patients or birds; (8) rarely, medical and nursing staff may be infected directly from patients suffering from the disease (Olsson and Treuting, 1944; Meyer, 1965).

Features of human disease

Its *incidence* is not easy to determine because many mild and atypical cases pass unnoticed but, in the UK, there has been a continual annual increase of proven cases since 1962 (when 37 were reported in England and Wales) apart from a temporary fall in 1977/78, in spite of the implementation of the Importation of Captive Birds Order 1976 (*Figure 11.13*) (Public Health Laboratory Service, 1973; Communicable Disease Report, 1980). Among cases of pneumonic disease in Sweden ornithosis was responsible for 6 to 11 per cent (Fransén, 1969; Jernelius *et al.*, 1975).

The incubation period is usually about ten days but ranges from four to 14 days.

Symptoms vary from those of a slight, non-specific, febrile flu-like illness to a severe infection with high fever, intense headache and rigors in which pleuritic pain, haemoptysis, giddiness and mental disturbance may occur. The older the patient the more severe the disease is likely to be.

Abnormal physical signs in the lungs are not prominent in many cases but crepitations may be heard and sometimes there is evidence of lobar consolidation.

The chest radiograph is abnormal in most, but not all, cases. The appearances, which are commonly more extensive than the physical signs suggest, may be those of lobar or segmental consolidation (usually unilateral), patchy pneumonic consolidation or bilateral linear infiltration, and, rarely, cases of pleural effusion (*Figure 11.14*). They are not pathognomonic in any way nor proportional to the severity of the illness, and may not resolve until more than a month after the patient has returned to health (Anderson, 1973); Jernelius *et al.*, 1975).

The pathological appearances are those of a desquamative pneumonia with Levinthal, inclusion bodies in alveolar and monocytic cells.

Diagnosis is often difficult and sporadic cases are frequently missed but the infection should be considered in all cases of non-bacterial pneumonia and of unexplained fever, especially as it is sometimes severe and even fatal. The most important finding is a four-fold rise in titre or a single titre above 1:80 of antibodies to the complement-fixing antigen of *Chlamydia* group B which distinguishes the disease from pneumonia due to Q fever (*see* next section), mycoplasma, viruses and legionnaires' disease which it may closely resemble (Byrom, Walls and Mair, 1979). However, if the psittacosis antigen employed for the test is of sub-optimal, strength it may not detect antibody and thus may fail to identify the disease. This can be overcome by employing an ether-extracted antigen (Dane and Pattison, 1974).

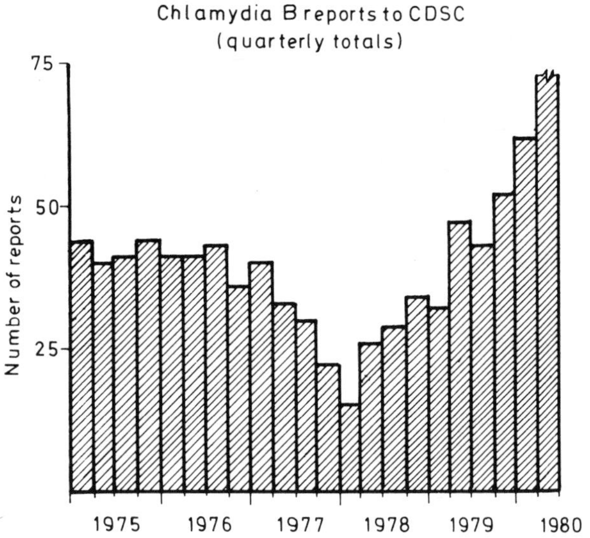

Figure 11.13 Numbers of cases of Chlamydia B *infections reported quarterly since 1975. Most have occurred in S.W. England but in the 1979/80 period the numbers in N.W. Thames, East Anglia and Northern Ireland have increased (*Communicable Disease Report, *1980. With the Editor's permission). Note: total in final column incomplete by three weeks*

It is important that, in its early stage, the illness in farmers and bird fanciers should not be confused with acute extrinsic allergic 'alveolitis' in which pleural effusion does not occur. Discovery of radiographic abnormality some time after recovery from a mild infection may raise the question of tuberculosis or bronchial carcinoma.

Complications are rare but can be serious. Fulminant, fatal psittacosis has been reported to present with acute renal failure and evidence of pancreatitis (Byrom, Walls and Mair, 1979). Valvar heart disease may occur (Ward and Ward, 1974) and pericarditis, myocarditis and endocarditis are well recognized (Byrom, Walls and Mair, 1979).

Prevention is difficult if there is unchecked importation of sick birds. In Britain birds can be isolated and premises disinfected under the Psittacosis and Ornithosis Order 1953, and all imported exotic birds are now placed in quarantine for 35 days. Sick birds must be destroyed and the disease confirmed by autopsy. Dead birds should be soaked in disinfectant, autopsy performed in a biohazard cabinet, and protective clothing, gloves and masks worn by the operators (Keymer, 1973). Laboratory based surveillance of all identified cases of human disease (which can only be confirmed in the laboratory) would greatly help control.

It should be noted that the antibiotic of choice in the treatment of disease in both birds and man is chlortetracycline which should be started early and continued until the infection is eradicated.

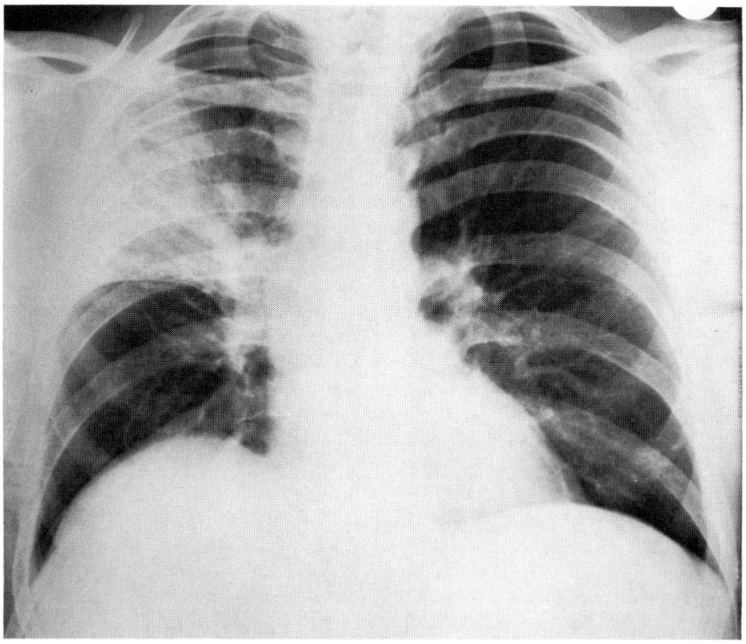

Figure 11.14 Chlamydia B *pneumonia. Partial consolidation of right upper lobe. Man aged 52 with a history of cough, lassitude, diarrhoea and fever for one week. No pathogenic organisms grown from the sputum. Initial chlamydial complement fixation titre 1:160 rising to 1:320 in one month. Complete recovery with tetracycline treatment. Pigeon breeder who kept 20 racing birds one of which was sick shortly before he became ill. (Dr J. P. Anderson's case reproduced with permission)*

RICKETTSIAL INFECTION

Q Fever

This is an acute infectious disease caused by *Coxiella (Rickettsia) burnetti* which derived its title from the original 'query' about its cause. In most cases it results from direct or indirect contact with infected animals. However, cows, sheep and goats which harbour the organism show no evidence of ill health and, though it may be present in high concentration in their udders, it does not interfere with milk production (Laing Brown, 1973). Furthermore, they give birth to normal young but the birth fluids and placenta contain enormous numbers of organisms which contaminate litter, hides and fleeces and can survive in dust for long periods (Hart, 1973).

The distribution of the disease is world wide. It is predominantly occupational and usually acquired by inhalation of contaminated aerosols; less often, by drinking infected milk. People at risk are: (1) farmers and shepherds and their families; (2) veterinary surgeons and their assistants; (3) stockyard workers; (4) employees of abattoirs and knackers' yards handling infected carcasses; (5) workers manufacturing fertilizers made from animal products; (6) medical and veterinary laboratory technicians; and (7) pathologists and post-mortem room attendants dealing with fatal human cases (McCallum, Marmion and Stoker, 1949; Johnson and Kadull, 1966; Hart, 1973). Dusty, contaminated straw used in packing cases was held responsible for an outbreak of disease involving 28 individuals in an art school (Harvey, Forbes and Marmion, 1951) and two members of a film crew and a doctor were infected after handling straw (Q fever 1976–7).

In Britain there were about 59 laboratory confirmed cases per year between 1967 and 1974, 117 in 1976 and 98 in 1977 (Q fever 1976–7). Antibodies to the organism have been detected in 29 per cent of abattoir workers, 20 per cent of veterinary surgeons, 13 per cent of farmers but only 1.9 per cent of town dwellers (Ramsay and Emond, 1978). In the USA Q fever is widely distributed but only 26 states require mandatory notification of human disease, and the diagnosis is unlikely to be made in some states which apparently lack the necessary laboratory capabilities. Serological surveys of dairy cattle have indicated that the percentage of infected cows has steadily increased in the past three decades. Hence, consideration should be given to the possibility of Q fever in all cases of obscure non-specific pneumonias (D'Angelo, Baker and Schlosser, 1979). In Bulgaria a

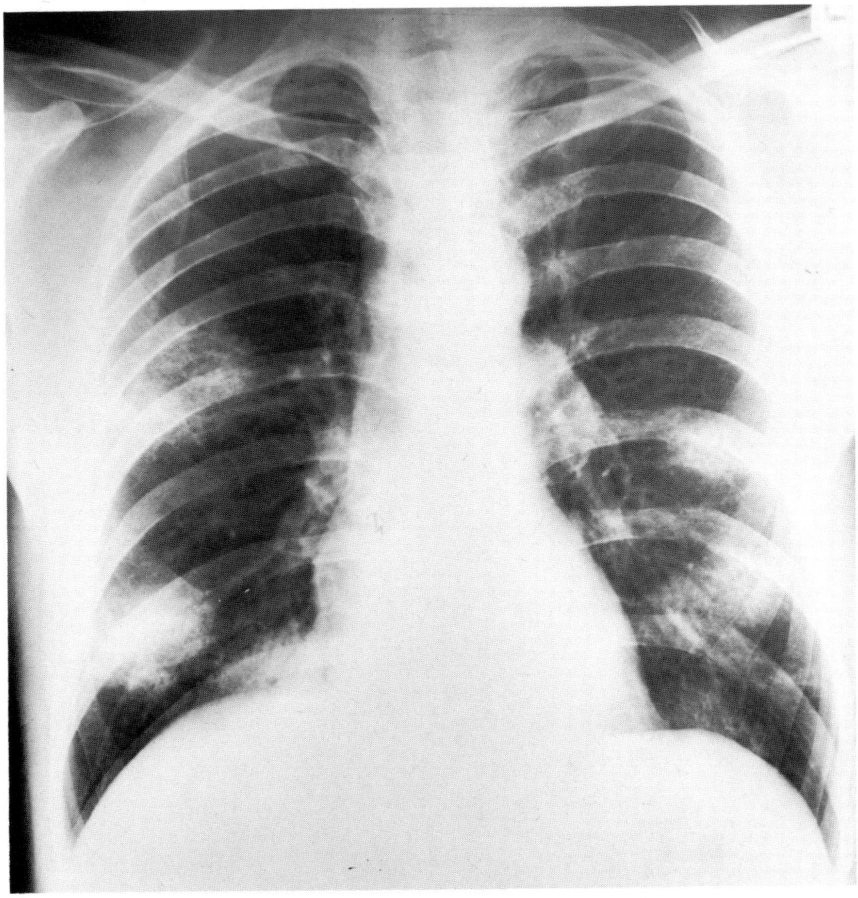

Figure 11.15 Q fever. Rounded opacities due to segmental consolidation. These appearances, especially if associated with signs of linear collapse seen in the left costophrenic angle, are very suggestive of this disease. (See Figure 11.16.) *(Courtesy of Dr J. K. Millar and the Editor of* Clinical Radiology*)*

remarkably high prevalence of antibodies has been reported in dustmen, obstetricians and midwives (Ganchev, Serbezov and Alexandrov, 1977).

The pathology is that of a non-specific, desquamative pneumonia.

Clinically there is fever ranging from 30 to 40.5 °C, severe sweats, shivering, backache and, in at least half the patients, troublesome cough occasionally with blood streaked sputum. Examination of the chest is either negative or reveals only localized evidence of consolidation. Lymphadenopathy and neck stiffness are occasionally present.

The chest radiograph is abnormal in most cases (87 per cent) and though the appearances are not pathognomonic, they are commonly associated with Q fever. In particular they consist of multiple round, segmental opacities of ground glass density, some 5 to 10 cm in diameter, situated usually in the lower zones (*Figure 11.15*); and linear collapse, again mainly in the lower zones (*Figure 11.16*). There may be evidence of complete or partial lobar collapse-consolidation and, in a few cases, pleural effusion. On average the abnormalities resolve in 30 days but may take up to 70 days (Millar, 1978).

Diagnosis depends on awareness of the disease, the patient's occupation and the radiographic appearances but is only proven by a four-fold or greater increase in the titre of complement fixing antibodies to the organism or by culture, though this should rarely be necessary and may expose laboratory technicians to risk of infection (Laing Brown, 1973).

Acute disease must be differentiated from influenza, brucellosis which presents almost identical symptoms and is similarly prevalent in farming communities, psittacosis, glandular fever, and *Mycoplasma pneumoniae* and respiratory virus infections. Investigations of a case of suspected brucellosis should always include Q fever antibodies (Laing Brown, 1973).

Complications are rare. But subacute bacterial endocarditis may occur on a previously damaged valve, and infection of an ischaemic ventricular aneurysm has been reported (Willey *et al.*, 1979).

Prevention is difficult as the infection in animals does not affect their health or productivity. Spread of disease via milk is, of course, prevented by pasteurization.

VIRUS INFECTION

Smallpox handlers' lung

A pneumonic illness with bilateral patchy low-density, radiographic opacities has been reported in nurses and others in close contact with smallpox patients (Howat and Arnott, 1944; Morris Evans and Foreman, 1963). As the illness may be followed by multiple, widespread, calcified pulmonary lesions similar to those which may be seen following chickenpox it is more likely to have been a modified smallpox pneumonia than a form of extrinsic allergic 'alveolitis' (Ross *et al.*, 1974). Smallpox is now said to have been eliminated throughout the world.

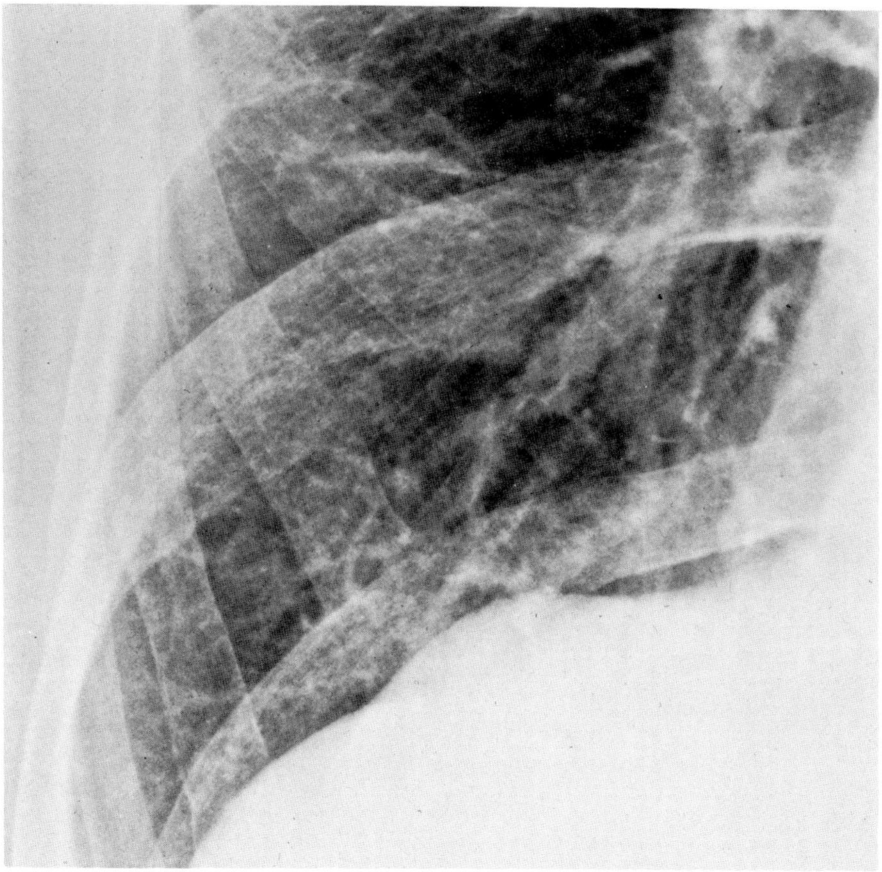

Figure 11.16 Linear collapse in Q fever. This is the only radiographic abnormality in some cases but is commonly seen during the resolution of areas of consolidation. (Courtesy of Dr J. K. Millar and the Editor of Clinical Radiology*)*

MYCOTIC INFECTIONS

Aspergillosis

Disease due to the *Aspergillus* species is related in the main, either to a lack of resistance in immunologically compromized patients or to an allergic response with asthma in atopic individuals. Occupational pulmonary aspergillosis is uncommon. Extrinsic allergic 'alveolitis' due to *A. clavatus* in malt workers has been referred to already. The *Aspergillus* sp. is ubiquitous in nature and is found in decaying vegetation, in grain, hay and straw and in farm buildings, and is it is a fairly common cause of disease in many species of birds, it may be present in their droppings. High levels of contamination by the spores may, therefore, be encountered by farm workers, threshers, millers, pigeon fanciers, poultry tenders, aviary workers and hair sorters. Chronic granulomatous disease which closely resembles cavitary tuberculosis occasionally occurs in individuals in these fields of activity in the absence of underlying disease or atopy (Hildick-Smith, Blank and Sarkany, 1964).

Diagnosis may be difficult as isolation of so ubiquitous an organism as *Aspergillus* from the sputum, even with proper laboratory precautions, does not establish the diagnosis, although repeated isolation makes it likely and the presence of large numbers of mycelia in mucous sputum 'plugs', almost certain. Serum precipitins to *Aspergilli* are found in the majority of cases of bronchopulmonary aspergillosis. However, the histological proof of lung biopsy may be necessary.

Histoplasmosis

This disease, which is primarily of respiratory origin, is caused by inhalation of the microconidia of the dimorphic fungus *Histoplasma capsulatum* and occurs in temperate and tropical climates: in particular, the eastern and central USA, Central, and South America, Mexico, South and South-West Africa. However, it is found in at least 60 countries and, though not indigenous to Britain, appears to be endemic in Europe (Ajello, 1971). It is, perhaps, the most important occupational pulmonary mycosis.

H. capsulatum is a soil-inhabiting, filamentous fungus which readily breaks up into minute particles if the soil is disturbed and these may become airborne. Its growth and sporulation are favoured by enrichment of the soil with the droppings or guano of birds and bats so that it has a predilection for their habitats. It is found in soil with substantial accumulation of droppings in and around chicken houses, under the roosts of gregarious birds such as starlings and ings inhabited by bats. In the USA the term 'blackbird' includes starlings which are mainly congregated in enormous numbers in the southern States, red-winged blackbirds, cowbirds and grackles—relatives of the mina bird (Chick *et al.*, 1980). The organism has been shown to survive in known contaminated soil for four to six years after being first isolated (di Salvo and Johnson, 1979), but it is unusual to find it in guano from a roosting site less than three years old (Chick *et al.*, 1980). Interestingly, birds are not infected by the organisms because their body temperature does not favour its reproduction, but they may harbour it in their feathers and thus contaminate their nests and other areas. By contrast, bats, which have a lower body temperature, may be infected and their faeces are not only a nutrient for fungal growth but may be infectious (Goodwin and Des Prez, 1978). Hence, though the distribution of the fungus is predominantly rural, it is found in cities; for example, in the soil of a tree-lined shopping area in Washington DC (Emmons, 1961).

The soil apart, contaminated deposits of bird or bat droppings may occur in chicken houses, silos, barns and attics of old buildings in both town and country; and outbreaks of histoplasmosis have followed the clearing of accumulated droppings from such places and from belfries, towers, civic buildings, the girders and pillars of bridges and the ground beneath (Dean *et al.*, 1978; Goodwin and Des Prez, 1978; Sorley *et al.*, 1979). Large collections of bat guano are particularly common in caves, disused mines, mine shafts, old ruins and hollow trees.

Therefore, occupations in which there is likely to be a risk of histoplasmosis in endemic areas include farm workers and their families, poultry keepers, gardeners and horticulturists using guano as a fertilizer, construction workers, bulldozer drivers, workers demolishing derelict buildings, bridge maintenance workers, ornithologists, geologists, spelaeologists, archaeologists and medical laboratory technicians handling cultures of the organism. Recent outbreaks of acute histoplasmosis in South Carolina and Louisiana have been associated with the clearing of bamboo cane fields (which were blackbird roosting sites) for pipe laying or construction work (di Salvo and Johnson 1979; Storch *et al.*, 1980), and with the felling of a giant oak tree (Ward *et al.*, 1979). Campbell (1980) has pointed out that demolition and construction work in city areas contaminated by bird or bat droppings may cause extensive outbreaks of disease and sporadic cases of severe pulmonary infection in passers-by who may live elsewhere. Bulldozing of positive bird roost sites is particularly apt to cause epidemics of disease (Chick *et al.*, 1980).

Most reported outbreaks of histoplasmosis have been due to acute pulmonary disease but an outbreak of chronic disease was recently observed in southern Kentucky following excavation of a substantial 'blackbird' roosting site (Latham *et al.*, 1980).

Cave sickness—so-named by Washburn, Tuohy and Davis (1948)—has been shown to be caused by *H. capsulatum* from the dust of bat guano in cave explorers in the USA (Lottenberg *et al.*, 1979), Venezuela (Campins *et al.*, 1956), South Africa (Murray *et al.*, 1957) and Rhodesia (Dean, 1957). *H. capsulatum* var. *duboisii*, which is widely distributed between the Sahara and Kalahari deserts, was probably responsible for cases on the African continent. Acute pulmonary disease due to this variant was reported in a white mining engineer in Ghana (Duncan, 1958). Dean (1975) has most plausibly suggested that the fatal 'Curse of the Pharaohs' suffered by Lord Carnarvon and others involved in the exploration of the tomb of Tutankhamun in 1923 was in fact histoplasmosis, for, during this period, the entrance to the tomb passages was guarded by a temporary open-grill iron door through which bats passed freely for temporary domicile.

Pathologically the microscopical appearances are those of epithelioid granulomas similar to tuberculosis but in which *H. capsulatum* can be identified by the periodic acid Schiff stain, and acid fast bacilli are absent.

Clinically histoplasmosis may be asymptomatic, a benign or widely disseminated and fatal acute disease, or a chronic lung disease. Its severity appears to depend on intensity of exposure. Fatal disease is uncommon.

Acute disease may be a mild illness with cough, chest pain, haemoptysis, fever, night sweats and joint pains. In the more severe cases there may be evidence of localized lung consolidation and endocarditis and meningitis may occur in disseminated disease. Chronic disease is marked by lassitude, low grade fever, productive cough and occasional haemoptysis.

Radiographically the appearances are identical to various stages of tuberculosis. In acute disease there may be multiple small or blotchy opacities or 'infiltrates', more sharply defined round opacities, scattered linear opacities, and signs of segmental consolidation and bilateral hilar node enlargement. Single or multiple cavitary lesions may also occur in asymptomatic and acute disease (Chick and Bauman, 1974; Davies and Sarosi, 1978). This last appearance may be mistaken for a lung tumour (Goodwin, Owens and Snell, 1976). In reinfection-type acute disease in patients who have retained an active immune response widespread miliary opacities are more commonly seen (Goodwin and Des Prez, 1978). Acute disease either resolves completely or undergoes fibrosis and calcification resulting in a single dense opacity or in multiple, small, 'buckshot' opacities. Rarely a single opacity enlarges gradually over a few years due to concentric layers of collagen being added to a healed primary focus. This so-called *histoplasmoma* may closely imitate a neoplasm but a central nidus or concentric rings of calcification are often present (Goodwin and Des Prez, 1978).

Chronic disease resembles fibro-cavernous tuberculosis.

Diagnosis depends on the occupational history and culture of *H. capsulatum* from the sputum or the histological features on biopsy. Rising titres of complement fixing antibodies in successive sera strongly suggest active disease. A positive histoplasmin skin test, however, only indicates remote or recent exposure and is not diagnostic. Differentiation from tuberculosis, psittacosis, coccidioidomycosis, tularaemia or tumour of the lung may be necessary according to what features the disease presents.

In Britain the possibility of an individual having contracted histoplasmosis while working in an occupational hazard in an endemic area should be remembered. Occasional cases have arisen from imported contaminated fomites (Ajello, 1971).

Prevention is difficult. Personal protection in the form of lightweight masks and protective clothing may be of some use when exposure is suspected. Known blackbird and chicken roosting sites should not be unnecessarily disturbed. When an area of soil is known or thought to be contaminated by the fungus it should be thoroughly treated with a 3 per cent solution of formalin before being disturbed (Storch *et al.*, 1980). So far as possible geologists, spelaeologists, ornithologists and archaeologists who are likely to visit bird or bat infested locations in endemic areas should be histoplasmin positive.

Coccidioidomycosis

Like histoplasmosis this is a disease of respiratory origin. It has acute primary and chronic forms which may be mild or disseminated and fatal. It is caused by inhalation of arthrospores of *Coccidioides immitis*, a soil-inhabiting fungus endemic to semi-arid regions of the USA and South America, which varies in virulence and antigenicity. It is apparently restricted to the western hemisphere and is unknown in Europe (Drutz and Catanzaro, 1978). Important factors in infection are long, dry summers, mild winters, a light soil productive of much dust which contains the spores, and windy conditions to scatter the dust. A widespread epidemic of coccidioidomycosis recently occurred in California following airborne dispersal of arthrospores by a high velocity dust storm (Flynn *et al.*, 1979).

Persons at risk in endemic areas are agricultural workers (including tractor drivers), cotton pickers, cotton gin and compress operators, grape pickers, road and construction workers and laboratory technicians. Anthropology, archaeology, geology and civil engineering students — particularly in California — have been affected by minor epidemic disease; and museum personnel handling unearthed specimens may be at risk (Werner *et al.*, 1972; Drutz and Catanzaro, 1978). In addition, it is important to recognize that transportation of contaminated material (as in the case of a cotton mill employee working with Californian cotton who had never been near the endemic areas) and laboratory infection may cause isolated cases of disease outside endemic areas (Gehlbach, Hamilton and Conant, 1973).

The histopathology consists of granulomatous lesions in which the fungus is readily demonstrated by periodic acid Schiff or Gomori stains.

Acute disease varies from a mild influenza-like illness to a severe pneumonic disease with intense pleuritic pain, cough, haemoptysis, myalgia and sometimes pleural effusion. Dissemination may occur early or late in about 0.5 per cent of cases due to haematogenous spread of sporangiospores. Negroes, Mexicans and Filipinos are particularly susceptible. Lesions develop in skin, bone and visceral organs.

Chronic disease follows acute disease in 2 to 8 per cent of cases and is usually symptomless, though cough and haemoptysis may occur. Sometimes, however, it is complicated by pleural effusion, empyema or spontaneous pneumothorax due to rupture of a cavity (Emmons *et al.*, 1977).

The *radiographic appearances* in acute disease are those of scattered patchy opacities often with bilateral hilar node enlargement. In chronic disease cavities, often single, which are usually thin-walled and may contain fluid, are seen. Occasionally there are miliary shadows.

Diagnosis depends on occupational history, isolation of the fungus in culture or its demonstration in sputum, pus or tissue sections. It may be necessary to differentiate the disease from tuberculosis, histoplasmosis or carcinoma of lung.

Prevention. In California guide-lines have been set for dealing with potential occupational exposures (Schmelzer and Tabershaw, 1968).

North American blastomycosis

This is a systemic fungal infection which originates in, and may be confined to, the respiratory tract. The causal organism is *Blastomyces dermititidis* the origin of which is uncertain but is thought to be from a restricted distribution in soil and organic debris. Infection in both man and animals is believed to result from inhalation of conidia in dust (Emmons *et al.*, 1977). Although the disease is most common in the North American continent a substantial number of cases occur in South America and Africa, and a few in the Middle East and India. It is believed not to occur in Europe but infection due to *B. dermatitidis* has been reported in a French Tunisian and in an individual in Poland, neither of whom were ever in North America (Drouhet *et al.*, 1968; Kowalska *et al.*, 1976).

It is difficult to prove occupational origin in individual cases but acute blastomycosis in a professional horticulturist was traced to *B. dermatitidis* isolated from pigeon manure which he had used as a fertilizer and subsequently stored in a hot house (Sarosi and Serstock, 1976). The disease is most prevalent in people with occupations involving contact with the soil and wooded areas. These include farmers, farm workers, labourers, construction workers, gardeners, oil field workers, woodmen, miners and heavy equipment workers (Veterans' Administration Cooperative Study on Blastomycosis, 1964). Some affected persons in cities have regularly visited remote rural areas (Sarosi, 1979). An outbreak of disease in the members of four families was associated with their cooperative effort to build a cabin on a wooded lake side (Tosh *et al.*, 1974). Laboratory technicians may be infected from agar plate cultures. The highest incidence of blastomycosis in the world is in the Mississippi region of the USA.

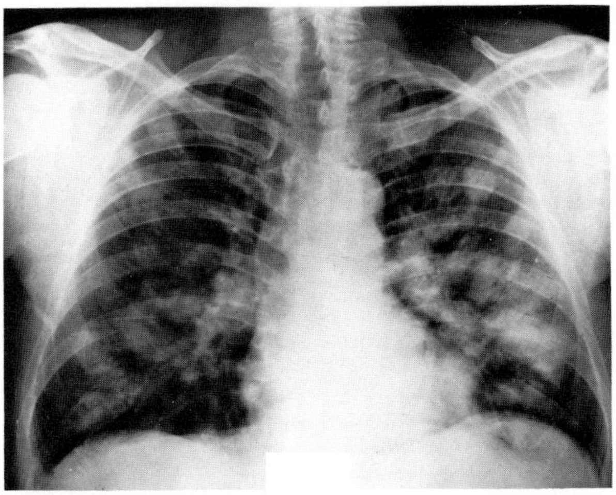

(a)

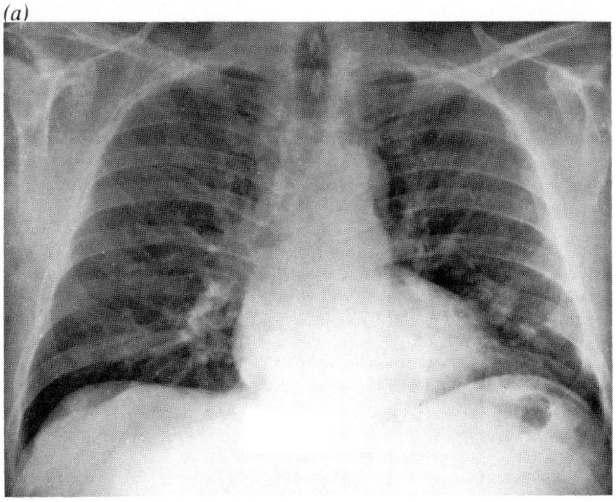

(b)

Figure 11.17 (a) Multiple ill-defined, round opacities due to acute blastomycotic pneumonia in a 52 year old man who assisted in building a lakeside log cabin. He developed fever, photophobia, arthralgia and persistent cough with sputum from which, after digestion with 10 per cent KOH, B. dermatitidis *was cultured. The blastomycin skin test was positive. (b) The radiographic changes resolved spontaneously and, although his health returned to normal within a few weeks, some opacities indicative of healed granulomas were still present in the left lower lung field seven years later. (Permission of Dr G. A. Sarosi and the Editor of* Radiology*)*

Like tuberculosis the disease takes three forms: *acute or primary, subacute or post-primary* and *chronic* (Sarosi and Davies, 1979). The acute phase consists of proliferative epithelioid granulomas with giant cells and radiographic changes indicative of pulmonary infiltration or consolidation which may take a multiple nodular form (*Figure 11.17*). This stage may resolve spontaneously or progress to post-primary disease which is occasionally miliary and fatal. But subacute disease is usually mild and not always preceded by an obvious primary illness. Chronic disease is clinically and radiographically identical to chronic tuberculosis; skin, bones and other organs may be affected (Baum and Schwarz, 1959; Laskey and Sarosi, 1978).

Diagnosis rests on occupational history, and identification of *B. dermatitidis* in the sputum digested with 10 per cent KOH or by culture of the organism. It may have to be differentiated from pneumonic and other granulomatous pulmonary disease (including histoplasmosis and coccidioidomycosis), nodular pneumoconiosis and carcinoma of the lung.

Cryptococcosis (torulosis)

This mycosis, which is both pulmonary and systemic, is caused by *Cryptococcus neoformans.* The lung disease is often mild but may be pneumonic, sometimes with pleural effusion, and severe. Occasionally solitary nodules containing the fungus are found in the lungs, Strains of varying virulence are often present in old pigeon nests and in accumulated guano under pigeon roosts, on buildings and on window ledges in cities, and in stables and barns in rural areas. It is probable, therefore, that the disease may occur in people whose occupations involve disturbing these deposits, such as demolition and farm workers (Emmons *et al.*, 1977).

The chest radiographic shows unilateral or bilateral, blotchy opacities or, on occasion, a solitary opacity. The fungus can be identified in or cultured from the sputum, and a complement fixation test for antigen is helpful but false negative results are fairly common.

Sporotrichosis

This occurs throughout the world in both temperate and tropical climates and is caused by *Streptothrix schenkii.* Granulomatous and pyogenic lesions are usually confined to the skin and superficial lymph nodes and only rarely affect the lungs but when they do the disease is clinically and radiographically indistinguishable from tuberculosis.

The fungus grows in soil, vegetation and rotting mine timbers. Hence, lung disease has been reported in farm workers, nursery men and miners (Baum *et al.*, 1969; Zvetina, Rippon and Daum, 1978).

OIL GRANULOMA (LIPOID PNEUMONIA)

Oils have some importance as an uncommon cause of

occupational lung disease and of pulmonary disease of non-occupational origin which may give rise to diagnostic difficulty in individuals exposed to a pneumoconiosis risk.

Aspiration of milk, olive oil, cod liver oil and mineral paraffin oil used as a laxative or in nasal drops has been known for years as a cause of lipoid pneumonia in the young, elderly and chronically sick. Oily nose drops are no longer widely used but are still available. Occasionally the disease has been caused by poppy seed oil as a bronchography medium.

Mineral oils are the chief cause of lipoid pneumonia in industry. They are used extensively as lubricants and cutting fluids and, in fluid or spray form, for turning, milling and grinding operations. They are employed in drop forging, metal rolling, in the jute and rope industry, as a base for synthetic fibre finishers and in high speed dental drills. Their physical character varies from thin spindle oil to thick, heavy oils according to the purpose for which they are required. Many of these operations are capable of producing a fine oil mist or vapour. Mineral oils have also found use as vehicles for spraying insecticides and other agents.

Lung disease caused by inhalation of mineral oil sprays was described by Pendergrass (1942) in a metal turner and by Proudfit, van Ordstrand and Miller (1950) in a man using a spray to lubricate cash registers. Subsequently, oil granuloma has been reported in workers exposed to mineral oil sprays used for insect extermination (Seidel, 1959) and cleaning aircraft (Foe and Bigham, 1954), and generated by compressed air jets applied to machine parts for removal of surface oil (Weissman, 1951). Exposure to burning animal and vegetable fats over a prolonged period during the testing of fire extinguishers on flash fires has, apparently, caused the disease (Oldenburger *et al.*, 1972); and oil pneumonitis followed aspiration of diesel oil contaminated sea water by survivors from torpedoed ships in both World Wars (Weissman, 1951). Increased linear opacities have been described in the chest radiographs of workers exposed to oil mists arising from the cold water reduction of mineral-oilcoated, hot-rolled strip steel, but the significance of this observation is uncertain (Jones, 1961)

More recent studies of men exposed to oil mists in machine shops, however, have not revealed any attributable respiratory symptoms, impairment of lung function or radiographic abnormality (Hendricks *et al.*, 1962; Ely *et al.*, 1970; Goldstein Benoit and Tyroler, 1970; Pasternack and Ehrlich, 1972; Welter, 1978).

There are a number of possible reasons for these differences in disease potential including differing work conditions over the years and the methodology of investigation. The comparative responses of the human respiratory tract to different mineral oils do not seem to be known so that some may be more harmful than others. Again, oil in work atmospheres may be present either in the droplet phase (mist) or vapour phase. The life span of droplets, which usually range from about 1 to 5 μm in diameter, depends largely on the boiling point of the oil. Those having high boiling points (and high molecular weights) persist as a fine aerosol for a long time whereas those with low boiling points have a fleeting existence — a few milliseconds. Furthermore increase in temperature from 20 (for example) to 37 °C, as may occur between ambient and tidal air, shortens droplet life dramatically. These points, incidentally, have an important bearing on methods of sampling oil in the atmosphere (Muir and Emmett, 1976; Davies, 1977). Oils with a very short droplet life (such as kerosene) are unlikely to offer a threat to the lungs unless present in enormous concentration but those with higher boiling points and longer life may be potentially harmful. However, little seems to be known about the effect on the lungs of oil in the vapour phase. In principle, therefore, it appears that mineral oils are only likely to cause lung disease if present in the atmosphere in high concentration or if their boiling points are in excess of about 300 °C.

Today the occupational circumstances which might cause oil granuloma of lungs are prolonged exposure to a long-life oil mist; a single sudden, accidental exposure to very high concentrations of oil droplets; and immersion in and aspiration of oil contaminated water.

PATHOLOGY

Droplets averaging 2.5 μm have been shown to pass through the nasal passages of mice exposed for up to four days to an oil mist and those which reach the alveoli are quickly taken up by alveolar macrophages and transported

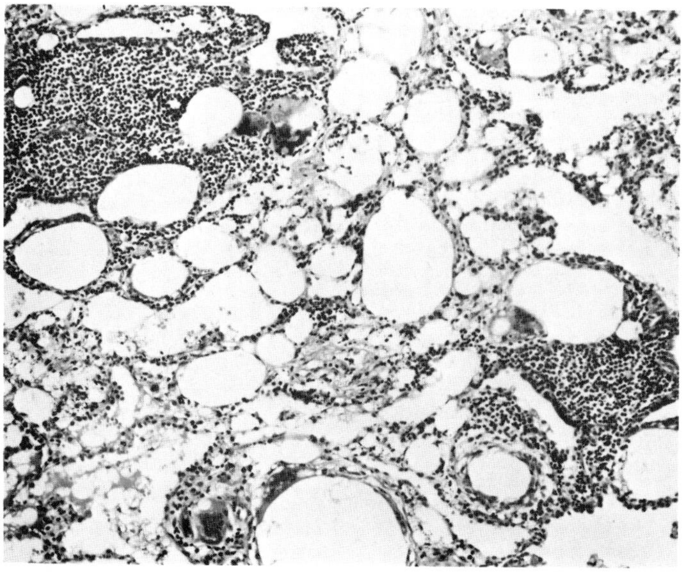

Figure 11.18 Microsection of Stage III oil granulomas due to aspiration of mineral oil. Foreign body giant cells are present in some areas and there is some early, loose, collagenous fibrosis. The enlarged alveolar spaces were occupied by oil globules dissolved out during fixing but clearly demonstrated by Sudan in frozen section; osmium tetroxide stain negative. (Original magnification ×160. H and E stain)

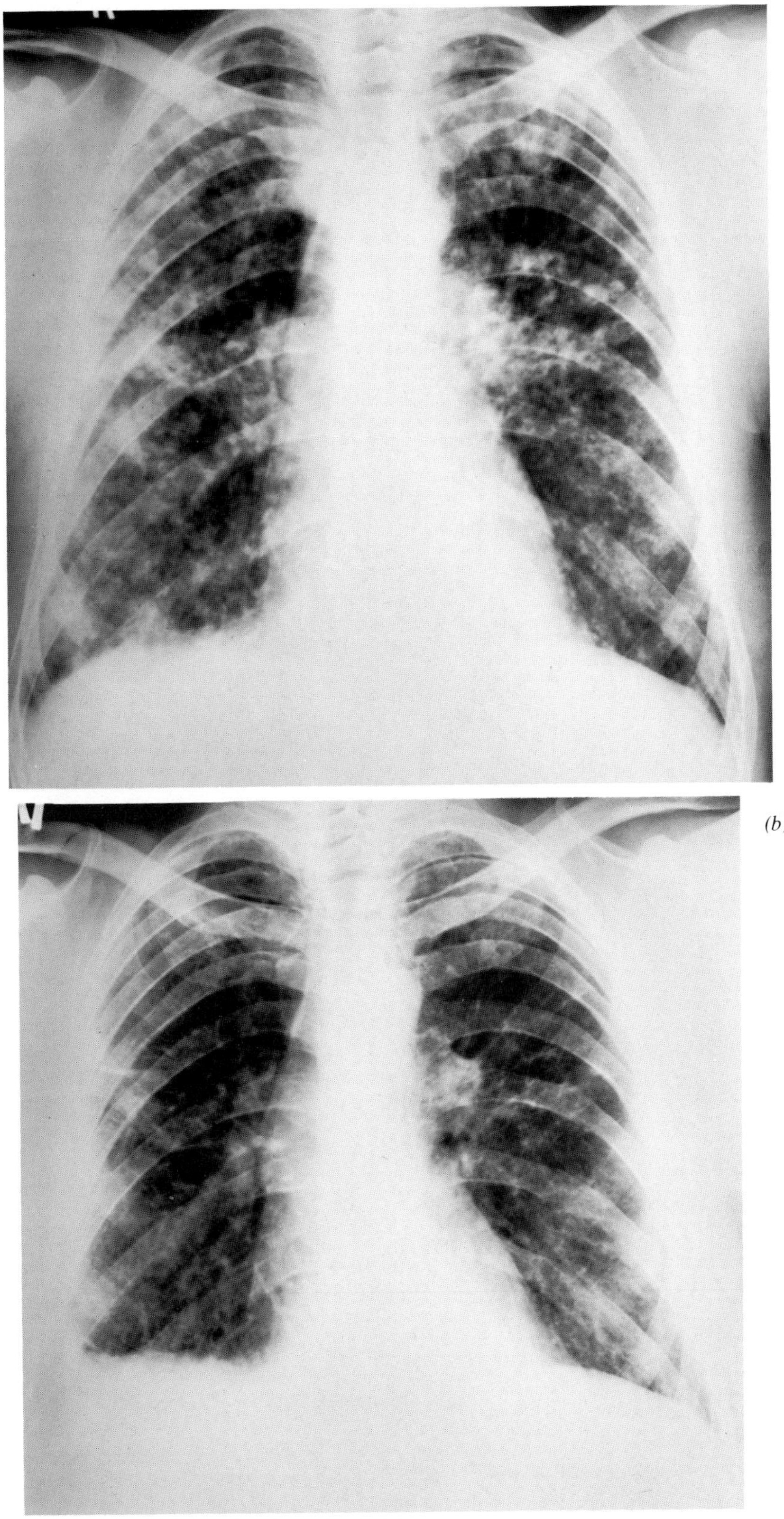

(a)

(b)

Figure 11.19 (a) Multiple opacities due to accidental aspiration of diesel oil aerosol. (b) Appearances seven years later with evidence of residual fibrosis. Coal miner exposed underground to a hot oil mist from sudden accidental leakage of a diesel engine. Initially coal pneumoconiosis wrongly diagnosed but lipoid pneumonia later confirmed by biopsy to pulmonary connective tissue and lymph nodes (Shoskes, Banfield and Rosenbaum, 1950).

The gross appearances of the lungs in man are those of a diffuse interstitial pneumonia or a localized dense fibrotic mass which often occupies the upper part of the lung.

The development of lesions is probably similar whether they are due to mineral, animal or vegetable oils and it has been subdivided into four stages by Wagner, Adler and Fuller (1955).

Stage I Haemorrhagic bronchopneumonia in which macrophages and giant cells quickly appear and take up oil droplets.

Stage II Numerous oil-laden macrophages in the alveoli the walls of which are epithelialized and thickened by infiltration of lymphocytes and plasma cells, and by reticulin proliferation. Oil-bearing macrophages are present in the lymphatics, lymphoid follicles are hyperplasic and there is endarteritis obliterans.

Stage III Development of loose collagenous fibrosis of the alveolar walls in which globules of oil and oil-containing macrophages are enmeshed and some loss of alveolar pattern. Numerous giant cell granulomas resembling tubercles are present. Endarteritis is prominent, and disruption of elastic fibres and bronchiolectasis are usual (*Figure 11.18*).

Stage IV Normal lung architecture is obliterated by dense fibrosis in which there are areas of hyaline degeneration and necrosis. Arterioles are completely occluded and bronchioles degenerated and flattened. Globules of oil are pooled in the fibrous tissue but granulomas have disappeared.

Exactly how mineral and other oils cause these changes is not fully understood.

Inhalation of shellac in sprays used in the furniture trade and in hair sprays appears to have caused disease similar to stages III and IV lipoid pneumonia (Hirsch and Russell, 1945; McLaughlin, Bidstrup and Konstam, 1963). This is discussed further in the next section.

Oil can only be identified in frozen sections as it is dissolved out in formalin-fixed and stained microsections. Vegetable and cod liver oils stain scarlet with Sudan IV and black with osmium tetroxide whereas mineral oil is paler red with Sudan IV and is *not* stained by osmium tetroxide (Wagner, Adler and Fuller, 1955).

CLINICAL FEATURES

Symptoms and abnormal physical signs are absent in most cases but occasionally cough, sputum, breathlessness on effort and unilateral or bilateral basal crepitations may be present. There may be restriction of ventilation and reduction in gas transfer and, on effort, Pa_{O_2} without airflow obstruction (Weill *et al.*, 1964). In cases of accidental aspiration of an oil-water mixture the features may be those of 'shock lung' with sequelae caused by the oil.

RADIOGRAPHIC APPEARANCES

These are disparate. There may be small discrete opacities either in groups or widespread throughout both lung fields having, in some cases, a miliary appearance (*Figure 11.19*). In other cases there are irregular opacities similar to those of DIPF in the lower halves of the lung fields; or, again, single or multiple large opacities. A single opacity is usually associated with medicinal oil aspiration (*Figure 8.45*), and multiple large opacities are most likely to result from massive aspiration of oil-contaminated water (*Figure 11.20*).

DIAGNOSIS

A thorough occupational history and enquiry into the use of oily nasal drops or laxatives are essential. And the possibility of aspiration of diesel oil should be considered in any case of pneumonic disease following immersion in the sea or water in ships' holds or factory vessels.

Repeated identification of oil-laden macrophages in sputum stained with Sudan IV or with benzpyrene caffeine examined by fluorescence microscopy strongly suggests the diagnosis (Weill *et al.*, 1964). Though oil-containing macrophages are occasionally seen with chronic inflammatory lung disease and histiocytosis X the history and other features of the disease should readily distinguish them.

The radiographic appearances are neither specific nor very helpful: discrete opacities may be mistaken for pneumoconiosis (*Figure 11.19*), sarcoidosis, tuberculosis and other causes of such opacities (*see Table 5.2*). Large opacities are likely to be mistaken for eevidence of primary or secondary neoplasia or interpreted as PMF (*Figure 8.45*).

Lung biopsy may be needed to establish diagnosis.

In many cases some degree of spontaneous resolution of disease may occur but with treatment, may be complete.

TREATMENT

If still exposed to an oily atmosphere the individual should be removed from it without delay.

Oral prednisolone causes a striking resolution of disease: oil-containing macrophages increase in the sputum and oil deposits in the lungs are reduced (Ayvazian *et al.*, 1967) (*Figure 11.20*).

PREVENTION

Oil aerosols in machine shops and other factory situations are greatly reduced or eliminated by enclosure of processes, automation and efficient exhaust ventilation systems. These methods usually keep the atmospheric concentrations below the recommended TLVs. Periodic medical examinations should be carried out. In other circumstances, however, it is difficult to prevent accidental exposure.

The possibility that carcinoma of the lung might be related to prolonged exposure to mineral oil mists is referred to briefly in Chapter 14.

LUNG DISEASE ASSOCIATED WITH HAIR SPRAYS

Aerosol hair sprays contain three essential components: the propellant, solvents and other ingredients and the active agent.

The propellants commonly used are fluorochlorohydrocarbons (trade name, Freons) which are gases at room

(a)

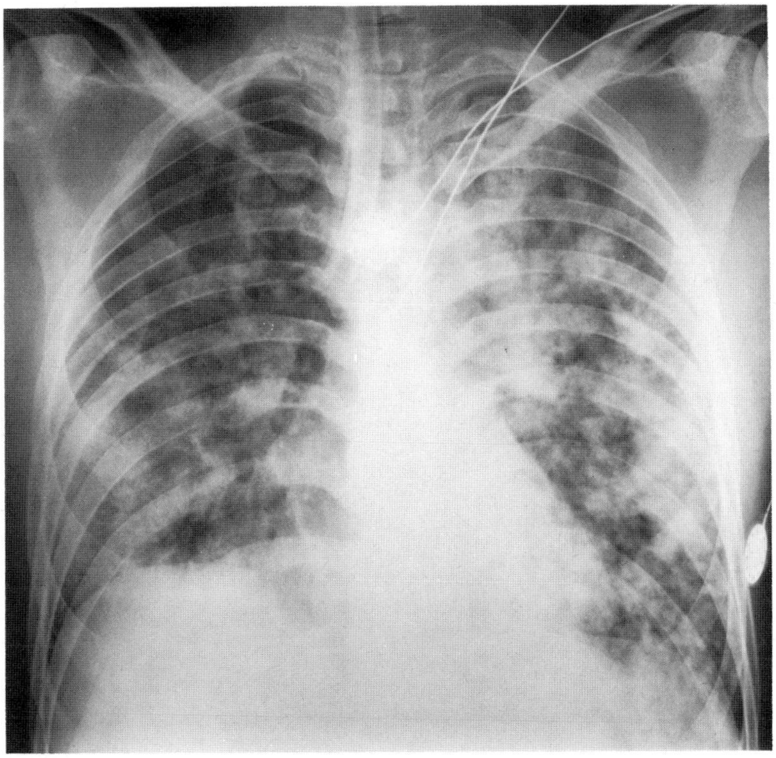

Figure 11.20 Acute aspiration lipoid pneumonia. The case of a marine engineer who, on entering a ship's ballast tank to investigate a pump failure, was overcome by an oxygen depleted atmosphere and fell unconscious, face down, into a mixture of sea water and diesel oil. He was quickly rescued and recovered consciousness in a few minutes. After about four hours, during which he appeared to suffer little ill-effect, he became acutely ill with fever, cough and severe dyspnoea and was admitted to intensive care. (a) Film taken in supine position. In spite of clinical improvement substantial radiographic abnormality persisted but gradually resolved with prednisolone treatment. (b) Twelve months later (standard film, erect) some abnormal shadows remain in the right cardiophrenic angle and left mid zone. Lung function at this time: mild decrease in FEV_1, FVC and TLC with moderate reduction of RV and gas transfer. (Dr J. B. Wilkinson's case reproduced with permission)

(b)

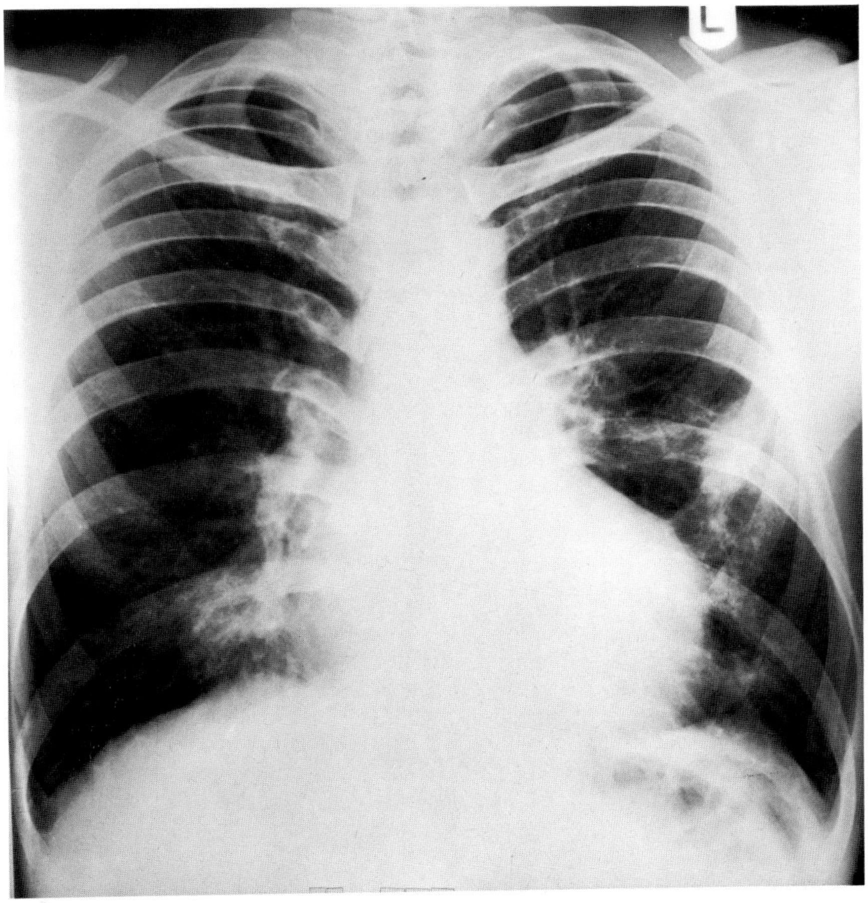

temperature and virtually inert so that they do not react with other materials in the canister. Vinyl chloride is also added in some preparations (Gay *et al.*, 1975) (*see* next section).

Solvents and other ingredients include ethyl alcohol, aromatic oils, castor oil and lanolin or its derivatives.

Active agents

(1) Polyvinylpyrrolidone (PVP).
(2) Polyvinyl acetate (PVA) and a co-polymer PVP-PVA.
(3) Shellac. Dewaxed shellac mixed in some preparations with castor oil and aromatic oils. Sometimes combined with one of the polyvinyls.
(4) Dimethyl hydantoin-formaldehyde resin.
(5) Modified polyacrylic acid resin.
(6) Lanolin.

The possibility that inhalation of hair sprays may be responsible for lung disease was suggested by Bergmann, Flance and Blumenthal in 1958 and thought to be due to persistence of macromolecules of PVP or its co-polymers in the lungs. It was thus considered to be a 'storage' disorder or '*thesaurosis*'. But the existence of a cause-and-effect relationship has since been widely disputed on the grounds that other causes of disease have not been satisfactorily excluded in individual cases and that, in general, surveys of exposed populations and animal studies have not confirmed its existence.

Hairdressers, both male and female, and 'beauticians' are occupationally exposed but, in the home, women may frequently use, and children play with hair sprays. Hence, exposure is very widespread.

The size distribution of the spray aerosols is evidently important in regard to their ability to reach the gas exchanging region of the lungs but reported data are widely and remarkably contradictory. At one extreme more than 50 per cent of particles were in excess of 35 μm (Brunner *et al.*, 1963); in between, there are reports of a mass median diameter of 7.8 μm (Swift, Zuskin and Bouhuys, 1976), 50 per cent of particles being smaller than 8.5 μm (Draize *et al.*, 1959) and of 20 per cent being less than 3 μm (Ripe *et al.*, 1969). At the other extreme the majority of particles were under 2 μm diameter (McLaughlin, Bidstrup and Konstam, 1963). Undoubtedly these discrepancies were due to differences in sampling and sizing techniques.

Microscopically, disease attributed to hair sprays has been variously described as DIPF with hilar lymphadenopathy (Bergmann, Flance and Blumenthal, 1958; Bergmann *et al.*, 1962; McLaughlin, Bidstrup and Konstam, 1963), sarcoid-type granulomas (Bergmann *et al.*, 1962) or foreign body granulomas (Gowdy and Wagstaff, 1972; Gebbers *et al.*, 1980). In some cases the features have been those of a desquamative fibrosing 'alveolitis'. Intracytoplasmic, PAS-positive granules observed in macrophages in lung tissue and in lymph nodes have been thought to be diagnostic of PVP particles (Bergmann *et al.*, 1962) but similar PAS-staining granules may be seen in sarcoid and other granulomas, and chemical analysis has failed to demonstrate PVP. Brunner *et al.* (1963) discounted PVP as a cause of lung disease. But a characteristic infrared absorption spectrum of PVA, not seen in normal lungs, has been reported in a case of alleged 'hairspray lung' by Ripe *et al.* (1969) who pointed out that whereas PVP is water-soluble PVA is only slightly so and is precipitated in the presence of water into plastic droplets ranging from 0.1 to 20 μm diameter. In theory, therefore, PVA is likely to be precipitated on airway walls and could be more injurious than PVP. PVP and PVA are apparently eliminated by the kidney when their molecular weights are less than 20 000 but are retained when these are 60 000 to 70 000 (Gebbers *et al.* 1980).

It has been argued, however, that many of these cases are, in fact, examples of sarcoidosis (Herrero, Feigelson and Becker, 1965; Schepers, 1962) though this does not appear to be true of them all.

The possibility that oily or fatty substances in PVP and 'mixed' sprays might give rise to granulomatous and fibrotic lesions seems to have received little or no attention. The patient described by McLaughlin, Bidstrup and Konstam (1963), in whom sarcoidosis was apparently excluded, was exposed to shellac-based sprays. Inhalation of shellac in the furniture trade is known to have caused a fibrosing lung disease presumed to be due to its high fatty acid content and related oils (Hirsch and Russell, 1945) (*see* previous section). Shellac consists of lac (which is a resinous material obtained from insects of the Coccidae family, *Laccifer lacca*) in a solvent which, in hair lacquers, is often an oil as indicated already. Lac itself is highly purified and consists essentially of complex fatty acids but no insect remains. It seems likely, therefore, that disease associated with shellac inhalation may be an oil granuloma and not, as was suggested in the first edition of this book, a possible example of extrinsic allergic 'alveolitis' due to insect protein.

It is improbable that the relatively inert and insoluble Freons, which resist chemical transformation and absorption of water, are responsible for disease but some suspicion may attach to vinyl chloride (*see* p. 401).

EPIDEMIOLOGY

Radiographic surveys of 2155 hairdressers in Britain, the USA, Italy and Germany revealed only 12 possible cases (Cambridge, 1973). However, a study of 500 students and graduate beauticians in the USA compared with controls matched for age, smoking habits and geographic locality is reported to have shown unspecified abnormalities of the chest radiographs, reduced VC and gas transfer, and atypical cells in the sputum; but no quantitative or other details are given (Frank, 1975). Nonetheless, the incidence of the disease—if it exists as a specific entity—is evidently very low.

EXPERIMENTAL OBSERVATIONS

Following brief exposure to various hair sprays by volunteers transient changes in their maximal expiratory flow-volume curves were observed by Zuskin and Bouhuys (1974) but the presence of abnormal airways function was not confirmed by Cohen (1976) and Friedman *et al.* (1977). Acute exposure of non-smokers to a hair spray aerosol, however, resulted in short-lived impairment of tracheal mucociliary transport which lasted under three hours whereas similar inhalation of Freon propellant alone had no effect (Friedman *et al.*, 1977).

Exposure of various species of animals to hair spray aerosols has failed to provoke pulmonary disease (Calandra and Kay, 1958; Draize *et al.*, 1959; Giovacchini *et al.*, 1965; Lowsma, Jones and Prendergast, 1966). After almost continuous exposure of guinea pigs for five days a week for 12 months to hair spray particles ranging from 0.6 to 1.2 μm diameter, there were no histopathological changes other than progressive lymphoid infiltration which, however, was also observed in a control group of animals maintained during the same period (Cambridge, 1973). But the possibility that a granulomatous response can be induced in animals treated previously with Freund's adjuvant raises the question of hypersensitivity (Gialdroni, Grassi and Clini, 1964) for which at present, however, there appears to be no convincing evidence in man. Although, in one case it appears that pulmonary infiltration which had cleared when exposure ceased reappeared when use of hair spray was resumed and disappeared yet again when it was once more stopped (Bergmann, 1973).

Storage of PVP does not seem to have been established in any of the reported cases of 'thesaurosis' but was shown to occur in the reticulo-endothelial system following intravenous injection, as was discovered when PVP was used some years ago as an inert plasma substitute.

CLINICAL FEATURES

Affected individuals may complain of cough and breathlessness, sometimes with mild pyrexia, but others are symptomless. Abnormal physical signs are few or absent.

The chest radiograph may show patchy bilateral infiltrates, fine linear opacities, a clear DIPF pattern or the appearances of lobar consolidation — the least frequently reported abnormality. After the use of sprays has ceased the radiographic appearances have returned to normal rapidly or within six months in most cases (suggesting that the sprays might have been the cause) but, in a few, resolution has taken about two years (Ripe *et al.*, 1969; Gowdy and Wagstaff, 1972).

Lung function tests have been described in very few cases and, on the whole, have shown little abnormality, but impairment of gas transfer was reported in cases with radiographic evidence of DIPF (Garibaldi and Caprotti, 1964).

CONCLUSION

When all the available evidence, much of which is circumstantial, is considered, inhalation of hair sprays has evidently not been proven to be a specific cause of lung pathology though they remain under suspicion in some cases. As 'storage' or accumulation of PVP or co-polymers in the lungs has not been demonstrated the term 'thesaurosis' is distracting and best abandoned.

Lung disease in individuals exposed to hair spray aerosols may be due to:

(1) unrelated and coincidental disease — possibly the most common explanation;
(2) lipoid pneumonia if there has been heavy exposure to oily shellac or lanolin preparations;
(3) some ingredient other than oils or fatty acids which is not the active agent or propellant;
(4) possibly PVA or vinyl chloride.

Hypersensitivity to any particular ingredient has not so far been demonstrated.

In attempting diagnosis the presence of PAS-positive granules in lung tissue is of no help, but staining for mineral and vegetable oils might be (*see* previous section).

If, in the individual patient, known causes of lung disease can be confidently excluded he or she should be advised to avoid further exposure whether at work or in the home.

Finally, as the use of hair sprays is so widespread and there is still a question as to whether they can occasionally cause disease more detailed and carefully controlled investigations than has been carried out so far seems desirable to establish once and for all whether we are faced with a rare, but real, disease or an illusion (Bergmann, 1973).

POLYVINYL CHLORIDE LUNG DISEASE

Polyvinyl chloride (PVC) has been used extensively in the plastics industry for some 30 years or more. It is produced by the polymerization of vinyl chloride monomer (VCM) (CH_2:CHCl)—a gas at normal temperature—under pressure at 40 to 70 °C. Polymerization does not normally proceed beyond about 95 per cent conversion so that some 5 to 6 per cent of monomer remains and is returned to the gas holders. However, because VCM has a strong affinity for PVC it is difficult to remove it all. PVC is dried in continuous driers and the resultant powder may contain about 50 ppm of VCM (Barnes, 1976). VCM is also used as a propellant in some aerosol sprays and as a refrigerant.

An association between prolonged exposure in the PVC production process and acro-osteolysis, Raynaud's disease, scleroderma, hepatomegaly with elevated alkaline phosphatase, and angiosarcoma of the liver is now well known although only apparent in recent years (Lilis *et al.*, 1975; Sakabe, 1975; Suciu *et al.*, 1975). Vinyl chloride monomer has been regarded as the responsible agent even in workers exposed only to PVC dust. Pulmonary disease, however, has rarely been described

Uses of PVC

Manufacture of floor coverings, imitation leather, a wide variety of plastic goods and synthetic fibres.

Sources of exposures

During production of VCM and PVC, drying and bagging of PVC and in the initial stages of plastics manufacture in which PVC particles are generally less than 5 μm diameter. High concentrations of VCM may be produced by hair spray or insecticide canisters in confined spaces (Gay *et al.*, 1975).

Experimentally

Inhalation of VCM and PVC by animals is reported to cause lung fibrosis (Frongia, Spinazzola and Bucarelli, 1974; Prodan *et al.*, 1975) although PVC is not apparently cytotoxic to alveolar and peritoneum macrophages *in vitro* (Styles and Wilson, 1973).

Epidemiological and clinical data

Some reduction in air flow which was related to age and duration of exposure to VCM and PVC in a processing plant and not thought to be wholly explained by smoking in workers aged 40 years or more has been reported by Miller *et al.* (1975), although prolonged exposure to the dust of PVC powder does not appear to be associated with impairment of ventilatory function (Chivers, Lawrence-Jones and Paddle, 1980). Asthma following exposure to fume from hot, PVC soft-wrap film is most probably caused by other agents and not by PVC (*see* Chapter 12, epoxy resin hardness).

Lilis *et al.* (1975) described an increased prevalence of irregular and small, rounded radiographic opacities mainly in the middle and lower lung fields of workers exposed to PVC and VCM but the significance of these changes is uncertain and still to be evaluated. However, their presence was associated with peripheral circulatory abnormalities.

Two cases of granulomatous disease with some collagen formation demonstrated by lung biopsy in men who were exposed to PVC dust have been described: one had shovelled the powder for a year in a plastics factory; the other had worked for 13 years in the bagging area of a polymerization plant. The chest radiographs showed either blotchy, irregular opacities or 'diffuse micronodular' opacities. PVC was extracted with a solvent from lung tissue in the one case and, in the other, electron microscopy revealed oval bodies about 0.3 to 0.4 μm in size identical to particles of PVC powder in the pulmonary macrophages (Szende *et al.*, 1970; Arnaud *et al.*, 1978).

There is some evidence that disease caused by PVC is an immune complex disorder initiated by the adsorption of vinyl chloride or a metabolite onto tissue or plasma protein (Ward *et al.*, 1976).

Conclusions

The evidence collected so far does not seem to provide incontrovertible proof that PVC or VCM are responsible for the patterns of lung disorders described, but it is suggestive and requires further investigation. Long-term observation of workers who have had prolonged exposure is clearly indicated. DIPF might, perhaps, follow granulomas.

Strict hygiene control in VCM polymerization plants and in the use of PVC powder for the manufacture of plastics, has been in force for a few years past because of the risk of serious extrapulmonary disease, so that the likelihood of new cases of lung disease occurring is now probably small. However, regular medical surveillance with ventilatory function tests and full size chest radiographs, in addition to other screening tests, is essential.

THERMOSETTING RESINS

A thermosetting resin containing methylene aminoacetonitrile and resorcinol used in the rubber tyre industry has been reported to cause laryngotracheobronchitis and pneumonic disease which improved during periods away from work and recurred on return. Airflow obstruction or reduced gas transfer was found in about one-third of exposed workers and chest radiographs showed bilateral blotchy opacities which cleared rapidly on cessation of exposure but returned with re-exposure in about one-quarter of cases. Biopsy revealed localized DIPF with cellular infiltration in one case.

The fact that a minority of exposed persons are affected and that disease may not occur for several weeks or months after initial contact but recurs rapidly on re-exposure suggests an allergic pathogenesis (doPico *et al.*, 1975).

TRIMELLITIC ANHYDRIDE (TMA)

This chemical is used extensively in the manufacture of plasticizers, alkyl resins for surface coatings applied to heated pipes, and paints, and as a curing agent for epoxy resins. Workers exposed to TMA vapour or dust in these processes or during its manufacture may develop three different respiratory syndromes:

(1) Rhinitis and immediate asthma after weeks or years of exposure (*see* Chapter 12).
(2) Late (non-immediate) or dual asthma frequently worse at night, also after prolonged exposure, with troublesome cough, haemoptysis, dyspnoea, malaise, rigors and myalgia (so-called 'TMA flu').
(3) Rhinorrhoea with occasional epistaxis, cough, wheezing and dyspnoea on the first heavy exposure followed by recovery in about eight hours.

The second syndrome, which has some of the features of extrinsic allergic 'alveolitis', may be of mild or moderate severity or potentially fatal with extensive bilateral opacities in the lower halves of both lung fields, like those of oedema, and is sometimes associated with anaemia of haemolytic or normochromic type, hypoxaemia and apparently *increased* gas transfer. This is referred to as the *TMA pulmonary disease-anaemia syndrome*. Lung biopsy has demonstrated alveolar wall congestion, intra-alveolar haemorrhages, and dense proteinaceous fluid, non-specific injury of alveolar walls and metaplasia of Type 11 cells but no inflammatory reaction (Rice *et al.*, 1977; Zeiss *et al.*, 1977; Ahmad *et al.*, 1979; Herbert and Orford, 1979; Patterson *et al.*, 1979).

TMA appears to act as a hapten which combines with autologous respiratory tract proteins resulting in an antibody response to these newly formed antigenic complexes. Subjects with immediate asthma and rhinitis give a Type 1 skin reaction on testing with TMA haptenized human serum albumin (TM–HSA) and have TMA–HSA-specific IgE antibodies. IgG and IgA antiTM–HSA antibodies are also present in patients with the pulmonary disease-anaemia syndrome but, at present, their significance is uncertain. The third type of TMA lung disease is not associated with any immunological changes (Patterson *et al.*, 1979; Zeiss *et al.*, 1980).

Asthma, whether of immediate or late type, may be sufficiently severe to impel the worker to leave the industry because renewed episodes may be provoked by entering parts of the factory away from the TMA source. As a rule complete recovery from the second type of illness with clearing of the chest radiograph occurs within a few weeks but in the severely ill appropriate supportive measures are needed and corticosteroids recommended. Iron treatment of anaemia is also required in some cases. Symptoms may recur on re-exposure.

EPOXY RESIN CURING MATERIAL

Epoxy resins are formed by chemical reaction of epoxy compounds (cyclic ethers or alkylene oxides) with one of a variety of curing agents to produce mechanically strong polymers which have a wide application as surface coatings, laminates, adhesive covering for electronic circuits and the like. There are many epoxy compounds and although an occasional case of pulmonary oedema following exposure is thought to have occurred, they have a low order of toxicity and appear to be insignificant as a cause of lung disease (Hine and Rowe, 1963); but they are an important cause of contact dermatitis (Malten and Zielhuis, 1964), and their decombustion at high temperatures (as by welding) evolves nitrogen dioxide (*see* Chapter 13). However, as described in the previous section, the inhalation of 'fumes' of the curing agent *trimellitic anhydride* used to activate epoxy compounds may cause significant respiratory disease.

POLYMER FUME FEVER

This is an influenza-like disorder, similar in many respects to metal fume fever (*see* p. 454), caused by pyrolysis products of tetrafluorethylene (TFE) resins: notably polytetrafluorethylene (PTFE — trade names: Fluon, Teflon and Halon) and polyvinyl fluoride.

PTFE resin is produced by controlled polymerization of TFE emulsion under pressure. It is then moulded in sintering ovens or by pressure processes. Physiologically it is inert and causes neither irritation nor allergic sensitization of body tissues. However, if heated to between 315 and 375 °C a particulate consisting, probably, of polymer chain fragments is evolved. Above 380 °C small amounts of the toxic gases hexafluoropropylene and octafluoroisobutylene are produced and at temperatures in excess of 500 °C (when the rate of pyrolysis increases) perfluoroisobutylene and carbonyl fluoride, which are also toxic, are formed. These toxic compounds can cause pulmonary oedema in animals (Harris, 1951; Okawa and Polakoff, 1974).

PTFE resins are used extensively for most modern plastics products including insulation materials, electrical components, bearings, gaskets, piping, coatings for wires, chemical vessels and non-stick cooking utensils, and in dirt-repellent starch sprays.

There is no hazard to health unless the polymer is subjected to heat in excess of 300 °C. This may occur in a variety of circumstances: the operation of moulding and extruding machines, high-speed machining of components, welding of metal coated with PTFE or attached to PTFE resin blocks, ironing clothes sprayed with polymer-starch mixture for prolonged periods, and smoking cigarettes contaminated with the polymer either by direct contact or by particles suspended in the workplace atmosphere. The temperature in the burning zone of a cigarette exceeds 800 °C (Touey and Mumpower, 1957; Harris, 1959; Adams, 1963; Lewis and Kerby, 1965; Williams and Smith, 1972; doPico *et al.*, 1973; Kuntz and McCord, 1974).

CLINICAL FEATURES

There is always a delay of some hours — often about three or four — between exposure to the 'fume' or particulate before symptoms develop.

Usually the first complaint is discomfort or an oppressive sensation in the chest and breathlessness with or without cough. General malaise, joint pains, rigors, sweating and pyrexia up to about 40 °C and tachycardia follow. Physical signs in the lungs are either absent or there may be a few scattered crepitations and the chest radiograph is normal. Recovery is complete in one to two days.

The illness is frequently regarded as influenza or some other acute infection by both patient and doctor unless there are recurrences. Hence, 'polymer fume fever' should be borne in mind in cases of 'pyrexia of unknown origin'.

The fundamental pathogenesis of the symptoms is not known. Unlike metal fume fever, to which tolerance is quickly acquired on repeated exposures and equally rapidly lost when exposure ceases during weekends or holidays, polymer fume fever seems to occur without regard to previous exposure (Kuntz and McCord, 1974; Malten and Zielhuis, 1964).

However, disease is not always so innocuous and pulmonary oedema may occasionally follow exposure to polymer subjected to high temperatures; for example, during welding. This is marked by respiratory distress and the physical and radiographic signs of oedema of the lungs. Recovery is rapid and no fatalities seem to have been reported (Robbins and Ware, 1964; Evans, 1973). Furthermore, DIPF appears to have followed numerous attacks of polymer fume fever caused by PTFE on cigarettes contaminated at work (Capodaglio, Monarco and de Vito, 1961; Williams, Atkinson and Patchefsky, 1974). Hence, although polymer fume fever is a benign and transient disorder in most instances continued observation of workers who have suffered multiple episodes is probably desirable.

It is likely that many cases of polymer fume fever and occasional cases of pulmonary oedema are overlooked.

PREVENTION

Enclosure and ventilation of the manufacturing processes, good housekeeping and prohibition of smoking where PTFE is cut, machined or processed are now general, and there is little hazard to health. Analysis of soluble fluoride levels in the urine is a helpful index of toxicity in workers who may have mild symptoms of polymer fume fever. The normal range is 0.098 to 2.19 mg/l (Okawa and Polakoff, 1974). Accidental, exposure to toxic pyrolysis products may occur in other circumstances from time to time.

PARAQUAT POISONING

Paraquat (known in Britain as Gramoxone which is concentrated and Weedol which is dilute, and in the USA as Orthoparaquat, Orthodualparaquat and Orthospot) is a bipyridyl herbicide which is used on a global scale in more than 130 countries. Its value in food production is due to its ability to destroy weeds on contact with their green parts while becoming harmless in the soil due to adsorption on to clay minerals (Conolly, 1975).

Paraquat is well known as a cause of serious lung disease which is commonly, but not invariably, fatal. The majority of cases have been due to ingestion of the liquid accidently from unmarked bottles or with suicidal intent (Bullivant, 1966; Campbell, 1968), and the possibility of absorption by routes other than the gastro-intestinal tract has been regarded, on the whole, as unimportant (Swan, 1969; Fairshter and Wilson, 1975). Certainly direct inhalation into the lungs from sprays is improbable as the particle size range appears to be too large (Kimburgh, 1974; Levin *et al.*, 1979), although paraquat mist drifting into a garden from nearby agricultural spraying operations has apparently caused non-fatal lung disease (George and Hedworth-Whitty, 1980). But absorption through intact or abraded skin and entry into the circulation can occur and is facilitated if paraquat is combined with a surface active 'wetting' agent as is usually the case (McDonagh and Martin, 1970; Jaros, 1978; Levin *et al.*, 1979). Hence, although paraquat has occasionally been drunk accidently by agricultural or horticultural workers the chief occupational hazard is percutaneous absorption of spray solution.

The severity of the *clinical presentation* following the ingestion of paraquat appears to depend on the dose taken, 20 to 40 mg/kg probably being fatal (Conolly, 1975). There is vomiting, abdominal pain, diarrhoea and burning, reddening and ulceration of the mouth and pharynx. With massive doses death may occur within a few hours in coma and cardiorespiratory failure but, in those who survive, longer acute kidney and liver damage occurs. In milder cases lung disease with bilateral or unilateral crepitations and pneumonic-type or small round radiographic opacities develop in two to five days. This is often followed by progressive fibrosis but in some cases the disease appears to resolve completely with supportive treatment only (Conolly, 1975; Higenbottam *et al.*, 1979). Disease following percutaneous absorption is likely to be less severe than that following intestinal absorption. Cases due to the former can be distinguished by a lack of reddening and ulceration of mouth and pharynx and gastro-intestinal disturbance, and by the presence of erythema and burning of the area of contaminated skin sometimes with ulceration.

Jaros (1978) described a fatality following exposure of the skin of an agricultural worker to concentrated paraquat which leaked from a container on to his neck, back and legs. Six days later he had respiratory distress which rapidly worsened. The chest radiograph showed multiple, small and occasional coalescent opacities. Pulmonary oedema and necrotizing 'alveolitis' were present at post mortem. Levin *et al.* (1979) have reported the case of ten workers who sprayed weeds in a vineyard with Gramoxone. One had balanced a leaky spray reservoir on his shoulder resulting in a burnt area of skin with ulceration, subsequent dyspnoea, cyanosis, crepitations, bilateral ill-defined opacities in the chest radiograph and rapid deterioration to death in respiratory failure (*Figure 11.21*). Of the other nine who were less heavily exposed but whose trousers were always soaked with spray below the knees with burning and redness of the underlying skin, none had distinctive symptoms but six had a reduced gas transfer. In three of these in whom the reduction was greatest there were 'increased basal markings' in the chest radiograph. Lung biopsy in two men showed medial hypertrophy of pulmonary arteries with evidence of fresh and organized thrombi and, in one, DIPF. The remaining three cases showed no abnormality. It is possible that mild lesions may regress completely.

Apparently patients who survive an episode of paraquat poisoning do not have clinically significant residual pulmonary damage although occasionally there are irreversible radiographic changes (Fitzgerald *et al.*, 1979).

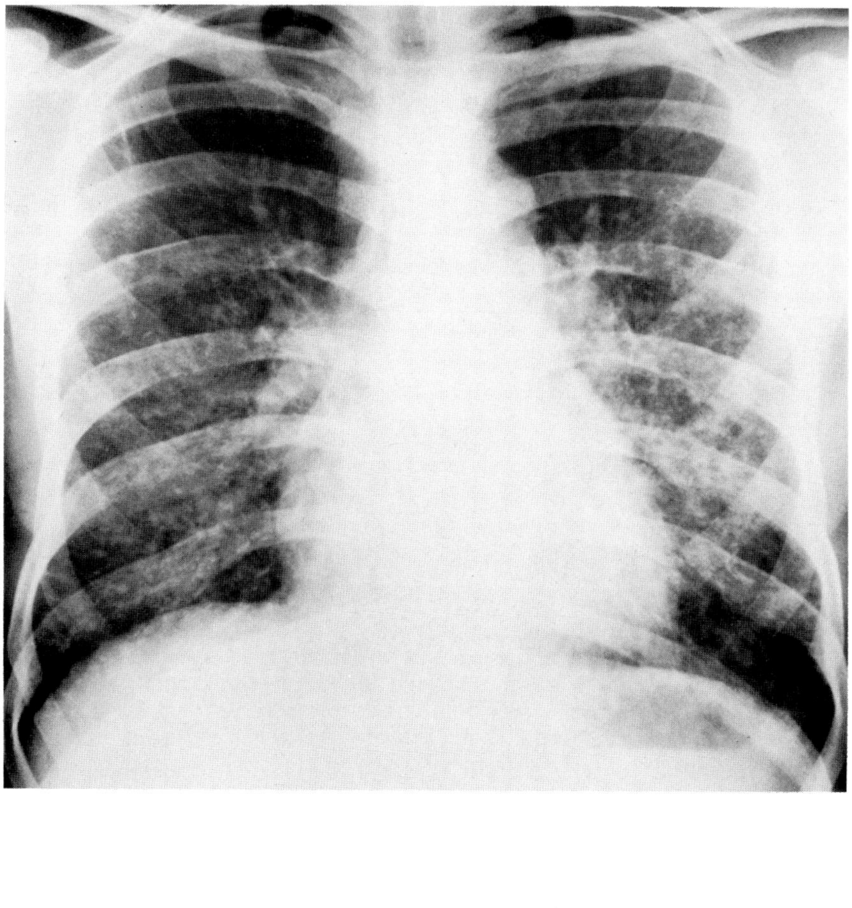

Figure 11.21 Bilateral soft opacities following percutaneous absorption of paraquat from a leaky spray reservoir. Man in good health two weeks earlier (see text). (By permission of Levin and colleagues and the Editors of Thorax*)*

PATHOLOGY

Two distinct phases are recognizable. The first, a destructive phase, consists of swelling and fragmentation of the alveolar epithelium followed by alveolar oedema and an acute inflammatory exudate. In the second, which is proliferative, there is a diffuse cellular *intra-alveolar* — not mural — fibrosis. This becomes dense and obliterates the pulmonary architecture. Medial hypertrophy of muscular pulmonary arteries which may contain organizing thrombi is often present (Smith and Heath, 1975; Thurlbeck and Thurlbeck, 1976; Fitzgerald *et al.*, 1979) (*Figure 11.22*).

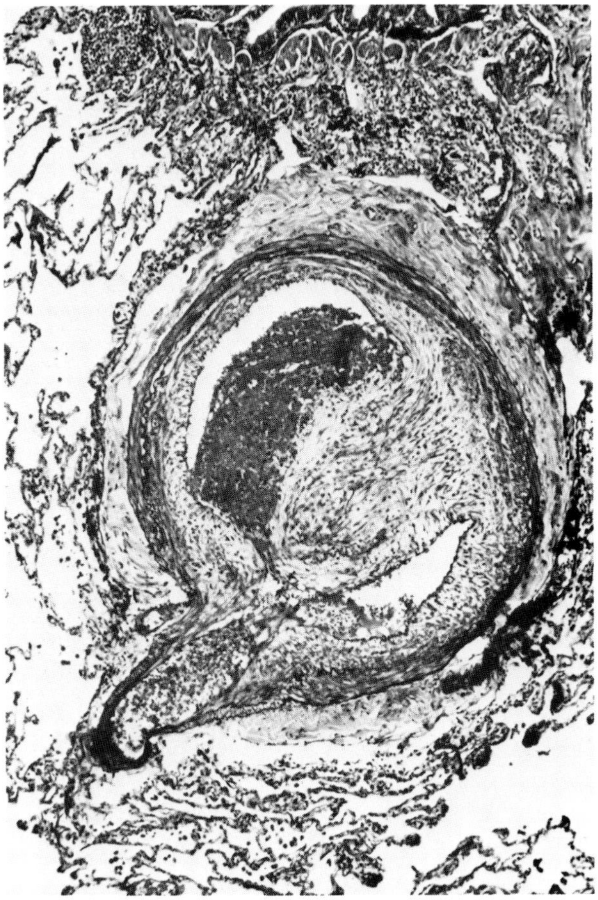

Figure 11.22 Biopsy of lung from the same patient as Figure 11.21 *showing a pulmonary artery with muscular hyperplasia and recent organizing thrombus. (Original magnification × 30. Elastic van Giesen.) (By permission of Levin and colleagues and the Editors of* Thorax*)*

Levin *et al.* (1979) were able to reproduce changes in the pulmonary arteries of rats whose skin had been painted at weekly intervals with a paraquat solution which were identical to those in human lungs. They attributed these lesions in both man and animals, not to chronic hypoxia (Smith and Heath, 1975), but to paraquat itself absorbed in low dosage through the skin over a prolonged period in contrast to the extensive alveolar changes caused by high ingested doses.

DIAGNOSIS

This depends upon the clinician being aware that paraquat poisoning may occasionally occur occupationally from percutaneous absorption. A careful history is, therefore, required. The skin of arms, shoulders, legs and feet must be inspected for 'burns', erythema and ulceration or abrasions; and also the mouth and pharynx to exclude the possibility of ingestion. Other acute pulmonary disorders must, of course, be excluded.

Measurement of plasma paraquat concentrations may be of value in assessing the severity and predicting the outcome of poisoning (Proudfoot, *et al.*, 1979).

TREATMENT

Gastric lavage and large doses of fuller's earth used in cases of paraquat poisoning by ingestion are unlikely to be relevant in lung disease. As paraquat generates superoxide — a reactive form of oxygen — which may be the toxic agent and which is normally inactivated by the enzyme superoxide dismutase, administration of this enzyme intravenously and by nebulized aerosol has been suggested (Saltzman and Fridovich, 1973). The inflammatory reaction in the lungs may possibly be reduced by large doses of beclomethasone or prednisolone (Davies and Conolly, 1975). The use of oxygen therapy, however, might well make the superoxide destructive process worse and thus endanger life (Rebello and Mason, 1978).

PREVENTION

Education of workers in the use of paraquat sprays, avoidance of spillage or leakage of concentrated paraquat (for example, when decanting) and wearing of protective clothing and impervious footwear during spraying operations.

ORGANIC INSECTICIDES

CHLORINATED CAMPHENE (TOXAPHENE)

This is a waxy material containing chlorine. When ingested it causes acute stimulation of the central nervous system in man and animals. It is used against cotton worms and other pests.

Inhalation may cause bilateral pneumonic disease which ranges radiographically from the appearances of pulmonary oedema to widespread miliary opacities in the middle and lower zones (Warraki, 1963). The underlying cause is not known.

Recovery is usually complete by eight weeks.

ORGANOPHOSPHATES

Chief among these are *parathion* and *malathion* which may be absorbed via the skin, gastro-intestinal tract or the lungs. They cause an excessive cholinergic effect by inhibiting the enzyme acetylcholinesterase at nerve endings. This results in excessive sweating and salivation, meiosis, bradycardia, increased peristalsis and bronchial secretions and, in some cases, pulmonary oedema of sudden onset which, if not treated promptly, is likely to be fatal (Bledsoe and Seymour, 1972). It is imperative, therefore, to anticipate the possibility of development of lung disease.

Those who are at risk from these chemicals are farm workers during and after spraying crops, and, occasionally, employees involved in their manufacture and transport.

Treatment consists primarily in inhibiting excessive cholinergic activity with atropine.

Pyrethrum has been referred to already (p. 386), as a possible cause of extrinsic allergic 'alveolitis'.

DIMETHYL SULPHATE $(CH_3)_2SO_4$

This organic ester is used extensively as a solvent of mineral oils and as a methylating agent in the perfume, dye and pharmaceutical industries. It is highly toxic and vesicant both as a liquid and a vapour, and, in the presence of water or moisture hydrolyses readily to sulphuric acid and methyl alcohol. Its effects are comparable to phosgene (*see* p. 480).

Exposure is likely to occur as result of accidental spillage, breakage or leakage of bottles or vessels containing the liquid, or when transferring the liquid from one container to another.

Symptoms are usually delayed for about six to 24 hours after exposure. Swelling of the face, eyelids and fauces due to severe oedema and vesication of all exposed or unprotected parts of the body occurs. There is pyrexia up to about 37.8 °C (100°F), tachycardia or bradycardia, dysphagia, respiratory distress with severe cough, bronchospasm and, commonly, the clinical and radiographic signs of pulmonary oedema which may be fatal. Hepatitis, nephritis, analgesia, convulsions and coma may also occur (Littler and McConnell, 1955; Haswell, 1960; Fasset, 1963; Browning, 1965).

Speedy application of treatment with oxygen, corticosteroids and antibiotics results in complete recovery in a few days but all drugs which are central nervous system depressants must be avoided. Inhalation of steam is helpful in relieving initial respiratory distress. Prior to the antibiotic era death from pneumonia was common.

Intermittent exposure to low concentrations of the vapour may be associated with persistent tracheitis.

Preventive measures include education of employees, good ventilation, closed handling systems, provision of airline respirators and protective clothing when entering a contaminated zone, and decontamination of spillages with a dilute alkali.

REFERENCES

Adams, W. G. F. (1963). Polymer fume fever due to inhalation of fume from polytetrafluorethlene. *Trans. Assoc. ind. med. Offrs* **13**, 20–21

Ahmad, D., Morgan, W. K. C., Patterson, R., Williams, T. and Zeiss, C. R. (1979). Pulmonary haemorrhage and haemolytic anaemia due to trimellitic anhydride. *Lancet* **2**, 328–330

Ajello, L. (1971). Coccidioidomycosis and histoplasmosis. A review of their epidemiology and geographical distribution. *Mycopath. Mycol. appl.* **45**, 221–230

Allen, D. H., Basten, A., Williams, G. V. and Woolcock, A. J. (1975). Familial hypersensitivity pneumonitis. *Am. J. Med.* **59**, 505–514

Allen, D. H., Basten, A. and Woolcock, A. J. (1977). Studies of cell-mediated and humoral immunity in bird breeder's hypersensitivity pneumonitis. *Am. Rev. resp. Dis.* **115** (2), 45 (Abstract)

Allen, D. H., Basten, A., Woolcock, A. J. and Guinan, J. (1977). HL-A and bird breeder's hypersensitivity pneumonitis. *Mongr. Allergy* **11**, 45–54

Anderson, J. P. (1973). Ornithosis in Somerset. Experience in the South Somerset clinical area 1964—71. *Postgrad. med. J.* **49**, 533–534

Anderson, J. P. and Bridgewater, F. A. J. (1968). Ornithosis in a chest clinic practice. *Br. J. Dis. Chest* **62**, 115–166

Anderson, D. C., Stoesz, P. A. and Kaufmann, A. F. (1978). Psittacosis outbreak in employees of a turkey-processing plant. *Am. J. Epidemiol.* **107**, 140–148

Arnaud, A., DeSanti, P. P., Garbe, L., Payan, H. and Charpin, J. (1978). Polyvinyl chloride pneumoconiosis. *Thorax* **33**, 19–25

Ávila, R. (1971). Extrinsic allergic alveolitis in workers exposed to fish meal and poultry. *Clin. Allergy* **1**, 343–346

Ávila, R. and Lacey, J. (1974). The role of *Pencillium frequentans* in suberosis (respiratory disease in workers in the cork industry). *Clin. Allergy* **4**, 109–117

Ávila, R. and Villier, T.G. (1968). Suberosis. Respiratory disease in cork workers. *Lancet* **1**, 620–621

Ayvazian, L. F., Steward, D. S., Merkel, C. G. and Frederick, W. W. (1967). Diffuse lipoid pneumonitis successfully treated with prednisone. *Am. J. Med.* **43**, 930–934

Banaszak, E. F., Thiede, W. H. and Fink, J. N. (1970). Hypersensitivity pneumonitis due to contamination of air conditioners. *New Engl. J. Med.* **183**, 271–276

Banham, S. W., Lynch, P. and Boyd, G. (1978). Environmental and constitutional factors determining hypersensitivity to avian antigens in pigeon fanciers. *Thorax* **33**, 674

Barbee, R. A., Callies, Q., Dickie, H. A. and Rankin, J. (1968). The long term prognosis in farmer's lung. *Am. Rev. resp. Dis.* **97**, 223–231

Barboriak, J. J. Sosman, A. J. and Reed, C. E. (1965). Serological studies in pigeon breeder's disease. *J. Lab. clin. Med.* **65**, 600–604

Barnes, A. W. (1976). Vinyl chloride and the production of PVC. *Proc. R. Soc. Med.* **69**, 277–280

Barrowcliff, D. F. and Arblaster, P. G. (1968). Farmer's lung: a study of an early acute fatal case. *Thorax* **23**, 490–500

Basich, J.E., Resnick, A. and Fink, J.N. (1980). Hypersensitivity pneumonitis and legionnaires' disease. *Am. Rev. resp. Dis.* **121**, 885–887

Baum, G. L., Donnerberg, R. L., Stewart, D., Mulligan, W. J. and Putnam, L. R (1969). Pulmonary sporotrichosis. *New Engl. J. Med.* **280**, 410–413

Baum, G. L. and Schwarz, J. (1959). North American blastomycosis. *Am. J. med. Sci.* **238**, 661–684

Beaudry, C. and Laplante, L. (1973). Severe allergic pneumonitis from hydrochlorothiazide. *Ann. intern. Med* **78**, 251–253

Benson, M. K., Lancaster-Smith, M. J., Perrin, J., Holborrow, E. J. and Pepys, J. (1972). Serum immunoglobulins, autoantibodies and avian precipitins in adult coeliac disease. *IXth Internat. Congr. Gastroenterol., Paris* 1972. Abstract, p. 398

Bergmann, M. (1973). Thesaurosis: Illness or Illusion? *Chest* **64**, 153–154

Bergmann, M., Flance, I. J. and Blumenthal, H. (1958). Thesaurosis following inhalation of hair spray. *New Engl. J. Med.* **258**, 472–476

Bergmann, M., Flance, I. J., Cruz, P. T., Klam, N., Aronson, P. R., Joshi, R. A. and Blumenthal, H. T. (1962). Thesaurosis due to inhalation of hair spray. report of 12 new cases including 3 autopsies. *New Engl. J. Med.* **266**, 750–755

Berrens, L., de Ridder, G. and de Boer, F. (1977). Longitudinal studies of immunological parameters in farmer's lung. *Scand. J. resp. Dis.* **58**, 205–214

Berrens, L., Guikers, C. L. H. and van Dijk, A. (1974). The antigens of pigeon breeder's disease and their interaction with human complement. *Ann. N.Y. Acad. Sci.* **221**, 153–162

Berrill, W. T., Eade, O. E., Fitzpatrick, P. F., Hyde, I., McLeod, W. M. and Wright, R. (1975). Bird fancier's lung and jejunal villous atrophy. *Lancet* **2**, 1006–1008

Berrill, W. T. and Van Rood, J. J. (1977) HLA-DW6 and avian hypersensitivity. *Lancet* **2**, 248–249

Bhattacharjee, J.W., Saxena, R.P. and Zaidi, S.H. (1980). Experimental studies on the toxicity of bagasse. *Environ. Res.* **23**, 68–76

Bice, D.E., McCarron, K., Hoffman, E.O. and Salvaggio, J.E. (1977). Adjuvant properties of *Micropolyspora faeni. Int. Arch. Allergy Appl. Immunol.* **55**, 267–274

Bishop, J. M., Melnick, S. C. and Raine, J. (1963). Farmer's lung: studies of pulmonary function and aetiology. *Q. Jl Med.* **32**, 257–258

Björnsson, O. (1960). Quoted by Staines, F.H. and Forman, J. A. S. (1961). A survey of 'farmer's lung'. *J. Coll. gen. Practnrs Res. Newsl.* **4**, 351–382

Blackman, E. (1969). Observations on the development of silica cells of the leaf sheaf of wheat (*Triticum aistium*). *Can. J. Bot.* **47**, 827–848

Bledsoe, F. H. and Seymour, E. Q. (1972). Acute pulmonary oedema associated with parathion poisoning. *Radiology* **103**, 53–56

Boren, M. N., Moore, V. L., Abramoff, P. and Fink, J. N. (1977). Pigeon breeder's disease. Antibody response of man against a purified component of pigeon dropping extract. *Clin. Immun. Immunopath.* **8**, 108–115

Boros, D. L. and Warren, K. S. (1973). The bentonite granuloma: characterization of model system for infectious and foreign body granulomatous inflammation using soluble mycobacterial histoplasma and schistoma antigens. *Immunology* **24**, 511–529

Bourne, W. R. P. (1975). Birds and hazards to health. *Practitioner* **215**, 165–171

Boyd, D. H. A. (1971). The incidence of farmer's lung in Caithness. *Scott. med. J.* **16**, 261–262

Boyd, G., Madkour, M., Middleton, S. and Lynch, P. (1977). Effect of smoking on circulating antibody levels to avian protein in pigeon breeder's disease. *Thorax* **32**, 651

Boyer, R. S., Klock, L. E., Schmidt, C. D. Hyland, L., Maxwell, K., Gardner, R. M. and Renzetti, Jr., A. D. (1974). Hypersensitivity lung disease in the turkey raising industry. *Am. Rev. resp. Dis.* **109**, 630–635

Brachman, P. S., Plotkin, S. A., Bumford, F. H. and Atchinson, M. M. (1960). An epidemic of inhalation anthrax: the first in the twentieth century. II Epidemiology. *Am. J. Hyg.* **72**, 6–23

Bradford, J. K., Blalock, J. B. and Wascom, C. M. (1961). Bagasse disease of the lungs. *Am. Rev. resp. Dis.* **84**, 582–585

Braun, S. R., doPico, G. A., Tsiatis, A., Horvath, E., Dickie, H. A. and Rankin, J. (1979). Farmer's lung disease: Long term clinical and physiological outcome. *Am. Rev.resp. Dis.* **119**, 185–191

Bringhurst, L. S., Byrne, R. N. and Gershon-Cohen, J. (1959). Respiratory disease of mushroom workers. *J. Am. med. Ass.* **171**, 15–18

Browning, E. (1965). *Toxicity and Metabolism of Industrial Solvents*, pp. 713–717. Amsterdam, London and New York; Elsevier

Brunner, M. J., Giovacchini, R. P., Wyatt, J. P., Dunlap, F. E. and Calandra, J. C. (1963). Pulmonary disease and hair spray polymers; a disputed relationship. *J. Am. med. Ass.* **184**, 851–857

Buchanan, T. M., Faber, L. C. and Feldman, R. A. (1974). Brucellosis in the United States, 1960–1972. An abattoir-associated disease. *Medicine* **53**, 403–413

Buechner, H. A. (1962). Bagassosis: a true pneumoconiosis. *Ind. Med. Surg.* **31**, 311–314

Buechner, H. A. (1968). Quoted by Seabury *et al.* (1968)

Buechner, H. A. Aucoin, E., Vignes, A. J. and Weill, H. (1964). The resurgence of bagassosis in Louisiana. *J. occup. Med.* **6**, 437–442

Buechner, H. A., Prevatt, A., Thompson, J. and Blitz, O. (1958). Bagassosis — a review, with further historical data, studies of pulmonary function and results of adrenal steroid therapy. *Am. J. Med.* **25**, 234–247

Bullivant, C. M. (1966). Accidental poisoning by paraquat: report of two cases in man. *Br. med. J.* **1**, 1272–1273

Bureau, M. A., Fectau, C., Patriquin, H., Rola-Pleszczynski, M., Masse, S. and Begin, R. (1979). Farmer's lung in early childhood. *Am. Rev. resp. Dis.* **119**, 671–675

Butcher, B. T., Jones, R. N., O'Neill, C. E., Glindmeyer, H. W., Diem, J. E., Dharmarajan, V., Weill, H. and Salvaggio, J. E. (1977). Longitudinal study of workers employed in the manufacture of toluene diisocyanate. *Am. Rev. resp. Dis.* **116**, 411–421

Byrom, N. P., Walls, J. and Mair, H. J. (1979) Fulminant psittacosis. *Lancet* **1**, 353–356

Calandra, J. and Kay, J. A. (1958). The effects of aerosol hair sprays on experimental animals. *Proc. scient. Sect. Toilet Goods Ass.* **30**, 41–44

Caldwell, J. R., Pearce, C. E., Spencer, C., Leder, T. and Waldman, R. H. (1973). Immunologic mechanisms in hypersensitivity pneumonitis. *J. Allergy clin. Immun.* **52**, 225–230

Calvanico, N. J., Ambegaonkar, S. P., Schlueter, D. P. and Fink, J. N. (1980). Immunoglobulin levels in bronchoalveolar lavage fluid from pigeon breeders. *J. Lab. clin. Med.* **96**, 129–140

Cambridge, G. W. (1973). Inhalation toxicity studies. *Aereosol Age* **18**, 32–68

Campbell, C. C. (1980). Histoplasmosis outbreaks. Recommendations for mandatory treatment of known microfoci of *H. capsulatum* in soils. *Chest* **77**, 6–7

Campbell, I. A. Cockcroft, A. E., Edwards, J. H. and Jones, M. (1979). Humidifier fever in an operating theatre, *Br. med. J.* **2**, 1036–1037

Campbell, J. M. (1932). Acute symptoms following work with hay. *Br. med. J.* **2**, 1143–1144

Campbell, S. (1968). Death from paraquat in a child. *Lancet* **1**, 144

Campins, H., Zubillaga, C., Lopez, L. G. and Dorante, M. (1956). An epidemic of histoplasmosis in Venezuela. *Am. J. trop. Med. Hyg.* **5**, 690–695

Cancella, de Carvalho (1959). Suberose. Alteraçoes pulmonares relacionadas com a inalação de poeiras de cortiça. Dissertaçao de Dontoramento, Lisboa

Capodaglio, E., Monarco, G. and de Vito, G. (1961). Sindrome respiratio da malazione di composi fuori alifatici nella preparzione del politetra-fluoretilene. *Rass. Med. ind.* **30**, 124–139

Carlson, J. E. and Villaveces, J. W. (1977) Hypersensitivity pneumonitis due to pyrethrum. *J. Am. med. Ass.* **237**, 1718–1719

Carrol, K. B., Pepys, J., Longbottom, J. L., Hughes, D. T. D. and Benson, H. G. (1975). Extrinsic allergic alveolitis due to rat serum proteins. *Clin. Allergy* **5**, 443–456

Castleden, L. I. M. and Hamilton-Paterson, J. L. (1942). Bagassosis. An industrial lung disease. *Br. med. J.* **2**, 478–480

Cangini, G. (1951). Casidi bagassosi in Italia. *Lotta c. tuberc.* **21**, 300

Černý, Z. (1976). Tularaemia infection rate and evaluation of the risk of the infection being contracted by workers of sugar refineries processing sugar-beet from areas of its endemic incidence. *Čslká Epidem. Mikrobiol. Immun.* **25**, 39–49. (*Abstracts Hyg.* 1976 **51**, 878)

Chan-Yeung, M., Grzybowski, S. and Schonell, M. E. (1972). Mushroom worker's lung. *Am. Rev resp. Dis.* **105**, 819–822

Chandra, S. and Jones, H. E. (1972). Pigeon fanciers' lung in children. *Archs Dis. Childh.* **47**, 716–718

Channel, S., Blyth, W., Lloyd, M., Weir, D. M., Amos, W. M. G., Littlewood, A. P., Riddle, H. F. V. and Grant, I. W. B. (1969). Allergic alveolitis in maltworkers. *Q. Jl Med.* **38**, 351–376

Charles, J., Bernstein, A., Jones, B., Jones, D. J., Edwards, J. H., Seal, R. M. E. and Seaton, A. (1976). Hypersensitivity pneumonitis after exposure to isocyanates. *Thorax* **31**, 127–136

Chick, E. W. and Bauman, D. S. (1974). Acute cavitary histoplasmosis — fact or fiction. *Chest* **65**, 479–480

Chick, E. W., Flanigan, C., Gompton, S. B., Pass III, T., Gayle, C., Hernandez, C., Pitzer, F. R. and Austin, Jr. E. (1980). Blackbird roosts and histoplasmosis. An increasing medical problem? *Chest* **77**, 584–585

Chivers, C. P., Lawrence-Jones, C. and Paddle, G. M. (1980). Lung function in workers exposed to polyvinyl chloride dust. *Br. J. industr. Med.* **37**, 147–151

Christensen, L. T., Schmidt, C. D. and Robbins, L. (1975).

Pigeon breeder's disease — a prevalence study and review. *Clin. Allergy* **5**, 417–430

Cochrane, C. G. (1971). Mechanisms involved in the deposition of immune complexes in tissues. *J. exp. Med.* **134** (Suppl.), 75–89

Cohen, B. M. (1976). Peripheral airway responses to acute hair spray exposure. *Am. Rev. resp. Dis.* **113** (Suppl.), 123

Cohen, H. I., Merigan, T. C., Kosek, J. C. and Eldridge, F. (1967). Sequoiosis. *Am. J. Med.* **43**, 785–794

Communicable Disease Report 1980. Week 23, page 1

Conolly, M. E. (1975). Paraquat poisoning. *Proc. R. Soc. Med.* **68**, 441

Cooper, I. A. and Greenaway, T. M. (1961). Farmer's lung: a case report. *Med. J. Aust.* **2**, 980–981

Cotton, D. J. and Dosman, J. A. (1978). Grain dust and health. III. Environmental factors. *Ann. intern. Med.* **89**, 420–421

Craig, D. B. and Donevan, R. E. (1970). Mushroom worker's lung. *Can. med. Ass. J.* **102**, 1289–1293

Craveri, R., Guicciardi, A. and Pacini, N. (1966). Distribution of thermophilic actinomycetes in compost for mushroom production. *Ann. di Microbiol.* **16**, 111–113

Cross, T. and Unsworth, B. A. (1976). Farmer's lung: a neglected antigen. *Lancet* **1**, 958–959

Cross, T. and Unsworth, B. A. (1977). List of actinomycete names: alternative proposals for the Genus *Thermoactinomyces*. *Actinomycetes and related organisms* **12**, 6–11

Cullen, G. A. (1974). Veterinary diagnosis of psittacosis. *Proc. R. Soc. Med.* **67**, 733

Cuthbert, O. D., Brostoff, J., Wraith, D. G. and Brighton, Q. D. (1979). 'Barn allergy': asthma and rhinitis due to storage mites. *Clin. Allergy* **9**, 229–236

Dane, D. S. and Pattison, J. R. (1974). Psittacosis. *Lancet* **1**, 135

D'Angelo, L. J., Baker, E. F. and Schlosser, W. (1979). Q fever in the United States, 1948–1977. From the Centers for Disease Control. *J. infect. Dis.* **139**, 163–165

Darke, C. S., Knowelden, J., Lacey, J. and Ward, A. M. (1976). Respiratory disease of workers harvesting grain. *Thorax* **31**, 293–302

Davies, C. N. (1977). Atmospheric concentrations of oil mist. *Ann. occup. Hyg.* **20**, 91–92

Davies, D. S. and Conolly, M. E. (1975). Paraquat poisoning — possible therapeutic approach. *Proc. R. Soc. Med.* **68**, 442

Davies, R. (1979). Allergic lung disease. *Br. J. hosp. Med.* **22**, 136–150

Davies, S. F. and Serosi, G. A. (1978). Acute cavitary histoplasmosis. *Chest* **73**, 103–105

Dean, A. G., Bates, J. H., Sorrels, C., Sorrels, T., Germany, W., Ajello, L., Kaufman, L., McGrew, C. and Fitts, A. (1978). An outbreak of histoplasmosis at an Arkansas courthouse, with five cases of probable reinfection. *Am. J. Epidem.* **108**, 36–46

Dean, G. (1957). Cave disease. *Cent. Afr. J. Med.* **3**, 79–81

Dean, G. (1975). The curse of the Pharaohs. *Wld Med.* **10** (18), 17–21

Dew, J., Mawson, K., Ellman, P. and Brough, D. (1960). Ornithosis in two railway guards: an occupational hazard. *Lancet* **2**, 18–19

de Week, A. L., Gutersohn, J. and Bütikofer, E. (1969). La maladie des laveurs de fromage ('Käsenwascherkranheit'): une forme particulière du syndrome du poumon du fermir. *Schweiz. med. Wschr.* **99**, 872–876

Di Salvo, A. F. and Johnson, W. M. (1979). Histoplasmosis in South Carolina: support for the microfocus concept. *Am. J. Epidemiol.* **109**, 480–492

Dickerson, M. S., Bilderback, W. R. and Pessarra, L. W. (1976). Ornithosis (chlamydiosis) outbreaks in Texas. *Texas med. J.* **72**, 57–61

Dickie, H. A. and Rankin, J. (1958). Farmer's lung: an acute granulomatous interstitial pneumonitis occurring in agricultural workers. *J. Am. med. Ass.* **167**, 1069–1076

Diment, J. A. and Pepys, J. (1977). Avian erythrocyte agglutination tests with the sera of bird fanciers. *J. clin. Path.* **30**, 29–34

Dinda, P., Chatterjee, S. S. and Riding, W. D. (1969). Pulmonary function studies in bird breeder's lung. *Thorax* **24**, 374–378

Dizon, G. D., Almonte, J. B. and Anselmo, J. E. (1962). Bagassosis and silicosis in the Philippines. *J. Philipp. med. Ass.* **38**, 865–872

doPico, G. A., Layton, Jr., C. R., Clayton, J. W. and Rankin, J. (1973). Acute pulmonary reaction to spray starch with soil repellant. *Am. Rev. resp. Dis.* **108**, 1212–1215

doPico, G. A., Rankin, J., Chosy, L. W., Reddan, W. G., Barbee, R. A., Gee, B. and Dickie, H. A. (1975). Respiratory tract disease from thermosetting resins. Study of an outbreak in rubber tire workers. *Ann. inten. Med.* **83**, 177–184

Draize, J. H., Nelson, A. A., Newburger, S. H. and Kelley, E. A. (1959). Inhalation toxicity studies of six types of aerosol hair sprays. *Proc. scient. Sect. Toilet Goods Ass.* **31**, 28–32

Drouhet, E., Enjalbert, L., Planques, J., Bollinelli, R., Moreau, G. and Sabatier, A. (1968). A propos d'un cas de blastomycose a localisations multiples chez un francais d'oridine Tunisienne guerison par l'amphotericine B. *Bull. Soc. Path. Exot.* **61**, 202–210

Drutz, D. J. and Catanzaro, A. (1978). Coccidioidomycosis. Parts I and II. *Am. Rev. resp. Dis.* **117**, 559–585 and 727–772

Duncan, J. T. (1958). Tropical African histoplasmosis. *Trans. R. Soc. trop. Med. Hyg.* **52**, 468–474

Dutkiewicz, J. (1978). Exposure to dust-borne bacteria in agriculture. I. Environmental studies. *Archs envir. Hlth* 250–259

Edwards, J. H. (1976). A quantitative study on the activation of the alternative pathway of complement by mouldy hay dust and thermophilic actinomycetes. *Clin. Allergy* **6**, 19–25

Edwards, J. H. (1978). Methodology involved in fractioning *Micropolyspora faeni* antigens. *J. Allergy clin. Immun.* **61**, 233–234

Edwards, J. H., Baker, J. T. and Davies, B. H. (1974). Precipitin test negative farmer's lung — activation of the alternative pathway of complement by mouldy hay dust. *Clin. Allergy* **4**, 379–388

Edwards, J. H., Barboriak, J. J. and Fink, J. N. (1970). Antigens in pigeon breeder's disease. *Immunology* **19**, 729–734

Edwards, J. H., Fink, J. N. and Barboriak, J. J. (1969). Excretion of pigeon serum proteins in pigeon droppings. *Proc. Soc. exp. Biol.* **132**, 907–911

Edwards, J. H., Griffiths, A. J. and Mullins, J. (1976). Protozoa as sources of antigen in 'humidifier fever'. *Nature* **264**, 438–439

Edwards, C. and Luntz, G. (1974). Budgerigar-fancier's lung: a report of a fatal case. *Br. J. Dis. Chest* **68**, 57–64

Edwards, J. H., Wagner, J. C. and Seal, R. M. E. (1976). Pulmonary responses to particulate materials capable of activating alternative pathway of complement. *Clin. Allergy* **6**, 155–164

Edwards, J. H., Wagner, J. C. and Seal, R. M. E. (1980). Production of granulomata by organic dusts deposited endotracheally. *8th International Conf. on Sarcoidosis and Granulomatous Disease*. Edited by W. Jones Williams and B. H. Davies, pp. 99–103. Cardiff; Alpha Omega Publishing

Effler, D., Roland, F. and Redding, R. A. (1976) The P blood group system in pigeon breeder's disease. *Chest* **70**, 719–725

Ely, T. S., Pedley, S. F., Hearne, F. T. and Stille, W. T. (1970). A study of mortality, symptoms, and respiratory function in humans occupationally exposed to oil mist. *J. occup. Med.* **12**, 253–261

Elman, A. J., Tebo, T., Fink, J. N. and Barboriak, J. J. (1968). Reactions of poultry against chicken antigens. *Archs envir. Hlth* **17**, 98–100

Emanuel, D. A., Lawton, B. R. and Wenzel, F. J. (1962). Maple bark disease. Pneumonitis due to *Coniosporium corticale*. *New Engl. J. Med.* **266**, 333–337

Emanuel, D. A., Wenzel, F. J. and Lawton, B. R. (1966). Pneumonitis due to *Cryptostroma corticale* (Maple bark disease). *New Engl. J. Med.* **274**, 1413–1418

Emanuel, D. A., Wenzel, F. J. and Lawton, B. R. (1975). Pulmonary mycotoxicosis. *Chest* **67**, 293–297

Emanuel, D. A., Wenzel, F. J., Bowerman, C. I. and Lawton, B. R. (1964). Farmer's lung. Clinical pathologic and immunologic study of twenty four patients. *Am. J. Med.* **37**, 392–401

Emmons, C. W. (1961). Isolation of *Histoplasma capulatum* from soil in Washington, DC. *Publ. Hlth Rep.* **76,** 591–596

Emmons, C. W., Binford, C. H., Utz, J. P. and Kwon-Chung, K. J. (1977). *Medical Mycology*, 3rd edition. Philadelphia; Lea and Febiger

Enticknap, J. B., Galbraith, N. S., Tomlinson, A. J. H. and Elias-Jones, T. F. (1968). Pulmonary anthrax caused by contaminated sacks. *Br. J. ind. Med.* **25,** 72–74

Evans, E. A. (1973). Pulmonary edema after inhalation of fumes from polytetrafluoroethylene (PTFE). *J. occup. Med.* **7**, 599–601

Evans, W. V. and Seaton, A (1979). Hypersensitivity pneumonitis in a technician using Pauli's reagent. *Thorax* **34,** 767–770

Fairshter, R. D. and Wilson, A. F. (1975). Paraquat poisoning: manifestations and therapy. *Am. J. med* **59,** 751–753

Farant, J. P. and Moore, C. F. (1978). Dust exposure in the Canadian grain industry. *Am. ind. Hyg. Ass. J.* **39,** 177–194

Fassett, D. W. (1963). Esters. In *Industrial Hygiene and Toxicology, Vol. II*, edited by F. A. Patty, pp. 1927–1930. New York, London; Interscience

Faux, J. A., Hendrick, D. J. and Anand, B. S. (1978). Precipitins to different avian serum antigens in bird fancier's lung and coeliac disease. *Clin. Allergy* **8,** 101–108

Faux, J. A., Wide,L., Hargreave, F. E., Longbottom, J. L. and Pepys, J. (1971). Immunological aspects of respiratory allergy in budgerigar (*Melopsittacus undulatus*) fanciers. *Clin. Allergy* **1,** 149–158

Fawcitt, R. (1938). Occupational diseases of the lungs in agricultural workers. *Br. J. Radiol.* **11,** 378–392

Feldman, H. A. and Sabin, A. B. (1948). Pneumonitis of unknown aetiology in a group of men exposed to pigeon excreta. *J. clin. Invest.* **27,** 533

Fergus, C. L. (1964). Thermophilic and thermotolerant moulds and actinomycetes of mushroom compost during peak heating. *Mycologia* **56,** 267–284

Festenstein, G. N., Lacey, J., Skinner, F. A., Jenkins, P. A. and Pepys, J. (1965). Self heating hay and grain in Dewar flasks, and the development of farmer's lung antigens. *J. gen. Microbiol.* **41,** 389–407

Fink, J. N., Banaszak, E. F., Barboriak, J. J., Hensley, G. T., Kurup, V. P., Scanlon, G. T., Schlueter, D. P., Sosman, A. J., Thiede, W. H. and Unger, G. F. (1976) Interstitial lung disease due to contamination of forced air systems. *Ann. intern. Med.* **84**, 406–413

Fink, J. N., Banaszak, E. A., Thiede, W. H. and Barboriak, J. J. (1971). Interstitial pneumonitis due to hypersensitivity to an organism contaminating a heating system. *Ann. intern. Med.* **74,** 80–83

Fink, J. N., Hensley, G. T. and Barboriak, J. J. (1969). An animal model of a hypersensitivity pneumonitis. *J. Allergy* **46,** 156–161

Fink, J. N., Moore, V. L. and Barboriak, J. J. (1975). Cell-mediated hypersensitivity in pigeon breeders. *Int. Archs Allergy appl. Immun.* **49,** 831–836

Fink, J. N. and Schlueter, D. P. (1978). Bathtub refinisher's lung: An unusual response to toluene diisocyanate. *Am. Rev. resp. Dis.* **118**, 955–959

Fink, J., Tebo, T. and Barboriak, J. J. (1969). Characterization of human precipitating antibody to inhaled antigens. *J. Immun.* **103**, 244–251

Fitzgerald, G. R., Barnville, G., Gibney, R. T. N. and Fitzgerald, M. X. (1979). Clinical radiological and pulmonary function assessment in 13 long-term survivors of paraquat poisoning. *Thorax* **34**, 414–415

Flaherty, D. K., Iha, T., Chmelik, F., Dickie, H. and Reed, C. E. (1975). HLA-8 in farmer's lung. *Lancet* **2**, 507

Flynn, N. M., Hoeprich, P. D., Kawachi, M. M., Lee, K. K., Lawrence, R. M., Goldstein, E., Jordan, G. W., Kundargi, R. S. and Wong, G. A. (1979). An unusual outbreak of windborne coccidioidomycosis. *New Engl. J. Med.* **301**, 358–361

Foe, R. B. and Bigham, Jr., R. S. (1954). Lipid pneumonia following occupational exposure to oil spray. *J. Am. med. Ass.* **155**, 33–34

Frank, R. (1975). Are aerosol sprays hazardous? *Am. Rev. resp. Dis.* **112**, 485–489

Frankland, A. W. and Lunn, J. A. (1965). Asthma caused by the grain weevil. *Br. J. ind. Med.* **22,** 157–159

Fransén, H. (1969). Ornithosis in Stockholm. *Scand. J. infect. Dis.* **1**, 61–66

Fredericks, W. (1978). Antigens in pigeon dropping extracts. *J. Allergy clin. Immun.* **61,** 221–223

Friedman, M., Dougherty, R., Nelson, S. R., White, R. P., Sackner, M. A. and Wauner, A. (1977) Acute effects of an aerosol hair spray on tracheal mucociliary transport. *Am. Rev. resp. Dis.* **116**, 281–286

Friend, J. A. R., Gaddie, J., Palmer, K. N. V., Pickering, C. A. C. and Pepys, J. (1977). Extrinsic allergic alveolitis and contaminated cooling-water in a factory machine. *Lancet* **1,** 297–300

Frongia, N., Spinazzola, A. and Bucarelli, A. (1974). Lesioni polmonari sperimentali da inalazione prolungata di polveri di PVC in ambiente di lavaro. *Medna Lav.* **65,** 321–342

Fuller, C. J. (1953). Farmer's lung: a review of present knowledge. *Thorax* **8**, 59–64

Ganado, W. (1965). Human brucellosis — some clinical observations. *Scott. med. J.* **10,** 451–460

Ganchev, N., Serbezov, V. and Alexandrov, E. (1977). Incidence of Q fever in two inadequately investigated occupational groups. *J. Hyg. Epidem. Microbiol. Immun.* **21,** 405–411

Ganguly, S. K. and Pal, S. C. (1955). Early bagassosis. *J. Indian med. Ass.* **34**, 253–254

Garibaldi, R. and Caprotti, M. (1964). Ricerche cliniche su un gruppo di soggetti esposti alla inalazione di lacche nebulizzate per capelli. *Medna Lav.* **55,** 424–433

Gay, B. W., Lonneman, W. A., Bridbord, K. and Moran, J. B. (1975). Measurements of vinyl chloride from aerosol sprays. *Ann. N.Y. Acad. Sci.* **246,** 286–295

Gebbers, J-O., Burkhardt, A., Tetzner, C., Rüdiger, H. W. and Von Wichert, P. (1980). Haarspray-Lunge. Klinische und morphologische Befunde. *Schweiz. med. Woch.* **110,** 610–615

Gehlbach, S. H., Hamilton, J. D. and Conant, N. F. (1973). Coccidioidomycocis. An occupational disease in cotton mill workers. *Archs intern. Med.* **131**, 254–255

George, M. and Hedworth-Whitty, R. B. (1980). Non-fatal lung disease due to inhalation of nebulised paraquat. *Br. med. J.* **280,** 902

Ghose, T., Landrigan, P., Killeen, R. and Dill, J. (1974). Immunopathological studies in patients with farmer's lung. *Clin. Allergy* **4**, 119–129

Gialdroni, C., Grassi, G. and Clini, V. (1964). Sulla possibilita di indurre sperimentalmente reazioni sarcoid-similia livello del pulmone. *Minerva Pneumonol.* **3,** 170–175

Giovacchini, R. P., Becker, G., Brunner, M. and Dunlop, F. E. (1965). Pulmonary disease and hair spray polymers: effects of long-term exposure of dogs. *J. Am. med. Ass.* **193,** 298–299

Goldstein, D. H., Benoit, J. N. and Tyroler, H. A. (1970). An epidemiological study of oil mist exposure. *Archs envir. Hlth* **21,** 600–603

Goldstein, R. A. and Janicki, B. W. (1974). Immunologic studies in nitrofurantoin induced pulmonary disease. *Med. Ann. Distr. Columbia* **43**, 115–119

González de Vega, N., Zamora, A., Cano, M. and Fernández Castany, A. (1966). Nuestra experiencia personal sobre la bagazosis en Espana Enferm. *Tórax* **15,** 215–237

Goodwin, R. A. and Des Prez, R. M. (1978). Histoplasmosis. *Am. Rev. resp. Dis.* **117,** 929–956

Goodwin, R. A., Owens, F. T. and Snell, J. D. (1976). Chronic pulmonary histoplasmosis. *Medicine* **55,** 413–452

Gourley, C. A. and Braidwood, G. D. (1971). The use of dust respirators in the prevention of recurrence of farmer's lung. *Trans. Soc. occup. Med.* **21,** 93–95

Gowdy, J. M. and Wagstaff, M. J. (1972). Pulmonary infiltration due to aerosol thesaurosis. *Archs envir. Hlth* **25,** 101–108

Grant, I. W. B., Blackadder, E. S., Greenberg, M. and Blyth, W.

(1976). Extrinsic allergic alveolitis in Scottish maltworkers. *Br. med. J.* **1**, 490–493

Grant, I. W. B., Blyth, W., Wardrop, V. E., Gordon, R. M., Pearson, J. C. G. and Mair, A. (1972). Prevalence of farmer's lung in Scotland. A pilot survey. *Br. med. J.* **1**, 530–534

Greatorex, F. B. and Pether, J. V. S. (1975). Use of serologically distinct strain of *Thermoactinomyces vulgaris* in the diagnosis of farmer's lung disease. *J. clin. Path.* **28**, 1000–1002

Greatorex, F. B. and Pether, J. V. S. (1976). Farmer's lung: a neglected antigen. *Lancet* **1**, 1134

Gregory, P. H. and Waller, S. (1951). *Cryptostroma corticale* and sooty bark disease of sycamore. (Acerpseudoplantanus:) *Trans. Br. mycol. Soc.* **34**, 579–597

Gregory, P. H., Lacey, J., Festenstein,G. N. and Skinner, F. A. (1963). Microbial and biochemical changes during moulding of hay. *J. gen. microbiol.* **33**, 147–174

HM Chief Inspector of Factories (1969). Annual report

Hansen, P. J. and Penny, R. (1974). Pigeon breeder's disease. A study of cell-mediated immune response to pigeon antigens by the lymphocyte culture technique. *Int. Archs Allergy appl. Immun.* **47**, 498–507

Hapke, E. J., Seal, R. M. E., Thomas, G. D., Hayes, M. and Meek, J. C. (1968). Farmer's lung. *Thorax* **23**, 451–468

Hargreave, F. E., Pepys, J. and Holford-Strevens, V. (1968). Bagassosis. *Lancet* 1, 619–620

Hargreave, F. E., Pepys, J., Longbottom, J. L. and Wraith, D. G. (1966). Bird breeder's (fancier's) lung. *Lancet* **1**, 445–449

Harper, L. O., Burrell, R. G., Lapp, J. L. and Morgan, W. K. C. (1970). Allergic alveolitis due to pituitary snuff. *Ann. intern. Med.* **73**, 581–584

Harries, M. G., Burge, P. S. and O'Brien, I. M. (1980). Occupational type bronchial provocation tests: testing with soluble antigens by inhalation. *Br. J. industr. Med.* **37**, 248–252

Harrington, J. M. (1975). Some occupational health hazards for hospital staff. *Proc. R. Soc. Med.* **68**, 94–95

Harris, D. K. (1951). Polymer-fume fever. *Lancet* **2**, 1008–1011

Harris, D. K. (1959). Some hazards in the manufacture and use of plastics. *Br. J. ind.Med.* **16**, 221–229

Hart, R. J. C. (1973). The epidemiology of Q fever. *Postgrad. med. J.* **49**, 535–538

Harvey, M. S., Forbes, G. B. and Marmion, B. P. (1951). An outbreak of Q fever in East Kent. *Lancet* **2**, 1152–1157

Haslam, P., Lukoszek, A. and Turner-Warwick, M. (1979). T cell responsiveness in extrinsic allergic alveolitis. (Personal communication)

Haswell, R. W. (1960). Dimethyl sulfate poisoning by inhalation. *J. occup. Med.* **2**, 454–455

Hearn, C. E. D. (1968). Bagassosis: An epidemiological, environmental and clinical survey. *Br. J. ind. Med.* **25**, 267–282

Hearn, C. E. D. and Holford-Strevens, V. (1968). Immunological aspects of bagassosis. *Br. J. ind. Med.* **25**, 238–292

Henderson, R. J., Hill, D. M., Vickers, A. A., Edwards, J. M. B. and Tillett, H. E. (1975). Brucellosis and veterinary surgeons. *Br. med. J.* **1**, 656–659

Hendrick, D. J., Faux, J. A., Anand,B., Piris, J. and Marshall, R. (1978b). Is bird fancier's lung associated with coeliac disease? *Thorax* **33**, 425–428

Hendrick, D. J., Faux, J. A. and Marshall, R. (1978a). Budgerigar-fancier's lung: the commonest variety of allergic alveolitis in Britain. *Br. med J.* **2**, 81–84

Hendrick, D. J., Marshall, R., Faux, J. A. and Krall, J. M. (1980). Positive 'alveolar' responses to antigen inhalation provocation tests: their validity and recognition. *Thorax* **35**, 415–427

Hendricks, N. V., Linden, N. J., Collings, G. H., Dooley, A. E., Garrett, J. T. and Rather, Jr. J. B. (1962). A review of exposure to oil mist. *Archs envir. Hlth* **4**, 139–145

Hensley, G. T., Garancis, J. C., Cherayil, G. D. and Fink, J. N. (1969). Lung biopsies in pigeon breeder's disease. *Archs Path.* **87**, 572–579

Herbert, F. A. and Orford, R. (1979). Haemorrhagic pneumonitis due to inhalation of resins containing trimellitic anhydride. *Chest* **76**, 546–551

Herrero, E. U., Feigelson, H. and Becker, A. (1965). Sarcoidosis in a beautician. *Am. Rev. resp. Dis.* **92**, 280–283

Higenbottam, T., Crome, P., Parkinson, C. and Nunn, J. (1979). Further clinical observations on the pulmonary effects of paraquat ingestion. *Thorax* **34**, 161–165

Hildick-Smith, G., Blank, H. and Sarkany, I. (1964). *Fungus Diseases and their Treatment*, pp. 334–339. London; J. and A. Churchill Ltd.

Hine, C. H. and Rowe, V. K. (1963). Epoxy compounds. In *Industrial Hygiene and Toxicology, Vol. II*, edited by Patty, F. A., pp. 1593–1654. New York, London; Interscience

Hinson, K. F. (1970). Diffuse pulmonary fibrosis. *Human Path.* **1**, 275–288

Hirsch, E. F. and Russell, H. B. (1945). Chronic exudative and indurative pneumonia due to inhalation of shellac. *Archs Path.* **39**, 281–286

Hodges, G. R., Fink, T. N. and Schlueter, D. P. (1974). Hypersensitivity pneumonitis caused by a contaminated cool-mist vapouriser. *Ann. intern. Med.* **85**, 501–504

Hoffman, W. (1946). Die Dreschkranheit. *Schweiz. med. Wschr.* **76**, 988–990

Holford-Strevens, V. (1971). Quoted by J. Lacey (1971a), q.v.

Hood, J. and Mason, A. M. S. (1970). Diffuse pulmonary disease with transfer defect occurring with coeliac disease. *Lancet* **1**, 445–448

Howat, H. T. and Arnott, W. M. (1944). Outbreak of pneumonia in smallpox contacts. *Lancet* **2**, 312

Hugh-Jones, M. E. and Austwick, P. K. C. (1967). Epidemiological studies of bovine mycotic abortion. *Vet. Rec.* **81**, 273–276

Hunter, D. and Perry, K. M. A. (1946). Bronchiolitis resulting from the handling of bagasse. *Br. J. ind. Med.* **3**, 64–74

Hyde, H. A. (1972). Atmospheric pollen and spores in relation to allergy. *Clin. Allergy* **2**, 153–179

Jackson, E. and Welch, K. M. A. (1970). Mushroom worker's lung. *Thorax* **25**, 25–30

Jamison, C. S. and Hopkins, J. (1941). Bagassosis — A fungus disease of the lung. *New Orl. med. Surg. J.* **93**, 580–582

Jaros, F. (1978). Acute percutaneous paraquat poisoning. *Lancet* **1**, 275

Jernelius, H., Pettersson, B., Schvarcz, J. and Vahlne, A. (1975). An outbreak of ornithosis. *Scand. J. infect. Dis.* **7**, 91–95

Jimenez-Diaz, C., Lahoz, C. and Canto, G. (1947). The allergens of mill dust. Asthma in millers, farmers and others. *Ann. Allergy* **5**, 519–525

Johnson, C. L., Bernstein, I. L., Gallagher, J. S., Bonventre, P. F. and Brooks, S. M. (1980). Familial hypersensitivity pneumonitis induced by *Bacillus subtilis*. *Am. Rev. resp. Dis.* **122**, 339–348

Johnson, N. E. and Kadull, P. J. (1966). Laboratory-acquired Q fever:a report of fifty cases. *Am. J. Med.* **41**, 391–403

Jones, J. G. (1961). An investigation into the effects of exposure to an oil mist on workers in a mill for the cold reduction of steel strip. *Ann. Occup. Hyg.* **3**, 264–271

Jones Williams, W. (1967). The pathology of sarcoidosis. *Hosp. Med.* **2**, 21–27

Joyce, J. C. and Kneafsey, D. (1955). Farmer's lung. *J. Irish med. Assoc.* **37**, 313–315

Katila, M–L. and Mäntyjärvi, R. A. (1978). The diagnostic value of antibodies to the traditional antigens of farmer's lung in Finland. *Clin. Allergy* **8**, 581–587

Kawai, T., Salvaggio, J., Lake, W. and Harris, J. O. (1972). Experimental production of hypersensitivity pneumonitis with bagasse and thermophilic actmomycete antigen. *J. Allergy clin. Immun.* **50**, 276–288

Keymer, I. F. (1972). The unsuitability of non-domesticated animals as pets. *Vet. Rec.* **91**, 373–381

Keymer, I. F. (1973). Psittacosis. *Lancet* **2**, 1436

Keymer, I. F. (1974). Psittacosis. *Proc. R. Soc. Med.* **67**, 733–735

Kimborough, R. D. (1974). Toxic effects of the herbicide paraquat. *Chest* **65** (Suppl.), 655–675

Korenblat, P., Slavin, R., Winzenburger, P., Marks, E. and Wenneker, M. D. (1977). Gerbil keeper's lung — a new form of hypersensitivity pneumonitis. *Ann. Allergy.* **38**, 437 (Abstract)

Kowalska, M., Hanski, W., Bielunska, S., Gawkowska-Turyczyn, M. (1976). North-American blastomycosis and possibilities of its occurrence in Poland. *Przegl. Derm.* **63,** 641–674

Kuntz, W. D. and McCord, C. P. (1974). Polymer-fume fever. *J. occup. Med.* **16,** 480–482

Kurup, V. P., Barboriak, J. J. and Fink, J. N. (1975). *Thermoactinomyces candidus,* a new species of thermophilic actinomycetes. *Int. J. syst. Bacteriol.* **25,** 150–154

Kuster, E. and Locci, R. (1964). Taxonomic studies of the genus *Thermoactinomyces. Int. Bull. Bact. Nomencl. Taxon.* **14,** 109–114

Lacey, J. (1969). Bagassosis. *Rothamsted Experimental Station Report for 1968.* Part 1, p. 133

Lacey, J. (1971a). *Thermoactinomyces sacchari* sp. nov., a thermophilic actinomycete causing bagassosis. *J. gen. Microbiol.* **66,** 327–338

Lacey, J. (1971b). Personal communication

Lacey, J. (1980). The microflora of grain dusts. In *Occupational Lung Disease — Focus on Grain Dust and Health.* Ed. J. A. Dosman and D. J. Cotton, pp. 417–440. Academic Press

Lacey, J. and Lacey, M. E. (1964). Spore concentrations in the air of farm buildings. *Trans. Br. mycol. Soc.* **47,** 547–552

Laing Brown, G. (1973). Clinical aspects of 'Q' fever. *Postgrad. med. J.* **49,** 359–541

Lancaster-Smith, M. J., Benson, M. K. and Strickland, I. D. (1971). Coeliac disease and diffuse interstitial lung disease. *Lancet* **1,** 473–476

Lancaster-Smith, M. J., Swarbrick, E. T., Perrin, J. and Wright, J. T. (1974). Coeliac disease and autoimmunity. *Postgrad. med. J.* **50,** 45–48

Laskey, W. and Sarosi, G. A. (1978). The radiological appearance of pulmonary blastomycosis. *Radiology* **126,** 351–357

Latham, R. H., Kaiser, A. B., Dupont, W. D. and Dan, B. B. (1980). Chronic pulmonary histoplasmosis following the excavation of a bird roost. *Am. J. Med.* **68,** 504–508

Leachman, R. D. and Yow, E. M. (1958). The epidemiology of psittacosis and report of a turkey-borne outbreak. *Archs intern. Med.* **102,** 537–543

Leading article, (1975). *Lancet* **1,** 436–438

Lehrer, S. B., Turner, E., Weill, H. and Salvaggio, J. E. (1978). Elimination of bagassosis in Louisiana paper manufacturing plant workers. *Clin. Allergy* **8,** 15–20

Levin, P. J., Klaff, L. J., Rose, A. G. and Ferguson, A. D. (1979). Pulmonary effects of contact exposure to paraquat: a clinical and experimental study. *Thorax* **34,** 150–160

Lewis, C. E. and Kerby, G. R. (1965). An epidemic of polymer-fume fever. *J. Am. med. Ass.* **191,** 375–378

Lilis, R., Anderson, H., Nicholson, W. J., Daum, S., Fischbein, A. S. and Selikoff, I. J. (1975). Prevalence of disease among vinyl chloride and polyvinyl chloride workers. *Ann. N.Y. Acad. Sci.* **246,** 22–40

Littler, T. R. and McConnell, R. B. (1955). Dimethyl sulphate poisoning. *Br. J. indust. Med.* **12,** 54–56

Lottenberg, R., Waldman, R. H., Ajello, L., Hoff, G. L., Bigler, W. and Zellner, S. R. (1979). Pulmonary histoplasmosis associated with exploration of a bat cave. *Am. J. Epidemiol.* **110,** 156–161

Lowsma, H. B., Jones, R. and Prendergast, J. (1966). Effects of respired polyvinyl pyrrolidone aerosols in rats. *Toxic. appl. Pharmac.* **9,** 571–582

Lunn, J. A. (1966). Millworker's asthma. Allergic responses to the grain weevil (Sitophiles granaries). *Br. J. ind. Med.* **23,** 149–152

Lunn, J. A. and Hughes, D. T. D. (1967). Pulmonary hypersensitivity to the grain weevil. *Br. J. ind. Med.* **24,** 158–161

MacCallum, F. O., Marmion, B. P. and Stoker, M. G. P. (1949). Q fever in Great Britain: isolation of *Rickettsia burneti* from an indigenous case. *Lancet* **2,** 1026–1027

McDonagh, B. J. and Martin, J. (1970). Paraquat poisoning in children. *Archs Dis. Childh.* **45,** 425–427

McKendrick, G. D. W., Davies, J. and Dutta, T. (1973). A small outbreak of psittacosis. *Lancet* **2,** 1255

McLaughlin, A. I. G., Bidstrup, P. L. and Konstam, M. (1963). The effect of hair lacquer sprays on the lungs. *Food Cosmet. Toxicol.* **1,** 171–188

Madsen, D., Klock, L. E., Wenzel, F. J., Robbins, J. L. and Schmidt, C. D. (1976). The prevalence of farmer's lung in an agricultural population. *Am. Rev. resp. Dis.* **13,** 171–174

Maesen, F. P. V. (1972). *Pigeon breeder's lung.* N. Vuitgeverij Winants, Heerlen, Hasselt

Mahon, W. E., Scott, D. J., Ansell, G., Manson, G. L. and Fraser, R. (1967). Hypersensitivity to pituitary snuff with miliary shadowing in the lungs. *Thorax* **22,** 13–20

Malten, K. E. and Zielhuis, R. L. (1964). *Industrial Toxicology and Dermatology in the Production and Processing of Plastics.* Elsevier Monographs

Mann, P. G. H. (1975). Scope and benefits of pet keeping. In *Pet Animals and Society,* edited by R. S. Anderson, pp. 1—39. Br. small animal Vet. Ass.; Balliere Tindall

Mann, P. G. and Richens, E. R. (1973). Aspects of human brucellosis. *Postgrad. med. J.* **49,** 523–525

Mansmann, R. A. and Osborn, B. I. (1971). Hypersensitivity pneumonitis to chickens in horses. *J. Allergy clin. Immun.* **51,** 103

Marx, J. J., Wenzel, F. J., Roberts, R. C., Gray, R. L. and Emanuel, D. A. (1973). Migration inhibition factor and farmer's lung antigens. (Abstract) *Clin. Res.* **21,** 852

Marx, J. J. and Flaherty, D. K. (1976). Activation of the complement sequence by extracts of bacteria and fungi associated with hypersensitivity pneumonitis. *J. Allergy Clin. Immun.* **57,** 328–334

Marx, Jr. J. J., Kettrick-Marx, M. A., Mitchell, P. D. and Flaherty, D. K. (1977). Correlation of exposure to various respiratory pathogens with farmer's lung disease. *J. Allergy clin. Immun.* **60,** 169–173

Medical Research Council Symposium (1977). Humidifier fever. *Thorax* **32,** 653–663

Metzger, W. J., Patterson, R., Fink, J., Semerdjam, R. and Roberts, M. (1976). Sauna-takers disease. *J. Am. med. Ass.* **236,** 2209–2211

Meyer, K. F. (1965). Psittacosis-lymphogranuloma venereum agents. In *Viral and Rickettsial Infections of Man,* edited by F. L. Horsfall and I. Tamm, p. 1006. Philadelphia; Lippincott

Millar, J. K. (1978). The chest film findings in 'Q' fever — a series of 35 cases. *Clin. Radiol.* **29,** 371–375

Miller, A., Teirstein, A. S., Chuang, M., Selikoff, I. J. and Warshaw, R. (1975). Changes in pulmonary function in workers exposed to vinyl chloride and polyvinyl chloride. *Ann. N.Y. Acad. Sci.* **246,** 42–52

Miller, G. J., Hearn, C. E. D. and Edwards, R. H. T. (1971). Pulmonary function at rest and during exercise following bagassosis. *Br. J. ind. Med.* **28,** 152–158

Miyagawa, T., Ochi, T. and Takahashi, H. (1978). Hypersensitivity pneumonitis with antibodies to *Cryptococcus neoformans. Clin. Allergy* **8,** 501–509

Molina, C. (1976). *Broncho-pulmonary immunopathology.* Edinburgh, London and New York; Churchill Livingstone, (Translated by J. Pepys)

Moore, V. (1978). Humoral and cellular immunologic aspects of hypersensitivity pneumonitis. *J. Allergy clin. Immun.* **61,** 210–213

Moore, V. L., Fink, J. N., Barboriak, J. J., Ruff, L. L. and Schlueter, D. P. (1974). Immunologic events in pigeon breeder's disease. *J. Allergy clin. Immun.* **53,** 319–328

Moore, V. L. and Fink. J. N. (1975). Immunologic studies in hypersensitivity pneumonitis-quantitative precipitins and complement-fixing antibodies in symptomatic and asymptomatic pigeon breeders. *J. Lab. clin. Med.* **85,** 540–545

Morgan, D. C., Smyth, J. T., Lister, R. W. and Pethybridge, R. J. (1973). Chest symptoms and farmer's lung: a community survey. *Br. J. indust. Med.* **30,** 259–265

Morgan, D. C., Smyth, J. T., Lister, R. W., Pethybridge, R. J., Gilson, J. C., Callaghan, P. and Thomas, G. O. (1975). Chest symptoms in farming communities with special reference to farmer's lung. *Br. J. indust. Med.* **32,** 228–234

Morris Evans, W. H. and Foreman, H. M. (1963). Smallpox handler's lung. *Proc. R. Soc. Med.* **56,** 274–275

Morris, J. S., Read, A. E., Jones, B., Cotes, J. E. and Edwards, J. H. (1971). Coeliac disease and lung disease. *Lancet* **1,** 754

Muir, D. C. F. and Emmett, P. C. (1976). Methods for determination of the atmospheric concentrations of oil mist. *Ann. occup. Hyg.* **19,** 89

Murray, J. F., Lurie, H. I., Kaye, J., Komins, C., Borok, R. and Way, M. (1957). Benign pulmonary histoplasmosis (cave disease) in South Africa. *S. Afr. Med. J.* **31,** 245–253

Nash, E. S., Vogelpoel, L. and Becker, W. B. (1967). Pigeon breeder's lung — a case report. *S. Afr. med. J.* **41,** 191–193

Newman Taylor, A., Pickering, C. A. C., Turner-Warwick, M. and Pepys, J. (1978). Respiratory allergy to a factory humidifier contaminant present as pyrexia of undetermined origin. *Br. med. J.* **2,** 94–95

Newman Taylor, A. J., Taylor, P., Bryant, D. H., Longbottom, J. L. and Pepys, J. (1977). False positive complement fixation tests with respiratory virus preparations in bird fanciers with allergic alveolitis. *Thorax* **32,** 563–566

O'Brien, I. M., Bull, J., Creamer, B., Sepulveda, R., Harries, M., Bunge, P. S. and Pepys, J. (1978). Asthma and extrinsic allergic alveolitis due to *Merulius lacrymans. Clin. Allergy* **8,** 535–542

Okawa, M. T. and Polakoff, P. L. (1974). Occupational Health Case Reports — No. 7. Teflon. *J. occup. Med.* **16,** 350–355

Oldberger, D., Maurer, W. J., Beltaos, E. and Magnin, G. E. (1972). Inhalation lipoid pneumonia from burning fats. A newly recognised industrial hazard. *J. Am. med. Ass.* **222**, 1288–1289

Oliver, P. O. (1979). Medical hazards at sea. *Br. J. hosp. Med.* **22,** 615–618

Olsson, B. J. and Treuting, W. L. (1944). An epidemic of a severe pneumonitis in the Bayon region of Louisiana. 1. Epidemiological study. *Publ. Hlth Rep. (Wash.)* **59,** 1299–1311

Panasenko, V. T. (1967). Ecology of microfungi. *Bot. Rev.* **33,** 189–215

Parratt, D. and Boyd, G. (1976). Farmer's lung: a neglected antigen. *Lancet* **1,** 1294

Parratt, D., Nielsen, K. H., Boyd, G. and White, R. G. (1975). The quantitation of antibody in farmer's lung syndrome using a radioimmunoassay. *Clin. exp. Immun.* **20,** 217–225

Parrot, W. F. and Blyth, W. (1980). Another causal factor in the production of humidifier fever. *J. Soc. occup. Med.* **30,** 63–68

Parry, W. H. and Mason, K. D. (1972). Psittacosis in pet shops: an occupational hazard. *Community Med.* **128,** 209–210

Pasternack, B. and Ehrlich, L. (1972). Occupational exposure to an oil mist atmosphere. A 12 year mortality study. *Archs envir. Hlth* **25**, 286–294

Patterson, R., Addington, W., Banner, A. S., Byron, G. E., France, M., Herbert, F. A., Nicotra, M. B., Pruzansky, J. J., Rivera, M., Roberts, M., Yawn, D. and Zeiss, C. R. (1979). Antihapten antibodies in workers exposed to trimellitic anhydride fumes: a potential immunopathogenetic mechanism for the trimellitic anhydride pulmonary disease-anaemia syndrome. *Am. Rev. resp. Dis.* **120,** 1259–1267

Patterson, R., Roberts, M., Roberts, R. C., Emanuel, D. A. and Fink, J. N. (1976). Antibodies of different immunoglobulin classes against antigens causing farmer's lung. *Am. Rev. resp. Dis.* **114,** 315–324

Paturau, J. M. (1969). *By-products of the Cane Sugar Industry*. Amsterdam; Elsevier

Pauli, B., Gerber, H. and Schatzmann, U. (1972). Farmer's Lung beim pferd. *Path. Microbiol.* **38,** 200–214

Pearsall, H. R., Morgan, E. H., Tesluk, H. and Beggs, D. (1960). Parakeet dander pneumonitis. Acute psittaco-kerato-pneumoconiosis. *Bull. Mason Clin.* **14,** 127–137

Pendergrass, E. P. (1942). Some considerations concerning the roentgen diagnosis of pneumoconiosis and silicosis. *Am. J. Roent.* **48,** 571–594

Pepys, J. (1969). *Hypersensitivity Diseases of the Lungs due to Fungi and Organic Dusts.* Basel: Karger

Pepys, J. (1977). Clinical and therapeutic significance of patterns of allergic reactions of the lungs to extrinsic agents. *Am. Rev. resp. Dis.* **116,** 573–588

Pepys, J. (1978). Antigens and hypersensitivity pneumonitis. *J. Allergy clin. Immun.* **61,** 201–203

Pepys, J. and Jenkins, P. A. (1965). Precipitin (FLH) test in farmer's lung. *Thorax* **20,** 21–35

Pestalozzi, C. (1959). Febrile Gruppener Krankungen in einer Modellschreinerei durch Inhalation von mit Schimelpilzen Kontaminiertem Befeuchterwasser ('Befeuchterfieber'). *Schweiz. med. Wschr.* **89,** 710–713

Pether, J. V. S. and Greatorex, F. B. (1976). Farmer's lung disease in Somerset. *Br. J. indust. Med.* **33,** 265–268

Pickering, C. A. C., Moore, W. K. S., Lacey, J., Holford-Strevens, V. C. and Pepys, J. (1976). Investigation of a respiratory disease associated with an air-conditioning system. *Clin. Allergy* **6,** 109–118

Pickles, W. N. (1944). The country doctor and public health. *Publ. Hlth* **58,** 2–5

Pierce, A. K., Nicholson, D. P., Miller, J. M. and Johnson, R. L. (1968). Pulmonary function in bagasse worker's lung disease. *Am. Rev. resp. Dis.* **97,** 561–570

Pimentel, J. C. (1970). Furrier's lung. *Thorax* **25,** 387–398

Pimentel, J. C. (1973). A granulomatous lung disease produced by bakelite. *Am. Rev. resp. Dis.* **108,** 1303–1310

Pimentel, J. C. and Ávila, R. (1973). Respiratory disease in cork workers ('suberosis'). *Thorax* **28,** 409–423

Pirie, H. M., Dawson, C. O., Breeze, R. G., Wiseman, A. and Hamilton, J. (1971). A bovine disease similar to farmer's lung: extrinsic allergic alveolitis. *Vet. Rec.* **88,** 346–350

Plessner, M. M. (1960). Une maladie des trieurs de plumes: la fièvre de canard. *Archs Mal. prof. Méd. trav.* **21,** 67–69

Plotkin, S. A., Brachman, P. S., Utel, M., Bumford, F. H. and Atchison, M. M. (1960). An epidemic of inhalation anthrax, the first in the twentieth century. *Am. J. Med.* **29,** 992–1001

Prodan, L., Suciu, I., Pislaru, V., Ilea, E. and Pascu, L. (1975). Experimental chronic poisoning with vinyl chloride (monochloroethene). *Ann. N.Y. Acad. Sci.* **246,** 159–163

Proudfit, J. P., van Ordstrand, H. S. and Miller, C. W. (1950). Chronic lipid pneumonia following occupational exposure. *Ind. Hyg. occup. Med.* **1,** 105–111

Proudfoot, A. T., Stewart, M. S., Levitt, T. and Widdop, B. (1979). Paraquat poisoning: significance of plasma-paraquat concentrations. *Lancet* **2,** 330–332

Public Health Laboratory Service (1973). Notes and news. *Br. med. J.* **3,** 704

Purtilo, D. T., Bonica, A. and Yang, J. P. S. (1978). Bird fancier's lung and coeliac disease. *Lancet* **1,** 1357–1358

Q fever (1976–7). *Br. med. J.* **2,** 900

Ramsay, A. M. and Emond, R. T. D. (1978). *Infectious Diseases.* 2nd edn. p. 113. London: Wm. Heinemann Medical Books Ltd

Rankin, J., Kobayashi, M., Barbee, R. A. and Dickie, H. A. (1967). Pulmonary granulomatoses due to inhaled organic antigens. *Med. Clins N. Am.* **51,** 459–482

Rebello, G. and Mason, J. K. (1978). Pulmonary histological appearances in fatal paraquat poisoning. *Histopath* **2,** 53–66

Reed, C. E., Sosman, A. and Barbee, R. A. (1965). Pigeon breeder's lung. *J. Am. med. Ass.* **193,** 261–266

Renaud, J., Pétavy, A. F., Duriez-Vauchelle, T., Guillot, J. and Coulet, M. (1979). Analyse antigénique des acariens du fromage et vue d'une étude de la maladie des fromagers. *Rev. fr. Mal. resp.* **7,** 441–447

Reyes, C. N., Emanuel, D. A., Roberts, R. C., Marx, Jr., J. J. and Wenzel, F. J. (1976). The histopathology of farmer's lung (60 consecutive cases). *Am. J. clin. Path.* **66,** 460–461 (Abstract)

Reynolds, H. Y., Fulmer, J. D., Kazmierowski, J. A., Roberts, W. C., Frank, M. M. and Crystal, R. G. (1977). Analysis of cellular and protein content of broncho-alveolar lavage fluid from patients with idiopathic pulmonary fibrosis and chronic hypersensitivity pneumonitis. *J. clin. Invest.* **59,** 165–175

Rice, D. L., Jenkins, D. E., Gray, J. M. and Greenberg, S. D. (1977). Chemical pneumonitis secondary to inhalation of epoxy pipe coating. *Archs envir. Hlth,* **32,** 173–177

Riddle, H. F. V. (1974). Prevalence of respiratory and sensitization by mould antigens among a group of malt workers. *Br. J. indust. Med.* **31,** 31–35

Riddle, H. F. V., Channell, S., Blyth, W., Weir, D. M., Lloyd, M., Amos, W. M. G. and Grant, I. W. B. (1968). Allergic alveolitis in a maltworker. *Thorax* **23,** 271–280

Ripe, E., Hanngren, A., Holmgren, A. and Johansson, I. (1969). Thesaurosis? — Analysis of a case. *Scand. J. resp. Dis.* **50,** 156–167

Robbins, J. J. and Ware, R. L. (1964). Pulmonary edema from Teflon fumes. *New Engl. J. Med.* **271,** 360–361

Roberts, R. C., Wenzel, F. J. and Emanuel, D. A. (1976). Precipitating antibodies in a midwest dairy farming population toward the antigens associated with farmer's lung disease. *J. Allergy and clin. Immun.* **57**, 518–524

Robinson, T. J. (1976). Coeliac disease with farmer's lung. *Br. med. J.* **1**, 745–746

Rodey, G. E., Fink, J., Koethe, S., Schlueter, D., Witkowski, J., Bettonville, P., Rimm, A. and Moore, V. (1979). A study of HLA-A, B, C and DR specificities in pigeon breeder's disease. *Am. Rev. resp. Dis.* **119,** 755–759

Ross, P. J., Seaton, A., Foreman, H. M. and Morris Evans, W. H. (1974). Pulmonary calcification following smallpox handler's lung. *Thorax* **29,** 659–665

Sakabe, H. (1975). Bone lesions among polyvinyl chloride production workers in Japan. *Ann. N.Y. Acad. Sci.* **246,** 78–79

Sakula, A. (1967). Mushroom worker's lung. *Br. med. J.* **3**, 708–710

Saltzman, H. A. and Fridovich, I. (1973). Oxygen toxicity. Introduction to a protective enzyme: superoxide dismutase. *Circulation* **48**, 921–923

Salvaggio, J., Arquembourg, P., Seabury, J. and Buechner, H. (1969). Bagassosis IV. Precipitins against extracts of thermophilic actinomycetes in patients with bagassosis. *Am. J. Med.* **46,** 538–544

Sarosi, G. A. (1979). Personal communication

Sarosi, G. A. and Davies, S. F. (1979). Blastomycosis. *Am. Rev. resp. Dis.* **120,** 911–938

Sarosi, G. W. and Serstock, D. (1976). Isolation of *Blastomyces dermatitidis* from pigeon manure. *Am. Rev. resp. Dis.* **114,** 1179–1183

Scadding, J. G. (1967). *Sarcoidosis.* p. 160. London; Eyre and Spottiswoode

Schatz, N., Patterson, R., Fink, J., Moore, V., Rodey, G., Cunningham, A., Roberts, M. and Harris, K. (1976). Pigeon breeder's disease. III. A study of a family exposed to doves. *Clin. exp. Immun.* **24,** 33–41

Schepers, G. W. H. (1962). Thesaurosis versus sarcoidosis. *J. Am. med. Ass.* **181**, 635–637

Scherrer, M., Imhof, K., Weickhardt, W. and Lebek, G. (1978). Befeuchterfieber in einer Giesserei. *Revue Suisse Med. (Praxis).* **67**, 1855–1861

Schlueter, D. P., Fink, J. N. and Henley, G. T. (1972). Wood pulp worker's disease: a hypersensitivity pneumonitis caused by *Alternaria. Ann. intern. Med.* **77,** 907–914

Schmelzer, L. L. and Tabershaw, I. R. (1968). Exposure factors in occupational coccidioidomycosis. *Am. J. publ. Hlth* **58,** 107–113

Schorlemmer, H. W., Edwards, J. H., Davies, P. and Allison, A. C. (1977). Macrophage responses to mouldy hay dust, *Micropolyspora faeni* and zymosan by the alternative pathway. *Clin. exp. Immun.* **27**, 198–207

Schulz, K. H., Felton, G. and Hausen, B. M. (1974). Allergy to the spores of *Pleurotus florida. Lancet* **1,** 29

Schuyler, M. R., Thigpen, T. P. and Salvaggio, J. E. (1978). Local pulmonary immunity in pigeon breeder's disease. *Ann. intern. Med.* **88**, 355–358

Seabury, J., Salvaggio, J., Buechner, H. and Kunder, V. G. (1968). The pathology of the acute and chronic stages of farmer's lung. *Thorax* **23,** 469–489

Seabury, J., Salvaggio, J., Buechner, H. and Kunder, V. G. (1968). Bagassosis III. Isolation of thermophilic and mesophilic actinomycetes and fungi from mouldy bagasse. *Proc. Soc. exp. Biol. Med.* **129,** 351–360

Seal, R. M. E. (1975). Pathology of extrinsic allergic bronchiolo-alveolitis. In *Alveolar Interstitium of the Lung. Prog. resp. Res.*, pp. 66–73, edited by H. Herzog, F. Basset and R. Georges

Seal, R. M. E., Edwards, J. H. and Hayes, M. (1975). The response of the lung to inhaled antigens. *Prog. resp. Dis.* **8,** 125–129

Seal, R. M. E., Hapke, E. J., Thomas, G. O., Meek, J. C. and Hayes, M. (1968). The pathology of the acute and chronic stages of farmer's lung. *Thorax* **23,** 469–489

Seidel, J. (1959). Mucolylitic aerosol therapy for lipid pneumonia. *J. Am. med. Ass.* **171,** 1810–1813

Sennekamp, J., Niese, D., Stroehmann, I. and Rittner, C. (1978). Pigeon breeder's lung lacking detectable antibodies. *Clin. Allergy* **8**, 305–310

Sennekamp, J., Rittner, C. and Vogel, F. (1977). HLA-B8 in pigeon fancier's lung. *Lung* **154,** 148–149

Sheffer, A. L., Rocklin, R. E. and Goetzl, E. J. (1975). Immunologic components of hypersensitivity reactions to cromolyn sodium. *New Engl. J. Med.* **293,** 1220–1224

Shelley, E., Dean, G., Collins, D. Dinah, R., Evans, J. and McHardy, J. (1979). Farmer's lung: a study in North-West Ireland. *J. Irish med. Ass.* **72,** 261–264

Shoshkes, M., Banfield, W. G. and Rosenbaum, S. J. (1950). Distribution, effect and fate of oil aerosol particles retained in the lungs of mice. *Archs ind. Hyg. occup. Med.* **1,** 20–35

Smith, P. and Heath, D. (1975). The pathology of the lung in paraquat poisoning. *J. clin. Path.* **28** (Suppl.) 9, 81–93

Smyth, J. T., Adkins, G. E., Lloyd, M., Moore, B. and McWhite, E. (1975). Farmer's lung in Devon. *Thorax* **30,** 197–203

Sodeman, W. A. and Pullen, R. L. (1943). Bagasse disease of the lungs. *N. Orleans med. Surg.* **95,** 558–560

Sodeman, W. A. and Pullen, R. L. (1944). Bagasse disease of the lungs. *Archs intern. Med.* **73,** 365–374

Sorley, D. L., Levin, M. L., Warren, J. W., Flynn, J. P. G. and Gerstenblith, J. (1979). Bat-associated histoplasmosis in Maryland bridge workers. *Am. J. Med.* **67,** 623–626

Spector, W. G. (1971). The cellular dynamics of granulomas. *Proc. R. Soc. Med.* **64,** 941–942

Spector, W. G. and Heesom, N. (1969). The production of granulomata by antigen-antibody complexes. *J. Path.* **98,** 31–39

Staines, F. H. and Forman, J. A. S. (1961). A survey of 'farmer's lung'. *J. Coll. gen. Practnrs Newsl.* **4,** 351–382

Stewart, C. J. (1974). Mushroom worker's lung — two outbreaks. *Thorax* **29**, 252–257

Stewart, C. J. and Pickering, C. A. C. (1974). Mushroom worker's lung. *Lancet* **1,** 317

Stiehm, E. R., Reed, C. E. and Tooley, W. H. (1967). Pigeon breeder's lung in children. *Pediatrics* **39,** 904–915

Stokes, P. L., Asquith, P., Holmes, G. K. T., Mackintosh, P. and Cooke, W. T. (1972). Histocompatibility antigens associated with adult coeliac disease. *Lancet* **2,** 162–164

Stokes, T. C. Turton, C. W. G. and Turner-Warwick, M. T. (1981). A study of immunoglobulin G subclasses in patients with farmer's lung. *Clin. Allergy* **11**, 201–207

Storch, G., Burford, J. G., George, R. B., Kaufman, L. and Ajello, L. (1980). Acute histoplasmosis. Description of an outbreak in Northern Louisiana. *Chest* **77**, 38–42

Styles, J. A. and Wilson, J. (1973). Comparison between *in vitro* toxicity of polymer and mineral dusts and their fibrogenicity. *Ann. occup. Hyg.* **16,** 241–250

Suciu, I., Prodan, L., Ilea, E., Paduraru, A. and Pascu, L. (1975). Clinical manifestations in vinyl chloride poisoning. *Am. N.Y. Acad. Sci.* **246**, 53–69

Swan, A. A. B. (1969). Exposure of spray operators to paraquat. *Br. J. indust. Med.* **26,** 322–329

Sweet, L. C., Anderson, J. A., Callies, Q. C. and Coates, Jr. E. O. (1971). Hypersensitivity pneumonitis related to a home furnace humidifier. *J. Allergy clin. Immun.* **48,** 171–178

Swift, D. L., Zuskin, E. and Bouhuys, A. (1976). Respiratory deposition of hair spray aerosol and acute lung function changes. *Am. Rev. resp. Dis.* **113** (Suppl.) 96

Szende, B., Lapis, K., Nemes, A. and Pinter, A. (1970). Pneumoconiosis caused by the inhalation of polyvinyl chloride dust. *Medna Lav.* **61**, 433–436

Tebo, T. H., Fredericks, W. W. and Roberts, R. C. (1977). The antigens of pigeon breeder's disease. II. Isolation and characterisation of antigen PDE_1. *Int. Archs Allergy appl. Immun.* **54,** 553–559

Tebo, T. H., Moore, V. L. and Fink, J. N. (1977). Antigens in pigeon breeder's disease. *Clin. Allergy* **7,** 103–108

Terho, E. O. and Lacey, J. (1979). Microbiological and serological studies of farmer's lung in Finland. *Clin. Allergy* **9,** 43–52

Terho, E. O., Lammi, S., and Heinonen, O. P. (1980). Seasonal variation in the incidence of farmer's lung. *Int. J. Epidemiol.* **9,** 219–223

Tewksbury, D. A., Wenzel, F. J. and Emanuel, D. A. (1968). An immunologic study of maple bark disease. *Clin. exp. Immunol.* **3,** 857–863

Thurlbeck, W. M. and Thurlbeck, S. M. (1976). Pulmonary effects of paraquat poisoning. *Chest* **69,** 276–280

Törnell, E. (1946). Thresher's lung. *Acta med. scand.* **125,** 191–219

Tosh, F. E., Hammerman, K. J., Weeks, R. J. and Sarosi, G. A. (1974). A common source epidemic of North American blastomycosis. *Am. Rev. resp. Dis.* **109,** 525–529

Touey, G. P. and Mumpower, R. C. (1957). Measurement of the combustion-zone temperature of cigarettes. *Tobacco, N.Y.* **144,** 18–22

Towey, J. W., Sweany, H. C. and Huron, W. H. (1932). Severe bronchial asthma apparently due to fungus spores found in maple bark. *J. Am. med. Ass.* **99,** 453–459

Treuhaft, M. W., Roberts, R. C., Hackbarth, C., Emanuel, D. A. and Marx, Jr. J. J. (1979). Characterization of precipitin response to *Micropolyspora faeni* in farmer's lung disease by quantitative immunoelectrophoresis. *Am. Rev. resp. Dis.* **119,** 571–578

Turner-Warwick, M. (1980). Immunological features of allergic alveolitis. *Proc. Nara Symposium on Sarcoidosis and other Granulomatous Diseases,* Japan (In press)

Turton, C. W. G., Morris, L. M., Lawler, S. D. and Turner-Warwick, M. (1978). HL-A in cryptogenic fibrosing alveolitis. *Lancet* **1,** 507–508

Vallery-Radot, P. and Giroud, P. (1928). Sporomycose des pelleteurs de grains. *Bull. Soc. méd. Hop. Paris* **52,** 1632–1645

van Toorn, D. W. (1970). Coffee workers' lung. *Thorax* **25,** 399–405

Veteran's Administration Cooperative Study (1964). Blastomycosis: a review of 198 collected cases in Veteran Administration Hospitals. *Am. Rev. resp. Dis.* **89,** 659–672

Viswanathan, R., de Monte, A. J. H., Shivpuri, D. N., Venkitasubramanian, T. A., Tandon, H. D., Chandrusekhars, S., Jain, S. K., Gupta, I. M., Singh, P., Gambhie, K. K., Randhawa, H. S. and Singh, V. N. (1963). Bagassosis. *Indian J. med. Res.* **51,** 563–633

Voisin, C., Tonnel, A. B., Lahoute, C., Robin, H. and Aerts, C. (1979). *Proc. International Congress on Resp. Dis.* (In press)

Wagner, J. C., Adler, D. I. and Fuller, D. N. (1955). Foreign body granulomata of the lungs due to liquid paraffin. *Thorax* **10,** 157–170

Ward, A. M., Udnoon, S., Watkins, J., Walker, A. E. and Darke, C. S. (1976). Immunological mechanisms in the pathogenesis of vinyl chloride disease. *Br. med. J.* **1,** 936–938

Ward, C. and Ward, A. M. (1974). Acquired valvular heart-disease in patients who keep pet birds. *Lancet* **2,** 734–736

Ward, J. I., Weeks, M., Allen, D., Hutchenson, Jr., R. H., Anderson, R., Fraser, D. W., Kaufman, L., Ajello, L. and Spickard, A. (1979). Acute histoplasmosis: clinical, epidemiologic and serologic findings of an outbreak associated with exposure to a fallen tree. *Am. J. Med.* **66,** 587–595

Warraki, S. (1963). Respiratory hazards of chlorinated camphene. *Archs envir. Hlth* **7,** 253–256

Warren, C. P. W. (1977). Extrinsic allergic alveolitis: a disease commoner in non-smokers. *Thorax* **32,** 567–569

Warren, C. P. W. and Tse, K. S. (1974). Extrinsic allergic alveolitis owing to hypersensitivity to chickens — significance of sputum precipitins. *Am. Rev. resp. Dis.* **109,** 672–677

Warren, C. P. W., Tse, K. S. and Cherniack, R. M. (1978). Mechanical properties of the lung in extrinsic allergic alveolitis. *Thorax* **33,** 315–321

Washburn, A. M., Tuohy, J. H. and Davis, E. L. (1948). Cave sickness. A new disease? *Am. J. publ. Hlth* **38,** 1521–1526

Weill, H., Buechner, H. A., Gonzales, E., Herbert, S. J., Aucoin, E. and Ziskind, M. M. (1966). Bagassosis: A study of pulmonary function in 20 cases. *Ann. intern. Med.* **64,** 737–747

Weill, H., Ferrans, V. J., Gay, R. M. and Ziskind, M. M. (1964). Early lipoid pneumonia. Roentgenological, anatomic and physiologic characteristics. *Am. J. Med.* **36,** 370–376

Weinberger, S. E., Kelman, J. A., Elson, N. A., Young, Jr. R. C., Reynolds, H. Y., Fulmer, J. D. and Crystal, R. G. (1978). Bronchoalveolar lavage in interstitial lung disease. *Ann. intern. Med.* **89,** 459–466

Weiss, N. S. and Soleymani, D. A. (1971). Hypersensitivity lung disease caused by contamination of an air conditioning system. *Ann. Allergy* **29,** 154–156

Weissman, H. (1951). Lipoid pneumonia: a report of two cases. *Am. Rev. Tuberc.* **64,** 572–576

Welter, E. S. (1978). Manufacturing exposure to coolant-lubricants. *J. occup. Med.* **20,** 535–538

Wenzel, F. J. and Emanuel, D. A. (1967). The epidemiology of maple bark disease. *Archs envir. Hlth* **14,** 385–389

Wenzel, F. J., Emanuel, D. A., Lawton, B. R. and Magnin, G. E. (1964). Isolation of the causative agent of farmer's lung. *Ann. Allergy* **22,** 533

Werner, S. B., Pappagianis, D., Heindl, I. and Mickel, A. (1972). An epidemic of coccidioidomycosis among archeology students in Northern California. *New Engl. J. Med.* **286,** 507–512

Willey, R. F., Matthews, M. B., Pleutherer, J. F. and Marmion, B. P. (1979). Chronic cryptic Q-fever infection of the heart. *Lancet* **2,** 270–272

Williams, J. V. (1963). Inhalation and skin tests with extracts of hay and fungi in patients with farmer's lung. *Thorax* **18,** 182–196

Williams, N. and Smith, F.K. (1972). Polymer fume fever. An elusive diagnosis. *J. Am. med. Ass.* **219,** 1587–1589

Williams, N., Atkinson, W. and Patchefsky, A. S. (1974). Polymer-fume fever: not so benign. *J. occup. Med.* **16,** 519–522

Williams, P. L., Sable, D. L., Mendez, P. and Smyth, L. T. (1979). Symptomatic coccidioidomycosis following a severe natural dust storm. *Chest* **76,** 566–570

Wüthrich, B. and Keiser, G. (1970). Das Käsewascherasthma Abgrenzung gegenuber die Käsewascherdrankei. *Schweiz. med. Wschr.* **100,** 1108–1111

Yoshida, K. and Maybank, J. (1978). Physical and environmental characteristic of grain dusts. In *Grain Dust and Health. III Environmental factors,* edited by D. J. Cotton and J. A. Dosman. *Ann. intern. med.* **89,** 420–421

Zaidi, S. H., Dogra, R. K. S., Shanker, R. and Chaudra, S. V. (1971). Experimental farmer's lung in guinea pigs. *J. Path.* **105,** 41–48

Zeiss, C. R., Levitz, D., Chacon, R., Wollonsky, P., Patterson, R. and Pruzansky, J. (1980). Quantitation and new antigenic determinant specificity of antibodies induced by inhalation of trimellitic anhydride in man. *Int. Arch. Allergy appl. Immunol.* **61,** 380–388

Zeiss, C. R., Patterson, R., Pruzansky, J. J., Miller, M., Rosenberg, M. and Levitz, D. (1977). Trimellitic anhydride-induced airway syndromes. Clinical and immunological studies. *J. Allergy clin. Immunol.* **60,** 96–103

Zuskin, E. and Bouhuys, A. (1974). Acute airway response to hair spray preparations. *New Engl. J. Med.* **290,** 660–663

Zvetina, J. R., Rippon, J. W. and Daum, V. (1978). Chronic pulmonary sporotrichosis. *Mycopathologia* **64,** 53–57

12 Occupational Asthma (including Byssinosis)

DEFINITION

Although there is no generally agreed definition of asthma, that based on the recommendation of the Ciba Guest Symposium Report (1959) which is practical, accurate and widely accepted as follows:

'Asthma is a disorder of function characterized by widespread partial obstruction of the airways which varies in severity, is reversible either spontaneously or as a result of treatment, and is not due to cardiovascular disease.'

This definition, which implies wide variations in resistance to intrapulmonary air flow (usually) over short periods of time, has the advantage of conveying the concept not of a 'disease' but of the patterns of response of the 'target-organs'—the lungs—mediated by many different provoking factors via a variety of intermediate pathways.

Asthma falls into two subgroups: *'extrinsic' asthma* due to specific external allergens; and *cryptogenic (or 'intrinsic') asthma* in which no external agency is evident. Occupational asthma, therefore, is caused by some specific extrinsic agent or agents in the form of dust, fume or vapour in an industrial environment. Byssinosis fulfils this definition of extrinsic asthma and is, therefore, considered in this chapter.

Though wheezing is a common feature of asthma it is not a criterion of the definition nor, therefore, of diagnosis, and is absent in some cases. Similarly, episodic dyspnoea though usual, may be slight or absent; and, on occasion, airflow obstruction may persist for long periods—weeks or even months.

PREVALENCE

It is impossible to give an overall indication of the prevalence of occupational asthma. It varies widely between different countries, different industries, with the nature of the causal agent and according to the numbers of workers exposed. It has been estimated that about 2 per cent of all cases of asthma are occupational (Introna, 1966). In Japan, some 15 per cent of asthma in adult males is believed to be occupational (Kobayashi, 1974). Among exposed workers, however, only a minority develop asthma. In recent years there has been a steady increase in potential asthma-provoking agents in industry and this can be expected to continue for the foreseeable future. The range of substances known to be responsible is very large as *Tables 12.1* to *12.6*, which make no claim to be complete, show.

PREDISPOSING FACTORS

Atopic individuals tend to develop allergy more readily than non-atopics after short periods of exposure and with low concentrations of the responsible agent.

Atopy can be defined as an ability to produce IgE antibodies readily on contact with common environmental allergens encountered in everyday life (Pepys, 1973). It can be identified by performing skin prick tests with a few of these allergens—for example, grass pollen and the house-dust mite. A 3mm weal to these allergens with a negative control constitutes atopy irrespective of the presence or absence of disease. Defined in this way atopy is present in about 25 to 35 per cent of unselected populations, though the prevalence is lower after 50 years of age (Barbee *et al.*, 1976; Davies, 1979).

In some industries there is a clear increase in the risk of sensitization in atopic workers: for example, those exposed to grain dust, biological detergents, platinum salts and locusts (*see* later under appropriate headings). Although occupational asthma due to other causes often develops in apparently non-atopic individuals the role of atopy in these cases has still to be adequately assessed.

The development of asthma may also be influenced by whether exposure to the offending agent is continuous or intermittent.

TABLES OF VARIOUS CAUSES OF OCCUPATIONAL ASTHMA

Table 12.1 Grains, Flour, Plants and Gum

Sensitizing agent	*Type of asthma*			*Other**	*Occupation*	*References*
	Immediate	*Late*	*Not specified*			
Wheat	–	–	+		Millers	Duke, 1935
Buckwheat	–	+	–		Bakers	Ordman, 1947
Grain	+	+	–	Systemic	Farmers and grain handlers	Skoulas, Williams and Merriman, 1964 Tse *et al.*, 1973 Warren, Cherniack and Tse, 1974
Grain	+	+	–	Recurrent, nocturnal	Farmer	Davies, Green and Schofield, 1976
Grain	+	+	–		Grain elevator workers	Chan-Yeung, Wong and Maclean, 1979
Flour	–	–	+		Bakers	Popa, George and Gavanescu, 1970
Flour	–	–	+		Bakers	Björkstén *et al.*, 1977
Flour	+	+	+		Bakers	Hendrick, Davies and Pepys, 1976
Hops (*Humulus lupulus*)	+	–	–	Urticaria	Brewery chemist	Newark, 1978
Tamarind seeds (*Tamarindus indica*)	–	+	–	Systemic	Millers (sizing agent)	Tuffnell and Dingwell-Fordyce, 1957
Green and roasted coffee beans	–	+	–	Rhinitis, dermatitis	Workers exposed to bean dust	Bernton, 1973 Lehrer, Kerr and Salvaggio, 1978 Žuškin, Valić and Skuric, 1979
Castor beans	+	+	–	Nocturnal	Millers and neighbourhood	Figley and Elrod, 1928
Castor beans	–	+	–	Nocturnal	Chemist	Bernton, 1923
Castor beans	+	+	–		Farmers and gardeners (fertilizer)	Small, 1952
Castor beans	+	+	–	Nocturnal	Coffee bean baggers and handlers	Figley and Rawlings, 1950
Maiko—tuberous roots of devil's tongue	+	–	–		Millers and neighbourhood	Shichijo *et al.*, 1951
Tea fluff	+	–	–		Tea sifting and packing	Uragoda, 1970
Gum acacia	–	–	+		Mould making in sweet factory	Spielman and Baldwin, 1933
Gum acacia	–	–	+		Printer	Bohner, 1941
Gum acacia	+	–	–		Printer	Sprague, 1942
Gum acacia	–	+	–		Printer	Fowler, 1952
Gum acacia	+	+	–		Drug manufacturer	Burge *et al.*, 1978b
Gum tragacanth	–	–	+		Sweet maker (ingested gum)	Brown and Creper, 1947
Gum tragacanth	–	–	+	Prolonged	Gum manufacturer	Gelfand, 1943
Strawberry pollen	–	–	+		Strawberry grower	Kobayashi, 1974
Tobacco dust	+	–	–		Cigarette factory workers	Valić, Beritić and Butković, 1976
Wool	+	–	–		Workers in woollen industry	Moll, 1933

*Nocturnal, recurrent and prolonged asthma and non-respiratory effects
Note: late = non-immediate

Table 12.2 Insects, Animal Products, Fungi and Other Agents

Sensitizing agent	*Type of asthma*			*Other**	*Occupation*	*References*
	Immediate	*Late*	*Not specified*			
INSECTS ETC.						
Beetles (Coleoptera)	+	–	–		Zoological museum curator	Sheldon and Johnston, 1941
Locusts	+	–	–		Laboratory workers	Frankland, 1953
Locusts	–	–	+		Laboratory workers	Joly, 1963
Locusts	+	–	–	Urticaria, rhinitis	Laboratory workers and schoolchildren	Burge *et al.*, 1979a
Cockroaches	+	–	–		Laboratory workers and others	Bernton, McMahon and Brown, 1972
Crickets	+	+?	–		Field contact	Harfi, 1980
Bee moths	+	–	–		Fish bait breeders	Stevenson and Mathews, 1967
Housefly maggots (*Musca domesticus*)	–	–	+		Anglers Anglers	Buisseret, 1978 Frankland, 1978
Grain weevil (*Sitophilus granarius*)	–	–	+		Laboratory workers	Frankland and Lunn, 1965
	+	–	–		Mill workers	Lunn, 1966
Grain storage mites	+	–	–	Rhinitis	Farm workers Farm workers	Cuthbert *et al.*, 1979 Davies, Green and Schofield, 1976
Grain storage mites	–	+	–	Recurrent nocturnal	Grain and flour mill workers, bakers	Wraith, Cunnington and Seymour, 1979
Mexican bean weevil (*Zabrotes subfasciatus*)	–	–	+		Pea and bean sorters	Wittich, 1940
Moths and butterflies					General population	Kino and Oshima, 1978
	+	+	–	Nocturnal	Entomologists	Randolph, 1934
Carmine (*coccus cactus*)		+	–		Cosmetic manufacturer/ dye maker	Burge *et al.*, 1979b
Silkworms	+	–	–		Silk worm sericulturers	Kobayashi, 1974
LABORATORY AND OTHER ANIMALS						
Rats and mice	+	–	–		Laboratory workers	Newman Taylor, Longbottom, and Pepys, 1977
Rats, mice and others	–	–	+		Laboratory workers	Lincoln, Bolton and Garrett, 1974
Rats, mice, guinea pigs and rabbits	–	–	+			Ohman, Lowell and Bloch, 1975
Rats	–	–	+		Laboratory workers	Frankland, 1974
Sea squirt fluid	–	+	–	Nocturnal	Oyster and pearl gatherers	Jyo *et al.*, 1980
OTHERS						
Avian proteins	–	+	–		Bird fancers	Hargreave and Pepys, 1972
Feathers	–	+	–	Systemic	Feather pickers	Plessner, 1960
Prawns	+	+	–		Prawn processing	Gaddie *et al.*, 1980
Oysters	–	+	–		Oyster shuckers	Jyo *et al.*, 1980
Pearl shell dust	–	–	+			Shioda *et al.*, 1973
Contaminated water (amoebae and other organisms)	–	+	–	Alveolitis	Stationery manufacture	Friend *et al.*, 1977 Newman Taylor, Longbottom and Pepys, 1977 Medical Research Council, 1977
Contaminated water (amoebae and other organisms)	–	+	–	Monday symptoms	Printing shop workers	Pickering *et al.*, 1976
FUNGI						
Alternaria and *aspergillus* spp.	+	+	–		Bakers	Klaustermeyer, Bardana and Hale, 1977

Table 12.2 (continued)

Sensitizing agent	*Type of asthma*			*Other**	*Occupation*	*References*
	Immediate	*Late*	*Not specified*			
Spores of *Cladiosporium, Verticillium* and *Paecilomyces*	+	+	–		Farm workers during harvesting	Darke *et al.*, 1976
Merulius lacrymans	+	+	–		Domestic	O'Brien *et al.*, 1978
Mushroom spores	–	–	+		Mushroom cultivator	Kobayashi, 1974

Table 12.3 Woods

Sensitizing agent	*Type of asthma*			*Other**	*Occupation*	*References*
	Immediate	*Late*	*Not specified*			
Western red cedar (*Thuja plicata*)	+	+	–		Wood workers	Chan-Yeung *et al.*, 1973
Western red cedar (*Thuja plicata*)	+	+	–	Prolonged	Wood workers	Chan-Yeung, 1977
Western red cedar (*Thuja plicata*)	–	+	–	Nocturnal and prolonged	Timber millers, joiners and carpenters	Gandevia and Milne, 1970
Western red cedar (*Thuja plicata*)	–	+	–		Carpenters	Pickering, Batten and Pepys, 1972
Cedar of Lebanon (*Cedrus libani*)	–	+	–	Nocturnal	Carpenters Carpenters	Greenberg, 1972 Sosman *et al.*, 1969
Iroko (*Chlorophora excelsa*)	+	–	–		Carpenters	Pickering, Batten and Pepys, 1972
South African boxwood	+	–	–	Systemic		Harvey Gibson, 1905
South African boxwood	+	+	–	Nocturnal	Shuttle makers	Hay, 1907
Mansonia	–	+	–	Systemic		Bridge, 1935
Oak	+	–	–		Sawmiller	Sosman *et al.*, 1969
Mahogany	+	+	–		Patterns maker	Sosman *et al.*, 1969
Abiruana	–	+	–	6-week recovery		Booth, Le Foldt and Moffitt, 1976
Cocabolla (*Dalbergia retusa*)	–	–	+	Rhinitis, dermatitis	Wood finishers	Eaton, 1973
Kejaat (*Pterocarbus angblensis*	+	+	–	Rhinitis, nocturnal	Wood machinist	Ordman, 1949
California redwood (*Sequoia sempervirens*)	+	+	–		Carpenter	Chan-Yeung and Abboud, 1976
California redwood (*Sequoia sempervirens*)	–	+	–		Woodworkers	doPico, 1978
Ramin (*Gonystylus bancanus*)	–	+	–	'Alveolitis'	Woodworker	Howie, Boyd and Moran, 1976
African zebrawood (*Microberlinia*)	+	–	–		Woodworker	Bush, Yunginger and Reed, 1978

Table 12.4 Metals, Chemicals including Soldering Fluxes, and Dyes

Sensitizing agent	*Types of asthma*			*Other**	*Occupation*	*References*
	Immediate	*Late*	*Not specified*			
METALS						
Boranes	+	+	−	Prolonged		(*See* Chapter 13)
Chromic acid	−	+	−	Dermatitis	Chrome plater	Joules, 1932
Potassium chromate and dichromate	−	+	−		Chrome polisher	Card, 1935
Potassium dichromate	−	+	−		Cement workers	Fueki *et al.*, 1972
Sodium bichromate	−	+	−		Chrome plater	Fueki *et al.*, 1972
Platinum salts	+	+	−		Platinum refiners	Hunter, Milton and Perry, 1945
Platinum salts	+	+	−	Rhinitis, conjuncti-vitis	Platinum refiners	Parrot *et al.*, 1969
Platinum salts	+	+	−	Urticaria	Platinum refiners	Pickering, 1972
Platinum salts	+	−	−	Dermatitis	Platinum refiners	Pepys, Pickering and Hughes, 1972
Chloroplatinic acid	−	+	−	Nocturnal	Platinum chemist	Cleare *et al.*, 1976
Nickel sulphate	−	+	−		Nickel plater	McConnell *et al.*, 1973
Nickel carbonyl	−	−	+	Löffler's syndrome	Chemical engineer	Sunderman and Sunderman, 1961
Vanadium and vanadium pentoxide	−	−	+		Gas turbine cleaners	Browne, 1955
Vanadium and vanadium pentoxide	−	+	−	Nocturnal	Boiler cleaners	Williams, 1952
Cobalt	+	−	−		Tungsten carbide grinder	Bruckner, 1967 (*see* Chapter 13)
Stainless steel (chromium and nickel)	+	+	−	Eczema	Welders	Keskinen *et al.*, 1980
CHEMICALS						
Persulfate salts	−	+	−	Dermatitis, rhinitis	Chemical workers	Baur, Fruhmann and von Liebe 1979
Fluorine	−	+	−		Aluminium pot room workers	Mudttum, 1960
Formalin	−	−	+		Match maker	Vaughan, 1939
Formalin	+	−	−		Laboratory worker	Sakula, 1975
Formalin	−	+	−		Phenolic resin moulder	Schoenberg and Mitchell, 1975
Formalin	−	+	−	Recurrent	Nurses	Hendrick and Lane, 1977
Tannic acid	+	−	−	Rhinitis, urticaria	Sunburn spray	Johnston *et al.*, 1951
Paraphenylene diamine	+	+	−		Fur dyers	Silberman and Sorrell, 1959
Dimethyl ethanolamine	+	−	−		Paint sprayer	Vallieres *et al.*, 1977
Amino-ethyl-ethanolamine	+	+	−		Aluminium cable soldering	Pepys and Pickering, 1972
Amino-ethyl-ethanolamine	−	+	−	Prolonged	Aluminium cable soldering	Sterling, 1967
Ethylene diamine	+	+	−		Rubber, shellac manufacturers; photography	Gelfand, 1963, Lam and Chan-Yeung, 1980
Triethyl tetramine	−	+	−		Aircraft fitter	Fawcett, Newman Taylor and Pepys, 1977
Chloramine T	+	+	−		Brewery workers	Bourne, Flindt and Walker, 1979
Phthalic anhydride	+	+	−		Paint manufacturer, tool setter, plastic moulder	Kern, 1939, Fawcett, Newman Taylor and Pepys, 1977

Table 12.4 (continued)

Sensitizing agent	*Types of asthma*			*Other**	*Occupation*	*References*
	Immediate	*Late*	*Not specified*			
Trimellitic anhydride	+	+	–		Chair sprayer	Fawcett, Newman Taylor and Pepys, 1977 (*see* Chapter 11)
Trimellitic anhydride	+	+	–	Systemic	Chemical workers	Zeiss *et al.*, 1977
Colophony (pine resin)	+	+	–	Nocturnal	Electronics manufacturer	Burge *et al.*, 1978
Colophony (pine resin)	+	+	–		Electronics manufacturer and hot melt gluer	Fawcett, Newman Taylor and Pepys, 1976
Polyether alcohol + poly-propylene glycol	+	–	–		Solderer	Stevens, 1976
Furan-based, resin binder systems (furfuryl alcohol)	–	+	–	Rhinitis, lacrimation	Foundry mold maker	Cockcroft *et al.*, 1980
Polyvinyl chloride vapour (phthalic anhydride)	+	+	–	Increased by smoking	Meat wrappers (PVC soft-wrap film)	Sokol, Aelony and Bell, 1973
Polyvinyl chloride vapour (phthalic anhydride)	–	–	+		Meat wrappers	Falk and Portnoy, 1976
Polyvinyl chloride vapour (phthalic anhydride)	+	+	–		Meat wrappers	Andrasch *et al.*, 1976
Tetrachlorphthalic anhydride	–	+	–	Severe systemic	Epoxy resin manufacturers	Schleuter *et al.*, 1978
REACTIVE DYES						
Levafix brilliant yellow	+	–	–		Dye weighers	Alanko *et al.*, 1978
Drimaren brilliant yellow	+	–	–		Dye weighers	Alanko *et al.*, 1978
Drimaren brilliant blue	+	–	–		Dye weighers	Alanko *et al.*, 1978
Cibachrome brilliant scarlet	+	–	–		Dye weighers	Alanko *et al.*, 1978
Persulphate and henna	+	+	–		Hairdressers	Pepys, Hutchcroft and Breslin, 1976

Table 12.5 Drugs and Enzymes

Sensitizing agent	*Type of asthma*			*Other**	*Occupation*	*References*
	Immediate	*Late*	*Not specified*			
DRUGS						
Psyllium	+	–	–		Laxative manufacturer	Busse and Schoenwetter, 1975
Methyl dopa	–	+	–	Nocturnal	Manufacturer	Harries *et al.*, 1979
Salbutamol intermediate	–	+	–		Manufacturer	Fawcett, Pepys and Erooga, 1976
Amprolium HCl	+	–	–		Poultry feed mixer	Greene and Freedman, 1976
Dichloramine	–	–	+		Manufacturer	Popa *et al.*, 1969b
Piperazine dihydrochloride	–	+	–	Prolonged recovery	Process worker and chemist	Pepys, Pickering and Loudon, 1972
Spiramycin	–	+	–		Manufacturing engineer	Davies and Pepys, 1975
Penicillins	–	+	–	Recurrent nocturnal	Manufacturer	Davies, Hendrick and Pepys, 1974
Phenylglycine acid chloride	+	–	–		Ampicillin manufacture	Kammermeyer and Mathews, 1973

Table 12.5 (continued)

Sensitizing agent	Type of asthma			Other*	Occupation	References
	Immediate	Late	Not specified			
Tetracycline	+	–	–		Encapsulator	Menon and Das, 1977
Tetracycline	+	–	–		Ingestion	Fawcett and Pepys, 1976
Sulphathiazole	–	–	+		Manufacturer	Popa *et al.*, 1969b
Sulphonechloramides, chloramine T and halazone	+	–	+		Manufacturers and neighbourhood	Feinberg and Watrous, 1945
Gentian powder	–	–	+		Pharmacists	Kobayashi, 1974
Phosdrin (organophosphate insecticide)	+	+	–		Manufacturers	Weiner, 1961
ENZYMES						
Trypsin	+	–	–		Process worker	Zweiman *et al.*, 1967
Trypsin	+	–	–		Plastic polymer production	Colten *et al.*, 1975
Pancreatic extracts	+	–	–		Parents of fibrocystic children	Dolan and Myers, 1974
Pancreatic extracts	–	–	+		Pharmaceutical manufacturer	Pilat, Popa and Tecoulesco, 1967
Bromelin	+	–	–		Process worker and messenger	Galleguillos and Rodriguez, 1978
Flaviastase	+	–	–		Pharmacists	Pauwels *et al.*, 1978
Papain	+	+	–		Food technologists	Milne and Brand, 1975
	+	+	–		Laboratory technician,	Tarlo *et al.*, 1978
	+	+	–		packer	Flindt, 1978
Bacillus subtilis	–	+	–		Detergent manufacturer	Flindt, 1969
Bacillus subtilis	–	–	+		Detergent manufacturer	Greenberg, Milne and Watt, 1970
Bacillus subtilis	–	–	+		Detergent manufacturer	Newhouse *et al.*, 1970
Bacillus subtilis	+	+	–	Recurrent	Detergent manufacturer	Mitchell and Gandevia, 1971
Bacilus subtilis	+	+	–		Detergent manufacturer	Pepys *et al.*, 1969
Fungal α-amylase	+	–	–		Enzyme manufacturer	Flindt, 1979

Table 12.6 Isocyanates

Sensitizing agent	Type of asthma			Other*	Occupation	References
	Immediate	Late	Not specified			
Toluene diisocyanate (TDI)	+	+	–	Nocturnal	TDI use	Brugsch and Elkins, 1963
Toluene diisocyanate (TDI)	+	+	–		TDI manufacture	Butcher *et al.*, 1976
Toluene diisocyanate (TDI)	+	–	–		Office workers—source in neighbouring factory	Carroll, Secombe and Pepys, 1976
Toluene diisocyanate (TDI)	+	+	–	Nocturnal	Plastics factory	Fuchs and Valade, 1951
Toluene diisocyanate (TDI)	–	–	+		Foam manufacture	Gandevia, 1964
Toluene diisocyanate (TDI)	+	+	–	Nocturnal fever	Tinners in electronics industry	Paisley, 1969

Table 12.6 (continued)

Sensitizing agent	Type of asthma			Other*	Occupation	References
	Immediate	Late	Not specified			
Toluene diisocyanate (TDI)	+	+	–		Foam manufacture	Glass and Thom, 1964
Toluene diisocyanate (TDI)	+	+	–	Nocturnal attacks	Toy maker	Sweet, 1968
Toluene diisocyanate (TDI)	+	+	–		TDI manufacture	Weill *et al.*, 1975
Toluene diisocyanate (TDI)	+	+	–		Boat builder, refrigerator manufacturer, printers, laminators, tinners and insulators	Pepys *et al.*, 1972; O'Brien *et al.*, 1979a and b
Hexamethylene diisocyanate (HDI)	–	+	–		Car sprayers, paint testers	O'Brien *et al.*, 1979a
Diphenylmethane diisocyanate (MDI)	–	+	–		Laminators; Printers; Rigid foam insulators	O'Brien *et al.*, 1979a; Munn, 1965; Longley, 1964
Diphenylmethane diisocyanate (MDI)	–	+?	–		Polyurethane foam manufacture	Tanser, Bourke and Blandford, 1973
Naphthalene diisocyanate (NDI)	+	+	–	Associated with smoking	'Rubber' workers	Harries *et al.*, 1979b
	–	–	+		Chemist	Munn, 1965

DURATION OF EXPOSURE

An allergic reaction does not occur on first exposure. The latent interval during which sensitization occurs varies from a few weeks to many years. In some industries sensitization occurs mainly within the first one to three years (for example, platinum refineries and locust handlers). High labour turnover (as in the electronics industry) reduces the incidence of sensitization (Perks *et al.*, 1979).

When asthma first develops some years after an employee entered an industry it is easy to understand that an occupational origin may be completely overlooked.

SMOKING

This is occasionally a determining factor as, for example, in the case of grain handlers' asthma.

TYPES OF ASTHMA

Distinct patterns emerge in sensitized workers following simulated occupational exposures in hospital, though these are brief and unlike prolonged and repetitive exposures at work (Pepys and Hutchcroft, 1975). However, careful

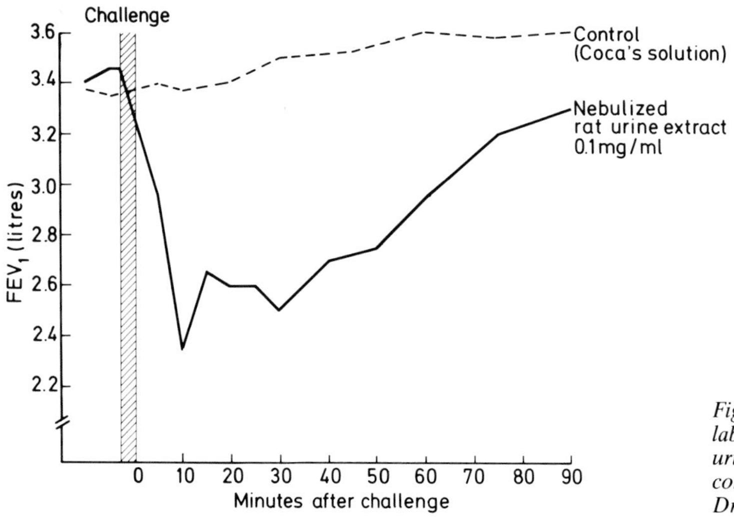

Figure 12.1 Immediate asthmatic reaction in animal laboratory technician challenged with an extract of rat urine nebulized for 3 min. Coca's control solution contains sodium chloride and bicarbonate. (Courtesy of Dr P. S. Burge)

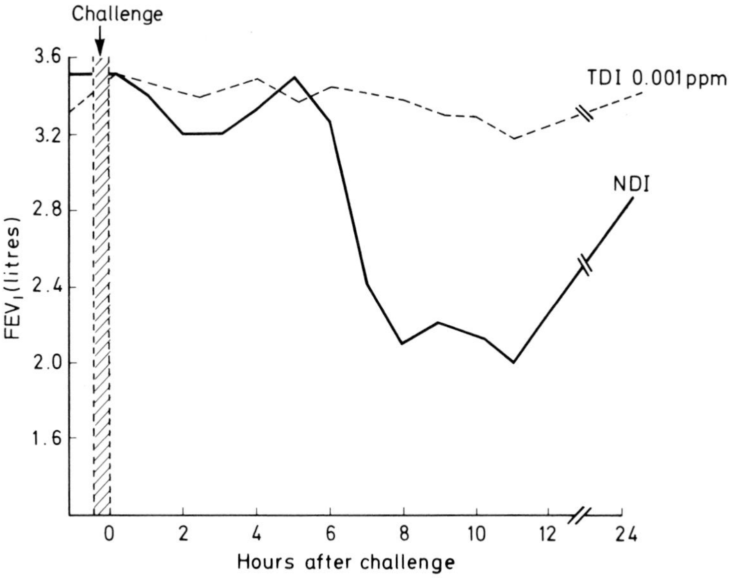

Figure 12.2 Non-immediate (late) reaction to inhalation challenge with naphthalene diisocyanate (NDI) for 60s. No reaction with similar exposure to toluene diisocyanate (TDI). (Courtesy of Dr P. S. Burge. Adapted from Thorax *1979* **34**, *762 with permission of the Editor)*

analysis of the respiratory responses that follow bronchial provocation tests, both with occupational agents and non-occupational allergens, has established the following basic asthmatic patterns.

IMMEDIATE

Typically this develops within minutes of exposure or bronchial provocation tests, is maximal at approximately ten to 20 min and recovers in one and a half to two hours (*Figure 12.1*). Wheeze and chest 'tightness' are almost always present.

LATE ('NON-IMMEDIATE')

This occurs in different forms. Most commonly it starts several hours after exposure, is maximal at about four to eight hours and recovers within 24 hours (*Figure 12.2*). But it may begin in about one hour and recover in three to four hours ('*intermediate*'). Or again, it may commence in the early hours of the morning with a tendency, in some cases, to recur about the same time on a number of successive nights following a single exposure or challenge (*recurrent late asthma*) (Newman Taylor *et al.*, 1979) (*Figure 12.3*). It is important to recognize that wheeze is often slight or absent; and that, in some cases, the only symptoms may be cough, a little yellow sputum and mild breathlessness, but, in others, there may be influenza-like symptoms with fever.

The term 'non-immediate' was introduced to avoid the implication that 'late' necessarily corresponds with late, Type III, hypersensitivity (Pepys and Hutchcroft, 1975), or refers to asthma developing in later life.

DUAL (OR COMBINED)

That is, the occurrence of both immediate and late types of asthma (*Figure 12.4*). To what extent dual reactions occur under normal work conditions, however, is uncertain.

All these forms of asthma may show considerable variation or fluctuation in one individual or in different individuals exposed to the same allergen. The development of an immediate reaction within minutes of handling the responsible material at work and rapid recovery when exposure ceases is strongly in favour of an occupational

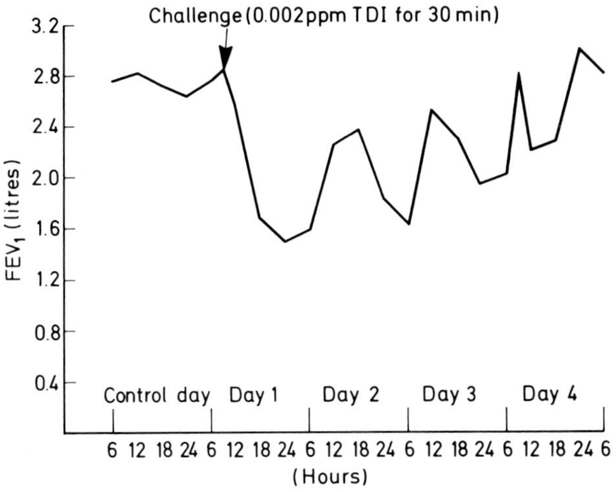

Figure 12.3 Recurrent, chiefly nocturnal, asthmatic reaction following single provocation with toluene diisocyanate 0.002 ppm for 30 min. (Courtesy of Dr P. S. Burge)

origin. But the commencement of late asthma at night—especially if it is recurrent or continues into weekends—may cause the diagnosis to be overlooked. Similarly, persistence of breathlessness, often without wheezing for several days after leaving work or during the early part of a holiday, may not be identified with work conditions. Furthermore, asthmatic reactions are frequently provoked by other causes, such as exercise and upper respiratory infections, in individuals with occupational asthma.

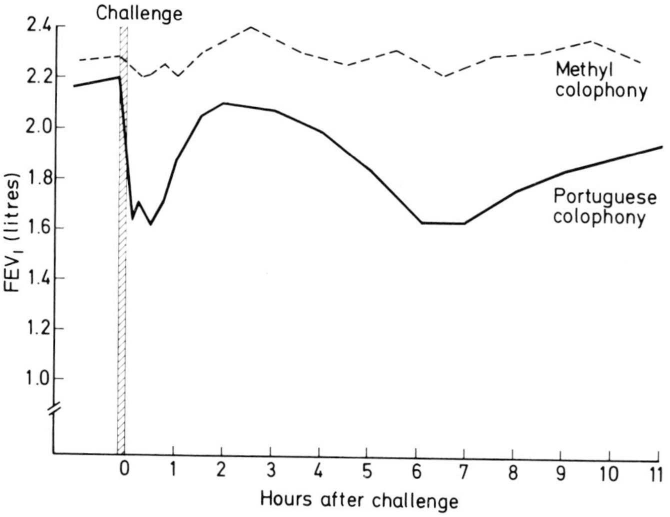

Figure 12.4 Combined immediate and non-immediate (dual) asthmatic reaction to Portuguese colophony fume (lower curve). No reaction on similar exposure to fume of methyl colophony, a substitute flux (upper curve). Five minute challenge time to both. (Courtesy of Dr P. S. Burge)

PHYSIOLOGICAL PATTERNS OF OCCUPATIONAL ASTHMA

Recurring physiological patterns can be demonstrated by prolonged measurements of daily maximum, minimum and mean PEFR at work and at home (*see* Investigation). However, in performing such tests it is important to note that diurnal variations of function occur in both normal and asthmatic individuals. In non-asthmatics the variation is less than 10 per cent but in asthmatics is 20 per cent or more. Lowest values are found either in the morning only ('morning dip') or in the morning and the evening ('double dip'). Although regular patterns are most frequently seen in asthmatics they also occur in some bronchitis subjects with wheeze. The 'morning dip' is characteristic of asthma and the 'double dip' tends to be more frequent in bronchitis (Connolly, 1979).

Four different patterns of asthmatic reactions have been defined which are, apparently, largely determined by the cumulative effect of repeated exposure and the time taken for recovery.

(1) *Progressive deterioration throughout the working week* Symptoms and reduction in ventilation are more severe at the end of the week than at the beginning and recovery takes one to three days. Provided that recovery is substantial within two to three days the weekly pattern is regular but if it takes three days and a late reaction occurs on the first day back at work the record on that day is the best of the week (the 'Monday best' pattern) (*Figure 12.5*). A morning dip may not develop until late in the week or it may be present throughout the week and on Sundays (*Figures 12.6a* and *b*).

(2) *Similar deterioration on each work day* Symptoms develop during each working shift but improve rapidly on leaving work so that recovery is virtually complete before the next work day.

(3) *Progressive deterioration week by week* This develops if the recovery period takes more than three days and the individual returns to work at the beginning of each week while his lung function is still reduced. A gradual decline in PEFR occurs until a state of 'fixed' airflow obstruction is reached. On withdrawal from exposure recovery may not begin for about ten days and, on occasion, may last for as long as three months. This pattern appears to be particularly associated with asthma due to wood dusts and diisocyanates but occurs with other substances (*Figure 12.7*).

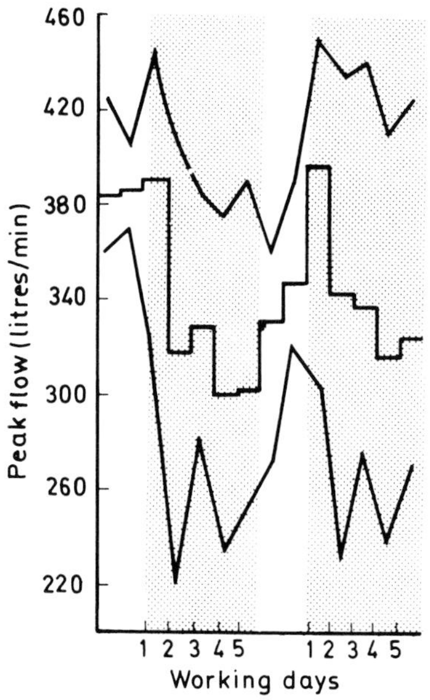

Figure 12.5 PEFR record of solderer exposed to colophony flux fume in an electronics factory. Maximum, mean and minimum daily results shown. The record exemplifies: (1) wide diurnal variations of function in both working weeks; and (2) progressive deterioration with each working day and a three day recovery period at the weekend—the 'Monday best' pattern. (Courtesy of Dr P. S. Burge. Adapted from Thorax *with permission of the Editor)*

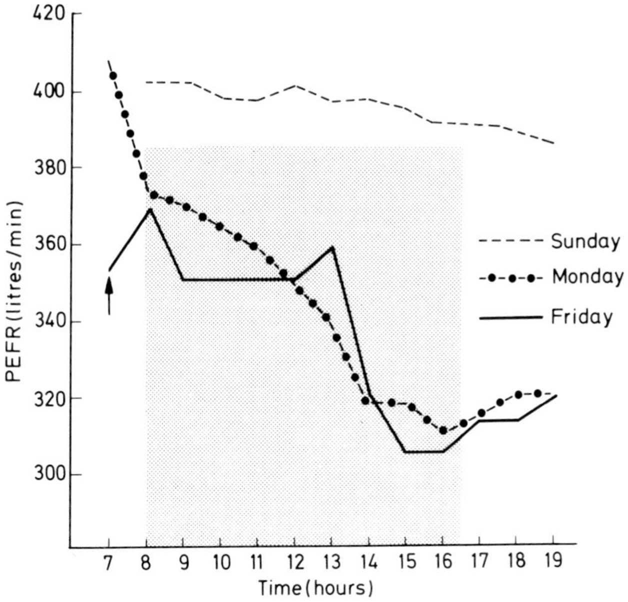

Figure 12.6(a) Hourly PEFR of a solderer exposed to colophony flux fume in an electronics factory recorded on Monday and Friday of the working week. There is an immediate fall in flow rate on morning shortly after starting work compared with Sunday at home and a progressive deterioration until leaving work. A 'morning dip' (arrowed) is apparent on Friday which obscures the initial fall in flow rate at work. In this subject the decline in function is similar on each working day. (Stippled area: working day.) (Courtesy of Dr P. S. Burge. Adapted from Thorax *with permission of the Editor)*

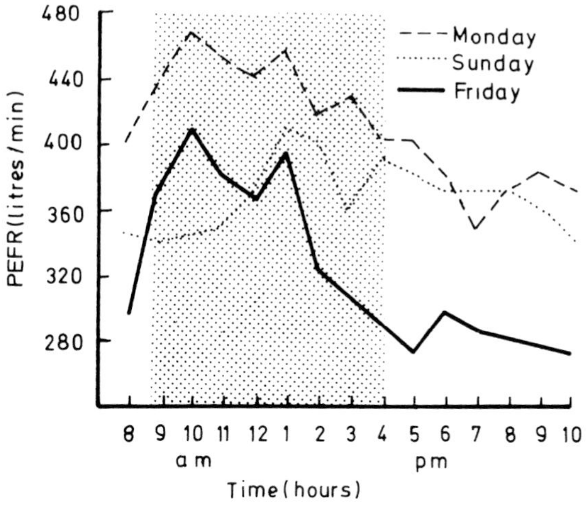

Figure 12.6(b) Plot of hourly PEFR in an electronics production line inserter exposed to colophony solder flux fume. Sunday record at home shows a morning dip and exaggerated 'normal' diurnal variation. Morning dip has lessened by Monday morning but a late asthmatic reaction starts just before leaving work. By Friday of same working week morning dip and late asthmatic reaction are pronounced. This record shows progressive deterioration with work exposure and a three-day recovery pattern. (By courtesy of Dr P. S. Burge and the Editor of Thorax*)*

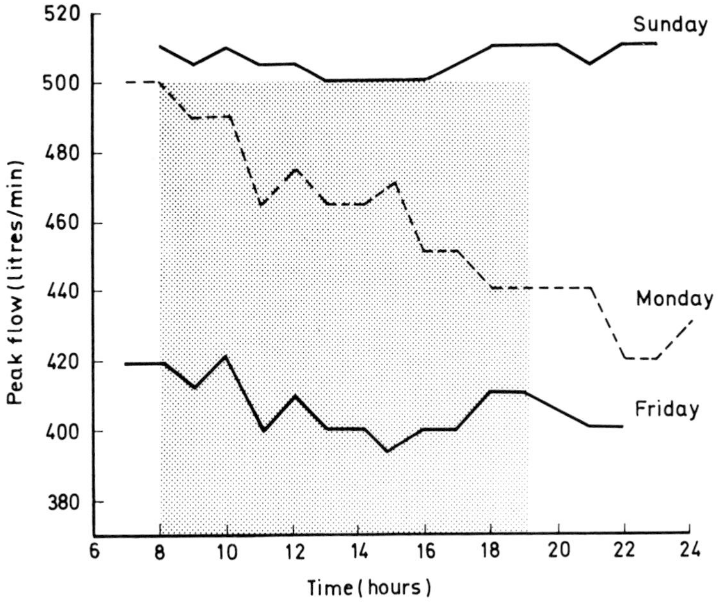

Figure 12.7 'Fixed' airflow obstruction developing at the end of a working week in a worker with platinum asthma. Exposure to end-product chlorplatinic acid from scrap recovery of oil catalysts. Prick test negative. Sunday record at home. (Courtesy of Dr P. S. Burge)

(4) *Maximal deterioration on the first day of the week* This pattern in which recovery occurs during the remainder of the week is only occasionally encountered in occupational asthma. It is a specific feature of 'humidifier fever' proper, polymer fume fever and byssinosis which, however, is *not* characterized by fever.

Correlation between the clinical patterns of asthma and immunological, pharmacological and neurological findings is poor (Turner-Warwick, 1978). The underlying mechanisms are thus incompletely understood and are beyond the scope of this chapter to discuss in detail but those which may be involved are mentioned briefly.

POSSIBLE MECHANISMS OF PATHOGENESIS

TYPE I HYPERSENSITIVITY

This may be mediated by IgE antibody or, in non-atopic subjects, by short-term sensitizing IgG antibody (IgG-STS). It is commonly associated with immediate asthmatic reactions and is prevented by pre-treatment with sodium cromoglycate which inhibits histamine release from mast cells.

Allergens which may provoke this response include grain dusts, animal products, insect proteins, *B. subtilis* enzymes, gum acacia and castor oil bean.

TYPE III HYPERSENSITIVITY

To what extent this reaction is a cause of asthma is uncertain. Although the time relationships of late asthma may suggest a Type III response there is, in general, a lack of correspondence of specific precipitating antibodies and Type III skin reactions to the responsible agent. Late asthma is also prevented by sodium cromoglycate. This suggests the possibility that an IgE mediated reaction, which, as just stated, is suppressed by the drug, may be necessary to initiate the late reaction (Turner-Warwick, 1978).

ACTIVATION OF COMPLEMENT VIA THE ALTERNATIVE PATHWAY

It is possible that this may be responsible in some cases but to what extent is not known.

HAPTEN LINKAGE WITH PROTEINS

Substances of small molecular weight may act as haptens and form complete allergens. Examples include metallic salts, isocyanates and aminoethanolamine. Immediate, late and dual asthmatic responses occur.

IRRITATION

Many of the agents which cause occupational asthma may act as non-specific irritants in high concentrations: for example, isocyanates, chlorine, formaldehyde, phthalic anhydride and colophony. Acute massive exposure may cause an asthmatic attack in a worker on first exposure. Such exposure, however, may result in permanent sensitization and subsequent provocation of asthma by very low concentrations (for example, isocyanates). In addition, inhalation of inert dusts by asthmatic individuals may stimulate a non-specific attack so that immediate asthma at work may not necessarily be caused by a specific allergen in the industry in question.

NON-IMMUNOLOGICAL RELEASE OF HISTAMINE

Histamine, a bronchoconstrictor, is released from mast cells in asthma of immunological origin but also in byssinosis in which immunological factors have not so far been identified. It appears that reactivity of the airways to an inhaled allergen depends not only upon sensitivity to the allergen itself but also on the degree of their non-specific, non-allergic responsiveness to histamine and cholinergic agents such as methacholine (Cockcroft *et al.,* 1979; Casterline, 1980). However, a correlation between reactivity to the asthma-provoking substance and to histamine is not always good—as is the case, for example, with soldering flux fumes (Burge *et al.,* 1980)—suggesting that the substance is acting as a specific sensitizer. There is reason to believe that increased bronchial reactivity may be a consequence rather than a predisposing factor in occupational asthma and that differences in the time of onset and severity of non-immediate reactions may to some extent reflect differences in airways reactivity when the test is performed (Lam, Wong and Chan-Yeung, 1979) (*see* p. 427).

RECURRENT NOCTURNAL ASTHMA

The factors responsible for this phenomenon following a single exposure to the causal agent are not understood (Newman Taylor *et al.,* 1979).

INVESTIGATION

SKIN REACTIONS

The prick test technique should always be used because it does not induce sensitization whereas the intradermal method introduces larger quantities of allergen which may cause dangerous anaphylaxis.

Although an immediate positive reaction to the test agent indicates Type I allergy it does not necessarily establish that this agent is the cause of the asthma, and correlation between a positive skin test and asthma is, on the whole, poor. For example, whereas positive weal and flare reactions to minute concentrations of ammonium tetrachlorplatinate correlate well with occupational asthma, in other situations (such as locust sensitivity) specificity is low. In fact in some types of occupational asthma skin tests are negative while inhalation provocation tests are positive to the offending agent. However, in some cases positive skin reactions may precede the development of asthma. The sensitivity and specificity of each skin testing solution requires to be thoroughly investigated.

Both immediate and late (Type III) skin reactions may occur in some cases of dual asthma.

SEROLOGY

In general, testing for specific antibodies is of little help. But specific IgE antibody has been found against *Bacillus subtilis* enzymes used in washing powders, complex salts of platinum, TDI, MDI, trimellitic anhydride, phthalic anhydride and avian proteins in individuals with asthma who have been exposed to these agents. Precipitating antibodies are probably only evidence of exposure and not necessarily of an allergic response. However, IgE antibodies and precipitins are present in some cases of dual asthma (Pepys and Hutchcroft, 1975). The radioallergosorbent test (RAST) is a sensitive method for detecting IgE antibodies (Baldo and Turner, 1975).

INHALATION BRONCHIAL PROVOCATION TESTS

These provide the most accurate means of demonstrating the occupational origin of asthma and of identifying the responsible agent when this is uncertain or difficult to establish as may happen if there is exposure to several recognized causes of asthma; and further, they enable previously unsuspected sensitizing substances to be identified. However, provocation tests do not differentiate between asthma caused by non-specific irritation and that due to a specific immunological reaction. This is an important point in view of the heightened response asthmatic individuals may have to non-specific irritants (Turner-Warwick, 1978).

Bronchial provocation testing is potentially dangerous. Tests should, therefore, be carried out by experience personnel with the worker in hospital conditions, and only one test should be performed each day. The first challenge should be very short after which the subject is observed for 24 hours with regular measurements of ventilatory function (FEV_1 or PEFR) in case a late or nocturnal asthmatic reaction occurs. Initially it may be necessary to use minute concentrations of some substances: for example, in the case of TDI, 0.005 ppm, which can be gradually increased on subsequent test days. Care must be taken not to exceed the concentrations which are likely to be met with at work. Hence, it may be advisable to monitor the levels which are normally encountered in the factory before deciding the test dose to be used.

There are two approaches to provocation testing. For some biological materials (for example, enzyme detergents, animals and insects) a freeze-dried extract can be prepared and diluted for inhalation by nebulization. However, this method is unsuitable for most small molecular weight industrial chemicals for which simulated occupational type provocation tests are preferable. These can be done by painting solutions (such as polyurethane varnishes, formaldehyde and cold adhesives) onto a surface; by heating materials which give off a fume or gas (such as colophony in soldering flux or diphenylmethane diisocyanate—MDI): or by creating a dust by tipping the substance from one tray to another. It is often necessary to dilute dusts with non-irritant materials, such as dried lactose: for example, 40 mg of platinum salt in 1 kg of lactose tipped from one tray to another produces atmospheric concentrations of the salt close to the recommended TLV. Whichever method is used control exposures to the diluents or solvents of the test agent must be also made to ensure that the observed reaction is specific. The concentration of the test agent in the surrounding air or in the patient's breathing zone can be determined by appropriate instruments. (*Figures 12.8* and *12.9*).

Inhalation tests with histamine or methylcholine have been used to detect non-specific bronchial hyper-reactivity for a few years past but they are time consuming and individual subjects show considerable variability of response. Exercise or isocapnic hyperventilation during inhalation of cold air (–10 to –20 °C) have been suggested as simpler and more reliable methods of provoking bronchospasm and of separating asthmatics from normal subjects who exhibit little response to these procedures (Leading article, 1980).

Immediate asthmatic reactions are prevented by sodium

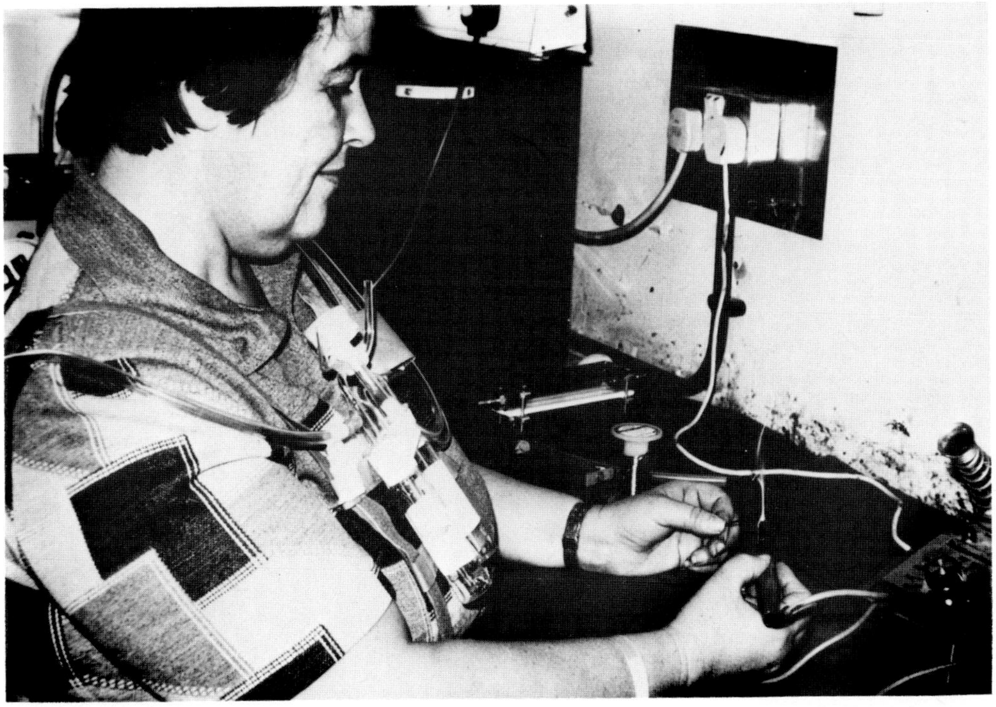

Figure 12.8 Inhalation challenge with colophony solder flux fume produced by the insertion of an electrode (seen in the patient's right hand) at a temperature of 350 °C into the flux. Note apparatus worn by the patient for determining fume concentration in the breathing zone. (Courtesy of Dr P. S. Burge)

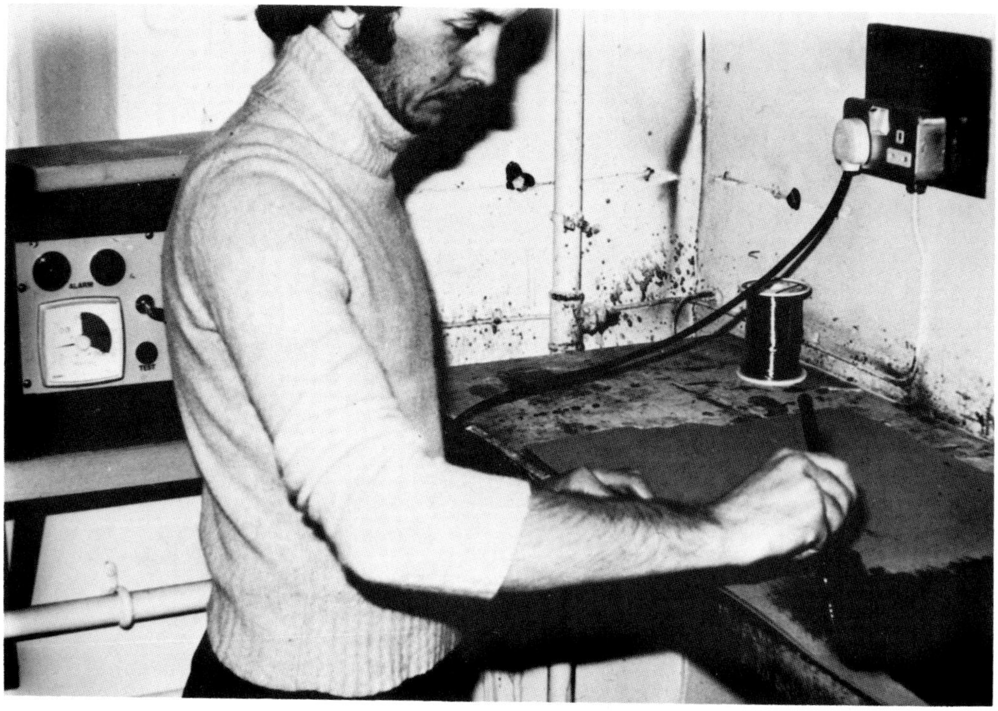

Figure 12.9 Inhalation challenge with TDI. Polyurethane varnish mixed with its activator is being brushed on to a wooden surface. Note instrument on the left is analysing fume concentration in the ambient air. (Courtesy of Dr P. S. Burge)

cromoglycate and reversed by the inhalation of isoprenaline, but are unaffected by systemic or inhaled corticosteroids. Late (non-immediate) reactions are only partially affected by isoprenaline but are inhibited by inhalation of sodium cromoglycate and by systemic or inhaled corticosteroids (Pepys and Hutchcroft, 1975).

PROLONGED MEASUREMENTS OF PEFR AT HOME AND AT WORK

Measurement of lung function before and after a work shift is the simplest method of providing objective confirmation of occupational asthma. However, it is a very insensitive method of making a diagnosis as many reactions occur in the evening and at night at home; and, as already stated, lung function is often depressed at the beginning of the day in some asthmatics ('morning dip') (*Figures 12.6a* and *b*). Thus, measurements of lung function are needed at home in the evenings, at weekends and often during holidays. Two weeks is the shortest useful record in most cases and occasionally it may be necessary to continue measurements for four to eight weeks.

The simplest and most practical method is to measure PEFR by Wright's peak flow meter or peak flow gauge at regular intervals and record the results. The worker can be shown how to do this himself. To obtain valid records he must continue in his normal working conditions during the test period: that is, he must be subjected to repeated unsupervised exposures to the agent or process which is suspected of causing his asthma. However, in the case of individuals with very severe symptoms bronchial provocation tests are safer and to be preferred.

In order to establish the *absence* of occupational asthma in a worker with normal PEFR values records taken over a two week period at work should show a less than 20 per cent diurnal variation. If the individual's PEFR is reduced tests should be continued for at least ten days away from work followed by a minimum of another two weeks at work so that the possibility of an unusually long recovery period can be identified (*Figure 12.10*). If the subject is receiving

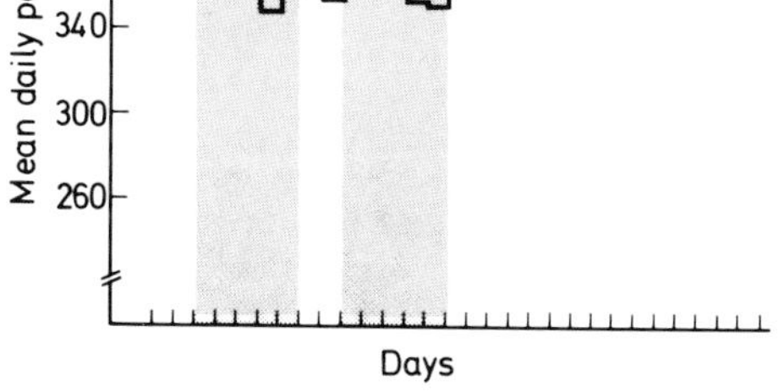

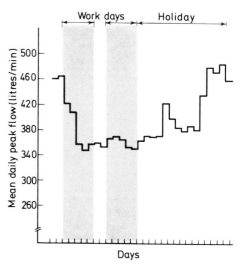

Figure 12.10 Printer exposed to TDI and MDI. 'Fixed' airflow obstruction with no improvement at weekends. Recovery is not complete until about ten days away from exposure. (Courtesy of Dr P. S. Burge)

bronchodilator drugs these should be recorded and the dose not varied either at work or at home during the period of investigation. And corticosteroids and sodium cromoglycate which may block changes in function must be withheld.

The results of this mode of investigation (which correlate well with bronchial provocation tests) are capable of making a specific diagnosis of occupational asthma though they do not identify the offending substance. This can be achieved by subsequent bronchial provocation tests. Moreover, they are particularly useful for confirming that probable non-occupational asthma is in fact unrelated to work conditions, and for verifying the results of earlier negative bronchial provocation tests (Burge, O'Brien and Harries, 1979).

In carrying out tests of airways obstruction in investigating asthma it is important to bear in mind that diurnal variations occur. As indicated earlier (p. 424), most regular patterns take one of two forms: the lowest values are found either in the morning ('morning dip') or both in the morning and evening ('double dip'). Regular patterns are most frequently seen in asthmatics but are also observed in some bronchitics with wheeze. If PEFR readings are taken only twice daily the magnitude of the diurnal variation may be underestimated (Connolly, 1979).

DIAGNOSIS

This rests chiefly on the clinician's awareness of the different patterns of asthma, of the wide variety of industrial exposures capable of inducing asthma, and, above all, on the taking of a detailed clinical and occupational history. And, in addition to occupational sources, possible contact with sensitizing agents in hobby activities and other domestic circumstances must be remembered and recorded.

Occupation should not be overlooked in atopic persons with asthma in which no extrinsic factor is readily identifiable; and care must be taken to exclude an unsuspected occupational cause in cases of 'intrinsic' asthma (which occurs most commonly in non-atopic individuals) before the asthma is regarded as cryptogenic (Davies, 1979).

It is important also to bear in mind how asthmatic patterns may vary in the one individual. Immediate reactions may be followed on some, but not all, occasions by a period of apparent normality with more persistent symptoms a few hours later; or late asthma may occur on some days and a dual response on others. The continuation of symptoms, especially breathlessness without wheeze, during a weekend or into a holiday period does not exclude a diagnosis of occupational asthma. But, in such cases, some improvement is usually apparent during two to three weeks away from work (*Figure 12.10*).

The diagnosis of recurrent nocturnal asthma may be difficult and recognized only by its cessation when the individual is on holiday or away from work; but in some cases it cannot be made with certainty without inhalation testing with the suspected agent (Newman Taylor *et al.*, 1979). Confusion with nocturnal cardiac asthma is possible at the outset.

In some cases, owing to the similarity of the time of onset and the symptoms, late (non-immediate) asthma may be difficult to differentiate from acute extrinsic allergic 'alveolitis'. This is particularly likely to occur in farm workers and bird fanciers in whom the presence of relevant precipitins may wrongly suggest a diagnosis of extrinsic allergic 'alveolitis' (*see* Chapter 11).

PROGNOSIS

In many cases asthmatic symptoms appear to cease if there is no further exposure but in some prolonged disabling asthma may ensue in the absence of further contact with the offending substance. Some instances of such protracted asthma may be due to cross-reactivity with other 'non-occupational' allergens (*see* Insects of the Orthoptera Order).

PREVENTION

This involves a number of considerations.

(1) Efficient hygienic control of processes involving known sensitizing materials, though complete enclosure is not always possible. Reduction of exposure levels in this way, for example, has dramatically reduced the proportion of workers becoming sensitized in the enzyme detergent industry (Juniper *et al.*, 1977). However, there are as yet few studies in which exposure levels of potential asthma-provoking substances have been related to subsequent development of sensitization. Sensitized workers who react to exceedingly low concentrations of a substance may still be affected in conditions of good hygienic control.

(2) Substitution by an innocuous or less harmful material. But the possibility that the substitute might also prove to have sensitizing potential has always to be borne in mind. For example, diphenylmethane diisocyanate (MDI), which has been used to replace toluene diisocyanate (TDI), may cause sensitization in some workers.

(3) Personal protection of the sensitized worker. This may be practical in special circumstances. For example, the use of an airline respirator and complete protective clothing has enabled laboratory workers sensitized to animals to continue their work.

(4) Identification of susceptible workers. Ideally atopic individuals identified by prick testing for common allergens could be prevented from entering processes carrying a known asthma risk. But this may mean the exclusion of more than 30 per cent of potential workers, and, furthermore, as described already, a substantial proportion of non-atopic individuals become sensitized.

(5) Periodic medical examinations. In order to detect early sensitization before asthma develops the identification of specific antibodies or positive skin tests is required but, at present, this is only possible in the case of a few substances—for example, platinum salts and *B. subtilis* enzymes. However, a routine clinical history or an unexpected fall in FEV_1 or PEFR may reveal the development of asthma at an early stage.

TREATMENT

Individuals with established asthma should be removed from exposure to the reponsible process. If it is impractical to move an affected person elsewhere in the factory, treatment with sodium cromoglycate should be tried and its effect observed by his recording his own PEFR with a peak flow meter or gauge at regular intervals for 24 hours. But, should this succeed, long-term medical supervision is still required. In some cases in which there is sensitization to very low concentrations of the offending agent the only solution may be to leave the industry.

Hyposensitization is difficult to achieve and is rarely successful.

EXAMPLES OF OCCUPATIONAL ASTHMA

It is not possible to discuss all known causes of occupational asthma. Many of these, the occupations at risk and the types of asthma which occur (when known) are listed in *Tables 12.1* to *12.6*. But a few important examples illustrating particular points with additional references are briefly described. Byssinosis, which in the terms of the widely adopted definition is a form of asthma, is discussed in more detail.

GRAIN AND FLOUR DUST

Asthma associated with grain dust has been well known since Rammazini's day. There is, as already described in Chapter 11, p. 375, a wide range of organic and inorganic materials in grain dusts which vary importantly according to whether the grain is encountered at harvest time or under differing conditions of storage, handling and transportation. Among the organic constituents there is a large number which may be potentially allergenic and, thus, possible causes of asthma—including flour itself.

Persons likely to be exposed are farm workers during harvest time and when handling stored grain in the winter months, grain elevator workers, millers, dockers (occasionally), bakers and pastry cooks.

Both immediate and late asthma may follow exposure to grain dust or uncontaminated flour even in the absence of skin reactivity to aqueous extracts of the dust. Precipitins to flour have been found in asthmatic bakers (Hendrick, Davies and Pepys, 1976; Chan-Yeung, Wong and MacLean, 1979). Recurrent nocturnal asthma may follow a single exposure to grain dust (Davies, Green and Schofield, 1976).

The atopic state of the worker seems to be important. A significant correlation between cutaneous reactivity to grain dust and wheezing when exposed to it has been observed in grain handlers; and wheezing and airflow obstruction are more prevalent among atopic than non-atopic workers (doPico *et al.*, 1977). Cigarette smoking is another important factor—whether synergistic or additive—in the pathogenesis of chronic respiratory disease in these workers (doPico, 1979). But grain dust also appears to act as a non-specific airways irritant. Increased non-specific bronchial reactivity to inhaled histamine by comparison with non-exposed control subjects has been demonstrated in non-atopic, life-long non-smoking, grain handlers (Mink *et al.*, 1980) who are also reported to have an increased prevalence of chronic bronchitis—that is, mucus hypersecretion— without respiratory disability or reduction in FEV_1/FVC though with significant reduction of mean values of MMFR and maximum expiratory flow rate at 50 per cent of VC (Gerrard *et al.*, 1979; Dosman *et al.*, 1980).

It is of interest that there is *in vitro* evidence that aqueous extracts of airborne grain dusts can activate both alternative and classic complement pathways in man (Olenchock, Mull and Major, 1980).

Clearly there are a number of unsolved questions concerning the effect of complex grain dusts on the human respiratory tract but, apart from dust control and other hygiene measures, it is probable that respiratory symptoms in workers who regularly handle grain or flour can be substantially reduced if they are non-smoking, non-atopic subjects (doPico, 1979).

STORAGE MITES ('BARN ALLERGY')

Infestation of grain and flour and also hay, straw and a large variety of stored food and vegetable products by storage mites is important and widespread. The mites comprise a wide range of families and species but, in general, members of the Acaridae and Glycyphagidae are the most common (Griffiths *et al.*, 1976; Wraith, Cunnington and Seymour, 1979). They may cause rhinitis and asthma in grain workers, flour millers, bakers, farmers and their wives, workers in food stores, housewives and others. The asthma may be of immediate, non-immediate or recurrent nocturnal type (Davies, Green and Schofield, 1976; Cuthbert *et al.*, 1979; Ingram *et al.*, 1979; Wraith, Cunnington and Seymour, 1979). In the UK the species most commonly found are *Acarus siro, Tyrophagus putrescentiae, Glycyphagus domesticus* and *Lepidoglyphus destructor.* Skin prick tests with extracts of these mites, which appear to be allergenically similar, are positive in a high proportion of exposed persons with and without asthma. Cross reactivity between these species probably occurs but not with the house mite (*Dermatophagoides pteronyssinus*) which, on present evidence, is antigenically distinct. If confirmed, this is important because hyposensitization with *Dermatophagoides* vaccines will be unlikely to benefit patients whose asthma is due to storage mites (Wraith, Cunnington and Seymour, 1979).

The necessity of distinguishing between acute extrinsic allergic 'alveolitis' and 'barn allergy' in farm workers is referred to in Chapter 11. If prick tests with extracts of the common species of storage mites are positive, relief of symptoms with sodium cromoglycate points to 'barn allergy' (Cuthbert *et al.*, 1979).

WOOD DUSTS

A large number of hard woods may cause asthma although, until recently, they were generally regarded as non-specific respiratory irritants. Some—Western red cedar, for example—are being used in increasing quantities in indoor and outdoor construction work. Immediate asthma may occur, but late, often nocturnal with bouts of coughing, and dual reactions appear to be more common and may sometimes persist for days or even weeks after cessation of exposure (Gandevia and Milne, 1970; Chan-Yeung, 1977). In many cases there is a long latent period from the time of first working with the wood and the development of symptoms, but red cedar asthma usually develops in the early months of exposure and affected workers tend to leave the industry (Chan-Yeung *et al.*, 1978). Because the asthma frequently occurs at night its relationship to occupation is readily overlooked.

Specific precipitins and skin test reactions to the individual woods are infrequently reported to be positive and further investigation is obviously needed. In the case of red cedar (*Thuja plicata*), however, its major non-volatile component, plicatic acid, appears to be the responsible allergen as judged by bronchial challenge tests (Chan-Yeung, 1977). Extracts of the dust cause direct release of histamine by lung tissue '*in vitro*' (Evans and Nicholls, 1974).

ENZYMES

As *Table 12.5* shows, a variety of enzymes are capable of causing asthma when inhaled.

Until recently the proteolytic enzymes Alcalase and Maxatase from *Bacillus subtilis* which are used in detergent washing powders have been the most important. Occupational exposure may occur among workers handling drums or paper sacks of the enzyme concentrates and during preparation and packing of the diluted powders (Flindt, 1969; Pepys *et al.*, 1969; Greenberg, Milne and Watt, 1970); and the risk of sensitization may also be present during their use in processes in the baking, brewing, fish, silk and leather industries. Asthma caused by enzyme washing powders in the home has rarely been encountered (Belin *et al.*, 1970) and the preparation of the enzyme particles in granulated form in latter years has reduced the likelihood. However, the possibility cannot be entirely excluded especially in atopic subjects.

Atopic individuals are more readily affected than non-atopics. Positive skin prick tests to the washing powder enzymes Alcalase, Maxatase and subtilisin A have demonstrated immediate-type allergy which correlates well with the presence of circulating IgE (Pepys *et al.*, 1973; How and Cambridge 1971). Late skin reactions to *B. subtilis* proteinase, Alcalase, Maxatase and subtilisin A which appeared to be of Arthus type have also developed in a few sensitized workers but biopsy of the test areas has not indicated evidence of Type III hypersensitivity nor of activation of complement. They appear to be mediated by high levels of specific IgE antibodies (Zetterström, 1978). Although precipitins are present in some cases they do not correlate with exposure, symptoms or prick test reactions; and they are also found in non-exposed individuals (Flindt, 1969). They are thought to be due to non-specific interaction between components of the crude enzyme and serum proteins similar to or identical with, α-globulins (How and Cambridge, 1971). In short, asthma associated with the manufacture of enzyme washing powders is both immediate (IgE mediated) and non-immediate. Dijkman (1973) has described dual asthmatic reactions following inhalation provocation tests with Maxatase in detergent factory workers; and the occurrence of recurrent nocturnal episodes after a single exposure to Alcalase is on record (Mitchell and Gandevia, 1971).

Encapsulation of the enzyme powder, hygienic control of production processes, and medical surveillance of employees have appreciably reduced the incidence of asthma and enabled sensitized persons to continue at work without developing respiratory symptoms. But the combination of accidental spillage and highly sensitive individuals may give rise to occasional cases. Routine prick tests with standardized, freeze-dried Alcalase and Maxalase are invaluable for the early diagnosis of allergy in individuals who have not developed clinical symptoms (How and Cambridge, 1971; Flindt, 1978). TLV levels have been gradually reduced over the years.

There appears to be little risk of peripheral lung disease or chronic obstructive airways disease being caused by washing powder enzymes as handled at present, though there is evidence of loss of pulmonary elastic recoil in some individuals with earlier exposures in the industry (Weill, Waddell and Ziskind, 1971; Biological Effects of Proteolytic Enzyme Detergents, 1976; Musk and Gandevia, 1976; Juniper *et al.*, 1977).

Because the allergenic potential of *B. subtilis* proteinase may persist after heat treatment, Flindt (1979) has suggested that the allergenic potential of proteolytic enzymes in general is related primarily to their large molecular weights rather than to their proteolytic properties. This is supported by his finding that workers had developed asthma and rhinitis, associated with positive skin prick tests, not only after handling the proteolytic enzyme, papain, but also after handling the non-proteolytic enzyme, fungal α-amylase (ex *Aspergillus oryzae*).

As α-amylase is used in flour milling and the bakery industry the possibility of sensitization of those exposed to it should be considered.

ISOCYANATES

The production of *polyurethanes* for the manufacture of fibres, plastics, elastomers, adhesives, surface coatings and flexible and rigid foams involves isocyanates which react with a variety of compounds containing active hydrogen atoms. The isocyanates are made by the reaction of amines with phosgene, and the four most important are toluene diisocyanate (TDI), and diphenylmethane diisocyanate (MDI), naphthalene diisocyanate (NDI) and hexamethylene diisocyanate (HDI) (Buist and Lowe, 1965). Of these TDI is by far the most significant commercially and toxicologically, its major use being in the manufacture of the foams. However, although the others have a more limited use, they have all been reported as occasionally causing respiratory symptoms (*see Table 12.6*).

TDI and HDI are highly volatile and vaporize readily, but the volatility of MDI used for urethane surface coatings is much lower. TDI, in the undistilled form employed for polyurethane manufacture, is a dark brown liquid.

Exposure to TDI vapour may occur in the following occupational situations: during its production; in the vicinity of foam-producing machines; during spraying and moulding operations; accidental leakage or spillage of liquid TDI during bulk or drum handling, or drum emptying; leakage from pumps; during disposal of TDI waste and welding polyurethane-covered wires (Pepys *et al.*, 1972). It is encountered with increasing frequency in non-occupational circumstances: for example, when polyurethane products are burned or during the use of polyurethane varnish with a TDI activator (Pepys *et al.*, 1972).

High concentrations of vapour (as may occur in major accidental spillage) cause rhinitis, pharyngitis, breathlessness, chest tightness, cough, wheezing and crepitations (Hama, 1957) and in severe cases there may be pulmonary oedema or bronchopneumonia. More commonly, low concentrations are encountered. In the first few months of exposure many workers complain of upper respiratory tract irritation which is usually transient although some complain of cough and wheezing towards the end of the day and at night. As the cough may predominate and there is a small amount of sputum, 'bronchitis' is often diagnosed rather than asthma.

Immediate, late and dual type asthma may develop even in response to very low concentrations of TDI (less than 0.001 ppm) (O'Brien *et al.,* 1979b). The physiological patterns have been well demonstrated by observing PEFR hourly or two-hourly in exposed workers between waking and sleeping. Important features include a tendency for some workers to be worse at the end of the working week and to deteriorate steadily week by week while at work. Recovery after leaving exposure commonly takes several days, occasionally as long as ten weeks. It is also clear that measurement of lung function before and after a working shift may miss a late reaction at home or a 'fixed' state of airflow obstruction which may persist in some workers for days or even weeks (*Figures 12.3* and *12.10*) (Burge, O'Brien and Harries, 1979). Slowness of recovery is not necessarily related to the severity of the asthma.

Asthma is believed to develop in about 5 per cent of workers regularly exposed to TDI, and most have been non-atopic. Individual susceptibility seems to vary greatly but once sensitization has occurred exposure to minute concentrations may provoke severe asthmatic episodes—a situation which may be permanent. Smoking does not seem to influence the symptoms.

The underlying cause of isocyanate asthma is not understood. Specific reaginic and complement-fixing antibodies to TDI have been found in some affected people (Butcher *et al.,* 1977a; Karol, Ioset and Alarie, 1978; Karol *et al.,* 1979) and lymphocyte transformation has been observed (Bruckner *et al.,* 1968). However, these results have not been confirmed by other investigators and negative findings with plasma histamine and complement in TDI-sensitive workers suggest that an immunological mechanism may not be involved. Furthermore, TDI reactive individuals have non-specific irritability of their airways. It has been suggested, therefore, that impairment of β-adrenergic receptors may play an important part in TDI reactivity (Butcher *et al.,* 1979). But failure to detect TDI-specific antibodies may be due to difficulties in the preparation of hapten-conjugated test antigens containing exposed tolyl groups because of the tendency of TDI to cross-link protein molecules; for it is the presence of the tolyl and not the isocyanate group on test antigens which appears to be decisive (Karol, Ioset and Alarie, 1978; Karol and Alarie, 1980).

Apart from the rare occurrence of pulmonary oedema due to high concentrations of TDI following accidental spillage, acute extrinsic allergic 'alveolitis' may sometimes occur and is discussed briefly in Chapter 11 (p. 386). Reduced values of VC and Kco compared with a control group have been reported in workers after prolonged exposure to isocyanates in plastics production, and it is suggested that this may indicate DIPF (Pham *et al.,* 1978). However, there is no proof of this and prolonged follow-up studies are evidently necessary.

There are no relevant radiographic abnormalities except in cases of pulmonary oedema or acute extrinsic allergic 'alveolitis'.

Rigorous hygienic measures are required in all isocyanate processes but in some it may be impossible to prevent low concentrations from entering the work place air. There is debate about an appropriate TLV.

Sensitization to the other isocyanates, HDI and NDI, is less common but may, nonetheless, be important. NDI, hitherto thought to be safer than TDI, may cause immediate and non-immediate asthma, when used as a hot curing agent in the manufacture of rubber, in workers who are irresponsive to TDI and NDI (Harries *et al.,* 1979a) (*Figure 12.2*).

DRUGS

The manufacture of a large number of diverse drugs, including pancreatic extracts, may cause asthma which, in many instances is either of late or dual type (*Table 12.5*). In some instances the asthma may be recurrent as exemplified in *Figure 12.3.* Oral administration of the offending drug (especially penicillins) has induced asthmatic attacks in affected workers. Hence, a drug to which an individual has become sensitized occupationally should not be used therapeutically. Davies and Pepys (1975) observed that a non-atopic worker who developed late asthma following exposure to spiramycin also had asthmatic attacks after eating eggs. In the UK and elsewhere spiramycin is often fed to poultry to improve rearing standards and consequently is present in low concentration in the eggs. Non-immediate asthma, with delayed positive skin tests, due to spiramycin has been reported in a non-atopic chicken breeder who handled poultry feed containing the antibiotic (Paggiaro, Loi and Toma, 1979).

METALS

Asthma caused by occupational exposure to metals or their salts is fairly uncommon. Affected individuals are often non-atopic.

CHROMIUM

The salts are usually responsible. Skin prick tests may be positive and specific antibody present. Welding of stainless steel may cause immediate and non-immediate asthma due, probably, to chromium in the fume, though nickel may also be contributory (Keskinen, Kalliomäki and Alanko, 1980).

NICKEL

The sulphate has caused immediate and late (non-immediate) asthma with a positive prick test in a non-atopic nickel plater. Nickel carbonyl has been shown to cause both asthmatic episodes and pulmonary eosinophilia (Löffler's syndrome) in a chemical engineer (*see Table 12.4*).

PLATINUM

The complex salts ammonium hexachloroplatinate and potassium tetrachloroplatinate are most commonly implicated. They are potent sensitizers and sensitization is related to the number of chlorine atoms present. Refinery workers exposed to dusts or sprays of the salts are chiefly affected but personnel working in electroplating processes, photography, the manufacture of fluorescent screens, emission control systems for cars and catalysts for agricultural fertilizers, and in the oil refining industry may also be at risk (*Figure 12.7*). Rhinitis and urticaria frequently accompany the asthma, and this triad is often referred to as 'platinosis'.

In most cases sensitization develops in six to 12 months but it may occur within ten days or be delayed for as long as 25 years. Wives may also be sensitized by dust from their husbands' clothes. Although the incidence of platinum asthma is not known for certain it is apparently uncommon.

Sensitivity is considered to be allergic and not toxic or irritant in origin because: there is a period of exposure without symptoms; only a proportion of those exposed become sensitized; and affected individuals are sensitive to extremely minute amounts of the salts. This is confirmed by the fact that specific IgE antibody has been demonstrated by a radioallergosorbent test in skin prick-positive individuals and by the passive transfer of Type I allergy to antibody to the complex salts to both man and monkey with sera from sensitized workers (Cromwell *et al.*, 1979; Pepys *et al.*, 1979). However, platinum asthma may occur with negative prick tests. Atopic individuals fare worse than non-atopics and tend to leave the industry early.

VANADIUM

Vanadium in the form of the pentoxide and vanadate are reported to cause wheezing, tightness in the chest and dyspnoea on effort some six to 24 hours after exposure (Williams, 1952; Browne, 1955). It is likely that these symptoms indicate asthma in some cases, possibly non-immediate and prolonged (*see* Chapter 13, pp. 470–472).

SOLDERING FLUXES

Fumes or vapours from fluxes containing amino-ethyl-ethanolamine or colophony (pine resin) can cause immediate, late and dual type asthma. This may worsen steadily during the working week and recover partially or completely at weekends (*Figures 12.6a* and *12.11*). Most affected workers experience wheeze and breathlessness at home in the evenings and about a third are awakened on some nights by breathessness. The combination of a three-day recovery period and development of late asthma on Mondays may result in a 'Monday best' pattern and a 'morning dip' with pronounced diurnal variation on Sundays (*Figures 12.5* and *12.6b*) (*see* p. 425). Prick tests with antigen from colophony in the flux are uniformly negative (Burge *et al.*, 1979c; Burge, O'Brien and Harries, 1979).

These fluxes are widely used in the electronics and related industries. In the case of colophony only a small proportion of workers—usually those who are atopic—are affected, commonly some months after first exposure but sometimes, not for more than a decade. In this situation it is easy to miss the occupational origin of the asthma. Asthma may be caused by one type of colophony but not by another (*Figure 12.4*). Asthmatic symptoms persist in some colophony-sensitized workers after they have left occupational exposure. This may be due to the use of colophony esters

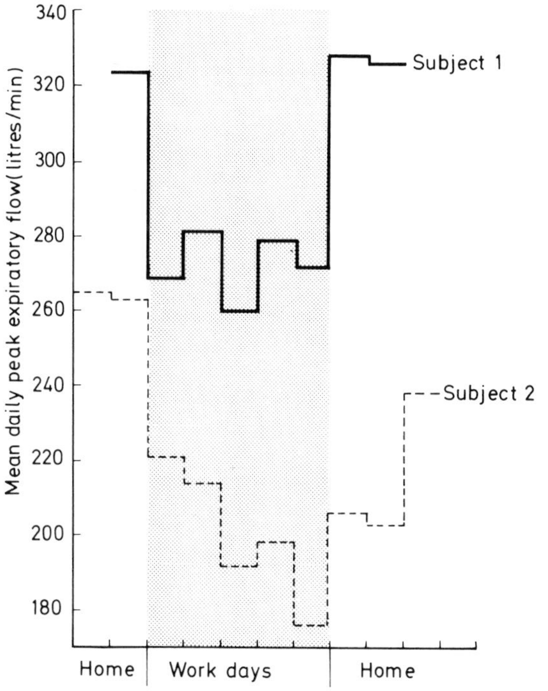

Figure 12.11 Different patterns of asthma in two electronics workers exposed to colophony solder flux. Subject 1 *recovers completely at the weekend.* Subject 2 *worsens progressively during the week and shows little improvement at the weekend. (Courtesy of Dr P. S. Burge)*

and amber oil (*Pinus* sp.) for flavouring of cigarette tobacco (Burge *et al.*, 1978a).

Polypropylene glycol and alkylaryl polyether alcohol in soft solder flux may cause immediate asthma shortly after first exposure.

It has, however, to be noted that isocyanates liberated from the polyurethane coating of wires during soldering are sometimes the cause of asthma in solderers (Pepys *et al.*, 1972).

EPOXY RESIN HARDENERS

Epoxy resins which are extensively used in the plastics industry, in the insulation of electrical wiring and coils and for metal coatings do not themselves cause asthma but the agents used for curing or hardening may. These include *phthallic anhydride, trimellitic anhydride* and *triethylene tetramine*. Their vapour is evolved during the curing process or if the combined resin and hardener are subjected to heat. One or more of these substances may be responsible for sensitization in an individual worker (*Figure 12.12*).

Asthma which has been associated with heat sealing and cutting of PVC soft wrap film and thermally activated price tag labels (so-called *'meat wrappers' asthma'*) is more likely to be due to phthalic anhydride or to the irritant effects of other products of pyrolysis, such as hydrogen chloride, from additives which constitute about 30 per cent by weight of the film rather than to sensitization to PVC itself (Pauli *et al.*, 1980; *Table 12.4*). However, the incidence of reactive bronchospasm among meat wrappers during and after work

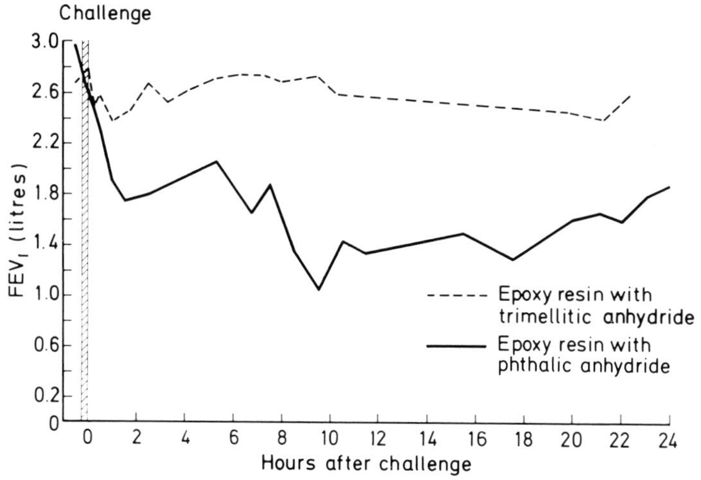

Figure 12.12 Asthma, which is 'dual' and prolonged, provoked by phthalic anhydride but not by trimellitic anhydride. (Courtesy of Dr P. S. Burge)

is low, and there is, apparently, no major respiratory hazard (Krumpke, Finley and Martinez, 1979).

The effects which may follow exposure to trimellitic anhydride are discussed in more detail in Chapter 11.

INSECTS OF THE ORTHOPTERA ORDER

This is a large Order but some members of its different families are bred or used for research or teaching purposes in technical institutions and schools: in particular, the migratory and desert locust (*Locusta migratoria* and *Schistocerca gregaria* respectively), stick insects (*Carausius morosus*) and cockroaches (*Leucophaea madera* Fabricius in the USA and *Blatella germanica* Linnaeus in the UK). Thus, individuals who may be in contact with them include entomologists, laboratory scientists and handlers, field workers, teachers, students and schoolchildren in biology classes.

A survey of 117 laboratory workers locusts showed that 28 per cent had asthma which improved when they were away from work at weekends. Sensitization tended to occur within the first three years of exposure and atopy predisposed to the development of symptoms. Specific anti-locust antibodies correlated both with exposure and with asthma.

Skin prick tests with locust antigens were found to be positive in 28 of 100 consecutive patients attending a hospital allergy clinic who had no contact with locusts. Positive tests correlated with atopy in general and *Dermatophagoides pteronyssinus* (house dust mite) reactions in particular suggesting that there are cross-reacting antigens between locusts and the house dust mite. Indeed, antisera to a mixture of locust extracts and antisera to *D. pteronyssinus* show lines of identity in precipitin tests (Edge and Burge, 1980). Hence, it is possible that cross-reactivity could be responsible for continued asthmatic symptoms after occupational exposure to locusts has ceased, and for sensitizing asymptomatic schoolchildren and laboratory workers to the house dust mite thus increasing the likelihood of their developing asthma in the future (Burge *et al.*, 1979a).

The terms 'locust' and 'grasshopper', incidently, are used in the USA for any member of the Acrididae family.

Crickets have been recorded as causing immediate and, possibly, non-immediate asthma (Harfi, 1980). Cockroaches are known to be a potent cause of immediate asthma and Frankland (1953), in fact, suggested the possibility of cross-reactivity with locust antigens (Bernton, McMahon and Brown, 1972). Insects of other Orders are also known to cause asthma (Feinberg, Feinberg and Benaim-Pinto, 1956; Perlman, 1958) (*Table 12.2*).

Thus, insects are a source of powerful allergens of which a number of components are common to various species and to *D. pteronyssinus*.

FORMALDEHYDE (Formalin)

Formaldehyde has numerous applications. It is used in the chemical and plastics industries for the manufacture of paraformaldehyde and melamine, phenol and urea formaldehyde resins, bakelite, artificial amber and celluloid; in the textile industry for hardening and mordanting fibres; for the destruction of anthrax spores in wool, skins and leather; in the tanning industry; for vulcanization processes in the rubber industry; and as a bactericide and preservative of anatomical and pathological specimens. Paraformaldehyde is readily depolymerized liberating formaldehyde when heated and in the presence of alkalis and acids. Phenol formaldehyde and melamine formaldehyde liberate formaldehyde vapour when heated; and urea formaldehyde which is employed as a wood glue, moulding resin and for cavity-wall insulation may also release the vapour. Formalin (a 40 per cent solution of formaldehyde in water with some added alcohol to prevent polymerization to paraformaldehyde) is used as a disinfectant and embalming fluid.

Formaldehyde is very soluble in water, is intensely irritant to the respiratory tract, skin and conjunctivae, and acute exposure causes cough, breathlessness and conjunctivitis. However, asthma associated with lower levels of exposure, is uncommon but has occurred in workers in the formaldehyde-using industries and among pathologists, embalmers, anatomists, zoologists, nurses, and laboratory technicians. It may be immediate or non-immediate and, occasionally, of recurrent nocturnal type following a single exposure (Newman Taylor *et al.*, 1979). Among workers on a production line using phenol formaldehyde 45 per cent complained of wheeze, shortness of breath and chest tightness compared with 7 per cent in an unexposed control population. Reduction in FEV_1 and FEV_1/FVC per cent correlated significantly with length of exposure, the effect being greatest after more than five years' exposure (Schoenberg and Mitchell, 1975). In general, however, only a minority of exposed individuals appear to develop asthmatic symptoms, and there is a prolonged symptom-free period following first exposure before asthma develops.

There are three possible ways by which formaldehyde vapour may cause asthma:

(1) Irritation of airways in a subject with previously established asthma.
(2) An immunological reaction. Precipitating antibodies have been reported in a majority of workers in an electronics factory exposed to a formaldehyde resin and who developed asthma on bronchial challenge with the vapour (Leading article, 1979).
(3) Direct release of histamine from lung tissue. The formaldehyde-containing compound, dimethyl-hydatoinformaldehyde, has been shown to provoke histamine-release '*in vitro*' (Nicholls, 1976).

BYSSINOSIS

The term 'byssinosis' (βϑσσος = flax and the linen made from it), introduced by Proust in 1877 and first employed in Great Britain by Oliver (1902), embraces a gradation of respiratory symptoms due to exposure to the dust of cotton, flax, soft hemp and, to a limited degree, sisal which range from acute dyspnoea with cough and reversible breathlessness and chest tightness on one or more days of a working week to (it is believed) permanent respiratory disability due to irreversible airflow obstruction.

Although cotton and flax have been used in the manufacture of textiles since times of antiquity, byssinosis does not seem to have been recognized or, possibly, to have existed until the introduction of mechanized processes in the early nineteenth century (Patissier, 1822). In 1831 Kay described respiratory disease, which appeared to differ from 'bronchitis', in cotton workers in Lancashire where most of the British cotton industry was concentrated but Greenhow, in 1860, seems to have given the first clear description of the symptom pattern now usually associated with byssinosis; namely, that of late-onset asthma worse at the beginning of the working week than at the end, and an increased severity of symptoms on the first day at work after a longer period of absence than a weekend.

Byssinosis was generally overlooked in Britain until surveys of the cotton industry were started about 30 years ago. The disorder was then thought to be mostly confined to Lancashire cotton workers (Schilling, 1956) and flax workers in Northern Ireland (Smiley, 1951) where it is commonly known as 'poucey chest' ('poucey' is a dialect word meaning dirty or nasty). But it was subsequently reported to occur in Scotland (Smith *et al.*, 1962), Holland, Germany, Sweden, the USA, Egypt, Greece, India and Taiwan (Bouhuys *et al.*, 1967a), Spain (Bouhuys *et al.*, 1967b), Belgium (Tuypens, 1961), Australia (Gandevia and Milne, 1965a) and Israel (Chwat and Mordish, 1963).

At this point it is important to note that other symptoms have been described and may still occur following exposure to cotton, flax or hemp because they are distinct from byssinosis. They are referred to respectively as *mill fever, weavers' cough* and *mattress makers' fever*.

MILL FEVER (FACTORY FEVER)

This is characterized by slight fever, cough, malaise, rigors and rhinitis which occur in some workers on *first contact* with cotton, flax, soft hemp or kapok dust. The symptoms, which are mild, usually last a few hours or, sometimes, days but cease as exposure continues (Greenhow, 1860; Arlidge, 1892; Gill, 1947; Uragoda, 1977). Its prevalence among new workers is not accurately known but assessments varying from 10 to 80 per cent have been made (Doig, 1949; Harris *et al.*, 1972; Uragoda, 1977). The cause is uncertain but may be due to endotoxins of contaminating Gram-negative bacteria in the vegetable dusts and in mill air (Rylander and Lundholm, 1978) (*see* p. 442).

Whether or not mill fever predisposes to the subsequent development of byssinosis is not known but, according to Gill (1947), byssinosis does not occur in the absence of a preceding history of mill fever.

WEAVERS' COUGH

This was an acute respiratory illness identical with late asthma, but accompanied by fever and malaise, in workers machining cotton yarns treated with flour paste or tamarind seed extract and was believed to be due to contaminating fungi (Collis, 1915). However, as indicated in *Table 12.1*, tamarind extract appears to have been responsible in some of these cases. Acclimatization does not occur and both new and old workers are equally affected. The asthma may last for months (Vigliani, Parmeggiani and Sassi, 1954).

MATTRESS MAKERS' FEVER

Acute symptoms occurred from one to six hours after starting work and consisted of fever, rigors, malaise, nausea and vomiting but none of the features of asthma. The cause was attributed to contamination of cotton by the Gram-negative bacillus *Aerobacter cloacae,* and the disease may well have been a form of extrinsic allergic 'alveolitis' (Neal, Schneiter and Caminita, 1942).

SOURCES OF EXPOSURE

Cotton (*Gossypium* spp)

The chief sources of dust production occur in the ginnery where seeds are removed from the cotton after picking in a special machine, the 'gin'; in the 'mixing room' during opening of bales of cotton; in the 'blow room' where the cotton is beaten and blown to eliminate dust and short fibres; and in the 'cardroom' where carding engines comb the fibres and remove dirt and defective material. The fibres are then gathered and twisted into fine strands for spinning. Other dusty operations are 'stripping', which consists of removing dust and cotton fibre adherent to the wire teeth of the carding engine, and 'grinding' (sharpening) the teeth.

Airborne dust consists of broken cotton fibres, bracts (thin, brittle leaves surrounding the stem of the cotton boll which cannot be separated from the cotton), pericarps, bacteria, fungi and minerals. Particles vary from 3.8 cm (1½ inches) in length to less than 2 μm diameter. The larger airborne particles visible to the naked eye consist mainly of broken cotton fibres up to 2.5 cm in length—which are apparently innocuous—and fragments of plant debris too large to enter the lungs which are known as *fly*. 'Coarse' grade cotton produces more dust than the 'fine' grade when the fibres are long. Although, in general, there has been less dust in spinning than in carding rooms there may be a risk of increased concentrations in spinning and winding rooms equipped with high speed machines.

Flax (*Linum usitatissimum*)

Although the industry has contracted owing to substitution of synthetic fibres, flax is still used (often with hemp) to manufacture linen (an Old English word for flax) and yarn for rope, twine, thread, hosepipes, tarpaulins, fishing nets and clothing. In Britain this industry is confined to Northern Ireland and Scotland.

Until the early 1960s flax fibre was separated from the woody parts of the plant (that is, 'retting') by a putrefactive process but this has subsequently been replaced by a chemical method.

Bales of flax are first opened and small bundles separated out by hand, mixed, and then passed into a machine which combs out and straightens the fibres and eliminates dirt ('hackling'). Tow produced during 'hackling' or received in bales is passed through a carding machine to be opened and agitated. All these processes are dusty but carding particularly so.

Fibres are next further straightened on 'drawing frames' and then formed into slivers of uniform thickness, twisted and wound on to bobbins. Much fine dust is produced. The yarn is then spun dry, half-dry or wet; only dry spinning gives off substantial amounts of dust. Winding, twisting and cabling of rope causes significantly smaller dust concentrations than opening, hackling, carding and spinning (Smith *et al.*, 1969).

Hemp

(Soft hemp, *Cannabis sativa;* also known as English or Irish hemp. Hard hemp or Manilla hemp, *Musa textiles;* Mauritius hemp, *Furcraea gigantea*)

It appears that only soft hemp, which is a stem fibre unlike the others which are leaf fibres, is associated with the development of byssinosis. It is used in the manufacture of rope and yarn.

After the hemp plant has been 'retted' it is dried, beaten (batted) to remove wood particles, 'hackled' and baled (Bouhuys *et al.*, 1967b). Until recently this was a flourishing industry in Callosa de Segura in Spain, but is now in rapid decline due to the increased use of synthetic fibres.

Batting and hackling are very dusty activities, but dust concentrations during cabling, twisting and polishing rope are low (Smith *et al.*, 1969).

Jute

(Fibre from bark of *Corchorus capsularis* and *C. oliterius*)

This is grown mainly in India and Pakistan and is used in the manufacture of carpets, felt, wadding and, in combination with flax, in various types of cloth. Retted jute is received by the mill in bales, the opening of which is dusty; mixing grades of fibres, carding and drawing fibre are also dusty processes.

Sisal

(Fibre from the leaves of *Agave sisalana*)

Sisal is employed chiefly in rope manufacture. The leaves are decorticated and brushed—a very dusty process—and the resulting fibre baled. Opening the bales and carding fibre also produce much dust.

Kapok

(a cotton-like fibre from the fruits of the tropical tree, *Ceiba pentandra*)

The tree grows in the Philippines, Indonesia, Thailand, India, Sri Lanka and East and West Africa. Its pods are husked by hand and then ginned manually or mechanically. Machinery, collecting and bagging are dusty processess (Uragoda, 1977).

Coir

This is a fibre obtained from husks of the coconut (*Cocos nucifera*)

It is used in the manufacture of brushes, rope, twine, nets, sacks and matting. Sri Lanka is the chief producer and it is imported by many countries but especially Great Britain, West Germany and Japan. The husks are retted in brackish water, milled and then mechanically teased, twisted and hackled according to the purpose for which it is required (Uragoda, 1975).

Rayon

(generic term for synthetic fibre produced from cellulose)

No untoward effects have been observed among workers in rayon spinning mills (Tiller and Schilling, 1958; Berry *et al.*, 1973).

NATURAL HISTORY OF BYSSINOSIS

As stated earlier byssinosis is a particular form of extrinsic asthma caused in some exposed workers by cotton, flax, hemp or, to a lesser extent, sisal dust with resultant breathlessness, tightness or oppression in the chest and objective evidence of airways obstruction over progressively longer periods of the working week, and which may be prevented or reduced by certain drugs (*see later*, p. 443). Thirty years ago Gill (1947) stated that established byssinosis is characterized by 'asthma-like nocturnal attacks'. Byssinotic symptoms do not apparently result from exposure to coir, kapok and jute (Uragoda, 1975; Žuškin, Valić and Bouhuys, 1976; Uragoda, 1977).

In most cases byssinosis does not develop until there has been ten or more years' exposure to cotton flax or hemp, and it is unusual under five years. There is some evidence that it is not more prevalent among atopic than non-atopic workers (Bouhuys, 1966) but surveys of large numbers of employees using a method of defining atopy like that described earlier (p. 415) do not appear to have been reported. However, asthmatic individuals, who react severely to cotton dust, and others who develop symptoms shortly after starting work almost certainly leave the industry at an early stage (Harris *et al.*, 1972).

The stages of byssinosis are sufficiently well defined to allow of subdivision on clinical grounds and the schema of clinical grades suggested by Schilling *et al.* (1963) is widely used.

Clinical grades

For clarity, these are prefixed by 'C' to distinguish them from the functional ('F') grades referred to in the next section.

Grade C½ Occasional tightness of the chest on the first day of the working week.
Grade C1 Tightness of the chest and/or difficulty in breathing on each first day only of the working week.
Grade C2 Tightness of the chest and/or difficulty in breathing on the first and other days of the working week.
Grade C3 Grade C2 symptoms accompanied by evidence of permanent respiratory disability from reduced ventilatory capacity.

The early symptoms cease completely when the worker is removed from exposure to the relevant vegetable fibre. Progression to more severe symptoms appears to be very variable. Some workers do not seem to progress beyond the early stages and never develop permanent respiratory disability, whereas others reach this stage within a few years. Some workers, however, never have symptoms of airways obstruction. To a large extent these differences are related to smoking habits (*see* Prevalence). Symptomatology is discussed further on pp. 443–444.

Functional grades

Theoretically, the immediate, or acute, effect of exposure to dust can be determined by measuring FEV_1 before and at the end of a working shift on the first working day after a period (usually a weekend) away from work. The difference between these values is the basis of the grading system suggested by Bouhuys, Gilson and Schilling (1970). An FEV_1 value below 80 per cent of predicted normal is taken as abnormal. When an abnormal value is recorded the test should be repeated after administration of a bronchodilator. It is, of course, necessary that the prediction data are valid for the populations examined. The grades are as follows.

Grade F0 (F = Function.) No demonstrable acute effect of the dust on ventilatory capacity; no evidence of chronic ventilatory impairment.
Grade F½ Slight acute effect of dust on ventilatory capacity; no evidence of chronic ventilatory impairment.
Grade F1 Moderate acute reduction of ventilatory impairment.
Grade F2 Evidence of slight to moderate irreversible impairment of ventilatory capacity.
Grade F3 Evidence of moderate to severe irreversible impairment of ventilatory capacity.

Data for each worker must also include his age, the nature and duration of his work, smoking habits and the presence of other respiratory disease.

It should be pointed out, however, that a system such as this is, on the whole, limited to specially controlled investigations. There are a number of reasons for this. For the purposes of routine medical examination in the clinic and factory, the error which may occur between repeated FEV_1 readings is likely to be significant and misleading; and it is impossible to estimate a residual acute effect due to exposure to cotton or similar dusts in the presence of chronic airways obstruction which is particularly likely to be present in smokers. Furthermore, it is not clear whether any difference is implied between 'chronic' and 'irreversible' ventilatory impairment in these grades.

A similar gradation of symptoms and impairment of ventilatory capacity also occurs among flax and soft hemp workers (Mair *et al.*, 1960; Elwood *et al.*, 1965) but in sisal workers, apart from a group in the brushing departments of Tanzanian factories (Mustafa *et al.*, 1978), the effects are usually absent or mild and transient (Velvart, 1971, 1972).

INCIDENCE AND PREVALENCE

Byssinosis occurs throughout the world where cotton, flax and soft hemp fibres are processed but cotton dust is most commonly responsible. Jute does not cause the symptoms associated with byssinosis though mild changes in ventilatory function have been described in workers milling the fibre (Gandevia and Milne, 1965b; Valić and Žuškin, 1971).

The prevalence of disease in cotton workers varies according to the quality and quantity of 'responsible' dust in their work environment. Plant debris and other foreign matter (that is '*cotton trash*') associated with cotton fibre appear to be the source of the agent or agents which cause byssinosis, and 'medium' to 'coarse' dust from this source may be encountered in the separation of cotton from lint (the ginning process), opening of the stripping and grinding of carding machines. In general, the prevalence of all grades of byssinosis is proportional to the total concentration of dust of 'medium' and 'coarse' cotton less 'fly' (that is, coarse waste cotton), and to duration of exposure (Žuškin and Valić, 1972). *Figure 12.13* shows the effect of the exclusion of 'fly' from total dusts.

Prevalence among cotton ginnery workers in tropical countries has been reported to be 20 per cent in the Sudan (Khogali, 1971) and 38 per cent in Egypt (El Batawi, 1962). In England between 1963 and 1966 the total prevalence of byssinosis grades C½ and C2 was 26.9 per cent and was higher in 'coarse' than in 'medium' cotton mills (Molyneux and Tombleson, 1970). Among cardroom workers in

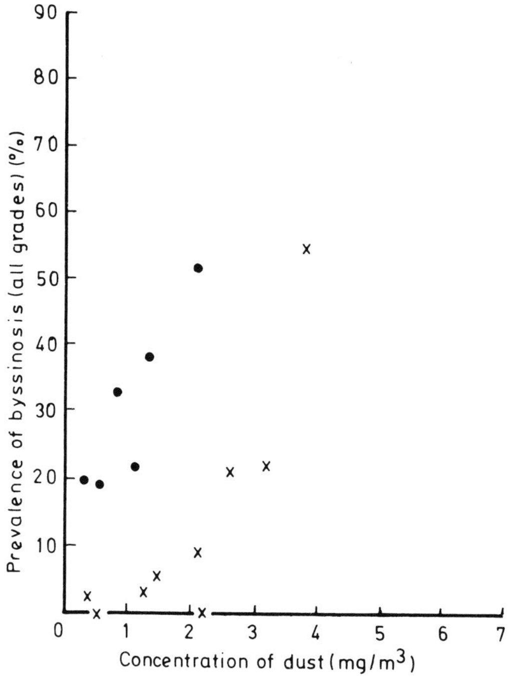

Figure 12.13 Prevalence of byssinosis (all grades); (●) plotted against total dust less fly, (x) plotted against total dust. (By courtesy of The British Occupational Hygiene Society)

Holland a prevalence of 17 per cent was reported (Lammers, Schilling and Walford, 1964) and in the USA, 25 per cent (Žuškin *et al.*, 1969).

Byssinosis is associated with dust concentration and years of exposure, apparently more so in women, and there is also an association between the incidence of new cases and dust levels. The highest prevalence occurs among strippers and grinders and the lowest in ring spinners (Berry, Molyneux and Tombleson, 1974). Expressing dust exposure in terms of a time-weighted dust measurement (that is, dust concentration = length of exposure or mg years/m^3) it has been reckoned that approximately 10 per cent of workers exposed to 0.5 mg/m^3 of cotton dust for 40 years will have byssinosis (Fox *et al.*, 1973). Prevalence is higher in men than in women but whether this is a true sex difference or an occupational difference is not known; certainly more men than women smoke (*Figures 12.14a* and *b*). Among spinners in Holland and the USA prevalence has been reported to be 1.6 and 12 per cent respectively (Lammers, Schilling and Walford, 1964; Žuškin *et al.*, 1969). In cotton seed (non-textile) mills in which levels of respiratory and total dust were high prevalence has been found to be low although there was a mean decline in ventilatory function over a working shift, but not on Fridays (Jones *et al.*, 1977). Possible explanations of dissimilar prevalences of byssinosis between jobs are variations between dust at different stages in cotton processing and, in part, differences between dust levels experienced by individual workers and dust sampling results as is exemplified by strippers and grinders who move continuously over a large working area (Berry, Molyneux and Tombleson, 1974) (*Figure 12.14b*). The differences reported for operatives working on similar processes in various countries may be due to dissimilar work conditions and dust composition and concentrations.

In flax workers byssinosis was apparently equally prevalent in all parts of the mill, and lower grade symptoms were common in those over 35 years of age (Mair *et al.*, 1960; Carey *et al.*, 1965). A prevalence of 22.9 per cent was recently reported in Egyptian flax workers (Noweir *et al.*,

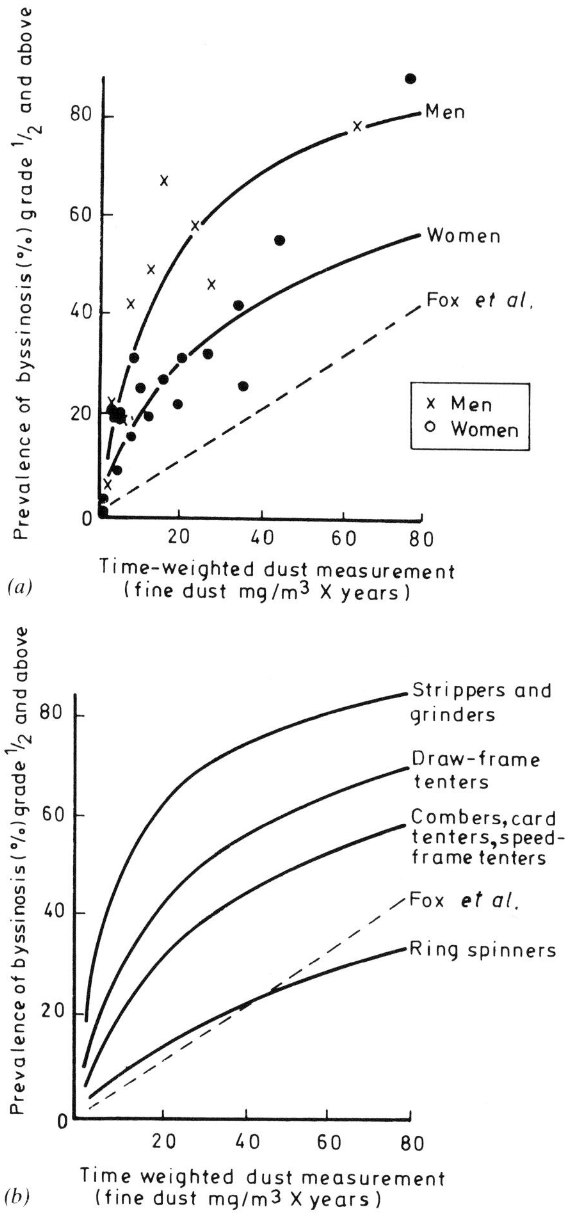

Figure 12.14 (a) Prevalence of byssinosis in the UK related to time-weighted dust measurement (that is, dust concentration × length of exposure). The curves which are fitted for both sexes by taking the logit of prevalence as linearly related to the logarithm of time-weighted dust show prevalence for given dust levels compared with that of Fox et al. *(1973) (broken line) in which the sexes are combined. (b) Prevalence of byssinosis related to time-weighted dust measurements, occupation and adjusted smoking in each sex separately. The proportions of smokers were 56 per cent of women and 76 per cent of men. (Dust concentrations referred to were measured during the period of the survey only, but earlier conditions were most probably more dusty). (Courtesy of Mr. M. G. Berry and the Editor of* Br. J. ind. Med.*)*

1975). Substantially more airflow obstruction was observed in Spanish hemp workers over 50 years of age than in a control population (Bouhuys *et al.*, 1969); and chronic airflow obstruction was reported in about 56 per cent of Czechoslovakian hemp workers (Velvart, 1971). However, since the biological retting of flax and hemp has been replaced by a chemical process byssinosis in these workers has been virtually eliminated.

EFFECTS OF SMOKING

Smokers have a greater incidence of byssinosis and loss of ventilatory function at all levels of dust exposure, and also show a greater tendency to develop byssinosis with increasing dust exposure than non-smokers. Among cotton workers smokers have significantly more byssinosis of each grade than non-smokers after dust concentration and length of exposure are allowed for (Elwood *et al.*, 1965; Bouhuys *et al.*, 1967b; Fox *et al.*, 1973; Merchant *et al.*, 1973a; Berry, Molyneux and Tombleson, 1974). A similar effect has been observed in flax and Tanzanian sisal workers (Smith *et al.*, 1962; Carey *et al.*, 1965; Noweir *et al.*, 1975; Mustafa *et al.*, 1978). However, in Spanish hemp workers there appears to be no clear evidence of an interaction between smoking and work exposure in regard to annual decline of FEV_1 (Bouhuys and Žuškin, 1976).

Fox *et al.* (1973) and Berry, Molyneux and Tombleson (1974) found that the prevalence of 'chronic bronchitis' (MRC definition) is unrelated to dust concentrations but Merchant *et al.* (1972) concluded that byssinosis and 'chronic bronchitis' (mucus hypersecretion) are both influenced by cotton dust exposure and cigarette smoking. Evidence of bronchitis, however, is not always present (Imbus and Suh, 1973). In Australian cotton mill workers the prevalence of productive cough and impairment of respiratory function was not found to be specifically attributable to exposure to cotton dust and was less than that observed in current cigarette smokers (Field and Owen, 1979).

Conclusion

It appears, therefore, that even allowing for individuals who leave the relevant textile industry because of respiratory troubles only a minority of exposed personnel ever develop byssinosis of any grade and that most of these are smokers.

PATHOLOGY

No specific abnormalities have been identified. Grey-black, macular pigmentation may be present in the lungs but there is no fibrosis. In cotton workers, cotton fibres, which are highly birefringent when viewed by polarized light, are occasionally seen. Round or oval bodies up to 10 μm diameter with a central black core surrounded by a yellowish coating which stains positively for iron may also be present (so-called 'byssinosis bodies'), but they have no diagnostic significance (Gough, 1959).

A post-mortem study (without control cases) of 43 British cotton workers diagnosed as having byssinosis during life revealed the following: no significant emphysema in 27 (63 per cent) but a varying amount of centrilobular emphysema in ten (23 per cent) and panlobular type in six (14 per cent) (Edwards *et al.*, 1975). Smoking habits were known in all but nine of the 43 cases: 'significant' emphysema was present in four of 17 life-long non-smokers, and in nine of 17 smokers (Rooke, 1981). Microscopy showed occasional minimal fibrosis but no granulomas or any other evidence of extrinsic allergic 'alveolitis', and the pulmonary blood vessels were unremarkable. But mucous gland hyperplasia and hypertrophy of smooth muscle (expressed as the airway wall formed by muscle) were observed in lobar but not in segmental bronchi: findings consistent with asthma. Takizawa and Thurlbeck (1971) found that the amount of bronchial smooth muscle in chronic bronchitics with no history of wheezing was the same as that in non-bronchitics but that in chronic bronchitics who had suffered bouts of wheezing the muscle was increased in amounts comparable to those seen in known asthmatics. However, it is likely that varying degrees of muscle hyperplasia will be present in chronic bronchitics according to the varying intensities of bronchospasm these patients may have; and, before valid specific inferences can be drawn from the presence of muscle hyperplasia, a frequency distribution curve of muscle proportions in bronchi obtained from random autopsies and from patients with chronic bronchitis is required (Thurlbeck, 1976). To these could be added patients with byssinosis but, unfortunately, the accuracy of this diagnosis in individual subjects during life is by no means certain depending, as it so often does, on subjective criteria.

A more recent retrospective study of the lungs of 49 cotton textile workers in the USA with smoking habits and appropriate control cases revealed a significant association between cotton dust exposure and mucous gland hyperplasia and goblet cell metaplasia, but none with emphysema; nor was there any significant or consistent difference in pigmentation between cotton and non-cotton workers. It was concluded that irreversible airflow obstruction and morphological emphysema in textile workers are most probably related to smoking and not to the occupational exposure (Pratt, Vollmer and Miller, 1980).

The quantitative and qualitative features of mast cells in the tracheobronchial tree do not seem to be known but in other asthmatic patients their numbers are apparently decreased and the prevalence of degranulated and disrupted cells increased (Salvato, 1961).

In view of an early report of an excess of systemic hypertension in heavily exposed cotton operatives (Schilling, Goodman and O'Sullivan, 1952) it is of interest that left ventricular weights in the subjects described by Edwards *et al.* (1975) did not substantiate this.

Rüttner, Spycher and Engeler (1968) described widespread pulmonary fibrosis in a cotton mill worker but this appears to have been the end result of sarcoidosis, and the incidental finding of cotton fibres by electron microscopy and of 'byssinosis bodies' does not, *de facto,* imply a causal relationship.

PATHOGENESIS

The potential of vegetable textile fibres to produce byssinosis ranges from potent to negligible in this order: cotton, flax, soft hemp and sisal. There is controversy in regard to the effect of sisal which, in general, appears to be minimal. Slight reduction in ventilatory capacity in sisal ropeworkers has been attributed to lubricant additives used as fibre softeners and not to sisal dust (Baker *et al.*, 1979).

Cotton and the other vegetable dusts have been conveniently classified by Gilson *et al.* (1962) into size grades: 'coarse'—greater than 2 mm; 'medium'—2 mm down to 7 μm; and 'respirable' less than 7 μm.

Cotton plant parts consist of bract, leaf, vein material, petiole, capsule, cotyledon and pericarp (which includes exocarp, mesocarp and endocarp). The potential for cotton trash to produce fine particulate material is determined by the friability of its components. Bract—the leaf-like structure which enfolds the cotton boll—and wood fragments are the most friable and thus, the most abundant 'respirable' (less than 10 μm) components of raw cotton; and lint and seed coat are the least friable (Morey, 1979). But cotton dust and trash contain bacteria, fungi, fragments of other plants (such as weeds and grasses), and inorganic material from the soil. The range of organic chemical contents is, therefore, enormous: it includes carbohydrates, proteins, lipids, amines, lignins, tannins, phenolic pigments, terpenes, terpinoid alcohols, carbonyl compounds and epoxides. However, bract is believed to contain the active agent, or agents, which cause the airways obstruction of byssinosis, although the bioactivity of bark and stem dusts which account for 25 per cent of the 'respirable' dust is not known (Wakelyn *et al.*, 1976; Morey, 1979).

But of all the compounds in cotton dust only those which are water-soluble cause byssinosis and, in fact, the bioactivity of cotton is greatly reduced by washing and steaming before processing (Merchant *et al.*, 1973b and 1974; Imbus and Suh, 1974). It is interesting to note that in the early days of the cotton industry in Lancashire cotton was washed and dried before being carded, and carding engines were designed for washed cotton (Aitken, 1795; Chapman, 1904).

The ventilatory capacity of workers with symptoms of byssinosis falls when they are exposed to cotton dust during a working day, but it also falls—although to a lesser degree—under similar conditions in workers who do not have byssinosis (*Figure 12.15*) (Berry *et al.*, 1973). It was originally believed that byssinosis is closely related to overall dustiness (Roach and Schilling, 1960) but it has been shown more recently that the 'respirable' and 'medium' components of the total dust correlate most significantly with the prevalence of respiratory symptoms (Molyneux and Berry, 1971).

Because Bouhuys (1970) found that cotton and hemp workers who develop chest tightness and dyspnoea after exposure have reduced FEV_1, maximum expiratory flow rate and VC, but no significant fall of specific conductance, whereas men with no symptoms following exposure do not exhibit change in FEV_1, maximum expiratory flow rate and VC, but do have a significant reduction of specific conductance, it appears that the first type of response results from the action of the dust on smaller airways, and the second, from its action on larger airways.

An interesting feature of the production of the disorder is revealed by an observation in cotton cardroom workers. Those who have been away from dust exposure for longer than a weekend (that is, for two weeks) show a significantly higher first FEV reading and a significantly lower final FEV reading than is usual on the day of return to work; whereas, in workers without byssinosis, the first reading is little different from usual although the final reading is significantly lower (McKerrow and Molyneux, 1971) (*Figure 12.16*).

The mechanism by which cotton and other vegetable fibre dusts cause narrowing of airways is not understood. A number of hypotheses have been suggested the most important of which are as follows:

(1) non-immunological local release of histamine in the lungs;
(2) an antigen–antibody reaction;
(3) bacterial endotoxins;
(4) fungous enzymes.

However, whichever (if any) of these is correct the responsible agency is known to be water-soluble.

Local histamine release

Symptoms identical to the 'Monday feeling' may occur with

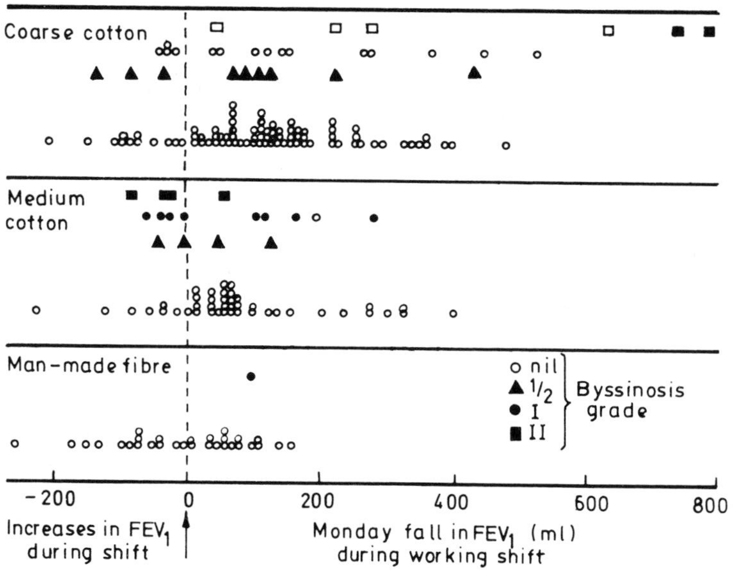

Figure 12.15 This shows the effect mill dust type has in determining the difference in Monday fall in FEV_1 among workers without byssinosis, the negligible mean fall in FEV_1 in man-made fibre mills and that the Monday fall of FEV_1, was related to symptoms of byssinosis only in the coarse-cotton mills. The relationship between Monday fall in FEV_1 and byssinosis is weak. (By courtesy of Berry et al., *1973, and the Editor of the* British Journal of Industrial Medicine*)*

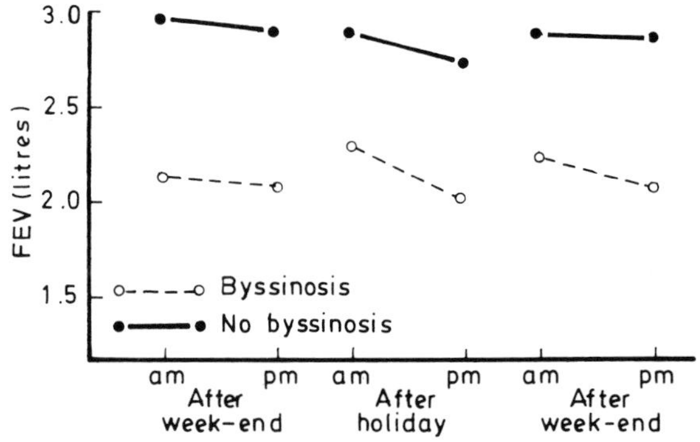

Figure 12.16 Change in $FEV_{0.75}$ *on Mondays in male cardroom workers before the holiday, immediately after the holiday, and one week later. (By permission of the President, International Conference on Respiratory Diseases in Textile Workers, Alicante, 1968)*

similar changes in lung function in healthy volunteers by inhalation challenge in the laboratory with cotton dusts or aerosols of aqueous extracts. The response begins after ten to 15 minutes and lasts some hours, though repeat challenge after 24 hours has no effect (McKerrow and Molyneux, 1971; Bouhuys, 1976). Changes in function include decreased FEV_1 and VC, increased airways resistance, maximum expiratory flow/volume curves, without any fall of gas transfer (*see* p. 444). Washed cotton dust, with similar physical properties, produces neither symptoms nor physiological changes on inhalation, suggesting that washing removes the causal agent (McDermott, Skidmore and Edwards, 1971). It was postulated that the agent might be a histamine-liberating substance in the cotton dust since histamine is a well-known powerful bronchoconstrictor and, although the amount of histamine in cotton is minute, extracts of cotton, flax and hemp dusts have been shown to release histamine from human lung tissue *in vitro* (Bouhuys, Lindell and Lundin, 1960; Nicholls, Nicholls and Bouhuys, 1966; Hitchcock, Piscitelli and Bouhuys, 1973). Histamine-releasing activity of various extracts is measured by adding them to guinea pig, rat, pig or human lung tissue or to smooth muscle preparations or porcine platelets (Ainsworth, Newman and Harley, 1979). However, until the agent which causes byssinosis is established these techniques are of limited value for the assessment of the byssinosis-producing potential of cotton and other vegetable dusts (Nicholls and Skidmore, 1975).

Aqueous extracts of Western red cedar wood, fungal spores and dimethylhydantoin formaldehyde resin also cause direct histamine release *in vitro* (Evans and Nicholls, 1974; Battigelli *et al.*, 1976; Nicholls, 1976).

However, there appears to be no correlation between the response of individuals, or groups of individuals, and dust concentration when this exceeds about 1 mg/m^3. There are two possible explanations for this. First, low solubility of the bronchoconstrictive substance may allow it to be eliminated with the dust before it can be dissolved out; or second, the amount of the substance (histamine, for example) which can be released by the lungs may be limited in any one individual (McDermott, Skidmore and Edwards, 1971).

Just as the bronchoconstrictor effect of histamine aerosol inhaled by human volunteers is potentiated by the β-adrenergic receptor blocking agent, propranolol, and prevented by atropine, the effect of challenge inhalations of hemp dust is similarly potentiated and inhibited by these drugs (Bouhuys, 1971). Furthermore, estimation of 24 hour excretion of the histamine metabolite 1-methyl-4-imidazole acetic acid in the urine is significantly increased in healthy volunteers following inhalation of cotton dust, but there is no increase after the inhalation of washed cotton dust (McDermott, Skidmore and Edwards, 1971).

These observations suggest that the acute changes of lung function provoked in normal persons might be due to histamine release from the lungs, and the unusually low final FEV values on the first day back at work after a holiday in workers without byssinosis are consistent with the possibility of an increase in histamine reserves during the holiday (McKerrow and Molyneux, 1971) and the successive decrease in the asthmatic response during the working week has been attributed to tachyphylaxis due to depletion of endogenous histamine (Nicholls, Nicholls and Bouhuys, 1966). A variety of the many chemical compounds in cotton flax and hemp dust have been suggested as the cause of byssinosis by stimulating the release of histamine but none has yet been positively identified to be the responsible agent (Textile Research Institute, 1978).

The weaknesses in this hypothesis are that direct histamine-release alone does not satisfactorily explain the time relationships of byssinosis nor does the immediate response provoked by bronchial challenge in healthy volunteers (*Figure 12.17*) usually occur in 'natural byssinosis'; this may represent 'mill fever' with little or no fever or a non-specific response. Indeed, apart from the mildness of the constitutional symptoms (which may reflect the size of the challenge dose), it closely resembles 'humidifier fever' (*see* Chapter 11 and *Figure 11.12*) as does the lack of response 24 hours later. However, histamine may be released indirectly by other mechanisms because the Monday fall in FEV_1 can be reduced by antihistamines (Bouhuys, 1963).

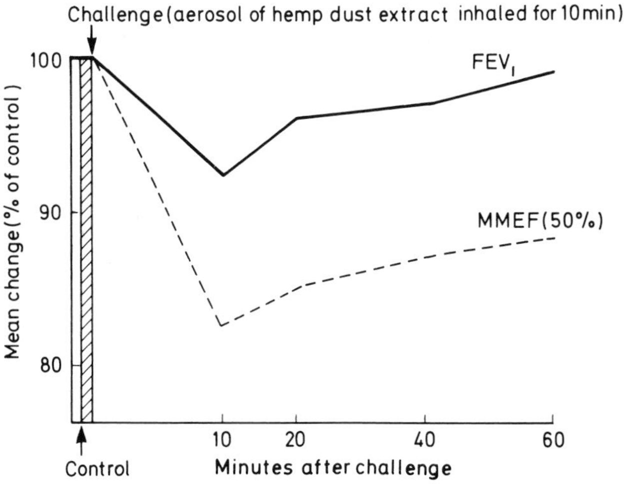

Figure 12.17 Mean acute changes in FEV_1 *and MMEF (50 per cent) following challenge with hemp dust extract in healthy volunteers. (Adapted with permission from Zuskin and colleagues, 1975 and the Editor of* British Journal of Industrial Medicine*)*

Antigen–antibody reaction

Precipitating IgG antibody against an antigen in cotton is

present in cotton workers and unexposed persons: its titre is highest in workers with byssinosis, lower in those without byssinosis and lowest in the unexposed subjects. It has been suggested that the symptoms of byssinosis are caused either directly by a late Arthus type reaction in the walls of airways or indirectly by the reaction liberating a pharmacologically active substance. The fact that symptoms of Grades C1 and C2 byssinosis disappear while the worker is still exposed to the dust is explained on the grounds that, as long as exposure continues, antibody is progressively removed from the circulation leaving insufficient to produce a reaction; whereas after a period away from the dust, during which antibody is not removed, its titre has increased by the time the worker is re-exposed (Massoud and Taylor, 1964). The presence of precipitins in control subjects may have been due to antibodies to other antigens cross-reacting with cotton antigens.

Subsequently, Taylor, Massoud and Lucas (1971) demonstrated that the precipitin titre is greatest at the beginning of the working week than at the end, and is increased after returning from a week's holiday. Titration of precipitin before and after challenge inhalation of cotton antigen by byssinosis and non-byssinosis cardroom workers, revealed smaller titres six hours after inhalation than before. Although 'Monday' symptoms were reproduced by inhalation of antigen, reduction in FEV_1 did not occur (Massoud, Taylor and Lucas, 1971). But evidence of antibody production in normal subjects and increases of Ig levels after ten days were not confirmed (Popa *et al.*, 1969a; Edwards *et al.*, 1970); and more recently Edwards and Jones (1974) found the reaction of the so-called 'byssinosis antigen' to be remarkably non-specific. However, Kamat *et al.* (1979) have reported a significant increase in serum IgG and fall in IgD and IgM in workers with byssinosis which were not found in those with 'chronic bronchitis' though the explanation of these findings remains to be established.

The fact that some workers similarly exposed to cotton or hemp dusts experience severe chest tightness with substantial reduction of FEV whereas others are in no way affected, appears to support the allergic hypothesis. On the other hand, intradermal tests with cotton dust extracts are completely negative in some studies of workers with byssinosis (Voisin *et al.*, 1966) or a high proportion of positive reactions have occurred in controls as well as in exposed workers with and without respiratory symptoms (Cayton, Furness and Maitland, 1952). This might suggest that byssinosis is not simply an allergic phenomenon. However, a more recent investigation of cotton, flax, hemp and jute workers has shown that, although immediate skin reactions were seldom seen, delayed reactions were often present in those both with and without 'byssinotic' symptoms, but were generally absent in normal subjects in other industries (Popa *et al.*, 1969a). These results, if confirmed, give some support to the possibility that Type III (Arthus) reactivity plays a part in pathogenesis though this is contradicted by the lack of correlation between the pattern of respiratory symptoms, lung histology and radiographic appearances which characterize byssinosis and extrinsic allergic 'alveolitis'.

There is also evidence that atopic workers in cotton seed crushing mills have a greater bronchoconstrictor response to cotton dust aerosol than non-atopics. This suggests that atopy is an important risk factor in the development of byssinosis and indicates the importance of identifying atopic workers (Jones *et al.*, 1980).

Bacterial endotoxins and fungous enzymes

There is good evidence that 'mill fever' (*see* p. 435) which may occur in workers in cotton, flax, hemp and grain mills and which is similar to 'humidifier fever' (*see* p. 384) is caused by the inhalation of the endotoxins of bacterial or other organisms growing in these materials (Pernis *et al.*, 1961; Rylander and Lundholm, 1978) (*see also* Chapter 11, Microflora of grain dusts). This has raised the question that byssinosis might also be caused by endotoxins especially as it was reported to occur in workers in factories where flax and hemp were biologically retted (during which bacteria and fungi might be expected to flourish) but not in those where these fibres were chemically retted with alkali (Bouhuys, Hartogensis and Korfage, 1963; Bouhuys *et al.*, 1967b).

Both bacteria and fungi are present in baled cotton and thus in the mill atmosphere. Gram-negative chromogenic bacteria (mainly of the Enterobacter genus) are much more prevalent than fungi and, although among the many species of fungi which have been isolated *T. vulgaris* and *M. faeni* may be widespread, they are seldom as abundant as other species: in particular *Penicillium* spp., *Cladosporium* spp. and *Aspergillus* spp. However, the relative abundance of different species of actinomycetes, fungi and bacteria in cotton mills remains to be established (Lacey, 1977; Rylander and Lundholm, 1978) (*see* Microflora of Grain, p. 375, Chapter 11).

Cumulative exposures to airborne bacteria, protease content of airborne dust and concentration of 2 to 4 mm particles in cotton cardroom air correlate significantly with byssinotic symptoms (Cinkotai and Whitaker, 1978). Cavagna, Foa and Vigliani (1969) found a better correlation between byssinosis prevalence and concentration of airborne endotoxins than with the total amount of dust; and inhalation of an aerosol of purified endotoxin by healthy subjects and patients with chronic bronchitis caused a significant reduction of FEV_1 in a minority of both groups.

Activation of the alternative complement pathway

Endotoxins can activate the alternative pathway yielding C3a and C5a which are capable of releasing histamine directly or indirectly by mobilizing leucocytes rich in histamine (Rylander and Snella, 1976). Recruitment of polymorph leucocytes to the surfaces of airways of hamsters and guinea pigs has been demonstrated following the inhalation of aerosols of cotton mill and trash dust extracts, and of the different strains of Gram-negative bacteria cultured from cotton (Kilburn *et al.*, 1973; Rylander and Lundholm, 1978); and polymorph leucocytosis occurs in human beings exposed to cotton dust (Pernis *et al.*, 1961; Merchant *et al.*, 1975). It is interesting, therefore, that cotton extracts—the most active of which were endotoxins—have also been found to activate the alternative pathway in fresh normal human serum and consume complement proteins in a dose-response manner. As the half-life of Factor B (C3PA) of the alternative pathway is, apparently, 75 hours' synthesis and replenishment of complement protein levels might be expected to occur in workers when away from exposure to dust at weekends and would thus explain that the greatest severity of their asthmatic symptoms is at the start of the working week (Wilson *et al.*, 1976; Wilson *et al.*, 1980).

Proteolytic enzyme activity, probably of fungous origin, has been demonstrated in cotton dust and the concentration of enzymes in the work room air correlates better than dust levels with airflow obstruction in cotton workers (Braun *et al.*, 1973). Fungal spores isolated from cotton dust have been shown to release histamine from lung tissue *in vitro* (Battigelli *et al.*, 1976). However, there is no clear evidence to date that fungal spores or enzymes are responsible for byssinosis; in fact, byssinosis-type symptoms do not occur in wool mills where airborne enzymes are abundant (Kováts and Bugyi, 1968; Cinkotai, 1976).

Although some organisms in the microflora of cotton and other vegetable fibres and, possibly, their endotoxins or enzymes appear to be the cause of 'mill fever' and 'mattress makers' fever' it is difficult to explain how the same agents could also cause byssinosis. But the possibility that they might activate complement by the alternative pathway in some individuals but not in others remains to be investigated.

The effect of drugs

As stated earlier antihistamines may reduce the Monday fall in ventilatory capacity in individuals with byssinosis but the influence of salbutamol, beclomethasone and sodium cromoglycate on the ventilatory response to cotton dust in mill workers with and without byssinosis has recently been investigated.

Salbutamol, which inhibits both immediate and late asthmatic reactions and is also a bronchodilator, was the most effective drug; but whether this was due to the bronchodilator effect or to suppression of antigen-induced histamine release was not determined. Beclomethasone caused improvement in ventilation in byssinotic workers but whether this was due to its ability to suppress late, possibly IgG mediated, asthmatic reactions or to a non-specific effect is not known. Sodium cromoglycate, which relieves immediate IgE-mediated asthma and suppresses histamine release from mast cells, achieved a significant effect only after three hours and was less active than the other two drugs (Fawcett *et al.*, 1978). Sodium cromoglycate has also been shown to block the effect of inhalation challenge with hemp dust extract in healthy subjects but the protection is shortlived (Žuškin and Bouhuys, 1977).

It is difficult to interpret the significance of these observations but the results do not contradict the possibilities that some form of antigenic mechanism or direct or indirect histamine release might be involved in the production of byssinosis.

Susceptibility to byssinosis

Flax workers whose fathers had been exposed occupationally to flax dust (especially if they had had byssinosis) are apparently less likely to develop byssinotic symptoms than fellow workers whose fathers had no such history (Noweir, Amine and Osman, 1975). Although the histocompatibility antigen, HLA-B27, is significantly more common in individuals with flax byssinosis it is not necessary for the development of byssinosis in these workers and its presence may be associated with other genes (Middleton *et al.*, 1979). There is a strong suggestion, but no more, that cotton workers who have had mill fever are more prone to develop byssinosis than those who have not (Gill, 1947).

IS BYSSINOSIS DISTINCT FROM OTHER FORMS OF BRONCHIAL ASTHMA?

Byssinosis has been regarded as a separate entity on the following grounds (Schilling, 1956; Bouhuys, 1976):

(1) Most asthmatics are hypersensitive to histamine but this is 'not a regular finding in byssinosis' (Bouhuys, 1967).
(2) A large proportion of textile workers may be affected by byssinosis but in other forms of asthma the number of workers affected is usually very small.
(3) The symptoms of byssinosis are delayed (that is, are not immediate) and improve during the working week.
(4) Skin tests with dust extracts correlate poorly with byssinosis by comparison with skin tests in atopic asthma.

However, the prevalence of byssinosis in different industries varies greatly and may be extremely low in comparable processes (Field and Owen, 1979). The pattern of grades C1 and C2 byssinosis is consistent with late asthma, and recovery on subsequent days of the working week also occurs in some other forms of occupational asthma (for example, 'humidifier fever', *see* Chapter 11); and, as indicated earlier, may be mediated via the alternative complement pathway. Lack of correlation with skin test reactions in other forms of occupational asthma is also fairly common because of difficulty in making appropriate preparations of some industrial agents. The clinical concept of byssinosis was established in the 1950s before the patterns of late (non-immediate) asthma and their wide variations were generally recognized; furthermore, it is by no means certain that *irreversible* airflow obstruction is an integral part of byssinosis. Hence, although the underlying mechanism of byssinosis is not fully understood its general features are those of late asthma, but recovery during the working week largely differentiates it from the majority of other occupational asthmas.

SYMPTOMS

The symptoms of byssinosis, which are distinct from those of 'mill fever', have already been summarized in Clinical grades (p. 437). Acute symptoms consist of chest tightness and breathlessness (Grades C½ to C2) which develop during the afternoon of the work day, although in severe cases they occur a few hours after starting work in the morning. Cough and wheezing may also be complained of but in many cases they are slight or absent, although wheeze may be heard in some on auscultation. The expression '*tightness*', incidentally, is commonly used to refer to the sensation of breathlessness experience by patients with lower airways disease, especially asthma, which has a vague but more 'internal' localization than the 'inability to get in enough air' associated with cardiac, neurological and other lung diseases (Widdicombe, 1979).

The 'Monday feeling' of Grade C½, consisting of chest tightness alone, occurs only on some Mondays (or first day back at work). Subsequently, breathlessness and fatigue, sometimes with cough, are complained of on every Monday in addition to chest tightness (Grade C1) but cease completely on the Tuesday. Grade C1 symptoms are best exempified in the words of a cotton stripper and grinder who had been exposed to cotton dust for ten years (Schilling, 1950).

> Monday is a different day to me. Getting to 11 o'clock I feel tight in the chest and short of wind, but I have no cough. Towards 5.30 I feel done and struggle for breath and I can't walk at my ordinary speed. I am a dead horse on Mondays, but could fell a bull on Tuesdays.

In many workers there may be no further progression of symptoms during their work in the textile industry, and when they leave, symptoms cease completely leaving no residual disability.

Grade C2 is characterized by a gradual progression of symptoms. Chest tightness and breathlessness increase in severity and, although usually worse on Mondays, are present on other days of the week. There may be some cough. These symptoms, like Grade C1 symptoms, disappear when exposure to dust ceases. Once again, a cotton operative's own words are of interest (Schilling, 1950).

> I first noticed Monday feeling about 15 years ago, and at first I only got it on Mondays, but now I get it every day and I don't think there is much difference between my condition on Monday and other days of the week. Now I am always short of breath on exertion.

Some workers with Grade C2 symptoms are believed to progress gradually to Grade C3 in which chest tightness and breathlessness on effort are present every day and may be severe enough to prevent them continuing their work. Although some relief may be experienced when they leave the industry this is incomplete and respiratory disability is permanently established.

Grade C3 byssinosis and chronic obstructive bronchitis

Although chronic bronchitis in the sense of mucous hypersecretion is often associated with byssinosis (Imbus and Suh, 1973), a state of irreversible (that is, non-asthmatic) airflow obstruction in textile workers which is *primarily* attributable to vegetable fibre dust and not to smoking is much less certain. But a study of a large number of male and female textile workers over the age of 45 matched with control subjects for age, sex and smoking habits suggested that there is an excess of chronic cough, wheeze, dyspnoea and persistent ventilatory impairment in the workers compared with controls. Work in textile mills was the chief variable affecting the prevalence of the symptoms but smoking was an additional significant variable related to all these features except dyspnoea (Bouhuys *et al.*, 1977). However, the pathological studies referred to earlier (p. 439) do not support the notion that ireversible airflow obstruction is an ultimate stage of byssinosis.

PHYSICAL SIGNS

As a rule there are no abnormal signs in grades C½ to C2 byssinosis though expiratory wheeze is sometimes present. Breath sounds may be impaired in some individuals with grade C3 symptoms.

INVESTIGATIONS

Lung function

There is a progressive reduction of ventilatory capacity (as indicated by FEV_1 and an increase of airways resistance throughout the working day in Grades C1 and C2 byssinosis, and also some unevenness of distribution of inspired gas (McKerrow *et al.*, 1958; Cotes, 1979). Decline in FEV_1 may occur during the working day without respiratory symptoms (Imbus and Suh, 1973). Maximum mid-expiratory flow (MMF) is also reduced and may be more sensitive in detecting airflow obstruction than FEV_1. Closing volume is a less sensitive, unreliable and more time-consuming test (Fairman *et al.*, 1975; Žuškin *et al.*, 1975). Observations by Field and Owen (1979) in Australia indicate that a fall in MMF occurs early in a shift and is consistent with constriction of distal airways whereas reduction in FEV_1 and PEFR, which is indicative of involvement of larger airways, occurs later and more gradually. These authors also found that the Monday morning fall in MMF was rarely accompanied by chest symptoms in contrast to the reported findings in Europe and North America which they suggest are due to extraneous factors. These functional changes are reversible on quitting exposure. Gas transfer remains within normal limits (Žuškin *et al.*, 1975).

The most practical tests for routine use in industry, however, are FEV_1 or PEFR.

Radiographic appearances

Byssinosis is not characterized by any abnormality of the chest radiograph.

Intradermal tests

Intradermal prick tests are usually negative with the cotton extracts which have been tried and are, therefore, of no help in identifying byssinosis in cotton workers.

DIAGNOSIS

Ideally the diagnosis of Grades C½ to C2 rests on:

(1) A history of industrial exposure to cotton, flax or soft hemp dust
(2) A typical history of these clinical grades.
(3) Fall in FEV_1 or MMF during the working day or the working week.

In clinical practice the objective evidence of ventilatory function at the time of the symptoms is not always available and the diagnosis then depends entirely on the reliability of the patient's history. Hence, the technique of eliciting the history is all important. It is essential, first, to allow him to relate his story without interruption and for the physician to ask leading questions only later in the examination; to start with leading questions ('Is your chest tight on Mondays?', for example) may result in false affirmative answers and wrong diagnosis. Every effort should be made to measure FEV_1 or PEFR before, during and after a working shift and, if possible, at regular intervals during a weekend or holiday period. However, the influence of diurnal variation on ventilatory capacity, both in healthy individuals and chronic bronchitics, must be taken into account.

In smokers with chronic obstructive bronchitis grade C1 and C2 byssinosis may be identified by an enhanced reduction in FEV_1, PEFR or MMF during a working shift.

The diagnosis of Grade C3 disease is said to depend on the work history, a history of progressive development of the clinical grades of byssinosis, and evidence of irreversible airflow obstruction. But in patients with chronic obstructive bronchitis the diagnosis is impossible for, even if the patient's declared memory of having had Grade C1 and C2 symptoms in the past is reliable, this cannot establish the co-existence of Grade C3 byssinosis. Although epidemiological evidence has shown that chronic respiratory disability is significantly more common among textile workers than among control subjects, this is of little practical help for diagnosis in individual patients. Grades C½ to C2 byssinosis cannot be confused with chronic obstructive bronchitis (MRC Definition, 1965).

To summarize

(1) The acute respiratory and constitutional symptoms of variable intensity of 'mill fever' and 'mattress makers' fever' are separate from byssinosis and the distinction has to be borne in mind. The occasional use of term 'Monday Fever' for Grade C1 byssinosis is both incorrect and confusing.
(2) Byssinosis Grades C½ to 2 behave as 'late' asthma possibly preceded by a mild 'immediate' stage (chiefly a slight reduction in FEV_1 or MMF) in some cases.
(3) The immediate asthmatic response in healthy persons on bronchial challenge with textile dust extracts or visiting a mill may not be relevant to 'natural' byssinosis in susceptible textile workers.
(4) Grade C3 byssinosis is an uncertain entity. It appears probable that it represents irreversible airflow obstruction associated chiefly with smoking.
(5) The features of extrinsic allergic 'alveolitis' are absent.

PROGNOSIS (*see* Addendum, p. 453)

Cotton workers without byssinosis who have the greatest Monday fall in FEV are most likely to develop byssinosis subsequently (Berry *et al.*, 1973).

Complete symptomatic and functional recovery from Grade C½ and C1 disease occurs when the worker leaves the industry and, in general, this is true of Grade C2 disease, although slight to moderate 'irreversible' impairment of ventilatory capacity is present in some individuals (Grade F2), and may be related to smoking.

TREATMENT

Workers with Grades C1 and C3 byssinosis should be removed from areas of dust exposure.

The prophylactic effects of antihistamines, salbutamol, beclomethasone and sodium cromoglycate have already been referred to. However, their use as a therapeutic measure is no substitute for prevention.

PREVENTION

Prevention depends upon the cooperation of engineering and medical disciplines.

Dust control

The most effective preventive measure is the replacement of natural by synthetic fibres. Although this has been achieved to some extent in Europe and the USA it is small by comparison with the world increase in cotton production; and, while the production of flax has declined that of hemp has not changed significantly.

Plant already in existence in established factories should be enclosed as far as is practicable and subjected to local exhaust ventilation; that is, cotton gins and opening and mixing and carding machines. But removal of dust is often inefficient due to unsatisfactory design, application and maintenance of equipment. The difficulty has been accentuated in recent years by rising production demands requiring a great increase in the speed of carding machines and, consequently, of the dust output. A proportionately greater demand, therefore, has been placed upon ventilation systems. Effective methods of water washing and steam treatment of raw cotton before processing are under active investigation.

General ventilation is also necessary and recirculated air must be efficiently filtered. Dust should be removed from machines, mill floors, ventilation equipment and other surfaces by vacuum cleaners.

Where sporadically large concentrations of dust occur (for example, stripping and grinding of carding machines) the operatives should wear efficient respirators.

Dust control measures and sampling techniques are related to current TLVs which are under review since the composition and biological activity of textile dusts can vary significantly in different processing operations so that a series of dust levels may be needed.

Suggested methods of control

(1) Spraying of ripening cotton with bacteriocides and fungicides.
(2) Treatment of raw cotton with gaseous hydrogen chloride or acetic acid as acids has been found to inactivate the active component in cotton bracts and dust.

Medical surveillance of workers

Pre-employment examination

All prospective employees in vegetable textile industries should be examined. Examinations should include a questionnaire similar to that of the Medical Research Council with additional details of atopic family history, personal history of allergy and asthma, physical examination, FEV_1, PEFR or MMF and a chest radiograph. Investigation of atopic status by skin prick tests to common allergens should be done in each case, and atopic subjects probably excluded.

It is advisable that moderate to heavy cigarette smokers and persons with chronic or recurrent respiratory disease should be placed in low- or no-risk areas; but in practice, in the case of the smokers, there is probably little chance of achieving this. Individuals with a FEV_1 less than 60 per cent of the predicted normal value should not be exposed to dust.

There is at present no practical immunological method of detecting individual susceptibility.

Periodic medical examinations

These serve two purposes: to identify workers who develop a pronounced reaction to the dust; and to provide a biological assessment of the efficiency of dust control and sampling in specific processes.

During the first month of his employment the worker's FEV_1 should be recorded before and after six hours of commencing his shift on the first day of a working week. If a significant decrease occurs he should be transferred to a less dusty area.

Systematic clinical examination and recording of FEV_1, PEFR or MMF should be done annually in all exposed workers. Those who are prone to develop substantial disability can be identified by comparing the annual fall of their FEV_1 with the predicted normal value after the effects of diurnal variation and cigarette smoking are allowed for. They should be moved to a no-risk area as soon as this is recognized.

REFERENCES

Ainsworth, S. K., Newman, R. E. and Harley, R. A. (1979). Histamine release from platelets for assay of byssinogenic substances in cotton mill dust and related materials. *Br. J. ind. Med.* **36,** 35–42

Aitken, J. (1795). *A Description of the Country from Thirty to Forty miles around Manchester.* Republished 1968. David and Charles; Newton Abbott

Alanko, K., Keskinen, H., Björkstén, F. and Ojanen, S. (1978). Immediate-type hypersensitivity to reactive dyes. *Clin. Allergy* **8,** 25–31

Andrasch, R. H., Bardana, Jr., E. J., Koster, F. and Pirofsky, B. (1976). Clinical and bronchial provocation studies in patients with meatwrapper's asthma. *J. Allergy clin. Immunol.* **158,** 291–298

Arlidge, J. J. (1892). The Hygiene, Disease and Mortality of Occupations, pp. 354–358. London; Percival and Co

Baker, M. D., Irwig, L. M., Johnston, J. R., Turner, D. M. and Bezuidenhout, B. N. (1979). Lung function in sisal ropemakers. *Br. J. ind. Med.* **36,** 216–219

Baldo, B. A. and Turner, K. J. (1975). The radioallergosorbent test (RAST). Its significance in clinical and experimental allergy. *Med. J. Aust.* **2,** 871–874

Barbee, R. A., Liebowitz, M. D., Thompson, H. C. and Burrows, B. (1976). Immediate skin reactivity in a general population sample. *Ann. intern. Med.* **84,** 129–133

Battigelli, M. C., Fischer, J. J., Craven, P. L. and Foarde, K. K. (1976). The etiology of byssinosis. *Am. Rev. resp. Dis.* **113,** 100 (Abstract)

Baur, X., Fruhmann, G. and von Liebe, V. (1979). Occupational asthma and dermatitis after exposure to dusts of persulfate salts in two industrial workers. *Respiration,* **38,** 144–150

Belin, L., Falsen, E., Hoborn, J. and André, J. (1970). Enzyme sensitisation in consumers of enzyme-containing washing powder. *Lancet* **2,** 1153–1157

Bernton, H. S. (1923). On occupational sensitisation to the castor bean. *Am. J. med. Sci.* **165,** 196–202

Bernton, H. S. (1973). On occupational sensitization—a hazard to the coffee industry. *J. Am. med. Ass.* **223,** 1146–1147

Bernton, H. S, McMahon, T. F. and Brown, H. (1972). Cockroach asthma. *Br. J. Dis. Chest* **66,** 61–66

Berry, G., McKerrow, C. B., Molyneux, M. K. B., Rossiter, C. E. and Tombleson, J. B. L. (1973). A study of the acute and chronic changes in ventilatory capacity of workers in Lancashire cotton mills. *Br. J. ind. Med.* **30,** 25–36

Berry, G., Molyneux, M. K. B. and Tombleson, J. B. L. (1974). Relationship between dust level and byssinosis and bronchitis in Lancashire cotton mills. *Br. J. ind. Med.* **31,** 18–27

Biological Effects of Proteolytic Enzyme Detergents. (1976). Report of symposium. Medical Research Council, UK and Soap and Detergent Industries Association, UK. *Thorax,* **31,** 621–634

Björkstén, F., Backman, A., Järvinen, K. A. J., Lehti, H., Savilahti, E., Syvänen, P. and Kärkkäinen, T. (1977). Immunoglobin E specific to wheat and rye flour proteins. *Clin. Allergy* **7,** 473–483

Bohner, C. B. (1941). Sensitivity to gum acacia, with a report of ten cases of asthma in printers. *J. Allergy* **12,** 290–294

Booth, B. H., Le Foldt, R. H. and Moffitt, E. M. (1976). Wood dust hypersensitivity. *J. Allergy clin. Immun.* **57,** 352–357

Bouhuys, A. (1963). Prevention of Monday dyspnoea in byssinosis: a controlled trial with an antihistamine drug. *Clin. pharmac. Ther.* **4,** 311–314

Bouhuys, A. (1966). Asthma and byssinosis. *Rev. Allergy* **22,** 473–476

Bouhuys, A. (1967). Response to inhaled histamine in bronchial asthma and in byssinosis. *Am. Rev. resp. Dis.* **95,** 89–93

Bouhuys, A. (1970). Byssinosis in textile workers. In *Pneumoconiosis. Proceedings of the International Conference.* Johannesburg, 1969, edited by H. A. Shapiro, pp. 412–416. Cape Town; Oxford University Press

Bouhuys, A. (1971). Byssinosis. *Archs envir. Hlth* **23,** 405–407

Bouhuys, A. (1976). Byssinosis: scheduled asthma in the textile industry. *Lung* **154,** 3–16

Bouhuys, A., Barbero, A., Schilling, R. S. F. and van de Woestijne, K. P. (1969). Chronic respiratory disease in hemp workers. *Am. J. Med.* **46,** 526–537

Bouhuys, A., Gilson, J. C. and Schilling, R. S. F. (1970). Byssinosis in the textile industry. *Archs envir. Hlth.* **21,** 475–478

Bouhuys, A., Hartogensis, F. and Korfage, H. J. H. (1963). Byssinosis prevalence and flax processing. *Br. J. ind. Med.* **20,** 320–323

Bouhuys, A., Heaphy, L. J. Jr., Schilling, R. S. F. and Welborn, J. W. (1967a). Byssinosis in the United States. *New Engl. J. Med.* **277,** 170–175

Bouhuys, A., Lindell, S. E. and Lundin, G. (1960). Experimental studies in byssinosis. *Br. med. J.* **1,** 324–326

Bouhuys, A., Lindell, S. E., Roach, S. A. and Schilling, R. S. F. (1967b). Byssinosis in hemp workers. *Archs envir. Hlth* **14,** 533–544

Bouhuys, A., Schoenberg, J. B., Beck, G. J. and Schilling, R. S. F. (1977). Epidemiology of chronic lung disease in a cotton mill community. *Lung* **154,** 167–186

Bouhuys, A. and Žuškin, E. (1976). Chronic respiratory disease in hemp workers. A follow-up study, 1967–1974. *Ann. intern. Med.* **84,** 398–405

Bourne, M. S., Flindt, M. L. H. and Walker, J. M. (1979). Asthma due to industrial use of chloramine. *Br. med. J.* **2,** 10–12

Braun, D. C., Scheel, L. D., Tuma, J. and Parker, L. (1973). Physiological response to enzymes in cotton dust. *J. occup. Med.* **15,** 241–244

Bridge, J. C. (1935). *Annual Report of the Chief Inspector of Factories*, p. 60. London; His Majesty's Stationery Office

Brown, E. B. and Creper, S. B. (1947). Allergy (asthma) to ingested gum tragacanth. *J. Allergy* **18,** 214–216

Browne, R. C. (1955). Vanadium poisoning from gas turbines. *Br. J. ind. Med.* **12,** 57–59

Bruckner, H. C. (1967). Extrinsic asthma in a tungsten carbide worker. *J. occup. Med.* **9,** 518–519

Bruckner, H. C., Avery, S. B., Stetson, D. M., Dodson, V. M. and Ranayne, J. J. (1968). Clinical and immunological appraisal of workers exposed to diisocyanates. *Archs envir. Hlth* **16,** 619–625

Brugsch, H. G. and Elkins, H. B. (1963). Toluene diisocyanate (TDI) toxicity. *New Engl. J. Med.* **268,** 353–357

Buisseret, P. (1978). Seasonal asthma in an angler. *Lancet* **1,** 668 (letter)

Buist, J. M. and Lowe, A. (1965). The chemistry of polyurethanes and their applications. *Ann. occup. Hyg.* **8,** 143–162

Burge, P. S., Edge, G., O'Brien, I. M., Harries, M. G. and Pepys, J. (1979a). Occupational asthma, rhinitis and urticaria in a research establishment breeding locusts. *Thorax* **34,** 415

Burge, P. S., Harries, M. G., O'Brien, I. M. and Pepys, J. (1978a). Respiratory disease in workers exposed to solder flux fumes containing colophony (pine resin). *Clin. Allergy* **8,** 1–14

Burge, P. S., Harries, M. G., O'Brien, I. M. and Pepys, J. (1978b). Occupational asthma in the manufacture of Pondrax due to sensitivity to gum acacia. In preparation

Burge, P. S., Harries, M. G., O'Brien, I. and Pepys, J. (1980). Bronchial provocation studies in workers exposed to fumes of electronic soldering fluxes. *Clin. Allergy* **10,** 137–149

Burge, P. S., O'Brien, I. M. and Harries, M. G. (1979). Peak flow rate records in the diagnosis of occupational asthma due to colophony. *Thorax* **34,** 308–316

Burge, P. S., O'Brien, I. M., Harries, M. G. and Pepys, J. (1979b). Occupational asthma due to inhaled carmine. *Clin. Allergy* **9,** 185–189

Burge, P. S., Perks, W. H., O'Brien, I. M., Burge, A., Hawkins, R., Brown, D. and Green, M. (1979c). Occupational asthma in an electronics factory: a case control study to evaluate aetiological factors. *Thorax* **34,** 300–307

Bush, R. K., Yunginger, J. W. and Reed, C. E. (1978). Asthma due to African zebrawood (*Microberlinia*) dust. *Am. Rev. resp. Dis.* **117,** 601–603

Busse, W. W. and Schoenwetter, W. F. (1975). Asthma from Psyllium in laxative manufacture. *Ann. intern. Med.* **83,** 361–362

Butcher, B. T., Jones, R. N., O'Neil, C. E., Glindmeyer, H. W., Diem, J. E., Dharmarajan, V., Weill, H. and Salvaggio, J. E. (1977). Longitudinal study of workers employed in the manufacture of toluene-diisocyanate. *Am. Rev. resp. Dis.* **116,** 411–421

Butcher, B. T., Karr, R. M., O'Neil, C. E., Wilson, M. R., Dharmarajan, V., Salvaggio, J. E. and Weill, H. (1979). Inhalation challenge and pharmacologic studies of toluene diisocyanate (TDI)—sensitive workers. *J. Allergy clin. Immunol.* **64,** 146–152

Butcher, B. T., Salvaggio, J. E., Weill, H. and Ziskind, M. M. (1976). Toluene diisocyanate (TDI) pulmonary disease: Immunologic and inhalation challenge studies. *J. Allergy clin. Immunol.* **58,** 89–100

Card, W. I. (1935). A case of asthma sensitivity to chromates. *Lancet* **2,** 1348–1349

Carroll, K. B., Secombe, C. J. P. and Pepys, J. (1976). Asthma due to non-occupational exposure to toluene di-isocyanate. *Clin. Allergy* **6,** 99–104

Casterline, C. L. (1980). Irritable airways. Early indicator of occupational lung disease. *Chest* **77,** 2–3

Cavagna, G., Foa, V. and Vigliani, E. C. (1969). Effects in man and rabbits of inhalation of cotton dust or extracts and purified endotoxins. *Br. J. ind. Med.* **26,** 314–321

Cayton, H. R., Furness, G. and Maitland, H. B. (1952). Studies in cotton dust in relation to byssinosis. Part II. Skin tests for allergy with extracts of cotton dusts. *Br. J. ind. Med.* **9,** 186–196

Chan-Yeung, M. (1977). Fate of occupational asthma. A follow-up study of patients with occupational asthma due to Western Red Cedar (*Thuja plicata*). *Am. Rev. resp. Dis.* **116,** 1023–1029

Chan-Yeung, M. and Abboud, R. (1976). Occupational asthma due to California redwood. (*Sequoia sempervirens*) dusts. *Am. Rev. resp. Dis.* **114,** 1027–1031

Chan-Yeung, M., Ashley, M. J., Willson, G., Dorken, E. and Grzybowski, S. (1978). A respiratory survey of cedar mill workers I. Prevalence of symptoms and pulmonary function abnormalities. *J. occup. Med.* **20,** 323–327

Chan-Yeung, M., Barton, G. M., Maclean, L. and Grzybowski, S. (1973). Occupational asthma and rhinitis due to Western Red Cedar (*Thuja plicata*). *Am. Rev. resp. Dis.* **108,** 1094–1102

Chan-Yeung, M., Wong, R. and Maclean, L. (1979). Respiratory abnormalities among grain elevator workers. *Chest* **75,** 461–467

Chapman, S. J. (1904). *The Lancashire Cotton Industry.* Manchester University Press

Chwat, M. and Mordish, R. (1963). Byssinosis investigations into cotton plants in Israel. 14th International Conference in Occupational Health, Madrid, 1963. *Int. Congr. Series No. 62,* pp. 572–573. Amsterdam; Excerpta Medica

Ciba Guest Symposium Report (1959). Terminology, definitions, and classification of chronic pulmonary emphysema and related conditions. *Thorax* **14,** 286–299

Cinkotai, F. F. (1976). The size-distribution and protease content of airborne particles in textile mill card rooms. *Am. indust. Hyg. Ass. J.* **37,** 234–238

Cinkotai, F. F. and Whitaker, C. J. (1978). Airborne bacteria and the prevalence of byssinotic symptoms in 21 cotton spinning mills in Lancashire. *Ann. occup. Hyg.* **21,** 239–250

Cleare, J. J., Hughes, E. G., Jacoby, B. and Pepys, J. (1976). Immediate (Type I) allergic responses to platinum compounds. *Clin. Allergy* **6,** 183–195

Cockcroft, D. W., Cartier, A., Jones, G., Tarlo, S. M., Dolovich, J. and Hargreave, F. E. (1980). Asthma caused by occupational exposure to a furan-based binder system. *J. Allergy clin. Immunol.* **66,** 458–463

Cockcroft, D. W., Ruffin, R. E., Frith, P. A., Cartier, A., Juniper, E. F., Dolovich, J. and Hargreave, F. E. (1979). Determinants of allergen-induced asthma: dose of allergen, circulating IgE antibody concentration, and bronchial responsiveness to inhaled histamine. *Am. Rev. resp. Dis.* **120,** 1053–1058

Collis, E. L. (1915). The occurrence of an unusual cough among weavers of cotton cloth. *Proc. R. Soc. Med.* **8,** (Part 2) 108–112

Colten, H. R., Polakoff, P. L., Weinstein, S. F. and Strieder, D. (1975). Immediate hypersensitivity to hog trypsin resulting from industrial exposure. *J. Allergy clin. Immunol.* **55,** 130 (abstract 148)

Connolly, C. K. (1979). Diurnal rhythms in airway obstruction. *Br. J. Dis. Chest* **73,** 357–366

Cotes, J. E. (1979). *Lung function. Assessment and Application in Medicine,* 4th edition. Oxford and Edinburgh; Blackwell

Cromwell, O., Pepys, J., Parish, W. E. and Hughes, E. G. (1979). Specific IgE antibodies to platinium salts in sensitized workers. *Clin. Allergy.* **9,** 109–117

Cuthbert, O. D., Brostoff, J., Wraith, D. G. and Brighton, W. D. (1979). 'Barn allergy': asthma and rhinitis due to storage mites. *Clin. Allergy* **9,** 229–236

Darke, C. S., Knowelden, J., Lacey, J. and Ward, A. M. (1976). Respiratory disease of workers harvesting grain. *Thorax* **31,** 294–302

Davies, R. J. (1979). Allergic lung disease. *Br. J. hosp. Med.* **22,** 136–150

Davies, R. J., Green, M. and Schofield, N. McC. (1976). Recurrent nocturnal asthma after exposure to grain dust. *Am. Rev. resp. Dis.* **114,** 1011–1019

Davies, R. J., Hendrick, D. J. and Pepys, J. (1974). Asthma due to inhaled chemical agents—ampicillin, benzyl penicillin, 6 amino penicillanic acid and related substances. *Clin. Allergy* **4,** 227–247

Davies, R. J. and Pepys, J. (1975). Asthma due to inhaled chemical agents—the macrolide antibiotic spiramycin. *Clin. Allergy* **5,** 99–107

Dijkman, J. H. (1975). Observation on biphasic bronchial reactions due to inhalation of enzymes of *Bacillus subtilis. Clin. Allergy* **1,** 25–31

Doig, A. T. (1949). Other lung diseases due to dust. *Postgrad. Med J.* **25,** 639–649

Dolan, T. F. and Myers, A. (1974). Bronchial asthma and allergic rhinitis associated with inhalation of pancreatic extracts. *Am. Rev. resp. Dis.* **110,** 812–813

doPico, G. A. (1978). Asthma due to dust from redwood (*Sequoia sempervirens*). *Chest* **73,** 424–425

doPico, G. A. (1979). Grain dust and health. *Chest* **75,** 416–417

doPico, G. A., Reddan, W., Flaherty, D., Tsiatis, A., Peters, M. E., Roa, P. and Rankin, J. (1977). Respiratory abnormalities among grain handlers. A clinical, physiologic and immunologic study. *Am. Rev. resp. Dis.* **115,** 915–927

Dosman, J. A., Cotton, D. J., Graham, B. L., Li, R. K. Y., Froh, F. and Barnett, G. D. (1980). Chronic bronchitis and decreased forced expiratory flow rates in lifetime non-smoking grain workers. *Am. Rev. resp. Dis.* **121,** 11–16

Duke, W. W. (1935). Wheat hairs and dust as a common cause of asthma among workers in wheat flour mills. *J. Am. med. Ass.* **105,** 957–958

Eaton, K. K. (1973). Respiratory allergy to exotic wood dust. *Clin. Allergy* **3,** 307–310

Edge, G. and Burge, P. S. (1980). Immunological aspects of allergy to locusts and other insects. *Clin. Allergy* **10,** 347

Edwards, C., Macartney, J., Rooke, G. and Ward, F. (1975). The pathology of the lung in byssinotics. *Thorax* **30,** 612–623

Edwards, J. H. and Jones, B. M. (1974). Immunology of byssinosis: a study of the reactions between the isolated byssinosis 'antigen' and human immunoglobulins. *Ann. N.Y. Acad. Sci.* **221,** 59–63

Edwards, J. H., McCarthy, P., McDermott, M., Nicholls, P. J. and Skidmore, J. W. (1970). The acute physiological, pharmacological and immunological effects of inhaled cotton dust in normal subjects. *J. Physiol.* **208,** 63–64

El Batawi, M. A. (1962). Byssinosis in the cotton industry in Egypt. *Br. J. ind. Med.* **19,** 126–130

Elwood, P. C., Pemberton, J., Merrett, J. D., Carey, G. C. R. and McAulay, I. R. (1965). Byssinosis and other respiratory symptoms in flax workers in Northern Ireland. *Br. J. ind. med.* **22,** 27–37

Evans, E. and Nicholls, P. J. (1974). Histamine release by Western red cedar (*Thuja plicata*) from lung tissue *in vitro*. *Br. J. ind. Med.* **31,** 28–30

Fairman, R. P., Hankinson, J., Imbus, H., Lapp, N. L. and Morgan, W. K. C. (1975). Pilot study of closing volume in byssinosis. *Br. J. ind. Med.* **32,** 235–238

Falk, H. and Portnoy, S. (1976). Respiratory tract illness in meat wrappers. *J. Am. med. Ass.* **235,** 915–917

Fawcett, I. W., Merchant, J. A., Simmonds, S. P. and Pepys, J. (1978). The effect of sodium cromoglycate, beclomethasone diproprionate and salbutamol on the ventilatory response to cotton dust in mill workers. *Br. J. Dis. Chest* **72,** 29–38

Fawcett, I. W., Newman Taylor, A. J. and Pepys, J. (1976). Asthma due to inhaled chemical agents, fumes from 'multicore' soldering flux and colophony resin. *Clin. Allergy* **6,** 577–585

Fawcett, I. W., Newman Taylor, A. J. and Pepys, J. (1977). Asthma due to inhaled chemical agents—epoxy resin systems containing phthalic anhydride, trimellitic anhydride and triethylene tetramine. *Clin. Allergy* **7,** 1–14

Fawcett, I. W. and Pepys, J. (1976). Allergy to a tetracycline preparation. *Clin. Allergy* **6,** 301–303

Fawcett, I. W., Pepys, J. and Erooga, M. A. (1976). Asthma due to 'Glycyl compound' powder—an intermediate in production of salbutamol. *Clin. Allergy* **6,** 405–409

Feinberg, A. R., Feinberg, S. M. and Benaim-Pinto, C. (1956). Asthma and rhinitis from insect allergens. *J. Allergy* **28,** 437–444

Feinberg, S. M. and Watrous, R. M. (1945). Atopy to simple chemical compounds—Sulfonechloramides. *J. Allergy* **16,** 209–220

Field, G. B. and Owen, P. (1979). Respiratory function in an Australian cotton mill. *Bull. europ. physiopath. resp.* **15,** 455–468

Figley, K. D. and Elrod, R. M. (1928). Endemic asthma due to castor bean dust. *J. Am. med. Ass.* **90,** 79–82

Figley, K. D. and Rawling, F. A. (1950). Castor bean: an industrial hazard as a contaminant of green coffee dust and used burlap bags. *J. Allergy* **21,** 545–553

Flindt, M. L. H. (1969). Pulmonary disease due to inhalation of derivatives of *Bacillus subtilis* containing proteolytic enzymes. *Lancet* **1,** 1177–1181

Flindt, M. L. H. (1978). Health and safety aspects of working with enzymes. *Process Biochem.* **13,** 3–7

Flindt, M. L. H. (1979). Allergy to α-amylase and papain. *Lancet* **1,** 1407–1408

Fowler, P. B. S. (1952). Printer's asthma. *Lancet* **2,** 755–757

Fox, A. J., Tombleson, J. B. L., Watt, A. and Wilkie, A. G. (1973). A survey of respiratory disease in cotton operatives. Part II Symptoms, dust estimations and the effect of smoking habit. *Br. J. ind. Med.* **30,** 48–53

Frankland, A. W. (1953). Locust sensitivity. *Ann. Allergy* **11,** 445–453

Frankland, A. W. (1974). Rat asthma in laboratory workers. In *Allergology*, edited by Y. Yamamura *et al.*, p. 123. Amsterdam; Excerpta Medica

Frankland, A. W. (1978). Maggots causing allergic complaints in fishermen. *Proceedings of the Third Charles Blackley Symposium on the Clinical Aspects of Allergic Disease,* M.A.A.R.A., p. 24 (abstract)

Frankland, A. W. and Lunn, J. A. (1965). Asthma caused by the grain weevil. *Br. J. ind. Med.* **22,** 157–159

Friend, J. A. R., Gaddie, J., Palmer, K. N. V., Pickering, C. A. C. and Pepys, J. (1977). Extrinsic allergic alveolitis and contaminated cooling-water in a factory machine. *Lancet* **1,** 297–299

Fuchs, S. and Valade, P. (1951). Étude clinique et expérimentale sur quelques cas d'intoxication par le Desmodur T (diisocyanate de toluylène 1-2-4 et 1-2-6). *Archs Mal. prof. Med. trav.* **12,** 191–200

Fueki, R., Kuramoti, G., Togawa, M., Kobayashi, S., Shichijo, K., Kikaki, Y. and Okawa, A. (1972). Studies on cement asthma. *Jap. J. Allerg.* **21,** 665–669 (Japanese)

Gaddie, J., Legge, J. S., Friend, J. A. R. and Reid, T. M. S. (1980). Pulmonary hypersensitivity in prawn workers. *Lancet,* **2,** 1350–1353

Galleguillos, F. and Rodriguez, J. C. (1978). Asthma caused by bromelin inhalation. *Clin. Allergy* **8,** 21–24

Gandevia, B. (1964). Respiratory symptoms and ventilatory capacity in men exposed to isocyanate vapour. *Australas. Ann. Med.* **13,** 157–166

Gandevia, B. and Milne, J. (1965a). Ventilatory capacity changes on exposure to cotton dust and their relevance to byssinosis in Australia. *Br. J. ind. Med.* **22,** 295–304

Gandevia, B. and Milne, J. (1965b). Ventilatory capacity on exposure to jute dust and the relevance of productive cough and smoking to the response. *Br. J. ind. Med.* **22,** 187–195

Gandevia, B. and Milne, J. (1970). Occupational asthma and rhinitis due to Western red cedar (*Thuja plicata*) with special reference to bronchial reactivity. *Br. J. ind. Med.* **27,** 235–244

Gelfand, H. H. (1943). The allergenic properties of vegetable gums. A case of asthma due to tragacanth. *J. Allergy* **14,** 203–217

Gelfand, H. H. (1963). Respiratory allergy due to chemical compounds encountered in the rubber, lacquer, shellac and beauty culture industries. *J. Allergy,* **34,** 374–381

Gerrard, J. W., Mink, J., Cheung, S-S, C., Tan, L. K-T. and Dosman, J. A. (1979). Nonsmoking grain handlers in Saskatchewan: airways reactivity and allergic status. *J. occup. Med.* **21,** 342–346

Gill, C. I. C. (1947). Byssinosis in the cotton trade. *Br. J. ind. Med.* **4,** 48–55

Gilson, J. C., Stott, H., Hapwood, B. E. C., Roach, S. A., McKerrow, C. B. and Schilling, R. S. F. (1962). Byssinosis: the acute effect on ventilatory capacity of dusts in cotton ginneries, cotton, sisal and jute mills. *Br. J. ind. Med.* **19,** 9–18

Glass, W. I. and Thom, N. G. (1964). Respiratory hazard associated with toluene di-isocyanate in polyurethane foam production. *N. Z. med. J.* **63,** 642–647

Gough, J. (1959). Occupational pulmonary disease. In *Modern Trends in Pathology,* p. 273. London; Butterworth

Greenberg, M. (1972). Respiratory symptoms following brief exposure to Cedar of Lebanon (*Cedra libani*) dust. *Clin. Allergy* **2,** 219–224

Greenberg, M., Milne, J. F. and Watt, A. (1970). Survey of workers exposed to dusts containing derivatives of *Bacillus subtilis*. *Br. med. J.* **2,** 629–633

Greene, S. A. and Freedman, S. (1976). Asthma due to inhaled chemical agents: amprolium hydrochloride. *Clin. Allergy* **6,** 105–108

Greenhow, H. (1860). Third report of the Medical Officer of the Privy Council. Sir John Simon, p. 152

Griffiths, D. A., Wilkin, D. R., Southgate, B. J. and Lynch, S. M. (1976). A survey of mites in bulk grain stored on farms in England and Wales. *Ann. appl. Biol.* **82,** 180–184

Hama, G. M. (1957). Symptoms of workers exposed to isocyantes. *Arch. ind. Hyg.* **16,** 232–233

Harfi, H. A. (1980). Immediate hypersensitivity to cricket. *Ann. Allergy* **44,** 162–163

Hargreave, F. E. and Pepys, J. (1972). Allergic respiratory reactions in bird fanciers provoked by allergen inhalation tests. *J. Allergy clin. Immunol.* **50,** 157–173

Harries, M. G., Burge, P. S., Samson, M., Newman Taylor, A. J. and Pepys, J. (1979a). Isocyanate asthma: respiratory symptoms due to 1,5-naphthylene di-isocyanate. *Thorax* **34,** 762–766

Harries, M. G., Newman Taylor, A., Wooden, J. and MacAuslan, A. (1979b). Bronchial asthma due to alpha-methyldopa. *Br. med. J.* **1,** 1461

Harris, T. R., Merchant, J. A., Kilburn, K. H. and Hamilton, J. D. (1972). Byssinosis and respiratory diseases in cotton mill workers. *J. occup. Med.* **14,** 199–206

Harvey Gibson, R. J. (1905). Poisonous wood in shuttle making. *Annual Report of the Chief Inspector of Factories and Workshops*, p. 380. London; HMSO

Hay, J. (1907). Conditions of the workers employed in the manufacture of shuttles from African boxwood. *Annual Report of the Chief Inspector of Factories and Workshops*, p. 266–268. London; HMSO

Hendrick, D. J., Davies, R. J. and Pepys, J. (1976). Baker's asthma. *Clin. Allergy* **6,** 241–250

Hendrick, D. J. and Lane, D. J. (1977). Occupational formalin asthma. *Br. J. indust. Med.* **34,** 11–18

Hitchcock, M., Piscitelli, D. M. and Bouhuys, A. (1973). Histamine release from human lung by a component of cotton bracts and by compound 48/80. *Archs envir. Hlth* **26,** 177–182

How, M. J. and Cambridge, G. W. (1971). Prick-tests and serological tests in the diagnosis of allergic reactivity to enzymes used in washing products. *Br. J. indust. Med.* **28,** 303–307

Howie, A. D., Boyd, G. and Moran, F. (1976). Pulmonary hypersensitivity to Ramin (*Gonystylus bancanus*). *Thorax* **31,** 585–587

Hunter, D., Milton, R. and Perry, K. M. A. (1945). Asthma caused by the complex salts of platinum. *Br. J. indust. Med.* **2,** 92–98

Imbus, H. R. and Suh, M. W. (1973). Byssinosis: a study of 10,133 textile workers. *Archs envir. Hlth* **26,** 183–191

Imbus, H. R. and Suh, M. W. (1974). Steaming of cotton to prevent byssinosis—a plant study. *Br. J. indust. Med.* **31,** 209–219

Ingram, C. G., Jeffrey, I. G., Symington, I. S. and Cuthbert, O. D. (1979). Bronchial provocation studies in farmers allergic to storage mites. *Lancet* **2,** 1330–1332

Introna, F. (1966). L'asma bronchiale allergica come malatta professionale. *Minerva Med.* **86,** 176–181

Johnston, T. G., Cazort, A. G., Marvin, H. N., Pringle, R. B. and Sheldon, J. M. (1951). Bronchial asthma, urticaria and allergic rhinitis from tannic acid. *J. Allergy* **22,** 494–499

Joly, P. (1963). Localisation et signification biologique de la substance provoquant des accidents allergiques chez les personnes exposées à un contact prolongé avec les grand Acridiens (*Locusta migratoria*). *C. r. Séanc. Soc. Biol.* **157,** 2299–2300

Jones, R. N., Butcher, B. T., Hammond, Y. Y., Diem, J. E., Glindmeyer III, H. W., Lehrer, S. B., Hughes, J. M. and Weill, H. (1980). Interaction of atopy and exposure to cotton dust in the bronchoconstrictor response. *Br. J. industr. Med.* **37,** 141–146

Jones, R. N., Carr, J., Glindmeyer, H., Diem, J. and Weill, H. (1977). Respiratory health and dust levels in cotton-seed mills. *Thorax* **32,** 281–286

Joules, H. (1932). Asthma from sensitization to chromium. *Lancet* **2,** 182–183

Juniper, C. P., How, M. J., Goodwin, B. F. J. and Kinshott, A. K. (1977). *Bacillus subtilis* enzymes: a 7-year clinical epidemiological and immunological study of an industrial allergen. *J. Soc. occup. Med.* **27,** 3–12

Jyo, T., Katsutani, T., Tsuboi, S., Kohmoto, K., Otsuka, T. and Oka, S. (1980). Hoya (Sea-Squirt) Asthma. In *Occupational Asthma*. Ed. by C. A. Frazier, pp. 209–228. New York; van Nostrand Reinhold Company

Kamat, S. R., Taskar, S. P., Tyer, E. R., Naik, M. and Kamat, G. R. (1979). Discrimination between byssinosis and chronic bronchitis in cotton mill workers by serum immunoglobulin patterns. *J. Soc. occup. Med.* **29,** 102–106

Kammermeyer, J. K. and Mathews, K. P. (1973). Hypersensitivity to phenylglycine acid chloride. *J. Allergy clin. Immunol.* **52,** 73–84

Karol, M. H. and Alarie, Y. (1980). Antigens which detect IgE antibodies in workers sensitive to toluene diisocyanate. *Clin. Allergy* **10,** 101–109

Karol, M. H., Ioset, H. H. and Alarie, Y. C. (1978). Tolyl-specific IgE antibodies in workers with hypersensitivity to toluene di-isocyanate. *Am. ind. Hyg. Ass. J.* **39,** 454–458

Karol, M. H., Sandberg, T., Riley, E. J. and Alarie, Y. (1979). Longitudinal study of tolyl-reactive IgE antibodies in workers hypersensitive to TD1. *J. occup. Med.* **21,** 354–358

Kay, J. P. (1831). Observations and experiments concerning molecular irritation of the lungs as one source of tubercular consumption; and on spinner's phthisis. *North Engl. med. Surg. J.* **1,** 348–363

Kern, R. A. (1939). Asthma and allergic rhinitis due to sensitisation to phthalic anhydride. *J. Allergy* **10,** 164–165

Keskinen, H., Kalliomäki, P-L. and Alanko, K. (1980). Occupational asthma due to stainless steel welding fumes. *Clin. Allergy* **10,** 151–159

Khogali, M. (1971). A population study in cotton ginnery workers in the Sudan. In *International Conference on Respiratory Diseases in Textile Workers, Allicante, Spain*, 1968, p. 79. Barcelona

Kilburn, K. H., Lynn, W. S., Tres, L. C. and McKenzie, W. N. (1973). Leucocyte recruitment through airway walls by condensed vegetable tannins and quercetin. *Lab. Investig.* **28,** 55–59

Kino, T. and Oshima, S. (1978). Allergy to insects in Japan. 1. The reaginic sensitivity to moth and butterfly in patients with bronchial asthma. *J. Allergy clin. Immunol.* **61,** 10–16

Klaustermeyer, W. B., Bardana, Jr., E. J., and Hale, F. C. (1977). Pulmonary hypersensitivity to *Alternaria* and *Aspergillus* in baker's asthma. *Clin. Allergy* **7,** 227–233

Kobayashi, S. (1974). Occupational asthma due to inhalation of pharmacological dusts and other chemical agents with some reference to other occupational asthma in Japan. *Allergology*, edited by Y. Yamamura *et al.*, p. 124–132. Amsterdam; Excerpta Medica

Kováts, F. and Bugyi, B. (1968). *Occupational Mycotic Diseases of the Lung*, pp. 193–195. Budapest; Akadémiai Kiadó

Krumpe, P. E., Finely, T. N. and Martinez, N. (1979). The search for expiratory obstruction in meat wrappers studied on the job. *Am. Rev. resp. Dis.* **119,** 611–618

Lacey, J. (1977). Micro-organisms in air of cotton mills. *Lancet* **2,** 455–456

Lam, S. and Chan-Yeung, M. (1980). Ethylenediamine-induced asthma. *Am. Rev. resp. Dis.* **121,** 151–155

Lam, S., Wong, R. and Chan-Yeung, M. (1979). Non-specific bronchial reactivity in occupational asthma. *J. Allergy clin. Immunol.* **63,** 28–34

Lammers, B., Schilling, R. S. F. and Walford, J. (1964). A study of byssinosis; chronic respiratory symptoms and ventilatory capacity in English and Dutch cotton workers, with special reference to atmospheric pollution. *Br. J. ind. Med.* **21,** 124–134

Leading article. (1979). Formaldehyde toxicity. *Lancet* **2,** 620–621

Leading article. (1980). Cold air to detect bronchial hyperreactivity. *Lancet* **1,** 1395–1396

Lehrer, S. B., Karr, R. M., Salvaggio, J. E. (1978). Extraction and analysis of coffee beans allergens. *Clin. Allergy* **8,** 217–226

Lincoln, T. A., Bolton, N. E. and Garrett, A. S. (1974). Occupational allergy to animal dander and sera. *J. occup. Med.* **16,** 465–469

Longley, E. O. (1964). Methane di-isocyanate. A respiratory hazard. *Archs envir. Hlth* **8,** 898

Lunn, J. A. (1966). Millworkers asthma: Allergic responses to the grain weevil (*Sitophilus granarius*). *Br. J. ind. Med.* **23,** 149–152

McConnell, L. H., Fink, J. N., Schlueter, D. P. and Schmidt, M. G. (1973). Asthma caused by nickel sensitivity. *Ann. intern. Med.* **78,** 888–890

McDermott, M., Skidmore, J. W. and Edwards, J. (1971). The acute physiological, immunological and pharmacological effects of inhaled cotton dust in normal subjects. In *International Conference on Respiratory Disease of Textile Workers, Alicante, Spain,* 1968, pp. 133–136. Barcelona

McKerrow, C. B., McDermott, M., Gilson, J. C. and Schilling, R. S. F. (1958). Respiratory function during the day in cotton workers: a study in byssinosis. *Br. J. ind. Med.* **15,** 75–83

McKerrow, C. B. and Molyneux, M. K. B. (1971). The influence of previous dust exposure on the acute respiratory effects of cotton dust inhalation. In *International Conference on Respiratory Diseases in Textile Workers. Alicante, Spain,* 1968, pp. 95–101. Barcelona

Mair, A., Smith, D. H., Wilson, W. A. and Lockhart, W. (1960). Dust disease in Dundee textile workers. An investigation into chronic respiratory disease in jute and flax industries. *Br. J. ind. Med.* **17,** 272–278

Massoud, A. and Taylor, G. (1964). Byssinosis antibody to cotton antigens in normal subjects and in cotton card-room workers. *Lancet* **2,** 607–610

Massoud, A., Taylor, G. and Lucas, F. (1971). Bronchial challenge with cotton plant antigen in byssinosis. *International Conference on Respiratory Diseases in Textile Workers.* Alicante, Spain, 1968, pp. 124–132. Barcelona

Medical Research Council. (1977). Humidifier fever. *Thorax* **32,** 653–663

Menon, M. P. S. and Das, A. K. (1977). Tetracycline asthma. *Clin. Allergy* **7,** 285–290

Merchant, J. A., Halprin, G. M., Hudson, A. R., Kilburn, K. H., McKenzie, W. N., Hurst, D. J. and Bermazohn, P. (1975). Responses to cotton dust. *Archs envir. Hlth* **30,** 222–229

Merchant, J. A., Kilburn, K. H., O'Fallon, W. M., Hamilton, J. D., and Lumsden, J. C. (1972). Byssinosis and chronic bronchitis among cotton textile workers. *Ann. intern. Med.* **76,** 423–433

Merchant, J. A., Lumsden, J. C., Kilburn, K. H., O'Fallon, W. M., Ujda, J. R., Germino, V. H. and Hamilton, J. D. (1973a). An industrial study of the biological effects of cotton dust and cigarette smoke exposure. *J. occup. Med.* **15,** 212–221

Merchant, J. A., Lumsden, J. C., Kilburn, K. H., Germino, V. H., Hamilton, J. D., Lynn, W. S., Byrd, H. and Baucom, D. (1973b). Pre-processing cotton to prevent byssinosis. *Br. J. ind. Med.* **30,** 237–247

Merchant, J. A., Lumsden, J. C., Kilburn, K. H., O'Fallon, W. M., Copeland, K., Germino, V. H., McKenzie, W. N., Baucom, D., Curran, P. and Stilman, J. (1974). Intervention studies of cotton steaming to reduce biological effects of cotton dust. *Br. J. ind. Med.* **31,** 261–274

Middleton, D., Logan, J. S., Magennis, B. P. and Nelson, S. D. (1979). LHA frequencies in flax byssinosis patients. *Br. J. ind. Med.* **36,** 123–126

Milne, J. and Brand, S. (1975). Occupational asthma after inhalation of dust of the proteolytic enzyme, papain. *Br. J. ind. Med.* **32,** 302–307

Mink, J. T., Gerrard, J. W., Cockcroft, D. W., Cotton, D. J. and Dosman, J. A. (1980). Increased bronchial reactivity to inhaled histamine in non-smoking grain workers with normal lung function. *Chest* **77,** 28–31

Mitchell, C. A. and Gandevia, B. (1971). Respiratory symptoms and skin reactivity in workers exposed to proteolytic enzymes in the detergent industry. *Am. Rev. resp. Dis.* **104,** 1–12

Moll, H. H. (1933). Occupational asthma with reference to wool sensitivity. *Lancet* 1340–1342

Molyneux, M. K. B. and Berry, G. (1971). The correlation of cotton dust exposure with prevalence of respiratory sysmptoms. In *Proceedings 2nd International Conference on Respiratory Diseases in Textile Workers. (Byssinosis), Alicante, Spain,* pp. 177–183

Molyneux, M. K. B. and Tombleson, J. B. L. (1970). An epidemiological study of respiratory symptoms in Lancashire mills. 1963–1966. *Br. J. ind. Med.* **27,** 225–234

Morey, P. R. (1979). Botanically what is raw cotton dust? *Am. ind. Hyg. Ass. J.* **40,** 702–708

Mudttum, O. (1960). Bronchial asthma in the aluminium industry. *Acta Allerg.* **15,** 208–221

Munn, A. (1965). Hazards of isocyanates. *Ann. occup. Hyg.* **8,** 163–169

Musk, A. W. and Gandevia, B. (1976). Loss of pulmonary recoil in workers formerly exposed to proteolytic enzyme (alcalaze) in the detergent industry. *Br. J. ind. Med.* **33,** 158–165

Mustafa, K. Y., Lakha, A. S., Milla, M. H. and Dahoma, U. (1978). Byssinosis, respiratory symptoms and spirometric lung function tests in Tanzanian sisal workers. *Br. J. ind. Med.* **35,** 123–128

Neal, P. A., Schneiter, R. and Caminita, B. H. (1942). Report on acute illness among rural mattress makers using low grade, stained cotton. *J. Am. med. Ass.* **119,** 1074–1082

Newhouse, M. L., Tagg, B., Pocock, S. J. and McEwan, A. C. (1970). An epidemiological study of workers producing enzyme washing powders. *Lancet* **1,** 689–693

Newman Taylor, A. J., Davies, R. J. Hendrick, D. J. and Pepys, J. (1979). Recurrent nocturnal asthmatic reactions to bronchial provocation tests. *Clin. Allergy* **9,** 213–219

Newman Taylor, A., Longbottom, J. L. and Pepys, J. (1977). Respiratory allergy to urine proteins of rats and mice. *Lancet* **2,** 847–849

Newmark, F. M. (1978). Hops allergy and terpene sensitivity: an occupational disease. *Ann. Allergy* **41,** 311–312

Nicholls, P. J. (1976). Release of histamine from lung tissue *in vitro* by dimethylhydantoinformaldehyde resin and polyvinyl pyrrolidone. *Br. J. ind. Med.* **33,** 127–129

Nicholls, P. J., Nicholls, G. R. and Bouhuys, A. (1966). Histamine release by compound 48/80 and textile dusts from lung tissue *in vitro.* In *Inhaled Particles and Vapours,* 11, pp. 69–74. Oxford and New York; Pergamon

Nicholls, P. J. and Skidmore, J. W. (1975). Comparative study of the smooth muscle contractor activity of airborne dusts and of dustiness in cotton flax and jute mills. *Br. J. ind. Med.* **32,** 289–296

Noweir, M. H., Amine, E. K. and Osman, H. A. (1975). Epidemiological investigation of the role of family susceptibility and occupational and family histories in the development of byssinosis among workers exposed to flax dust. *Br. J. ind. Med.* **32,** 297–301

Noweir, M. H., El-Sadik, Y. M., El-Dakhakhny, A. and Osman, H. A. (1975). Dust exposure in manual flax processing in Egypt. *Br. J. ind. Med.* **32,** 147–154

O'Brien, I. M., Bull, J., Creamer, B., Sepelveda, R., Harries, M., Burge, P. S. and Pepys, J. (1978). Asthma and extrinsic allergic alveolitis due to *Merulius lacrymans. Clin. Allergy* **8,** 535–542

O'Brien, I. M., Harries, M. G., Burge, P. S., Pepys, J. (1979a). Di-isocyanate induced asthma. 1. reactions to TDI, MDI, HDI and histamine. *Clin. Allergy* **9,** 1–6

O'Brien, I. M., Newman Taylor, A. J., Burge, P. S., Harries, M. G., Fawcett, I. W., Pepys, J. (1979b). Toluene di-isocyanate induced asthma. II. bronchial provocation and reactivity studies. *Clin. Allergy* **9,** 7–16

Ohman, J. L., Lowell, F. C. and Bloch, K. J. (1975). Allergens of mammalian origin. Characterisation of allergens extracted from rat, mouse, guinea pig and rabbit pelts. *J. Allergy clin. Immunol.* **55,** 16–24

Olenchock, S. A., Mull, J. C. and Major, P. C. (1980). Extracts of

airborne grain dusts activate alternative and classical complement pathways. *Ann. Allergy* **44,** 23–28
Oliver, T. (1902). *Dangerous Trades,* p. 273. London; Murray
Ordman, D. (1947). Buckwheat allergy. *S. Afr. med. J.* **21,** 737–739
Ordman, D. (1949). Wood dust as an inhalant allergen. Bronchial asthma caused by kejaat wood (*Pterocarpus angolensis*). *S. Afr. med. J.* **23,** 973–976
Paggiaro, P. L., Loi, A. M., Toma, G. (1979). Bronchial asthma and dermatitis due to spiramycin in a chick breeder. *Clin Allergy* **9,** 571–574
Paisley, D. P. G. (1969). Isocyanate hazard from wire insulation: An old hazard in a new guise. *Br. J. ind. Med.* **26,** 79–81
Parrot, J. L., Hébert, R., Saindelle, A., Ruff, F. (1969). Platinum and platinosis. *Archs envir. Hlth* **19,** 685–691
Patissier, P. (1822). *Traité des Maladies des Artisans.* Paris
Pauli, G., Bessot, J. C., Kopferschmitt, M. C., Lingot, G., Wendling, R., Ducos, P. and Limasset, J. C. (1980). Meat wrapper's asthma: identification of the causal agent. *Clin. Allergy* **10,** 263–269
Pauwels, R., Devos, M., Callens, L. and Van der Straeten, M. (1978). Respiratory hazards from proteolytic enzymes. *Lancet* **1,** 669 (letter)
Pepys, J. (1973). Immunopathology of allergic lung disease. *Clin. Allergy* **3,** 1–22
Pepys, J. (1977). Allergy to platinum compounds. Chapter 7 in *Platinum Group Metals.* Report of the Sub-Committee on Platinum Group Metals of the committee on Medical and Biologic Effects of Environmental Pollutants, p. 105. National Academy of Sciences
Pepys, J., Hargreave, F. E., Longbottom, J. L., Faux, J. (1969). Allergic reaction of the lungs to enzymes of *Bacillus subtilis. Lancet* **1,** 1181–1184
Pepys, J. and Hutchcroft, B. J. (1975). Bronchial provocation tests in etiologic diagnosis and analysis of asthma. *Am. Rev. resp. Dis.* **112,** 829–859
Pepys, J., Hutchcroft, B. J. and Breslin, A. B. X. (1976). Asthma due to inhaled chemical agents—persulphate salts and henna in hairdressers. *Clin. Allergy* **6,** 399–404
Pepys, J., Parish, W. E., Cromwell, O. and Hughes, E. G. (1979). Passive transfer in man and the monkey of Type I allergy due to heat labile and heat stable antibody to complex salts of platinum. *Clin. Allergy* **9,** 99–108
Pepys, J. and Pickering, C. A. C. (1972). Asthma due to inhaled chemical fumes—aminoethyl ethanolamine in aluminium soldering flux. *Clin. Allergy* **2,** 197–204
Pepys, J., Pickering, C. A. C., Breslin, A. B. X. and Terry, D. S. (1972). Asthma due to inhaled chemical agents—tolylene diisocyanate. *Clin. Allergy* **2,** 225–236
Pepys, J., Pickering, C. A. C. and Hughes, E. G. (1972). Asthma due to inhaled chemical agents—complex salts of platinum. *Clin. Allergy* **2,** 391–396
Pepys, J., Pickering, C. A. C. and Loudon, H. W. G. (1972). Asthma due to inhaled chemical agents—piperazine dihydrochloride. *Clin. Allergy* **2,** 189–196
Pepys, J., Wells, I. D., D'Souza, M. F. and Greenberg, M. (1973). Clinical and immunological responses to enzymes of *Bacillus subtilis* in factory workers and consumers. *Clin. Allergy* **3,** 143–160
Perks, W. H., Burge, P. S., Rehahn, M. and Green, M. (1979). Work related respiratory disease in employees leaving an electronics factory. *Thorax* **34,** 19–22
Perlman, F. (1958). Insects as inhalant allergens. *J. Allergy* **29,** 302–328
Pernis, B., Vigliani, E. C., Cavagna, G. and Finulli, M. (1961). The role of bacterial endotoxins in occupational diseases caused by inhaling vegetable dusts. *Br. J. ind. Med.* **18,** 120–129
Pham, Q. T., Cavelier, C., Mereau, P., Mur, J. M. and Cicolella, A. (1978). Isocyanates and respiratory function: a study of workers producing polyurethene foam moulding. *Ann. occup. Hyg.* **21,** 121–129
Pickering, C. A. C. (1972). Inhalation tests with chemical allergens: complex salts of platinum. *Proc. R. Soc. Med.* **65,** 272–274
Pickering, C. A. C., Batten, J. C. and Pepys, J. (1972). Asthma due to inhaled wood dusts: Western red cedar and iroko. *Clin. Allergy* **2,** 213–218
Pickering, C. A. C., Moore, W. K. S., Lacey, J., Holford-Strevens, V. C. and Pepys, J. (1976). Investigation of a respiratory disease associated with an air-conditioning system. *Clin. Allergy* **6,** 109–118
Pilat, L., Popa, V. and Tecoulesco, D. (1967). L'allergie professionelle aux hormones protéiques dans l'industrie pharmaceutique. *Rev. franç. Allergie.* **7,** 153–160
Plessner, M. (1960). Une maladie des trieurs de plumes: La fièvre de canard. *Arch. Mal. prof.* **21,** 67–69
Popa, V., Gavrilescu, N., Preda, N., Teculescu, D., Plecias, M. and Cîrstea, M. (1969a). An investigation of allergy in byssinosis: sensitisation to cotton, hemp, flax and jute antigens. *Br. J. ind. Med.* **26,** 101–108
Popa, V., George, S. A. and Gavanescu, O. (1970). Occupational and non occupational respiratory allergy in bakers. *Acta Allerg.* **25,** 159–177
Popa, V., Teculescu, D., Stănescu, D. and Gavrilescu, N. (1969b). Bronchial asthma and asthmatic bronchitis determined by simple chemicals. *Dis. Chest* **56,** 395–404
Pratt, P. C., Vollmer, R. T. and Miller, J. A. (1980). Epidemiology of pulmonary lesions in nontextile and cotton textile workers: a retrospective autopsy analysis. *Archs. environ. Med.* **35,** 133–137
Prime, F. J. (1960). Peak flow meter. *Br. med. J.* **1,** 423 (letter)
Proust, A. (1877). *Traité d'Hygiène Publique et privée,* pp. 171–174. Paris; Masson
Randolph, H. (1934). Allergic response to dust of insect origin. *J. Am. med. Ass.* **103,** 560–562
Roach, S. A. and Schilling, R. S. F. (1960). A clinical and environmental study of byssinosis in the Lancashire cotton industry. *Br. J. ind. Med.* **17,** 1–9
Rooke, G. B. (1981). The pathology of byssinosis. *Chest* (To be published)
Rüttner, J. R., Spycher, M. A. and Engeler, M-L. (1968). Pulmonary fibrosis induced by cotton fibre inhalation. *Path. Microbiol.* **32,** 1–14
Rylander, R. and Lundholm, M. (1978). Bacterial contamination of cotton and cotton dust and effects on the lung. *Br. J. industr. Med.* **35,** 204–207
Rylander, R. and Snella, M-C. (1976). Acute inhalation toxicity of cotton plant dusts. *Br. J. ind. Med.* **33,** 175–180
Sakula, A. (1975). Formalin asthma in hospital laboratory staff. *Lancet* **2,** 816 (letter)
Salvato, G. (1961). Mast cells in bronchial connective tissue of man: their modifications in asthma and after treatment with the histamine liberator 48/80. *Int. Arch. Allergy appl. Immunol.* **18,** 348–358
Schilling, R. S. F. (1950). Byssinosis. *Br. med. Bull.* **7,** 52–56
Schilling, R. S. F. (1956). Byssinosis in cotton and other textile workers. *Lancet* **2,** 261–265
Schilling, R., Goodman, N. and O'Sullivan, J. (1952). Cardiovascular disease in cotton workers. Part II. A clinical study with special reference to hypertension. *Br. J. ind. Med.* **9,** 146–156
Schilling, R. S. F., Vigliani, E. C., Lammers, B., Valic, F. and Gilson, J. C. (1963). A report on a Conference on Byssinosis. (14th International Conference on Occupational Health. Madrid, 1963). pp. 137–144. *Int. Congr. Series.* No. 62. Amsterdam; Excepta Medica
Schleuter, D. P., Banaszak, E. F., Fink, J. N. and Barboriak, J., (1978). Occupational asthma due to tetrachlorphthalic anhydride. *J. occup. Med.* **20,** 183–188
Schoenberg, J. B. and Mitchell, C. A. (1975). Airway disease caused by phenolic (phenol-formaldehyde) resin exposure. *Archs envir. Hlth* **30,** 574–577
Sheldon, J. M. and Johnston, J. H. (1941). Hypersensitivity to beetles (Coleoptera). *J. Allergy* **12,** 493–494
Shioda, K., Hamada, A., Mitani, K. and Matsuda, M. (1973).

Asthma caused by dust from pearl shell. In *Occupational Bronchial Asthma, Society of Occupational Allergy,* pp. 242–250. Tokyo; Asakura-Shoten

Silberman, D. E. and Sorrell, A. H. (1959). Allergy in fur workers with special reference to paraphenylene diamine. *J. Allergy* **30,** 11–18

Skoulas, A., Williams, N. and Merriman, J. E. (1964). Exposure to grain dust. II. A clinical study of the effects. *J. occup. Med.* **6,** 359–372

Small, W. S. (1952). Increasing castor bean allergy in southern California due to fertiliser. *J. Allergy* **23,** 406–415

Smiley, J. A. (1951). The hazards of rope making. *Br. J. ind. Med.* **8,** 265–270

Smith, D. H., Lockhart, W., Mair, A. and Wilson, W. A. (1962). Flax workers byssinosis in East Scotland. *Scott. med. J.* **7,** 201–211

Smith, G. F., Coles, G. V., Schilling, R. S. F. and Walford, J. (1969). A study of rope workers exposed to hemp and flax. *Br. J. ind. Med.* **26,** 109–114

Sokol, W. N., Aelony, Y. and Beall, G. N. (1973). Meat-wrapper's asthma. *J. Am. med. Ass.* **226,** 639–641

Sosman, A. J., Schlueter, D. P., Fink, J. N. and Barboriak, J. J. (1969). Hypersensitivity to wood dust. *New Engl. J. Med.* **281,** 977–980

Spielman, A. D. and Baldwin, H. S. (1933). Atopy to acacia (gum arabic). *J. Am. med. Ass.* **101,** 444–445

Sprague, P. H. (1942). Bronchial asthma due to sensitivity to gum acacia. *Can. med. Ass. J.* **47,** 253

Sterling, G. M. (1967). Asthma due to aluminium soldering flux. *Thorax* **22,** 533–537

Stevens, J. J. (1976). Asthma due to soldering flux: A polyether alcohol-polypropylene glycol mixture. *Ann. Allergy* **36,** 419–422

Stevenson, D. D. and Mathews, K. P. (1967). Occupational asthma following inhalation of moth particles. *J. Allergy* **39,** 274–283

Sunderman, F. W. and Sunderman, Jr., F. W. (1961). Löffler's syndrome associated with nickel sensitivity. *Archs intern. Med.* **107,** 405–408

Sweet, L. C. (1968). Toluene-diisocyanate asthma. *Univ. Mich. med. Cent. Bull.* **34,** 27–29

Takiszawa, T. and Thurlbeck, W. M. (1971). Muscle and mucous gland size in the major bronchi of patients with chronic bronchitis, asthma and asthmatic bronchitis. *Am. Rev. resp. Dis.* **104,** 331–336

Tanser, A. R., Bourke, M. P. and Blandford, A. G. (1973). Isocyanate asthma: respiratory symptoms caused by diphenylmethane di-isocyanate. *Thorax* **28,** 596–600

Tarlo, S. M., Shaikh, W., Bell, B., Cuff, M., Davies, G. M., Dulovich, J. and Hargreave, F. E. (1978). Papain induced allergic reactions. *Clin. Allergy* **8,** 207–213

Taylor, G., Massoud, A. A. E. and Lucas, F. (1971). Studies in aetiology of byssinosis. *Br. J. ind. Med.* **28,** 145–151

Textile Research Institute. (1978). Chemical composition of cotton dust and its relation to byssinosis; a review of the literature. Regulatory Technical Information Centre. T. F. Cooke, Director. Report No. 1. Textile Research Institute. Box 625. Princeton, New Jersey 08540

Thurlbeck, W. M. (1976). *Chronic Airflow Obstruction in Lung Disease, Vol. V,* pp. 54–55. *Major Problems in Pathology.* Philadelphia, London, Toronto; W. B. Saunders

Tiller, J. R. and Schilling, R. S. F. (1958). Respiratory function during the day in rayon workers. *Trans. Ass. ind. med. Offrs.* **7,** 161–162

Tse, K. S., Warren, P., Janusz, M., McCarthy, D. S. and Cherniack, R. M. (1973). Respiratory abnormalities in workers exposed to grain dust. *Archs envir. Hlth* **27,** 74–77

Tuffnell, P. G. and Dingwall-Fordyce, I. (1957). An investigation into the acute respiratory reaction to the inhalation of tarmarind seed preparations. *Br. J. ind. Med.* **14,** 250–252

Turner-Warwick, M. (1978). *Immunology of the Lung.* London; Edward Arnold

Tuypens, E. (1961). Byssinosis among cotton workers in Belgium. *Br. J. ind. Med.* **18,** 117–119

Uragoda, C. G., (1970). Tea maker's asthma. *Br. J. ind. Med.* **27,** 181–182

Uragoda, C. G. (1975). A clinical and radiographic study of coir workers. *Br. J. ind. Med.* **32,** 66–71

Uragoda, C. G. (1977). An investigation into the health of kapok workers. *Br. J. ind. Med.* **34,** 181–185

Valić, F., Beritić, D. and Butković, D. (1976). Respiratory response to tobacco dust exposure. *Am. Rev. resp. Dis.* **113,** 751–755

Valić, F. and Žuškin, E. (1971). A comparative study of respiratory function in female non-smoking cotton and jute workers. *Arch. envir. Hlth* **23,** 359–364

Vallieres, M., Cockcroft, D. W., Taylow, D. M., Dolovich, J. and Hargreave, F. E. (1977). Dimethyl ethanolamine-induced asthma. *Am. Rev. Resp. Dis.* **115,** 867–871

Vaughan, W. T. (1939). *The Practice of Allergy,* p. 677. St. Louis; C. V. Mosby Co

Velvart, J. (1971). Respiratory symptoms and changes in lung function in workers handling hemp, flax and sisal in Czechoslovakia. In *Proceedings of the International Conference on Respiratory Disease In Textile Workers (Byssinosis). Alicante, Spain,* 1968, pp. 55–58

Velvart, J. (1972). Schadigung der Atemwege durch Staubeinwirkung von Sisal. *Int. Arch. Arbeitsmed.* **30,** 213–222

Vigliani, E. C., Parmeggiani, L. and Sassi, C. (1954). Studio de un epidemia di bronchite asmatica fra gli operai di una tessitura di cotone. *Med. Lav.* **45,** 349–378

Voisin, C., Jacob, M., Furon, D. and Lefebre, J. (1966). Aspects cliniques et allergologiques des manifestations asthmatiques observées chez 114 ouvriers de filatures de coton. *Poumon Coeur.* **22,** 529–538

Wakelyn, P. J., Greenblatt, G. A., Brown, D. F. and Tripp, V. W. (1976). Chemical properties of cotton dust. *Am. ind. Hyg. Assoc. J.* **37,** 22–31

Warren, P., Cherniack, R. M. and Tse, K. S. (1974). Hypersensitivity reactions to grain dust. *J. Allergy clin. Immunol.* **53,** 139–149

Weill, H., Salvaggio, J., Neilson, A., Butcher, B. and Ziskind, M. (1975). Respiratory effects in toluene di-isocyanate manufacture: a multidisciplinary approach. *Environ. Hlth Perspect.* **11,** 101–108

Weill, H., Waddell, L. C. and Ziskind, M. (1971). A study of workers exposed to detergent enzymes. *J. Am. med. Ass.* **217,** 425–433

Weiner, A. (1961). Bronchial asthma due to organic phosphate insecticides. *Ann. Allergy* **19,** 397–401

Widdicombe, J. G. (1979). Dyspnoea. *Bull. europ. physiopath. resp.* **15,** 437–440

Williams, H. (1952). Vanadium poisoning from cleaning oil fired boilers. *Br. J. ind. Med.* **9,** 50–55

Wilson, M. R., Arroyave, C. M., Nakamura, R. M., Vaughan, J. H. and Tan, E. M. (1976). Activation of the alternative complement pathway in systemic lupus erythematosus. *Clin. exp. Immunol.* **26,** 11–20

Wilson, M. R., Sekul, A., Ory, R., Salvaggio, J. E. and Lehren, S. B. (1980). Activation of the alternative complement pathway by extracts of cotton dust. *Clin. Allergy* **10,** 303–308

Wittich, F. W. (1940). Allergic rhinitis and asthma due to sensitization to the Mexican bean weevil. (*Zabrotes subfasciatus* Boh). *J. Allergy* **12,** 42–45

Wraith, D. G., Cunnington, A. M. and Seymour, W. M. (1979). The role and allergenic importance of storage mites in house dust and other environments. *Clin. Allergy* **9,** 545–561

Zeiss, C. R., Patterson, R., Pruzansky, J. J., Miller, M. M., Rosenberg, M. and Levitz, D. (1977). Trimellitic anhydride-induced airway syndromes: Clinical and immunologic studies. *J. Allergy clin. Immunol.* **60,** 96–103

Zetterström, O. (1978). Dual skin test reactions and serum antibodies to subtilisin and *Aspergillus fumigatus* extracts. *Clin. Allergy* **8,** 77–91

Žuškin, E. and Bouhuys, A. (1977). Protective effect of disodium cromoglycate against airway constriction induced by hemp dust extract. *J. Allergy clin. Immunol.* **57,** 473–479

Žuškin, E. and Valić, F. (1972). Respiratory symptoms and ventilatory function changes in relation to length of exposure to cotton dust. *Thorax* **27,** 454–458
Žuškin, E., Valić, F., Butković, D. and Bouhuys, S. (1975). Lung function in textile workers. *Br. J. ind. Med.* **32,** 283–288
Žuškin, E., Valić, F. and Bouhuys, A. (1976). Byssinosis and airway responses due to exposure to textile dust. *Lung* **154,** 17–24
Žuškin, E., Valić, F. and Skurić, Z. (1979). Respiratory function in coffee workers. *Br. J. ind. Med.* **36,** 117–122
Žuškin, E., Wolfson, R. L., Harpel, G., Welborn, J. W. and Bouhuys, A. (1969). Byssinosis in carding and spinning workers. *Archs envir. Hlth* **19,** 666–673
Zweiman, B., Green, G., Mayock, R. L. and Hildreth, E. A. (1967). Inhalation sensitisation to trypsin. *J. Allergy* **39,** 11–16

Addendum

Byssinosis

In a recent survey of respiratory symptoms in 2528 flax mill workers in Northern Ireland, Elwood, McAulay and Elwood (1982) found no evidence that byssinosis is a cause of excess mortality and, consequently, they suggest that it is also unlikely to be responsible for serious long-term morbidity.

Elwood, P.C., McAulay, I.R. and Elwood, J.H. (1982). The flax industry in Northern Ireland twenty years on. *Lancet* **1**, 1112–1114

13 Non-neoplastic Disorders due to Metallic, Chemical and Physical Agents

The various topics in this chapter are considered under the broad categories of metals, chemical agents and physical—mainly pressure change—effects. Metals and chemicals may occur in the form of fumes, gases, vapours, smokes or dusts; and some may exist in more than one of these physical states. Occupational pulmonary oedema and welding are summarized briefly at the end of the chapter.

METALS AND METALLOIDS

Metalloids are elements which have some of the properties of metals and others of non-metals: for example, antimony, boron, carbon and selenium.

METAL FUME FEVER

This is a fairly common non-specific, benign, self-limiting acute illness which resembles an attack of malaria. It has been variously known as *brass founders' ague, welders' ague, copper fever, Monday fever* and *the smothers.* It is caused chiefly by fumes of zinc, copper and magnesium and, less often, by those of aluminium, antimony, iron, manganese and nickel.

It occurs in welding, galvanizing and smelting operations and in the arc-air gouging process involving these metals especially under enclosed or poorly ventilated conditions (Sanderson, 1968). Thus, it is most commonly encountered among shipyard and other metal workers, and foundry men. Sculptors working in metal may be affected. Copper *dust* from the polishing of copper plates and from other sources may produce an identical syndrome but the term 'metal fume fever' cannot properly be applied to it (Gleason, 1968).

The illness commences a few hours after exposure and consists of thirst, dry cough, dry throat, nausea, headache, rigors, profuse sweating, fatigue, aching in the chest and pains in the limbs. Temperature rises to 38.9 °C (102°F) or higher, and there is polymorphonuclear leucocytosis. Recovery is usually complete in 24 hours and the man is able to return to work. No permanent damage occurs.

A curious feature of this syndrome, which may have an immunological explanation, is that men who are continuously exposed acquire a tolerance which, however, is lost after a short period away from work so that it recurs on the first day back at work—'Monday fever'. The underlying cause is not understood but is probably related to the minute size—under 1 μm diameter—of fume particles which enables them to reach the alveoli in large numbers; and the production of endogenous pyrogens has also been held responsible (Pernis *et al.*, 1961).

With a proper occupational history, the diagnosis should be evident, but the symptoms of acute cadmium inhalation poisoning are initially identical. As the prognosis of the two disorders is quite different it is most important that cadmium poisoning should be suspected in welders in whom the symptoms persist with fever and severe chest pain after 24 hours (*see* Cadmium, p. 457). Influenza may be wrongly diagnosed.

Treatment is symptomatic.

Polymer fume fever, the features of which are identical apart from the fact that tolerance of exposure does not develop, is referred to in Chapter 11.

ALUMINIUM ('ALUMINIUM LUNG')

The term 'aluminium lung' refers to lung fibrosis attributed to two different inhalable materials: on the one hand, fumes from the smelting of *bauxite,* hydrous aluminium oxide, $A1_2OH_x$ on the other, metallic aluminium dust. Unfortunately this and another commonly used term—'aluminosis' —beg the question of pathogenesis which has not yet been solved. Fibrosis associated with exposure to bauxite fume is often known as *Shaver's disease;* Shaver jointly described the association in 1947.

Bauxite is the ore from which aluminium is smelted or extracted by electrolysis when *alumina* (aluminium oxide, Al_2O_3) is dissolved in molten *cryolite* (sodium aluminium fluoride, Na_3AlF_3). Impurities in bauxite include quartz, cristobalite and hematite in some deposits, and clay minerals such as kaolinite, halloysite and chlorite. *Corundum*, being a naturally crystallized oxide of aluminium, is not usually classed with bauxite. Artificial corundum—or synthetic emery—is manufactured from bauxite.

Aluminium is used not only in metal alloys (such as duralumin), in wrapping foils and refractory materials, but in finely divided form for explosives and fireworks (when it is known as 'pyro'), and, in a coarser form, for paints and ink.

Sources of exposure

Artificial corundum production

Ground, calcined bauxite is the chief raw material. It is mixed with coke (to reduce some of the oxide) and iron and fused in an electric furnace with movable carbon electrodes at a temperature of about 2000 °C, although the temperature in the neighbourhood of the electrodes is nearer 4000 °C (Finlay, 1950). At temperatures around 2000 °C a white fume which consists of 35 to 64 per cent alumina and 16 to 54 per cent 'silica' is evolved (Jephcott, 1950). The quartz and clay minerals yield alumina-glass but some cristobalite will escape melting (*see* Chapter 2). The particle size of the fume is less than 1 μm and generally ranges from 0.5 μm to 0.02 μm (Hatch, 1950). Men who developed lung disease operated the furnaces or worked above them on overhead storage bins and cranes (Shaver and Riddell, 1947; Hagen, 1950). Curiously, no lung disease appears to have occurred over the many years during which this process was used before the Second World War when, at a time of greatly increased production, Shaver's cases occurred (Drinker and Hatch, 1954). But an identical 'outbreak' of pulmonary fibrosis was observed among Korunschmelzerns in similarly overloaded German plants about the same time. This, and Shaver's cases, were attributed by Gärtner (1952) to 'amorphous silica' with the clay mineral mullite as a 'contributory' factor (*see also* Chapter 9, pp. 311 and 317).

Preparation and use of aluminium powders

There are two sorts of powder: a *flake type*, the particle size of which may be as small as 0.6 μm, prepared in a stamp or ball-mill from the cold metal or foil; and a *granular type* made from molten metal. Stearine (a mixture of fatty acids prepared by hydrolysis of fats), paraffin or spindle oil is usually added to the flake variety as a lubricant to permit separation of the particles.

Flake powder of particularly small particle size to which stearine is not added ('pyro') is employed in the manufacture of explosives, incendiary devices and fireworks. Many of the early cases of fibrosis attributed to aluminium exposure were reported in Germany during the Second World War (Goralewski, 1940; Goralewski and Jaeger, 1941; Barth, Frik and Scheidemandel, 1956). There have also been similar reports among workers in stamping-mills in the UK and Sweden where, for a period, stearine was either reduced in quantity or replaced by mineral oil (Ahlmark, Bruce and Nyström, 1960; Mitchell *et al.*, 1961; McLaughlin *et al.*, 1962). In the preparation of powder for paint manufacture the aluminium particles are large and mixed with considerable quantities of stearine.

Pathology

The pathology appears to be similar in workers who have been exposed to bauxite fume or to metallic aluminium dust.

The lungs are indurated and grey-black, and the pulmonary pleura is thickened, often with numerous underlying air blebs. Emphysematous bullae are common. When the lungs are cut, radiating bands or dense areas of grey-black fibrous tissue are seen predominantly in the upper and middle zones. Silicotic nodules are absent. In some cases scar emphysema may be severe.

Microscopically, there is cellular infiltration with thickening of alveolar walls, macrophages in the air spaces and interstitial alveolar wall fibrosis in which particles of dust may be evident. Giant cells with clefts, possibly occupied by cholesterol crystals, are fairly numerous. In places, the histological features are those of the 'mural' type of fibrosing 'alveolitis' (Wyatt and Riddell, 1949; Mitchell *et al.*, 1961). Obliteration of alveolar spaces by fibrosis may be widespread but the elastic framework of the walls can be recognized. Bronchioles and alveoli which survive in fibrotic areas are lined by epithelial cells and may be much dilated giving a 'honeycomb' appearance. Obliterative endarteritis and perivascular fibrosis may be present in or near the fibrosis (Wyatt and Riddell, 1949). No evidence of silicotic nodules, sarcoid-type granulomas or lipoid pneumonia has been found in recorded cases. However, multiple foreign body granulomas, with no evidence of hypersensitivity, believed to be caused by aluminium fume have been described in a welder; but he had also been exposed to other occupational respiratory hazards including work in cedar saw mills and rock crushing (Chen *et al.*, 1978).

Ash of the lungs from some workers exposed to bauxite fume contains a high percentage of alumina and 'silica' of particle size as low as 0.02 μm and in proportions similar to those present in furnace fumes (Jephcott, 1950). Chemical and energy dispersive X-ray (EDAX) analysis of the lungs of workers exposed to aluminium powders has confirmed the presence of aluminium, and specific staining for aluminium with auramine may identify particles of the metal (Mitchell *et al.*, 1961; Chen *et al.*, 1978).

Pathogenesis

The question which requires an answer is two-fold: does metallic aluminium cause the fibrosis or is some associated agent responsible?

In the first place, there is a notable lack of lung fibrosis among workers exposed to aluminium dusts. No evidence of disease has been found in men in aluminium reduction plants (Medical Research Council, 1936; Kaltreider *et al.*, 1972), in potteries where alumina has replaced flint for biscuit placing (Posner and Kennedy, 1967), and in stamp-mills producing aluminium powders for paint and ink manufacture (Crombie, Blaisdell and MacPherson, 1944), although in this case the authors did not state whether stearine was added or not. A survey of men polishing duralumin aeroplane propellers discovered no evidence of fibrosis, but the dust they inhaled was chiefly that of the aluminium oxide abrasive employed and not metallic aluminium (Hunter *et al.*, 1944). Furthermore, the inhalation of metallic aluminium and aluminium oxide dusts for the treatment of silicosis over some years did not, apparently, cause any ill effects (Crombie, Blaisdell and MacPherson, 1944; Bamberger, 1945; Kennedy, 1956). Granular metallic powder usually has a coating of aluminium oxide.

Where fibrosis has been ascribed to metallic dust this has, in most cases, been flake aluminium in which stearine has been wholly or partly replaced by mineral oil or wax (Goralewski, 1947; Ahlmark, Bruce and Nyström, 1960; Mitchell *et al.*, 1961), although an exception to this apparently occurred in an aluminium stamper who used only stearine-containing powders (McLaughlin *et al.*, 1962). In Britain lung disease attributable to aluminium exposure does not appear to have been seen before 1959 and its subsequent occurrence has been thought to be due to the use of mineral oil instead of stearine in the stamping process (Jordan, 1961; Mitchell *et al.*, 1961).

It has been suggested that an aluminium oxide covering of granular particles and a stearine coating of flake particles prevent metallic aluminium from exerting a fibrogenic effect. But Corrin (1963) showed that three separate samples of stamped aluminium coated with stearine, coated with mineral oil or uncoated by defatting with acetone were all capable of causing prominent collagenous, nodular fibrosis of similar severity in rat lungs. Fat stains were negative though many of the macrophages in animals treated with stearine-coated and oil-coated powders were periodic acid Schiff positive. As defatted aluminium caused equally severe fibrosis it seems unlikely that either stearine or mineral oil contributed to fibrogenesis (*see* Chapter 11). These findings appear to contradict the hypothesis and are at odds with the industrial experience but the large dose of dust administered to the animals may have allowed sufficient concentrations of aluminium to escape from the stearine and oil coatings to cause fibrosis. By contrast granular aluminium powders caused a negligible effect in the rat lung.

The question as to whether lung fibrosis is caused by bauxite smelting fumes, and, if so how, has not been satisfactorily answered. Although Gärtner (1952) was 'inclined to implicate' amorphous silica he did not furnish proof of its presence. Initially the smelting process forms some mullite ($3Al_2O_3$. 2 SiO_2) from associated clay minerals and by the combination of alumina with free silica. But mullite dissociates into corundum and free silica at about 1810 °C. And as free silica melts at about 1723 °C it will be in the liquid phase some of which is vapourized but, on cooling, will convert—in part at least—to cristobalite (*see* Chapter 2). It is most probable, therefore, that a variable quantity of finely divided cristobalite, possibly coated with amorphous silica, is present in the fume (Bloor, 1979). However, metallic aluminium burnt in air evolves γ-Al_2O_3 (Finlay, 1950) which has been shown to cause fibrosis in the rat lung whereas α-Al_2O_3 does not (Stacy *et al.*, 1959). But as γ-Al_2SO_3 converts to α-Al_2SO_3 between 1000 and 1200 °C it is unlikely to survive in the fume cloud and, therefore, to offer any hazard to bauxite smelters.

There is no evidence that immunological reactivity is involved in pathogenesis in man but, on the basis of experiments using pure aluminium implanted into the lungs of mice which provoked infiltration of lymphocytes and plasma cells and diffuse fibrosis, Greenburg (1977) has suggested that the metal may act as an antigen in a hypersensitivity reaction. But neither single nor multiple intradermal injections of aluminium chlorhydrate in rabbits cause any reaction or granuloma formation and, unlike beryllium sulphate, it does not produce macrophage inhibition factor nor lymphocyte stimulation *in vitro* (Kang *et al.*, 1977).

To summarize: 'Aluminium lung' in man is an enigma. More than one cause may operate.

(1) Fibrosis related to aluminium fume in bauxite smelting is probably due to cristobalite in which case it is a form of silicosis.
(2) It is uncertain that metallic aluminium itself causes fibrosis as the apparent effects of uncoated metal in man and animals are contradictory. An immunological mechanism, though possible, has not been demonstrated.
(3) Although apparently not fibrogenic in rats the stearine or oil coating of flake aluminium might, perhaps, be so in man.

Whatever the truth may be, however, pulmonary fibrosis associated solely with aluminium processes is rare.

The use of aluminium silicate clays in the manufacture of refractory ceramics and bricks and the possibility of cristobalite being produced under some conditions is referred to in Chapter 9, p. 317.

Clinical features

In most cases, fibrosis develops gradually over a period of years and respiratory symptoms are usually absent until it is well established, when breathlessness on effort and cough—often without sputum—are complained of. In advanced cases, dyspnoea is severe and chest pain, associated with spontaneous pneumothorax and loss of weight, may occur. In some instances, however, symptoms develop and disease advances with remarkable rapidity after only one or two years' exposure (Mitchell *et al.*, 1961), especially in workers exposed to fume among whom spontaneous pneumothorax, which may be bilateral and recurrent, is a common complication (Riddell, 1950).

The abnormal physical signs of established disease are those of fibrosis of the upper parts of the lungs, often with deviation and distortion of the trachea, and, possibly, pneumothorax.

Lung function tests reveal a restrictive pattern without significant fall in gas transfer (Mitchell *et al.*, 1961).

Radiographic abnormality precedes the onset of symptoms in most cases by some years. The earliest change appears to be widening of the mediastinal shadows at hilar level, although the reason for this is not clear. Fine linear and discrete opacities appear later in the upper zones and then throughout the lung fields. There may be evidence of spontaneous pneumothorax (Shaver, 1948; Riddell, 1950). In other cases, evidence of fibrosis commences in the apical regions and progresses to large irregular opacities with adjacent distortion of the trachea and, occasionally, of the oesophagus as displayed by barium swallow (Goralewski, 1950; Mitchell *et al.*, 1961). These appearances are obviously indistinguishable from those of fibrocaseous tuberculosis. Signs of scar emphysema with distortion of the diaphragm may be present.

There is apparently no increased liability to tuberculosis.

Treatment

If the chest radiograph reveals evidence suggestive of disease the worker should be removed from exposure in the hope that progressive fibrosis may not occur.

Prevention

Exhaust ventilation to remove fume and, in the case of dust, enclosure of machinery or, if this is not practicable, personal protection of the worker in enclosed suits supplied with compressed air are required.

ANTIMONY TRICHLORIDE AND PENTACHLORIDE

Metallic antimony is discussed in Chapter 6.

Antimony trichloride is produced by the interaction of chlorine with antimony or by dissolving antimony trisulphide with hydrochloric acid. Antimony pentachloride is formed by reaction of molten antimony trichloride with chlorine. Both are used for 'blueing' steel and colouring aluminium, pewter and zinc and as catalysts in organic synthetic processes. They are highly toxic substances which may cause pulmonary oedema (Gudzovskii, 1971; Cordasco and Stone, 1973).

BORANES

The boranes are hydrogen compounds—boron hydrides—of boron (B) and those usually encountered in industry, *diborane, pentaborane* and *decaborane,* are highly toxic. Diborane is the most important in relation to lung disease and its toxicity has been compared to that of phosgene (Krackow, 1953).

Diborane (B_2H_6), a gas under ordinary conditions, produces great heat on hydrolysis igniting spontaneously in moist air and, on this account, is used in high energy fuels for rockets and high-flying aircraft. It is also employed in some welding processes, in the manufacture of fungicides and bactericides, and for polymerizing catalysts. It may be capable of producing an exothermic reaction in the lungs.

Acute, subacute and chronic effects are described (Lowe and Freeman, 1957; Cordasco *et al.*, 1962). *Acute illness* follows exposure to high concentrations and is a clinical syndrome similar to metal fume fever (*see* p. 454) with breathlessness, chest tightness, non-productive cough and wheezing which occurs in about one to 24 hours and lasts in most cases for three to five days. However, unlike metal fume fever, radiographic signs of bilateral pneumonic consolidation may develop but resolve in a few days. In the *subacute phase* cough, chest tightness, headache and drowsiness are most prominent. *Chronic disease* which follows recurrent low level exposure consists of unproductive cough, wheeze—which may be increased by exercise—and dyspnoea on effort which may occasionally last as long as two to three years before finally ceasing. Where ventilatory function tests have been done they have indicated a fairly severe degree of airflow obstruction which ultimately recovers.

The effects of pentaborane and decaborane are predominantly neurological: they include headache, drowsiness, muscle spasms and fasciculation but cough, chest tightness and inspiratory crepitations may be present in some patients.

Treatment of acute disease may require oxygen and corticosteroids, and bronchodilators will be necessary for more protracted airways obstruction.

Preventive measures include special conditions of storage, handling and processing, the use of respiratory protective equipment and informing personnel about the nature of the hazard.

Metallic boron is non-toxic.

CADMIUM

Cadmium metal or its compounds may either be inhaled or ingested, but only the results of inhalation which occur in industry are relevant here.

Freshly generated cadmium fumes (cadmium oxide) are so toxic that at one time they were considered as a possible weapon of chemical warfare. Fume, produced when the metal burns in air, is orange-brown in colour and tends to settle as a fine dust on cold surfaces. The metal melts at 321 °C (610°F) and boils at 767 °C (1800°F).

Uses and sources of exposure

Cadmium is highly resistant to corrosion and is used in antifriction metal alloys for engine bearings, for electroplating iron and steel, in the plates of nickel–cadmium storage batteries, in brazing and soldering alloys, wires and rods; in copper alloys for cables and trolley wires, in electrical capacitors, as cadmium sulphide and sulphoselenide in the preparation of pigments for paints, ceramics, glass, plastics and leather; in pesticides and veterinary medicines, and as a neutron absorber in atomic reactors. It is worth noting that both cadmium and beryllium are used in the manufacture of non-sparking tools.

Any of these processes is a potential source of exposure to dust or fume. Exposure to fume may also occur during the smelting and refining of zinc, lead and copper ores in which cadmium is present; during the recovery of scrap metal containing cadmium, and occasionally outside industry as in the use of cadmium alloys by sculptors in metal and by enthusiasts in metallist hobbies.

Oxyacetylene burning and welding of cadmium-plated metal and silver brazing have proved to be especially hazardous (Beton *et al.*, 1966; Blejer and Caplan, 1971) because they are often carried out in enclosed or ill-ventilated places. The fume is freshly generated and the risk is frequently unsuspected. Silver brazing is a form of high temperature welding in which metal is joined by the application of heat from 985 to 1650 °C (1800 to 3000°F) with a silver alloy filler (commonly containing cadmium) which melts at about 428 °C (800°F). Cadmium-plated metals may resemble galvanized (zinc-plated) metals and be mistaken for them. A simple test for the detection of cadmium is to heat gently a *small* spot of the metal with the welding rod when the film formed in the presence of cadmium is golden-yellow but is smokey-grey if zinc is present (Blejer and Caplan, 1971). High frequency and gas soldering of cadmium-containing metal produce cadmium smoke of minute particle size.

The danger is heightened by the fact that concentrations of cadmium fume or dust sufficient to cause severe illness or death do not give rise to any early warning symptoms. Therefore, any process which may evolve cadmium fume or dust in the vicinity of a worker's 'breathing zone' must be regarded as potentially dangerous; that is, any form of heating, brazing, welding, soldering or grinding of cadmium-containing metals (Blejer and Caplan, 1971).

Cadmium fume consists of minute particles up to about 0.1 μm diameter which form aggregates with overall diameters which may be as large as 25 μm. Cadmium oxide and chloride dusts are soluble in mildly acid conditions and body fluids, but cadmium sulphides and seleno-sulphides are relatively insoluble.

Smokers are exposed to low concentrations of cadmium because some of the cadmium content of tobacco passes into the smoke and, though many foods contain measurable amounts of cadmium which are poorly absorbed from the gastro-intestinal tract, cigarette smoke appears to be the chief non-industrial source of cadmium accumulation in the body—especially in heavy smokers. However, the quantity of cadmium in the smoke is very small: on average a cigarette contains 1 μg of cadmium about 15 per cent of which is absorbed by the smoker (Nandi *et al.*, 1969; Lewis *et al.*, 1972).

Absorption and excretion

Cadmium fume is readily soluble in slightly acid media and so is rapidly absorbed into the blood following inhalation. The dust tends to be of larger particle size, to be less soluble and to follow the routes of dust elimination from the lungs (*see* Chapter 3), although some solution evidently occurs. In the alkaline-battery industry only 20 per cent of particles were found to be of 'respirable' size (Adams, Harrison and Scott, 1969). The total quantity of cadmium in the lungs, therefore, is significantly less than that found in the liver, kidneys, pancreas and thyroid of exposed persons. The liver and the kidneys are believed to contain more than 50 per cent of the total body burden (Lane and Campbell, 1954; Friberg, 1957; Hirst *et al.*, 1973; Piscator, 1976). The biological half-life of cadmium in man is not known for certain but, in the kidney, it has been calculated to vary, from 17 to 33 years and, in the liver, to be less than seven years (Webb, 1975). Excretion occurs mainly through the kidney and cadmium tends to accumulate in the cortex (Smith, Smith and McCall, 1960).

Cadmium blood levels

In unexposed non-smokers cadmium is usually less than 0.5 μg/100 ml and in unexposed smokers, under 1 μg/100 ml (Lauwerys, 1980). In workers currently exposed to cadmium oxide dust or fume levels may vary from 1 to 10 μg/100 ml (90 to 890 nmol/l) (Cernick and Sayers, 1975). When exposure has ceased a significant fall in blood cadmium usually occurs (Welinder, Skerfving and Henricksen, 1977); but the rate of fall probably depends on the body burden of the metal (Lauwerys, 1980). Increased blood cadmium correlates significantly with elevated serum β_2-microglobulin (Iwao, Tsuchiya and Sakurai, 1980) (*see* Effect on the kidneys).

Pathology and pathogenesis

Acute disease

This is caused chiefly by freshly generated fume and is a 'chemical pneumonia' with oedema. It is estimated that a cumulative total exposure of 2500 mg/m^3 of cadmium oxide fume over five hours or 5 mg/m^3 over an eight hour period could be lethal (British Occupational Hygiene Society Committee on Hygiene Standards, 1977).

Respiratory tract The trachea and bronchi are congested and inflamed. Petechiae may be present in the pulmonary pleura. The lungs are voluminous and massively oedematous with blood-tinged fluid which is also found in the airways. Oedema is less pronounced if the patient has suvived a week or more.

Microscopically, the alveoli and terminal airways are filled with proteinaceous fluid, and large areas of intra-alveolar haemorrhage may be seen. There may be partial hyaline membrane formation (Blejer and Caplan, 1971). The alveolar walls are thickened by oedema and may contain many lymphocytes and neutrophils and a number of fibroblasts. There are hyperplasia and metaplasia of alveolar epithelial cells with much desquamation but in some cases many alveolar spaces are completely filled by masses of cuboidal cells (Patterson, 1947; Christensen and Olsen, 1957; Beton *et al.*, 1966). The type of appearance varies according to intensity of exposure and the time the patient survives. If he recovers, these lesions resolve completely.

Experimentally, cadmium has a similar effect to ozone (*see* p. 480) in animals in that there is initial desquamation of Type I pneumocytes followed by proliferation of Type II pneumocytes, and a striking increase in vascular permeability (Steele and Wilhelm, 1967; Carrington and Greene, 1970; Palmer, Snider and Hayes, 1975).

Kidneys Toxic nephrosis occurs in cases of heavy exposure. Microscopically there is widespread cortical necrosis, occlusion of the glomerular vessels by thrombi and tubular damage which may be extensive and severe (Beton *et al.*, 1966).

Chronic disease

This may result from repeated short exposures to moderate or low concentrations of cadmium oxide fume or of cadmium oxide, sulphide and stearate dusts over a prolonged period of time (Smith, Smith and McCall, 1960; Bonnel, 1965; Friberg, 1971).

Effect on the lungs Emphysema of both panlobular and centrilobular type found at post mortem in a small number of cadmium-exposed individuals has been attributed to cadmium (Baader, 1952; Lane and Campbell, 1954; Gough, 1960; Smith, Smith and McCall, 1960; Gough, 1968). Mild peribronchiolar fibrosis has also been described (Baader, 1952). However, no post-mortem studies with long exposures to cadmium compared with those of appropriate matched controls appear to have been done.

The question of so-called 'cadmium emphysema' is discussed in the next section.

An excess mortality from cancer of the lung among workers in one cadmium smelting plant has been reported by Lemen *et al.* (1976) but in this retrospective study comparison was made with mortality rates for the total white male population of the USA, and details of smoking habits and tumour histology were not analysed. As lung cancer has not previously been linked with cadmium exposure in man further investigation is obviously necessary to clarify the matter, but, at present, there is no adequate evidence from which to conclude that there is any relationship between cadmium and human cancer (British Occupational Hygiene Society Committee on Hygiene Standards, 1977).

Effects on the kidneys Normal *urinary excretion of cadmium* is about 2 μg or less a day, certainly under 5 μg a day, but in some individuals none is detectable (Webb, 1975; Lauwerys, 1980). These levels increase with occupational exposure to cadmium (Welinder, Skerfving and Henriksen, 1977). But a high level (which reflects the body burden of cadmium) is not necessarily associated with impaired renal function (Lauwerys, 1980). Unfortunately, urinary cadmium may be expressed in a number of ways: for example, μg/100 ml, μg/l, μg/l creatinine and nmol/l. Standardization is, thus, needed to avoid confusion (Kazantzis, 1980).

At a certain critical level of cadmium accumulation in the renal cortex—estimated to be about 200–250 ppm (Roels *et al.*, 1979)—dysfunction with increased urinary excretion of plasma proteins may occur. The proteinuria consists of low molecular weight (LMW) proteins (less than 40 000), β_2-microglobulin, α_2-microglobulin (retinol binding protein) and post-γ-protein; and also high molecular weight (HMW) proteins (higher than 40 000) such as albumin, transferrin and IgG which may signify glomerular damage (Bernard *et al.*, 1979). Increase of urinary β_2-microglobulin, a highly sensitive test of renal tubular dysfunction, has been regarded as important evidence of cadmium intoxication. To place this in perspective brief consideration must be given to the significance of β_2-microglobulin.

This protein is normally synthesized by most types of body cell and is present in normal serum in a mean concentration of 1.8 mg/l. During filtration through the kidney, being of small size, it undergoes almost complete reabsorption by the tubules so that its maximal daily excretion in the urine is only about 0.1 per cent of the total amount filtered—about 350mg/day. Elevation of serum β_2-microglobulin may result from: (1) reduced glomerular filtration rate; (2) increased synthesis; (3) both. Increased *synthesis* may be associated with carcinomatosis, certain lymphomas, chronic lymphatic leukaemias, multiple myeloma, rheumatoid arthritis, systemic lupus erythematosus, sarcoidosis and alcoholic liver damage. Increased *excretion* occurs in chronic pyelonephritis, reflux nephropathy even in the absence of infection, and a variety of interstitial nephropathies including those caused by phenacetin and salicylates (Schardijn *et al.*, 1979). Both symptomatic and asymptomatic urinary tract infections are common in general practice. Thus, it is evident that increased urinary excretion of β_2-microglobulinaemia is not *specific* evidence of chronic cadmium intoxication. Furthermore, standardization of the methods for estimating this protein and more information about its levels in the general population are needed (Kazantzis, 1980).

Interpretation of urinary β_2-microglobulin excretion as an index of cadmium intoxication can, therefore, be summarized as follows. (1) If excretion is slightly or moderately raised disorders which are known to cause increased serum β_2-microglobulin must first be excluded. In addition, a rise in urinary β_2-microglobulin is not necessarily due to impairment of tubular function but may be the result of increased blood β_2-microglobulin exceeding the renal threshold (Iwao, Tsuchiya and Sakutai, 1980). (2) If, in the absence of evidence of other relevant disorders, the level of excretion is consistently very high (that is, in excess of 1000 μg/l) and there is an increase of total protein or amino acid excretion permanent renal damage due to cadmium can probably be assumed (Kazantzis, 1980). At present it is not known whether, or to what extent, cadmium workers in whom only increased excretion of β_2-microglobulin is detectable will ultimately develop clinical proteinuria or other evidence of renal damage (British Occupational Hygiene Society Committee on Hygiene Standards, 1977).

β_2-microglobulin, is not detectable by standard clinical urinalysis but is identified by electrophoresis and, more accurately, by radioimmunoassay (Welinder, Skerfving and Henriksen, 1977). High levels of the enzyme carbonic anhydrase C, which are additional evidence of tubular dysfunction, may also be found in the urine by radioimmunoassay either in the presence or in the absence of β_2–microglobulin (Taniguchi *et al.*, 1979).

Once kidney damage is established there is an increased daily excretion of cadmium coincident with proteinuria (Lauwerys *et al.*, 1974; Webb, 1975; Welinder, Skerfving and Henricksen, 1977). Ultimately, the Fanconi Syndrome may develop in some cases and occasionally, as a consequence, secondary hyperparathyroidism and its effects including renal calculi and osteoporosis (Ahlmark *et al.*, 1960). After prolonged industrial exposure renal dysfunction may range from slight, asymptomatic tubular damage to severe atrophy: the former has been shown to be reversible in animals when exposure ceases (Piscator and Axelsson, 1970). In general, however, clinically detectable renal changes are of a minor order.

The renal aspect of the matter has been dwelt upon because it is the chief, and often only, evidence of cadmium intoxication.

Other effects Yellow pigmentation of the teeth is seen in some cases and mild hypochromic anaemia, believed to be due to iron deficiency and increased red cell destruction, may occur (Cotter and Cotter, 1951; Friberg, 1957).

In spite of the accumulation of cadmium in the liver cirrhosis or other chronic hepatic disorders do not seem to have been reported, nor does liver function appear to be adversely affected (Piscator, 1976). This may be due to cadmium combining with the low-molecular weight protein, metallothionein, which probably exerts a protective effect (Webb and Etienne, 1977). The underlying reason for the toxicity of cadmium is believed to be inhibition of certain tissue enzyme systems (in the kidney, those regulating tubular reabsorption) which depend upon the presence of copper, cobalt and zinc ions (Kendrey and Roe, 1969; Mustafa *et al.*, 1971).

The question of 'cadmium emphysema'

Some 20 years ago it was concluded, on the basis of clinical, lung function and radiographic changes in some workers exposed to cadmium that cadmium dust or fume causes emphysema (Friberg, 1950; Bonnell, 1955; Kazantzis, 1956; Bonnell, Kazantzis and King, 1959; Smith, Smith and McCall, 1960; Holden, 1965). Baader (1951) claimed that six of eight exposed workers had emphysema though the diagnosis rested solely on undefined clinical and radiographic findings. The fact that centrilobular or panlobular types of emphysema have been found post mortem in a small number of cadmium workers has, somewhat surprisingly, been taken as proof of a causal relationship (*see* previous section)—a belief now widely held.

But there were a number of important deficiencies in the data which led to this conclusion (Leading article, 1973):

(1) Definitions and the means of detecting emphysema were imprecise. For example, an increase in RV/TLC was taken as specific evidence of emphysema by Friberg (1950).
(2) Information on the smoking habits of the workers studied was lacking.
(3) Decline in lung function due to age was not allowed for, especially in investigations in which workers with short exposure were compared with those with long exposure.
(4) The fact that other observers had found no evidence of lung damage in some workers with prolonged exposure (Princi, 1947; Potts, 1965; Tsuchiya, 1967) was not taken into account.

Hence, it is necessary to consider the evidence of more recent investigations.

Lung function Stănescu *et al.* (1977) studied 18 workers who had experienced significant cadmium exposure over an average period of 32 years and a control group of 20 non-exposed workers matched for age, height, weight and smoking habits. The urinary excretion of cadmium and cadmium blood levels were greater in the exposed workers than in the controls and the excretion of urinary proteins, singificantly higher. Lung volumes, specific airways conductance (SGaw), maximal expiratory flow rate, closing volume, elastic recoil and single breath gas transfer showed no significant difference between the two groups; and standard PA and lateral chest films and full tomograms did not distinguish between them. The authors concluded that these results do not support the concept that cadmium causes emphysema. Similarly, Telescu and Stănescu (1970) found no functional or radiographic evidence of emphysema in a group of Rumanian cadmium workers.

In a group of workers exposed to high concentrations of airborne cadmium Smith *et al.* (1976) found no significant reduction in FEV_1 or maximal mid-expiratory flow rate compared with control subjects though they did observe some reduction in FVC, the significance of which is uncertain.

Chemical investigations The quantity of cadmium found in the lungs is lower than that in other organs but its presence in emphysematous lungs is consistent with, but not proof of, a causal relationship; whereas its absence from such lungs offers no proof either way. The content of lung tissue and liver has been found to be significantly higher in patients with no occupational exposure dying of severe emphysema compared with control subjects who died from other causes (Lewis, Lyle and Miller, 1969; Hirst *et al.*, 1973). This has been attributed to inhalation of cadmium in cigarette smoke. But as cadmium constitutes less than 10^{-5} parts by weight of the smoke among the many other possible pathogenic agents the smoke contains it does not seem plausible to regard this as the chief cause of smoking-related emphysema (Leading article, 1973). Indeed, Lewis *et al.* (1972) showed that, after standardizing for smoking habits, people who died of chronic bronchitis and emphysema did not have more cadmium in their tissues than those who died of other causes. It is, therefore, probably only a marker of cigarette smoke inhaled. And, although Chowdhury and Louria (1976) reported that cadmium inhibits the α_1-antitrypsin content of human plasma and its trypsin inhibiting capacity *in vitro*—observations which they suggested offered an explanation for emphysema seen in some cadmium workers—Bernard *et al.* (1977) found no reduction in α_1-antitrypsin nor of trypsin inhibiting capacity in the blood of workers with cadmium intoxication.

Post-mortem studies As indicated earlier very few post-mortem cases have been reported and no control-matched studies of substantial numbers of ex-cadmium workers appear to be on record. Even so it is difficult to see how post-mortem findings could provide the answer to this question.

Animal experiments These have not helped to resolve the problem. Although emphysema-like lesions have been produced in different species the doses administered by intratracheal injection or inhalation have been high relative to human experience, and the lesions have not borne a close resemblance to human emphysema. Moreover, not all observers have been able to induce these changes with cadmium (Thurlbeck, 1976). In this connection it is also worth noting that acute cadmium pneumonia and oedema in man were not followed by physiological or radiographic evidence of emphysema over four and a half years' observation (Townshend, 1968).

Conclusion The sum of evidence to date, therefore, gives little or no support to the view that exposure to cadmium fume or dust causes emphysema in man, and the presence of emphysema in cadmium workers during life or post mortem would seem to be fortuitous.

Clinical features

Acute disease

There are no symptoms during exposure. They are delayed for several hours, commonly starting when the man has returned home and retired to bed, and are identical to those

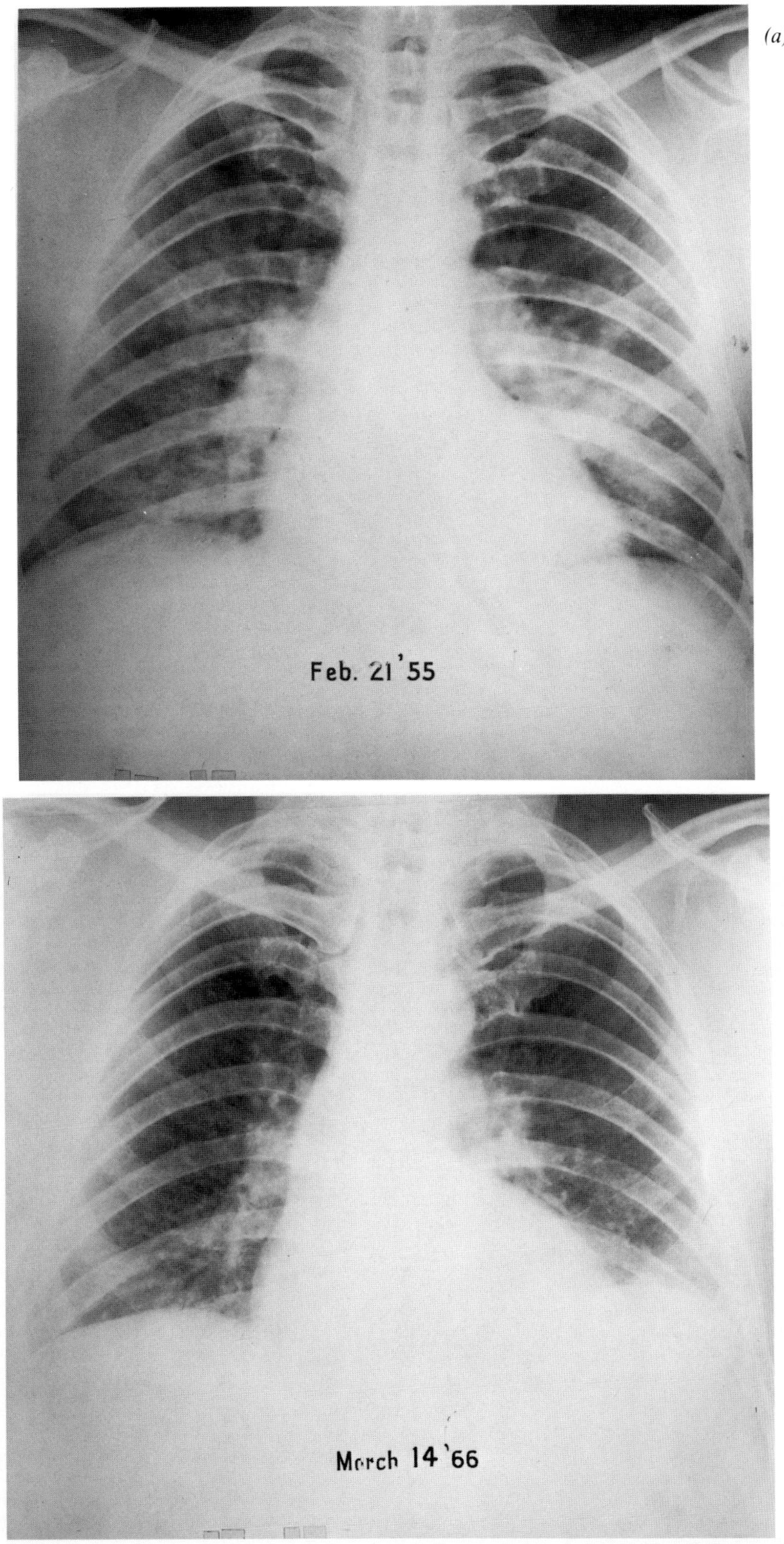

(a)

(b)

Figure 13.1 (a) Appearances of acute chemical pneumonia (pulmonary oedema) one week after heavy exposure to cadmium fume. Two months later the radiograph was normal. (b) No evident abnormality (emphysema or hyperinflation) 11 years after the incident. Case of a welder and sheet metal worker in a small ill-ventilated workshop who failed to remove the cadmium coating from the metal surface before welding. He developed intense burning pain in the chest, severe cough, vomiting and dyspnoea but was symptom-free in three weeks. No evidence of chronic respiratory disease during the rest of his life. He was a pinbowling enthusiast until shortly before his death from a non-respiratory illness. (Courtesy of Dr A.J. Karlish) of 'metal fume fever' (*see* p. 454) with the addition, in some cases, of abdominal cramps and diarrhoea. He may feel well enough to return to work the following day. But some 12 to 36 hours later there is dyspnoea, severe chest pain with a sense of precordial constriction (which may be mistaken for myocardial infarction), persistent cough with frothy sputum which may be bloodstained, wheeze, weakness and malaise (Beton *et al.*, 1966).

On examination of severely ill patients there is fever, central cyanosis, restlessness and the signs of pneumonia or pulmonary oedema. There may be mild proteinuria and toxic liver damage may be suggested by increased serum glutamic oxylactic transaminase (SGOT) and bilirubin levels (Blejer and Caplan, 1971). Pronounced loss of weight occurs in patients who survive some days.

The chest radiograph reveals the appearances of pulmonary oedema which usually resolve in a week or two but may not disappear completely for two or three months (Evans, 1960; Karlish, 1960; Townshend, 1968) (*Figure 13.1*).

Complete recovery is usually rapid with appropriate treatment, although a mortality rate of 15 to 20 per cent due to respiratory failure was reported by Bonnell (1965), and fatalities still occur due in most cases to failure to make the diagnosis (Patwardhan and Finckh, 1976). In some of these death is caused by acute renal failure. In those who recover there are no sequelae, and later deterioration of ventilatory function (FEV_1 and FVC) and gas transfer over a period of years does not seem to occur (Townshend, 1968).

Chronic disease

Symptoms of chronic intoxication usually develop over a period of years. They include tiredness, lassitude and loss of weight. Some degree of breathlessness on exertion with little cough or sputum is said to occur (Bonnell, 1965) but its significance is doubtful. Anosmia with watery nasal discharge is an uncommon complaint (Adams and Crabtree, 1961). Later the symptoms of nephrolithiasis and, ultimately, of chronic renal failure occasionally develop though renal failure as a cause of death is exceptional. Bone pains due to osteomalacia appear to be rare.

Yellow pigmentation of the teeth and anaemic pallor are sometimes seen.

Lung function tests and chest radiographs may or may not suggest emphysema, but if emphysema is present it is almost certainly coincidental (*see* last section). Changes indicative of intrapulmonary fibrosis are not seen. Although radiographic 'evidence suggestive of pulmonary fibrosis' has been described in a few cases by Smith *et al.* (1976) the significance of this observation is not clear. Scott *et al.* (1976) reported that a restrictive functional defect was more common in cadmium workers than in control subjects but they found no radiographic evidence of fibrosis.

Proteinuria, though often slight, is usually present and can be crudely detected by precipitation with a 3 per cent solution of sulphosalicylic acid or 25 per cent trichloracetic acid, but not by boiling. However, a more sensitive, though practical, semiquantitative method which identifies both LMW and HMW urinary proteins is sodium dodecyl sulphate-polyacrylamide gel electrophoresis (SDS–PAGE) (Bernard *et al.*, 1979); and, as mentioned earlier, β_2-microglobulin can be detected by radioimmunoassay. Proteinuria is accompanied by increased urinary cadmium. There may also be evidence of a multiple tubular malabsorption defect. In general, this is slight and not associated with any disability but, in some cases after prolonged exposure, there is significant renal glycosuria, abnormal aminoaciduria, hypercalcuria, hyperchloraemic acidosis and impaired concentration of urine.

Piscator (1978) has suggested that renal glomerular function in cadmium workers is better evaluated by estimating serum creatinine levels as serum β_2-microglobulin levels may give false positive results.

Rarely, there may be clinical and radiographic evidence of osteomalacia.

Blood cadmium in venous and capillary blood is much in excess of 'normal' levels (less than 1 μg/100 ml in smokers and non-smokers) and is an indication of intensity of recent exposure. A useful method for determining blood cadmium has been described by Cernik and Sayers (1975).

Diagnosis

Acute disease

The two most important requirements are a detailed occupational history from the patient or a workmate, and an awareness by the physician of the existence of this disorder and the work conditions which may give rise to it.

It is imperative that the diagnosis is made promptly and that the illness is not mistaken for harmless 'metal fume fever'. If symptoms persist—especially fever and severe chest pain—after 24 hours (when those of 'metal fume fever' have ceased) in a man with an appropriate or suspicious work history, acute poisoning must be suspected. A worker who has previously experienced 'metal fume fever' and is unaware of recent exposure to cadmium fume may wrongly attribute his symptoms to 'metal fume fever' and not seek medical advice until the delayed effects of cadmium are established. It should be noted that the other most commonly mistaken diagnoses are broncho-pneumonia, virus pneumonia, influenza and, occasionally, myocardial infarction.

Chronic disease

Diagnosis rests on the following:

(1) Known exposure to cadmium.
(2) Increased urinary excretion of cadmium (normal range 1 to 5 μg per day.
(3) Persistently and substantially high urinary β_2-microglobulin levels (that is, in excess of 1000 μg/l).
(4) Exclusion of other causes of raised β_2-microglobulin excretion.
(5) Increase of total urinary protein, and, possibly, aminoaciduria and other evidence of malabsorption.

The value of cadmium concentration in blood and urine as an indication of the *intensity* of past exposure is uncertain (Lauwerys, Buchet and Roels, 1976).

Serum and urinary calcium may be raised in some cases as a result of secondary hypoparathyroidism due to chronic renal failure, but this is a consequence of disease and not a diagnostic feature.

Treatment

Acute chemical pneumonia and pulmonary oedema

First aid
(1) Warmth and rest.
(2) Administration of oxygen.
(3) The patient must be warned against any exertion.

In hospital
(1) Warmth and rest must be continued for several days over the period when delayed-onset pulmonary oedema may occur.
(2) Oxygen administered by intermittent positive pressure ventilation.
(3) Removal of bronchial exudates by suction tube. In many cases elective tracheostomy with a large cuff endobronchial tube is indicated.
(4) Corticosteroids. Early administration greatly improves the prognosis. In severely ill patients they should be given intravenously for a few days and thereafter in the form of prednisolone by mouth until recovery is established.
(5) Chelating agents. Calcium ethylenediamine tetracetic acid (EDTA) by the intravenous route has been recommended by some authorities but is regarded by Friberg (1971) as undesirable. If it is used the dose must be strictly controlled and renal function frequently checked. The reason for this is that it is nephrotoxic in combination with cadmium. The maximal recommended dose is 2.5 g/4.5 kg bodyweight, and for each 4.5 kg is 170 mg/hour, 330 mg/day or 1670 mg/week. No more than two such courses with a one-week interval should be given (Blejer and Caplan, 1971). Dimercaprol (BAL) is contraindicated.
(6) Analgesics may be required for chest pain but morphine or other respiratory depressants should be avoided or given only in small doses.
(7) A bronchodilator drug may give additional relief if wheezing is pronounced.
(8) A broad spectrum prophylactic antibiotic is probably desirable.

Chronic disease

The worker should be removed permanently from exposure to cadmium and, in most cases this is all that is necessary. But occasionally anaemia or renal malabsorption may require treatment. The use of EDTA should be avoided as it may worsen renal damage.

Prevention

General hygiene measures
(1) The potential hazard of cadmium exposure and the processes and materials which can cause it should be made clear to all likely to be concerned. Brazers and welders should be familiarized with the orange-brown appearance of cadmium fume and warned of the danger of overheating cadmium–silver solders. A warning label should be firmly attached to all cadmium-containing materials and, whenever possible, cadmium-free silver-alloy fillers made available for silver brazing.
(2) Efficient exhaust ventilation must be applied to alloying and refining furnaces, to all dusty operations and, whenever practicable, to welding and similar processes involving cadmium alloys. During oxyacetylene burning, welding or brazing in confined spaces where exhaust ventilation is impossible or when carried on outdoors (where dangerous concentrations of fume may still occur in workers' breathing zones) appropriate respirators must be worn. Men working in the vicinity of fume-producing processes should also have respirator protection.
(3) The concentration of cadmium dust or fume in environmental and 'breathing zone', air should be monitored periodically and the results recorded.
(4) Workers should not be allowed to eat, drink or smoke in workplaces where cadmium fume or dust may be present, and they should not take working clothes home.

Medical surveillance In addition to routine clinical examination screening of urine at regular intervals for β_2-microglobulin is probably of value if the employee has been exposed for ten years or more, but not otherwise (Adams, 1980). Urine is collected in metal-free polythene containers and part is refrigerated at –20 °C for β_2-microglobulin analysis. Cadmium levels should also be determined. If proteinuria persists the work environment needs to be carefully surveyed. It would seem undesirable, however, to remove workers from exposure simply because a certain arbitrary limit of β_2-microglobulin is exceeded. This decision should rest on careful assessment of the features of each case (Kazantzis, 1980).

Regular assessment of ventilatory function—preferably at six-monthly intervals—is recommended by the British Occupational Hygiene Society Committee on Hygiene Standards (1977).

Pre-employment examination of prospective entrants to processes in which there may be significant cadmium fume or dust should exclude those with a past history or current evidence of renal disease, and those with anaemia or chronic respiratory disease.

Threshold limit values These have been reviewed in various countries in recent years and levels lowered since 1976 (American Conference of Governmental Hygienists; British Occupational Hygiene Society Committee on Hygiene Standards, 1977; Health and Safety Executive, 1976). Recommended standards consist of 'ceiling values' or 'long-term exposure values'.

'Ceiling values' aim to prevent the hazard of acute disease though a Special Short-Term Exposure List of a specified concentration for a maximum of ten minutes in a working shift is preferred by the BOHS Committee. For long-term exposures different levels are suggested according to whether dusts are of 'respirable' or 'non-respirable' size.

CHROMIUM

Metallic chromium is used extensively in the production of various alloys with nickel and molybdenum, cobalt, vanadium and niobium; and also in the chromate industry. Chromium plating is carried out by depositing chromium from a solution of chronic acid by electrolysis. Hexavalent sodium dichromate is employed in leather tanning, and other chromates are used for various purposes such as pigments for paints and ceramics, and mordants or fixatives in dyeing. Chromium may occasionally be present in arc welding fumes.

Chromite mining is referred to in Chapter 7.

Effects

Chromium, its chromates and dichromates, and chromic acid are all capable of causing asthma and dermatitis; indeed chromium is a potent sensitizer (*see Table 12.4*) (Hicks, Hewitt and Lam, 1979). Inhalation of high concentrations of chromic acid causes intense irritation of the upper and lower respiratory tracts with cough, dyspnoea, chest pain and radiographic changes (Meyers, 1950.)

A significant excess of carcinoma of the lung has been reported among chromium platers and chromate workers (*see* Chapter 14).

COBALT

Cobalt is used for a variety of purposes and appears to be the cause of lung disease associated with the hard metal industry. Three types of disorder are attributed to it: *acute*, in the form of asthma; *subacute,* fibrosing 'alveolitis'; and *chronic,* in the form of progressive DIPF—*Hard Metal Disease*.

Cobalt (Co) is a silvery blue-white metal with magnetic properties which is obtained when copper is extracted from its ore. Various grades of cobalt powder are manufactured and the extra-fine grade is used in the manufacture of hard metal. The particles are rod shaped with a mean diameter of 1.4 μm and a length about ten or 20 times greater but they break down during milling (Payne, 1979).

It has a wide range of uses in industry, medicine and nuclear weapons, but its industrial applications only are considered here.

Industrial uses

(1) *Metallic alloys* (a) In combination with aluminium, nickel and other alloys to produce permanent magnets for the electrical and electronic industries. (b) In combination with nickel, chromium and molybdenum in the production of Vitallium for joint prostheses in orthopaedic surgery. (c) In the manufacture of high speed steels.

(2) *Tungsten carbide (hard-metal)* This synthetic metal, which possesses exceptional properties of resistance to heat and wear and a hardness only slightly less than that of diamond, was first introduced in Germany in the 1920s and in the UK and the USA a decade later. Because its hardness increases with rising temperature the metal is used for high-speed cutting tools and drills which can operate at temperatures up to about 1090 °C, and in armour plating, bullets and the nose cones of armour piercing shells.

Tungsten carbide is produced by blending and heating tungsten (wolfram) and carbon in an electric furnace. It is then mixed and finely ground in a ball-mill with cobalt in quantities varying from 3 to 25 per cent in order to form a matrix for the tungsten carbide crystals. Other metals—such as chromium, nickel, titanium and tantulum—may be added according to the properties required in the final product. All these constituents are in a finely divided state having a mean diameter of about 1.5 μm (Coates and Watson, 1971). The powdered metal is next pressed into ingots or particular shapes. After pressing, it is fused (or sintered) in an electric furnace at approximately 1000 °C, and the product finally heated to about 1500 °C (cobalt melts at 1495 °C). All these processes and dry grinding, drilling and finishing of hard-metal products, and cleaning equipment may be dusty if exhaust ventilation is inadequate. However, drilling and grinding operations usually require special coolant fluids in which varying amounts of cobalt dissolve and accumulate, and which form a fine aerosol spray. Lung disease appears to be more common in 'wet' (coolant-using) areas where cobalt occurs in ionized form but in lower concentrations than in 'dry' areas where it is non-ionized (Sjögren *et al.*, 1980).

(3) In the china, glass, paint and glaze industries as a clear blue pigment.

(4) As a catalyst in the chemical and oil industries.

Respiratory effects

Acute

Pulmonary oedema This occasionally follows exposure to high concentrations of cobalt fume: for example during melting and pouring the metal into moulds.

Asthma Exposure to cobalt dust alone (as can occur during the milling of cobalt metal) may cause either asthma or itching of the skin with urticaria and erythematous papules, or both. After a variable period in the hard metal industry a small proportion of exposed workers develop asthma. The asthma, which is of late (non-immediate) type (*see* Chapter 12), occurs towards the end of the day's work or in the evening and is associated with chest tightness and productive cough. It ceases during the weekend and holidays but usually recurs on the first day back at work. It responds to bronchodilators and is cured by removal from exposure. In general, it does not develop until workers have been exposed for between six to 18 months. The chest radiograph in most cases shows no abnormality but appearances similar to those of acute or subacute fibrosing 'alveolitis' may develop in a small number (Bruckner, 1967; Tolot *et al.*, 1970; Coates *et al.*, 1973; Sjögren *et al.*, 1980).

Reduction of FEV_1 during the course of a working week with recovery when absent from work is apparently fairly common in tungsten carbide workers (Alexanderson, 1979).

Subacute

Fibrosing 'alveolitis' Cough which is usually non-productive, dyspnoea on exertion, loss of weight, crepitations at the lung bases and linear or ill-defined rounded opacities with prominent hilar shadows on the chest radiograph develop within a year or less and usually after only a few years in the hard metal industry. Complete resolution occurs in some cases when exposure ceases but is incomplete in others. These changes may recur on re-exposure which, if repeated, might lead to progressive fibrosis.

The histological appearances are those of desquamating fibrosing 'alveolitis'. Alveolar walls are thickened and infiltrated with lymphocytes, plasma cells and macrophages, and alveolar lining cells (Type I pneumocytes) are swollen and many exfoliated. Granulomatous foci have also been reported (Joseph, 1968). Crystals identified as tungsten carbide by X-ray diffraction have been found in the macrophages (Miller *et al.*, 1953; Lundgren and Öhman, 1954; Scherrer *et al.*, 1970; Coates and Watson, 1973); and cobalt has been identified in the mediastinal lymph nodes of some workers (Sjögren *et al.*, 1980).

Chronic

Hard metal disease This was first described as an abnormal radiographic appearance by Jobs and Ballhausen (1940) in Germany. Occasional cases of progressive DIPF occur in susceptible workers after some years in the hard metal industry: the time varies from two to 25 years but is usually in excess of ten years. Cases have been reported in Britain (Bech, Kipling and Heather, 1962), Europe (Jobs and Ballhausen, 1940; Reber and Burckhardt, 1970; Scherrer *et al.*, 1970), Sweden (Lundgren and Öhman, 1954; Ahlmark, Bruce and Nyström, 1960), Czechoslovakia and Russia (Bech, Kipling and Heather, 1962), Australia (Joseph, 1968) and the USA (Miller *et al.*, 1953; Coates and Watson, 1971 and 1973).

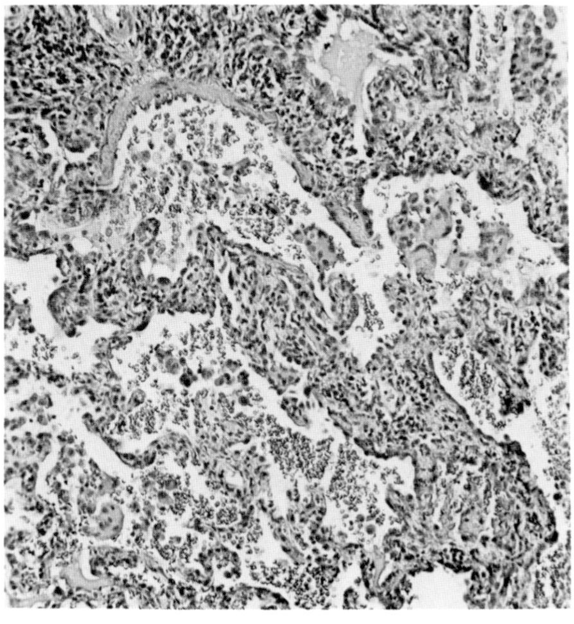

Figure 13.2 Microsection of the lung of a man who worked for two years in the final grinding process of tungsten carbide. There is pronounced interstitial cellular infiltration, fibrosis of alveolar walls and some metaplasia of alveolar lining cells. Large cells, many of which are multinucleated, lie free in the alveolar spaces. (Original magnification × 175, reproduced at × 87.5; H and E stain; courtesy of Dr E. Osborne Coates, Detroit, and the Editor of Annals of Internal Medicine*)*

The gross appearances of the lungs are those of widespread DIPF often with honeycomb cysts; and the histological features, those of fibrosing 'alveolitis' of mural type (*see* Chapter 4). Collagen and elastic tissue are prominent in the alveolar walls and a moderate number of mononuclear cells—apparently Type II pneumocytes—and some multinucleated cells of histiocytic type may be present in the alveolar spaces (*Figure 13.2*). Sarcoid-type granulomas are not seen. Electron microscopy reveals swelling of Type I cells with the formation of numerous microvilli and groups of crystals identifiable as tungsten carbide within macrophages and their lysosomes and in alveolar walls. Cobalt, however, is only occasionally identifiable (Coates and Watson, 1971 and 1973).

Effect on the myocardium

The possibility that prolonged exposure to high concentrations of cobalt dust in the hard metal industry may occasionally, and incidentally, result in fatal cardiomyopathy has been suggested (Barborik and Dusek, 1972; Kennedy, Dornan and King, 1981). In excessive quantities cobalt is, of course, a known myocardial poison.

Pathogenesis

The mechanism responsible for asthma is obscure but inhalation challenge with powdered cobalt has been shown to provoke chest tightness and wheezing with itching of the skin after one hour whereas, with powdered tungsten, there was no response (Coates *et al.*, 1973). In patients with allergic dermatitis due to metallic cobalt skin patch tests with the powdered metal are positive but negative with other metals (Schwarz *et al.*, 1945). This test has been found to be positive in hard metal workers with both fibrosing 'alveolitis' and skin sensitization (Sjögren *et al.*, 1980).

Particulate cobalt metal is strikingly toxic to the lungs of experimental animals when inhaled or injected by the intratracheal route. It results in haemorrhagic oedema, obliterative bronchiolitis and proliferation and desquamation of alveolar cells (Harding, 1950; Schepers, 1955a), whereas particulate tungsten metal, tantulum and titanium alone are relatively innocuous (Delahant, 1955; Schepers, 1955b, c; Kaplun and Mezencewa, 1960). Dust mixtures containing tungsten, titanium and cobalt cause a more pronounced effect than cobalt alone (Kaplun and Mezencewa, 1960). Finely divided cobalt, but not tungsten carbide, is toxic to normal human leucocytes *in vivo,* particularly in patients with fibrosing 'alveolitis' (Coates and Watson, 1971).

However, there is no correlation between the quantity of cobalt in human lungs and the severity of disease although tungsten and titanium are usually present (Bech, Kipling and Heather, 1962; Coates and Watson, 1971). But there is a similar lack of correlation in beryllium disease (Chapter 10). The high solubility of cobalt in biological fluids undoubtedly allows it to escape from the lungs. In ionized form it combines readily with proteins and amino acids and thus could conceivably act as a hapten capable of promoting immunological reactions both in the lungs and the skin (Harding, 1950; Heath, Webb and Caffrey, 1969; Rae, 1975; Sjögren *et al.*, 1980).

The failure of some metal-to-metal cobalt-chromium-molybdenum hip arthroplasties owing to necrosis of bone, muscle and joint capsule adjacent to the prosthesis has been attributed to the release of cobalt due to metal attrition; and a similar observation has been made in bone fixed with such fracture plating (Halpin, 1975; Jones *et al.,* 1975). The tissues adjacent to the prostheses often show a granulomatous reaction and tissue destruction (Rae, 1975). In these instances skin patch tests with cobalt were positive whereas those with nickel and chromium were negative, but a high incidence of allergy to chromium has also been found in some patients with metal-to-metal prostheses (Benson, Goodwin and Brodyoff, 1975). Particulate cobalt and cobalt–chromium alloy have been shown to be cytotoxic to macrophages *in vitro* whereas chromium, molybdenum and titanium are not; and they are also strongly haemolytic to human erythrocytes but chromium, molybdenum and titanium are only feebly so (Rae, 1975 and 1978).

Thus, whereas tungsten is apparently inert, cobalt, whether free or in alloy form, is allergenic and cytotoxic and may be capable of provoking release of a fibrogenic agent from macrophages.

Although, unfortunately, few immunological studies appear to have been done in reported cases of hard metal disease the following points are consistent with its being a specific entity—probably due to cobalt—and not a coincidental fibrosing 'alveolitis':

(1) Relationship of development of disease to exposure.

(2) The average size range of the metallic particles is of the order of 1.2 to 1.9 μm (McDermott, 1971) so that a large proportion are capable of reaching the alveoli. Tungsten and associated metals are usually present in affected lungs though of course, this does not establish proof of a causal relationship. The frequent absence of cobalt has been explained.

(3) The reported association of subacute disease with positive cobalt patch tests.

(4) Despite the fact that the number of recorded cases and apparent incidence of the disease are very small in relation to the numbers of workers exposed—in one American series, nine out of 1500 (Coates and Watson, 1971)—the clinical features and pathology appear to be similar in all.

(5) The allergenic potential and cytotoxicity of cobalt.

Though the exact mode of causation remains to be established, the features of reversible, or partly reversible, subacute disease and of progressive fibrosis are closely akin to those of extrinsic allergic 'alveolitis'.

Clinical features

The clinical, physiological and radiographic features are similar to those of DIPF from other causes, which is predominant in the lower halves of the lungs (*Figure 13.3*). In a few cases the disease has been fatal due to cardiorespiratory

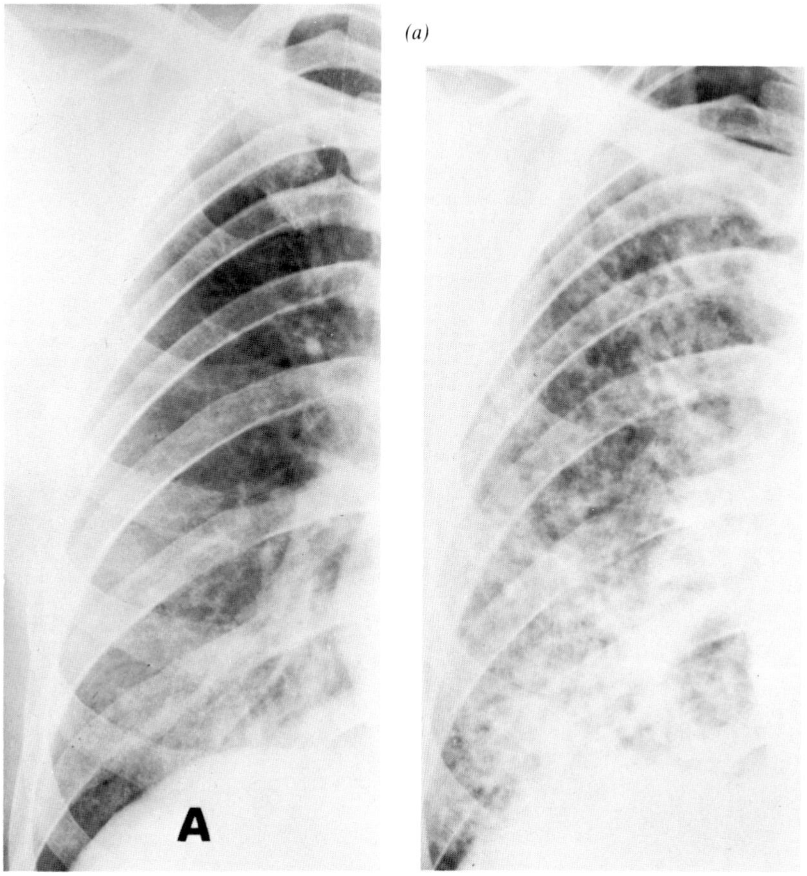

Figure 13.3 Radiographs of a man who worked with soft and hard tungsten carbide for four years. Fine linear opacities (ILO Category 's') are present in the lower half of the lung field in (a). Film (b), taken ten years later, shows coarse linear and round opacities with some suggestion of 'honeycombing'. (By courtesy of Dr E. Osborne Coates and the Editor of Annals of Internal Medicine*)*

failure. As the atomic number of tungsten is 74 it might be expected that small dense radiographic opacities would be seen if sufficient dust is stored in the lungs but this seems rarely to have been described. No investigations of circulating antibodies appear to have been reported but hyperglobulinaemia is recorded (Miller *et al.*, 1953).

Diagnosis

A detailed occupational history is essential for identifying the cause of the asthma and in the diagnosis of the subacute and chronic forms of hard metal disease. Identification of tungsten by lung biopsy confirms exposure and may imply the association of cobalt but does not prove the lung pathology to be that of hard metal disease. Other possible causes must be excluded.

The value of cobalt patch tests in diagnosis of the subacute and progressive types of disease has still to be determined. Tests of lymphocyte transformation and leucocyte inhibition factor in response to cobalt might be of help (Christiansen, 1979; Mayor, Merritt and Brown, 1980).

Concentrations of cobalt in the blood and urine appear to correlate well with levels of exposure (Alexandersson, 1979).

Treatment

Asthma is relieved by bronchodilators but is cured when the worker ceases to be exposed. The desquamative fibrosing 'alveolitis' stage of the disorder responds to treatment with corticosteroids. Prompt diagnosis is, therefore, paramount. On recovery the worker should not return to exposure. Chronic disease is not amenable to treatment.

Prevention

Dust from the various processes in the preparation of hard-metal and the finishing of products should be reduced to a minimum by efficient exhaust ventilation of the high-velocity, low-volume type locally applied as in the machining of beryllium alloys (Chapter 10) (McDermott, 1971). And the environmental air, both breathing-zone and general, should be monitored. As far as possible, coolant liquids with the lowest capacity for dissolving cobalt should be used.

Periodic medical examination including chest radiographs and tests of ventilatory function should be done yearly, and atopic subjects should be excluded from work involving potential exposure. Workers who develop contact skin sensitivity and whose cobalt patch test is positive should probably be removed from exposure (Sjögren *et al.*, 1980).

COPPER

Copper as a potent cause of metal fume fever in workers exposed to finely divided oxide (for example, melting the metal in electric furnaces) is referred to earlier in this chapter.

Vineyard sprayers' lung

Lung disease which appears to be related to the use of copper sulphate as an anti-mildew spray has been described in Portuguese vineyard workers (Pimentel and Marques, 1969; Villar, 1974).

A solution of 1 to 2 per cent copper sulphate neutralized with hydrated lime and known as Bordeaux mixture is sprayed periodically on vines by manual or mechanical means. After prolonged exposure some workers develop dyspnoea on effort and bilateral, irregular and rounded opacities in their chest radiographs.

Examination of the lungs reveals green-blue patches on their surfaces and, on section, dark blue rounded and coalescent areas in all lobes. Microscopically, the appearances include lymphocytic infiltration and diffuse fibrosis of alveolar walls, foreign body granulomas which stain for copper and, at a later stage, fibrohyaline nodular lesions which tend to coalesce. Similar changes have been produced in guinea pigs with Bordeaux mixture.

The nature and pathogenesis of vineyard sprayers' lung has still to be elucidated.

An excess of carcinoma of lung is believed to occur in vineyard sprayers but this requires confirmation (Villar, 1974).

LITHIUM HYDRIDE (LiH)

This is a respiratory irritant gas which causes violent sneezing and coughing when microgram quantities are dispersed in air (Spiegl *et al.*, 1956). It is used in the atomic energy industry, experimentally as a rocket fuel propellent because of its exothermic properties, as a reducing agent in the organic chemical industry and as a convenient means of transporting hydrogen.

It has been reported to have caused pulmonary oedema of rapid onset in a worker who entered a tank to investigate a gas leak. Intensive care treatment resulted in rapid recovery in about 48 hours. Other cases have occurred (Cordasco *et al.*, 1965).

MANGANESE

Exposure to manganese dust may occur in the mining and crushing of *pyrolusite* ore and in some of the processes in which the dioxide is used. These include the manufacture of 'dry' electric batteries, extensive applications in the chemical industry, and for colouring glass. Metallic manganese is an important ingredient in a variety of alloys, in particular manganese steel.

Metal fume fever may follow exposure to nascent manganese dioxide fume, and an unduly high incidence of pneumonia is said to have been associated with exposure to high concentrations of dust. Manganese dioxide causes necrosis and haemorrhage in the lungs of mice, and the disease in man may be a chemical pneumonia (Lloyd Davies, 1946; Lloyd Davies and Harding, 1949; Morichau-Beauchant, 1964).

A syndrome similar to Parkinson's disease which may develop as a result of heavy exposure to manganese dust has rarely been seen in the UK in recent years.

MERCURY

This silvery, metallic liquid has a boiling point of 357 °C and vaporizes at room temperature. The smaller the globules the higher the vaporization rate becomes. The vapour is odourless.

Lung disease caused by mercury is uncommon but serious and sometimes fatal. In industry it is usually due to exposure in confined spaces.

Mercury is used in the electrical industry for the manufacture of mercury vapour lamps, transformers, rectifiers and dry cell batteries; in the chemical industry in electrolytic processes and in the manufacture of pharmaceuticals and fungicides; in metallurgy for the production of amalgams of silver, gold, tin and copper; and in the manufacture and repair of thermometers, barometers, manometers and vacuum pumps. Mercury-steam boilers and mercury-arc rectifiers are also used in power generation.

Thus, accidental exposure in industry may result from spillage in the production of thermometers and manometers, and in laboratories and dental surgeries; from rupture of mercury-vapour boilers and contamination by 'blown' manometers in generator plants; and from cleaning out tanks used for chemical electrolysis (Christensen, Krogh and Nielsen, 1937; King, 1954; Teng and Brennan, 1959; Tennant, Johnston and Wells, 1961; Milne, Christophers and de Silva, 1970; Merfield *et al.*, 1976). But accidental exposure to mercury vapour has also been reported in the home from the heating of mercury or mercury-containing materials on stoves and has caused fatalities in children (Campbell, 1948; Mathes *et al.*, 1958; Hallee, 1969).

Pathology

The lungs of individuals who die within a day or two show severe tracheobronchitis with stratification of the epithelium of bronchioles, pulmonary oedema with proteinaceous exudate in the alveolar spaces and well-developed hyaline membranes. Small numbers of lymphocytes and large mononuclear cells are present in the alveolar walls and there are early proliferative changes of the lining and interstitial cells. At about three weeks, however, fairly extensive DIPF is present with early evidence of 'honeycombing', striking hyperplasia of alveolar lining cells many of which are atypical, and persistence of hyaline membrane (Liebow, 1975) (*Figure 13.4*). Mild DIPF has also been demonstrated some five months after exposure (Hallee, 1969).

Some of the inhaled mercury is exhaled and the rest, apparently removed rapidly from the lungs. Experimental observations in monkeys and rabbits indicate that about 80 per cent of the mercury in the blood is in the erythrocytes leaving little free in the plasma (Berlin, Fazackerley and Nordberg, 1969). Urinary excretion of the metal correlates poorly with the quantity absorbed (Teisinger and Fiserova-Bergerova, 1965).

Clinical features

Symptoms do not usually develop until about one to four

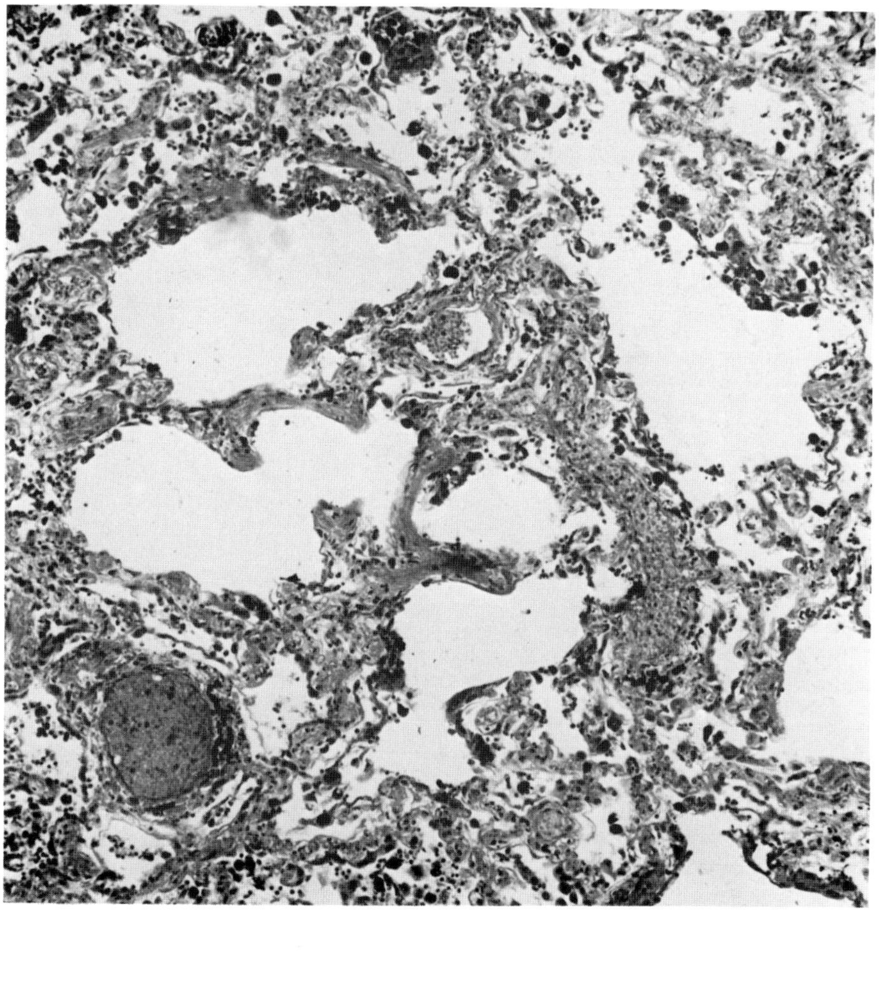

Figure 13.4 Interstitial and intra-alveolar fibrinous oedema caused by mercury vapour with cellular infiltration, desquamation of alveolar lining cells and some hyaline membrane formation. Approximately two weeks after exposure. (Original magnification × 160, H and E stain.) (Courtesy of the late Professor A. A. Liebow)

hours after exposure. They include initial tightness and soreness of the chest followed by shivering, profuse sweating, fever, persistent cough, severe breathlessness and restlessness. In addition there may be crampy abdominal pains and diarrhoea. The severity of the symptoms varies according to the degree of exposure.

Bilateral inspiratory crepitations are present at the lung bases in most cases.

The chest radiograph reveals bilateral 'soft' opacities similar to those of pulmonary oedema which are most prominent in the lower halves of the lung fields.

In severe cases death may occur in 48 to 72 hours though sometimes the patient may survive a week or two but, with prompt treatment, complete recovery is the rule. However, DIPF may occasionally develop.

Diagnosis

This depends chiefly on a history of exposure and on the symptoms. Estimation of blood mercury may be of value if whole blood and not serum is analysed; levels of urinary mercury, due to their great variability, are probably unhelpful.

Differentiation from bacterial and viral pneumonia is imperative.

Treatment

Corticosteroids should be started as soon as possible even in individuals who may not seem severely affected. Oxygen and other supportive measures will usually be required.

NICKEL

Nickel is used extensively in the production of nickel-based alloys including ferro–nickel, in the manufacture of steel, in nickel electroplating and in glass, enamels and ceramics. It may occur in some welding fumes. High purity nickel is obtained from the decomposition of nickel carbonyl in the Mond process.

Acute effects

Asthma

Nickel, which is well known as a cause of allergic dermatitis has been reported to cause late-type asthma which ceases at weekends and recurs on Mondays in the nickel plating industry and in the production of nickel carbonyl. In one case it was reproduced over a period of five hours by a single bronchial challenge with $NiSO_4$; gas transfer was not affected. Löffler's syndrome is also recorded in association with both asthma and dermatitis (Sunderman and Sunderman, 1961; McConnell *et al.*, 1973) (*see Table 12.4*).

Chemical pneumonia and pulmonary oedema

These may follow exposure to nickel carbonyl. Nickel carbonyl ($Ni(CO)_4$) is a heavy, colourless, unstable liquid which is vapourized at 43 °C. The vapour is highly toxic.

Acute disease caused by inhalation of the vapour has two phases: *immediate,* consisting of nausea, vomiting and severe headache which usually recovers fairly quickly; and *delayed,* the onset of which may vary from ten to 36 hours—occasionally up to eight days—after exposure, consisting of paroxysmal coughing, breathlessness, chest tightness, substernal pain, and extreme weakness. The clinical and radiographic signs of pulmonary oedema and patchy bilateral consolidation develop.

Following heavy exposure death may occur in a few days when the lungs at post mortem show haemorrhagic oedema with areas of consolidation some of which may contain fibrinoid and be necrotic. Otherwise recovery, though slow, is complete (Sunderman and Kincaid, 1954).

Treatment requires the use oxygen and corticosteroids. The value of chelating agents is doubtful.

Chronic effects

It is by no means certain that there are any. But DIPF with honeycomb cysts has been described in a few nickel workers exposed to $Ni(CO)_4$ and, although this was attributed to 'chronic pulmonary inflammation' it is possible that nickel may have been responsible. Both nickel and copper were present in the lungs (Jones Williams, 1958). Experimentally, animals which survive exposure to $Ni(CO)_4$ develop severe extensive lung fibrosis (Barnes and Denz, 1950).

Carcinoma of lung

The possibility of nickel or nickel carbonyl being carcinogenic is referred to in Chapter 14.

OSMIUM

Metallic osmium has a limited use in industry for certain alloys and in the chemical industry. It is innocuous but when heated, as in annealing, or at room temperature it evolves osmic acid, or osmium tetroxide (OsO_4) which is used as a tissue fixative in electron microscopy. Osmium tetroxide is intensely irritant and toxic and, if inhaled even in small amounts, causes severe acute laryngo-tracheobronchitis with chest tightness and bronchospasm (McLaughlin, Milton and Perry, 1946). However, because the vapour is so irritant, this is of rare occurrence. But accidental exposure to high concentrations would undoubtedly cause acute pulmonary oedema.

Prevention consists of good ventilation and storage of osmic acid in sealed containers.

SELENIUM COMPOUNDS

Selenium is a semi-metal, or metalloid, with similar properties to sulphur. It is widely distributed in small quantities in igneous rocks, volcanic material and glacial drifts, chiefly in the form of metallic selenides or in combination with sulphur. It is obtained largely as a by-product of processes involving selenium-containing sulphide minerals.

Selenium is most extensively used in the manufacture of metal plate rectifiers, photoelectric cells and other electronic devices. It is also employed as an additive to alloys steels, to decolorize poor grade green glass, in insecticides and with cadmium to produce orange and maroon pigments.

Elemental selenium is believed to be harmless to man but it burns readily in air producing dark red selenium dioxide fume which is irritant and toxic. Hydrogen selenide gas, which may be evolved when the metal comes in contact with acid or water, is also dangerous.

Selenium dioxide (SeO_2)

Exposure to fume which smells of garlic may occur when selenium is added to furnaces or ladles and under other conditions of heating when it may also take the form of a light powder. Inhalation causes upper and lower respiratory tract irritation with cough and substernal pain and, in large amounts, may result in non-fatal pulmonary oedema. In addition, gastric irritation and epigastric pain after meals and, occasionally haematuria may occur. But no chronic pulmonary effects appear to have been reported.

Hydrogen selenide (selenium anhydride, H_2Se)

Contact with this gas is less likely to arise in industry than exposure to selenium dioxide but it appears to be more toxic. Acute intoxication has occurred in laboratory workers and as a result of industrial accidents in processes where selenium is present, for example: heating copper, zinc or lead; the production of glass; and roasting pyrites. Accidental leakage from cylinders of the gas has caused acute respiratory disease (Schecter *et al.*, 1980).

The symptoms are similar to those caused by sulphur dioxide. Initially there is watering of the eyes and nose, sneezing, cough and chest tightness which recover fairly quickly. These are followed after about six to eight hours by the symptoms and signs of pulmonary oedema often during the night. Severe dyspnoea with violent coughing, pneumomediastinum and subcutaneous emphysema have been reported 18 hours after exposure and were associated with severe obstructive and restrictive functional defects which slowly improved, though some impairment was still present three years later (Schecter *et al.*, 1980). However, fatal cases have not been described and this may be attributable to hydrogen selenide being rapidly oxidized to elemental selenium on mucosal surfaces.

Treatment includes oxygen, diurectics and, probably, corticosteroids and antibiotics.

Prevention involves careful control of selenium-using processes, provision of goggles and respirators and storage of selenium away from acids and water (Clinton, 1947; Glover, 1970).

TITANIUM TETRACHLORIDE

This is referred to in Chapter 6 (p. 127). It is highly irritant and, due possibly to the production of hydrochloric acid within the lungs, may cause severe pulmonary oedema.

VANADIUM

Vanadium (atomic number, 23) is found in combination with other elements in igneous and sedimentary rocks and in some petroleum deposits because of the fossilized remains of sea squirts of the tunicate family and sea cucumbers whose normal blood consists, in part, of vanadium.

Sources of exposure and uses

Vanadium ore is first crushed and dried ('inactive ore'), finely ground in a ball mill ('active ore') and roasted; it is then mixed with sulphuric acid and the resulting precipitate, which is dried, is vanadium pentoxide. This is packed in bags. The roasting and bagging processes tend to produce most dust, grinding and crushing, rather less.

Vanadium-bearing slags, produced on a large scale during the manufacture of steel from titaniferous magnetite, are becoming an increasingly important source of vanadium in some countries (for example, South Africa and the USSR). Other important sources of vanadium-containing dusts are furnace residues from oil refineries, soot from oil-fired boilers and slags from the production of ferrovanadium (Williams, 1952). The soot is ground and treated with sodium hydroxide and slag is crushed, extracted with water, neutralized with sulphuric acid and filtered. In addition to vanadium, carbon dust is also produced by these processes. Deposit formed on heat-exchanger tubes of gas turbines contains some 11 to 20 per cent of vanadium (Browne, 1955); its removal gives rise to much dust.

Carnotite ($K_2O.2UO_3.V_2O_5.3H_2O$), a uranium-containing vanadium mineral found in South Australia and Colorado and Utah in the USA, forms the cementing material of sandstones and, being disseminated through them, must be mined with them. After mining it is milled and processed on a large scale as a uranium source. Mining and milling may thus carry a quartz risk, but the chief potential hazard to health lies in the production of radon decay products (Archer *et al.*, 1962) (*see* Chapter 14).

Vanadium metal is used extensively for metal alloys; ferrovanadium and molybdenum-vanadium steels, and vanadium bronze and brass. Vanadium pentoxide and ammonium vanadate (NH_4VO_3) are used as catalysts in the manufacture of various chemicals and ammonium vanadate and other vanadium salts are also employed in inks, dyeing processes, paints, insecticides, photographic developer and glass production.

Pathology

Acute bronchitis and pneumonitis or bronchopneumonia may follow heavy exposure to vanadium pentoxide dust and fume. The pneumonic lesions are usually patchy but they may be widespread and confluent.

Wyers (1946) suggested on the grounds of alleged abnormalities in chest radiographs of vanadium-exposed workers (but without the benefit of pathological examination of lungs) that permanent lung changes—interpreted as fibrosis—were caused by vanadium pentoxide, but Sjöberg (1950) and Williams (1952) did not confirm this. In fact, no pathological studies appear to be on record which demonstrate fibrosis in human lungs attributable to vanadium. However, mild cases of silicosis due to the presence of small quantities of quartz in the dust of dry sedimented dross seem to have occurred, though mining of the ore and exposure to metallic vanadium appear to be harmless.

Rabbits exposed to low concentrations of vanadium pentoxide for more than eight months showed no evidence of lung fibrosis, and no fibrosis resulted after its injection into the peritoneum of guinea pigs (Sjöberg, 1950).

Symptoms and physical signs

Exposure to fairly high concentrations of vanadium pentoxide dust (such as may result from the soot and bottom ash of oil-fired boilers in ships and electricity generating stations, from furnace residues of oil refineries and from slags from the production of ferrovanadium) causes intense irritation of the nose and eyes with lacrimation, sore throat and persistent, often violent cough. The cough develops a few hours after exposure and persists for seven to ten days. It is often accompanied by wheeze which may last two or three days (Lewis, 1959; Zenz and Berg, 1967). On examination, this is not always present but transient crepitations and wheezes may follow re-exposure. Sometimes wheezing is pronounced and associated with dyspnoea on exertion—in fact, it appears to be a late (non-immediate) asthmatic reaction (*see* Chapter 12). Bronchoscopy reveals diffuse hyperaemia of the mucosa of the trachea and bronchi with some viscid mucus. In the absence of pneumonic disease the patient is afebrile (Sjöberg, 1950). Both symptoms and signs clear completely (Zenz and Berg, 1967). Signs of bronchopneumonic consolidation may develop, however, following intense exposure.

Although chronic cough (Dutton, 1911) and dyspnoea (Wyers, 1946) have been attributed to vanadium exposure, there was no satisfactory evidence of a causative relationship. In Dutton's cases pulmonary tuberculosis appears to have been responsible. Prospective studies of vanadium workers have not shown that the presence of chronic cough, breathlessness and abnormal physical signs can be ascribed to this cause, although 'bronchitis with bronchospasm' appear to be enhanced by repeated exposure to europium-activated yttrium orthovanadate (Sjöberg, 1950; Vintinner *et al.*, 1955; Tebrock and Mackle, 1968). Furthermore, the assertion, sometimes made, that prolonged exposure to the dust of vanadium compounds causes chronic bronchitis and emphysema is not substantiated by available evidence (Sjöberg, 1950; Williams, 1952; Zenz and Berg, 1967). It should, perhaps, be noted that smoking habits have been largely ignored in most reports.

It is possible that hypersensitivity may play some part in the disease process for a positive skin reaction to a patch test with 2 per cent sodium vanadate has been observed after 48 hours in some cases although this did not correlate very well with the severity of the illness, and eosinophilia was not a feature (Sjöberg, 1950). In general, the test appears to be negative (Lees, 1980).

Tiredness and lassitude due to anaemia was at one time thought to occur in vanadium workers but this has not been confirmed (Hudson, 1964); on the contrary, it appears rather to stimulate haemopoiesis. Dyspnoea from this cause, therefore, can be discounted.

Vanadium is present in the urine of exposed workers of whom a small number develop a greenish-black furring of the tongue. The fur, which contains vanadium, may, however, indicate no more than inhalation of vanadium dust through the mouth (Hudson, 1964; Lees, 1980).

Lung function

No difference in VC between exposed subjects and controls was found by Sjöberg (1950) and Vintinner *et al.* (1955) did not observe any significant impairment of other spirometric values. Kiviluoto (1980) found no significant difference in ventilatory function compared with matched controls in a group of vanadium pentoxide production workers exposed to concentrations ranging from 0.1 to 3.9 mg/m^3 for an average of 11 years.

Zenz and Berg (1967) reported that, although volunteers exposed to 0.25 mg/m^3 of vanadium pentoxide for eight hours complained of cough within 24 hours which ceased in seven to ten days, the values of their ventilatory function tests over a period of weeks did not fall below pre-exposure values even when exposure was repeated. However, men exposed to 523 μg/m^3 time-weighted average of respirable dust ($<$ 10 μm) containing 15.3 per cent of vanadium from the bottom ash of oil-fired boilers developed a pronounced fall in FEV_1, FVC and FMF in 24 hours which did not fully return to normal in eight days, though four weeks after exposure there were no residual defects (Lees, 1980). This author suggests that transient loss of function is not attributable simply to reflex bronchial reaction to irritation by an inert dust (Lees, 1980).

Radiographic appearances

Appearances of unilateral or bilateral pneumonic consolidation or, possibly, small areas of segmental collapse may be present after heavy exposure. Otherwise no abnormality is seen. Wyers (1946) reported fine linear markings ('X-ray reticulation') in three cases with low level exposure but the validity of this observation—which has never been confirmed (Williams, 1952; Tebrock and Mackle, 1968)—is most doubtful. Discrete opacities have not been described (*see* Chapter 6).

Diagnosis

Because the symptoms and signs are identical to those of an acute upper and lower respiratory infection it is necessary to identify recent exposure to vanadium pentoxide dust or fume, and to exclude viral or bacterial infection. In the absence of pneumonia lack of fever supports the diagnosis. Detection of vanadium in the blood and urine is proof of exposure.

The possibility of non-immediate vanadium-induced asthma should be borne in mind.

As vanadium does not cause any permanent radiographic abnormality there can be no confusion with pneumoconiosis or other forms of lung disease. If this is not understood abnormal radiographic shadows in a worker known to have been exposed to vanadium dust or fume in the past may be wrongly attributed to this cause and the responsible disease thus overlooked.

Prognosis

No permanent pulmonary damage appears to be attributable to exposure to vanadium pentoxide. Pneumonia usually recovers completely with appropriate treatment but, occasionally, after heavy exposure, it may be fatal.

Treatment

Apart from bronchopneumonia to which the standard principles apply, treatment is symptomatic.

Prevention

Efficient, well-fitting respirators for exposed personnel are essential. Routine annual spirometry and quantitative analysis of urinary vanadium as an index of the amount absorbed have been suggested (Lees, 1980).

ZINC

Zinc oxide fume has been referred to earlier as a potent cause of metal fume fever. In general, zinc salts are not harmful to the lungs but zinc chloride smoke is an important exception.

Zinc chloride is employed in galvanizing iron, oil refining, dry batteries and taxidermy, and has been used for smoke bombs in war time and for fire fighting exercises. Normally it is rarely hazardous, but if encountered in confined spaces the smoke can be lethal. Acute oedema and chemical pneumonia occur and may progress to dense DIPF with fatal pulmonary heart disease within a few weeks. The radiographic changes are those of pulmonary oedema or patchy irregular consolidation (Evans, 1945; Whitaker, 1945; Milliken, Waugh and Kadish, 1963).

Prevention includes the wearing of respiratory protective equipment and protective clothing.

ZIRCONIUM TETRACHLORIDE ($ZrCl_4$)

This is produced in the chlorination process for the preparation of zirconium. It reacts violently with water and is usually found in gaseous form. It is on record as causing severe pulmonary oedema (Cordasco and Stone, 1973).

NON-METALLIC GASES

Many of these gases are irritant to mucous membranes and so are capable of causing inflammation of airways or pulmonary oedema if a sufficient concentration is inhaled. A highly soluble gas (ammonia, for example) gives rise to immediate and intense irritation of eyes, nose and upper respiratory tract which impels the exposed individual to make a prompt escape if he can. In these circumstances only small amounts of the gas reach the lower respiratory tract, and the lungs are little, if at all, affected. But if escape is impossible or the concentration of the gas is high sufficient quantities may reach the alveoli to provoke pulmonary oedema. An irritant gas of low solubility (such as nitrogen dioxide or phosgene), on the other hand, has no, or only a minor, irritant effect on the upper respiratory tract so that the worker may inhale considerable amounts before leaving the contaminated area, and its effects on the lungs may be delayed for a number of hours. Gases of intermediate solubility (such as chlorine) cause pulmonary oedema if exposure is fairly prolonged or concentration is high. In some instances—especially if the noxious gas is a respiratory depressant (for example, hydrogen sulphide and methyl bromide)—pulmonary oedema may be due to hypoxia of the lung rather than to direct assault by the gas on alveolar membranes.

In general, non-fatal cases of acute pulmonary damage from exposure to a noxious gas appear to recover completely although secondary patchy pneumonia may occur during recovery resulting on occasion in small areas of permanent segmental fibrosis. However, no prolonged follow-up studies of substantial numbers of severe gassing accidents seem to have been reported.

ACETALDEHYDE (ETHANAL, $CH_3.CHO$)

This volatile, colourless liquid with a strong pungent odour is produced by oxidation of ethylene gas. Its main use is as an intermediary in the production of a large number of chemicals, but it is also used in the manufacture of synthetic resins, plastics, synthetic rubber and disinfectants. It is highly irritant to the respiratory tract and is narcotic.

Low concentrations cause irritation of the eyes and hypersecretion of the upper respiratory and bronchial mucus. High concentrations cause headache, stupor and acute pulmonary oedema which may not develop for some 24 hours.

Treatment, in most cases, consists simply of the relief of symptoms but, if there is suspicion of exposure to high concentrations, observation for development of pulmonary oedema should be maintained for at least 48 hours.

Prevention depends upon good ventilation, avoidance of spillages, and protective goggles and clothing.

ACROLEIN (ACRYLIC ALDEHYDE, CH_2:CHCHO)

This is an oily liquid produced by catalytic oxidation of propylene. In the liquid state it presents little hazard but, as it has a high vapour pressure it may quickly form dangerous concentrations of a colourless, pungent, irritating gas.

It is used in the manufacture of plastics, textile finishes, acrylates, synthetic fibres and pharmaceuticals, and may be evolved when oils and fats containing glycerol are heated to high temperatures such as may occur in the production of soap, fatty acids and linseed oil, and during the reduction of animal fats.

Because the gas is so irritating serious intoxication is rare as it is impossible to tolerate its effects for more than a brief period. But accidental leakages or spillages from vessels or pipes may cause inhalation of high concentrations by workers before they can make their escape. This is followed by productive cough, shortness of breath, chest tightness and the signs of pulmonary oedema.

Treatment with oxygen, corticosteroids and an antibiotic must be commenced as soon as possible as there is a risk of permanent lung damage.

AMMONIA

Ammonia is a colourless, highly soluble, extremely irritant alkaline gas. It is used extensively in industry. Very large quantities are employed in the manufacture of soil fertilizers and in the pharmaceutical and chemical industries. Its other important uses include: refrigeration, the manufacture of plastics and explosives, oil refining and as an additive to furnaces to inhibit oxidation.

In most instances exposure to the gas occurs as a result of rupture or leakage of tanks or other containers, fractured pipes or valve failures. The general public may also be affected if transporter tanks are involved in road or rail accidents (Caplin, 1941; Kass *et al.*, 1972; Walton, 1973; Sobonya, 1977).

Because of its high solubility ammonia causes chemical burns of eyes, skin, oropharynx and upper respiratory tract. There is severe burning pain in the mouth and throat followed quickly by a feeling of suffocation with cough, copious watery sputum and difficulty in breathing. With exposure to high concentrations death occurs from asphyxia due to obstructive laryngeal oedema; with lower exposures the severity of symptoms varies.

In death shortly after exposure the post-mortem appearances are those of severe laryngeal and pulmonary oedema with haemorrhage (Walton, 1973). In patients who survive for some days bacterial infection supervenes, and terminal pneumonia due to *Nocardia asteroides* has been described (Sobonya, 1977). Many who survive acute disease recover completely, though slowly, but others may be left with bronchiectasis (which may be severe and widespread) and fibrous obliteration of small airways (Kass *et al.*, 1972; Sobanya, 1977).

Clinically, the heavily exposed individual is in respiratory distress with blood stained sputum, cyanosis, stridor, loss of voice and fever; and, in addition, to the signs of pulmonary oedema, there are chemical burns of varying degree. The chest radiograph may show the features of pulmonary oedema but correlation between the severity of clinical disease and radiographic appearances seems to be poor; often there is no evident abnormality. Patients with no abnormal physical signs in the chest tend to recover in 24 hours whereas those with abnormal signs have a more protracted and complicated course. Thus, the clinical signs are the best guide to prognosis (Montague and MacNeil, 1980).

Treatment is a matter of urgency in severely affected individuals and often requires an intensive care regime. The complication of serious secondary pulmonary infection must be anticipated. Otherwise conservative medical treatment is usually sufficient.

CHLORINE

Chlorine is a greenish-yellow gas, two and a half times heavier than air, the toxic qualities of which were exploited in the First World War. It is used in the manufacture of innumerable chemicals varying from pharmaceuticals to plastics, and for disinfecting water. It is usually transported commercially by road, sea or rail as a liquid under pressure. Exposure may occur during a manufacturing process, from leakage of pipes or tanks, from accidental spillage during transportation or as a result of mixing chlorine bleach with an acid cleaner (Jones, 1952; Chasis *et al.*, 1947; Joyner and Durel, 1962; Kowitz *et al.*, 1967; Weill *et al.*, 1969). Swimming pool attendants may also be accidentally exposed when changing gas cylinders (Decker and Koch, 1978).

The injurious effects of the gas are thought to be due to its potent oxidative properties which liberate nascent oxygen—a protoplasmic poison—from water and to the fact that hydrochloric acid is formed (Kramer, 1967). The changes in the lungs may be those of oedema with some fibrin and the formation of hyaline membrane in alveoli and early bronchiolar damage and obstruction of small blood vessels by thrombi. Brief concentrations of 3 to 5 ppm of the gas appear to be tolerated without injury, but exposure to 5 to 8 ppm for a significantly long period may cause mild acute illness. Levels of 14 to 21 ppm are dangerous and when over 40 ppm acute pulmonary oedema occurs. The effects of exposure, however, depend not only on the concentration of gas but also on duration of exposure, and the presence or absence of pre-existing disease. The very young and the aged suffer more severely than healthy adults (Kramer, 1967).

Clinical features

Symptoms of over-exposure consist of smarting of the eyes, lacrimation, rhinorrhoea, severe persistent cough, dyspnoea, retrosternal chest pain and a sense of constriction. Nausea, epigastric pain and vomiting may also occur. In spite of the severity of the symptoms the patient usually recovers quickly when removed from the area of contamination. With higher concentrations of gas there is pink, frothy sputum, and restlessness, severe respiratory distress, central cyanosis, widespread coarse crepitations—often with wheezing—and low-grade fever (Beach, Sherwood Jones and Scarrow, 1969). The patient is critically ill for some 48 hours and, even with appropriate treatment it may be some weeks before dyspnoea on exertion finally ceases.

The chest radiograph of severely ill patients shortly after exposure shows the signs of pulmonary oedema which may occasionally be followed in a few days by bronchopneumonic consolidation. However, although both oedema and secondary infection are uncommon complications, death sometimes occurs (Flake, 1964; Beach, Sherwood Jones and Scarrow, 1969).

In fatal cases there is acute laryngo-tracheobronchitis and large quantities of frothy, bloody fluid in the lungs and airways. Microscopy shows massive pulmonary oedema, and some alveolar spaces filled with polmorphonuclear leucocytes and thrombosis in large proximal and central blood vessels. If death is delayed for 75 hours or so after exposure, hyaline membranes are present with fibrin in the capillary vessels (Weston *et al.*, 1972).

After clinical recovery there are no residual respiratory symptoms and lung function apparently returns to normal (Weill *et al.*, 1969), although in the first six months after exposure there may be some impairment of ventilatory function—chiefly in smokers—which by 12 months is very slight. But long-term follow-up of some victims of a severe gassing accident in the USA is in progress (Weill, 1980).

Occasionally the development of pulmonary oedema is delayed for up to two days after exposure.

Long-term exposure of chlorine gas workers to concentrations of less than 1 ppm is not associated with significant impairment of ventilatory function, but those who smoke have a lower maximum mid-expiratory flow rate than non-smokers (Chester, Gillespie and Krause, 1969).

Treatment

This is similar to that required for nitrogen dioxide poisoning with the exception of correction of methaemoglobulinaemia (*see* p. 479). A bronchodilator in nebulizer form is often recommended but may be unnecessary if corticosteroids are used. In healthy adults with mild poisoning, simple symptomatic treatment and oxygen at atmospheric pressure may be all that is needed. The case of intense exposure from which the individual cannot immediately escape is a medical emergency which demands prompt treatment of shock, coma and respiratory arrest.

Pre-employment medical examination of workers who may be exposed to a potential chlorine hazard should be done to exclude those with respiratory or cardiovascular disease.

HYDROGEN CHLORIDE (HYDROCHLORIC ACID)

This is evolved as a gas or vapour during the production of hydrochloric acid by various methods; in particular during decanting, the operation of pumps and the use of pouring frames. Accidental exposure may sometimes occur in the manufacture of dyes, fertilizers and textiles; in the rubber and ore refining industries; in fires, and during welding in an atmosphere containing halogenated hydrocarbons. But serious exposures are rare because the highly irritant nature of the vapour quickly warns the worker of its presence.

Inhalation of a substantial quantity of the vapour causes irritation of the upper respiratory tract, acute bronchitis, oedema of the glottis and pulmonary oedema.

HYDROGEN FLUORIDE (HYDROFLUORIC ACID, HF)

This is produced by the reaction of concentrated sulphuric acid and fluorspar (calcium fluoride). It is a colourless gas which smells a little like chlorine, is readily soluble in water and forms a dense white vapour in moist air. It is used in the production of fluorocarbons and inorganic fluorides, in the refining of certain metals, as a constituent of some types of welding electrodes, as a catalyst for electro-tinning of steel and in the chemical industry.

Hydrogen fluoride is highly irritant and toxic to the skin and mucous membranes and inhalation cause burning of the nose, mouth and throat which may be followed by pulmonary oedema and pneumonia, the symptoms and signs of which, however, may not develop for 12 to 24 hours. The oedema may be severe enough to cause asphyxia requiring the full resources of an intensive-care unit.

Preventive measures include special handling methods, exhaust ventilation and appropriate personal protection. Containers for transportation, duly labelled, are designed to avoid accidental spillage.

HYDROGEN SULPHIDE (SULPHURETTED HYDROGEN, H_2S)

This gas is classed as an asphyxiant because, following absorption from the lungs, it rapidly causes central respiratory paralysis. But it is also an irritant. It is encountered as a by-product in the manufacture of some chemicals and dyes; in the rayon, tannery and rubber industries; in petroleum refining; in areas of volcanic activity; in mines with sulphide ores; in sewers; and in the fishing and fish meal industries—in which, incidentally, ammonia may also be a hazard (Dalgaard *et al.*, 1972).

Exposure to concentrations greater than about 700 ppm (which are, usually, accidental) causes death from respiratory failure due to depression of medullary centres before the irritant effects in the lungs have time to develop. More prolonged exposure to lower levels (for example, 300 to 600 ppm) result in pain in the nose, throat and chest, cough, headache, and dizziness followed by pulmonary oedema which may be complicated by pneumonia.

Oedema is both inter- and intra-alveolar and haemorrhagic. There is widespread damage to Type I pneumocytes and, to a lesser extent, to capillary endothelial cells (Biesold, Bachofen and Bachofen, 1974).

Respiratory failure can be reversed by prompt artificial respiration after removing the subject from exposure, otherwise intensive treatment for toxic pulmonary oedema is required.

METHYL BROMIDE (BROMETHANE)

This gas ($CH_3.Br$) which has a low boiling point is used as a refrigerant, herbicide, fumigant insecticide, and in the manufacture of aniline dyes. It has also been employed as a fire extinguishing agent. Though one of the most toxic of the organic halides it gives little warning of its presence to the senses and disperses slowly. It is thus highly dangerous especially if encountered in enclosed spaces.

Inhalation of high concentrations of the gas cause acute bronchitis with frothy, bloodstained sputum, signs of pulmonary oedema sometimes with haemorrhagic pleural effusions. In addition, there may be convulsions with other neurological abnormalities and subsequent coma. In such cases prognosis is poor. With exposure to lower concentrations pulmonary involvement is unusual but may occur in milder form, and the abnormalities (giddiness, convulsions, ataxia, pyramidal and extrapyramidal signs, changes EEG and anuria) are confined to the central nervous system and kidneys. Symptoms and signs generally develop some two to four hours after exposure but are often insidious and may be delayed for about 48 hours.

Diagnosis depends on history of exposure. The presence of convulsions and prominent neurological signs, however, may distract attention from involvement of the lungs.

Treatment of individuals with pulmonary symptoms and signs includes immediate removal from exposure, oxygen, corticosteroids and bed rest. Seizures require the use of anticonvulsive agents (Johnstone, 1945; Rathus and Landy, 1961).

Prevention involves mixing some pungent substance which can be readily smelled with methyl bromide, the use of efficient halide detectors, efficient ventilation and, where necessary, the wearing of appropriate gas masks.

OXIDES OF NITROGEN

The oxides of nitrogen include nitrous oxide (N_2O), nitric oxide (NO), nitrogen dioxide (NO_2), nitrogen trioxide (N_2O_3) and nitrogen tetroxide (N_2O_4). Nitrous oxide, of course, is a harmless anaesthetic gas. The other oxides which may occur in industry originate as NO. Nitric oxide is fairly stable having a half-life of about 10 ppm/hour and, therefore, converts slowly to NO_2 (the situation in the case of explosions may be different) (Commins, 1972). Nitrogen dioxide may polymerize to N_2O_4 which is so unstable that it promptly dissociates to NO_2. These gases are often popularly, but incorrectly, referred to as 'nitrous fumes'. Nitrogen dioxide is a reddish-brown gas which is heavier than air, has an odour like domestic bleach and is the oxide of medical importance.

Nitrogen dioxide may be encountered in a wide variety of industrial situations: during the manufacture and use of nitric acid, and the manufacture of explosives; during welding electroplating and engraving; in the exhaust from metal cleaning processes; in forage tower silos; during shot-firing in mines and other blasting operations; from slow burning of gun-cotton and cordite and from the exhaust of diesel engines. Nitrogen dioxide is used as a constituent of jet engine and missile fuels. It has also occurred as an accidental contaminant of nitrous oxide for anaesthesia (Clutton-Brock, 1967).

The occurrence of nitrogen dioxide in metal welding and cutting is referred to in the section on welding p. 482.

The oxides of nitrogen and their effects on man and animals are comprehensively reviewed by the World Health Organization (1977).

Forage tower silos

The need for a reliable supply of bulk fodder for cattle in winter months led to the adoption of ensilage of grass or other green crops. This began on the European continent in the mid-nineteenth century and spread to Britain (Jenkins, 1884). At first, lined pits or adapted barns were used but the method was a failure owing to lack of understanding of the biological processes involved. The tower silo was introduced to the eastern counties of England from the USA at the beginning of this century (Hall, 1923). However, it was not generally adopted because of the expense involved, and above-ground clamps, later with devices for self-feeding of cattle, were in common use until the 1950s (Turner, 1953). Then, a new type of American tower silo with mechanical loading and distributing equipment came to Britain in the late 1950s and has been installed increasingly since, its stark outline in the countryside being a mark of agricultural change (*Figure 13.5*).

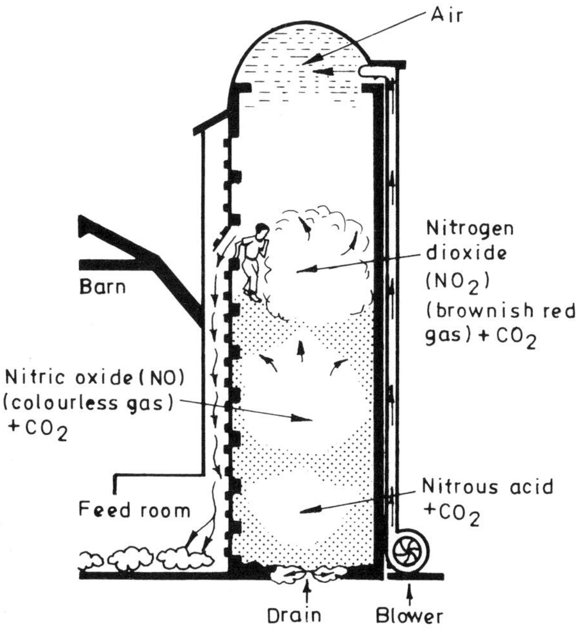

Figure 13.5 Diagram (not to scale) of a forage tower silo. (Adapted, with permission, from Ramirez and Dowell (1971) and the Editor of Annals of Internal Medicine*)*

Concentrations of nitrogen dioxide produced during the preparation of silage may be sufficiently high to cause death to a worker entering a silo (Grayson, 1956; Lowry and Schuman, 1956; Delaney, Schmidt and Stroebel, 1956; Desbaumes, 1968; *Farmer and Stockbreeder,* 1970).

Evolution of carbon dioxide—which is detected first (Commins, Raveney and Jesson, 1971)—and NO_2 begins a few hours after silo-filling commences, is maximal in one to two days and continues at a decreasing rate for a week or ten days (Lowry and Schuman, 1956). At the same time, the concentration of oxygen falls. The processes which underlie the production of these gases are not wholly understood but appear broadly to be as follows.

Carbohydrates in the crops yield acetic and lactic acids and CO_2 due to degradation by bacteria. The nitrate content of plants is derived chiefly from inorganic nitrates which are converted into nitrites by enzymatic action; it is increased by soils highly nitrated by fertilizers, by drought and by immaturity of the plants. The potential concentration of NO_2 is said to be roughly proportional to the amount of nitrate in the silage crop by some authors (Lowry and Schuman, 1956) but not by others (Commins, Raveney and Jesson, 1971). The nitrites react with the acids to form nitrous acid (HNO_2) which decomposes to water, NO and NO_2 as the temperature of the silage rises due to fermentation (Grayson, 1956). Temperatures 3½ feet (105 cm) below the silage surface may range from 40.6 to 57 °C (Delaney, Schmidt and Stroebel, 1956). Initially the concentration of NO is higher than that of NO_2 but later this situation is reversed and the ratio NO_2/NO rises (Commins, Raveney and Jesson, 1971). Some N_2O_4 is also evolved but breaks down rapidly to NO_2. According to the type of crop, its pH and moisture content, bacterial activity may, in addition, give rise to free ammonia, butyric acid and free amines.

The presence and concentrations of the gases vary widely in different towers but there is no evidence that those made of concrete slats are less likely to develop potentially dangerous concentrations, due to their porosity, than steel towers (Jesson, 1972).

Both CO_2 and NO_2, being about one and a half times heavier than air, are concentrated at or near the silage surface and in depressions. Dangerous amounts of gas may be present, not only for a few days after filling, but some months later if the silo has remained unopened. The silage surface and silo wall may be stained yellow-red and a similar coloured vapour may be seen above the surface. An open door in the discharge (or feed) chute permits the gases to flow down into an attached barn (*Figure 13.5*). A man entering the silo does so normally through a chute door above the silage surface. He climbs the vertical chute

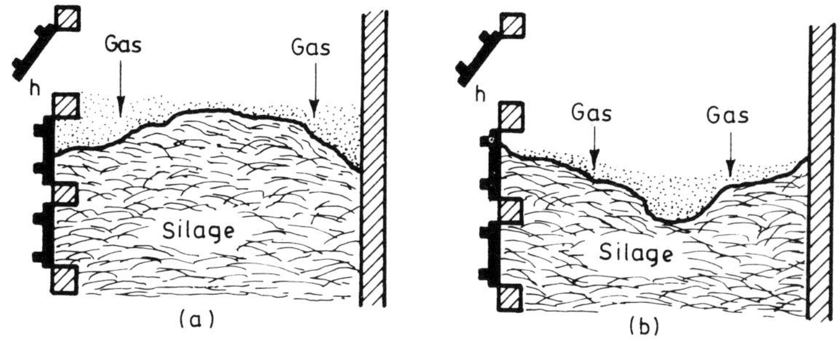

Figure 13.6 Diagram showing two different contours of the silage surface. Gas is likely to be encountered by the farm worker as he climbs on to a convex surface (a) from the hatch (h) or descends into a central concavity (b) disturbing pockets of NO_2 gas

ladder, opens one of the chute doorways at the appropriate height, climbs through the narrow opening and jumps on to the surface which may be a few feet below. If he becomes unwell due to the effects of accumulated gases he may be physically incapable of the effort necessary to retrace his path through the door and down the ladder. When the surface is convex he is more likely to encounter higher gas concentrations immediately on entry than when it is concave, but a concavity may also contain high concentrations (*Figure 13.6*). Levelling the silage surface, therefore, may be a dangerous procedure if the difference between its highest and lowest levels exceeds the height of a man (Jesson, 1972). When the surface is concave the peripheral concentration of gas may be too low at breathing level to be detected by smell and so cause a false sense of security on entry; while the higher concentrations at the surface and in depressions may make descent into a

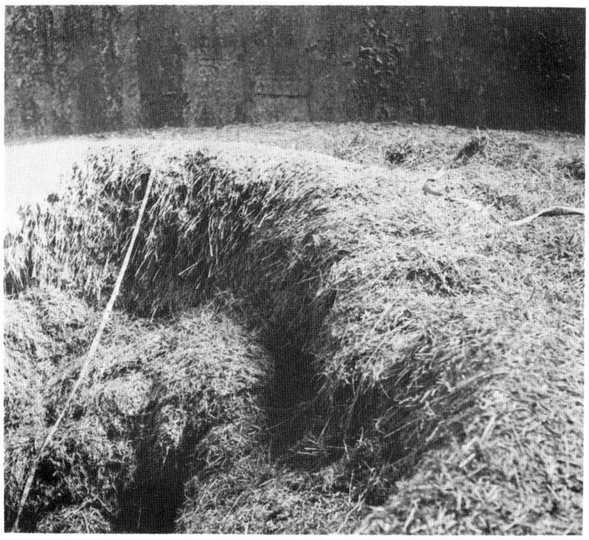

Figure 13.7 Photograph showing a concavity in the silage some five or six feet deep in the silage surface. The potential danger of the situation is evident. (By courtesy of Mr M. W. Jesson and the National Institute of Agricultural Engineering, Silsoe, Bedfordshire)

depression and its disturbance during levelling, or an accidental fall, especially hazardous (*Figure 13.7*). Furthermore, the movement of men in a tower disturbs the gases and may release gas trapped in the silage.

The presence of high CO_2 and low oxygen concentrations are important as they cause deep breathing which facilitates penetration of nitrogen dioxide to alveolar level and so enhances its effect (Commins, Raveney and Jesson, 1971). High concentrations of gas render a man helpless in two or three minutes (*Farmer and Stockbreeder*, 1970).

Respiratory illness due to nitrogen dioxide in silos is known as *silo fillers' disease*. Its potential seriousness and the increasingly widespread use of tower silos indicate the necessity for a general awareness of the risks involved.

Mining

Nitrogen dioxide is produced in varying degree by the firing of nitro-explosive charges in mines and from the exhaust of diesel haulage locomotives.

The regular use of 'exhaust gas conditioners' on diesel engines in British coal-mines greatly reduces the output of NO_2, and concentrations of the gas in the vicinity of these engines and in the driver's cab are usually well below the recommended TLV. The average concentration of nitrogen dioxide appears to be about 10 per cent of the nitrogen oxides in undiluted exhaust gases (Godbert and Leach, 1970).

Concentrations of gas from shot-firing only reach dangerous levels under conditions of imperfect detonation of charges or poor ventilation which may exist, for example, in tunnelling operations. Ventilation in most areas of coal-mines is good and serious pulmonary disease does not, therefore, occur. However, as there is some speculation that shot-firing in coal-mines might constitute a hazard to underground workers the matter must be discussed in a little more detail. If an effect were produced it would be most likely to occur in men ('deputies' and shot-firers) working on headings and in tunnels, although in British coal-mines it is the practice that they do not return to the working place for at least ten minutes after firing more than six charges, or at least five minutes after firing six or less.

Both NO and NO_2 are produced by the explosion, the former being present in larger quantity, and the production of these gases varies little with the different explosives used but those with a negative or near-negative oxygen balance give rise to smaller quantities of gas. The gases are evolved in the form of a bolus and the rate at which this travels away from the explosion and is dispersed is determined by the velocity of the ventilating air. As the bolus passes a given point the concentration of the gases rises rapidly and then gradually falls, and the further it travels from source the more the gases are diluted. Hence, peak concentrations are very brief and the men are not likely to be exposed to them because they are outside the area. There is, moreover, no evidence that such transient peak concentrations have any medical significance.

Thus, in general, coal-miners have not been exposed to the risk of developing acute disease (Kronenberger, 1959) though four possible cases of pulmonary oedema attributed to high exposure to shot-firing gases in 1960/1961 were reported by Kennedy (1972).

A variety of conditions influence the amount of oxides produced. They include the nature and quantity of explosive, the method of stemming and detonation, the area of the working place and the air volume. Therefore, although the concentrations vary from place to place those to which miners are subjected are uniformly low (Graham and Runnicles, 1943; Powell, 1961; Godbert and Leach, 1970). The average concentrations of mixed oxides for a whole working shift at the return end of the coal-face has been found to be 4 ppm (Graham and Runnicles, 1943), but may now be lower since the introduction of power loading in the 1960s. There is no satisfactory evidence to suggest that such concentrations are injurious to health, but the problem is currently (1980) under investigation in Britain by the National Coal Board.

Other occupational hazards

Firemen may be exposed to high concentrations of NO_2 from burning furnishings and fires in chemical plants. Due to inadvertent firing of the Reaction Control System in the Apollo–Soyuz spacecraft three American astronauts were exposed to NO_2 for about four minutes and developed acute pulmonary oedema the day after 'splashdown' (Hatton *et al.*, 1977).

Chemical effects

The severity of the effect of NO_2 depends mainly on its concentration and the duration of exposure to it, and is similar whatever its mode of origin. Unlike most water-soluble gases it is only feebly irritant to the upper respiratory tract. The reason for this is believed to be that, owing to its relatively low solubility, its conversion to HNO_2 and HNO_3—which are the cause of its harmful effects in the lungs—occurs slowly in water or humid air and is not maximal, therefore, until it reaches the peripheral airways and alveoli resulting in pulmonary oedema and chemical pneumonia (Pattey, 1963). Nitric acid apparently dissociates in the lungs into nitrates and nitrites resulting in local tissue damage and the formation of methaemoglobulin (Clutton-Brock, 1967), and methaemoglobulinaemia is known to follow exposure to high concentrations of NO_2.

Experimental observations

In animals

Short-term exposure of animals to 7 to 16 ppm of NO_2 causes endothelial damage with transudation of fluid into alveolar and air spaces, impairment of surfactant activity and airway closure (Dowell, Kilburn and Pratt, 1971). Oedema, haemorrhage, hyperinflation, desquamation of the respiratory epithelium and bronchopneumonia are produced by the inhalation of the higher oxides of nitrogen (Shiel, 1967). Long-term exposure of animals to 12 to 26 ppm of NO_2 has been reported to cause bronchiolar hyperplasia and mild centrilobular dilatation of alveoli (Freeman and Haydon, 1964); and some partial closure of terminal bronchioles by fibrosis and occasional attenuation and fracture of alveolar walls has been described many weeks after prolonged exposure to an average of 15 ppm of NO_2 had ceased (Freeman, Crane and Furiosi, 1969).

Drozdz, Kucharz and Szyja (1977) reported that guinea pigs exposed to 2 mg/m^3 NO_2 for 180 days develop emphysema-like lesions and reduction in collagen content of the lungs. But Kleinerman (1979) found that, in hamsters exposed to approximately 30 ppm NO_2—a high concentration—for 22 hours daily for three weeks, total collagen content decreased within four days but returned to normal in about 14 days, and that both collagen and elastin content were normal three weeks after exposure had been stopped. It has been suggested that alteration in collagen and elastin content and emphysema-like lesions in animals may be caused by enzyme activity but prolonged exposure of hamsters to 30 ppm NO_2 revealed no evidence of proteolytic enzyme activity (Kleinerman and Rynbrandt, 1976; Rynbrandt and Kleinerman, 1977). Interestingly, Kleinerman and Wright (1961) observed reversal of the lung lesions caused by single or multiple treatments of animals with nitrites.

In a series of '*in vitro*' experiments with 'macrophage-like cells' and sheep erythrocytes Davis *et al.* (1978) found no overall differences between the cytotoxic effects of pure coal-dust and samples onto which high levels of NO_2 had been adsorbed.

In man

To what extent (if at all) these and similar observations are relevant to man is uncertain. But some evidence of degradation of lung collagen, deduced from changes in urinary hydroxylysine glycosides, was observed in the Apollo astronauts who developed pulmonary oedema after short exposure to high concentrations of NO_2—average 250 ppm (510 mg/m^3) (Hatton *et al.*, 1977).

Healthy young men challenged with 5 ppm NO_2 for two hours a day developed a significant increase in airways resistance and decrease in alveolar–arterial oxygen pressure differences (Hackney and Linn, 1979); but young male non-smokers exposed to lower concentrations—0.62 ppm NO_2—for two hours showed no significant changes in pulmonary function, including no consistent alteration of closing volume or maximum expiratory flow rate at low lung volumes (FEV 75 per cent) (Folinsbee *et al.*, 1978). Though acute inhalation of NO causes some transient changes in lung function this gas is strikingly less toxic than NO_2 (World Health Organization, 1977).

Pathology

The gross appearances of the lungs in rapidly fatal cases following exposure to large concentrations of NO_2 are those of haemorrhagic oedema with watery blood-tinged fluid in the airways and patches of pneumonia; in patients who survive for a few weeks before finally succumbing there are small paplable nodules and haemorrhagic areas.

Microscopy of rapidly fatal cases shows, in addition to oedema, extensive damage of the respiratory epithelium which may be completely shed in the small bronchi and bronchioles; and in the later cases, generalized infiltration of alveolar walls with lymphocytes, numerous macrophages in alveolar spaces and bronchiolitis obliterans in various stages of organization which is responsible for the palpable nodules (McAdams, 1955; Darke and Warrack, 1958; Moskowitz, Lyons and Cottle, 1964). If the patient recovers, these lesions usually resolve completely, especially if he has been treated with corticosteroids (Moskowitz, Lyons and Cottle, 1964).

Clinical features

The absence of immediate and pronounced irritation of the upper respiratory tract allows the worker to inhale gas for some time without distress. Irritation of the throat does not apparently occur until concentration of the oxides of nitrogen reaches 60 ppm, and cough, not until it is 100 ppm (Pieters and Creyghton, 1951). Severe headache and dizziness which have sometimes been complained of by magazine attendants, 'deputies' and shot-firers in coalmines have been caused more by absorption of the nitroglycerin of explosives cartridges through the skin or by ingestion, or to the inhalation of carbon monoxide from an exploded charge than by nitrogen dioxide (Powell and Lomax, 1960). But dizziness may occur early in some cases of NO_2 exposure due to the production of systemic hypotension.

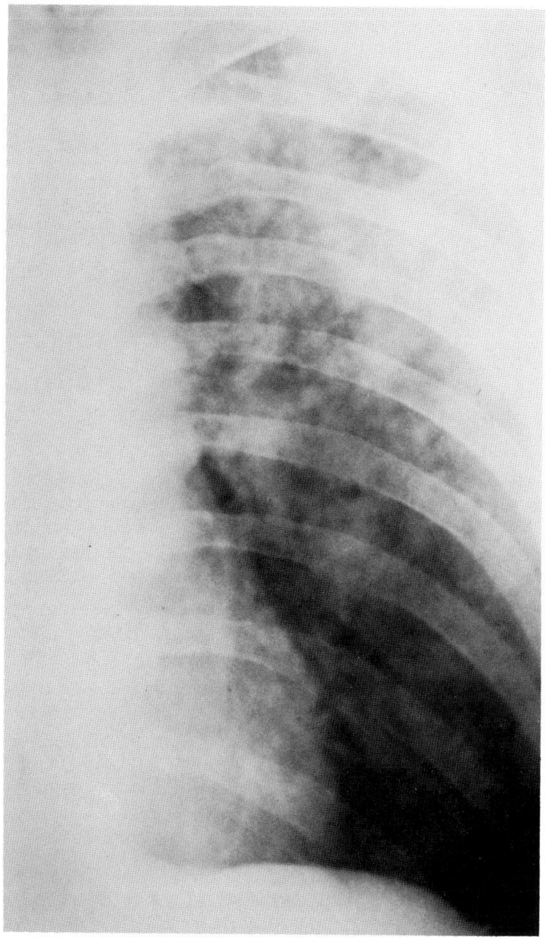

Figure 13.8 Confluent opacities which developed three to four weeks after exposure to high concentrations of nitrogen dioxide in a tower silo. The appearances in the right lung field were similar. Complete resolution and symptomatic recovery subsequently occurred. (Courtesy of Dr R. H. G. Greenspan, Connecticut)

The onset of respiratory symptoms is delayed for three to 30 hours after exposure (although some transient choking and tightness in the chest, and sometimes central chest pain with profuse sweating may occur during exposure) so that, in some cases, a man may return to work before becoming ill. However, in the mixed gas conditions which may be encountered in a tower silo a man may rapidly be rendered senseless.

The patient becomes acutely ill with paroxysmal cough, wheeze, frothy bloodstained sputum, nausea, vomiting, increasing dyspnoea, restlessness and anxiety. He is feverish (38.3 to 38.9 °C) and centrally cyanosed and there are widespread crepitations and polymorpholeucocytosis. There may be systemic hypotension and evidence of haemoconcentration due to intrapulmonary fluid loss; and the chest radiograph reveals the ill-defined, woolly opacities characteristic of pulmonary oedema. Death from respiratory failure may occur at this stage.

Patients who recover may pass into a latent period lasting *two to six weeks* during which time they continue to improve, and abnormal clinical and radiographic signs disappear, and then suddenly they relapse with a *second acute episode* similar to the first without having been re-exposed to the gas. The radiographic appearances consist either of small opacities (which have been mistaken for miliary tuberculosis) or confluent 'woolly' opacities (Becklake *et al.*, 1957) (*Figure 13.8*). The reason for this 'rebound' episode (which does not occur in every case) is uncertain: it may be due to recurrence of oedema provoked by a minor infection in lungs in which repair of previously damaged alveolar epithelial cells is incomplete. If this is so it is perhaps surprising that the phenomenon does not appear to be caused by any other toxic gas. It is also possible that it corresponds to the development of bronchio-alveolitis obliterans. However, recovery is usual with prompt treatment with corticosteroids, but irreversible bronchiolar fibrosis seems to have occurred in a few untreated cases (Moskowitz, Lyons and Cottle, 1964; Milne, 1969; Horvath *et al.*, 1978).

Hence, there are three distinct clinical stages:

(1) Acute oedema.
(2) A period of apparent recovery.
(3) Relapse in a second acute illness. This stage may develop even though the Stage 1 illness may have been mild.

Lung function during stages (1) and (3) shows variable abnormal patterns but vital capacity is much reduced, airways resistance increased, gas distribution uneven and gas transfer impaired. Serial tests during the delayed acute stage have shown normal elastic recoil and airflow resistance with reduction of dynamic compliance dependent on respiratory frequency, and hypoxaemia on exercise suggesting dysfunction of the small airways (Fleming, Chester and Montenegro, 1979). Although airways obstruction and reduction of gas transfer may be present for weeks or months after the chest radiograph has cleared it is rare to find any permanent abnormality of function (Becklake *et al.*, 1957; Ramirez-R. and Dowell, 1971; Jones, Proudfoot and Hall, 1973), but mild hyperinflation (Moskowitz, Lyons and Cottle, 1964) or airways obstruction have occasionally been reported though, in most of these cases, lung function values have not been recorded prior to exposure.

The chest radiograph clears quickly with treatment without evidence of residual lung damage.

Does exposure to nitrogen dioxide cause irreversible pulmonary damage?

This, in fact, poses two questions which must be considered separately.

(1) *Does acute disease with pulmonary oedema result in permanent lung damage?* As indicated in the previous section complete recovery is the rule in those cases of pulmonary oedema or bronchiolitis obliterans which have been followed for a sufficient length of time and is hastened by treatment with coricosteroids. But varying degrees of pulmonary dysfunction may persist in occasional cases due, possibly, to unresolved bronchiolitis. However, some follow-up studies can be criticized for being too short and lacking smoking histories and adequate clinical and physiological assessment (Horvath *et al.*, 1978).

(2) *Does intermittent, long-term exposure to low concentrations cause emphysema?* From his clinical and physiological investigation of 100 cases of coal-miners exposed to oxides of nitrogen during shot-firing underground, Kennedy (1972, 1974) contends that 'nitrous fumes' cause emphysema. However, there are some important deficiences in this study which put the validity of the conclusion in doubt: (a) the men investigated were not randomly selected and appear to have been referred because they had respiratory symptoms (McLintock, 1972); (b) there was no matched control group; (c) smoking habits were not taken into account; (d) the presence or absence of other pulmonary disease was not mentioned; (e) NO—which converts slowly to NO_2—and NO_2 were not monitored separately (Bergman, 1972). Similar criticisms apply to two other reports of workers exposed in non-mining occupations in which the same conjecture was advanced with the additional complication that the men had also been exposed to other toxic agents (Vigdortschik *et al.*, 1937; Kosmider *et al.*, 1972).

Because the open flames of gas cookers produce short-term peaks of NO_2 in cooking areas Keller *et al.* (1979a and b) investigated the prevalence of respiratory illness and ventilatory function ($FEV_{0.75}$ and FVC) in gas cooking compared with electric cooking households. They found no evidence that cooking with gas is associated with any excess of respiratory disease or impairment of lung function.

There is, then, no adequate proof to date that intermittent exposures to NO_2 cause emphysema, and the following two statements summarize current opinion on the matter.

(1) 'the literature on industrial exposure to oxides of nitrogen provides little useful data on the chronic or acute effects of low level exposures' (World Health Organization, 1977).

(2) 'presently, there is no conclusive evidence that long-term exposure to low levels of NO_2 leads to emphysema or chronic bronchitis in humans' (Horvath *et al.*, 1978).

However, comprehensive controlled, follow-up studies over a prolonged period of occupational groups exposed to NO_2 are necessary to provide an unequivocal and final answer to this question. It is to be hoped that the present National Coal Board investigation (referred to earlier) will contribute to this.

Diagnosis

Awareness of the pattern of illness caused by NO_2 and a detailed occupational and medical history will usually point to the diagnosis but it may be necessary to exclude myocardial infarction. It is vital that diagnosis is made without delay and that a second acute episode is not mistaken for pneumonia because failure to use appropriate corticosteroid treatment at this stage may be fatal. Even with immediate appropriate treatment mortality from acute disease may be as high as 30 per cent (Ramirez-R. and Dowell, 1971).

Acute farmers' lung may also occur as a result of disturbing mouldy material immediately below the silage surface while removing the top seal or unloading ('topping') of grass or grain (*see* Chapter 11, p. 376). The history is all important for differentiation. The risk of silo fillers' disease is associated with freshly filled silos and is, therefore, present during the harvest season; the worker may have noticed both the smell and yellow-red colour of the gas. Extrinsic allergic 'alveolitis' is most likely to occur in winter or spring due to moulding of the previous summer's harvest, and the signs of NO_2 gas will have been absent. The presence of methaemoglobinaemia may help to identify silo fillers' disease.

It is possible that widespread pulmonary fibrosis which has occasionally been attributed to silage gases in the past was in reality chronic extrinsic allergic 'alveolitis'.

Treatment

In all cases in which there has been a significant, or suspicion of significant, exposure to NO_2 admission to hospital for 48 to 72 hours is imperative. If signs of pulmonary oedema and respiratory distress develop corticosteroids should be commenced immediately and, in some patients oxygen, possibly with assisted ventilation, may be necessary. Steroid treatment should be continued for at least eight weeks to prevent relapse and the development of bronchiolitis obliterans (Horvath *et al.*, 1978). Other measures which may be needed are as follows:

(1) Antibiotics. Their use is indicated only if evidence of infection supervenes.
(2) Reconversion of methaemoglobulinaemia by an initial dose of methylene blue 2 mg/kg intravenously and subsequent doses titrated against the methaemoglobulin concentration in the blood (Prys-Roberts, 1967).
(3) Correction of haemoconcentration in some cases.
(4) The use of a vasopressor drug in the event of severe systemic hypotension.

The patient should be kept under observation for at least three months from the date of exposure.

Prevention

Good ventilation is the most important measure in any potential nitrogen dioxide hazard. Some welding processes can be subjected to exhaust ventilation techniques. Respirators used in enclosed spaces must be of approved type as some models are ineffective against NO_2.

Special measures apply to forage tower silos. These include:

(1) Thorough ventilation of the tower by use of the blower (*Figure 13.5*) for at least half an hour before entry (Jesson, 1972).
(2) A safety harness to which a rope can be attached should be worn and two workmates should be in attendance outside the tower.
(3) If it is necessary to enter a silo during filling (for example, to level the silage by hand), this should be done immediately after the last load and not left until the following day when gas may already have been evolved.

It has also been recommended that, after opening a chute door, the worker should immediately climb above it in order to be higher than any remaining gas which might escape. However, Jesson (1972) has shown that this manoeuvre cannot be relied upon and may be hazardous as the direction of air flow after the chute door is opened varies with wind direction.

Education of workers about the risks involved in their industry is important and there are recommended TLVs for NO_2 and NO.

OZONE

Ozone is a highly toxic gas and one of the most powerful oxidizing substances known. It is normally present in the atmosphere in minute quantities without any harmful effect, but it occurs in increased concentrations at high altitudes. Significant amounts may enter the cabins of aircraft at altitudes greater than 30 000 feet (9000 m) (Bennett, 1962; Young, Shaw and Bates, 1962). It is produced in lightning and high-tension, non-sparking, electrical discharges in air or oxygen. It is used in industry for sterilizing water, bleaching paper, flour and oils and deodorizing organic factory effluents by masking, but not destroying, the odour (Pattey, 1963).

The evolution of potentially dangerous levels of ozone from atmospheric oxygen by ultraviolet radiation produced by gas-shielded welding and arc-air gouging is referred to in the section on Welding and Similar Processes. Ultraviolet radiation from air-conditioning equipment and office photocopying machines may give rise to low levels but, in ordinary ventilated areas, these are unlikely to be harmful.

The effects of ozone on the lungs of experimental animals have been extensively investigated but they remain incompletely understood and their relevance to human beings uncertain (Cross *et al.*, 1976). Alveolar Type I cells are most vulnerable and undergo necrosis but Type II cells are remarkably resistant and proliferate to replace them even during continuous exposure to the gas (Stephens *et al.*, 1974; Castleman *et al.*, 1980); and Clara cells and alveolar macrophages are also stimulated though, with high concentrations of gas, the function of macrophages is inhibited (Huber *et al.*, 1971). It is also reported that prolonged exposure results in mild pulmonary fibrosis and high concentrations inhibit the activity of a variety of enzymes (Cross *et al.*, 1976).

There is suggestive evidence in man that elaboration of the enzyme superoxide dismutase protects the lungs of those chronically exposed to ozone-polluted, urban air (Hackney *et al.*, 1975).

Clinical features

Ozone is ten to 15 times more toxic than NO_2 (Stokinger, 1965).

Acute illness following heavy exposure (in excess of 2 ppm) is either rapid in onset consisting of severe headache, substernal pain and dyspnoea (suggesting myocardial infarction) or develops more slowly with irritation of the nose and eyes which may last for a day or so, with severe cough, bloodstained sputum, dyspnoea and fever. Symptoms, physical signs and radiographic appearances are those of pulmonary oedema. Exposures of from 5 to 20 ppm from one hour or more may be fatal (Kleinfeld, Giel and Tabershaw, 1957; Stokinger, 1965; EMAS, 1972).

Concentrations of 0.4 to 0.5 ppm inhaled for three hours a day for five days cause reduction of FVC and specific airways conductance in healthy human beings on the first three days but, subsequently, there are no significant differences and respiratory symptoms cease after the second day (Farrell *et al.*, 1979). In addition, with such concentrations there is no significant alteration in gas transfer or static compliance (Kerr *et al.*, 1975), though there may be transient changes with higher concentrations (Young, Shaw and Bates, 1964). Although levels less than 0.5 ppm have an inhibitory effect on acetylcholinesterase this is not apparently related to the presence of bronchoconstriction (as revealed by FEV_1 and maximal expiratory flow rates) which, at these concentations, occurs only in smokers (Fabbri *et al.*, 1979). Workers exposed to about 1 ppm or less complain of upper respiratory tract irritation, headache, tightness in the chest and wheezing (Challen, Hickish and Bedford, 1958).

Treatment

In cases of acute illness this is similar to that required for the effects of nitrogen dioxide, but methaemoglobulinaemia does not occur.

Prevention

Local exhaust ventilation is necessary where significant concentrations of the gas may occur but is unlikely to be adequate unless measures to screen off the ozone-producing source are taken (Frant, 1963).

PHOSGENE (CARBONYL CHLORIDE, $CO.Cl_2$)

This gas—used as a poison gas in the First World War—is

many times more toxic than chlorine, is about three and a half times heavier than air and has a sweet, pungent smell resembling new mown hay which, however, may not be detected at low concentrations.

Situations in which phosgene may cause poisoning are as follows: the chemical industry in which it is used as a chlorinating agent in the synthesis of organic compounds such as dyes; in the metallurgical industry for separation of certain metals by chlorination; during welding of metals cleaned with chlorinated hydrocarbons such as carbon tetrachloride and trichlorethylene which yield the gas when heated; the use of chlorinated hydrocarbons for fire fighting; and the use of paint removers such as methylene chloride in heated enclosed spaces (Gerritsen and Buschmann, 1960; Seidelin, 1961; Doig and Challen, 1964; English, 1964; Everett and Overholt, 1968). Although phosgene occurs in fires in which there is burning polyvinyl chloride (PVC) its quantitiy is very small and makes little or no contribution to the overall toxicity of the decomposition products (Wooley, 1971).

As phosgene is less soluble than chlorine and ammonia its effects fall chiefly on the alveoli and capillaries. Thus significant quantities of gas can be inhaled before any symptoms develop. At first there may be cough with some breathlessness and tightness in the chest but, with low concentrations, symptoms may be mild or absent. The symptoms and signs of pulmonary oedema and respiratory distress follow but often not until 24 to 48 hours after exposure. Collapse in hypovolaemic shock may occur with coma and death. The pathological changes include inter- and intra-alveolar oedema with sloughing of the bronchiolar mucosa.

Patients who survive recover completely over a period of one or two weeks and, as far as is known, have no permanent lung damage (Seidelin, 1961; English, 1964).

Prolonged exposure to minute concentrations of phosgene does not appear to have any adverse effects.

PHOSPHINE (HYDROGEN PHOSPHIDE, PH_3)

Exposure to this colourless gas which has the foul odour of rotten fish is uncommon and usually accidental and unexpected. It may occur under the following conditions: handling of hot phosphoric acid; processing of wet ferrosilicon metals due to the presence of metallic phosphides as impurities; production of acetylene; from aluminium phosphate stored under unsatisfactory moist conditions; welding of steel coated with phosphate rust-proofing; during the manufacture of phosphide agricultural insecticides and the striking surfaces of matchboxes with phosphorus sesquisulphide; and the use of calcium phosphide in the pyrotechnics industry. As a rule the offensive smell warns workers of its presence but the odour threshold is sufficiently high for dangerous concentrations to be unrecognized.

Inhalation of phosphine causes weakness, faintness, cough, dyspnoea and, in concentrations over about 300 ppm, pulmonary oedema which usually occurs in 24 hours but is occasionally delayed for a few days after exposure. Concentrations above 400 to 600 ppm are rapidly fatal with convulsions and coma (Pattey, 1963).

Treatment is similar to that for pulmonary oedema due to other toxic gases but absolute rest is necessary in seriously ill patients, and exposed individuals who do not appear to be seriously affected must be kept under close medical supervision for at least a week.

SULPHUR DIOXIDE (SO_2)

This gas, which is more than twice as heavy as air, is an intense respiratory irritant because it is first hydrated and then oxidized to sulphuric acid on mucosal surfaces. The most commonly encountered toxic gas, it is used extensively in the chemical and paper industries; and in bleaching, fumigation, refrigeration and preserving. It also occurs as a by-product of smelting sulphide ores and during the action of sulphuric acid on reducing agents. In the USA some 500 000 workers are believed to be at risk of exposure to acute sulphur dioxide inhalation (Charan *et al.,* 1979).

An accident involving five previously healthy men in the paper industry working inside or near a digester tank partly filled with wooden chips, and who were exposed to varying concentrations of the gas exemplifies the range of effects it can have. Two men inside the tank were able to climb out but died within five minutes in respiratory arrest and shock with pink frothy fluid around their mouths. The pharyngeal and laryngeal mucosa had a coagulated appearance and, microscopically, the superficial columnar epithelium was widely denuded. The lungs and airways were filled with pink, proteinaceous oedema fluid but there was no inflammation, cell infiltration and no disruption of alveolar walls. The three survivors outside the tank experienced tightness in the chest with intense dyspnoea, and soreness of eyes, nose and throat. Crepitations and rhonchi were heard in their lungs but chest radiographs were normal. One of these men subsequently developed irreversible airways obstruction with air trapping, hyperinflation and dyspnoea on slight exertion; and another (who was a smoker) had a mild degree of airflow obstruction four months after exposure. The third (a non-smoker), had no lung function abnormalities shortly after exposure or subsequently (Charan *et al.,* 1979).

As a rule most individuals who survive acute exposure recover completely.

In a recent study of paper pulp workers exposed frequently to low concentrations of sulphur dioxide gas and paper mill workers with no exposure there was no difference in mortality or specific cause of death between the two groups and little, if any, difference in pulmonary function values between them (Ferris, Puteo and Chen, 1979). And, in copper miners cumulative long-term, low exposure to the gas did not contribute to reduction in ventilatory capacity (Federspiel *et al.,* 1980). Low level exposure to sulphur dioxide is also referred to in Chapter 1 (Chronic Bronchitis).

WELDING AND SIMILAR PROCESSES

As a variety of potential respiratory hazards may exist in these processes it may be helpful to group them together in one section but, as the subject is large and complex, only a brief outline is attempted.

WELDING

This involves uniting pieces of metal or thermoplastic at joint faces which are rendered liquid or plastic by heat or pressure, or both. Other methods of metal jointing include brazing, braze welding and soldering (*see* Chapter 12, Soldering fluxes).

There are many types of welding which can be conveniently classified according to the sources of heat used (Challen, 1965).

Gas welding

This employs a fuel gas and oxygen or air which are piped separately to a blowpipe where they are mixed before combustion in a nozzle directed at the work surface. The most commonly used fuel gases are acetylene, natural gas and propane. Oxygen–gas mixtures burn at a higher temperature than air–gas mixtures: for example, oxygen–acetylene at 3260 °C and air-acetylene at 2325 °C; and oxygen–propane at 3000 °C and air–propane at 1950 °C. Welding of this type includes gas welding, braze welding, gas (oxygen) cutting and flame gouging.

Electric arc welding

Heat is generated by striking an arc between an electrode and the workpiece. The temperature may reach about 4000 °C and some molten metal is usually added to the join. This is achieved either by melting a separate 'filler' rod (non-consumable electrode process) or melting the electrode itself (consumable electrode process). An inert gas shield is often used to protect the weld area from the atmosphere. The gases employed are helium, argon or carbon dioxide. Other methods employ electrical resistance and not an arc.

(a) Non-consumable electrode processes These are carbon arc and inert gas tungsten-arc welding.

(b) Consumable electrode processes Here the electrode, the end of which is raised to melting point, is either uncoated and provided with an inert gas shield or covered by a flux coat which vaporizes in the arc to form a shielding gas and slag which reacts with the molten metal to protect the cooling weld. These processes include *inert-gas* (CO_2) *metal-arc welding, covered electrode metal arc welding,* CO_2*-flux arc welding* and *magnetic flux arc welding.* They may be semi-automatic or automatic.

A large number of different ingredients are employed in electrode coatings: for example, cellulose, metallic oxides and salts, 'silica' sometimes as diatomite, and a variety of silicates including asbestos, feldspar and mica.

(c) 'Plasma' arc welding The arc is formed at a small orifice through which hydrogen, helium, argon or nitrogen, or a mixture of these gases, flows. The arc 'plasma' consists of ionized gas at a temperature of about 24 000 °C which forms into a jet under the gas pressure and becomes an intense flame beyond the nozzle.

Fluxes commonly used are aluminium, calcium, iron and manganese silicates with small amounts of fluorspar, but less fume is evolved than in most other forms of welding.

Resistance welding

This involves the application of a powerful squeezing force to the components being welded while a strong, low voltage electric current flows through them generating heat at the interface. It includes *spot welding, flash welding* and *electro-slag welding.* Little fume production should occur unless components are layered with oil or coated with primer or with metallic or plastic coatings.

Metal coatings materials

Metal surfaces may be covered with rust proofing material or coated with plastic or synthetic resins as insulating layers. The metallic and resin composition of such coatings may be complex so that it is impossible to draw up a comprehensive list of potential local air contaminants when they are vaporized at welding temperatures (Steel, 1964).

POTENTIAL RESPIRATORY HAZARDS OF WELDING

The effects of all the substances listed are discussed either in this chapter or Chapters 6, 7, 11 or 12.

Gases

These usually occur in small amounts but in some circumstances substantial local concentrations may occur.

Oxides of nitrogen Nitrogen dioxide may be produced in significant concentrations by oxy-acetylene, oxy-propane and electric arc welding and by oxy-gas cutting due to the combination of oxygen and nitrogen caused by high temperatures (Roe, 1959). It is only potentially hazardous, however, when welding is done in enclosed and poorly ventilated spaces (Norwood *et al.*, 1966; Steel, 1968). The larger the current used in arc welding the more nitrogen dioxide is likely to be evolved and electrodes with a coating of high cellulose content give rise to above average amounts of the gas. In general, there is little likelihood of hazardous concentrations of gas occurring when these processes are carried out in 'open shop' conditions. Gas-shielded welding produces insignificant quantities of nitrogen dioxide (Roe, 1959; Morley and Silk, 1970).

Ozone This gas may be evolved in dangerous quantities from atmospheric oxygen due to ultraviolet radiation produced during inert gas-shielded welding with consumable or non-consumable electrodes and arc-air cutting (Sanderson, 1968). It is formed up to a distance of 1 m from the source of radiation of 1800 Å (180 nm) in gas-shielded welding (Frant, 1963). However, insignificant amounts appear to be produced by manual arc-welding (Doig and Challen, 1964).

Phosgene This may be evolved from metals degreased with chlorinated hydrocarbons such as trichlorethylene and carbon tetrachloride or if these vapours are present in the surrounding atmosphere.

Phosphine From metal coated with phosphate rust-proofing material.

Acrolein From alkyl and epoxy resin metal coatings.

Formaldehyde Similar to acrolein.

Isocyanates From polyurethane resin coatings.

Fumes

Zinc oxide From galvanized iron and zinc pigment primers—a potential cause of metal fume fever. Occasionally other metallic oxides may cause metal fume fever.

Iron oxide This, the chief metallic fume produced by welding, may cause siderosis which may regress after exposure has ceased (Garnusewski and Dobrzyński, 1967).

Cadmium and beryllium oxides These arise from welding of cadmium-plated material or cadmium or beryllium-containing alloys and may cause chemical pneumonia. As a rule their presence is unexpected and accidental.

Manganese oxides These may cause chemical pneumonia in high concentrations which, however, are an exceptional occurrence.

Chromium and nickel Welding of alloys containing these metals (stainless steel, for example) is unusual. They may cause asthma (*see* Chapter 12).

Vanadium pentoxide This may be evolved from vanadium-containing filler wires and cause chemical pneumonia or asthma.

Tetrafluorethylene resins If present in coating materials these may cause polymer fume fever.

Dusts

Lesions of 'mixed dust fibrosis' of microscopical or large conglomerate dimensions have occasionally been reported in arc welders (Morgan, 1962; Guidotti *et al.*, 1978). In view of the fact that iron oxide is non-fibrogenic (*see* Chapter 6), there are two possible explanations for this: the presence of some form of free silica in the welding fume or inhalation of free silica from another source.

The reactions which take place in the melt and adjacent to the arc of flux-coated electrodes are highly complex and poorly understood. Volatilization of silicates in consumable electrodes and of any free silica which might be formed occurs. Whether or not the free silica converts to cristobalite is uncertain for, owing to the relatively small volume of the high temperature mass at the welding point, the cooling rate of volatilized silica is likely to be too rapid for cristobalite to form. However, under some circumstances, it is conceivable that welding fume may occasionally contain amorphous-coated cristobalite of small particle size; but this is speculative (Bloor, 1980). If true, it might, perhaps, account for a few of the cases of 'mixed dust fibrosis'.

Exposure to free silica from some other source is the more likely explanation: either in some previous occupation or from processes in the vicinity of the welder's work (para-occupational), such as fettling and knocking out in foundry shops. Free silica has sometimes been identified in welders' lungs.

Welders (especially in shipyards and power stations) sometimes work in proximity to insulation workers or have to clear a work area of lagging material themselves. Thus, intermittent exposure to asbestos may occur.

TO SUMMARIZE

Airborne contaminants due to welding and related processes are determined by the composition of the electrode, flux, base metal and its coating and the shielding gas. Lung disorders associated with welding may be due to:

(1) *direct (occupational) exposure.* Metal fume fever, polymer fume fever, siderosis, pulmonary oedema or chemical pneumonia, asthma and, possibly, 'mixed dust fibrosis'.
(2) *indirect (para-occupational) exposure.* 'Mixed dust fibrosis' or silicosis in foundries and asbestosis or other asbestos-related disease in shipyards and power stations.

THE HEALTH OF WELDERS

The use of welding has increased greatly in recent years chiefly in the form of fusion welding with resistance welding being less common. Newer types of welding processes (not considered here) such as laser, electron beam and explosive welding, and welding under water and in outer space will, no doubt, expand in the future (Challen, 1974).

As welders work in so many different environments it is difficult to interpret the significance of exposure to welding processes in industrial situations with respect to respiratory disease. In fact, 'welders do not suffer from any specific disease due to their occupation that could be described as "welders' disease"' (Doig and Duguid, 1951). Hence, terms such as this and 'welders' lung' have little meaning and should be avoided.

An increased mortality (SMR) from pneumonia among welders, cutters and braziers has been reported, but it is likely that a proportion consisted of (unsuspected) cases of chemical pneumonia or oedema caused by one or other of the toxic fumes or gases (Doig and Challen, 1964; Challen, 1974).

There has been much speculation and controversy as to whether recurrent exposure to low concentrations of welding gases such as ozone and nitrogen dioxide causes irreversible impairment of lung function. In some studies none has been found but in others either obstructive or restrictive impairments have been reported. These disparate results have been due mainly to lack of control populations, unmatched controls, smoking habits unaccounted for, and exposure to other respiratory hazards such as free silica or asbestos (Challen, 1974). In brief, however, it can be fairly summarized that chronic simple bronchitis (mucous hypersecretion) is more common in working welders than in unexposed workers (Antti- Poika, Hassi and Pyy, 1977) but that there is no convincing or consistent evidence that chronic airflow obstruction is more prevalent in welders than in non-welders, though respiratory *symptoms*—that is, cough and sputum—may be increased in welders of older age (over 45 years) who smoke compared with smoking non-welders of similar age (Fogh, Frost and Georg, 1969; McMillan and Heath, 1979).

With regard to possible effects during the working day McMillan and Heath (1979) found in a study of electric arc welders in a naval dockyard that there were no significant acute changes in group mean lung function results in either the welders or control individuals, whether they were smokers or non-smokers, during the period of the shift although there was a positive correlation between a slight increase in residual volume over the shift period and the level of respirable fume to which the welders were exposed.

PREVENTION

(1) Education of welders in the potential risks and their avoidance.
(2) Good general and local exhaust ventilation.
(3) Wearing of respiratory protective equipment in confined spaces if these are not efficiently ventilated.
(4) Monitoring of welders' breathing zone for toxic fumes and gases.
(5) The value of periodic medical examination of welders in ordinary welding shops has been doubted on the grounds that they do not appear more likely to develop serious pulmonary disease than other workers (Antti-Poika, Hassi and Pyy, 1977). However, routine examinations are clearly desirable in processes in which there is a risk of asthma (*see* Chapter 12). Individuals with established chronic pulmonary disease should probably be excluded from welding.

FIRE SMOKE

Acute respiratory injury either with or without external burns has long been known to occur in victims of fires but chronic sequelae are unusual. Workers and other personnel may be caught in major conflagrations in factories, offices, mines, ships and aircraft; and firemen, unless protected by appropriate breathing apparatus, are at risk.

It is important to stress that respiratory injury may occur in the absence of burns. Immediately following exposure there is cough and soreness of the throat which recover quickly but, after an asymptomatic interval varying from eight to 24 hours, cough with thick tenaceous sputum, hoarseness of voice and central chest pain occur. In badly affected individuals there is severe breathlessness with bilateral fine, basal crepitations and widespread rhonchi. The clinical and radiographic features of pulmonary oedema are present at this stage in some, but not all, cases (Hampton, 1971). Secondary respiratory infection is particularly apt to develop and has been shown to occur after 24 hours in dogs exposed to high concentrations of wood smoke (Stephenson *et al.*, 1975).

Pathologically, the trachea and major airways are intensely hyperaemic with oedema in the submucosal layers, variable mucosal necrosis and fibrinous exudate with pronounced cellular infiltration. Pulmonary oedema is present in cases of severe exposure. These effects are due to the smoke and its various components and not to thermal burns (Hampton, 1971).

A wide variety of materials may be involved in fires including wood, wool, leather, cork and synthetic polymer foams—in particular PVC and polyurethane. The resulting products differ according to what extent they undergo combustion or pyrolysis. *Combustion* consists of thermal decomposition of organic material in an oxygen atmosphere; *pyrolysis* is thermal decomposition in an oxygen depleted atmosphere. Both occur to a varying degree in fires and, in general, the products of complete combustion are less harmful than those of incomplete combustion (Kimmerle, 1976). Thus, toxic gases which may occur in fires include carbon monoxide, the oxides of nitrogen, hydrogen chloride (from PVC), aldehydes and toluene diisocyanate 'smoke' which, at high temperatures, yields hydrogen cyanide. Release of phosgene from burning PVC, however, is negligible (Wooley, 1971; Stark, 1972; Wooley and Palmer, 1976). Hydrogen chloride gas, which is rarely encountered in industry under normal conditions, is highly irritant and may cause severe pulmonary oedema.

Firemen have been found to have no impairment of respiratory function one month after exposure to dense smoke, and a three-year study of firemen showed no increased annual loss of ventilatory function (Tashkin *et al.*, 1977; Musk, Peters and Wegman, 1977). The major, and apparently independent, factor in airways obstruction in firemen, in fact, is cigarette smoking but a few non-smokers may have symptomless dysfunction of the small airways, the significance of which is uncertain (Loke *et al.*, 1980). However, a study of 30 firemen examined immediately after and up to 18 months following severe smoke exposure showed 'a significant decrement' in FEV_1 and FVC which did not improve, accompanied by a high prevalence of non-specific respiratory symptoms throughout the follow-up period by comparison with matched controls. The authors suggest that impaired lung function may result more from repeated exposures than from a sudden decrease due to a specific exposure (Unger *et al.*, 1980). As this fire was in a warehouse where complex chlorinated hydrocarbons were stored it is likely that the men had substantial exposure to phosgene.

Surface burns and smoke inhalation together have a greater deleterious effect on lung function (FEV_1 and FVC) than either alone. This is probably due to the combination of airways inflammation, chest wall burns and increased lung water (subclinical pulmonary oedema). The likelihood of smoke-provoked pulmonary oedema developing may be enhanced by reduction in colloid osmotic pressure caused by loss of serum protein from the burns, and by therapeutic fluid replacement. The development of a restrictive spirometric defect within the first 12 hours of exposure is a more sensitive indication of pulmonary oedema than the chest radiograph (Whitener *et al.*, 1980).

Treatment

As smoke inhalation is potentially life-threatening

immediate action is required. Substantial doses of corticosteroids for a few days only with appropriate antibiotics are recommended in individuals with respiratory distress and also in those without if there has been heavy exposure. Oxygen may be required. Even if initially relatively symptomless all persons who have had significant exposure to smoke should be kept under medical surveillance for at least 48 hours (Hampton, 1971).

The combination of extensive surface burns and smoke inhalation is especially menacing and requires attention to colloid and crystalloid adjustment as well as cardiorespiratory resuscitation. In cases of smoke inhalation alone normal spirometry shortly after the accident excludes significant exposure (Whitener *et al.*, 1980).

Most patients who survive have no permanent lung damage although full recovery may not occur for some months. However, bronchial stenosis or bronchiectasis with airflow obstruction may occasionally follow (Kirkpatrick and Bass, 1979; Whitener *et al.*, 1980).

CHANGES IN AMBIENT PRESSURE AND ACCELERATION

The effects of environmental pressure changes on the lungs and on the body as a whole are complex and diverse. Hence, only a brief description of this topic as it affects the lungs will be given, but authoritative works which the reader should consult are referred to in this section.

A hyperbaric environment may cause lung damage either as a result of compression or of decompression to normal atmospheric pressure which at sea level is 760 mmHg or 1 atmosphere or 1 bar or 100 kN/m². Persons most likely to be affected, therefore, are divers, workers in compressed air in caissons, pressurized tunnels and sewers and, to a minor extent, patients and personnel in hyperbaric therapy units. But, under certain circumstances rapid ascent from sea level to high altitude in aircraft may cause decompression effects. Rarely, lung damage may follow strong acceleration forces, blast and blunt injury to the chest (*see Table 13.1*).

Although most diving and compressed air accidents are referred to specialized units attached, for example, to naval establishments, oil rig organizations and tunnelling contracts, general and chest physicians and radiologists may see cases in non-professional divers or in compressed air workers who have been inadequately decompressed, and also the sequelae of past incidents in such workers.

Types of diving can be summarized briefly as follows:

(1) Free or breath-holding diving with or without a simple snorkel tube.
(2) Scuba or aqualung diving (that is, self-contained underwater breathing apparatus). Compressed air automatically regulated for any depth supplied from a cylinder worn by the diver. Widely employed for commercial, military and naval purposes, in marine biology and sport.
(3) Standard or conventional diving. Copper helmet with an air line to the surface. Limited to underwater construction work such as bridges and harbours.
(4) Surface demand diving. Air or a mixture of breathing gases is piped from the surface to divers wearing scuba-type suits. Air normally limited to 50 m depth because of nitrogen narcosis.
(5) Bounce diving. The diver swims from a bell to which gas mixtures such as oxy-helium are piped from the surface. Used for short duration naval and commercial work such as the oil industry.
(6) Saturation diving. Divers remain at depth, sometimes for days, and their tissues are saturated with breathing gases in the bells or chambers. This enables repeated work sorties to be carried out at depth without change in pressure, and at the cost of only one final decompression.
(7) Caissons. These are static, pressurized, inverted boxes in which men can work on bridge piers and structural foundations under water. In tunnelling through clay or permeable rock underwater compressed air is used behind air-tight bulkheads to control water seepage.

Table 13.1 Physical Causes of Lung Damage (Excluding Radiation Injury)

PULMONARY DYSBARYSM
- (1) *Below sea level*
  - (a) Compression—*pulmonary barotrauma of descent* ('lung squeeze')
  - (b) Decompression—*pulmonary barotrauma of ascent* ('burst lung'). Ascent from diving and submarine escape
    —*acute respiratory decompression sickness* (the 'chokes'). Ascent from diving; too rapid emergence from compressed air work
- (2) *Above sea level*
  - Decompression—rapid ascent in unpressurized aircraft
    —emergency ejection of personnel from pressurized aircraft at altitude
    —failure of cabin pressure at altitude

ACCELERATION
- In aircraft

BLAST WAVE AND BLUNT INJURY

NEAR DROWNING

HIGH ALTITUDE

TERMINOLOGY (Elliott, Hallenbeck and Bove, 1974)

Dysbarism is the best generic term for any illness resulting from changes in environmental pressure. It includes barotrauma and decompression sickness.

Barotrauma consists of mechanical damage to the tissues directly caused by increased or decreased environmental pressure. Pulmonary barotrauma is the most important form of decompression barotrauma.

Decompression sickness consists of the various terms for illness which follows reduction of environmental pressure sufficient to cause the formation of bubbles from dissolved gases in the tissues. It includes acute respiratory decompression sickness—usually referred to by divers as the 'chokes'—which must be clearly distinguished from pulmonary barotrauma.

PULMONARY DYSBARISM (*Table 13.1*)

(1) Below sea level

Small changes in depth below sea level cause substantial pressure changes: at 33 feet (10 m) sea water exerts an additional pressure of 1 atmosphere on the diver—that is, a total pressure of 2 atmospheres; at 66 feet (20 m), 3 atmospheres; and so on for each similar increment of depth. Gas-containing spaces in the body are subject to Boyle's law and are thus compressible and distensible by pressure changes whereas the tissues of the body, which are composed chiefly of water, are virtually incompressible. Gas volume in the lungs at a depth of 33 feet in sea water is half that at sea level; at 99 feet (30 m), a quarter of the surface volume; and at 165 feet (50 m), one-sixth of the surface volume. A TLC of 6 l at the surface is, therefore, reduced to 1.5 l at 99 feet—that is, close to RV (Edmonds, 1976).

Pulmonary barotrauma

(a) Pulmonary barotrauma of descent ('lung squeeze') This is an uncommon event which may occur with breath-holding during descent if TLC approaches RV; with loss of surface pressure gas supply due to failure of a non-return valve in conventional and surface demand diving; and with failure to adjust the gas supply to rate of descent in conventional diving. During breath-holding at pressures greater than 100 psi (that is, at depth greater than 99 feet of sea water) there is a substantial shift of blood into the pulmonary venous bed. This and compression of the lungs approximately to RV causes pulmonary venous congestion, haemorrhage and oedema. Divers using open-circuit apparatus inhale gases at the same pressure as that of the environment and, thus, are not at risk from pulmonary barotrauma of descent (Edmonds, 1975).

The *clinical features* consist of haemoptysis, chest pain and haemorrhagic pulmonary oedema which can be fatal.

Treatment consists of oxygen, which initially may need to be 100 per cent, and fluid replacement. Intermittent positive pressure respiration may be required (Edmonds, 1975).

(b) Pulmonary barotrauma of ascent in water or after work in compressed air ('burst lung') Rapid reduction in pressure results in local expansion and trapping of air or gas in the lungs. If TLC is exceeded the limit of their elasticity is passed and patchy rupture of alveolar walls occurs. This is especially likely to happen during buoyant ascent and escape from submarines when it may be impossible for the individual to vent gases with sufficient speed to maintain equilibrium. Factors which contribute to these anatomical changes are:

(1) breath-holding during ascent, inadvertent coughing or sneezing, water inhalation and faulty apparatus;
(2) pre-existing lung pathology such as cysts, localized narrowing of airways (due, for example, to abnormal lymph nodes), mucus plugs, bronchioliths, asthma and unresolved respiratory infection;
(3) collapse of some small airways (bronchioles) in normal lungs due to pressure being lower inside their lumens than outside resulting in localized air trapping. In some individuals there is an innate reduction of compliance which predisposes their lungs to greater pressure stresses than the lungs of divers with normal compliance (Colebatch, Smith and Ng, 1976).

Pulmonary barotrauma is much less apt to occur after saturation diving and compressed air work in caissons or tunnels because of the gradualness of decompression in pressurized chambers.

Pathogenesis and clinical features

Rupture of alveoli in regions of trapped gas allows the gas to escape into lung tissue causing interstitial emphysema, pneumothorax and, by tracking centrally to the mediastinum, mediastinal emphysema, pneumopericardium and subcutaneous ('surgical') emphysema of the anterior triangle of the neck. Minute gas bubbles may pass through the lungs to the systemic circulation and cause arterial gas embolism of the brain, in particular via the basilar arteries.

In most cases, therefore, the presenting features which are of very rapid onset include mental disorientation (in approximately one-third), loss of consciousness (approximately one-third), and pulmonary signs are commonly absent. But if pulmonary barotrauma has occurred it is most likely to become apparent during gradual decompression to 1 atmosphere following therapeutic recompression as gas in the pleural or mediastinal spaces expands with resultant symptoms and signs. Pulmonary barotrauma in the absence of neurological signs is uncommon but its recognition is important in treatment management.

Symptoms immediately on surfacing consist of chest pain and expectoration of bloodstained froth or frank haemoptysis. If pneumothorax or severe mediastinal emphysema develop breathlessness of both pulmonary and cardiac origin may be moderate to intense. Subcutaneous emphysema at the root of the neck is diagnostic but is not present in all cases.

If radiography is available in the compression chamber the chest film may show multiple miliary opacities, mediastinal emphysema or pneumothorax and, occasionally, large basal intrapulmonary cysts (*Figure 13.9*). The miliary shadowing resolves in about 48 hours after recompression (Kidd and Elliott, 1975).

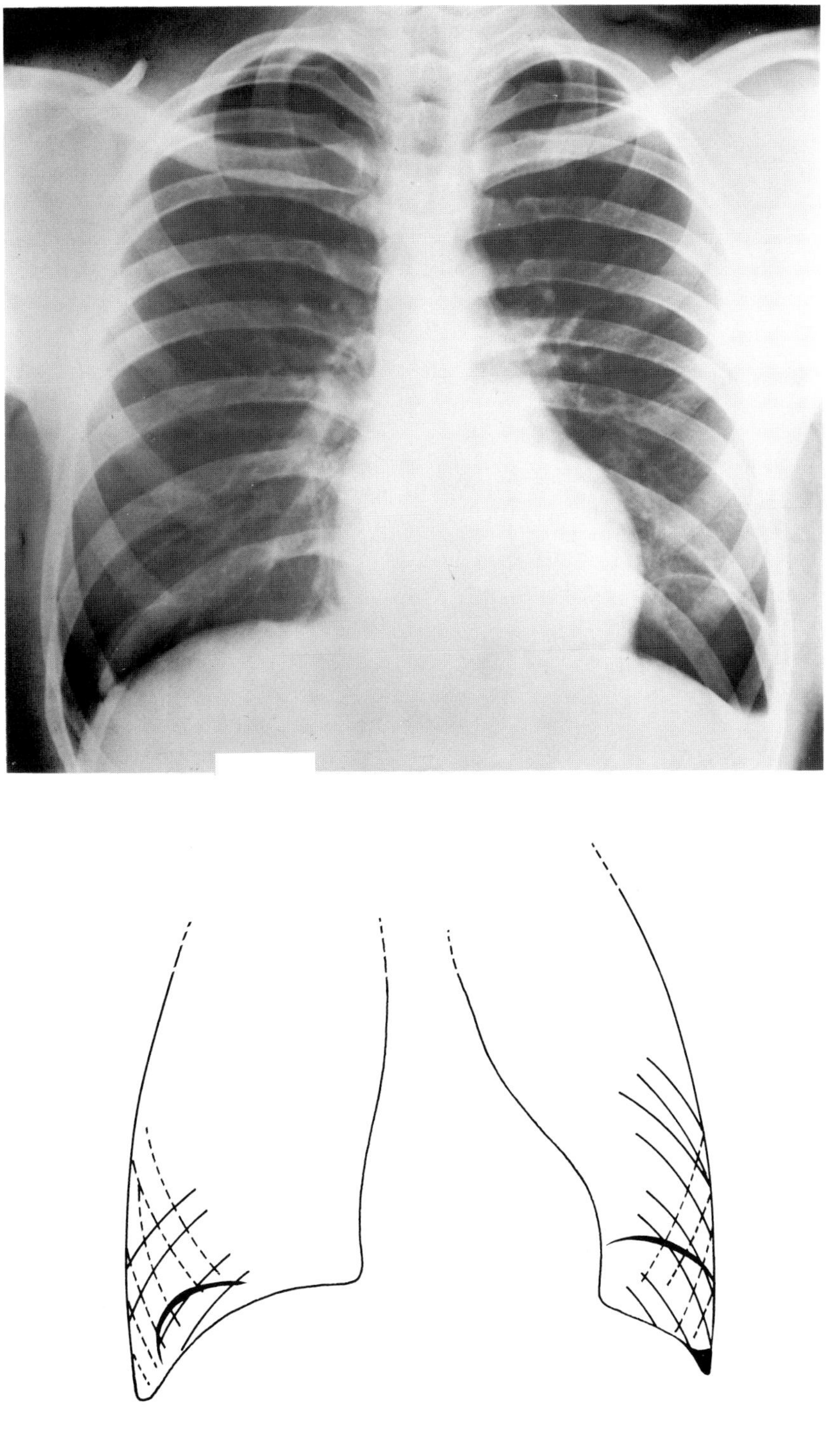

Figure 13.9 Bilateral basal thin-walled cysts following barotrauma of ascent in a diver. He complained of chest tightness during buoyant ascent from 6 atmospheres (4560 mmHg) and became unconscious shortly after surfacing but recovered rapidly on recompression. Initially his chest radiograph showed bilateral pneumothoraces, basal thin-walled cysts and probable pneumopericardium. Re-expansion and complete recovery occurred in approximately two weeks with bed rest. But the cysts were still present another two weeks later (this film) though, subsequently, they disappeared. (Reproduced by permission of Surgeon Commodore J. A. B. Harrison, Ministry of Defence)

Acute respiratory decompression sickness

Pathogenesis and clinical features The initial symptoms and signs of *decompression sickness* may develop within minutes of decompression or, more commonly, are delayed for several hours. The non-respiratory features consist of musculo-skeletal pains (the 'bends'), pruritis, lymphatic oedema of the skin, and a variety of neurological manifestations caused by localized central or peripheral involvement of the nervous system. These are well described by Elliott, Hattenbeck and Bove, 1974; Kidd and Elliott, 1975; and Strauss, 1976).

Acute respiratory decompression sickness (the 'chokes') characteristically consists of sudden retrosternal pain (a sharp 'catch') which is worsened or sometimes only present on maximal inspiration, and may first be experienced when the diver lights a cigarette on surfacing. Deep inspiration may cause paroxysmal coughing. In addition there is sweating, pallor apprehension and breathlessness with rapid, shallow breathing. Respiratory symptoms frequently *precede* the other features of decompression sickness often within minutes of severe decompression, although their onset may be delayed for some hours especially if limb bends have not been treated (Behnke, 1945; Kidd and Elliott, 1975; Strauss, 1979).

The factors which give rise to decompression sickness are:

(1) too rapid decompression from depth;
(2) sufficient gas in solution in the tissues to release harmful bubbles;
(3) personal idiosyncracy such as age, obesity, dehydration and 'hang-over'.

The formation of large gas bubbles in the lungs is responsible for the 'chokes' but the neurological changes, which are usually due to spinal cord or brain-stem damage, are apparently caused by obstruction of the epidural, vertebral venous system by bubbles with the production of venous infarcts (Elliott, Hallenbeck and Bove, 1974).

Diagnosis

(1) Pulmonary barotrauma is generally associated with relatively rapid ascent through water and is usually present immediately or within a few minutes after surfacing. It is uncommon in the absence of cerebral gas embolism. It may follow any compressed-gas dive whereas decompression sickness only occurs after a dive of sufficient depth or duration to permit substantial uptake of gas by body tissues. Thus, if a dive has been performed within the known limits of decompression safety, gas embolism due to pulmonary barotrauma is the more likely diagnosis (Elliott, Hallenbeck and Bove, 1974).
(2) The symptoms of acute respiratory decompression sickness are distinct from those of pulmonary barotrauma and their onset is delayed.
(3) The neurological symptoms and signs of barotrauma are almost immediate in onset and of cerebral type whereas those of decompression sickness are usually delayed and most commonly of spinal cord origin.
(4) The symptoms and signs of pulmonary barotrauma are distinct from those of acute respiratory decompression sickness and are diagnostic. But it must be noted that the absence of subcutaneous emphysema does *not* exclude pulmonary barotrauma.

Treatment

The treatment of both arterial gas embolism and decompression sickness (including the 'chokes') is immediate recompression, but in the few cases of pulmonary barotrauma in which there are no cerebral manifestations this is not necessary. However, these individuals must be kept under close observation within easy reach of a compression chamber so that they can be quickly recompressed if signs of neurological involvement develop. As diving accidents are apt to occur in remote areas the patient may have to be transferred some distance to the nearest chamber or hyperbaric therapeutic chamber in hospital. If an aircraft is needed it must either fly at low altitude or be pressurized to sea level cabin pressure. Uncontrolled ascent from sea level seriously worsens the patient's clinical condition.

The required technique for recompression and decompression varies in each case and codes of practice and therapeutic tables for divers and compressed air workers are specified in regulations in the UK, the USA and other countries (Bennett and Elliott, 1975; Kindwell, 1975; Miles and Mackay, 1976; Strauss, 1979).

In pulmonary barotrauma rest and sedation are required and in mild cases may be sufficient without recompresssion. In more severe cases inhalation of oxygen–helium mixtures relieves respiratory distress during decompression, and should be used whenever possible. Methyl prednisolone 5 mg/kg/24 hours in six equal doses has been recommended to reduce cerebral oedema and secondary infection. Pneumothorax may require thoracentesis especially when of tension type which may develop during decompression following therapeutic recompression. In decompression sickness correction of hypovolaemia may be needed.

Sequelae Recovery is usually complete but occasionally radiographic evidence of air cysts may persist (*Figure 13.9*). Diving and submarine escape training should not be permitted after an incidence of pulmonary barotrauma has occurred (Kidd and Elliott, 1975).

Prevention

(1) Awareness of the dangers and education of individuals at risk.
(2) Pre-employment medical examination with lung function tests and chest radiographs should exclude persons with a history of spontaneous pneumothorax and chest surgery, and those with chronic obstructive bronchitis or asthma, or with radiographic evidence of air cysts or bullae from diving or work in compressed air.
(3) All divers should have a standard chest radiograph and a record of FEV_1, FVC and FEFR annually.

    In the UK monthly medical examination of all workers in compressed air where tunnel pressures exceed 18 psi and re-examination of upper respiratory tract infections or any illness or injury causing more than three days absence from work are statutory requirements (Employment Advisory Service 1975). Both diving and compressed air work are subject to Special Regulations.
(4) Scuba diving must be avoided for 12 hours before and after diving or compressed air work; as must flying for more than three hours after exposure (Kindwell, 1975; Balldin, 1980).

(5) Smoking should be discouraged and should certainly not occur for at least two hours before diving.

(2) Above sea level

Atmospheric pressure at 5000 m is approximately 405.4 mmHg; at 10 000 m, 198.8 mmHg; and at 20 000 m, 41.5 mmHg. At normal, ground level, environmental pressure on aviator's tissues are fully saturated with gas so that the factors which determine his decompression risk are, in the main, rate of ascent and altitude reached. Rapid ascent in unpressurized aircraft, emergency ejection from a pressurized aircraft and failure of aircraft cabin pressure at high altitude subject pilots, aircrew and passengers to acute decompression effects.

Although a number of aircraft decompression accidents occur annually pulmonary barotrauma is uncommon, but may follow emergency ejection at high altitude. Decompression sickness may develop during ascent in unpressurized aircraft. The 'chokes' respond to recompression at ground level although the symptoms sometimes persist for a day or two. Non-respiratory features usually recover at ground level but migraine-like symptoms may occur.

ACCELERATION EFFECTS

The contribution of high acceleration (g) forces and breathing high concentrations of oxygen on pilots of high performance aircraft may result in areas of basal segmental or subsegmental lung collapse. Positive 'head-to-foot' g forces cause compression of the lung bases with decreased expansion and obstruction of some of the smaller airways. These changes are intensified by breathing an atmosphere of oxygen containing little or no diluent gas of low absorption coefficient (such as nitrogen or helium) which, on account of its being poorly absorbed, exerts a 'braking' effect on lung collapse. Reduced total barometric pressure respiratory infections and constriction of the chest during flight are contributory factors (Ernsting, 1960; Levy *et al.*, 1962; Karstens and Welch, 1971).

Cough, pleuritic pain and basal rhonchi occur but recover fairly quickly and radiographic evidence of basal collapse clears in about 48 hours. Recovery is facilitated by coughing and deep breathing exercises.

The addition of nitrogen or helium to the oxygen supply prevents collapse (Karstens and Welch, 1971). Pilots who fly high performance aircraft should be discouraged from smoking for some hours before 'take-off' and those with respiratory infections, 'grounded' until better (Levy *et al.*, 1962).

BLAST WAVE AND BLUNT TRAUMA EFFECTS

These include blast injuries in air from explosions in factories, ships and mines and other confined spaces; and in water where divers, seamen and armed forces personnel may be affected. Blunt trauma may be caused by falls into water from a height or blows on the chest wall. Alveolar rupture occurs due, probably to a shearing injury of the lungs rather than overinflation as is the case in 'burst lung'. In many cases, especially those of blast in water or blunt trauma, there may be no fracture of ribs or penetrating injury of the chest though ecchymosis over the area of impact is usual.

The effects of blast underwater are more pronounced than in air owing to the greatly increased pressure wave generated in underwater explosions caused by the relative incompressibility of water and the higher velocity of sound in water than in air. In addition to individuals who are immersed at the time of an explosion, pilots who fire their ejection seats to escape from submerged aircraft may be injured in this way.

Clinical features are cough, frothy bloodstained sputum or frank haemoptysis and crepitations in the lungs. As a rule multiple small opacities of so-called acinar-filling type appear within a few hours and are usually most prominent adjacent to the area of maximum impact. Subcutaneous emphysema, mediastinal emphysema, pneumothorax (often bilateral) and haemothorax may subsequently develop. Pulmonary oedema, delayed for some 24 to 48 hours is a common complication of blast injury (Fallon, 1940; Williams, 1942; Watt, 1977; Robertson, Lakshminarayan and Hudson, 1978).

Pathologically, the surface of the lungs is contused and large quantities of blood are present in the alveoli and airways.

Treatment includes bronchial aspiration, oxygen, corticosteroids as anti-inflammatory agents and prophylactic antibiotics. There is some controversy concerning the use of positive pressure ventilation (as is also the case in pulmonary barotrauma) because of the risk of inducing air embolism and surgical emphysema. But volume-cycled mechanical ventilation with positive end-expiratory pressure sufficient to maintain arterial oxygen pressure above 60 mmHg in a group of attempted suicide cases who had fallen 50 m into water did not provoke any incidents of air embolism (Robertson, Lakshminarayan and Hudson, 1978). Treatment of pneumothorax may be necessary.

Patients who recover usually do so without sequelae but some may have permanent, diffuse unilateral or bilateral pleural fibrosis. Occasionally empyema occurs.

NEAR DROWNING (Rivers, Orr and Lee, 1970)

That is, survival following a drowning episode in salt or fresh water usually as a result of successful resuscitative measures. In spite of apparently good recovery death may still occur some hours later from 'secondary drowning'. This consists of the development of pulmonary oedema, aspiration pneumonia, airflow obstruction, anoxaemia and acidosis.

Whether salt or fresh, water contains significant quantities of particulate matter such as diatoms and other inert or reactive materials. On reaching the alveoli it causes an influx of plasma-rich fluid from the capillaries with consequent oedema which, in turn, results in hypoxaemia and acidosis.

Secondary drowning is heralded by troublesome cough, frothy pink sputum, substernal and pleuritic pain, tachypnoea, cyanosis, widespread crepitations and, in some patients, high fever with leucocytosis. The multiple opacities of pulmonary oedema appear in the chest radiograph but are absent in about one-quarter of cases.

Treatment is that of pulmonary oedema with carefully controlled adjustment of blood volume, corticosteroids in high dosage for a limited period and antibodies.

A wide variety of occupations is obviously at risk from near drowning episodes (sometimes in exceptional and bizarre circumstances); including seamen, dock, quayside and oil-rig workers and bridge maintenance men.

HIGH ALTITUDE

Pulmonary oedema is one of the manifestations of illness which may occur at high altitude and which has become increasingly important in recent years because many more individuals in a variety of occupations are being transported to high mountain regions in a very short time.

The body's acute response to hypoxia at high altitude consists of hyperventilation and tachycardia with palpitations and is more pronounced on effort than at rest. These changes, which are relieved by oxygen, are the normal acclimatization reaction and they gradually pass off. However, when some individuals travel quickly to heights over 6500 feet (2000 m) they develop *acute mountain sickness, high altitude pulmonary oedema* or *cerebral oedema,* or a combination of these illnesses depending upon the altitude, rate of ascent and individual susceptibility. Although hypoxia and not change in atmospheric pressure is the primary cause, precisely how these effects are produced is an enigma. This section is chiefly concerned with a brief discussion of pulmonary oedema. For authoritative and more detailed accounts of high altitude disorders the reader should consult Heath and Williams (1981) and Green and Fletcher (1979).

ACUTE MOUNTAIN SICKNESS

This consists of headache, dizziness, shortness of breath, fatigue, malaise and vomiting which occur within a few hours of ascent. Drowsiness is common, periodic breathing may disturb sleep at night, and oliguria is usual. The illness occurs with increasing frequency at heights over 8000 feet (3000 m) if time is not taken for acclimatization. All age groups may be affected.

HIGH ALTITUDE PULMONARY OEDEMA

This rarely develops below 3500 m and most cases, which may be precipitated by physical exertion, tend to occur between 3000 and 4000 m in unacclimatized individuals. Onset is usually insidious taking between one to four days. Initially there is an irritating cough, undue breathlessness on moderate effort, chest tightness, headache and weakness and some creptitations may be detectable. Subsequently, cough becomes intractable, frothy bloody sputum is raised, there is low grade fever, and widespread crepitations and bubbling sounds are heard in the lungs. Symptoms are frequently worse at night, and confusion and delirium may occur. Descent to lower altitude brings rapid relief otherwise some cases are fatal.

The chest radiograph shows multiple large, soft, frequently confluent, bilateral opacities which are prominent in the hilar regions. The typical distribution of oedema due to left ventricular failure or uraemia is exceptional. Sometimes the changes may be predominantly unilateral (*Figure 13.10*). There is rupture of alveolar septa causing subpleural bullae, and peripheral air embolism may result from escape of air into the blood vessels.

The incidence is higher in young than in older people. It may be as high as 6 per cent in those under 21 years and as low as 0.4 per cent in those over 21 years (Hultgren and Marticorena, 1968). In Indian troops who were transported rapidly from low altitude to over 4000 m (13 000 feet) it varied from 2.3 to 15.5 per cent between the companies (Grover *et al.,* 1979). However, in view of the increased number of people now travelling to high altitude the average incidence may be higher in all age groups.

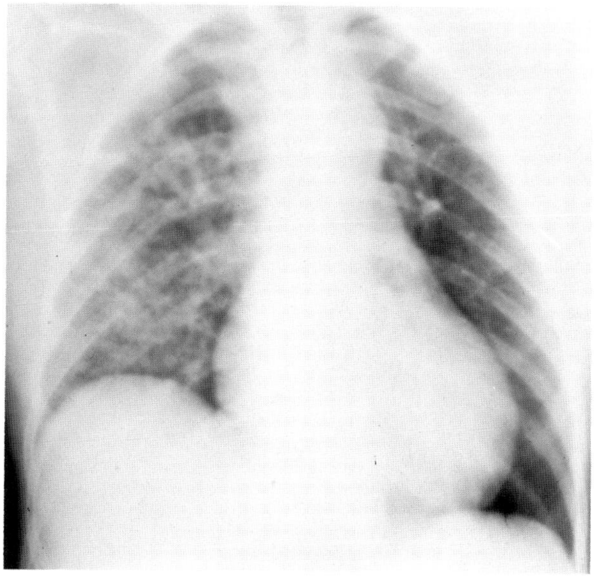

Figure 13.10 High altitude pulmonary oedema (largely unilateral) in a 52 year old female who developed typical mixed cerebral and pulmonary mountain sickness at 12 700 ft (3810 m). The lung fields were normal in a film taken five days later following removal to lower altitude. (Courtesy of Dr John Dickinson)

At post mortem the lungs show the features of congestion and oedema which is chiefly interstitial.

The *pathogenesis* of the oedema is obscure. Pulmonary hypertension is a normal response to hypoxia but individuals who have experienced recurrent episodes of high altitude pulmonary oedema have a greater than average increase in pulmonary arterial pressure (Hultgren, Grover and Hartley, 1971). There is also evidence that left ventricular dysfunction may play a part (Balasubramarian *et al.,* 1978). When rats are subjected to hypoxia and subatmospheric conditions approximating those at the summit of Mount Everest (height 8850 m and atmospheric pressure 250 mmHg) endothelial vesicles of oedema fluid appear in their alveolar walls and protrude into and obstruct the capillaries. These lesions are rapidly reversed by restoring normal atmospheric conditions and could explain the changes which occur in man (Heath, Moosavi and Smith, 1973).

CEREBRAL OEDEMA

This may occur at heights over 3500 m (11 500 feet) and is a very serious complication. There is severe headache, mental confusion, hallucinations and, in some cases, papillodema and localized neurological defects. If descent to lower altitude is not undertaken swiftly coma and death may follow.

Retinal haemorrhages, which are usually asymptomatic, may occur in 20 to 30 per cent of individuals at altitudes greater than 4500 m (Houston, 1976).

Acclimatization to high altitude requires continuous exposure but is lost as quickly as it is gained. So that, although an individual may remain at sea level for a few days before returning to altitude with little or no loss of acclimatization, high altitude pulmonary oedema (or another form of high altitude illness) is as likely to occur as on the occasion of his first ascent if his return is delayed for more than two weeks (Houston, 1975). This point is important for individuals who work regularly at high altitude.

OCCUPATIONS AT RISK

Both men and women in a wide variety of occupations may be subjected to occasional or repeated high altitude conditions. They include tunnellers, miners, civil engineers, geologists, journalists, personnel who man mountain observatories (such as the new Edinburgh University infrared telescope at 4250 m on the summit of Mauna Kea in Hawaii) and high altitude research stations, mountain rescue workers and armed forces personnel. In addition, an increasing number of tourists drive or are flown to high altitudes on trekking tours to such mountain ranges as the Himalayas, Andes, Rocky Mountains, Pyrenees, the Sierra Madre and other high altitude areas of interest. Skiers and other athletes may also be affected.

The highest mine in the world is the volcanic sulphur mine on Aucanquilcha in Chile at an altitude of approximately 6000 m. Active fumaroles contribute sulphur dioxide to the local atmosphere. The processing plant is situated at about 3500 m.

DIAGNOSIS

Differentiation may have to be made from pneumonia, heart failure and pulmonary embolism. Pain in the chest does not occur but may be present with pneumonia and pulmonary embolism which, unlike the other disorders, is of sudden onset.

TREATMENT

It must be stressed that high altitude pulmonary oedema in all but the mildest cases is a medical emergency. Without prompt action rapid worsening of oedema may occur with a fatal outcome within a few hours. The most important step is early descent which should be taken immediately if cough, inappropriate breathlessness, severe lassitude, and crepitations develop. A reduction of as little as 800 to 1000 m may be sufficient to reverse the oedema, which suggests that an increase of total atmospheric pressure itself may be beneficial (Grover *et al.*, 1979).

The method of descent will depend upon the terrain and its degree of accessibility or remoteness—carriage by porter or yak, by helicopter or other aircraft or by a motor vehicle—but, if possible, should not be postponed to await the arrival of transport from a distance. If he is able the affected individual should descend on foot. Temporarily oxygen may be life saving but is not to be considered as an alternative to descent. However, in severe cases and when immediate transportation is impossible oxygen supplied continuously or on demand with positive expiratory pressure from a simple portable apparatus such as that described by Feldman and Herndon (1977) may be decisive. Emergency oxygen equipment is, therefore, essential in all high altitude conditions.

The use of diuretics is controversial but may be justifiable in severe cases provided that there is constant observation for the development of hypovolaemia. Morphine may give relief but must be used with caution if there are any signs of cerebral oedema (Dickinson, 1979; Heath and Williams, 1981).

Table 13.2 Summary of Extrinsic Agents and Injuries which may cause Pulmonary Oedema

Inorganic	*Organic*	*Physical*
Ammonia	Acetaldehyde	Fire smoke
Antimony trichloride	Acrolein	Pulmonary barotrauma of descent and ascent
Antimony pentachloride	Chlorinated camphene	Blast
Cadmium	Dimethyl sulphate	Blunt trauma
Cobalt	Methyl bromide	Near drowning
Chlorine	Nickel carbonyl	High altitude
Hydrogen chloride	Organophosphates	
Hydrogen fluoride	Phosgene	
Hydrogen selenide	Polytetrafluorethylene	
Hydrogen sulphide	Toluene diisocyanate in high concentration	
Lithium hydride	Trimellitic anhydride	
Mercury vapour		
Nitrogen dioxide		
Ozone		
Phosphine		
Selenium dioxide		
Sulphur dioxide		
Titanium tetrachloride		
Zinc chloride		
Zirconium tetrachloride		

A worker known or suspected to have been exposed to any of these agents or conditions should be placed under close medical supervision for at least 72 hours even if there are no significant symptoms immediately after exposure

PREVENTION

(1) Awareness by physicians and exposed personnel of the dangers of rapid ascent to high altitude.
(2) Slow ascent to achieve acclimatization is the most important preventive measure.
(3) If time cannot be taken for acclimatization and in the case of unusually susceptible individuals, acetazolamide (Diamox) for two to three days before ascent has been recommended as it results in a significant reduction in symptoms due, possibly, to metabolic acidosis causing increased respiratory drive and arterial oxygen tension (Houston, 1976; Hackett, Rennie and Levine, 1976; Birmingham Medical Research Expeditionary Society Mountain Sickness Study Group, 1981). It has also been suggested that a low salt diet may be beneficial (Joosens, 1977).
(4) Continued vigilance for the early signs of high altitude pulmonary oedema and prompt descent if these develop.
(5) It should be borne in mind that because of individual susceptibility to develop acute mountain sickness high altitude pulmonary oedema may recur on return to altitude (Hackett and Rennie, 1976).

The occupational causes of acute pulmonary oedema referred to in the text are summarized in *Table 13.2*.

REFERENCES

Adams, R. (1980). β_2-microglobulin levels in nickel-cadmium battery workers. *Occupational Exposure to Cadmium,* pp. 41–42. Report on seminar: London, 20th March, 1980. London; Cadmium Association

Adams, R. G. and Crabtree, N. (1961). Anosmia in alkaline battery workers. *Br. J. ind. Med.* **18**, 216–221

Adams R. G., Harrison, J. F. and Scott, P. (1969). The development of cadmium-induced proteinuria, impaired renal function and osteomalacia in alkaline battery workers. *Q. Jl Med.* **38**, 425–443

Ahlmark, A., Bruce, T. and Nystrom, A. (1960). *Silicosis and Other Pneumoconioses in Sweden*, pp. 361–365; 371–373. London; Heinemann

Ahlmark, A., Axelsson, B., Friberg, L. and Piscator, M. (1960). Further investigations into kidney function and proteinuria in chronic cadmium poisoning. *Proc. 13th Internat. Congr. Occup. Hlth New York*, pp. 201–203

Alexandersson, R. (1979). Investigations of the effects of exposure to cobalt. VI Exposure, assimilation and pulmonary effect of cobalt in the tungsten carbide industry. Arbete och Hälsa (Vetenskaplig skriftserie). Stockholm; Arbetars-kyddsverket

Antti-Poika, M., Hassi, J. and Pyy, L. (1977). Respiratory disease in arc welders. *Int. Arch. occup. Envir. Hlth* **40**, 225–330

Archer, V. E., Magnuson, H. H., Holaday, D. A. and Lawrence, P. A. (1962). Hazards to health in uranium mining and milling. *J. occup. Med.* **4**, 55–60

Baader, E. W. (1951). Die chronische Kadmiumvergiftung. *Dtsch. Med. Wschr.* **76**, 484–487

Baader, E. W. (1952). Chronic cadmium poisoning. *Ind. Med. Surg.* **21**, 427–430

Balasubramanian, V., Mathew, O. P., Tiwari, S. C., Behl, A., Sharma, S. C. and Hoon, R. S. (1978). Alterations in left ventricular function in normal man on exposure to high altitude (3658m). *Br. Heart J.* **40**, 276–285

Balldin, U. I. (1980). Venous gas bubbles while flying with cabin altitudes of airliners or general aviation aircraft three hours after diving. *Aviat. Space environ. Med.* **51**, 649–652

Bamberger, P. J. (1945). Aluminium therapy in silicosis. *Ind. med. Surg.* **14**, 477–479

Barborik, M. and Dusek, J. (1972). Cardiomyopathy accompanying industrial cobalt exposure. *Br. Heart J.* **34**, 113–116

Barnes, J. M. and Denz, F. A. (1950). The effect of 2–3 dimercapto-propanol (BAL) on experimental nickel carbonyl poisoning. *Br. J. ind. Med.* **8**, 117–126

Barth, G., Frik, W. and Scheidemandel, H. (1956). Die Aluminiumlunge. Verlaufsbeobachtungen and Neuerkrankungen in der Nachkreigszeit. *Dt. med. Wschr.* **81**, 1115–1119

Beach, F. X. M., Sherwood Jones, E. and Scarrow, G. D. (1969). Respiratory effects of chlorine gas. *Br. J. ind. Med.* **26**, 231–236

Bech, A. O., Kipling, M. D. and Heather, J. C. (1962), Hard metal disease. *Br. J. ind. Med.* **19**, 239–252

Becklake, M. R., Goldman, H. I., Boxman, A. R. and Freed, C. C. (1957). The long-term effects of exposure to nitrous fumes. *Am. Rev. Tuberc.* **76**, 398–409

Behnke, A. R. (1945). Decompression sickness incident to deep sea diving and high altitude ascent. *Medicine* **24**, 381–402

Bennett, G. (1962). Ozone contamination of high altitude aircraft cabins. *Aerospace Med.* **33**, 969–973

Bennett, P. B. and Elliott, D. H. (1975). *The Physiology and Medicine of Diving and Compressed Air Work.* London; Bailliere, Tindall and Cassell

Benson, M. K. D., Goodwin, P. G. and Brodyoff, J. (1975). Metal sensitivity in patients with joint replacement arthroplastics. *Br. med. J.* **4**, 374–375

Bergman, I. (1972). Nitrous fumes and coal miners with emphysema. Discussion. *Ann. occup. Hyg.* **15**, 301

Berlin, M., Fazackerley, J. and Nordberg, G. (1969). The uptake of mercury in the brains of mammals exposed to mercury vapor and to mercuric salts. *Archs envir. Hlth* **18**, 719–729

Bernard, A., Goret, A. Buchet, J. P. Roels, H. and Lauwerys, R. (1979). Comparison of sodium dodecyl sulfate–polyacrylamide gel electrophoresis with quantitative methods for the analysis of cadmium-induced proteinuria. *Int. Arch. occup. envir. Hlth.* **44**, 139–148

Bernard, A., Roels, H. A., Buchet, J. P., Mason, P. L. and Lauwerys, R. (1977). α_1-antitrypsin level in workers exposed to cadmium. In *Clinical Chemistry and Chemical Toxicology of Metals*, edited by S. A. Brown, pp. 161–164 Amersterdam; Elsevier

Beton, D. C., Andrews, G. S., Davies, H. J., Howells, L. and Smith, G. F. (1966). Acute cadmium fume poisoning *Br. J. ind. Med.* **23**, 292–301

Biesold, J., Bachofen, M. and Bachofen, H. (1974). Pulmonary oedema due to hydrogen sulfide. *Swiss National Science Foundation* (3. 394–0. 74)

Birmingham Medical Research Expeditionary Society Mountain Sickness Study Group (1981). Acetazolamide in control of acute mountain sickness. *Lancet* **1**, 180–183

Blejer, H. P. and Caplan, P. E. (1971). *Occupational Health Aspects of Cadmium Fume Poisoning*, 2nd edition California; Bureau Occup. Hlth and Environ. Epidemiol.

Bloor, W. A. (1979). Personal communication

Bloor, W. A. (1980). Personal communications

Bonnell, J. A. (1955). Emphysema and proteinuria in men casting copper-cadmium alloys. *Br. J. ind. Med.* **12**, 181–195

Bonnell, J. A. (1965). Cadmium poisoning. *Ann. occup. Hyg.* **8**, 45–50

Bonnell, J. A., Kazantzis, G. and King, R. (1959). A follow-up study of men exposed to cadmium oxide fume. *Br. J. ind. Med.* **16**, 135–147

British Occupational Hygiene Society Committee on Hygiene Standards: Subcommittee on Cadmium. (1977). Hygiene standards for cadmium. *Ann. occup. Hyg.* **20**, 215–228

Browne, R. C. (1955). Vanadium poisoning from gas turbine. *Br. J. ind. Med.* **12**, 57–59

Bruckner, H. C. (1967). Extrinsic asthma in a tungsten carbide worker. *J. occup. Med.* **9**, 518–519

Campbell, N. S. (1948). Acute mercurial poisoning by inhalation of metallic vapour in an infant. *Can. med. Ass. J.* **58**, 72–75

Caplin, M. (1941). Ammonia-gas poisoning. *Lancet* **2**, 95–96

Carrington, C. B. and Green, T. J. (1970). Granular pneumocytes in early repair of diffuse alveolar injury. *Archs intern. Med.* **126**, 464–465

Castleman, W. L., Dungworth, D. L., Schwarz, L. W. and Tyler, W. S. (1980). Acute respiratory bronchiolotis. *Am. J. Path.* **98**, 811–827

Cernik, A. A. and Sayers, M. H. P. (1975). Application of blood cadmium determination to industry using a punched disc technique. *Br. J. ind. Med.* **32**, 155–162

Challen, P. J. R. (Ed.) (1965). *Health and Safety in Welding and Allied Processes* 2nd edition. (Institute of Welding), London and Woking: Unwin

Challen, P. J. R. (1974). Some news on welding and welders. *J. Soc. occup. Med.* **24**, 38–47

Challen, P. J. R., Hickish, D. E. and Bedford, J. (1958). An investigation of some health hazards in an inert-gas tungsten-arc welding shop. *Br. J. ind. Med.* **15**, 276–282

Charan, N. B., Myers, C. G., Lakshminarayan, S. and Spencer, T. M. (1979). Pulmonary injuries associated with acute sulphur dioxide inhalation. *Am. Rev. resp. Dis.* **119**, 555–560

Chasis, H., Zapp, J. A., Bannon, J. H., Whittenberger, J. L., Helm, J., Doheny, J. L. and MacLeod, C. D. (1947). Chlorine accident in Brooklyn. *Occup. Med.* **4**, 152–176

Chen, W., Monnat, R. J., Chen, M. and Mottet, N. K. (1978). Aluminium induced pulmonary granulomatosis. *Human Path.* **9**, 705–711

Chester, E. H., Gillespie, D. G. and Krause, F. D. (1969). The prevalence of chronic obstructive pulmonary disease in chlorine gas workers. *Am. Rev. resp. Dis.* **99**, 365–373

Chowdhury, P. and Louria, D. B. (1976). Influence of cadmium and other trace metals on human α-antitrypsin: an *in vitro* study. *Science* **191**, 480–481

Christensen, H., Krogh, M. and Nielsen, M. (1937). Acute mercury poisoning in a respiration chamber. *Nature (London)* **139**, 626

Christensen, F. C. and Olsen, E. C. (1957). Cadmium poisoning. *Archs ind. Hlth* **16**, 8–13

Christiansen, K. J. (1979). The correlation between prosthesis failure and metal sensitivity as determined by a new immunological technique. *J. Bone Jt Surg.* **61B**, 240

Clinton, M. (1947). Selenium fume exposure. *J. ind. Hyg. Toxicol.* **29**, 225–227

Clutton-Brock, J. (1967). Two cases of poisoning by contamination of nitrous oxide with higher oxides of nitrogen during anaesthesia. *Br. J. Anaesth.* **39**, 388–392

Coates, E. O., Jr., Sawyer, H. J., Rebusk, J. W., Kvale, P. H. and Sweet, L. W. (1973). Hypersensitivity bronchitis in tungsten carbide workers. *Chest* **64**, 390

Coates, E. O. and Watson, J. H. L. (1971). Diffuse interstitial lung disease in tungsen carbide workers. *Ann. intern. Med.* **75**, 709–716

Coates, E. O., Jr., and Watson, J. H. L. (1973). Pathology of the lung in tungsten carbide workers using light and electron microscopy. *J. occup. Med.* **15**, 280–286

Colebatch, H. J. H., Smith, M. M. and Ng, C. K. Y. (1976). Increased elastic recoil as a determinant of pulmonary barotrauma in divers. *Resp. Physiol.* **26**, 55–64

Commins, B. T. (1972). Personal communication

Commins, B. T., Raveney, F. J. and Jesson, M. W. (1971). Toxic gases in tower silos. *Ann. occup. Hyg.* **14**, 275–283

Cordasco, E. M., Cooper, R. W., Murphy, J. V. and Anderson, C. (1962). Pulmonary aspects of some toxic experimental space fuels. *Dis. Chest* **41**, 68–74

Cordasco, E. M., Kosti, H., Vance J. W. and Golden, L. N. (1965). Pulmonary edema of non-cardiac origin. *Archs envir. Hlth* **11**, 588–596

Cordasco, E. M. and Stone, F. D. (1973). Pulmonary oedema of environmental origin. *Chest* **64**, 182–185

Corrin, B. (1963). Aluminium pneumoconiosis II. Effect on the rat lung of intra-tracheal injections of stamped aluminium powders containing different lubricating agents and of a granular aluminium powder. *Br. J. ind. Med.* **20**, 268–276

Cotter, L. H. and Cotter, B. H. (1951). Cadmium poisoning. *Archs ind. Hyg.* **3**, 495–504

Crombie, D. W., Blaisdell, J. L. and MacPherson, G. (1944). Treatment of silicosis with aluminium powder. *Can. med. Ass. J.* **50**, 318–328

Cross, C. E., De Lucia, J., Reddy, A. K., Hussain, M. Z., Chow, C. and Mustafa, J. G. (1976). Ozone interactions with lung tissue. Biochemical approaches. *Am. J. Med.* **60**, 929–935

Dalgaard, J. B., Dencker, F., Fallentin, B., Hansen, P., Kaempe, B., Steensberg, J. and Wilhardt, P. (1972). Fatal poisoning and other health hazards connected with industrial fishing. *Br. J. ind. Med.* **29**, 307–316

Darke, C. S. and Warrack, A. J. N. (1958). Bronchiolitis from nitrous fumes. *Thorax* **13**, 327–333

Davis, J. M. G., Gormley, I. P., Collings, P., Ottery, J. and Robertson, A. (1978). Studies on the cytotoxicity of coal dust samples, including the effects of adsorbed nitrous fumes. *Institute of Occupational Medicine, Edinburgh. Final Report.* 6244–00/8/105

Decker, W. J. and Koch, H. F. (1978). Chlorine poisoning at the swimming pool: an overlooked hazard. *Clin. Toxicol.* **13**, 377–381

Delahant, A. B. (1955). An experimental study of the effects of rare metals on animal lungs. *Archs. ind. Hlth* **12**, 116–120

Delaney, L. T., Schmidt, H. W. and Stroebel, C. F. (1956). Silofillers' disease. *Proc. Staff Meet. Mayo Clin.* **31**, 189–198

Desbaumes, P. (1968). Intoxications mortelles par les gaz de fermentation de silos agricoles (oxyde de carbone et oxydes d'azote). *Arch. Tox.* **23**, 160–164

Dickinson, J. G. (1979). Severe acute mountain sickness. *Postgrad. med. J.* **55**, 454–458

Doig, A. T. and Challen, P. J. R. (1964). Respiratory hazards of welding. *Ann. occup. Hyg.* **7**, 223–229

Doig, A. T. and Duguid, L. N. (1951). *The Health of Welders.* London; HMSO

Dowell, A. R., Kilburn, K. H. and Pratt, P. C. (1971). Short term exposure to nitrogen dioxide. *Archs intern. Med.* **128**, 74–80

Drinker, P. and Hatch, T (1954). *Industrial Dust*, 2nd edition, pp. 50–51. London, New York, Toronto: McGraw-Hill

Drozdz, M., Kucharz, E. and Szyja, J. (1977). Effect of chronic exposure to nitrogen dioxide on collagen content in lung and skin of guinea pigs. *Envir. Res.* **13**, 369–377

Dutton, W. F. (1911). Vanadiumism. *J. Am. med. Ass.* **56**, 1648

Edmonds, C. (1976). Barotrauma. In *Diving Medicine*, edited by Richard H. Strauss, pp. 49–61. New York, San Francisco, and London; Grune and Stratton

Elliott, D. H., Hallenbeck, J. M. and Bove, A. A. (1974). Acute decompression sickness. *Lancet* **2**, 1193–1199

EMAS (1972). *Ozone. Notes of Guidance.* London; Chief Employment Medical Adviser, Health and Safety Executive

Employment Medical Advisory Service (1975). A report of the work of the Service for 1973 and 1974, pp. 13–14. Department of Employment. London; HMSO

English, J. M. (1964). A case of probable phosgene poisoning. *Br. med. J.* **1**, 38

Ernsting, J. (1960). Some effects of oxygen breathing in man. *Proc. R. Soc. Med.* **53**, 96–98

Evans, D. M. (1960). Cadmium poisoning. *Br. med. J.* **1**, 173–174

Evans, E. H. (1945). Casualties following exposure to zinc chloride smoke. *Lancet* **2**, 368–369

Everett, E. D. and Overholt, E. L. (1968). Phosgene poisoning. *J. Am. med. Ass.* **205**, 243–245

Fabbri, L., Mapp, C., Rossi, A., Sarto, F., Trevisan, A. and De Rosa, E. (1979). Pulmonary changes due to low level occupational exposure to ozone. *Med. Lav.* **4**, 307–312

Fallon, M. (1940). Lung injury in the intact thorax. *Br. J. Surg.* **28**, 39–49

Farmer and Stockbreeder (1970). Check on poison gas in tower silos. **84**, 11

Farrell, B. P., Kerr, H. D., Kulle, T. J., Sauder, L. R. and Young, J. L. (1979). Adaption in human subjects to the effects of inhaled ozone after repeated exposure. *Am. Rev. resp. Dis.* **119**, 725–730

Federspiel, C. F., Layne, J. T., Auer, C. and Bruce, J. (1980). Lung function among employees of a copper mine smelter: lack of effect of chronic sulfur dioxide exposure. *J. occup. Med.* **22**, 438–444

Feldman, K. W. and Herndon, S. P. (1977). Positive expiratory pressure for the treatment of high altitude pulmonary oedema. *Lancet* **1**, 1036–1037

Ferris, B. G. Jr., Puleo, S. and Chen, H. Y. (1979). Mortality and morbidity in a pulp and paper mill in the United States: a ten year follow-up. *Br. J. ind. Med.* **36**, 127–134

Finlay, G. R. (1950). In *Pneumoconiosis* (Sixth Saranac Symposium), edited by A.J. Vorwald, pp. 493–497. New York; Hoeber

Flake, R. E. (1964), Chlorine inhalation. *New Engl. J. Med.* **271**, 1373

Fleming, G. M., Chester, E. H. and Montenegro, H. D. (1979). Dysfunction of small airways following pulmonary injury due to nitrogen dioxide. *Chest,* **75**, 720–721

Fogh, A., Frost, J. and Georg. J. (1969). Respiratory symptoms and pulmonary function in welders. *Ann. occup. Hyg.* **12**, 213–218

Folinsbee, L. J., Horvath, S. M., Bedi, J. F. and Delehunt, J. C. (1978). Effect of 0.62 ppm NO_2 on cardiopulmonary function in young male non-smokers. *Envir. Res.* **15**, 199–205

Frant, R. (1963). Formation of ozone in gas-shielded welding. *Ann. occup. Hyg.* **6**, 113–125

Freeman, G. and Haydon, G. B. (1964). Emphysema after low-level exposure to NO_2. *Archs envir. Hlth* **8**, 125–128

Freeman, G., Crane, S. C. and Furiosi, N. J. (1969). Healing in rat lung after subacute exposure to nitrogen dioxide. *Am. Rev. resp. Dis.* **100**, 622–676

Friberg, L. (1950). Health hazards in the manufacturer of alkaline accumulators will special reference to chronic cadium poisoning. *Acta med. scand.* **138**, Suppl. 240, 7–124

Friberg, L. (1957). Deposition and distribution of cadmium in man in chronic poisoning. *Archs ind. Hlth* **16**, 27–29

Friberg, L. (1971). Cadmium, alloys, compounds. In *Encyclopedia of Occupational Health and Safety*, pp. 233–234. Geneva; International Labour Office

Garnusewski, Z. and Dobrzyński, W. (1967). Regression of pulmonary radiological changes in dockyard welders after cessation or decrease of exposure to welding fumes. *Polish med. J.* **6**, 610–613

Gärtner, H. (1952). Etiology of corundum smelter's lung. *Arch. ind. Hyg. occup. Med.* **6**, 339–343

Gerritsen, W. B. and Buschmann, C. H. (1960). Phosgene poisoning caused by the use of chemical paint removers containing methylene chloride in ill-ventilated rooms heated by kerosene stoves. *Br. J. ind. Med.* **17**, 187–189

Gleason, R. P. (1968), Exposure to copper dust. *Am. ind. Hyg. Ass. J.* **29**, 461–462

Glover, J. R. (1970). Selenium and its industrial toxicology. *Indust. med. Surg.* **39**, 50–54

Godbert, A. L. and Leach, E. (1970). *Research Report 265.* A preliminary survey of the pollution of mine air by nitrogen oxides from diesel exhaust gases. Sheffield; Safety in Mines Research Establishment

Goralewski, G. (1940). Zur Symptomatologie der Aluminium-Staublunge. *Arch. Gewerbepath. Gewerbehyg.* **10**, 384–408

Goralewski, G. (1947). Die Aluminiumlunge: eine neue Gewerbeerkrankung. *Z. ges. inn. Med.* **2**, 665–673

Goralewski, G. (1950). Die Aluminiumlunge. Eine klinische Studie. *Arbeitsmedizin.* **26**

Goralewski, G. and Jaeger, R. (1941). Zur Klinik, Pathologie und Pathogenese der Aluminiumlunge. *Arch. Gewerbepath. Gewerbehyg.* **11**, 102–105

Gough, J. (1960). Emphysema in relation to occupation. *Ind. Med. surg.* **29**, 283–285

Gough, J. (1968). The pathogenesis of emphysema. In *The Lung*, edited by A. A. Liebow and D. E. Smith, pp. 124–126. Baltimore; Williams and Wilkins

Graham, J. I. and Runnicles, D. F. (1943). Nitrous fumes from shot-firing in relation to pulmonary disease. In *Chronic Disease in South Wales Coal Miners.* Med. Res. Council Spec. Rep. Ser. No. 244, pp. 187–213

Grayson, R. R. (1956). Silage gas poisoning: nitrogen dioxide pneumonia, a new disease in agricultural workers. *Ann. intern. Med.* **45**, 393–408

Green, I. D. and Fletcher, R. F. (1979). Acute Mountain Sickness. Symposium held at the Medical School, University of Birmingham, 1978. *Postgrad. med. J.* **55**, 441–512

Greenburg, S. R. (1977). The pulmonary effects of pure aluminium in the Swiss mouse. *Lab. Invest.* **36**, 339

Grover, R. F., Hyers, T. M., McMurtry, I. F. and Reeves, J. T. (1979). High altitude pulmonary oedema. In *Pulmonary Oedema*, edited by Alfred P. Fishman and Eugene M. Renkin, pp. 229–240. Bethesda, Maryland; American Physiological Society

Gudzovskii, G. A. (1971). Antimony: alloys and compounds. *Encycl. Occup. Hlth Safety*, Vol. 1, pp. 112–114. Geneva; ILO

Guidotti, T. L., Abraham, J. L., DeNee, P. B. and Smith, J. R. (1978). Arc welders' pneumoconiosis: application of advanced scanning electron microscopy. *Archs envir. Hlth.* **33**, 117–124

Hackett, P. H., Rennie, D. and Levine, H. D. (1976). The incidence, importance and prophylaxis of acute mountain sickness. *Lancet* **2**, 1149–1155

Hackney, J. D. and Linn, W. S. (1979) Koch's postulates updated: a potentially useful application to laboratory research and policy analysis in environmental technology. *Am. Rev. resp. Dis.* **119**, 849–852

Hackney, J. D., Linn, W. S., Mohler, J. G., Pedersen, E. E., Breisacher, P. and Russo, A. (1975). Experimental studies on human health effects of air pollutants. 11. Four-hour exposure to ozone alone and in combination with other pollutant gases. *Archs envir. Hlth* **30**, 379–384

Hagen, J. (1950). Ueber Lungenveränderungen be Korund-schmelzern. *Dt. med. Wschr.* **75**, 399–400

Hall, A. D. (1923). Can silage be substituted for roots? *J. Fmr's Club*, March, 20–21

Hallee, T. J. (1969). Diffuse lung disease caused by inhalation of mercury vapor. *Am. Rev. resp. Dis.* **99**, 430–436

Halpin, D. S. (1975). An unusual reaction in muscle in association with a Vitallium plate: a report of possible metal hypersensitivity. *J. Bone Jt. Surg.* **57–B**, 451–453

Hampton, T. R. W. (1971). Acute inhalation injury. *J. R. naval Med. Service* **57**, 4–9

Harding, H. E. (1950). Notes on the toxicology of cobalt metal. *Br. J. ind. Med.* **7**, 76–78

Hatton, D. V., Leach, C. S., Nicogossian, A. E. and Di Ferrante, N. (1977). Collagen breakdown and nitrogen dioxide inhalation. *Archs envir. Hlth* **32**, 33–36

Hatch, T. F. (1950). In *Pneumoconiosis* (Sixth Saranac Symposium), edited by A. J. Vorwald, pp. 498–501, New York; Hoeber

Heath, D., Moosavi, H. and Smith, P. (1973). Ultrastructure of high altitude pulmonary oedema. *Thorax* **28**, 694–700

Heath, J. C., Webb, M. and Caffrey, M. (1969). The interaction of carcinogenic metals with tissues and body fluids. Cobalt and horse serum. *Br. J. Cancer* **23**, 153–166

Heath, D. and Williams, D. R. (1981). *Man at High Altitude.* 2nd edn. Edinburgh, London and New York; Livingstone Churchill

Hicks, R., Hewitt, P. J. and Lam, H. F. (1979). An investigation of the experimental induction of hypersensitivity in the guinea pig on material containing chromium, nickel and cobalt from arc welding fumes. *Int. Archs Allergy appl. Immunol.* **59**, 265–272

Hirst, R. N., Jr., Perry, H. M., Jr., Cruz, M. G. and Pierce, J. A. (1973). Elevated cadmium concentration in emphysematous lungs. *Am. Rev. resp. Dis.* **108**, 30–39

Holden, H. (1965). Cadmium fume. *Ann. occup. Hyg.* **8**, 51–54

Horvath, E. P., doPico, G. A. Barbee, R. A. and Dickie, H. A. (1978). Nitrogen dioxide-induced pulmonary disease. *J. occup. Med.* **20**, 103–110

Houston, C. S. (1975). Medical problems of high altitude. In *Medicine for Mountaineering*, 2nd edition. edited by James A. Wikerson, pp. 136–151. Seattle, Washington; The Mountaineers

Houston, C. S. (1976). High altitude illness. Disease with protean manifestations. *J. Am. med. Ass.* **326**, 2193–2195

Huber, G. L., Mason, R. J., La Force, M., Spencer, N. J., Gardner, D. E. and Coffin, D. L. (1971). Alteration in the lung following the administration of ozone. *Archs intern. Med.* **128**, 81–93

Hudson, T. G. F. (1964). *Vanadium, Toxicology and Biological Significance*. edited by E. Browning, Amersterdam, London, and New York; Elsevier

Hultgren, H. N., Grover, R. F. and Hartley, L. H. (1971). Abnormal circulatory responses to high altitude in subjects with a previous history of high-altitude pulmonary oedema. *Circulation* **44**, 759–770

Hultgren, H. N. and Marticorena, R. A. (1968). Epidemiologic observations of incidence of high altitude pulmonary edema. *Clin. Res.* **16**, 142

Hunter, D., Milton, R., Perry, K. M. A. and Thompson, D. R. (1944). Effect of aluminium and alumina on the lung in grinders of duralumin aeroplane propellers. *Br. J. ind. Med.* **1**, 159–164

Iwao, S., Tsuchiya, K. and Sakuria, H. (1980). Serum and urinary β-2-microglobulin among cadmium-exposed workers. *J. occup. Med.* **22**, 399–402

Jenkins, H. M. (1884). Report on the practice of ensilage. *Jl R. agric. Soc.* 2nd ser. **20**. 132–137

Jephcott, C. M. (1950). Chemical aspect of Shaver's disease. In *Pneumoconiosis.* (Sixth Saranac symposium), edited by A.J. Vorwald, pp. 489–493. New York; Hoeber

Jesson, M. W. (1972). *Removal of Gases from a Forage Tower Prior to Entry*. Rep. No. 3. Silsoe, Beds.; National Institute of Agricultural Engineering

Jobs, H. and Ballhausen, C. (1940). Quoted by Bech, A.O., Kipling, M. D. and Heather, J. C. (1962). Hard metal disease. *Br. J. ind. Med.* **19**, 239–252

Johnstone, R. T. (1945). Methyl bromide intoxication in a large group of workers. *Indust. med. Surg.* **14**, 495–497

Jones, A. T. (1952). Noxious gases and fumes. *Proc. R. Soc. Med.* **45**, 609–610

Jones, D. A., Lucas, H. K., O'Driscoll, M., Price, C. H. G. and Wibberley, B. (1975). Cobalt toxicity after McKee hip arthroplasty. *J. Bone Jt. Surg.* **57–B,** 289–296

Jones, G. R., Proudfoot, A. T. and Hall, J. T. (1973). Pulmonary effects of acute exposure to nitrous fumes. *Thorax* **28**, 61–65

Jones Williams, W. (1958). The pathology of the lungs in five nickel workers. *Br. J. ind. Med.* **15**, 235–242

Joosens, J. V. (1977). Acute mountain sickness. *Lancet* **1**, 139

Jordan, J. W. (1961). Pulmonary fibrosis in a worker using an aluminium powder. *Br. J. ind. Med.* **18**, 21–23

Joseph, M. (1968). Hard metal pneumoconiosis. *Australas. Radiol.* **12,** 92–95

Joyner, R. E. and Durel, E. G. (1962). Accidental liquid chlorine spill in a rural community. *J. occup. Med.* **4**, 152–154

Kaltreider, N. L., Elder, M. J., Cralley, L. V. and Colwell, M. O. (1972). Health survey of aluminium workers with special reference to fluoride exposure. *J. occup. Med.* **14**, 531–541

Kang, K., Bice, D., Hoffman, E., D'Amato, R. and Salvaggio, J. (1977). Experimental studies of sensitization to beryllium, zirconium and aluminium compounds in the rabbit. *J. Allergy clin. Immunol.* **59**, 425–436

Kaplun, Z. S. and Mezencewa, N. W. (1960). Experimentellstudie uber die toxische Wirkung von Staub bei der Erzengung von Sintermettallen. *J. Hyg. Epidem. Microbiol. Immunol.* **4**, 390–399

Karlish, A. J. (1960). Cadmium poisoning. *Br. med. J.* **1**, 173–174

Karstens, A. I. and Welch, B. E. (1971). Spacecraft atmospheres. In *Aerospace Medicine* 2nd edition, edited by Hugh W. Randel, pp. 668–669. Baltimore; The Williams and Wilkins Company.

Kass, I., Zamel, N., Dobry, C. A. and Holzer, M. (1972). Bronchiectasis following ammonia burns of the respiratory tract. *Chest* **62**, 282–285

Kazantzis, G. (1956). Respiratory function in men casting cadmium alloys. *Br. J. ind. Med.* **13**, 30–36

Kazantzis, G. (1980). *Occupational Exposure to Cadmium,* pp. 55–56 and 58–61. Report on Seminar: London, 20 March, 1980. London; Cadmium Association

Keller, M. D., Lanese, R. R., Mitchell, R. I. and Cote, R. W. (1979a). Respiratory illness in households using gas and electricity for cooking. 1. Survey and Incidence. *Envir. Res.* **19**, 495–503

Keller, M. D., Lanese, R. R., Mitchell, R. I. and Cote, R. W. (1979b). Respiratory illness in households using gas and electricity for cooking. 11. Symptoms and objective findings. *Envir. Res.* **19**, 504–515

Kendrey, G. and Roe, F. J. C. (1969). Cadmium toxicology. *Lancet* **1**, 1206–1207

Kennedy, A., Dornan, J. D. and King, R. (1981). Fatal myocardial disease associated with industrial exposure to cobalt. *Lancet* **1,** 412–414

Kennedy, M. C. S. (1956). Aluminium powder inhalations in the treatment of silicosis of pottery workers and pneumoconiosis of coal miners. *Br. J. ind. Med.* **13**, 85–99

Kennedy, M. C. S. (1972). Nitrous fumes and coal-miners with emphysema. *Ann. occup. Hyg.* **15**, 285–300

Kennedy, M. C. S. (1974). Nitrous fume poisoning in coal-miners. *Rev. Inst. Hyg. Mines* **29**, 167–174

Kerr, H. D., Kulle, T. J., McIlhany, M. L. and Swidersky, P. (1975). Effects of ozone on pulmonary function in normal subjects. *Am. Rev. resp. Dis.* **111**, 763–773

Kidd, D. J. and Elliott, D. H. (1975). Decompression disorders in divers. In *The Physiology and Medicine of Diving*, edited by P. B. Bennett and D. H. Elliott, pp. 471–494. London; Balliere Tindell and Cassell

Kimmerle, G. (1976). Toxicity of combustion products with particular reference to polyurethane. *Ann. occup. Hyg.* **19**, 269–273

Kindwell, E. P. (1975). Medical aspects of commercial diving and compressed air work. In *Occupational Medicine*, edited by C. Zenz, pp. 361–421

King, G. W. (1954). Acute pneumonitis due to accidental exposure to mercury vapor. *Ariz. Med.* **11**, 335

Kirkpatrick, M. B. and Bass, J. B. (1979). Severe obstructive lung disease and smoke inhalation. *Chest* **76**, 108–110

Kiviluoto, M. (1980). Observations on the lungs of vanadium workers. *Br. J. ind. Med.* **37,** 363–366

Kleinerman, J. (1979). Effects of nitrogen dioxide on elastin and collagen contents of lung. *Archs envir. Hlth* **34**, 228–232

Kleinerman, J. and Rynbrandt, D. (1976). Lung proteolytic activity and serum protease inhibition after NO_2 exposure. *Archs envir. Hlth* **31**, 37–41

Kleinerman, J. and Wright, G. W. (1961). The reparative capacity of animal lungs after exposure to various single and multiple doses of nitrite. *Am. Rev. resp. Dis.* **83**, 423–424

Kleinfeld, M., Giel, C. and Tabershaw, I. R. (1957). Health hazards associated with inert-gas-shielded metal arc welding. *Archs ind. Hlth* **15**, 27–31

Kosmider, S., Ludyga, K., Misiewicz, A., Drożdź, M. and Sagan, J. (1972). Experimentalle and klinische Untersuchungen über emphysembildende Wirkung der Stickstoffoxyde. *Zentrabl. Arbeitsmed.* **22**, 362–368

Kowitz, T. A., Reba, R. C., Parker, R. T. and Spicer, W. S. (1967). Effects of chlorine gas upon respiratory function. *Archs envir. Hlth* **14**, 545–558

Krackow, E. H. (1953). Toxicity and health hazards of boron hydrides. *Arch. ind. Hyg. occup. Med.* **8**, 335–339

Kramer, C. G. (1967). Chlorine. *J. occup. Med.* **9**, 193–196

Kronenberger, F. L. (1959). Bronchiolitis after shot-firing in a colliery. *Br. J. Dis. Chest* **53**, 308–313

Lane, R. E. and Campbell, A. C. P. (1954). Fatal emphysema in two men making a copper cadmium alloy. *Br. J. ind. Med.* **11**, 118–122

Lauwerys, R. (1980). *Occupational Exposure to Cadmium,* pp. 57–61. Report on Seminar: London, 20 March, 1980. London; Cadmium Association

Lauwerys, R. R., Buchet, J. P. and Roels, H. (1976). The relationship between cadmium exposure or body burden and the concentration of cadmium in blood and urine in man. *Int. Arch. occup. envir. Hlth* **36**, 275–285

Lauwerys, R. R., Buchet, J. P., Roels, H. A., Brouwers, J. and Stanescu, D. (1974). Epidemiological survey of workers exposed to cadmium. *Archs envir. Hlth* **28**, 145–148

Leading article. (1973). Cadmium and the lung. *Lancet* **2**, 1134–1135

Lees, R. E. M. (1980). Changes in lung function after exposure to vanadium compounds in fuel oil ash. *Br. J. ind. Med.* **37**, 253–256

Lemen, R. A., Lee, J. S., Wagoner, J. K. and Blejer, H. P. (1976). Cancer mortality among cadmium production workers. *Ann. N.Y. Acad. Sci.* **271**, 273–279

Lewis, C. E. (1959). The biological effects of vanadium exposure. II The signs and symptoms of occupational vanadium exposure. *Arch. industr. Hyg.* **19**, 497–503

Lewis, G. P., Lyle, H. and Miller, S. (1969). Association between elevated hepatic water-soluble protein-bound cadmium levels and chronic bronchitis and/or emphysema, *Lancet* **2**, 1330–1333

Lewis, G. P., Jusko, W. J., Coughlin, L. L. and Hartz, S. (1972). Contribution of cigarette smoking to cadmium accumulation in man. *Lancet* **1**, 291–292

Levy, P. M., Jaeger, E. A., Stone, R. S. and Douona, C. T. (1962). Aero-atelectasis: a respiratory syndrome in aviators. *Aerospace Med.* **33**, 988–994

Liebow, A. A. (1975). Definition and classification of interstitial pneumonias in human pathology. *Prog. Resp. Res.* **8**, 1–33. Basel; Karger

Lloyd-Davies, T. A. (1946). Manganese pneumonitis. *Br. J. ind. Med.* **3**, 111–135

Lloyd-Davies, T. A. and Harding, H. E. (1949). Manganese pneumonitis. *Br. J. ind. Med.* **6**, 82–90

Loke, J., Farmer, W., Matthay, R. A., Putman, C. E. and Walker Smith, G. J. (1980). Acute and chronic effects of fire fighting on pulmonary function. *Chest* **77**, 369–373

Lowe, H. J. and Freeman, G. (1957). Boron hydride (Borane) intoxication in man. *Arch. ind. Hlth* **16**, 523–533

Lowry, T. and Schuman, L. M. (1956). 'Silo-filler's disease'—a syndrome caused by nitrogen dioxide. *J. Am. med. Ass.* **162**, 153–160

Lundgren, K. D. and Öhman, H. (1954). Pneumokoniose in der Hartmetall-industrie. *Virchows. Arch. path. Anat. Physiol.* **325**, 259–284

McAdams, A. J. (1955). Bronchiolitis obliterans. *Am. J. Med.* **19**, 314–322

McConnell, L. H., Fink, J. N., Schlueter, D. P. and Schmidt, M. G. Jr. (1973). Asthma caused by nickel sensitivity. *Ann. intern. Med.* **78**, 888–890

McDermott, F. T. (1971). Dust in the cemented carbide industry. *Am ind. Hyg. Ass. J.* **32**, 188–193

McLaughlin, A. I. G., Kazantzis, G., King, E., Teare, R. J. and Owen, R. (1962). Pulmonary fibrosis and encephalopathy associated with inhalation of aluminium dust. *Br. J. ind. Med.* **19**, 253–263

McLaughlin, A. I. G., Milton, R. and Perry, K. M. A. (1946). Toxic manifestations of osmium tetroxide. *Br. J. ind. Med.* **3**, 183–186

McLintock, T. S. (1972). Discussion. *Ann. occup. Hyg.* **15**, 301

McMillan, G. H. G. and Heath, J. (1979). The health of welders in naval dockyards: acute changes in respiratory function during standardized welding. *Ann. occup. Hyg.* **22**, 19–32

Mathes, F. T., Kirschner, R., Yow, M. D. and Brennan, J. C. (1958). Acute poisoning associated with inhalation of mercury vapour. *Pediatrics* **22**, 675–688

Mayor, M. B., Merritt, K. and Brown, S. A. (1980). Metal allergy and the surgical patient. *Am. J. Surg.* **139**, 477–479

Medical Research Council (1936). Industrial Pulmonary Disease Committee. *Br. med. J.* **2**, 1273–1275

Merfield, D. P., Taylor, A., Gemmell, D. M. and Parish, J. A. (1976). Mercury intoxication in a dental surgery following unreported spillage. *Br. dent. J.* **141**, 179–186

Meyers, J. B. (1950). Acute pulmonary complications following inhalation of chromic acid mist. *Arch. ind. Hyg.* **2**, 742–747

Miles, S. and Mackay, D. E. (1976). *Underwater Medicine*, 4th edition, London; Adlard Coles Limited

Miller, C. W., Davies, M. W., Goldman, A. and Wyatt, J. P. (1953). Pneumoconiosis in the tungsten carbide tool industry. *Archs ind. Hyg.* **8**, 453–465

Milliken, J. A., Waugh, D. and Kadish, M. E. (1963). Acute interstitial pulmonary fibrosis caused by a smoke bomb. *Can. med. Ass. J.* **88**, 36–39

Milne, J. E. H. (1969). Nitrogen dioxide inhalation and bronchiolitis obliterans. *J. occup. Med.* **11**, 538–547

Milne, J., Christophers, A. and de Silva, P. (1970). Acute mercurial pneumonitis. *Br. J. ind. Med.* **27**, 334–338

Mitchell, J., Manning, G. B., Molyneux, M. and Lane, R. E. (1961). Pulmonary fibrosis in workers exposed to finely powdered aluminium. *Br. J. ind. Med.* **18**, 10–20

Montague, T. J. and MacNeil, A. R. (1980). Mass ammonia inhalation. *Chest*, **77**, 496–498

Morgan, W. K. C. (1962). Arc welders' lung complicated by conglomeration. *Am. Rev. resp. Dis.* **85**, 570–575

Morichau-Beauchant, G. (1964). Pneumonies manganiques. *J. fr. Méd. Chir. thorac.* **18**, 300–312

Morley, R. and Silk, S. J. (1970). The industrial hazard of nitrous fumes. *Ann. occup. Hyg.* **13**, 101–107

Moskowitz, R. L., Lyons, H. A. and Cottle, H. R. (1964). Silofiller's disease. *Am. J. Med.* **36**, 457–462

Mur, J-M., Mereau, P., Cavelier, C., Pham, Q. T. and Castet, P. (1979). Ateliers de fonderie et fonction respiratoire. *Arch. Mal. Prof.* **40**, 587–595

Musk, A. W., Peters, J. M. and Wegman, D. H. (1977). Lung function in firefighters: 1. A three-year follow-up of active subjects. *Am. J. publ. Hlth* **67**, 626–629

Mustafa, M. G., Cross, C. E., Munn, R. J. and Hardie, J. A. (1971). Effects of divalent metal ions on alveolar macrophage membrane adenosine triphosphatase activity. *J. Lab. clin. Med.* **77**, 563–571

Nandi, M., Jick, H., Slone, D., Shapiro, S. and Lewis, G. P. (1969). Cadmium content of cigarettes. *Lancet* **2**, 1329–1330

Norwood, W. D., Wisehart, D. E., Earl, C. A., Adley, F. E. and Anderson, D. E. (1966). Nitrogen dioxide poisoning due to metal cutting with oxyacetylene torch. *J. occup. Med.* **8**, 301–306

Palmer, K. C., Snider, G. L. and Hayes, J. A. (1975). Cellular proliferation induced in the lung by cadmium aerosol. *Am. Rev. resp. Dis.* **112**, 173–179

Patterson, J.C. (1947). Studies on the toxicity of inhaled cadmium. *J. ind. Hyg.* **29**, 294–301

Pattey, F. A. (1963). In *Industrial Hygiene and Toxicology. Vol. II*, Editors: David W. Fassett and Don. D. Irish, pp. 883–884. New York/London; Interscience Publishers; John Wiley and Sons

Patwardhan, J. R. and Finckh, E. S. (1976). Fatal cadmium fume pneumonitis. *Med. J. Aust.* **1**, 962–966

Payne, L. R. (1979). Personal communication

Pernis, E., Vigliani, G., Cavagna, G. and Finulli, M. (1961). Endogenous pyrogen in the pathogenesis of metal fume fever. Proc. X111 *Int. Congr. occup. Hlth, New York*. pp. 770–772

Pieters, H. A. J. and Creyghton, J. W. (1951). *Safety in the Chemical Laboratory*. London; Butterworths

Pimentel, J. C. and Marques, F. (1969). Vineyard sprayer's lung: a new occupational disease. *Thorax* **24**, 678–688

Piscator, M. (1976). Health hazards from inhalation of metal fumes. *Envir. Res.* **11**, 268–270

Piscator, M. (1978). Serum β_2-microglobulin in cadmium exposed workers. *Path. Biologie.* **26**, 321–323

Piscator, M. and Alexelsson, B. (1970). Serum proteins and kidney function after exposure to cadmium. *Archs envir. Hlth* **21**, 604–608

Posner, E. and Kennedy, M. C. S. (1967). A further study of china biscuit placers in Stoke-on-Trent. *Br. J. ind. Med.* **24**, 133–142

Potts, C. L. (1965). Cadmium proteinuria—the health of battery workers exposed to cadmium oxide dust. *Ann. occup. Hyg.* **8**, 55–61

Powell, M. (1961). Toxic fumes from shotfiring in coal mines. *Ann. occup. Hyg.* **3**, 162–183

Powell, M. and Lomax, A. (1960). The toxic effects of handling and firing explosives in coal mines. *Ann. occup. Hyg.* **2**, 141–151

Princi, F. (1947). A study of industrial exposures to cadmium. *J. ind. Hyg.* **29**, 315–320

Prys-Roberts, C. (1967). Principles of treatment of poisoning by higher oxides of nitrogen. *Br. J. Anaesth.* **39**, 432–438

Rae, T. (1975). A study of the effects of particulate metals of orthopaedic interest on murine macrophages *in vitro*. *J. Bone Jt. Surg.* **57–B**, 444–450

Rae, T. (1978). The haemolytic action of particulate metals. *J. Path.* **125**, 81–89

Ramirez-R., J. and Dowell, A. R. (1971). Silo-filler's disease: nitrogen dioxide-induced lung injury. *Ann. intern. Med.* **74**, 569–576

Rathus, E. M. and Landy, P. J. (1961). Methyl bromide poisoning. *Br. J. ind. Med.* **18**, 53–57

Reber, E. and Burckhardt, P. (1970). Über Hartmetallstaublungen in des Schweiz. *Respiration* **27**, 120–153

Riddell, A. R. (1950). Clinical aspects of Shaver's disease. In *Pneumoconiosis* (Sixth Saranac Symposium), edited by A.J. Vorwald, pp. 459–482. New York; Hoeber

Rivers, J. F., Orr, G. and Lee, H. A. (1970). Drowning. Its clinical sequelae and management. *Br. med. J.* **1**, 157–161

Robertson, H. T., Lakshminarayan, S. and Hudson, L. D. (1978). Lung injury following a 50-metre fall into water. *Thorax* **33**, 175–180

Roe, J. W. (1959). Gases and fumes produced in fusion welding and cutting. *Ann. occup. Hyg.* **2**, 75–84

Roels, H., Bernard, A., Buchet, J. P., Goret, A., Lauwerys, R., Chettle, D. R., Harvey, T. C. and Al Haddad, I. (1979). Critical concentration of cadmium in renal cortex and urine. *Lancet* **1**, 221

Rynbrandt, D. and Kleinerman, J. (1977). Nitrogen dioxide and pulmonary proteolytic enzymes. *Archs envir. Hlth* **32**, 165–172

Sanderson, J. T. (1968). Hazards of the arc-air gouging process. *Ann. occup. Hyg.* **11**, 123–133

Schardijn, G., van Eps, L. W. S. Swaak, A. J. G., Kager, J. C. G. M. and Persijn, J. P. (1979). Urinary β_2-microglobulin in upper and lower urinary-tract infections. *Lancet* **1**, 805–807

Schecter, A., Shanske, W., Stenzler, A., Quintilian, H. and Steinberg, H. (1980). Acute hydrogen selenide inhalation. *Chest* **77**, 554–555

Schepers, G. W. H. (1955a). The biological action of particulate cobalt metal. *Archs ind. Hlth* **12**, 127–133

Schepers, G. W. H. (1955b). The biological action of particulate tungsten metal. *Archs ind. Hlth* **12**, 134–136

Schepers, G. W. H. (1955c). The biological action of tantalum oxide. *Archs ind. Hlth* **12**, 121–123

Scherrer, M., Parambadathumalail, A., Burki, H., Senn. A. and Zürcher, R. (1970). Drei Falle von Hartmetallstaublunge. *Schweiz. med. Wschr.* **100**, 2251–2255

Schwarz, L., Peck, S. M., Blair, K. E. and Markuson, K. E. (1945). Allergic dermatitis due to metallic cobalt. *J. Allergy* **16**, 51–53

Scott, R., Paterson, P. J., Mills, E. A., McKirdy, A., Fell, G. S., Ottoway, J. M., Husain, F. E. R., Fitzgerald-Finch, O. P., Yates, A. J., Lemont, A. and Roxburgh, S. (1976). Clinical and biochemical abnormalities in coppersmiths exposed to cadmium. *Lancet* **2**, 396–398

Seidelin, R. (1961). The inhalation of hosgene in a fire extinguisher accident. *Thorax* **16**, 91–93

Shaver, C. G. (1948). Further observations of lung changes associated with the manufacture of alumina abrasives. *Radiology* **50**, 760–769

Shaver, C. G. and Riddell, A. R. (1947). Lung changes associated with the manufacture of alumina abrasives. *J. ind. Hyg. Toxicol.* **29**, 145–157

Shiel, O. M. F. (1967). Morbid anatomical changes in the lungs of dogs after inhalation of higher oxides of nitrogen during anaesthesia. *Br. J. Anaesth.* **39**, 413–424

Sjöberg, S. (1950). Vanadium pentoxide dust. *Acta med. scand. Suppl.* 238

Sjögren, I., Hillerdal, G., Anders, A. and Zetterström, O. (1980). Hard metal lung disease; importance of cobalt in coolants. *Thorax*, **35**, 653–659

Smith, J. P., Smith J. C. and McCall, A. J. (1960). Chronic poisoning from cadmium fume. *J. Path.* **80**, 287–296

Smith, T. J., Petty, T. L., Reading, J. C. and Lakshminarayan, S. (1976). Pulmonary effects of chronic exposure to airborne cadmium. *Am. Rev. resp. Dis.* **114**, 161–169

Smith, J. P., Smith, J. C. and McCall, A. J. (1960). Chronic poisoning from cadmium fume. *J. Path. Bact.* **80**, 287–296

Sobonya, R. (1977). Fatal anhydrous ammonia inhalation. *Human Path.* **8**, 293–299

Spiegl, C. J., Scott, J. K., Steinhardt, H., Leach, L. J. and Hodge, H. C. (1956). Acute inhalation toxicity of lithium anhydride. *Arch. ind. Hlth* **14**, 468–470

Stacy, B. D., King, E. J., Harrison, C. V., Nagelschmidt, G. and Nelson, S. (1959). Tissue changes in rats' lungs caused by hydroxides, oxides and phosphates of aluminium and iron. *J. Path. Bact.* **77**, 417–426

Stănescu, D., Veriter, C., Frans, A., Goncette, L., Roels, H., Lauwerys, R. and Brasseur, L., (1977). Effects on lung of chronic occupational exposure to cadmium. *Scand. J. resp. Dis.* **58**, 289–303

Stark, G. W. V. (1972). Smoke and toxic gases from burning plastics. *Trans. I. Mar. Eng.* **84**, 25–34

Steel, J. (1964). Health hazards in the welding and cutting of paint-primed steel. *Ann. occup. Hyg.* **7**, 247–251

Steel, J. (1968). Respiratory hazards in shipbuilding and ship repairing. *Ann. occup. Hyg.* **11**, 115–121

Steele, R. H., and Wilhelm, D. L. (1967). The inflammatory reaction in chemical injury II. *Br. J. exp. Path.* **48**, 592–607

Stephens, R. J., Sloan, M. A., Evans, M. J. and Freeman, G. (1974). Early response of lungs to low levels of ozone. *Am. J. Pathol.* **74**, 31–58

Stephenson, S. F., Esrig, B. C., Polk, H. C. Jr. and Fulton, R. L. (1975). The pathophysiology of smoke inhalation injury. *Ann. Surg.* **182**, 652–660

Stokinger, H. E. (1965). Ozone toxicology: a review of research and industrial experience, 1954–1964. *Archs envir. Hlth* **10**, 719–731

Strauss, R. H. (1979). Diving Medicine. *Am. Rev. resp. Dis.* **119**, 1001–1023

Sunderman, F. W. and Kincaid, J. F. (1954). Nickel poisoning. 11. Studies on patients suffering from acute exposure to vapors of nickel carbonyl. *J. Am. med. Ass.* **155**, 889–894

Sunderman, F. W. and Sunderman, F. W. Jr. (1961). Löffler's syndrome associated with nickel sensitivity. *Archs intern. Med.* **107**, 405–408

Taniguchi, N., Tanaka, M., Kishihara, C., Ohne, H., Kondo, T., Matsuda, I., Fujino, T. and Harada, M. (1979). Determination of carbonic anhydrase C and β_2-microglobulin by radioimmunassay in urine of heavy-metal-exposed subjects and patients with renal tubular acidosis. *Envir. Res.* **20**, 154–161

Tashkin, D. P., Genovesi, M. G., Chopra, S., Coulson, A. and Simmons, M. (1977). Respiratory status of Los Angeles fireman: One-month follow-up after inhalation of dense smoke. *Chest* **71**, 445–449

Tebrock, H. E., and Mackle, W. (1968). Exposure to europium-activated yttrium orthovanadate. *J. occup. Med.* **10**, 692-696

Teisinger, J. and Fiserova-Bergerova, V. (1965). Pulmonary retention and excretion of mercury vapors in man. *Ind. med. Surg.* **34**, 580–584

Telescu, D. B. and Stanescu, D. C. (1970). Pulmonary function in workers with chronic exposure to cadmium oxide fumes. *Int. Archs. Arbeitsmed.* **26**, 335–345

Teng, C. T. and Brennan, J. C. (1959). Acute mercury vapour poisoning. A report of four cases with radiographic and pathologic correlation. *Radiology* **73**, 354–361

Tennant, R., Johnson, H. J. and Wells, J. B. (1961). Acute bilateral pneumonitis associated with the inhalation of mercury vapour. *Conn. Med.* **25**, 106–109

Thurlbeck, W. H. (1976). *Chronic Airflow Obstruction in Lung Disease. Volume V. Major Problems in Pathology*, edited by James L. Bennington, pp. 303–304. Philadelphia, London, Toronto; W. B. Saunders

Tolot, F., Girard, R., Dortit, G., Tabourin, G., Galy, P. and Bourret, J. (1970). Manifestations pulmonaires des 'métaux durs': troubles irritatifs et fibrose (Enquête et observations cliniques). *Archs Mal. prof. Méd. trav.* **31**, 453–470

Townshend, R. H. (1968). A case of acute cadmium pneumonitis: lung function tests during a four-year follow-up. *Br. J. ind. Med.* **25**, 68–71

Tsuchiya, K. (1967). Proteinuria of workers exposed to cadmium fume. *Archs envir. Hlth* **14**, 875–880

Turner, C. (1953). Self-feeding of silage. *Agriculture* **60**, 358–359

Unger, K. M., Snow, R. M., Mestas, J. M. and Miller, W. C. (1980). Smoke inhalation in firemen. *Thorax* **35,** 838–842

Vigdortschik, N. A., Andreeva, E. C. Matussevitsch, I. Z., Nikulina, M. M., Frumina, L. M. and Stritor, V. A. (1937). The symptomatology of chronic poisoning with oxides of nitrogen. *J. ind. Hyg. Toxicol.* **19**, 469–473

Villar, T. G. (1974). Vineyard sprayers' lung. *Am. Rev. resp. Dis.* **110**, 545–555

Vintinner, F. J., Vallenas, R., Carlin, C. E., Weiss, R., Macher, C. and Ochoa, R. (1955). Study of the health of workers employed in mining and processing vanadium ore. *Arch. ind. Hlth.* **12**, 635–642

Walton, M. (1973). Industrial ammonia gassing. *Br. J. ind. Med.* **30**, 78–86

Watt, J. (1977). The role of the services in accident and disaster. *J. R. naval Med. Serv.* **63**, 117–125

Webb, M. (1975). Cadmium. *Br. med. Bull.* **31**, 246–250

Webb, M. and Etienne, A. T. (1977). Studies on the toxicity and metabolism of cadmium-thionein. *Biochem. Pharmacol.* **26**, 15–30

Weill, H. (1980). Unpublished observation

Weill, H., George, R., Schwarz, M. and Ziskind, M. (1969). Late evaluation of pulmonary function after acute exposure to chlorine gas. *Am. Rev. resp. Dis.* **99**, 374–379

Welinder, H., Skerfving, S. and Henriksen, O. (1977). Cadmium metabolism in man. *Br. J. ind. Med.* **34**, 221–228

Weston, J. T., Liebow, A. A., Dixon, M. G. and Rich, T. H. (1972). Untoward effects of exogenous inhalants on the lung. *J. Forensic Sc.* **17**, 199–279

Whitaker, P. H. (1945). Radiological appearances of the chest following partial asphyxia by a smoke screen. *Br. J. Radiol.* **18**, 396–397

Whitener, D. R., Whitener, K. M., Robertson, K. J., Baxter, C. R. and Pierce, A. K. (1980). Pulmonary function measurements in patients with thermal injury and smoke inhalation. *Am. Rev. resp. Dis.* **122,** 731–739

Williams, E. R. P. (1942). Blast effects in warfare. *Br. J. Surg.* **30**, 38–49

Williams, N. (1952). Vanadium poisoning from cleaning oil fired boilers. *Br. J. ind. Med.* **9**, 50–55

Wooley, W. D., (1971). Decomposition products of PVC for studies of fires. *Br. Polymer J.* **3**, 186–193

Wooley, W. D. and Palmer, K. N. (1976). Plastics in fires and toxic hazards. *Building Res. Estb. News* **37**, 12. London; HMSO

World Health Organization. (1977). Oxides of Nitrogen. *Environmental Health Criteria* 4. Geneva; WHO

Wyatt, J. P. and Riddell, A. C. R. (1949). The morphology of bauxite fume pneumoconiosis. *Am. J. Path.* **25**, 447–465

Wyers, H. (1946). Some toxic effects on vanadium pentoxide. *Br. J. ind. Med.* **3**, 177–182

Young, W. H., Shaw, D. B. and Bates, D. V. (1964). Presence of ozone in aircraft flying at 35 000 feet. *Aerospace Med.* **33**, 311–318

Young, W. A., Shaw, D. B. and Bates, D. V. (1964). Effect of low concentrations of ozone on pulmonary function in man. *J. appl. Physiol.* **19**, 765–768

Zenz, C. and Berg. B. A. (1967). Human responses to controlled vanadium pentoxide exposure. *Archs envir. Hlth* **14**, 709–712

14 Lung Cancer and Occupation

Interest in this complex topic and the question of occupational cancer in general has greatly increased in recent years. But as a detailed discussion of the problem is impossible in a chapter of this length five key points are made followed by a section on ionizing radiation and a tabular summary of other established and some suspected causes of occupational carcinoma of the lung (*Table 14.1*).

Firstly, tobacco smoke is established as the overwhelmingly dominant respiratory carcinogen in man but agents present in some occupations (ionizing radiation and certain minerals and chemicals) are known to cause lung cancer both in smokers and non-smokers though the risk is substantially greater in smokers — in short, a co-carcinogenic effect. This excess risk in smokers applies to all known industrial carcinogens. However, the available evidence indicates that industrial carcinogens are responsible for only a small proportion of lung cancers, for the occupational component of *all* cancers is estimated to be approximately 1 to 5 per cent (Higginson and Muir, 1976; Doll, 1977; Wynder and Gori, 1977; Higginson, 1980a)—possibly as much as 15 per cent in the USA (Cole, 1977). Nonetheless, this group, though a minority, is important. A recent report by Bridbord *et al.* (1978), which claims that some 30 per cent of all cancers which develop in the next few decades will probably be wholly or partly due to industrial carcinogens, has been strongly criticized as being based on evidence which is inadequate in a variety of important respects (Leading article, 1978; Abelson, 1979; Morgan, 1979). Higginson and Muir (1979) maintain that, on present knowledge, 'most cancers of presumed environmental aetiology cannot readily be ascribed to industrial exposures, either point-source or general'.

Secondly, epidemiological studies of cancer incidence in industry must have cohorts and mortality data (including hospital and post-mortem records) which are validly matched in all relevant respects and cover a sufficient period of time. This is important in view of the relatively low attack rate of carcinoma of the lung and the long interval between cessation of exposure and development of the tumour in most cases (Kotin, 1968).

Surveys in England and Wales have shown that, in spite of the fact that certain occupations are associated with a greater or lesser cancer risk than the general population average, almost 90 per cent of such variation disappears when comparison is made between individuals of similar habits and social class (Registrar General, 1978; Fox and Adelstein, 1978; Higginson, 1980a). (*See also* Epidemiology, Chapter 1.) The 88 to 90 per cent of cancers which are of non-occupational origin are related to so-called 'lifestyle' factors—'lifestyle' being understood as 'the total cultural, behavioural and dietary environment'. It is unlikely that carcinogenesis can be conceived of in terms of any single mechanism, though one may be overwhelmingly predominant. 'Thus, over 80 per cent of lung cancers in men would not occur in the absence of the cigarette habit. In this sense, cigarette smoking may be considered the *practical cause* without precluding a modulating role for other factors, including individual susceptibility' (Higginson, 1980b). At present there is some controversy regarding the 'lifestyle' concept of carcinogenesis—the opposing aspects of which are exemplified by Epstein and Swartz (1981) and Peto (1980)—but it is not appropriate to discuss this here.

Thirdly, although animal experiments may give advanced warning of possible carcinogenic potential in man, extrapolation of tumour induction in animals to man involves many pitfalls (such as doses of the suspected carcinogen administered, species response differences and spontaneously developing tumours) and is rarely valid in the absence of clear epidemiological confirmation in exposed workers (Morgan, 1978). Whether or not *in vitro* testing of bacterial mutagenesis in the presence of a suspected carcinogen will prove to be more validly applicable to man remains to be determined (Bridges and Fry, 1978). Although rigorous epidemiological methods are essential for detection of a cancer risk of low magnitude—as in respiratory cancers induced by ionizing radiation in some circumstances—'the alert clinician remains the most important source of leads to occupational cancer' (Archer, 1977; Cole, 1977).

Fourthly, most occupationally associated lung carcinomas are of squamous or epidermoid type but, in some instances, they are predominantly of adeno-carcinomatous or large cell type.

Fifthly, the importance of identifying an occupational origin of lung cancer lies in the fact that it can be prevented by elimination or hygienic control of the carcinogenic source. The role of periodic medical examination of personnel exposed to a potential carcinogen is discussed under 'Ionizing radiation' and it is equally applicable to the other cancer risks.

The relationship of the asbestos minerals to respiratory malignancy is referred to separately in Chapter 9.

IONIZING RADIATION

IN MINING

Airborne radioactivity may occur in mines even when no radioactive mineral is obviously present. This is due to diffusion of radon and thoron gases which originate respectively from uranium-238 and thorium-232 in igneous rocks. These elements are present in minute amounts in all rocks but local concentrations occur and, under these circumstances, significant airborne radioactivity is likely. Thus, the greatest concentrations are encountered in uranium mining but lower, and possibly important concentrations, may occur in other types of mine.

Uranium gives rise to decay chain products of which uranium-238 is the first member through a series of solid elements to radium-226 which decays to the gas radon-222 which, in turn, when in air rapidly gives rise to other isotopes—radon 'daughters'. The important members of the series in the present context are those which emit α-particles: namely, radon-222 (half-life 3.8 days) and the three radon daughters, polonium-218 (half-life 3.05 minutes), polonium-214 (half-life 26.8 minutes) and polonium-210 (half-life 19.4 years). Radon-222 leaks from rocks, fallen ore and soil and escapes into the air although concentrations at ground level are very low (Morgan, 1970). But in enclosed areas, such as mines, concentrations may be high because the gas has less chance to diffuse away, it may be carried into the workings by mine-waters from which it escapes, and ventilation is limited.

Thorium, also fairly abundant in the Earth's crust, is usually found in association with uranium. It decays into thoron gas (radon-220), thorium A (polonium-216), thorium-B (lead-212) and thorium C (bismuth-212). Of these thoron, thorium B and thorium C are α emitters.

When first formed, the decay products are single ionized atoms but they readily attach themselves to molecules of water vapour or to dust particles as 'cluster ions' (Chamberlain and Dyson, 1956). It has been calculated that their mean radioactivity diameter is about 0.25 μm in non-operational mines and about 0.4 μm diameter in operational mines (Davies, 1967). In this aerosol state, therefore, they can, on inhalation, penetrate to the trachea, bronchi and beyond, and be retained in the lungs.

Alpha-particles are positively charged helium nuclei with two protons and neutrons which have a greater mass than other radiation particles and great kinetic energy but, owing to their large mass and positive charge, have only feeble penetrating power. They cause dense ionization along their traverse paths which is maximal when their energy is nearly spent; that is, less than 2 MeV (MeV = million electron volts. One electron volt is the energy acquired by an electron when accelerated through a potential difference of 1 V). This occurs when they have passed through the bronchial mucosa and reached the basal cells. Their average penetrability is about 50 μm (Lea, 1955). Beta particles, being electrons, have greater penetrating capacity but less ionizing power. It is believed that ionization is the cause of malignant change in living cells.

For this reason inhaled α-particles are more important than β-particles—although high doses of the latter may induce lung tumours in experimental animals—and there is strong evidence that exposure of man to radon-222 and α-emitting radon daughters is responsible for a significantly increased risk of developing carcinoma of the lung. The radiation dose to the lungs of radon and thoron appears to be approximately similar (Albert, 1966).

URANIUM MINING

This is carried on in Canada (Saskatchewan), Australia (Queensland, Northern Territory and South Australia), the USA (Colorado, Arizona, New Mexico and Utah), South Africa (Witwatersrand), Czechoslovakia (Joachimstal) and the USSR. Like any other hard rock mining, the ore is extracted by deep mining or open pit methods.

The radiation environment of uranium mines is variable and complicated. Miners are exposed to external γ radiation and some β radiation, to airborne radon and radon daughters, and to rock dust. Of these the radon daughters present the most important risk. Other radiation sources are, in general, less than the prescribed occupational limits and do not require specific control.

Radon gas leaks continuously through rock surfaces into all the mine air spaces and may be carried some distances in mine waters before escaping. But owing to increased activity of radon daughters with 'residence time' of air in the mine, variations in mining activity, alterations in the rate of diffusion of radon into the air, and changes in ventilation rates, accumulation of radon and radon daughters is especially complex. Measurement of the composition and concentration of their mixtures at different sites underground is, therefore, necessary. High ventilation rates efficiently reduce radon daughter concentrations in the mine atmosphere but may increase dispersion of silica-containing dust (International Commission on Radiological Protection, 1977).

Mine rock also emits γ radiation. The exposure rate is low in tunnels and shafts but higher in workings, particularly those with ore lenses rich in uranium. Beta radiation is less important.

Ore dust containing members of the uranium decay series is dissipated in the air by mining operations and settles on various surfaces from which it may be resuspended by strong air currents or mechanical agitation. Concentrations vary widely with the site and moisture of the ore and with time, being about zero under inactive mining conditions but very high in the vicinity of blasting operations. The average concentrations of α activity in ordinary mining operations are usually less than 10 pCi m^{-3} (*see* later, this section) (International Commission on Radiological Protection, 1977).

Where ionizing radiation is present in non-uranium mines its characteristics in the environment are similar but levels are usually substantially lower.

Airborne radon was suggested as the cause of an excess of carcinoma of the lung in Schneeberg metal miners and Joachimstal uranium miners (Ludewig and Lorensen, 1924; Šikl, 1930). An increased frequency of undifferentiated bronchial carcinomas and mortality due to lung cancer in American uranium miners has been correlated with radiation exposure and found to be greater as the level of exposure increased (Saccomanno *et al.*, 1964; Archer and Lundin, 1967; Donaldson, 1969; Lundin *et al.*, 1969). A similar association between lung cancer and exposure to radon daughters has been observed in Czechoslovakian miners (Ševc, Kunz and Plaček, 1976).

To control radiation levels in mines the US Public Health Service introduced the *Working Level* (WL) unit which is defined as any combination of radon daughters in one litre of air that will result in the ultimate emission of 1.3×10^5 MeV/l of potential alpha energy. The measure of total exposure of miners is expressed as a *Working Level Month* (WLM): that is, inhalation for one working month (170 hours) of air containing a radon daughter concentration of 1 WL, or for two months' exposure to a concentration of 0.5 WL—and so on. Correlation between cancer mortality and radiation exposure in the American series just described occurred with exposures in excess of 120 WLM cumulative exposure (Archer, Wagoner and Lundin, 1973).

The International Commission on Radiological Protection (1977), on the other hand, adopted the *curie* (Ci) as the unit to express exposure limits and recommended that the operational limit for α activity in ore dust should be 70 pCi hl^{-1} (one curie, which is a unit of radioactivity, equals 3.7×10^{10} nuclear transformations/second). One WL is equivalent to 100 pCi l^{-1} of radon in radioactive equilibrium with its daughters.

Saccomanno *et al.* (1971) have confirmed an increased incidence of undifferentiated lung carcinomas with increasing radiation exposure compared with a control population matched for age and smoking habits. Where radiation exposure was high (that is, more than 1500 cumulative WLM) small cell undifferentiated tumours (WHO Classification 2B) accounted for more than half the total number. An average of 15.9 years elapsed from the commencement of mining to the development of cancer. The effect of radiation is to increase the small cell undifferentiated tumours in all age and cigarette smoking groups, but to decrease the squamous cell tumours which are related mainly to age. An excess of small cell tumours has also been observed in Joachimstal and South African uranium miners (Horáček, 1969; Webster, 1970). More recently, however, an increased frequency of all histological types of lung cancer has been reported in American and Czechoslovakian miners (Archer, Saccomanno and Jones, 1974; Horáček, Plaček and Ševc, 1977). In the Czechoslovakian miners the dose-effect relationship differs with different time distribution of exposure: lung cancer incidence per unit of exposure decreases with increase of exposure rate at higher cumulative exposures. This decrease is due chiefly to a decline in cancers of small cell undifferentiated type which are known to be more sensitive to the 'sterilizing' effect of radiation than cancers of epidermoid type (Kunz *et al.*, 1979).

There is a striking co-carcinogenic effect between cigarette smoking and radiation, the lung cancer rate being ten times greater among smoking uranium miners than non-smoking miners (Lundin *et al.*, 1969). And, although an excess of lung cancer also occurs in non-smokers, the 'induction-latent period' of the tumour in miners who smoke 20 or more cigarettes per day is shorter (Archer, Gillam and Wagoner, 1976). This relationship is consistent with a multiplicative rather than an additive effect (Doll, 1972).

CONTROL OF THE RADIATION HAZARD IN MINES

This rests essentially upon the amount of radon-222 and α-emitting radon daughters in air being kept as low as reasonably possible below maximum permissible concentrations or operational limits of exposure, but unanimous agreement on the levels of these concentrations has not yet been reached. Most authorities at present accept the WL unit and that no worker should have an exposure of more than 2 WLM in any consecutive three-month period and no more than 4 WLM in any consecutive 12-month period. This is equivalent to an average concentration of radon daughters of 0.3 WL over the working year (Duggan *et al.*, 1970). The International Commission on Radiological Protection (1977) has also recommended that the annual average concentration of radon-222 in equilibrium with short-lived daughters or any mixture of radon and daughters should not exceed 30 pCi l^{-1}. WLM dose conversion factors for radon daughters have been suggested by Walsh (1979).

Efficient ventilation of the mine is imperative. This can also be applied to working areas by portable air ducts and fans; and radon should be isolated or diverted from main air streams. Radon-bearing water must be prevented from flowing through mine workings by channelling it into pipes and conducting it away from work areas. Personal protective equipment may be used but respirators are not often practicable (International Commission on Radiological Protection, 1977).

Periodic determination of the concentration of radon and the short-lived radon daughters in mine air is required and the frequency of sampling will depend upon the geological characteristics of the region. This involves special equipment and techniques. Individual exposure may be monitored by personal film badges resembling those worn by X-ray workers, and careful records of radiation levels kept.

Pre-employment medical examination should exclude individuals with chronic lung disease or chronic nasal obstruction. Routine medical examination of miners and other exposed workers is recommended including a full size chest radiograph and lung function tests annually, and regular cytology of sputum. An experienced cytologist may be able to detect pre-cancerous metaplasia or the pre-invasive stage of carcinoma. Class II, Stage III metaplasia (WHO Classification) is said to be the last stage before malignancy supervenes (Saccomanno *et al.*, 1965, 1976). If these changes are observed removal of the miner (or other worker) from further exposure and cessation of smoking is advised. However, false positive and false negative results may occur. Hence, there is uncertainty concerning the sensitivity of such screening methods and whether or not they affect prognosis of cancer significantly. The question is currently under investigation at the Mayo Clinic (Fontana, 1977; Morgan, 1978).

All exposed personnel should be strongly encouraged not to smoke.

Methods of protection against radiation in industry generally are described by the Department of Employment (1971), the World Health Organization (1972), the International Commission on Radiological Protection (1977) and the National Radiological Protection Board (1977).

Before leaving the topic of uranium mining it must be remembered that the quartz content of many uranium-bearing rocks is high, so that miners are also exposed to a risk of silicosis. Some uranium miners exhibit a pattern of impaired lung function compatible with fibrotic changes and it has been suggested that α-particles may increase the fibrogenic effect of quartz (Trapp *et al.*, 1970); but this remains to be proved. Lung fibrosis has been induced in dogs by inhalation of an α-emitter (Sanders and Park, 1971).

MILLING URANIUM ORE

The crushing of the ore and the weighing and packing into drums of the extracted product carries a similar risk of airborne radioactivity and quartz-containing dust as mining the ore.

Preventive measures include enclosure of mills and weighing and packing machines, protective clothing, efficient exhaust ventilation, good 'house-keeping' and monitoring of the air. As soluble compounds are absorbed into the blood, deposited in bone and excreted via the kidney the uranium level in the urine should be determined regularly as part of periodic medical examination.

The burden of natural uranium in the lungs of exposed workers may be high or low according to the physical and chemical properties of the uranium aerosol and, possibly, physiological idiosyncrasy (Donaghue *et al.*, 1972).

OTHER TYPES OF MINING

Thorium mining

Thorium is largely obtained by surface offshore digging of monazite sands or open-pit mining methods. Under these conditions radiation levels are low. But in underground mine workings in igneous rock (for example, in granite) fairly high concentrations of thoron daughters have been observed (Albert, 1966).

Fluorspar mining

Fluorspar is the term used for the naturally occurring mineral which consists essentially of fluorite (CaF_2) with variable quantities of other associated minerals. It occurs in many geological environments: at one extreme, as an accessory mineral in igneous rocks; and, at the other, as replacements in carbonate rocks (*see* Chapter 7, p. 135). Fluorspar is mined extensively throughout the world. The major producing countries include Mexico, Spain, France, Italy, the UK, USA, South Africa and Canada (Notholt and Highley, 1975).

Miners in the Newfoundland mines, where the mineral occurs as veins in granite and rhyolite porphory, are reported to have a lung cancer rate about 29 times greater than expected. This excess has been attributed to exposure to radon and radon daughters with average levels of 2.5 to 10 WL in the mine air. But no radioactive ore bodies were detected in exposed rocks and it is probable that radon is carried into the workings by water (de Villiers and Windish, 1964). The prevalence of pneumoconiosis in these miners is low—1.93 per cent (Parsons *et al.*, 1964). The possibility of an associated silica risk is referred to in Chapter 7.

In the UK where the mines are in limestone districts of various ages estimated WLM per year exposure rates exceeded 4 WLM per year in two of 12 mines surveyed in 1973 and 1975. But very few miners are employed (Strong, Laidlaw and O'Riordan, 1975).

Metal mining

A threefold increased incidence of lung cancer attributed to radon daughters has been observed in a group of underground metal miners in the USA (Wagoner *et al.*, 1963). An excess has also been reported in miners in Swedish zinc, silver and lead mines where radon daughter levels were apparently high until the 1950s (Axelson and Rehn, 1971).

Tin mining

The geology of tin is referred to in Chapter 6. Because the ore occurs in acidic igneous rock bodies it is closely associated with uranium ores. The estimated exposure rate of radon daughters was found to be above the recommended 4 WLM per year limit in three of four Cornish tin-miners surveyed in 1975, although, as a result of improved ventilation, it was considerably below the estimates recorded in 1973 (Strong, Laidlow and O'Riordan, 1975).

Hematite mining

Investigation of iron ore miners in West Cumberland hematite mines where median concentrations of radon daughters were found to be between 0.15 and 2 WL revealed a mortality from carcinoma of the lung apparently 70 per cent higher than expected (Boyd *et al.*, 1970; Duggan *et al.*, 1970). But no radioactivity was identified in representative samples of exposed rocks and the radon source may be the underlying igneous series of Borrowdale Volcanics or mine water, as in the Newfoundland fluorspar mines. In 1973 the estimated WLM per year was slightly above the recommended level in two mines surveyed but, in one of those resurveyed in 1975, it was well below this level (Boyd *et al.*, 1970; Strong, Laidlow and O'Riordan, 1975).

It is unlikely that iron ore dust is carcinogenic (*see* Chapter 6).

Coal-mining

Although, in general, coal seams are less radioactive than other sedimentary rocks a local increase may be present especially if the seams are overlaid by igneous rocks. Soluble uranium salts in percolating groundwater are altered to an insoluble form in coal-beds so that the highest coal seam (that is, nearest the surface) in a series is often the most radioactive. Thorium may be present in zircons which occur in relatively high concentration in some coal measures (Parks, 1963; Ogden, 1974). Thus, it may be deduced that airborne activity of radon and thoron daughters in coal-mines is intermediate between levels of radioactivity which exist at the Earth's surface and in uranium mines. Duggan, Howell and Soilleux (1968) found median radon concentrations of 2 pCi l^{-1} in 12 British coal-mines compared with concentrations in excess of 100 pCi l^{-1} in uranium and other metalliferous mines. These results are similar to measurements made in American coal-mines. It is believed that from 0.1 to 1 per cent of all dust particles of respirable size in coal mines emit α particles in the lungs between deposition and clearance (Ogden, 1974). The level of radioactivity in coal-mines is not associated with lung cancer in the miners who, as described in Chapter 8 (p. 217), have a lower than expected incidence of the tumour.

Phosphate rock mining

Phosphate is found in all igneous and sedimentary rocks but is mined only when present in high concentrations. Deposits are worked chiefly by opencast and to some extent by underground mining methods. It occurs as fluorapatite ($Ca_5(PO_4)_3F$), or *apatite*, in igneous rocks and as other phosphates, known as *phosphorite*, in sedimentary rocks. Almost all sedimentary phosphates are uraniferous, concentrations being about one or two orders of magnitude higher than the average uranium concentration of the Earth's crust, and thorium is also present (O'Riordan *et al.*, 1972).

About 90 per cent of the world's phosphate rock production is used in the manufacture of phosphate fertilizers and the remainder, chiefly in the chemical industry. Phosphogypsum ($Ca\,SO_4.\,2H_2O$), or by-product gypsum, a waste product in the manufacture of phosphoric acid from phosphate rock, is often stock-piled near the plant and is used to a limited degree in plaster boarding.

No excess of lung cancer appears to have been reported in mine workers but people living near phosphogypsum stock-piles may be subjected to an increased risk (Walsh, 1979). Radiation from the use of by-product gypsum as a building material, however, is substantially below the dose limits recommended by the International Commission on Radiological Protection (O'Riordan *et al.*, 1972).

SURVEY OF VARIOUS BRITISH MINES BY THE NATIONAL RADIOLOGICAL PROTECTION BOARD

Apart from coal-mines and other mines already referred to in this chapter (fluorspar, tin and hematite) some of the following mines were surveyed in 1973 and 1975: ironstone, gypsum, limestone, calcspar (calcite), honestone (a sedimentary shale), fireclay, ball clay, lead, slate, barytes and salt. The estimated exposure rates of radon and radon daughters in 1973 were substantially below the recommended limit of 4 WLM/year in all but one limestone, one fireclay and one barytes mine. In 1975, with the exception of the same limestone mine, all these mines were well below the limit (Strong, Laidlow and O'Riordan, 1975).

OTHER POTENTIAL SOURCES OF EXPOSURE TO IONIZING RADIATION

Tunnels

Excessive levels of radon-222 may be present in the air of tunnels and underground chambers in igneous and some other rock formations and necessitate an efficient ventilatory system, possibly steel plate or concrete barriers, and regular monitoring of radioactivity (Lloyd, Pendleton and Downard, 1968).

Thorium extraction and industrial use

Alpha emitters may be present in thorium ore extracting plants (where a risk of silicosis may also exist as the quartz content of monazite sands is high) and in thorium refining. Little seems to be known of the concentrations which occur under various conditions but in two processing plants in India thoron concentrations were reported to be typically 50 to 500 pCi l^{-1} (Duggan, 1973). One survey of a thorium refinery did not reveal any evidence of radiation injury in a small number of long-term workers (Albert, 1966).

Other industries in which airborne thoron and daughters are present include the manufacture of gas mantles in which thorium nitrate is used, the production of magnesium-thorium alloys and the manufacture of refractory crucibles (thoria ware). Thorium is also important in the nuclear energy industry. High concentrations of thoron may be present close to the source (for example, tanks of thorium nitrate solution for the impregnation of gas mantle hose) but, due to its short half-life (55.3 seconds), gradients fall sharply within short distances (Duggan, 1973).

There appear to be no epidemiological studies from which evidence of an exposure risk relationship to thoron inhalation can be derived so that assessment of dose in individual conditions is essential. In some circumstances doses of inhaled thoron, thoron B and thoron C may be comparable (Duggan, 1973). A thoron WL has been defined by analogy with the radon WL as 'equivalent to the sum of the potential alpha energy of 100 pCi l^{-1} of each of the thoron daughters' (Kotrappa *et al.*, 1976).

No evidence of radiation injury to the lungs or other organs as a result of work with thorium in industry appears to have been reported (Tarasenko, 1972).

Atomic energy industry

Plutonium-239 which is produced, handled and stored in the nuclear power industry is an α emitter. Because of this, concern has been expressed about the effect that its insoluble particles may have when inhaled into the lungs. But, although the metal and its compounds are highly carcinogenic in experimental animals, no case of lung cancer which can be confidently attributed to plutonium has so far been reported in human beings. This is undoubtedly due to the stringent radiological protection measures and safety standards which have been applied since the early days of the industry (Medical Research Council, 1975; Mole, 1977).

There appear to be three clearance phases of plutonium from the lung at one, 30 and 500 days so that observation of pulmonary radioactivity in cases of accidental exposure

Table 14.1 Other Known or Suspected Causes of Occupational Cancer of the Lung

	Substance	*Processes*	*Remarks*	*References*
Established causes	Asbestos		Complication of asbestosis	*See* Chapter 9
	Arsenic trioxide, arsenates and arsenites	Copper, zinc and lead smelting Processing and packing arsenical pesticides	Inorganic arsenic is present in various metal ores	Hill and Faning (1948) Lee and Fraumeni (1969) Karatsune *et al.* (1974) Ott, Holder and Gordon (1974) Mabuchi, Lilienfeld and Snell (1980)
	Chloroethers (chloromethylmethyl ether and bis-chloromethyl ether)	Used in the chemical industry for organic solvents, bacteriocides, fungicides and cross-linking agents	Clear dose–response relationship Small-cell carcinoma a specific response to chloromethyl ethers	Figueroa, Raszkowski and Weiss (1973) Weiss and Boucot (1975) Lemen *et al.* (1976) Nelson (1976) Pasternack, Shore and Albert (1977) Weiss, Moser and Auerbach (1979)
	Chromates	Extraction of chromium and chromite ore Chromate production Chromate pigment industry	Sodium and potassium chromate and dichromate. Zinc chromate Downward prevalence trend in chemical industry due to improved hygiene	Baetjer (1950) Mancuso (1951) Bidstrup and Case (1956) Enterline (1974) Langard and Norseth (1975) Ohsaki *et al.* (1978) Hill and Ferguson (1979)
			Chromium content of lungs increases with length of exposure. Remains in lungs for many years after last exposure	Tsuneta *et al.* (1980)
	Coal carbonization volatiles	Carbonization of steel (iron and steel workers). Coking plants, gas workers	Carcinogen uncertain—benzpyrene, coal tar? Decline in tumour incidence in recent years	Lloyd (1971) Redmond *et al.* (1972) Redmond, Strobino and Cypess (1976) Davies (1977)
	Nickel dust and fume	Nickel refining, calcining, smelting and electrolysis Nickel carbonyl process Treatment of crude matte	Carcinogenic form of nickel not known May be nickel copper sulphide or copper oxide Risk eliminated in British (South Wales) nickel refinery in 1930s	Doll (1958) Morgan (1958) Pedersen, *et al.* (1973) Doll, Mathews and Morgan (1977) Kreyberg (1978) Lessard *et al.* (1978)
Suspected or uncertain causes	Benzpyrene and other polycyclic hydrocarbons. Aromatic amines?	Roofers and water-proofers working with hot pitch and asphalt	Similar to coal carbonization hazard, smoking habits not known	Hammond *et al.* (1976)
		Aluminium reduction workers	Volatiles from pitch-bonded anodes	Gibbs and Horowitz, (1979) Milham (1979)
		Oil refinery workers	Validity of control workers uncertain	Hanis, Stavraky and Fowler (1979)
	Beryllium and its compounds		Further studies are needed, possibly with review of expected lung cancer ratios	*See* Chapter 10

Table 14.1 (continued)

	Substance	Processes	Remarks	References
	Vinyi chloride	Polymerization workers Vinyl acetate copolymer. Vinylidene chloride copolymer	Initial exposure in most workers less than 15 years previously Details of smoking habits incomplete (Further investigation important. Unspecified exposure to other chemicals had occurred in one of the studies)	Waxweiler *et al.* (1976) Buffler *et al.* (1979)

should be continued for at least two years (Watts, 1974). Bronchopulmonary lavage is probably an important therapeutic measure in accidental inhalation as up to 85 per cent of inhaled insoluble particles can be removed (Brightwell, 1974).

OCCUPATIONAL EXPOSURE WITH NO KNOWN LUNG CANCER RISK

These include free silica (Chapter 7), coal-mine dust (Chapter 8), carbon black (Robertson and Ingalls, 1980), man-made fibres (Chapter 9) and mineral oil mists.

Mineral oils are well known to cause skin cancer in man but there is no consistent evidence to suggest that their inhalation is a cause of lung cancer either in man or in animals (Kennaway and Kennaway, 1947; Lushbaugh, Green and Redemann, 1960: Jones, 1961; Wagner, Wright and Stokinger, 1964; Ely *et al.,* 1970; Goldstein, Benoit and Tyroler, 1970; Decoufle, 1976). This may be explained by the fact that many oils which may occur in aerosol form in industrial processes have a brief droplet life and thus do not penetrate far into the lung airways (*see* Chapter 11, p. 396). However, it should, perhaps, be noted that follow-up of exposed workers for longer than about 20 years does not seem to have been reported.

Although there has been a suspicion of excess lung cancer in workers exposed to the *chloroprene* (2-chlorobutadiene) monomer which has a chemical structure similar to vinyl chloride and is used in the manufacture of synthetic rubber, this has not so far been substantiated but long-term investigation is continuing (Lloyd, 1976; Pell, 1978). The possibility that the toxic organism ester *dimethyl sulphate*—widely used as an industrial solvent (*see* Chapter 11)—may cause lung cancer in man has not been confirmed (Stokinger, 1974).

The question of cadmium and lung cancer is referred to in Chapter 13, p. 459.

REFERENCES

Abelson, P. H. (1979). Cancer—opportunism or opportunity. *Science* **206**, 11

Albert, R. E. (1966). *Thorium. Its Industrial Hygiene Aspects.* New York and London; Academic Press

Archer, V. E. (1977). Occupational exposure to radiation as a cancer hazard. *Cancer* **39,** 1802–1806

Archer, V. E., Gillam, J. D. and Wagoner, J. K. (1976). Respiratory disease mortality among young uranium miners. *Ann. N.Y. Acad. Sci.* **271**, 280-293

Archer, V. E. and Lundin, F. E., Jr. (1967). Radiogenic lung cancer in man: exposure-effect relationship. *Envir. Res.* **1**, 370–383

Archer, V. E., Saccomanno, G. and Jones, J. H. (1974). Frequency of different histological types of bronchogenic carcinoma as related to radiation exposure. *Cancer* **34**, 2056-2060

Archer, V. E., Wagoner, J. K. and Lundin, E. E. (1973). Lung cancer among uranium miners in the United States. *Hlth Phys.* **25**, 351–371

Axelson, O. and Rehn, M. (1971). Lung cancer in miners. *Lancet* **2**, 706–707

Baetjer, A. M. (1950). Pulmonary carcinoma in chromate workers. 1. A review of the literature and a report of cases. *Arch. Ind. Hyg. occup. Med.* **2**, 487–504

Bidstrup, P. L. and Case, R. A. M. (1956). Carcinoma of the lung in workmen in the bichromates-producing industry in Great Britain. *Br. J. ind. Med.* **13**, 260–264

Boyd, J. T., Doll, R., Faulds, J. S. and Leiper, J. (1970). Cancer of the lung in iron ore (hematite) miners. *Br. J. ind. Med.* **27**, 97–105

Bridges, J. W. and Fry, J. R. (1978). Mammalian short-term tests for carcinogens. In *Carcinogenicity Testing, Principles and Problems*, edited by A. D. Dayan and R. W. Brimblecome, pp. 29–52. Lancaster; MTP Press

Bridbord, K., Decoufle, P., Fraumeni, J. F., Hoel, D. G., Hoover, R. N., Rall, D. P., Saffiotti, U., Schneiderman, M. A. and Upton, A. C. (1978). Estimates of the fraction of cancer in the United States related to occupational factors. Report by National Cancer Institute, National Institute of Environment Health Sciences, National Institute for Occupational Safety and Health

Brightwell, J. (1974). The efficiency of bronchopulmonary lavage as a therapeutic procedure for removing insoluble radioactive particles from the lung. In *The Radiological Protection of People Exposed to Plutonium: Current Research at the National Radiological Protection Board.* National Protection Board. NRPB – R 31, pp 74–88

Buffler, P. A., Wood, S., Eifler, C., Suarez, L. and Kilian, D. J. (1979). Mortality experience of workers in a vinyl chloride monomer production plant. *J. occup. Med.* **21**, 195–203

Chamberlain, A. C. and Dyson, E. D. (1956) The dose to the trachea and bronchi from the decay products of radon and thoron. *Br. J. Radiol.* **29**, 317–325

Cole, P. (1977). Cancer and occupation: status and needs of epidemiological research. *Cancer* **39**, 1788–1791

Davies, C. N. (1967). In *Assessment of Airborne Radioactivity*, pp. 3–20. Vienna; Internat. Atomic Energy Agency

Davies, G. M. (1977). A mortality study of coke oven workers in two South Wales integrated steelworks. *Br. J. Ind. Med.* **34**, 291–297

Decoufle, P. (1976). Cancer mortality among workers exposed to cutting-oil mist. *Ann. N.Y. Acad. Sci.* **271**, 94–101

Department of Employment (1971). *Code of Practice for the Protection of Persons Exposed to Ionising Radiations in Research and Teaching.* London; HMSO de Villiers, A. J. and Windish, J. P. (1964). Lung cancer in a fluorspar mining community. I. Radiation, dust and mortality experience. *Br. J. ind. Med.* **21**, 94–109

Doll, R. (1958). Cancer of the lung and nose in nickel workers. *Br. J. ind. Med.* **15**, 217–223

Doll, R. (1972). The age distribution of cancer: implications for models of carcinogenesis. *Jl R. statist. Soc.* **134**, 133–155

Doll, R. (1977). Strategy for detection of cancer hazards in man. *Nature* **265**, 589–596

Doll, R. Mathews, J. D. and Morgan, L. G. (1977). Cancers of the lung and nasal sinuses in nickel workers: a reassessment of the period of risk. *Br. J. ind. Med.* **34**, 102–105

Donaghue, J. K., Dyson, E. D., Hislop, J. S., Leach, A. M. and Spoor, N. L. (1972). Human exposure to natural uranium. A case history and analytical results from some postmortem studies. *Br. J. ind. Med.* **29**, 81–89

Donaldson, A. W. (1969). The epidemiology of lung cancer among uranium miners. *Hlth Phys.* **16**, 563–569

Duggan, M. J. (1973). Some aspects of the hazard from airborne thoron and its daughter products. *Hlth Phys* **24**, 301–310

Duggan, M. J., Howell, D. M. and Soilleux, P. J. (1968). Concentrations of radon-222 in coal mines in England and Scotland. *Nature, Lond.* **219**, 1149

Duggan, M. J., Soilleux, P. J., Strong, J. C. and Howell, D. M. (1970). The exposure of United Kingdom miners to radon. *Br. J. ind. Med.* **27**, 106–109

Ely, T. S., Pedley, S. F., Hearne, F. T. and Stille, W. T. (1970). A study of mortality, symptoms and respiratory function in humans occupationally exposed to oil mist. *J. Occup. Med.* **12**, 253–261

Enterline, P. E. (1974). Respiratory cancer among chromate workers. *J. occup. Med.* **16**, 523–526

Epstein, S. S. and Swartz, J. B. (1981). Fallacies of lifestyle cancer theories. *Nature*, **289**, 127–130

Figueroa, W. G., Raszkowski, R. and Weiss, W. (1973). Lung cancer in chloromethyl ether workers. *New Engl. J. Med.* **288**, 1096–1097

Fontana, R. S. (1977). Early diagnosis of lung cancer. *Am. Rev. resp. Dis.* **116**, 399–402

Fox, A. J. and Adelstein, A. M. (1978). Occupational mortality: work or way of life? *J. epid. and Community Hlth* **32**, 73–78

Gibbs, G. W. and Harowitz, I. (1979). Lung cancer mortality in aluminium reduction plant workers. *J. occup. Med.* **21**, 347–353

Goldstein, D., Benoit, J. N. and Tyroler, H. A. (1970). An epidemiological study of oil mist exposure. *Arch. environ. Hlth* **21**, 600–603

Hammond, E. C., Selikoff, I. J., Lawther, P. L. and Seidman, H. (1976). Inhalation of benzpyrene and cancer in man. *Ann. N.Y. Acad. Sci.* **271**, 116–124

Hanis, N. M., Stavraky, K. M. and Fowler, J. L. (1979). Cancer mortality in oil refinery workers. *J. occup. Med.* **21**, 167–174

Higginson, J. (1980a). Proportion of cancers due to occupation. (IARC, WHO Review Committee). *Prev. Med.* **9**, 180–188

Higginson, J. (1980b). The environment and cancer. *Am. J. Med.* **69**, 811–813

Higginson, J. and Muir, C. S. (1976). The role of epidemiology in elucidating the importance of environmental factors in human cancer. *Cancer Detect. Prev.* **1**, 79–105

Higginson, J. and Muir, C. S. (1979). Environmental carcinogenesis: misconceptions and limitations to cancer control. *J. Nat. Cancer Inst.* **63**, 1291–1298

Hill, A. B., and Faning, E. L. (1948). Studies in the incidence of cancer in a factory handling inorganic compounds of arsenic 1. Mortality experience in the factory. *Br. J. ind. Med.* **5**, 1–6

Hill, W. J. and Ferguson, W. S. (1979). Statistical analysis of epidemiological data from a chromium chemical manufacturing plant. *J. occup. Med.* **21**, 103–110

Horáček, J. (1969). Der Joachimstaler Lungenkrebs nach dem zweiten Weltkreig (Bericht uber 55 Falle). *Z. Krebsforsch.* **72**, 52–56

Horáček, J., Plaček, V. and Ševc, J. (1977). Histological types of bronchogenic cancer in relation to different conditions of radiation exposure. *Cancer* **40**, 832–835

International Commission on Radiological Protection (1977). *Radiation Protection in Uranium and other Mines.* ICRP Publication 24. Oxford, New York, Frankfurt; Pergamon Press

Jones, J. G. (1961). An investigation into the effects of exposure to an oil mist on workers in a mill for the cold reduction of steel strip. *Ann. occup. Hyg.* **3**, 264–271

Karatsune, M., Tokudome, S., Shirakusa, T., Yoshida, M., Tokumitsu, Y., Hayano, T. and Seita, M. (1974). Occupational lung cancer among copper smelters. *Int. J. Cancer* **13**, 552–558

Kennaway, E. L. and Kennaway, N. M. (1947). A further study of the incidence of cancer of the lung and larynx. *Br. J. Cancer* **1**, 260–298

Kotin, P. (1968). Carcinogenesis of the lung: environmental and host factors. In *The Lung*, edited by A. A. Liebow and D. E. Smith, pp. 203–225. Baltimore; Williams and Wilkins

Kotrappa, P., Bhanti, D. P., Menon, V. P., Dhandayutham, R., Gohel, C. O. and Nambiar, P. P. V. J. (1976). Assessment of airborne hazards in the thorium processing industry. *Am. ind. Hyg. Assoc. J.* **37**, 613–616

Kreyberg, L. (1978). Lung cancer in workers in a nickel refinery. *Br. J. ind. Med.* **35**, 109–116

Kunz, E., Ševc, J., Plaček, V. and Horáček, J. (1979). Lung cancer in man in relation to different time distribution of radiation exposure. *Hlth Phys.* **36**, 699–706

Langård, S. and Norseth, T. (1975). A cohort study of bronchial carcinomas in workers producing chromate pigments. *Br. J. ind. Med.* **32**, 62–65

Lea, D. E. (1955). *Actions of Radiations on Living Cells*, 2nd edition, p. 25. London; Cambridge University Press

Leading article (1978). What proportion of cancers are related to occupation? *Lancet* **2**, 1238–1240

Lee, A. M. and Fraumeni, J. F. Jr. (1969). Arsenic and respiratory cancer in man: an occupational study. *J. Nat. Cancer Inst.* **42**, 1045–1052

Lemen, R. A., Johnson, W. M., Wagoner, J. K. Archer, V. E. and Saccomanno, G. (1976). Cytolytic observations and cancer incidence following exposure to BCME. *Ann. N.Y. Acad. Sci.* **271**, 71–80

Lessard, R., Reed, D., Naheux, B. and Lambert, J. (1978). Lung cancer in New Caledonia, a nickel smelting island. *J. occup. Med.* **20**, 815–817

Lloyd, J. W. (1971). Long-term mortality study of steelworkers. V. Respiratory cancer in coke plant workers. *J. occup. Med.* **13**, 53–68

Lloyd, J. W. (1976). Cancer risks among workers exposed to chloroprene. *Ann. N.Y. Acad. Sci.* **271**, 91–93

Lloyd, R. D., Pendleton, R. C. and Downard, T. R. (1968). Radioactivity within a tunnel in granitic rock. *Hlth Phys.* **15**, 274–276

Ludewig, P. and Lorensen, E. (1924). Untersuchungen der Grubenluft in den schneeberger Gruben auf den Gehalt and Radiumemanation. *Strahlentherapie.* **17**, 428–435

Lundin, F. E., Jr., Lloyd, J. W., Smith, E. M., Archer, V. E. and Holaday, D. A. (1969). Mortality of uranium miners in relation to radiation exposure, hard-rock mining and cigarette smoking—1950 through September 1967. *Hlth Phys.* **16**, 571–578

Lusbaugh, C. C., Green, J. W. and Redemann, C. R. (1960). Effects of prolonged inhalation of oil fogs on experimental animals. *Arch. ind. Hyg. occup. Med.* **1**, 237–247

Mabuchi, K., Lilienfeld, A. M. and Snell, L. M. (1980) Cancer and occupational exposure to arsenic: a study of pesticide workers. *Prev. Med.* **9**, 51–77

Mancuso, T. F. (1951) Occupational cancer and other health hazards in a chromate plant: of medical appraisal. II Clinical and toxicologic aspects. *Ind. med. Surg.* **20**, 293–407

Medical Research Council (1975). *The Toxicity of Plutonium.* London; HMSO

Milham, S. Jr. (1979). Mortality of aluminium reduction plant workers. *J. occup. Med.* **21**, 475–480

Mole, R. H. (1977). Anxieties and fears about plutonium. *Br. med. J.* **2**, 743–745

Morgan, A. (1970). Physical behaviour of radon and its daughters with particular reference to monitoring methods. In *Pneumoconiosis. Proceedings of the International Conference, Johannesburg, 1969,* edited by H.A. Shapiro, pp. 540–543. Cape Town; Oxford University Press

Morgan, J. G. (1958). Some observations on the incidence of respiratory cancer in nickel workers. *Br. J. industr. Med.* **15,** 224–234

Morgan, W. K. C. (1978). Screening for occupational cancer of the lung. *Chest* **74**, 239–241

Morgan, W. K. C. (1979). Industrial carcinogens: the extent of the risk. *Thorax* **34**, 431–433

National Radiological Protection Board. (1977). The work of the NRPB 1974/76. London; HMSO

Nelson, N. (1976). The chloroethers—occupational carcinogens: a summary of laboratory and epidemiology studies. *Ann. N.Y. Acad. Sci.* **271**, 81–90

Notholt, A. J. G. and Highley, D. E. (1975). Fluorspar. Mineral Dossier No. 1. Mineral Resources Consultative Committee. London; HMSO

Ogden, T. L. (1974). A method for measuring the working-level values of mixed radon and thoron daughters in coal-mine air. *Ann. occup. Hyg.* **17**, 23–34

Ohsaki, Y., Shosaku, A., Kimura, K., Tsuneta, Y., Mikami, H. and Murao, M. (1978). Lung cancer in Japanese chromate workers. *Thorax* **33**, 372–374

O'Riordan, M. C., Duggan, M. J., Rose, W. B. and Bradford, G. F. (1972). The radiological implications of using by-product gypsum as a building material. National Radiological Protection Board. Harwell. Oxon. NRCB-R7

Ott, M. G., Holder, B. B. and Gordon, H. L. (1974). Respiratory cancer and occupational exposure to arsenicals. *Archs envir. Hlth* **29**, 250–255

Parks, B. C. (1963). Origin, petrography and classification of coal. In *Chemistry of Coal Utilization.* Supplementary Vol, edited by H. H. Lowry, pp. 1–34. New York; John Wiley

Parsons, W. D., de Villiers, A. J., Bartlett, L. S. and Becklake, M. R. (1964). Lung cancer in a fluorspar mining community. 11. Prevalence of respiratory symptoms and disability. *Br. J. ind. Med.* **21**, 110–116

Pasternack, B. S., Shore, R. E. and Albert, R. E. (1977). Occupational exposure to chloromethyl ethers. *J. occup. Med.* **19**, 741–746

Pederson, E., Hogetveit, A. C. and Anderson, A. (1973). Cancer of respiratory organs among workers at a nickel refinery in Norway. *Int. J. Cancer* **12**, 32–41

Pell, S. (1978). Mortality of workers exposed to chloroprene. *J. occup. Med.* **20**, 21–29

Peto, R. (1980). Distorting the epidemiology of cancer: the need for a more balanced overview. *Nature* **284**, 297–300

Redmond, C. K. A., Ciocco, J. W., Lloyd, J. W. and Rush, H. W. (1972). Long-term mortality study of steelworkers. V1. Mortality from malignant neoplasms among coke oven workers. *J. occup. Med.* **14**, 621–629

Redmond, C. K., Strobino, B. R. and Cypess, R. H. (1976). Cancer experience among coke by-product workers. *Ann. N.Y. Acad. Sci.* **271**, 102–115

Registrar General (1978). Office of population censuses and surveys: occupational mortality. Decennial supplement for England and Wales, 1970–72. London; HMSO

Robertson, J. M. and Ingalls, T. H. (1980). A mortality study of carbon black workers in the United States from 1935 to 1974. *Arch. environ. Hlth* **35**, 181–186

Saccomanno, G., Archer, V. E., Saunders, R. P., James, L. A. and Beckler, P. A. (1964). Lung cancer of uranium miners in Colorado plateau. *Hlth Phys.* **10**, 1195–1201

Saccomanno, G., Archer, V. E. Auerbach, O., Kuschner, M., Saunders, R. P. and Klein, M. G. (1971). Histological types of lung cancer among uranium miners. *Cancer, Philad.* **27**, 515–523

Saccomanno, G., Archer, V. E., Saunders, R. P. Auerbach, O. and Klein, M. G. (1976). Early indices of cancer risk among uranium miners with reference to modifying factors. *Ann. N.Y. Acad. Sci.* **271**, 377–383

Saccomano, G., Saunders, R. P., Archer, V. E., Auerbach, O., Kuschner, M. and Beckler, P. A. (1965). Cancer of the lung: the cytology of sputum prior to the development of carcinoma. *Acta cytol.* **9**, 413–423

Sanders, C. L. and Park, F. J. (1971). Pulmonary distribution of alpha dose from $^{239}PuO_2$ and induction of neoplasia in rats and dogs. In *Inhaled Particles and Vapours, III,* Vol. 1, edited by W. H. Walton, pp. 489–497. Woking; Unwin

Ševc, J., Kunz, E. and Plaček, V. (1976). Lung cancer in uranium miners and long-term exposure to radon daughter products. *Hlth Phys.* **30**, 433–437

Šikl, H. (1930). Über den Lungenkrebs der Berglente in Joachimstal. (Tschechoslowakei). *Z. Krebsforsch.* **32**, 609–613

Stokinger, H. E. (1974). Carcinogen standard. *J. occup. Med.* **16**, 119–120

Strong, J. C., Laidlow, A. J. and O'Riordan, M. C. (1975). Radon and its daughters in various British mines. National Radiological Protection Board. Harwell, Oxon. NRPB-R39

Tarasenko, N. Ju. (1972). Thorium compounds. In *Encyclopaedia of Occupational Health and Safety. Vol. 11,* pp. 1404–1406. Geneva; International Labour Office

Tsuneta, Y., Ohsaki, Y., Kimura, K., Mikami, H., Abe, S. and Murao, M. (1980). Chromium content of lungs of chromate workers with lung cancer. *Thorax* **35**, 294–297

Trapp, E., Rehzetti, A. D., Jr., Kobayashi, T., Mitchell, M. M. and Bigler, A. (1970). Cardiopulmonary function in uranium miners. *Am. Rev. resp. Dis.* **101**, 27–43

Wagner, W. D., Wright, P. G. and Stokinger, H. E. (1964). Inhalation toxicology of oil mists. I. Chronic effects of white mineral oil. *Am. ind. Hyg. Assoc. J.* **25,** 158–168

Wagoner, J. K., Miller, R. W., Lundin, F. E., Jr., Fraumeni, J. F., Jr. and Haij, M. E. (1963). Unusual cancer mortality among a group of underground metal miners. *New Engl. J. Med.* **269**, 284–289

Walsh, P. J. (1979). Dose conversion factors for radon daughters. *Hlth Phys.* **36**, 601–609

Watts, L. M. (1974). Analysis of data on the clearance of insoluble compounds of plutonium in the lung. In *The Radiological Protection of People Exposed to Plutonium: Current Research at the National Radiological Protection Board,* pp. 103–115. National Radiological Protection Board, NRPB-R31

Waxweiler, R. J., Stringer, W., Wagoner, J. K. and Jones, J. (1976). Neoplastic risk among workers exposed to vinyl chloride. *Ann. N.Y. Acad. Sci.* **271**, 40–48

Webster, I. (1970). Bronchogenic carcinoma in South African gold miners. In *Pneumoconiosis. Proceedings of the International Conference, Johannesburg, 1969,* edited by H. A. Shapiro, pp. 572–574. Cape Town; Oxford University Press

Weiss, W. and Boucot, K. R. (1975). The respiratory effects of chloromethyl methyl ether. *J. Am. med. Ass.* **234**, 1139–1142

Weiss, W., Moser, R. L. and Auerbach, O. (1979). Lung cancer in chloroethyl ethers. *Am. Rev. resp. Dis.* **120**, 1031–1037

World Health Organization (1972). *Protection Against Ionizing Radiation: A Survey of Current World Legislation.* Geneva; WHO

Wynder, E. L. and Gori, G. B. (1977). Contribution of the environment to cancer incidence: an epidemiological exercise. *J. Natn. Cancer. Inst.* **58**, 825–832

Appendix

STOKES' LAW (Chapter 3)

This states that the fluid resistance experienced by a small sphere of radius 'a' moving at a uniform velocity 'v' through a fluid of viscosity 'η' is 6πaηυ. On being released a small sphere rapidly attains a constant (terminal) velocity and when falling at this speed the fluid resistance equals the gravitational force '*g*'. Thus:

$$\tfrac{4}{3}\pi a^3(\sigma - \rho)g = 6\pi a \eta v$$

where σ is the density of the spheres and ρ, the density of the fluid. Hence:

$$\mathbf{v} = \tfrac{2}{9}\,\frac{a^2(\sigma - \rho)g}{\eta}$$

In air $\sigma \approx \frac{\sigma}{800}$ and is neglected. The formula fails in air if the spheres are so small as to be comparable with the mean free path of the air molecules. It also fails in air and in liquids if the spheres are too large since the rate of fall then rises to such an extent that the velocities communicated to the fluid become large enough to introduce a fluid inertia effect. This results in the lines of fluid flow failing to close up on the lee side of the sphere as they do in viscous (Stokes) flow, so raising the fluid resistance. Therefore, larger spheres fall more slowly than is given by Stokes' law.

MAGNETOPNEUMOGRAPHY (Chapter 5)

This is a sensitive technique (of limited availability at present) for measuring the concentration and distribution in the lungs of magnetizable exogenous mineral dusts, which was developed following the observation that a weak magnetic field can be detected over the chests of some individuals with occupational dust exposure (Cohen, 1973). In essence it consists of applying a magnetic field to the whole thorax or to localized areas (Cohen, 1975; Kalliomäki *et al.*, 1976; Robinson and Freedman, 1979). This results in a short-lived, electronically detectable alignment of ferrimagnetic minerals in the lungs which is not, apparently, exhibited by paramagnetic minerals such as asbestos nor by endogenous iron. The content of these minerals in welding fume and iron and steel foundry dusts may be as much as 30 per cent (Kalliomäki *et al.*, 1979).

The technique has revealed significant accumulation of ferrimagnetic minerals in arc welders, foundry workers and to a lesser extent in coal miners before their presence is detectable radiographically (Kalliomäki *et al.*, 1976; Kalliomäki *et al.*, 1978a and b; Freedman, Robinson and Johnston, 1980). It may prove to be of value for the early detection of undue accumulation of dust in the lungs of groups of workers exposed to dusts which contain ferrimagnetic minerals.

POST-MORTEM PREPARATION OF LUNGS

FORMALDEHYDE FIXATION METHODS

After removal of the intact lungs, main bronchi and trachea formol-acetate solution (10 per cent formalin in 4 per cent sodium acetate) is run through a cannula into both main bronchi from a reservoir placed at a height of about 120 cm, or delivered at this pressure by an electric pump. When perfusion is complete the lungs are placed in a large vessel containing the same solution for at least 48 hours. This is the method of Gough and Wentworth.

Another method, employing formalin vapour, is used for research purposes especially where quantitative studies of the lung or examination of bronchial mucus (which is unaffected) is to be made; but it is not appropriate for routine use and also tends to cause some shrinkage of the lungs.

Silverton (1964) has made a detailed survey and comparison of these and similar methods which should be referred to.

Lungs prepared by these methods are best examined by cutting serial slices 1 to 3 cm thick in the sagittal plane (in some cases the coronal plane may be preferable). The slices can then be studied in order and the observations recorded both in writing and diagrammatically. When the lung is inspected in this way discrete, non-fibrotic dust macules are indistinguishable to touch from the surrounding lung and are not raised above the surface; by contrast, discrete, fibrotic dust lesions are firm, hard and 'nodular' to touch and are raised above the cut surface.

A *whole lung section* mounted on paper for permanent record is prepared by cutting 300 to 500 μm sections from slices about 4 cm thick and, after special processing which preserves the natural colours of the lung, attaching them to paper (Gough and Wentworth, 1960; Silverton, 1964). They are then covered with Cellophane or a layer of methacrylic resin. A modification of this method which permits more rapid preparation of sections has been described by Whimster (1969).

IMPREGNATION OF LUNG SLICES WITH BARIUM SULPHATE

This simple method, introduced by Heard, greatly improves the clarity of emphysema and DIPF, and does not mask dust pigmentation. It provides good specimens for demonstration and photography. The technique is as follows: 'A selected slice from the middle of the lung is lightly squeezed free of excess water and placed flat in a tray (25 × 30 cm) containing saturated aqueous barium nitrate at room temperature for one minute. It is pressed with the fingertips intermittently to encourage the solution to enter the depths of the slice. After squeezing, it is transferred to a tray of saturated aqueous sodium sulphate for one minute; a cloud of precipitated barium sulphate appears at this stage and the slice quickly whitens. It is then squeezed and washed briefly in running tap water to remove excess barium sulphate. One impregnation is sufficient as a rule. The reagents are used for several weeks and the supernatant is selected each time. The precipitate is retained to strengthen the solution when it is returned to the bottle.' (Heard, 1969).

PRESERVATION FOR ELECTRON MICROSCOPY

Bachofen, Weibel and Roos (1975) have developed an effective, practical method of injecting a fixative solution into the periphery of the lung within 30 minutes of death without opening the thorax. It achieves good preservation for at least eight hours. The solution consists of an isomolar mixture of 5 per cent glutaraldehyde and 0.025 g of indocyanine green in 19 ml of distilled water and 1 ml of pasteurized plasma protein.

ROUTINE OPTICAL MICROSCOPY

Routine examination of lung tissue requires sections about 6 to 7 μm thick and standard staining practice should include haematoxylin and eosin and van Giesen methods. The use of other stains is referred to in relevant places in the text. Search for asbestos and other ferruginous bodies is greatly facilitated by 30 μm sections.

IDENTIFICATION OF MINERALS IN THE LUNGS

Adequate discussion of this specialized subject is beyond the scope of this book but an understanding of results produced by various methods and their interpretation is essential if errors of deduction are to be avoided.

In general, there is no single property which defines a mineral. Thus, in order to identify a mineral species, or a variety of that species, a number of its characteristics must be established by different analytical methods. Deductions based on a single mineral characteristic are likely to be incorrect or misleading.

Accurate identification requires the determination of *chemical composition* and *crystalline structure*. Such detailed analysis, however, is neither necessary nor practical for routine purposes but is needed in problematical cases, in establishing whether or not a potentially hazardous mineral is present or not in an industrial material, and for research. The *morphology* of mineral particles gives additional helpful information but is not essential in their identification.

CHEMICAL ANALYSIS

Methods used include:

(1) standard gravimetric and volumetric analysis;
(2) electron and ion microprobe mass analysis (EMMA, IMMA);
(3) transmission and scanning electron microscopy (TEM, SEM) with energy-dispersive X-ray spectrometry (EDXA);
(4) back-scattered electron analysis;
(5) mass spectrography;
(6) X-ray fluorescence.

CRYSTALLOGRAPHY

Techniques employed include:

(1) infrared spectroscopy;
(2) X-ray and electron diffraction (XRD, ED);
(3) differential thermal analysis (DTA);
(4) polarized light microscopy.

Analysis of chemical composition, irrespective of the method used, does not identify a *specific* mineral. It cannot, for example, distinguish between sepiolite (meerschaum) and chrysotile; both are hydrous magnesium silicates yet are clearly dissimilar. X-ray diffraction analysis generally yields unequivocal results so far as identification of the mineral species is concerned. But the variety of some species cannot be positively identified by X-ray diffraction methods; in these circumstances the addition of chemical analysis is necessary. Infrared spectroscopy alone is not a definite analytical technique but it yields useful information on the type of chemical bonding present. Differential thermal analysis may be a valuable auxiliary to X-ray diffraction.

Polarized light microscopy

Polarized light is often used in routine microscopy of lung tissue in the hope of identifying the nature of any crystalline particles present. Although the application of petrological techniques can, in some cases, identify a mineral species, a properly equipped polarizing microscope with a graduated rotating stage for orientating the specimen with respect to the vibration direction of the incident light is necessary; or, alternatively, some means of rotating the polarizers with respect to the specimen. Moreover, the use of the petrological microscope (which is not usually available in medical laboratories) for identifying the mineral constituents of rocks requires knowledge of crystallography and crystal optics to interpret the observations made. Simple rule-of-thumb tests are inadequate.

Thus, if the examination of lung microsections is confined to observations with a 'medical' microscope to which crossed polars are simply added, the demonstration of birefringent particles in the tissues establishes no more than the presence of crystalline substances; it does *not* by itself identify the nature of the crystals.

PARTICLE MORPHOLOGY

This may be determined by:

(1) optical microscopy;
(2) TEM and SEM.

Morphology is not definitive of any mineral species because particles of minerals in many different mineral classes have similar shape and form. Also, used alone, it may mislead: as, for example, when sideways orientation of rolled-up forms of platy minerals, such as talc, are misinterpreted as fibres. Nonetheless, particle size and shape can give valuable information when crystal structure and composition are known.

Thus, specific minerals can be identified, often in minute quantity and small particle size, by appropriate combinations of these techniques. But it should be emphasized that careful appraisal of the findings is necessary; for the presence of an exogenous mineral in the lungs is *not necessarily* proof of a pathogenic relationship to existing disease even if the mineral is of a type known to be capable of fibrogenic or other pathogenic potential. However, the association of a particulate material with a specific lesion, especially if in close proximity, may indicate a need for further investigation (Abraham, 1978).

PROOF OF A CAUSAL RELATIONSHIP BETWEEN A SPECIFIC EXOGENOUS AGENT (INORGANIC OR ORGANIC) AND DISEASE

By modifying the principle of the postulates originally enunciated by Henlé and Koch a number of criteria for testing the validity of a suggested relationship can be applied. In the main, these rely on the identification of a specific suspect substance or agency, its consistent presence in the lungs (or in the lesions) in most diseases, thorough epidemiological investigation of the disease, and, where possible, production of similar disease in animals by the substance. However, additional influences–genetic, immunológical or physiological–may be involved. Also, extrapolation of animal experiments to man may sometimes lead to dubious, even inadmissable, conclusions.

A useful group of basic criteria for causation of chronic disease which should be satisfied is as follows (Surgeon General, Advisory Committee of the USPHS, 1964):

(1) The consistency of the association.
(2) The strength of the association.
(3) The specificity of the association.
(4) The temporal relationship of the association.
(5) The coherence of the association.

But in some circumstances particular difficulty may be encountered, or require to be recognized, in that the same clinical and pathological state may be produced by a variety of causal agencies. The fact that workers in any industry are not exempt from developing lung disorders which occur in the general population should not be lost sight of. Thus, in spite of their having had appropriate occupational exposure, lung disease in some individuals is not necessarily of occupational origin. Other factors may also have to be accounted for. For example: a single agent may produce different clinical and pathological responses in different conditions; and two or more agents or co-factors acting in conjunction may be required to cause disease (Evans, 1976).

REFERENCES

Abraham, J. L. (1978). Recent advances in pneumoconiosis: the pathologists' role in etiological diagnosis. In *The Lung, Structure, Function and Disease*. No 19, International Academy of Pathology. Edited by W. M. Thurlbeck and M-R. Abell, pp. 96–137. Baltimore; Williams and Wilkins

Bachofen, M., Weibel, E. R. and Roos, B. (1975). Postmortem fixation of human lungs for electron microscopy. *Am. Rev. resp. Dis.* **111,** 247–256

Cohen, D. (1973). Ferromagnetic contamination in the lungs and in other organs of the human body. *Science* **180,** 745–748

Cohen, D. (1975). Measurement of the magnetic fields produced by the human heart, brain and lungs. *Institute of Electrical and Electronics Engineers Transactions. Mag.* **11,** 694–700

Evans, A. S. (1976). Causation and disease: the Henle–Koch postulates revisited. *Yale J. biol. Med.* **49,** 175–195

Freedman, A. R., Robinson, S. E. and Johnston, R. F. (1980). Non-invasive magnetopneumographic estimation of lung dust loads and distribution in bituminous coal workers. *J. occup. Med.* **22,** 613–618

Gough, J. and Wentworth, J. E. (1960). Thin sections of entire organs mounted on paper. In *Recent Advances in Pathology,* 7th Edn, edited by C. V. Harrison. London; Churchill

Heard, B. . E. (1969). *Pathology of Chronic Bronchitis and Emphysema,* p. 9. London; J and A Churchill Ltd

Kalliomäki, P-L., Karp, P. J., Katila, T., Mäkipää, P. Tos-Savainen, A. (1976). Magnetic measurements of pulmonary contamination. *Scand. J. Work environ. Hlth* **4,** 232–239

Kalliomäki, P-L., Korhonen, O., Vaaranen, V., Kalliomäki, K. and Kuponen, M. (1978a). Lung retention and clearance of shipyard arc welders. *Int. Arch. occup. environ. Hlth* **42,** 83–90

Kalliomäki, P-L., Alanko, K., Korhonen, O., Mattson, T., Vaaranen, V. and Koponen, M. (1978b). Amount and distribution of welding fume lung contaminants among arc welders. *Scand. J. Work environ. Hlth* **4,** 122–130

Kalliomäki, P-L., Kalliomäki, K., Korhonen, O., Koponen, M., Sortti, V. and Vaaranen, V. (1979). Lung contamination among foundry workers. *Int. Arch. occup. environ. Hlth* **43,** 85–91

Robinson, S. E. and Freedman, A. P. (1979). Direct magnetopneumographic measurement of particle concentration and clearance in the lung. Frontiers of Engineering in Health Care. *Institute of Electrical and Electronics Engineers.* 183–188

Silverton, R. E. (1964). A comparison of formaldehyde fixation methods used in the study of pulmonary emphysema. *J. med. Lab. Technol.* **21,** 187–217

Surgeon General, Advisory Committee of the USPHS. (1964). *Smoking and Health.* PHS Pub. No. 1103, Washington, DC, Supt. of Doc. (Quoted by Evans, 1976)

Whimster, W. F. (1969). Rapid giant paper sections. *Thorax* **24,** 737–741

Index